MEDICAL ASSISTING SKILLS CDS QUICK LOCATOR

This is your link to **Delmar's Medical Assisting Skills** CD-ROMs, which are found on the inside back cover of this book.

Ⓐ = Administrative Skills CD-ROM
Ⓒ = Clinical Skills CD-ROM

W9-CNA-747

Text Chapter	Skills and Their Location on the CD-ROMs	Text Chapter	Skills and Their Location on the CD-ROMs
7	Ⓐ Legal Concepts	31	Ⓒ Removing Items
9	Ⓒ CPR	31	Ⓒ Wound Specimen
9	Ⓒ Heimlich	31	Ⓒ Bandaging
9	Ⓒ Accidental Poisoning	31	Ⓒ Dry Dressing
10	Ⓐ Patient Reception	31	Ⓒ Sutures/Staples
12	Ⓐ Telephone Skills	33	Ⓒ Safe Lifting
12	Ⓐ Telephone Messages	33	Ⓒ Safe Falling
13	Ⓐ Scheduling	33	Ⓒ Moist Heat
14	Ⓐ Records Management	33	Ⓒ Dry Heat
15	Ⓐ Parts of a Letter	33	Ⓒ Cold Treatment
15	Ⓐ Parts of the Envelope	33	Ⓒ ROM Exercises
15	Ⓐ Telephone Messages	33	Ⓒ Assisting with Crutches
15	Ⓐ Prescriptions	33	Ⓒ Elastic Bandaging
15	Ⓐ Medical Record	33	Ⓒ Splint
17	Ⓐ Patient Receipts	33	Ⓒ Arm Sling
17	Ⓐ Purchase Orders	33	Ⓒ Casting
17	Ⓐ Payroll Procedures	33	Ⓒ Cast Care
17	Ⓐ Banking	36	Ⓒ Oral Meds
19	Ⓐ Insurance Coding	36	Ⓒ Ear Meds
20	Ⓐ Pegboard Accounting	36	Ⓒ Eye Meds
20	Ⓐ Superbill, Ledger Card, Daily Log/Day Sheet	36	Ⓒ Skin/Topical Meds
22	Ⓒ Handwashing	36	Ⓒ Nasal Meds
22	Ⓒ Gloves and Gowns	36	Ⓒ Rectal Meds
22	Ⓒ Removing Items	36	Ⓒ Nebulized Meds
22	Ⓒ Sterile Gloves	36	Ⓒ Intradermal Injection
23	Ⓐ Medical Record	36	Ⓒ Subcutaneous Injection
24	Ⓒ Taking a Temperature	36	Ⓒ Intramuscular Injection
24	Ⓒ Taking a Pulse	36	Ⓒ Z-Track Injection
24	Ⓒ Counting Respirations	36	Ⓒ Vial
24	Ⓒ Taking a Blood Pressure	36	Ⓒ Ampule
24	Ⓒ Weighing	36	Ⓒ Mixing Meds
30	Ⓒ Clean Catch Urine	37	Ⓒ EKG
30	Ⓒ Testing Urine	40	Ⓒ Venipuncture
30	Ⓒ Collecting Nose, Throat, Sputum Specimens	42	Ⓒ Clean Catch Urine
30	Ⓒ Testing for Occult Blood	42	Ⓒ Testing Urine
30	Ⓒ Skin Puncture	43	Ⓒ Wound Specimen
30	Ⓒ Blood Glucose	44	Ⓒ Collecting Nose, Throat, Sputum Specimen
30	Ⓒ Oxygen Therapy	44	Ⓒ Occult Blood
30	Ⓒ Peak Expiratory Flow	44	Ⓒ Skin Puncture
31	Ⓒ Sterile Gloves	44	Ⓒ Blood Glucose
31	Ⓒ Handwashing	44	Ⓒ Wound Specimen
31	Ⓒ Gloves and Gowns	48	Ⓐ Résumé Writing

Delmar's COMPREHENSIVE

MEDICAL ASSISTING

Administrative and Clinical Competencies

Wilburta Q. Lindh, CMA

Marilyn S. Pooler, RN, CMA-C, MEd

Carol D. Tamparo, CMA-A, PhD

Joanne U. Cerrato, BS, MT (ASCP), MA

2nd Edition

DELMAR

THOMSON LEARNING

Australia Canada Mexico Singapore Spain United Kingdom United State

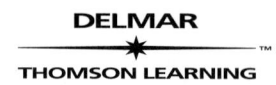

Delmar's Comprehensive Medical Assisting: Administrative and Clinical Competencies, 2nd Edition
by Wilburta Q. Lindh, Marilyn S. Pooler, Carol D. Tamparo, and Joanne U. Cerrato

Business Unit Director:
William Brottmiller

Executive Marketing Manager:
Dawn F. Gerrain

Production Coordinator:
John Mickelbank

Acquisitions Editor:
Maureen Muncaster

Executive Editor:
Cathy L. Esperti

Art/Design Coordinator:
Mary Colleen Liburdi

Senior Developmental Editor:
Elisabeth F. Williams

Project Editors:
David Buddle
Patricia Gillivan

Cover Design:
The Drawing Board

Editorial Assistants:
Jennifer Frisbee
Jill Korznat

For permission to use material from this text or product, contact us by
Tel   800-730-2214
Fax 800-730-2215
www.thomsonrights.com

Library of Congress Cataloging-in-Publication Data

Delmar's comprehensive medical assisting: administrative and clinical competencies / Wilburta Q. Lindh ... [et al.].—2nd edition
    p. cm.
  Includes bibliographical references and index.
  ISBN 0-7668-2418-7
  1. Medical assistants. 2. Physicians' assistants. I. Title: Comprehensive medical assisting. II. Lindh, Wilburta Q.
R728.8.D396   2001
610.69'53   dc21

2001032536

NOTICE TO THE READER

CONTENTS

For practice activities, these
icons tell you when to turn to
Delmar's Medical Assisting Skills
CD-ROMs in the back
of the book.

Ⓐ Administrative Skills CD-ROM

Ⓒ Clinical Skills CD-ROM

MANAGING AUTHORS

Wilburta (Billie) **Q. Lindh**, CMA, holds professor emeritus status at Highline Community College, Des Moines, Washington, and currently serves as program director and consultant to the Medical Assistant Program. She is a member of the SeaTac Chapter of the American Association of Medical Assistants (AAMA) and has lectured at AAMA seminars on the importance of communication. Lindh is co-author of *Therapeutic Communications for Allied Health Professions* published by Delmar. She has also co-authored *The Radiology Word Book* and *The Ophthalmology Word Book*, texts frequently used by transcriptionists. Lindh also authored the medical assistant chapter for *Guide to Careers in the Health Professions*.

Marilyn S. Pooler, RN, CMA-C, MEd, is a professor in the Medical Assisting Department at Springfield Technical Community College, Springfield, Massachusetts. Pooler has taught at Springfield for 24 years and previously served as chair of the Medical Assisting Department. She has served on the certifying board of the AAMA task force for test construction and is a member of the executive board of the New England Association of Allied Health Educators. She also is a site surveyor for AAMA, reviewing medical assisting programs at schools and colleges seeking accreditation.

Carol D. Tamparo, CMA-A, PhD, is Dean of Business and Allied Health at Lake Washington Technical College in Kirkland, Washington. Tamparo, who taught at Highline Community College in Des Moines, Washington, for 23 years, is a member of the SeaTac Chapter of the AAMA. Tamparo, a speaker at numerous AAMA seminars and educational conferences, is recognized as an expert on medical law, ethics, and bioethics. She is the co-author of *Diseases of the Human Body*; *Medical Law, Ethics, and Bioethics for Ambulatory Care*; and *Therapeutic Communications for Allied Health Professions*.

ACKNOWLEDGMENTS

The managing authors personally acknowledge the following people:

To my husband, who continually supports and assists in so many ways, thank you. To my family for support and encouragement, and to Laura, who provided expertise for some chapters, thank you. To the students, graduates, and fellow colleagues who challenge me to stay current with skills and up-to-date with technology, thank you.

Billie Q. Lindh

Thanks to my friends who were very supportive of my efforts, and a special thanks to my husband, Jud, for his patience and understanding during this endeavor.

Marilyn S. Pooler

To all my students in health care programs who keep me current, to my school administrators and family members who have been supportive of this project, and to the health care providers who patiently and lovingly cared for my mother in an assisted living Alzheimer's unit until her death in April 2001, my thanks and deepest regard and respect.

Carol D. Tamparo

A sincere thank you to Joanne Cerrato, former co-author, for her many invaluable contributions to the formation of the first edition of this text.

A special thank you to William Patten, MHS, MT (ASCP), for editing Unit 9, Laboratory Procedures. Bill is a laboratory supervisor at the Baystate Medical Center in Springfield, Massachusetts. He is a certified medical technologist and has a master's degree with a concentration in allied health education. He has 25 years of experience in the laboratory field. His responsibilities have included program director of a Committee on Allied Health Education and Accreditation (CAHEA)-approved medical technology program, Director of Education for the Department of Pathology at Baystate Medical Center, and, most recently, Service Coordinator for the Baystate Reference Laboratories. He is also a faculty member at a number of area academic institutions. He has taught phlebotomy, clinical chemistry, and other laboratory science courses during the past 10 years. He is a member of the American Society of Clinical Pathologists and has served as a site surveyor in the inspection process for the National Accrediting Agency for Clinical Laboratory Science (NAACLS) and the College of American Pathology (CAP).

REVIEWERS

Kaye Acton
Director of Medical Assisting
    Program
Alamance Community College
Graham, NC

Magdalena Andrasevits, NRCMA
Medical Assistant Program Director
Sanford-Brown College
North Kansas City, MO

Joseph DeSapio, RMA
Director of Facility and Library
    Resources
Medical Assisting Instructor
Ultrasound Diagnostic School
New York, NY

Eleanor K. Flores, RN, BSN, MEd
Briarwood College
Southington, CT

Tova Green
IVTC Fort Wayne
Fort Wayne, IN

Karen Jackson, NR-CMA
Medical Program Chair
Education America, Dallas Campus
Garland, TX

Barbara G. Kalfin, BS, AAS,
    CMA-C
Medical Assisting Extern Coordinator
Instructor, Medical Assisting Program
City College
Ft. Lauderdale, FL

Theresa Offenberger, PhD
Professor of Medical Assisting
Cuyahoga Community College
Cleveland, OH

Agnes Pucillo, LPN
Medical Assisting Program Director
Ultrasound Diagnostic School
Iselin, NJ

Patricia Schrull, RN, MBA, MEd,
    CMA
Program Director, Medical Assisting
    Program
Lorain County Community College
Elyria, OH

Janet Sesser, BS Ed. Admin., RMA,
    CMA
Corporate Director of Education,
    Allied Health
High-Tech Institute, Inc.
Phoenix, AZ

Kimberly A. Shinall, RN
President and CEO
KAS Enterprises
Virginia Beach, VA

Lois M. Smith, RN, CMA
Arapahoe Community College
Golden, CO

Susan Sniffin
Suffolk Community College
Great Neck, NY

Alisa M. Tetlow, RMA
Medical Assistant Program Director
Ultrasound Diagnostic School
Philadelphia, PA

Nina Thierer
Tidewater Technical Institute
Virginia Beach, VA

Fred Valdes, MD
Medical Department Chairman
City College
Ft. Lauderdale, FL

Sujana Wardell, RMA, RPT (AMT),
    AS
Program Director for Clinical and
    Administrative Medical Assisting
San Joaquin Valley College, Visalia
    Campus
Visalia, CA

Sally Wooten
Whitman Education Group
Miami, FL

Terri Wyman, CMA
Director of Health Information
    Specialties
Ultrasound Diagnostic School
Springfield, MA

CONTRIBUTORS

Sandra K. Anderson, MS
Chapter 11: *Computers in the Ambulatory Care Setting*

Julie B. Brown, RNC, MSN, CMA
Chapter 22: *Infection Control, Medical Asepsis, and Sterilization*

Barbara Dahl, CMA
Chapter 22: *Infection Control, Medical Asepsis, and Sterilization*, Chapter 31: *Assisting with Minor Surgery*, and Chapter 39: *Introduction to the Medical Laboratory*

Bonnie Lou Deister, MS, BSN, RN, CMA-C
Chapter 45: *The Medical Assistant as Office Manager* and Chapter 46: *The Medical Assistant as Human Resources Manager*

Walter R. English, MA, MT
Chapter 42: *Urinalysis*

Jeanette Girkin, EdD, CMA
Chapter 15: *Written Communications*

Mary K. Hickey
Chapter 12: *Telephone Techniques* and Chapter 17: *Daily Financial Practices*

Lynn B. Hoeltke, MBA, MT (ASCP), PBT, DLM
Chapter 40: *Phlebotomy: Venipuncture and Capillary Puncture*

Jan L. Johnson, MEd, CMA
Chapter 13: *Patient Scheduling* and Chapter 14: *Medical Records Management*

Benna Kisin, CMT
Chapter 15: *Written Communications*

Diane Klieger, RN, MBA, CMA
Chapter 30: *Examinations and Procedures of Body Systems* and Chapter 37: *Electrocardiography*

Kathy A. McCall, CMA-AC, BS, MA
Chapter 20: *Billing and Collections* and Chapter 21: *Accounting Practices*

Sharon Paff, AS, RMA (AMT)
Chapter 24: *Vital Signs and Measurements*, Chapter 25: *The Physical Examination*, and Chapter 30: *Examinations and Procedures of Body Systems*

Tom Palko, MEd, MCS, MT (ASCP)
Chapter 41: *Hematology*

Theresa Perry, MS, BS, CMA
Chapter 34: *Nutrition in Health and Disease*

Jane Rice, RN, CMA-C
Chapter 35: *Basic Pharmacology* and Chapter 36: *Calculation of Medication Dosage and Medication Administration*

Lisa Shimeld, MS
Chapter 44: *Specialty Laboratory Tests*

Sylvia Taylor, BS, CMA
Chapter 2: *Health Care Settings and the Health Care Team*

Virginia Lawless Thompson
Chapter 9: *Emergency Procedures and First Aid*

Ginny Torres, CMA
Chapter 19: *Medical Insurance Coding* and Chapter 23: *Taking a Medical History, the Patient's Chart, and Methods of Documentation*

Adrianne C. Williams
Chapter 33: *Rehabilitation and Therapeutic Modalities*

LIST OF PROCEDURES

PREFACE

The world of health care has changed rapidly over the past few years, and as we travel through the 21st century, health care professionals will encounter more challenges than ever before. As medical assistants you will be called on to do more and respond to an increasing number of clinical and administrative responsibilities, especially in this age of managed care. Now is the time to equip yourself with the skills you will need to excel in the field. Now is the time to maximize your potential, expand your base of knowledge, and dedicate yourself to becoming the best multifaceted, multiskilled medical assistant that you can be.

The new edition of *Delmar's Comprehensive Medical Assisting: Administrative and Clinical Competencies* will guide you on this journey. The word *comprehensive* is not used lightly here, for this text is part of a dynamic learning system that also includes two skills CD-ROMs and a workbook. Together, these learning tools conform to the standard and advanced areas of competence defined by AAMA's Role Delineation Study and AMT's Registered Medical Assistant Competency Inventory. They emphasize the importance of interpersonal communications in the medical environment. They explore changes in the health care setting including the development of standard precautions and the implications of managed care. This powerful learning system gives you an intimate look at the challenges you'll face and the opportunities you'll find as a medical assistant.

Unlike many texts, *Delmar's Comprehensive Medical Assisting*, 2nd edition, was written not just by one or two individuals but by many talented authors—experts who give you a sound and thorough understanding of the fundamentals. The text then moves beyond theory and develops all concepts in a real-life situation. What is it like to be working in the field? What are the problems you may encounter?

You'll discover common challenges faced by medical assistants through realistic scenarios woven into the chapter introductions. Case studies depict the ambulatory care setting where you, as a medical assistant, may very well be employed. Patient teaching tips provide practical advice. Proper documentation is emphasized.

How the Text Is Organized

Delmar's Comprehensive Medical Assisting, 2nd edition, presents a logical, in-depth review of all administrative and clinical competencies required of today's multi-skilled medical assistants—*in full color!*

- **Section I, General Procedures (Chapters 1 through 9)**, provides the groundwork for understanding the role and responsibilities of the medical assistant. Topics include the medical assisting profession, the health care team, history of medicine, therapeutic communications, coping skills for the medical assistant, legal and ethical issues, and emergency procedures and first aid.

- **Section II, Administrative Procedures (Chapters 10 through 21)**, provides up-to-date information on all administrative competencies required of medical assistants. Topics include creating the facility environment, computer use, telephone techniques, patient scheduling, medical records management, written communications, transcription, insurance and coding, managing facility finances, billing and collections, and accounting practices.

- **Section III, Clinical Procedures (Chapters 22 through 44)**, gives you a thorough understanding of all clinical, diagnostic, and laboratory procedures important to today's ambulatory care settings. Topics include medical asepsis, medical history, vital signs and measurements, physical examination, obstetrics and gynecology, pediatrics, male reproductive system, gerontology, body systems, assisting with minor surgery, diagnostic imaging, rehabilitation medicine, nutrition, pharmacology, medication calculations, EKG, safety guidelines, venipuncture, hematology, urinalysis, microbiology, and specialty tests.

- **Section IV, Professional Procedures (Chapters 45 through 48)**, examines the role of the medical assistant as office and human resources manager and provides tools and techniques to use when preparing for externship, medical assisting credentials, and employment.

- **Glossary** includes definitions of all key terms, with related chapter numbers indicated.

- **Two Medical Assisting Skills CDs—Administrative and Clinical**—are found on the inside back cover of this book. This interactive software challenges you to apply content, think critically, develop competency in skills, and improve your knowledge base.

How Each Chapter Is Organized

All chapters include similar features and presentation and function as building blocks to a comprehensive medical assisting education. However, each chapter is also a self-contained module and can be studied in any order or independently of other chapters in the text.

Each chapter contains:

- A listing of *key terms*
- *Role delineation components*, both standard and advanced
- An *outline of chapter*
- *Objectives*
- An *introduction* with a real-life scenario
- *Graphic icons, tables, and figures*
- *Full-color illustrations and photographs*
- *Procedures* with step-by-step instructions
- *Patient teaching tips*
- *Spotlight on AAMA Essentials through CAAHEP* boxes
- *Case studies with review questions*
- *Summary*
- *Review questions*
- *Bibliography* for further study

To receive the full value of *Delmar's Comprehensive Medical Assisting*, 2nd edition, it is important to understand the structure of the text and each chapter. Review the following information, plus "How to Use This Book" and "How to Use the Medical Assisting Skills CD-ROMs." Together, these materials will make your medical assisting education comprehensive and meaningful, providing you with the skills and understanding to enable you to practice your profession with confidence and competence.

EXTENSIVE TEACHING/LEARNING PACKAGE

The complete supplements package helps instructors efficiently manage time and resources and helps students to develop the necessary skills and competencies required by the demanding profession of medical assisting.

Instructor's Resource Kit

Order #0-7668-2419-5
This dynamic resource is a must-have for all instructors. This comprehensive three-ring binder includes:

Instructor's Guide. Complete with teaching strategies and learning concepts, this resource offers:

- Teaching/learning concepts
- Objectives and evaluation
- Instructional strategies

- Lesson plans
- Classroom activities

Computerized and Printed Testbank. Both electronic and printed testbanks are included, containing approximately 1,200 multiple choice questions.

PowerPoint Slides. The CD included in the *Instructor's Resource Kit* contains over 250 PowerPoint slides, making a backdrop with impact for your classroom presentations.

Medical Assisting CD-ROM. This is an innovative, comprehensive multimedia learning reference tool to enhance classroom presentations and increase student learning.

Instructor's Manual

Order #0-7668-2421-7
This compact resource is designed as a quick reference tool for classroom activity and instruction. Chapters include:

- Proficiency assessments
- Answers to text review questions
- Answers to text critical thinking questions
- Answers to workbook exercises
- Answers to workbook case studies

Student Workbook

Order #0-7668-2422-5
The workbook helps you learn and reinforce the essential competencies needed to become a successful, multiskilled medical assistant. Each chapter includes:

- Vocabulary builder exercises
- Learning review
- Investigation activity
- Case study
- Skills assessment checklist

HOW TO USE THIS BOOK

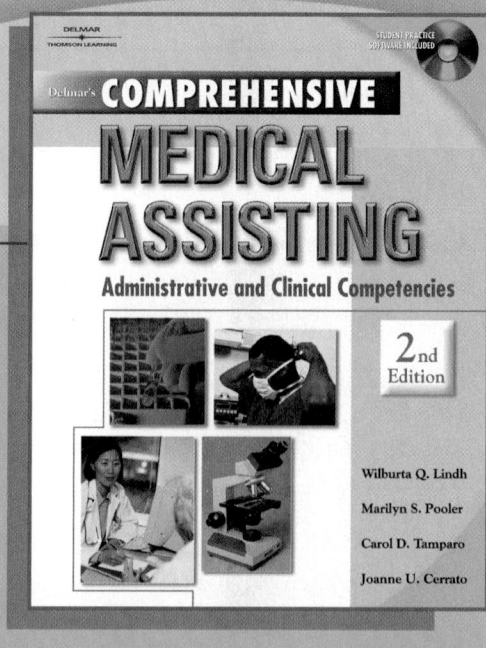

Delmar's *Comprehensive Medical Assisting: Administrative and Clinical Competencies, 2nd edition,* contains many features that make it an easy-to-use learning system. They include:

1 Key Terms

All key terms are listed at the beginning of each chapter. Within the text, the term is always boldfaced at its first occurrence for easy identification. Turn to the glossary for definitions of all key terms.

2 Chapter Outline

At the beginning of each chapter, you'll find an outline of all major headings. Review these headings of topic areas before you study the chapter. They are a road map to your understanding.

3 Objectives

Performance objectives test your knowledge of the key facts presented in the chapter. Use these objectives, together with review questions, to test your understanding of the chapter's content.

4 Role Delineation Components

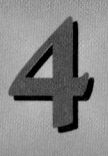

This opening list in each chapter keeps the focus on the medical assistant's actual job functions as defined by the accrediting bodies.

5 Real-Life Scenarios

The introductions to most chapters include an overview of the material *and* a real-life scenario based on two distinct ambulatory care settings and their physicians, medical assistants, and patients. Through these scenarios you'll come to understand some of the stimulating challenges faced by medical assistants and gain insight into how these challenges are overcome.

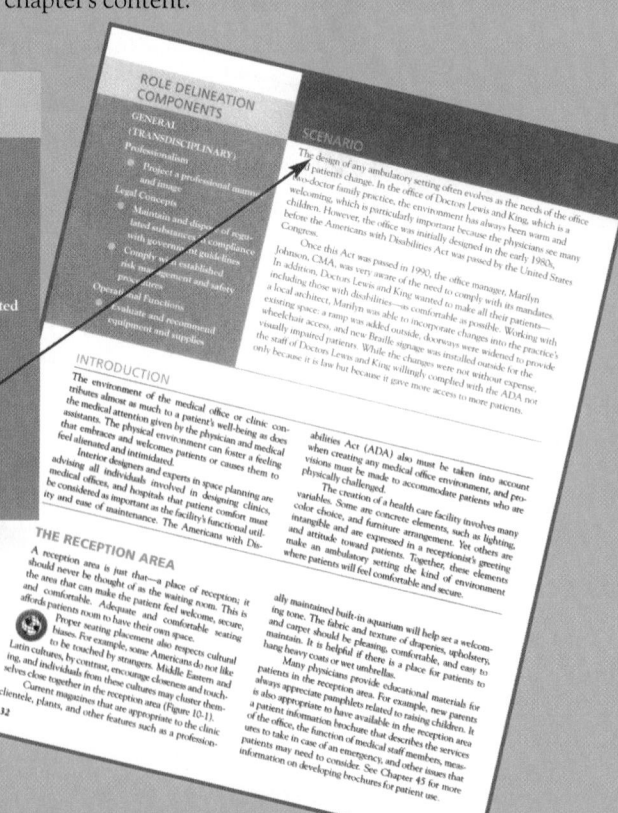

6 Patient Teaching Tips

This feature helps all current and future medical assistants anticipate patient concerns and provides sound suggestions for effective patient communication.

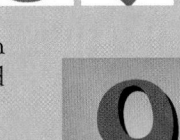

Patient Teaching Tip

Encourage patients to think of themselves as members of the health care team for they can provide information about their medical history. Use good communication skills to encourage the patient to describe symptoms and provide other information that is useful in diagnosis and treatment.

7 Icons

Graphic icons pinpoint information that relates to legal, safety, computer, managed care, and global or cultural issues.

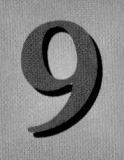

8 Procedures

Step-by-step procedures are now conveniently grouped together at the end of each chapter. They give detailed information on all important administrative, clinical, and general competencies as defined by AAMA and AMT.

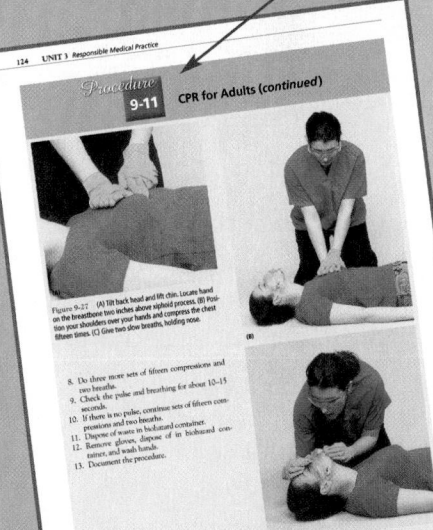

124 UNIT 3 Responsible Medical Practice

Procedure 9-11 CPR for Adults (continued)

Figure 9-27 (A) Tilt back head and chin. Locate hand on the breastbone two inches above xyphoid process. (B) Position your shoulders over your hands and compress the chest fifteen times. (C) Give two slow breaths, holding nose.

8. Do three more sets of fifteen compressions and two breaths.
9. Check the pulse and breathing for about 10–15 seconds.
10. If there is no pulse, continue sets of fifteen compressions and two breaths.
11. Dispose of waste in biohazard container.
12. Remove gloves, dispose of in biohazard container, and wash hands.
13. Document the procedure.

9 Spotlight on AAMA Essentials through CAAHEP

These psychology tips help you focus on the CAAHEP-mandated understandings required of medical assistants.

SPOTLIGHT ON AAMA ESSENTIALS THROUGH CAAHEP

- Recognizing a patient's cultural background is part of caring for the patient as a whole person.
- Human kindness often eliminates fear of the unknown.
- A positive attitude helps to lessen a negative feeling.

10 Web Activities

This new feature at the end of each chapter gives you practice navigating the Internet by suggesting online activities to help you begin to use those sites.

11 Case Studies

The case studies with accompanying review questions encourage a problem/solution approach. Use the case studies to put your knowledge into practice and arrive at a deeper understanding of the profession. Answers to the case studies are included as an appendix of the text.

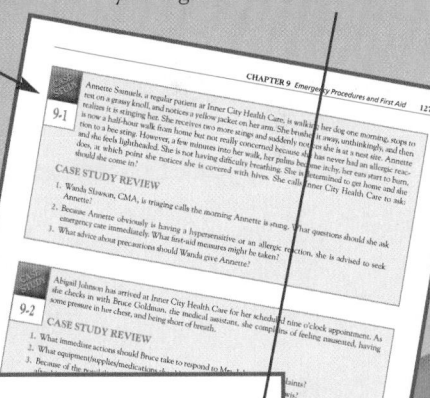

CHAPTER 9 Emergency Procedures and First Aid 127

12 Review Questions

Test your comprehension of the chapter with structured multiple choice questions and open-ended critical thinking questions that require you to combine an understanding of chapter material with your personal insight and judgment.

136 UNIT 4 Integrated Administrative Procedures

REVIEW QUESTIONS

13 Skills CDs Quick Locator

This invaluable tool inside the front cover tells you when to turn to your Skills CD-ROMs for practice activities that will strengthen your understanding of the chapter you are reading.

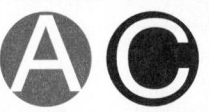

xxiii

HOW TO USE THE MEDICAL ASSISTING SKILLS CDs

The Skills CDs are designed to accompany **Delmar's Comprehensive Medical Assisting: Administrative and Clinical Competencies, 2nd edition,** so you can review and reinforce the important concepts you are learning in the textbook. By using these CDs, you'll challenge yourself and make your study of medical assisting concepts more effective and fun.

ADMINISTRATIVE SKILLS CD-ROM

The Administrative Skills CD-ROM is designed with you, the user, in mind. Several medical assistants lead you on a verbal guided tour through the medical office.

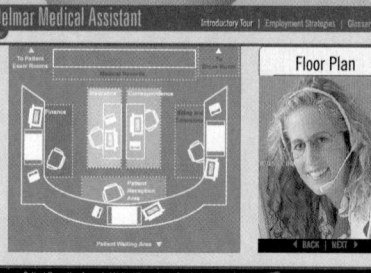

An introductory tour gives you an overview of the entire office. To navigate through the office, click on the area you wish to visit.

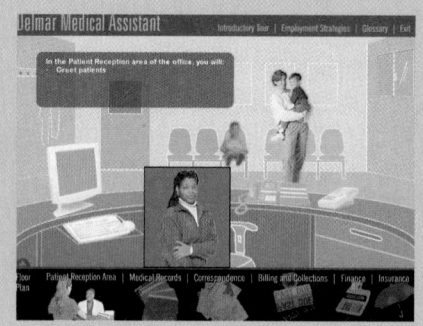

The medical assistant will give you an overview of the tasks and responsibilities associated with each area, and guide you through your many choices. In the patient reception area, for example, you may click on the active areas such as the computer, the phone, the answering machine, or the patient to branch into different content areas.

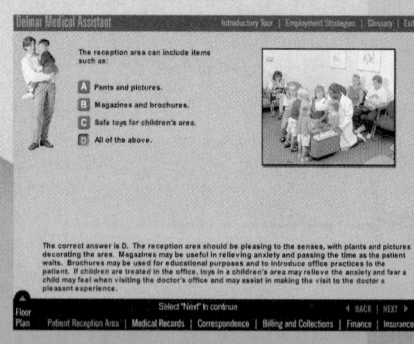

The medical assistant will give you instruction so you understand the various aspects of each area. Activities include multiple choice questions with correct and incorrect responses noted, scheduling appointments by dragging and dropping the information into the appointment book, filling out a message pad, and maintaining a telephone log.

In other areas such as billing and collections, you will be asked to complete a patient receipt by entering information into the correct area, fill out a daily log sheet, use the pegboard system, complete a super bill and ledger card by entering and highlighting information, complete a patient charge slip, write a check, and complete a deposit slip.

In the break room, you can test your knowledge of legal and ethical principles by completing a crossword puzzle.

A comprehensive glossary allows you to check your understanding of important key words and phrases.

CLINICAL SKILLS CD-ROM

The Clinical Skills CD-ROM is designed to be easy to use. It includes basic clinical skills used in medical assisting, a glossary of words used in the office, important infection control information, a help feature, and a tutorial that will assist you in using the CD-ROM.

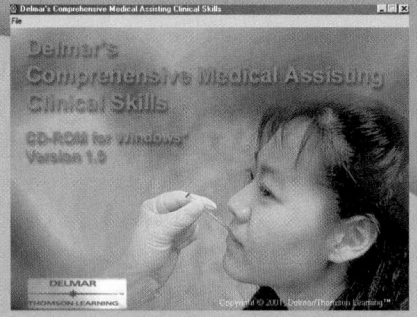

The skills menu lists each of the clinical skills contained on the CD-ROM. Click on the button of the skill you wish to study.

As you choose each skill, a menu will appear listing each of the sections included with the skill. By clicking on the buttons, you will navigate through the skill.

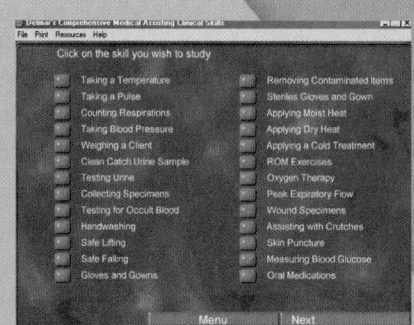

Clicking on the skills menu will take you to the main menu of skills you will be reviewing.

At any time you may return to this menu by clicking on the **Main Menu** button.

If you need to go back to the previous screen, just hit the **Previous** button.

The **Next** button takes you to the next step in the procedure.

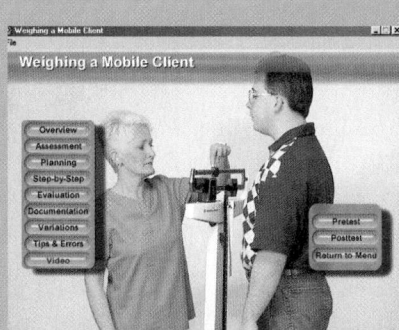

Each skill includes a pretest and a post-test section so you may enhance your learning by checking your knowledge before and after viewing the skill.

Each question on the pretest and post-test gives you a chance to answer correctly. You will be asked if that is the answer you want to go with, and you are able to change your answer. The correct answer will be displayed and your score will be tallied as you advance through the questions.

At the end, your final score with your percent rate for passing will be given. You are able to reset the questions and try again by simply clicking on the **Reset** button.

A glossary of terms is included to help you with your medical terminology. To find a term, just scroll down or use the buttons to advance you to the place in the alphabet where the word is found.

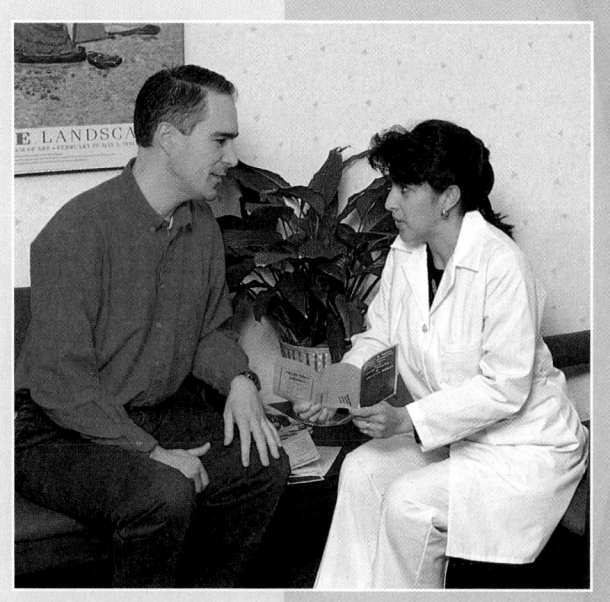

GENERAL PROCEDURES

Unit

1

INTRODUCTION TO MEDICAL ASSISTING AND HEALTH PROFESSIONS

Chapter 1

MEDICAL ASSISTING AS A PROFESSION

KEY TERMS

Accreditation
Ambulatory Care Setting
Attribute
Baccalaureate
Certification
Certified Medical Assistant (CMA)
Competency
Compliance
Credentialed
Disposition
Empathy
Externship
Facilitate
Improvise
Integrate
Internship
License
Licensure
Litigious
Practicum
Proprietary
Registered Medical Assistant (RMA)

OUTLINE

OBJECTIVES

The student should strive to meet the following performance objectives and demonstrate an understanding of the facts and principles presented in this chapter through written and oral communication.

1. Define the key terms as presented in the glossary.
2. Identify and discuss nine personal attributes that are important for a professional medical assistant to possess.
3. Discuss the history of medical assisting.
4. Describe the American Association of Medical Assistants and list its three major functions.
5. Explain accreditation, certification, and continuing education as they pertain to the professional medical assistant.
6. Identify the importance of the accreditation process to an educational institution.
7. Recall two methods to obtain recertification.
8. List five means of obtaining continuing education units. (*continues*)

OBJECTIVES (*continued*)

9. Describe the certifying agency that certifies medical assistants as registered medical assistants (RMA).
10. Describe the externship experience.
11. Recall two criteria for the selection of externship sites.
12. List three benefits of externship to student and site.
13. Describe the profession of medical assisting and analyze its career opportunities in relationship to your interests.
14. Differentiate among certification, licensure, and registration.
15. State the importance of understanding the scope of practice for the medical assistant.

ROLE DELINEATION COMPONENTS

GENERAL (TRANSDISCIPLINARY)

Professionalism

- **Project a professional manner and image**
- **Adhere to ethical principles**
- **Demonstrate initiative and responsibility**
- **Work as a team member**
- **Adapt to change**
- **Promote the CMA credential**
- **Enhance skills through continuing education**

Legal Concepts

- **Maintain confidentiality**
- **Practice within the scope of education, training, and personal capabilities**

INTRODUCTION

Historically, medical science has been fascinating to most people. Perhaps you have been drawn to medical assisting because you too are intrigued by medicine and want to learn about advances in health care and want to become involved in providing care to patients. More than likely you have a desire to help others.

Medical assistants have always played an integral role in physicians' offices and **ambulatory care settings** such as clinics and urgent care facilities, where health care services are offered on an outpatient basis. And now more than ever, because of the explosion of knowledge and high technology in medicine, medical assistants are involved in an ever-widening scope of clinical and administrative duties. With the medical assistant's expanded role has come the responsibility to become a well-educated and highly competent professional dedicated to providing the highest quality of health care.

Consumers of health care have become increasingly aware, primarily through the media, of the availability of the latest advances, techniques, and discoveries in medicine. They realize that they have a right for health care to be provided to them by educated, skilled, and competent professionals.

As you study to become a medical assistant, it is important for you to understand what a professional is. According to *Merriam-Webster's Collegiate Dictionary,* 10th edition, it is "one who has acquired a specialized body of knowledge, skills, and attitudes."

You will learn to **integrate,** or unify, your desire and need to help others with the knowledge, skills, and attitudes you acquire through your studies. By blending all of these, you will be able to provide patients with the best health care possible and learn what it means to be a professional medical assistant.

PERSONAL ATTRIBUTES OF THE PROFESSIONAL

There are certain characteristics or personal qualities that medical assistants should strive to cultivate. These are the **attributes** that identify a true professional; when caring for patients these qualities should come from the heart. They will enable the patient to trust you, the caregiver.

Empathy

To have **empathy** means to consider the patient's welfare and to be kind. It means stepping into the patient's place, discovering what the patient is experiencing, and then recognizing and identifying with those feelings.

Medical assistants should treat patients as they themselves would want to be treated. A visit to the doctor is often a time of fear and anxiety. Apprehension can be allayed tremendously when patients realize that their caregiver understands their feelings and desires to make their lives more pleasant and comfortable. See Figure 1-1.

It is important to realize that patients' health problems can have a profound effect on the caregiver. By maintaining a balanced outlook, medical assistants can safeguard themselves from becoming too emotionally involved with patient problems. Empathy is extremely important in the health care profession; however, emotionalism can cloud one's judgment.

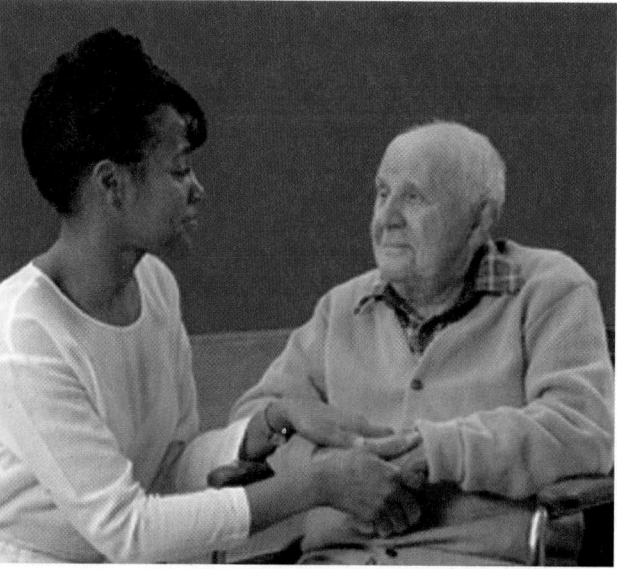

Figure 1-1 The medical assistant should have a friendly disposition and communicate empathy for the patient.

Attitude

A friendly, warm **disposition** and a sense of humor will help patients feel more at ease. A sincere affection for people can be conveyed by actions that **facilitate** open and honest communication. Your attitude should radiate genuine interest.

On occasion, difficult patients can test the tolerance level of the most experienced medical assistant because they seem never to be content with the care or services received. But no matter what the circumstances, patients should never be treated with disinterest or in an unfriendly manner. The medical assistant should always be pleasant and courteous.

When giving care to patients, do so unrestricted by your concerns about their attitudes, disease, race, religion, economic status, or sexual orientation.

As a member of the health care delivery team, the medical assistant needs to be cooperative and supportive of all other members, working with the team in an honest, open manner while keeping in mind the patient's right to privacy and confidentiality.

Dependability

When providing for a patient's well-being, it is important to focus attention on activities in the office or clinic environment that will demonstrate being well-organized, accurate, and responsive to the patient's needs.

Being dependable means that employer and coworkers rely on the medical assistant to be respectful of them, of patients, and of equipment and materials. Other members of the health care team will expect duties and responsibilities to be carried out responsibly. A dependable person interacts with coworkers in a supportive manner, is punctual, and limits absences from work.

Initiative

The willingness and ability to work independently shows initiative. A person with initiative is observant, notices work that needs to be done, and then takes action to complete those tasks without being told to do them. Employer and coworkers must be able to count on one another to anticipate patients' needs and be attentive to work that needs to be accomplished. The successful medical assistant will be ready to pitch in and recognize when others need assistance.

By asking appropriate questions and seeking information that will improve performance, medical assistants will demonstrate that they have the foresight and the "get up and go" needed to complete the numerous and varied tasks of the ambulatory care environment.

Flexibility

The ability to be adaptable is a trait that serves all professionals well. When caring for ill people, unexpected situations arise daily and medical assistants must be able to respond to a variety of situations (many of them emergencies and unanticipated) without losing a sense of equilibrium. Finding solutions to problems and developing alternative action plans demonstrates flexibility. To **improvise,** or solve problems that arise either routinely or spontaneously, is a characteristic worth nurturing.

Desire to Learn

A willingness to continually learn and grow is the mark of a true professional. With the growing technology in medicine, there is an ongoing necessity for constant learning. Medical assistants must be dedicated to high standards of performance, which can be accomplished by showing a desire to acquire information and by constantly updating their knowledge and skills. Keeping abreast of the latest diseases, treatments, procedures, and techniques can be achieved in a variety of ways, such as college courses, seminars, workshops, reading, and simply by being observant. The sharper the power of observation, the more the medical assistant will learn from physician, employer, and coworkers.

Physical Attributes

Appearance is important in patients' perceptions of the delivery of their care. Imparting the look of a professional requires an appearance that is clean and fresh and wholesome; in general, an appearance that reflects good health habits (Figure 1-2). Good personal hygiene practices, weight control, healthy-looking skin, hair, teeth, and nails all contribute to a professional appearance. Rest, good nutrition, regular exercise, and recreation all promote good health.

Female medical assistants should wear appropriate light daytime makeup. For the safety of both the professional and the patient, no necklaces or dangling earrings should be worn. The only jewelry worn should be single earposts or wedding rings. Hair should be neat and off the collar. Wear only clear, unchipped nail polish over short, manicured nails. Male medical assistants should be clean-shaven and have short hair. The only jewelry should be a wedding ring. Colognes, perfumes, and aftershave should not be worn at work. Tattoos should not be visible.

Patient care can place physical demands upon medical assistants. Lifting and moving patients is often required and the use of correct body mechanics will help minimize injuries to the back. While every reasonable accommodation is made for physically challenged medical assistants, to be mobile without assistance is important because medical assistants move about throughout the day while performing tasks and procedures. It is frequently necessary to bend, stoop, kneel, and crouch, especially when filing and retrieving patients' records, and for other tasks as well. Most procedures require that medical assistants have the ability to hear and see well for the accurate completion of tasks (Figure 1-3). Listening to blood pressures, taking a medical history, observing patients, performing phlebotomy, and identifying microorganisms under a microscope are some of the routine tasks and procedures performed daily in a medical facility. Manual dexterity is also needed for manipulating certain instruments and for entering data using a computer.

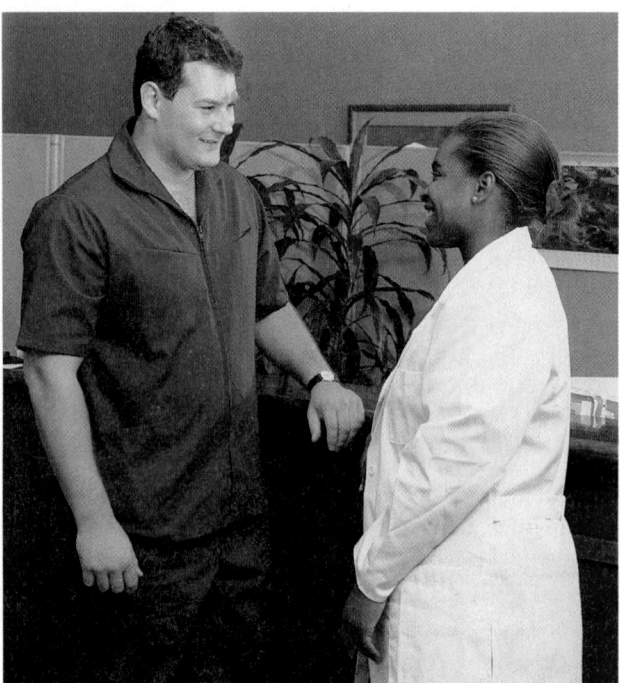

Figure 1-2   A professional, neat appearance makes patients feel at ease with their health care provider.

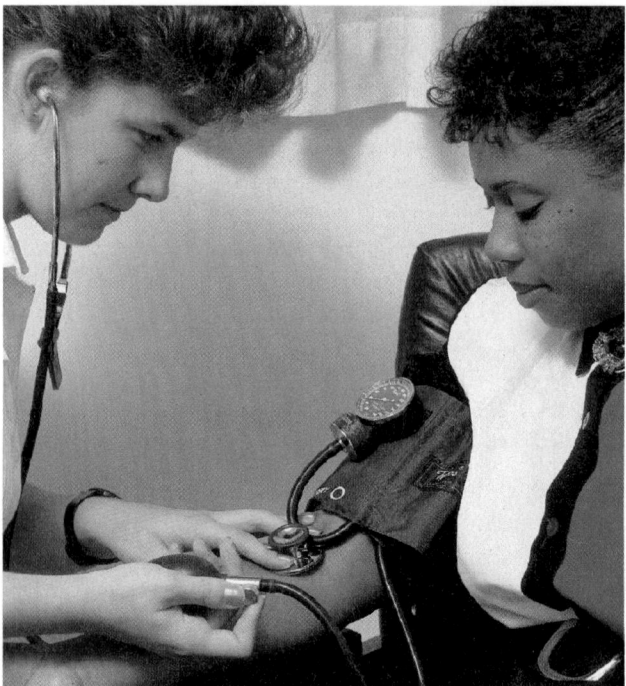

Figure 1-3   Measuring blood pressure is a task that requires the medical assistant to see and hear well.

Ability to Communicate

It is important that medical assistants learn to develop the ability to communicate well verbally and nonverbally with patients, staff, and other professionals.

Compliance with the physician's treatment plan is important for a positive outcome of patients' illnesses (Figure 1-4). Also, patients will feel more comfortable and less threatened in a medical office or ambulatory center that encourages staff to keep them informed.

Ethical Behavior

No discussion about personal attributes is complete without the mention of ethics. Ethics is a system of values each individual has that determines perceptions of right and wrong. Our life experiences mold this set of values, which is considered a personal code of ethics.

Medical ethics govern medical conduct or that behavior practiced as health care providers. These ethics involve relationships with patients, their families, fellow professionals, and society in general. Good ethical behavior will have a positive impact on the profession of medical assisting and on the medical community as well. By adhering to the medical assistants' Code of Ethics, we endeavor to elevate the profession to a position of dignity and respect. (A more in-depth discussion of this Code of Ethics can be found in Chapter 8.)

The personal qualities of empathy, healthy attitude, dependability, initiative, flexibility, the desire to learn, a wholesome physical presence, the ability to communicate well, and ethical behavior are some of the characteristics that any professional possesses and that medical assistants should strive to develop. When entering into the profession of medical assisting, it is important to learn more about these and other qualities and to begin to cultivate and refine them.

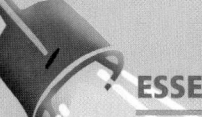

SPOTLIGHT ON AAMA ESSENTIALS THROUGH CAAHEP

- It is your attributes that enable others to trust you as their caregiver.
- A true professional behaves in an ethical manner.
- Continuing education should be an ongoing and life-enhancing experience.

HISTORICAL PERSPECTIVE OF MEDICAL ASSISTING

Historically, when physicians began their practices, it was common for them to hire individuals and train them on the job. Physicians originally hired nurses, but eventually they came to realize that nurses could not perform the variety of duties that are required in medical offices and ambulatory care centers. The nurse's role was limited to assisting the physician with clinical procedures, whereas the medical assistant's role was and is much broader and includes a large number of activities, procedures, and responsibilities, both administrative and clinical.

Today, with a much more informed patient comes the need for educated and credentialed medical assistants. Additionally, in today's litigious atmosphere, which makes health care providers vulnerable to malpractice suits, most employers recognize the importance of employing medical assistants who are professionally prepared through formal education. Employers want knowledgeable and dependable medical assistants so that physicians can focus their time and attention on the medical decisions, treatments, and techniques for which they have been educated and licensed. This leaves in the hands of the medical assistant, assisting the physician and the operation and management of the practice.

It was in 1978 that the profession of medical assisting was formally recognized by the United States Department of Education. Twenty-four years prior to this official recognition of the profession, a group of medical assistants gathered to establish a professional organization. With support, encouragement, and guidance from the American Medical Association (AMA), the American Association of Medical Assistants (AAMA) was founded in 1956 (Figure 1-5). The first president of the organization was Maxine Williams.

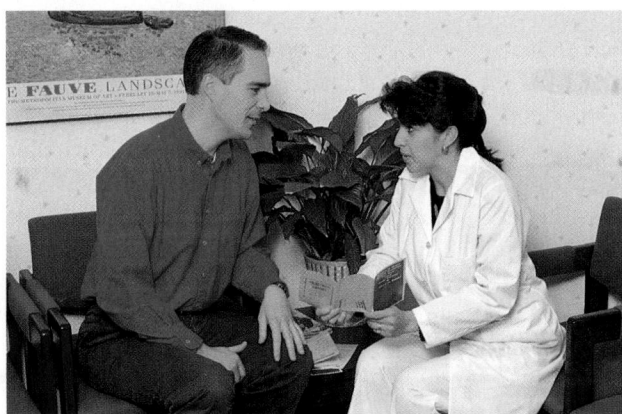

Figure 1-4 Patient education requires skill in communicating instructions to patients in language appropriate to their needs.

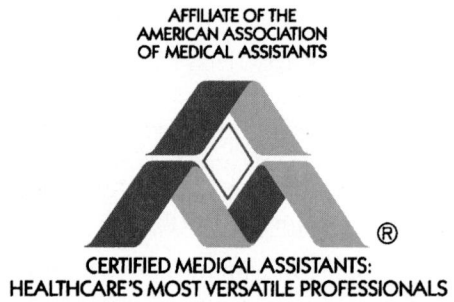

AFFILIATE OF THE
AMERICAN ASSOCIATION
OF MEDICAL ASSISTANTS

CERTIFIED MEDICAL ASSISTANTS:
HEALTHCARE'S MOST VERSATILE PROFESSIONALS

Figure 1-5 Logo of the American Association of Medical Assistants, a professional organization founded in 1956. (Courtesy of the AAMA)

In 1991, the AAMA's board of trustees approved the present definition of medical assisting:

> Medical Assisting is an allied health profession whose practitioners function as members of the health care delivery team and perform administrative and clinical procedures.

AMERICAN ASSOCIATION OF MEDICAL ASSISTANTS

The American Association of Medical Assistants has three major purposes:

1. Accreditation
2. Certification
3. Continuing education

Accreditation and certification standards were developed by the AMA and the AAMA through the Commission on Accreditation of Allied Health Education Programs (CAAHEP) for schools wishing assurance that their medical assistant programs are of the highest quality and satisfy CAAHEP criteria.

Accreditation

The AAMA works jointly with the AMA to define the essential components and appropriate standards of quality that educational institutions offer in their medical assistant curriculum. The United States Department of Education has approved the AAMA and AMA as an accreditation, or approving, body for educational programs for medical assistants. A medical assisting program that is accredited meets the standards as outlined in the *Standards and Guidelines for an Accredited Education Program for the Medical Assistant. Standards* are the minimum standards of quality used in accrediting programs that prepare individuals to enter the medical assisting profession. On-site review teams evaluate the program's compliance

with, or adherence to, the standards. All aspects of programs seeking accreditation status undergo scrutiny to ascertain the program's quality and to ensure continued compliance with the standards.

Certification

As the profession grew and developed, some states came to require special licensure or certification to perform certain tasks, and in other states health professionals were challenged by the skill and broad spectrum of the medical assistant's ability. To defend medical assistants whose right to practice clinical procedures was being challenged, the AAMA responded at their 1995 convention with the following policy, which became effective February 1, 1998:

> that any candidate for the AAMA Certification Examination be a graduate of a CAAHEP-accredited medical assisting program. This requirement would become effective February 1, 1998. Anticipated benefits of the recommendation are to: (1) safeguard the quality of care to the consumer; (2) ensure the CMA's role in the rapidly evolving health care delivery system; and (3) continue to promote the identity and stature of the profession.

For a three-year trial period beginning in March 1998, graduates of medical assisting programs accredited by the Accrediting Bureau of Health Education Schools (ABHES) with 12 months of full-time health work experience or 24 months of part-time health work experience were eligible to take the AAMA certification examination. Certification is voluntary, not mandatory, for medical assistants to practice, although the AAMA strongly urges those eligible to take the national certification examination. The exam measures professional competency at job entry level. Successful completion of the examination earns the individual the status of being certified and of being known as a certified medical assistant (CMA). The initials follow the individual's name. Conferring of the CMA status is referred to as being credentialed (Figure 1-6). It signifies recognition of competency by having attained a certain level of knowledge and skill.

In some areas of the United States, employers hire only certified medical assistants. The examination is offered twice yearly simultaneously at more than 200 test sites across the United States.

Recertification of the credential must be undertaken within five years from the date of certification in order to maintain current status as a CMA. Two routes are available to recertify. One is by accumulating approved continuing education hours, the other is by taking the certification examination again.

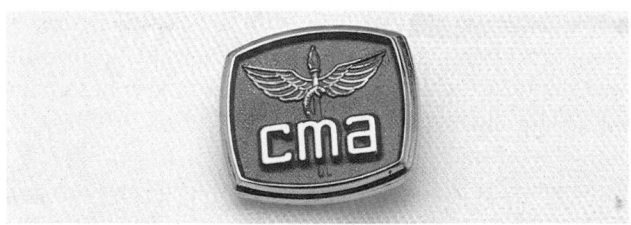

Figure 1-6 CMA pin awarded by the American Association of Medical Assistants upon successful completion of the national certification examination.

The status of a medical assistant's credentials (whether current or not current) is a public record available at the AAMA executive office, 20 N. Wacker Dr., Suite 1575, Chicago, IL 60606-2963. The AAMA Board of Trustees approved a policy change at the association's 1999 annual convention in Nashville. Effective January 1, 2003, all certified medical assistants who are employed or seeking employment *must* have current status as a CMA in order to use the credential. The mandatory current status for use of the CMA designation protects patients, employers, and the medical assistant's right to practice. Certification and recertification attest to the medical assistant's desire for professional development.

At one time, the credentials CMA-A (Certified Medical Assistant, Administrative); CMA-C (Certified Medical Assistant, Clinical); CMA-AC (Certified Medical Assistant, Administrative and Clinical); and CMA-Ped (Certified Medical Assistant, Pediatrics) were awarded to candidates who successfully passed specialty examinations in addition to the basic CMA examination.

While these specialty examinations have been phased out for newly graduated medical assistants, current medical assistants who have already earned these specialty credentials can maintain them and continue to be recertified through the Continuing Education Unit method.

Continuing Education

The AAMA vigorously encourages continuing education for all medical assistants. This can be accomplished through various means such as educational meetings, seminars, workshops, conventions, and the "Quest for Excellence," AAMA's series of home study courses for continuing education credit.

Membership in the AAMA is tri-level: local, state, and national. Educational meetings are held regularly at local and state meetings and conventions. The annual AAMA national convention provides an excellent forum for attaining knowledge through its educational offerings and for networking with other medical assistants.

Continuing an education is a lifelong process and serves as testimony to a commitment to professionalism.

REGISTERED MEDICAL ASSISTANT

The American Medical Technologists (AMT) is a national agency that certifies several different health professionals including medical assistants. In 1972, the AMT began offering and administering a national certification examination to medical assistants. The AMT offers a computerized examination year-round to qualified candidates. Upon successful completion of the examination, medical assistants receive a certificate designating them as **registered medical assistants (RMA).**

The association is similar to the AAMA. It has its own committees, conventions, bylaws, state chapters, officers, registrations, and revalidation examinations.

RMAs have been active in legislation to protect medical assistants, assuring improvement in medical assistant education, and providing for continuing education opportunities.

The RMA certification examination is given yearly in June and November at schools that have been accredited by the Accrediting Bureau of Health Education Schools (ABHES). To sit for the examination, applicants must have graduated from a medical assisting program accredited by ABHES or must meet certain experience requirements. AMT continuing education programs for renewal of the RMA credential also are available. The credential is awarded through the AMT (Figure 1-7). For more information, call 1-800-275-1268 or write to AMT, 710 Higgins Rd., Park Ridge, IL 60068.

EDUCATION OF THE PROFESSIONAL MEDICAL ASSISTANT

Formal education of medical assistants takes place in community and junior colleges as well as in **proprietary** schools. The AAMA has established educational requirements for program directors to follow for their programs to be considered accredited. These requirements were previously known as the DACUM Competencies. In 1997, in coordination with the National Board of Medical Examiners, educators, and practicing CMAs, the AAMA developed the Medical Assistant Role Delineation Chart, which is the occupational analysis of the medical assisting profession, and is included as an appendix of this

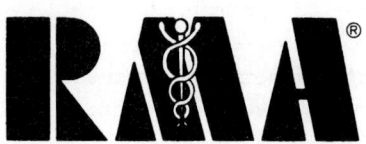

Figure 1-7 Logo of Registered Medical Assistant, representing a credential awarded by the American Medical Technologists Association.

text. In addition, the entry-level competencies that must be mastered by students in academic programs and the *Standards (formerly "Essentials") and Guidelines for an Accredited Education Program for Medical Assistants* will be revised to reflect the findings of the Role Delineation Study.

Educational institutions seeking accreditation for a medical assisting program must develop the curricula to these *Standards and Guidelines* to ensure the highest quality medical assistant education and employment preparedness.

While not a complete list, some of the administrative, general (transdisciplinary), and clinical courses include those shown in Table 1-1.

Another aspect of an educational medical assisting program is the **externship,** a period of time when students participate in a **practicum.** This provides an excellent opportunity to apply theory to practice.

Preparation for Externship

Externship, practicum, and internship are all terms used to define the transition period between the classroom and actual employment. An externship is planned and supervised by a coordinator from the medical assisting program and the health care facility that agrees to become a partner in the education and employability of the student.

Externship Sites. Sites for externship are chosen carefully to ensure that a variety of experiences is available for the student. The sites should provide the student with adequate administrative, clinical, and general experiences. The staff at the various sites must be willing to make a commitment to the medical assistant's education by spending appropriate time observing and instructing the student.

Benefits of Externship. The externship experience is mutually beneficial to the student and staff at the health care facility that is providing the educational experiences.

Some of the benefits to the student are the opportunity to:

- Apply classroom knowledge and skill in a real-world medical setting
- Recognize improvement in performance and knowledge
- Understand that there may be more than one acceptable method of performance
- Begin to establish a network of support through colleagues

Some of the benefits to the externship site are:

- Greater alertness of staff because of their educational responsibilities to the student
- Opportunity for staff to observe students who will soon be seeking employment
- Possibility that staff will learn more about the profession of medical assisting

Educational institutions that confer associate or baccalaureate degrees require general education courses for graduation in addition to the administration and clinical courses.

There are four-year institutions of higher learning that offer a **baccalaureate** degree to medical assistants who have graduated with an associate's degree from a community or junior college. The graduate is accepted as a third-year student and can obtain a baccalaureate degree in such areas as health care management or health care facility administrator.

Because there is a demand for medical assistant educators, some medical assistants take education courses to become allied health educators.

TABLE 1-1	TYPICAL ADMINISTRATIVE, GENERAL, AND CLINICAL COURSES IN AN ACCREDITED MEDICAL ASSISTING PROGRAM

Administrative Courses

Computer Applications
Manual Recording of Patients' Data
Scheduling Appointments
Maintaining Medical Records
Word Processing/Typewriting/Keyboarding
Billing/Collections/Managing Patients' Accounts
Coding/Insurance Claims
Telephone Triage
Personnel Management

General Courses

Anatomy and Physiology
Medical Terminology
Diseases
Patient Education
Medical Law and Ethics

Clinical Courses

Pharmacology/Administration of Medications
Assisting Techniques/Physical Examination
Assisting with Minor Surgery
Basic Laboratory Procedures/Routine Blood and Urine Testing
Cardiopulmonary Resuscitation

CAREER OPPORTUNITIES

Medical assistants have been described as health care's most versatile, multifaceted professionals. The fact that medical assistants possess a broad scope of knowledge and skills makes them ideal professionals for any ambulatory care setting. Indeed, owing to such versatility, medical assistants find employment in a variety of settings: offices, clinics, hospitals, medical laboratories, insurance companies, government agencies, pharmaceutical companies, and educational institutions. Although the range of employment opportunities continues to grow, in the past decade, about four out of five medical assistants were employed in physicians' offices and clinics. About one in five worked in offices of other health care practitioners, such as chiropractors, optometrists, and podiatrists. The outlook for employment for medical assistants is very promising. According to the AAMA, there are presently 1.3 million medical assistants in the work force. The United States Department of Labor Bureau of Statistics listed medical assisting as one of the fastest growing allied health professions for the years 1998–2008.

Increased employment opportunities for medical assistants result from the increased medical needs of an aging population, growth in the number of health care practitioners and their desire to hire the most qualified person for the task, increased diagnostic testing, greater volume and complexity of paperwork and computer information, managed care's emphasis on ambulatory care, and the insurance-mandated shorter stay of patients in hospitals.

REGULATION OF HEALTH CARE PROVIDERS

One way health care providers can be regulated is through the process of credentialing. Credentialing recognizes health care providers who are professionally and technically competent. Recognition comes from professional associations, certifying agencies, and the state or federal government. Regulation ensures:

- Competence of health care providers
- A minimum standard of knowledge, training, and skill
- The limiting of the performance of certain procedures to a specific occupation

Licensure, certification, and registration are three kinds of regulations/credentialing. See Table 1-2.

Scope of Practice

Medical assisting is not licensed as a profession; however, some states require that medical assistants be graduates of an accredited medical assisting program in order to work as medical assistants.

Two examples of licensed professions are medicine and nursing. A license regulates the activities of these professions by enacting laws that specify educational requirements and by defining the scope of practice. A license is conferred upon an individual who successfully completes specialized educational requirements and successfully passes an examination administered by the state in which the individual resides. The state grants a license to that individual to practice medicine or nursing. Licensure forbids anyone who is not licensed from performing activities that are designated by that particular license. For example, the law states that the physician's license allows diagnosing and prescribing treatment. If someone were to diagnose or prescribe without a license, that individual would be committing an illegal act and would be practicing medicine without a license, which is considered a felony.

There are state laws that govern the practice of medicine and nursing (medical practice acts, nursing practice acts), and many states have acts that give physicians the right to delegate certain clinical procedures to

TABLE 1-2	COMPARISON OF REQUIREMENTS FOR CERTIFICATION, LICENSURE, AND REGISTRATION		
	Certification	**Licensure**	**Registration**
Practice Requirement	Voluntary	Mandatory	Voluntary
Conferred by	Nongovernmental agency or professional association	Legislated by each state	Professional association
	If qualified and meets requirements	If qualified and meets requirements	Listed on an official roster
	Must pass examination	Must pass state examination	Passing examination not always required
How restrictive	Used by most professional associations	Most restrictive	Least restrictive

qualified allied health professionals. Because medical assistants are not required to be licensed, they are allowed to perform clinical procedures only under the supervision of the physician or other licensed health care professional who is granted the right and who delegates the specific clinical procedures to them.

In some states, including California, Washington, and others, unlicensed health care providers are required to have authorization from the state to perform allergy testing, venipuncture, and to give injections. A registration fee and mandatory training are required. In such circumstances, medical assistants or other health care providers would be breaking the law if they performed these procedures without registration and training.

In some states, authorization is required for unlicensed health care providers to expose patients to X rays.

Medical assistants do not perform procedures for which they have not been educated and trained. The AAMA's Role Delineation Chart in the appendices is an excellent reference source that identifies which clinical, administrative, and general (transdisciplinary) procedures medical assistants are educated to perform. However, due to the variability of state statutes, the medical assistant would be wise to check with the executive director of the AAMA if there is doubt regarding the legality of performing certain clinical procedures.

SUMMARY

Progress has been made in the advancement of the profession of medical assisting since the first group of medical assistants gathered to become organized and formed the American Association of Medical Assistants. For example, the number of certified medical assistants has exceeded 70,000 and continues to grow since certification began in 1963. The total number of medical assistants in the work force is 1.3 million and employment opportunities continue to grow. Educational requirements have become increasingly important. The AAMA continues to promote standards of excellence for its members, encouraging continuing education and awarding continuing education credits to members of AAMA via various means.

All of these factors are evidence of a strong professional perspective and should offer encouragement and support to any student or graduate of medical assisting.

Becoming a professional is a gradual process and cannot be learned in its entirety from a textbook. The challenge of becoming a professional medical assistant will require open-mindedness and a desire for continued learning and education, certification, and recertification of the CMA credential, and professional involvement through organizational participation.

As the scope of work done by medical assistants broadens and medical assistants seek and require formal education, the professional medical assistant will gain additional respect and be in even greater demand. Medical assistants must continuously pursue excellence, which is the hallmark of all professional behavior.

REVIEW QUESTIONS

Multiple Choice

1. Medical assisting has been recognized by the United States Department of Education as a profession since what year?
   a. 1956
   b. 1964
   c. 1978
   d. 1995
2. The AAMA was established as a professional organization in what year?
   a. 1945
   b. 1956
   c. 1962
   d. 1967
3. The "Quest for Excellence" is:
   a. a professional publication for medical assistants
   b. a code of professional behavior for medical assistants
   c. otherwise known as ethical behavior
   d. the AAMA's series of home study courses
4. The designation Registered Medical Assistant is awarded by:
   a. American Association of Medical Assistants (AAMA)
   b. Accrediting Bureau of Health Education Schools (ABHES)
   c. American Medical Association (AMA)
   d. American Medical Technologists (AMT)

5. Increased employment opportunities for medical assistants result from:
   a. decreases in diagnostic testing
   b. computers decreasing volume of paperwork
   c. managed care's emphasis on ambulatory care
   d. longer hospital stays for patients

Critical Thinking

1. For each personal attribute used in your textbook to describe a professional, identify individuals from your family, friends, church, or community who possess one or more of these traits.
2. Patients and physicians desire professional medical assistants who have had the benefit of a formal education to care and work for them. Discuss the impact of this education on patients and employers. Why is it important to both groups?
3. Discuss the importance of certification and recertification.
4. Differentiate among certification, licensure, and registration.
5. Describe externship and its benefits.

WEB ACTIVITIES

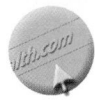

1. Visit the National Accrediting Agency for Clinical Laboratory Sciences (NAACLS) web site at http://www.naacls.org
   • What allied health professions other than medical technologist and clinical laboratory scientist are accredited by NAACLS?
   • Does NAACLS have a code of ethics for the medical assistant?
2. Visit the American Association of Medical Assistants web site at http://www.amaa-ntl.org
   • What allied health profession does the AAMA accredit?
   • What resources are available on the web for medical assistants interested in continuing education?
3. Visit the American Medical Technologists web site at http://www.amtl.com

REFERENCES/BIBLIOGRAPHY

Balasa, D. (2000). Securing the future for medical assistants to practice. *Professional medical assistant,* January/February 2000, 6–7.

Keir, L., Wise, B. A., & Krebs, C. (1998). *Medical assisting: Administrative and clinical competencies* (4th ed.). Albany, NY: Delmar.

Kinn, M. E., & Woods, M. A. (1999). *The medical assistant: Administrative and clinical* (8th ed.). Philadelphia: W. B. Saunders.

Merriam-Webster (1998). *Merriam-Webster's collegiate dictionary* (10th ed.). Springfield, MA: Author.

Prickett-Ramutkowski, B., Barrie, A., Keller, C., Dazarow, L., & Abe, C. (1999). *Medical assistant: A patient-centered approach to administrative and clinical competencies* (1st ed.). Princeton, NJ: Glencoe/McGraw Hill.

HEALTH CARE SETTINGS AND THE HEALTH CARE TEAM

KEY TERMS

Acupuncture
Allied Health Professionals
Ambulatory Care Setting
Fringe Benefit
Health Maintenance Organization (HMO)
Holistic
Independent Physician Association (IPA)
Integrative Medicine
Managed Care
Managed Care Operation
Managed Competition
Partnership
Preferred Provider Organization (PPO)
Sole Proprietorship
Triage

OUTLINE

Ambulatory Health Care Settings
　Individual and Group Medical
　　Practices
　Urgent Care Centers
　Managed Care Operations
**The Impact of Managed Care in
　the Health Care Setting**

The Health Care Team
　The Role of the Medical Assistant
　Health Care Professionals and
　　Their Roles
　Allied and Other Health Profes-
　　sionals and Their Roles
　The Role of Integrative or Alter-
　　native Health Care Therapies
　The Value of the Medical Assis-
　　tant to the Health Care Team

OBJECTIVES

The student should strive to meet the following performance objectives and demonstrate an understanding of the facts and principles presented in this chapter through written and oral communication.

1. Define the key terms as presented in the glossary.
2. Analyze the benefits and limitations of working in the different health care settings.
3. Assess the role and impact of managed care in the health care environment.
4. Identify and describe the three primary medical management models.
5. Describe the function of the health care team.
6. Discuss the role of the medical assistant in the health care team.
7. List and describe a minimum of twelve physician specialists.
8. List and describe a minimum of five nonphysician health care specialists.
9. List and describe a minimum of twelve allied health professionals.
10. Compare and contrast the types of nurses.
11. Critique alternative therapies and discuss their role in today's health care setting.

**GENERAL
(TRANSDISCIPLINARY)**

Professionalism

- Project a professional manner and image
- Adhere to ethical principles
- Demonstrate initiative and responsibility
- Work as a team member
- Promote the CMA credential

Communication Skills

- Serve as liaison

Legal Concepts

- Practice within the scope of education, training, and personal capabilities

INTRODUCTION

There are few professions in our society as rich and complex as the health care profession. In recent years, especially, the health care environment has been very much in flux as the profession seeks ways to provide quality care while containing costs. This effort to curtail costs has resulted in the rise of what is known as managed care, which, in turn, has spawned a number of medical models such as health maintenance organizations (HMOs) and preferred provider organizations (PPOs), two well-known managed care entities.

Many other types of physician networks and alliances are also being established as providers merge in order to give patients the best of care while controlling their costs. Ambulatory care settings, where services are provided on an outpatient basis, have become increasingly pivotal to consumer health care as insurers direct dollars away from hospitals and toward outpatient care.

Just as the medical setting continues to evolve to meet new societal needs, health care technology is ever-changing. Health care is a dynamic, stimulating industry that requires the medical assistant and other professionals to constantly develop new skills if they are to contribute to the team effort. The range of skills within the health care team is astonishing, and includes physicians, or medical doctors, in more than 25 specialties, more than 20 kinds of allied health professionals, and an increasing number of nontraditional alternative practitioners.

AMBULATORY HEALTH CARE SETTINGS

While medical assistants may work in a number of different environments, including laboratories or hospitals, most are employed in an **ambulatory care setting** such as a medical office (either a solo-physician or group practice), an urgent or primary care center, or a managed care organization such as an HMO.

Often, the medical assistant will choose to work in one setting rather than another based on interests, personality, and work preferences. For instance, the individual practice may provide medical assistants with the opportunity to use their full array of skills, while in urgent care centers, the work of the medical assistant may be more specialized in nature.

Medical assistants should also be aware of the three major forms of medical practice management and how they affect salary, benefits, and liability issues (Figure 2-1).

Individual and Group Medical Practices

For years, the most common form of medical office was the individual physician or group practice. Although this model now competes with a variety of other models such as urgent care centers and HMOs, many medical assistants will still find the individual or group practice a challenging place of employment.

Individual Practices. In the individual practice, also called the solo practice, one primary physician sees and treats all patients. While this type of arrangement is limited in the number of people it can serve, many patients feel secure in this kind of health care setting for they come to know and trust their doctor. Because they always see the same doctor, they feel their health care is being managed in a personal way. The solo-physician practice, however, can be an expensive arrangement, because one doctor must undertake the costs of office space, equipment, and personnel.

Group Practices. In today's managed care environment, group practices are attractive arrangements where two or more physicians can share the high costs of space, equipment, and personnel. The advantages of a group practice are not solely economic, however; physicians learn from and consult one another, while patients receive the benefit of this exchange of information and knowledge. Often, a group practice may have more than one office and some employees may be asked to travel between sites to cut overhead. Group practices may also be formed to offer specialized care, such as oncology or women's health care.

In most smaller group practices, patients may

FORMS OF MEDICAL PRACTICE MANAGEMENT

Medical assistants employed in ambulatory care settings or medical offices and clinics are likely to see three major forms of medical practice management. They are sole proprietorships, partnerships, and corporations.

Whatever form of management is chosen by physicians, they are responsible for the employees that serve with them. (Refer to the discussion of *respondeat superior* in Chapter 7.) Physician-employers and their medical assistants must have the kind of healthy working relationship where mutual trust and respect are apparent. The physician must understand the skill level of the medical assistant, and the medical assistant must feel secure enough to ask any questions necessary or admit any errors. Critical errors are often made when this trust does not exist between employer and employee. This causes a breakdown in the delivery of the best health care for patients.

Sole Proprietorships

In the past, many physicians preferred a solo practice. A solo practice entitles the physician or sole proprietor to hold exclusive right to all aspects of the medical practice or sole proprietorship, including profits and debts. If the business fails, the sole proprietor's personal property may also be attached.

A sole proprietorship may employ other physicians to participate in the practice. The employed physician(s) would be entitled to any employee fringe benefits such as health insurance and paid vacation, but the solo practitioner is not so entitled.

It is predicted that the business of practicing medicine may become more generalized and government regulated. Trends indicate more group practices and managed care facilities may gain dominance over the sole proprietorship form of management for physicians. The accelerating cost of maintaining an office has become more prohibitive for a physician in a sole proprietorship, especially the new-graduate physician.

Partnerships

When two or more physicians join together under a legal agreement to share in the total business operations of the practice, a partnership is formed. Several physicians who share a facility and practice medicine are often referred to as a group. Partners share expenses, income, debt, equipment, records, and personnel according to a predetermined agreement. Partners are liable for only their own actions, but may be liable for the whole amount of the partnership debts.

Corporations

Physicians may form a corporation, usually referred to as a professional service corporation. The physician shareholders are considered employees of the corporation. A corporation allows income and tax advantages to all employees. A variety of fringe benefits can be offered to the employees, which may include pension, profit-sharing plans, medical expense reimbursement, and life, health, and disability insurance. These benefits are separate from salary. Another advantage is that professional employees of a corporation are liable only for their own acts, and personal property cannot be attached in litigation. A sole proprietor may incorporate if the practice is large enough.

The health maintenance organization (HMO) is one type of corporation in which physicians often practice. Basically, physicians are employees of the HMO and are paid by various methods; physicians in the HMO usually serve as the primary care physician (PCP). In this situation, a referral from the PCP may be necessary before a patient can see a specialist or allied health professional.

Figure 2-1 Different forms of medical practice models and how they may affect the medical assistant.

request that they see the same physician for all appointments, although sometimes patients are assigned to the next available doctor. For emergencies, group practices have the staff and flexibility to ensure that there is always a doctor on call.

Urgent Care Centers

Urgent care centers are usually private, for-profit centers that provide services for primary care, routine injuries and illnesses, and minor surgery. Sometimes lab services and a radiology department are located on the premises. Physicians and other health care professionals in the center are often salaried employees, not owners who share in the profits, and often are associated with other medical facilities.

The pace in most urgent care centers is brisk and typically a number of doctors are working at one time. Patients may be requested to make appointments, but in some centers drop-ins are accepted, especially for emergencies.

Because these centers can see a higher volume of patients, usually for a lower cost than the traditional solo-physician or small group practice, some experts predict that ambulatory care settings will continue to grow as private practices decrease in number.

Managed Care Operations

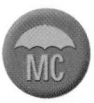 Health maintenance organizations, or HMOs, are probably the most familiar managed care operation. Originally, HMOs were

designed to provide a full range of health care services under one roof. More recently, the HMO without walls has become established, which is typically a network of participating physicians within a defined geographic area.

Originally, the HMO with walls was conceived to provide patients with comprehensive health care services at one facility. Today, as managed care and managed competition sweep the health care industry, other arrangements include the **preferred provider organization (PPO)**, where physicians network to offer discounts to employers and other purchasers of health insurance, and the **independent physician association (IPA)**, whose members agree to treat patients for an agreed-upon fee.

THE IMPACT OF MANAGED CARE IN THE HEALTH CARE SETTING

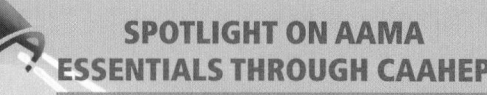

The emergence of **managed care** in today's society provides new administrative and clinical challenges to members of the health care team as they struggle to provide the best health care while working within limitations often imposed by insurance carriers. Virtually all health care settings, whether they are individual practices or urgent care centers, are experiencing the impact of managed care and **managed competition,** where physicians network and compete to serve patients better and more cost-efficiently.

Under managed care, critics charge, health care dollars have grown scarce, physicians must strive to provide the same quality for reduced reimbursement, preapprovals must be obtained for many services, and some services may be denied because they are not considered cost-effective.

Clinically, managed care may set limits on services or length of services. Second opinions are encouraged and sometimes required. In some systems, the patient selects a primary care physician, who is considered the gatekeeper and who must provide a referral for specialist care. Critics of managed care point out that restricting or denying services may lead to an increase in professional liability.

Administratively, paperwork and documentation have become increasingly important to assure proper reimbursement. While it is the patient's responsibility to understand the conditions of the insurance policy, these are often difficult to understand or interpret. The medical office or center must be fully aware of when a preapproval or treatment plan is required, when a second opinion is necessary for reimbursement, and of other clauses and restrictions that affect care and reimbursement for care.

At the same time, while managed care is challenging even the most resilient of providers, the very real need to keep costs down has also generated considerable creativity and energy among the health care profession as

SPOTLIGHT ON AAMA ESSENTIALS THROUGH CAAHEP

● Working as a team member and adapting to change makes a professional medical assistant stand out from others.

● Communication makes the difference between competency and negligence.

● Compassion and a caring attitude provide a positive experience for patients even when they are too ill to express their feelings.

physicians seek to use technology more efficiently, as they collaborate on new, cost-effective delivery methods, and as everyone involved in health care—insurers, providers, and patients—works together to contain costs by emphasizing prevention and lifestyle changes.

THE HEALTH CARE TEAM

In every kind of health care setting, the team concept is critical to the quality of patient care. A primary care physician is most likely the main source of health care for patients. From time to time, however, a specialist will be sought or recommended. A number of different allied health professionals, including the medical assistant, will supply additional health care as ordered by the physician. Increasingly, patients are looking outside traditional medicine for portions of their health care. While alternative care may not be covered by medical insurance, traditional and nontraditional health care practices are nonetheless blending in many areas. For example, **acupuncture** is becoming recognized as effective in the treatment of chronic pain. In whatever manner health care is sought, all members of this health care team must communicate, sometimes in person and sometimes just through the medical history and record, with one another to assure quality patient care.

The Role of the Medical Assistant

In the ambulatory care setting, a critical allied health professional is the medical assistant. The medical assistant, performing both administrative and clinical tasks under the direction of the physician, is an important link between patient and physician. The medical assistant serves in many capacities—receptionist, secretary, transcriptionist, bookkeeper, insurance coder and biller, patient educator, and clinical assistant. The latter requires the medical assistant to be able to administer injections and perform venipuncture, prepare patients for examinations, assist the physician with examinations and special procedures, and perform electrocardiography and various laboratory tests. Medical assistants *triage* and assess patient needs when scheduling appointments and tests. However, while medical assistants have a broad range of responsibilities, it is critical that they perform only within the scope of their training and personal capabilities and always function within ethical and legal boundaries and state statutes.

Because medical assistants are often the patient's first contact with the facility and its physicians, a positive attitude is important. They must be excellent communicators, both verbally and nonverbally, and project a professional image of themselves and their physician-employer. Medical assistants who believe in their work, who are proud of their career, and who convey compassion and caring provide a positive experience for patients who may be ill or in a great deal of discomfort.

Health Care Professionals and Their Roles

The public is often confused by the title *doctor*. The term implies an earned academic degree of the highest level in a particular area of study. Physicians have earned the MD or Doctor of Medicine degree. A doctorate in medicine and/or a license to practice allows a person to diagnose and treat medical conditions. The doctor of medicine candidate will attend four years of medical school after receiving a baccalaureate degree. An internship of one to two years follows in a hospital or major medical center. If a physician chooses to specialize, as many do, a residency

Patient Teaching Tip

Encourage patients to think of themselves as members of the health care team for they can provide invaluable information about their medical history. Use good communication skills to encourage patients to describe symptoms, identify their medications, and provide other information that is useful in diagnosis and treatment.

of two to five years in that specialty is required. In the medical field, the abbreviation *Dr.* is used and the title *doctor* is addressed to the person qualified by education, training, and licensure to practice medicine.

Other medical degrees include the Doctor of Osteopathy (DO), Doctor of Dentistry (DDS), Doctor of Optometry (OD), Doctor of Podiatric Medicine (DPM), Doctor of Chiropracty (DC), and Doctor of Naturopathy (ND). This group of doctors completes a different training regimen than that required for the Doctor of Medicine. The training is highly specialized and very specific but still grants the title of doctor upon completion, and when licensed, allows these health care professionals to diagnose and treat medical conditions.

In other nonmedical disciplines, the persons who have achieved a doctorate conferred by a college or university include the Doctor of Education (EdD) and the Doctor of Philosophy (PhD). Both the EdD and PhD have several areas of specialty.

Table 2-1 gives a selected listing of medical and surgical specialties, while Table 2-2 lists other health care specialists.

TABLE 2-1 SELECTED MEDICAL AND SURGICAL SPECIALTIES			
American Board of	**General Certificates**	**Subspecialty Certificates**	
Allergy & Immunology	Allergy & Immunology	Clinical & Laboratory Immunology	
Anesthesiology	Anesthesiology	Critical Care Medicine	Pain Management
Colon & Rectal Surgery	Colon & Rectal Surgery		
Dermatology	Dermatology	Clinical & Laboratory Dermatological Immunology	Dermatopathology Pediatric Dermatology
Emergency Medicine	Emergency Medicine	Medical Toxicology Pediatric Emergency Medicine	Sports Medicine Undersea & Hyperbaric Medicine
Family Practice	Family Practice	Geriatric Medicine	Sports Medicine

(continues)

TABLE 2-1 *(continued)*			
American Board of	**General Certificates**	**Subspecialty Certificates**	
Internal Medicine	Internal Medicine	Adolescent Medicine Cardiovascular Disease Clinical Cardiac Electrophysiology Clinical & Laboratory Immunology Critical Care Medicine Endocrinology, Diabetes & Metabolism Gastroenterology	Geriatric Medicine Hematology Infectious Disease Interventional Cardiology Medical Oncology Nephrology Pulmonary Disease Rheumatology Sports Medicine
Medical Genetics	Clinical Biochemical Genetics Clinical Cytogenetics Clinical Genetics (MD) Clinical Molecular Genetics Ph.D. Medical Genetics	Molecular Genetic Pathology	
Neurological Surgery	Neurological Surgery		
Nuclear Medicine	Nuclear Medicine		
Obstetrics & Gynecology	Obstetrics & Gynecology	Critical Care Medicine Gynecologic Oncology	Maternal & Fetal Medicine Reproductive Endocrinology
Ophthalmology	Ophthalmology		
Orthopaedic Surgery	Orthopaedic Surgery	Hand Surgery	
Otolaryngology	Otolaryngology	Otology/Neurotology Pediatric Otolaryngology	Plastic Surgery within the Head and Neck
Pathology	Anatomic Pathology & Clinical Pathology Anatomic Pathology Clinical Pathology	Blood Banking/Transfusion Medicine Chemical Pathology Cytopathology Dermatopathology Forensic Pathology	Hematology Immunopathology Medical Microbiology Molecular Genetic Pathology Neuropathology Pediatric Pathology
Pediatrics	Pediatrics	Adolescent Medicine Clinical & Laboratory Immunology Development-Behavioral Peds Medical Toxicology Neonatal-Perinatal Medicine Neurodevelopmental Disabilities Pediatric Cardiology Pediatric Critical Care Medicine Pediatric Emergency Medicine Pediatric Endocrinology	Pediatric Gastroenterology Pediatric Hematology- Oncology Pediatric Infectious Diseases Pediatric Nephrology Pediatric Pulmonology Pediatric Rheumatology Sports Medicine

Physical Medicine
    & Rehabilitation
	Physical Medicine
	    & Rehabilitation
		Pain Management
		Spinal Cord Injury Medicine
			Pediatric Rehabilitation
			    Medicine

Plastic Surgery	Plastic Surgery	Surgery of the Hand Plastic Surgery within the Head and Neck	
Preventive Medicine	Aerospace Medicine Occupational Medicine Public Health & General Preventive Medicine	Medical Toxicology Undersea & Hyperbaric Medicine Undersea Medicine	

Psychiatry & Neurology	Psychiatry
	Neurology
	Neurology with Special
	    Qualifications in Child
	    Neurology
		Addiction Psychiatry
		Child & Adolescent Psychiatry
		Clinical Neurophysiology
			Forensic Psychiatry
			Geriatric Psychiatry
			Neurodevelopmental
			    Disabilities
			Pain Management

Radiology	Diagnostic Radiology Radiation Oncology Radiological Physics	Neuroradiology Nuclear Radiology Pediatric Radiology	Vascular & Interventional Radiology
Surgery	Surgery	Pediatric Surgery Surgery of the Hand	Surgical Critical Care Vascular Surgery
Thoracic Surgery	Thoracic Surgery		
Urology	Urology		

Copyright 2000 American Board of Medical Specialties

TABLE 2-2 OTHER HEALTH CARE SPECIALISTS

Title	Degree	Function
Chiropractic Medicine	Chiropractors are licensed in their field of practice. They hold a degree of DC, or Doctor of Chiropractic.	Manipulative treatment of disorders originating from misalignment of the spinal vertebrae
Dentistry	Dentists are licensed in their field of practice, which can range from general to highly specialized. They hold the degree of DDS, or Doctor of Dental Surgery.	Diagnosing and treating diseases and disorders of the teeth and gums
Optometry	Optometrists are licensed in their field of practice. They hold the degree of OD, or Doctor of Optometry.	Measuring the accuracy of vision to determine if corrective lenses are needed
Osteopathy	Osteopaths are physicians who hold the title DO or Doctor of Osteopathy.	A therapeutic system that restores or preserves health through manipulation of the skeleton and muscles. Osteopaths also rely upon physical, medicinal, and surgical methods
Podiatry	Podiatrists are licensed in their field of practice. They hold the degree of DPM, or Doctor of Podiatric Medicine.	Diagnosing and treating diseases and disorders of the feet
Psychology	Psychologists are licensed in their field of practice. They hold the degree of PhD, or Doctor of Philosophy. (Some hold only a master's degree, or MA, and are not permitted to use the title *doctor*.)	Evaluating and treating emotional problems. These professionals give counseling to individuals, families, and groups

Allied and Other Health Professionals and Their Roles

In the health care team, allied health professionals bring specific educational backgrounds and a broad array of skills to the medical environment. Medical assistants are considered allied health professionals. Table 2-3 lists some of the allied health professionals recognized by the Commission on Accreditation of Allied Health Education Programs (CAAHEP) and other national accrediting bodies.

TABLE 2-3 ALLIED HEALTH PROFESSIONS

Occupation	Abbreviations	Job Description
Anesthesiologist Assistant	AA	Performs preoperative tasks, performs airway management and drug administration for induction and maintenance of anesthesia during surgery under direction of a licensed and qualified anesthesiologist
Athletic Trainer	AT	Provides a variety of services including injury prevention, recognition, immediate care, treatment, and rehabilitation after athletic trauma
Cardiovascular Technologist	CVT	Performs diagnostic exams under the direction of a physician in (1) invasive cardiology, (2) noninvasive cardiology, and (3) noninvasive peripheral vascular study
Clinical Laboratory Scientist	CLS	Develops data on the blood, tissues, and fluids of the human body by using a variety of precision instruments
Clinical Laboratory Technician *Associate Degree*	CLT	Performs all routine tests in a medical lab and is able to discriminate and recognize factors that directly affect procedures and results. Works under direction of pathologist, physician, medical technologist, or scientist
Clinical Laboratory Technician *Certificate*	CLT	Performs many routine uncomplicated procedures in medical lab where discrimination is clear and errors are few and easily corrected. Works under direction of pathologist, physician, medical technologist, or scientist
Cytotechnologist	CT	Works with pathologists to detect changes in body cells that may be important in early diagnosis of cancer or other diseases primarily through microscopic analysis

(continues)

TABLE 2-3 *(continued)*

Occupation	Abbreviations	Job Description
Diagnostic Medical Sonographer	DMS	Provides patient services using medical ultrasound under the supervision of a physician
Electroneurodiagnostic Technologist	EEG-T	Possesses the knowledge, attributes, and skills to obtain interpretable recordings of a patient's nervous system functions
Emergency Medical Technician—Paramedic	EMT-P	Recognizes, assesses, and manages medical emergencies of acutely ill or injured patients in prehospital care settings, working under the direction of a physician (often through radio communication)
Health Information Administrator	RRA	Manages health information systems consistent with the medical, administrative, ethical, and legal requirements of the health care delivery system
Health Information Technician	ART	Possesses the technical knowledge and skills necessary to process, maintain, compile, and report patient data
Medical Assistant	MA, CMA, RMA	Functions under the supervision of licensed medical professionals and is competent in both administrative/office and clinical/lab procedures
Medical Illustrator	MI	Creates visual material designed to facilitate the recording and dissemination of medical, biological, and related knowledge through communication media
Nuclear Medicine Technologist	NMT	Assists the nuclear medicine physician to make diagnostic evaluations of the anatomic or physiologic conditions of the body and to provide therapy with unsealed radioactive sources
Occupational Therapist	OT	Educates and trains individuals in the application of purposeful, goal-oriented activity in the evaluation, diagnosis, and/or treatment of loss of the ability to cope with the tasks of living and impairment due to physical injury, illness, or emotional disorder, congenital or developmental disability, or the aging process
Occupational Therapy Assistant	OTA	Directs an individual's participation in selected tasks to restore, reinforce, and enhance performance; facilitates learning of those skills and functions essential for adaptation and productivity; diminishes or corrects pathology; and promotes and maintains health (under the direction of an occupational therapist)
Ophthalmic Medical Technician or Technologist	OMT	Assists ophthalmologists to carry out diagnostic and therapeutic procedures
Orthotist/Prosthetist	OP	Orthotists design and fit devices to provide care to patients who have disabling conditions of the limbs and spine; prosthetists design and fit devices for patients who have partial or total absence of a limb
Perfusionist	PERF	Operates extracorporeal circulation equipment during any medical situation where it is necessary to support or temporarily replace the patient's circulation or respiratory functions
Physician Assistant (includes Surgeon's Assistant)	PA	Practices medicine under the direction and responsible supervision of a doctor of medicine or osteopathy; performs diagnostic, therapeutic, preventive, and health maintenance services in any setting in which the physician renders care
Radiation Therapist	RADT	Administers radiation therapy services to patients under the supervision of radiation oncologists
Radiographer	RT(R)	Provides patient services using imaging modalities, as directed by physicians qualified to order and/or perform radiologic procedures
Respiratory Therapist	RRT	Applies scientific knowledge and theory to practical clinical problems of respiratory care
Respiratory Therapy Technician	CRTT	Administers general respiratory care
Surgical Technologist	ST	Works as integral member of the surgical team, which includes surgeons, anesthesiologists, registered nurses, and other surgical personnel delivering patient care and assuming appropriate responsibilities before, during, and after surgery

Adapted from Health Professions Directory, 2000–2001, 28th ed. © American Medical Association, Chicago, IL

As a medical assistant, you may not work directly with all the identified allied health care professionals, but you are likely to have contact with many of them by telephone and written or electronic communication. Knowledge of the roles these health professionals play enables you to interact more intelligently with all members of the health care team.

In addition to the professionals listed in Table 2-3, you may encounter some or all of the following health care professionals in daily patient care.

Health Unit Coordinator (HUC). Health unit coordinators (HUC) perform nonclinical patient care tasks for the nursing unit of a hospital. This profession requires a self-motivated, mature individual who can handle the stress and hectic pace of coordinating personnel and their duties at the nurses' station. Also called unit secretary, administrative specialist, ward clerk, or ward secretary, a health unit coordinator receives on-the-job training with an emphasis on administrative office skills.

Medical Laboratory Technologist (MLT). Medical laboratory technologists physically and chemically analyze, as well as culture, urine, blood, and other body fluids and tissues. They work closely with physician specialists such as oncologists, pathologists, and hematologists. Knowledge of specimen collection, anatomy and physiology, biochemistry, laboratory equipment, asepsis, and quality control is essential. The American Society of Clinical Pathology (ASCP) is a professional organization that oversees credentialing and education in the medical laboratory professions. See Figure 2-2.

Nurses. The nursing profession is not listed in Table 2-3 because CAAHEP is not responsible for nurses' training and accreditation. Nurses are licensed by the state in which they practice. Although nurses' education and training are oriented to bedside care, some are employed in medical offices as clinical assistants, especially in offices where surgery is performed. Nurses play a number of roles on the health care team.

Registered Nurse (RN). In the United States, RNs are professionals who have completed at a minimum, a two-year course of study at a state-approved school of nursing and passed the National Council Licensure Examination (NCLEX-RN). They are licensed only by the state to practice. Employment settings most often include hospitals, convalescent homes, clinics, and home health care.

Licensed Practical Nurse (LPN). An LPN is a professional trained in basic nursing techniques and direct patient care. LPNs practice under the direct supervision of a registered nurse or physician and are employed in similar settings to RNs. Training includes completion of a state-approved program in practical nursing and successful completion of a national licensure examination.

Nurse Practitioner (NP). A nurse practitioner is a registered nurse who, by advanced education (usually a master's degree) and clinical experience in a branch of nursing, has acquired expert knowledge in a specific medical specialty. Nurse practitioners are employed by physicians in private practice or in clinics, and sometimes practice independently, especially in rural areas.

Registered Dietitian (RD). Registered dietitians have specialized training in the nutritional care of groups and individuals and have successfully completed an examination of the Commission on Dietetic Registration. Dietitians assist patients in regulating their diets. Although they are typically employed in hospitals and clinics, they can also be found working with the public in personal nutritional counseling. Education includes a baccalaureate degree with a major in dietetics, food and nutrition, or food service systems management plus completion of an approved internship. See Chapter 34, Nutrition in Health and Disease, for more information.

Pharmacist (RPh). Pharmacists are licensed by each state to prepare and dispense all types of medications as well as medical supplies related to medication administration. They may practice in hospitals, medical centers, and pharmacies. The minimum training for a pharmacist is a five-year baccalaureate degree; some pharmacists pursue a Doctor of Pharmacy degree (Pharm D), offered by major universities in the United States. Pharmacy technicians assist the pharmacist with preparation and administration

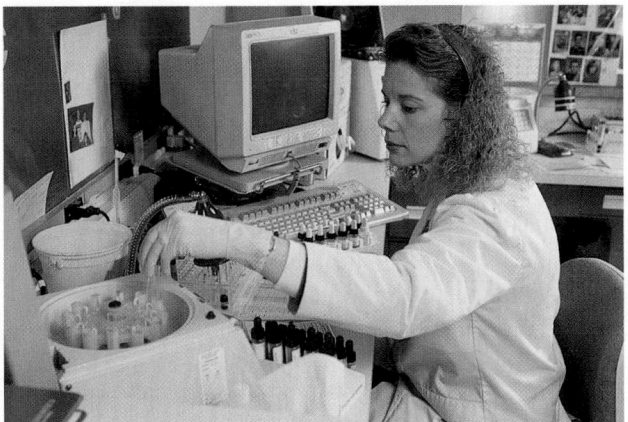

Figure 2-2 Medical technologists perform blood analyses and analyze and culture other body fluids as well. (Photo by Marcia Butterfield, courtesy of W. A. Foote Memorial Hospital, Jackson, MI)

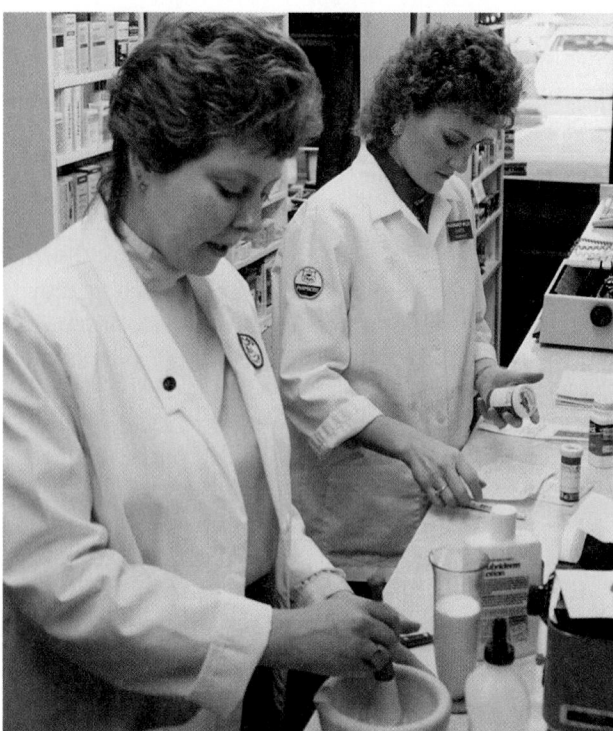

Figure 2-3 Pharmacy technicians prepare medications to be dispensed. (Courtesy of the Michigan Pharmacists Association and the Michigan Society of Pharmacy Technicians)

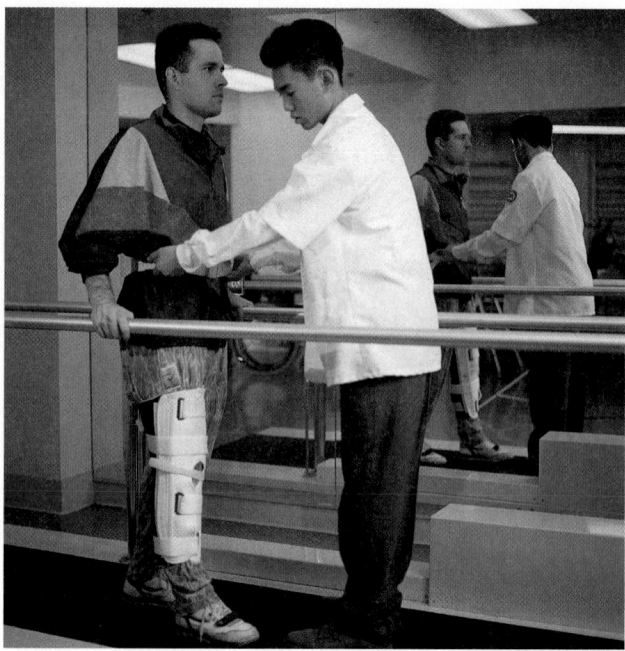

Figure 2-4 Physical therapists work with disabled and physically challenged individuals and with patients who require physical rehabilitation.

of medications, as well as perform receptionist and billing duties. Professional certification of pharmacy technicians varies from state to state and is administered by state pharmacy associations. See Figure 2-3.

Phlebotomist (LPT). Phlebotomists are trained in the art of drawing blood for diagnostic laboratory testing. Phlebotomists are also referred to as lab liaison technicians. Phlebotomists may be nationally certified and are employed in medical clinics, hospitals, and laboratories. Training consists of one to two semesters in a community college program or on-the-job training.

Physical Therapist (PT). Physical therapists are licensed professionals who assist in the examination, testing, and treatment of physically disabled or challenged people. They also assist in physical rehabilitation of patients following an accident, injury, or serious illness using special exercises, application of heat or cold, *ultrasound* therapy and other techniques. Educational requirements for a physical therapist are a minimum of a four-year baccalaureate degree (bachelor of science) or a special certificate course after obtaining the bachelor of science in a related field. Physical therapists must also successfully complete a state licensure examination. See Figure 2-4.

Physical Therapy Assistant (PTA). Physical therapy assistants are trained to use and apply physical therapy procedures such as exercise and physical agents under the supervision of a physical therapist. The physical therapy assistant is a graduate of an accredited associate of science degree program and must pass a licensure or registry examination in selected states.

The Role of Integrative or Alternative Health Care Therapies

Increasingly, integrative medicine or alternative forms of health care are being perceived as complements to traditional health care. As mentioned earlier, some nontraditional approaches, such as acupuncture, have been very successful in pain management or in reducing stress-related illnesses. For example, a patient being treated with medication for high blood pressure may also try to manage the hypertension with diet, exercise, and relaxation techniques. Sometimes this is considered a holistic approach to patient care, which takes into account the whole person.

While there is often controversy and confusion about the role of many alternative approaches, medical assistants should nonetheless be aware of the philosophy and intent of nontraditional therapies. Table 2-4 reviews some of the more common approaches.

TABLE 2-4	SELECTED EXAMPLES OF ALTERNATIVE APPROACHES TO HEALTH CARE
Type of Approach	**Description of Approach**
Acupuncture	A piercing of the skin by long needles into any of 365 points along twelve meridians that transverse the body. Each point is related to a particular organ. Acupuncture is often successful in managing pain and has been successfully used to treat drug dependency.
Biofeedback	A relaxation technique that uses monitoring devices to gain information about certain automatic body responses such as heart rate or blood pressure in order to help the patient gain some voluntary control over that function. Biofeedback is often used to treat hypertension and migraine headaches.
Holism	An approach that treats the whole body, mind, and spirit. A holistic practitioner considers the needs of the patient in all areas, including physical, emotional, social, spiritual, and economic.
Homeopathy	A method of treating disease by administering very dilute doses of remedies that are typically made from natural substances. In more massive doses, these remedies would produce symptoms of the disease being treated. This is in contrast to traditional allopathic medicine, which typically treats disease with remedies that produce effects different from those caused by the disease itself.
Hypnotherapy	An approach that encourages patients to enter a trance-like state in which they are more open to suggestion. The hypnotherapist makes verbal suggestions in the attempt to bring some desired behavior change.
Naturopathy	Naturopaths are licensed in their field of practice and hold the degree of ND, Doctor of Naturopathy. Naturopaths diagnose and treat patients using the relationship between mind/body/spirit and nature.
Therapeutic Touch	Therapeutic touch uses the hands to facilitate healing and to restore wholeness, harmony, and well-being to the patient. Often practiced by nurses, therapeutic touch is considered a modern interpretation of ancient healing practices. It is thought to be effective for producing relaxation, reducing pain, and promoting wound healing.

The Value of the Medical Assistant to the Health Care Team

With their broad range of competencies in both administrative and clinical areas, medical assistants are increasingly valued as health care team members. Medical assistants are the great communicators, serving as liaison between physician and hospital staff and between physician and any number of allied and other health professionals. Because they are the first providers to see or speak with patients, they undertake responsibility for directing, informing, and guiding patient care while establishing a professional and caring tone for the entire health care team. The value of a competent, professional, caring medical assistant is immeasurable in today's fast-paced and challenging health care environment.

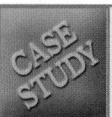

CASE STUDY

2-1

The number of sole proprietors is declining in this country.

CASE STUDY REVIEW

1. Identify at least five reasons for this decline.
2. Describe the impact, if any, this decline has on quality health care.

SUMMARY

The health care environment is a dynamic profession and one that changes rapidly in response to new technology and societal needs. In an effort to reduce the cost of health care, managed care has had and will continue to have a profound impact on all health care settings. A strong health care team is critical in the health care setting, as primary care physicians, specialists of all disciplines, and allied and other health professionals collaborate on the best way to provide patient care. Increasingly, selected alternative treatments may begin to complement traditional health care solutions. In almost any health care environment, but especially the ambulatory care setting, the medical assistant is a vital link in the team and is responsible for a range of responsibilities, both clinical and administrative.

REVIEW QUESTIONS

Multiple Choice

1. Medical assistants are employed for the most part in:
   a. hospitals
   b. nursing facilities
   c. ambulatory care settings
   d. insurance companies
2. A health maintenance organization is one kind of:
   a. managed care operation
   b. individual practice
   c. sole proprietorship
   d. hospital
3. With its emphasis on controlling costs, managed care is likely to affect:
   a. only hospitals
   b. all health care settings
   c. only physicians in private practice
   d. only patients
4. The health care team:
   a. should exclude the patient from being part of the team
   b. is only important in the hospital setting
   c. is made up of physicians and nurses
   d. is made up of physicians, nurses, allied and other health care professionals, patients, and sometimes a practitioner of nontraditional medicine
5. Integrative or alternative health care approaches:
   a. are increasingly accepted as complementary to traditional health care
   b. are always covered by insurance
   c. are not safe to practice
   d. are not important to understand
6. A medical assistant permitted by law to draw blood for diagnostic laboratory testing performs a procedure similar to those performed by a:
   a. health unit coordinator
   b. radiation therapist
   c. phlebotomist
   d. cytotechnologist
7. The distinct difference between the PA and the MA is that the PA:
   a. draws blood and gives injections
   b. practices medicine
   c. performs diagnostic services
   d. both b and c
8. Physicians just establishing their practice often seek to work with another physician in the same field. When expenses and profits are shared, this form of management is called a/an:
   a. HMO
   b. corporation
   c. sole proprietor
   d. group or partnership
9. Managed care may be identified as care that:
   a. offers unlimited services
   b. forbids second opinions
   c. establishes a primary care physician as gate-keeper
   d. offers protection to physicians against liability
10. An alternative approach to medicine that treats patients using the relationship between mind/body/spirit/and nature is:
    a. homeopathy
    b. holism
    c. acupuncture
    d. naturopathy

Critical Thinking

1. Evaluate the different health care settings and discuss the pros and cons of working in each setting.
2. From a patient point of view, which health care setting do you think offers more benefits? Why?
3. Review the three forms of medical management models. Which is probably the most advantageous from the physician's point of view? From the medical assistant's point of view?
4. Discuss the purpose of managed care. What impact is it having on health care?
5. What kinds of professionals make up the health care team?
6. Discuss the role of the medical assistant in the health care team. What qualities does the medical assistant need to possess?
7. If you were attending a family reunion and overheard a discussion about the title *doctor,* how would you clarify the situation? What are some examples of individuals who might be referred to as a doctor?
8. What organization recognizes allied health professionals?
9. Recall a few types of allied health professionals and, working in small groups, have each student create a scenario in which the medical assistant needs to coordinate with two or three allied professionals.
10. What role might alternative therapies play in the health care setting? Describe a few different alternative approaches and their philosophies.

WEB ACTIVITIES

Visit http://www.abms.org for the most current list of the American Board of Specialties. What does board certified mean? Who credentials a specialist? How is this different from the certification or registration of medical assistants?

REFERENCES/BIBLIOGRAPHY

American Board of Medical Specialties (1997). *The official ABMS directory of board certified medical specialists* (26th ed.). Evanston, IL: author.

Burton Goldberg Group (1995). *Alternative medicine*. Fife, WA: Future Medicine Publishing.

Health professions directory (27th ed.). (1999–2000). Chicago: American Medical Association.

Humphrey, D. D. (1996). *Contemporary medical office procedures* (2nd ed.). Albany, NY: Delmar.

Mosby's medical, nursing and allied health dictionary (5th ed.). (1998). St. Louis: Mosby-Year Book, Inc.

Smith, G. L., Davis, P. E., & Dennerll, J. T. (1999). *Medical terminology: A programmed systems approach* (8th ed.). Albany, NY: Delmar.

Stanfield, P. S. (1995). *Introduction to the health professions* (2nd ed.). Sudbury, MA: Jones & Bartlett Publishers.

Taber's cyclopedic medical dictionary (18th ed.) (1997). Philadelphia: F. A. Davis.

Warden, C. D. (1986). *Health care in the 1980s from a consumer's perspective*. Unpublished doctoral dissertation, Union Graduate School, Seattle, WA.

Weil, A. (1995). *Spontaneous healing*. New York: Alfred A. Knopf.

3

HISTORY OF MEDICINE

KEY TERMS

Acupuncture
Allopathic
Asepsis
Bubonic Plague
Malaria
Moxibustion
Pharmacopoeia
Pluralistic (Pluralism)
Septicemia
Typhus (Typhoid)
Yellow Fever

OUTLINE

Cultural Heritage in Medicine
Medical Specialists
Medical Education
Attitudes toward Illness

Medical Treatments
Significant Contributions to Medicine
New Frontiers in Medicine

OBJECTIVES

The student should strive to meet the following performance objectives and demonstrate an understanding of the facts and principles presented in this chapter through written and oral communication.

1. Define the key terms as presented in the glossary.
2. Discuss the effects of culture on medicine.
3. Identify the role of religion, magic, and science in medicine's history.
4. Describe how attitudes toward illness are manifested today.
5. Identify a minimum of three common medical treatments used in the past.
6. Recall a minimum of three theories/practices of ancient medicine still prevalent today.
7. Name and describe the historical roles of medical specialists.
8. Discuss the role of women in medicine.
9. Trace the progression of medical education.
10. Name at least five significant contributions to medicine.
11. Identify a minimum of three recent developments in medicine.

A historical overview of medicine must do more than identify a series of contributions by physicians. It must remind us that more than one discipline and more than one philosophy have contributed to medicine. This is perhaps more true now than ever as our world becomes smaller and our society becomes increasingly **pluralistic,** ethnically, culturally, and religiously.

CULTURAL HERITAGE IN MEDICINE

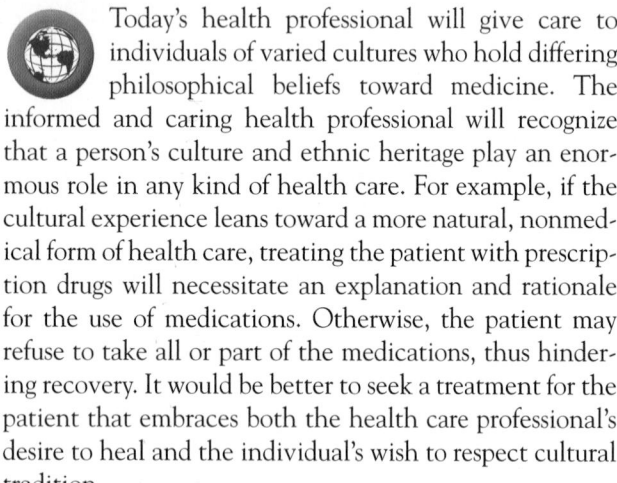

Today's health professional will give care to individuals of varied cultures who hold differing philosophical beliefs toward medicine. The informed and caring health professional will recognize that a person's culture and ethnic heritage play an enormous role in any kind of health care. For example, if the cultural experience leans toward a more natural, nonmedical form of health care, treating the patient with prescription drugs will necessitate an explanation and rationale for the use of medications. Otherwise, the patient may refuse to take all or part of the medications, thus hindering recovery. It would be better to seek a treatment for the patient that embraces both the health care professional's desire to heal and the individual's wish to respect cultural tradition.

In every society, medicine has been an important element for its people. From the earliest time, culture was an important influence on medicine, and modern day medicine is in many ways a reflection of this diverse and rich heritage.

It is certain that religion, magic, and science all played a vital part in the history of medicine. Religion was important because it was perceived that certain gods were to be called upon for a cure through ceremonies, prayers, and sacrifices. Magic was practiced because it was such an important part of many societies and was seen as an essential ingredient to chase away evil spirits. The importance of science was demonstrated in the use of plants and minerals for medicinal purposes. The use of plants and minerals is found throughout medicine's history. Unearthed clay tablets reveal hundreds of plants, minerals, and animal substances used for medicinal purposes in ancient Mesopotamia and Babylon. The Chinese **pharmacopoeia** was rich in the use of herbs.

Skeletal remains of prehistoric cultures show advanced stages of arthritis, a nearly toothless jaw and only a 20- to 40-year lifespan for humans. Skull bones reveal round holes (trephination) believed to be necessary to release the evil spirits thought to be causing a person's illness. Mesopotamian cultures believed that illness was a punishment by the gods for violation of a moral code. Ancient Egyptians believed the body was a system of channels for air, tears, blood, urine, sperm, and feces. All the channels were thought to come together in the rectum, and were thought to become easily clogged. Thus, emetics, enemas, and purges of the anus were common treatments. In ancient India, plastic surgery was practiced. Punishment for adultery was cutting off the nose, therefore allowing physicians many opportunities to practice and refine the art of nose reconstruction.

The ancient Chinese examined and carefully monitored the pulse in each wrist. It was believed that the pulse had hundreds of characteristics important in medical treatment. There were five methods of treatment to bring a person back to the right track. They were:

1. Cure the spirit.
2. Nourish the body.
3. Give medications.
4. Treat the whole body.
5. Use acupuncture and moxibustion.

Acupuncture is the piercing of the skin by long needles into any of 365 points along twelve meridians that transverse the body and transmit an active life force called "ch'i" (pronounced chee). Each of these spots is related to a particular organ. **Moxibustion** requires the use of a powdered plant substance that is made into a small mound on the person's skin and then burned, usually raising a blister.

Even today's **allopathic,** or traditional, physicians would agree that the first four methods of treatment from Chinese culture are excellent guidelines for health care. There is an increasing awareness, also, that acupuncture has a valid place in allopathic medicine, especially for the control of pain.

MEDICAL SPECIALISTS

Medicine's history gives early evidence of many "specialists" in the healing arts. They were known by various names—witch doctors, medicine men and women, shamans or healing priests, and physicians. These healers were more than ancestors of the modern physician, however, for they performed many functions that involved the welfare of the entire community or village. By today's standards, they were considered to be equivalent to spiritual advisers, social workers, counselors, and teachers.

While women were accepted as healers in primitive societies, later cultures reduced their status to that of being allowed to care only for women and to assist in childbirth. In any culture that granted women only secondary status, women are also considered unqualified to become physicians. In Chinese culture, the first reference to a female physician mentioned by name is in documents from the Han dynasty (206 B.C.–A.D. 220). In Muslim society, the reluctance of Arabic physicians to violate social taboo and touch the genitals of female strangers further encouraged relegating the practice of obstetrics and gynecology to midwives.

Women were not accepted as medical doctors in Western culture until the nineteenth and twentieth centuries. Italy granted women the status earlier than other cultures. In America, the first female physician was Elizabeth Blackwell, who was awarded her degree in 1849. While she was snubbed by the public, she soon earned the respect of her colleagues. When she refused to be absent from class when the male reproductive system was discussed, her fellow male students supported her actions.

From the earliest times, it appears that some payment was expected for medical services rendered. In many instances, the payment was dependent upon the status of the physician as well as the patient. At the same time, some cultures punished a physician who was not successful in treatment by forcing that physician to treat only those too poor to pay.

MEDICAL EDUCATION

During the rise of Christianity, emphasis was placed on the soul rather than the body; therefore, early Christian monks held great control over medicine. This is evidenced by St. Benedict of Nursia (480–554) who forbade the study of medicine. The care of the sick was encouraged, but only through prayer and divine intervention. Thus, Christ's healing mission was institutionalized in a fashion that was to control medical care almost completely for the next 500 years, until the seventh century.

At that time, however, the religion of Islam moved to preserve the classical learning that had been achieved in medicine, and practitioners were not only able to return to the same methods as those practiced by earlier Greeks and Romans, but medical study was now encouraged.

Medical education in established universities began in the ninth century. These universities included Salerno in southern Italy, the University of Montpelier in southern France, and the University of Paris. By the time the Renaissance was at its height in the midfifteenth century, the physician had become licensed, was receiving great status, and was attending the ill in a velvet bonnet and fur-trimmed cloak.

Art and science were more closely related during the Renaissance than at any other period of time. Michelangelo (1475–1564) spent years on careful human dissection and this anatomical detail is evident in his paintings in the Sistine Chapel in the Vatican in Rome. Leonardo da Vinci (1452–1519) made anatomical preparations from which he produced drawings representing the skeletal, muscular, nervous, and vascular systems. His accurate sketch of the spinal vertebrae went undiscovered for more than 100 years.

ATTITUDES TOWARD ILLNESS

Various attitudes prevailed toward the ill person. A sick person might be excused from daily activity, but was likely to be shunned if the disease was believed to be a punishment by the gods for mortal sin. This forced isolation may well have been beneficial to the community. In contrast, touching by Jesus was an important component of healing, as was the faith of the individual involved. The New Testament parable of the Good Samaritan helped establish a nexus between the early church and a concern for the sick. It was felt that though the body might be wasted and foul with disease, the purity of the soul guaranteed life everlasting. This was unlike the pagan religions that tended to abandon individuals thought to be ill because they were in disfavor with the gods.

Native Americans had various feelings about illness. The ill were treated with kindness among the Navaho and Cherokee, and some who recovered from serious illness were considered to have extraordinary powers. However, if a tribe was faced with famine, suicide by the aged and infirm was considered a highest form of bravery. The Eskimos put their elderly unprotected onto ice floes. Neither the Romans nor the Greeks treated the hopelessly ill or deformed, and unwanted infants were disposed of quickly or left to die.

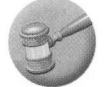
Some of these attitudes are seen even today. The Western medical community and the consumers it serves are heatedly debating the right to choose life or death and the ethics and legality of physician-assisted suicide, which is acceptable in many other cultures. Even with our vast knowledge of medicine and the disease process, many individuals are still very fearful of any illness they do not understand or that they perceive as threatening their health—AIDS is a good example. This fear is often accompanied by public ill treatment of the individuals suffering from certain diseases. For example,

SPOTLIGHT ON AAMA ESSENTIALS THROUGH CAAHEP

- Recognizing a patient's cultural background is part of caring for the patient as a whole person.
- Human kindness often eliminates fear of the unknown.
- A positive attitude helps to lessen a negative feeling.

Cuba quarantines everyone who tests positive for the human immunodeficiency virus (HIV), even if they show no signs of illness.

MEDICAL TREATMENTS

The writings of ancient Egypt reveal that when a woman suspected she was pregnant, she urinated over a mixture of wheat and barley seeds combined with dates and sand. If any of the grains sprouted, she was surely pregnant. If the wheat grew, she would have a boy. If the barley grew, it would be a girl. Urine is still used in modern tests to determine pregnancy.

Early medical treatments were often crude. For a sore throat, a physician might mix barley water, vinegar, and mulberry syrup for a gargle. Someone suffering with rheumatism might be given a prescription of chopped mice, lynx claws, and elk hooves. Rhubarb, senna, bitter apple, turpentine, camphor, and mercury were among the physicians' staples. Some physicians washed the instruments used in treating the ill; others scoffed at such a practice. **Malaria,** diphtheria, tuberculosis, **typhoid,** and dysentery were commonplace. Leprosy was prevalent and venereal diseases were rife. Smallpox was frequent in villages; sometimes the sufferer would be placed in a meat pickling vat and fumigated. The death toll from such diseases was particularly high among children. Finally in the eighteenth century, Edward Jenner made a great contribution to the prevention of disease by discovering a method of vaccination against smallpox.

Medicine progressed rapidly during the nineteenth century. Two very important discoveries occurred: anesthesia to alleviate pain during surgery and the realization that some bacteria cause disease. Once it had been proven that certain bacteria were causes of diseases and were transmissible agents responsible for contagion, greater care was taken to prevent that transmission. **Asepsis** became important to reduce the risk of infection. The Hungarian physician and obstetrician Ignaz Phillipp Semmeweis (1818–1865) was able to prove that physicians who came from an autopsy directly to the care of postpartum women, without scrubbing their hands and washing instruments, carried infection with them that often caused puerperal fever (**septicemia** following childbirth) and death to the new mothers.

The names of Louis Pasteur (1822–1895), Joseph Lister (1827–1912), and Robert Koch (1843–1910) are familiar to all bacteriologists. Louis Pasteur has sometimes been referred to as the father of preventive medicine as the result of his work in recognizing the relationship between bacteria and infectious disease (Figure 3-1). Joseph Lister revolutionized surgery because of his belief in Pasteur's theory of using carbolic acid as an antiseptic spray. He insisted that all instruments and physicians' hands be washed with the solution (Figure 3-2). Robert Koch used the culture-plate method for isolating bacteria

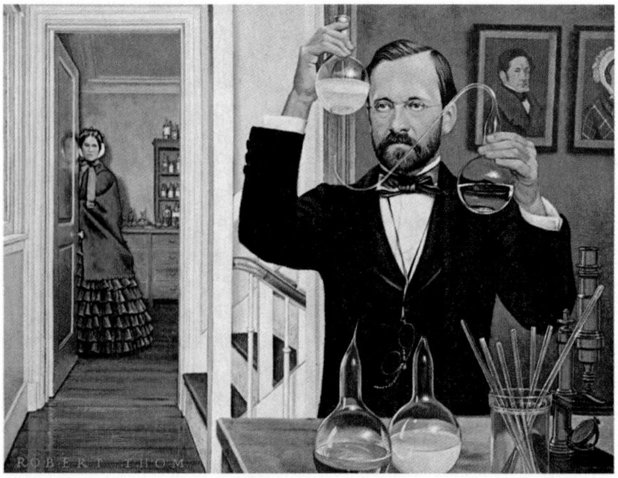

Figure 3-1 Louis Pasteur, the father of preventive medicine. (Courtesy Parke-Davis & Company, © 1957).

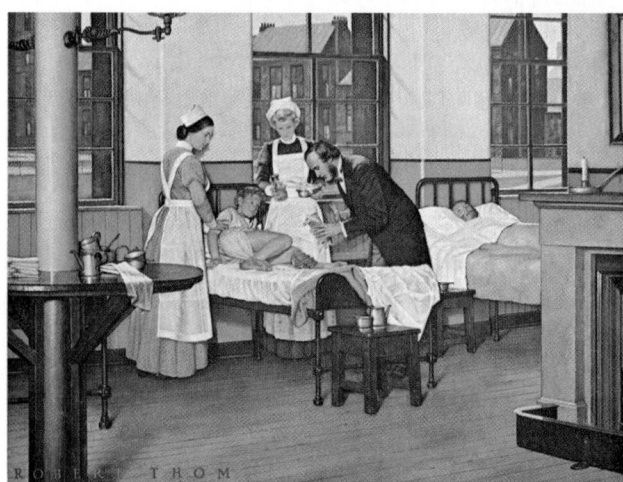

Figure 3-2 Joseph Lister revolutionized surgery by introducing antisepsis. (Courtesy Parke-Davis & Company, © 1957)

and demonstrated how cholera was transmitted by food and water. His discovery changed the way health departments cared for persons with infectious disease.

Fortunately, early in the twentieth century, society was finally liberated from many of the infectious and epidemic diseases that had scourged the human race for millennia. Smallpox vaccinations became common and causes of **yellow fever, typhus,** and **bubonic plague** were determined. Life expectancy increased. Tuberculosis became less frequent. In 1922, Frederick G. Banting and a medical student, Charles Best, were able to isolate and inject insulin into a fourteen-year-old boy who was dying of diabetes. Two weeks later, the boy was alive and alert. By 1923, insulin was available for general sale in pharmacies throughout the world. Antibiotics were discovered and the Salk and Sabin vaccines were found for poliomyelitis.

Yet, as we enter the twenty-first century, we are quite aware of the limitations of modern medicine. The rise of AIDS is a reminder that plagues are still possible. In developing countries torn with war and strife, cholera causes the deaths of thousands simply because there is no proper sanitation. In the microbial world, there are new, drug-resistant strains of malaria, tuberculosis, and other diseases that are not responding to known treatments. The challenge of medicine is as strong today as it was 100 years ago.

SIGNIFICANT CONTRIBUTIONS TO MEDICINE

Hippocrates (c. 460–c. 377 B.C.) is the physician most recall from the Greek culture (Figure 3-3). It is not known

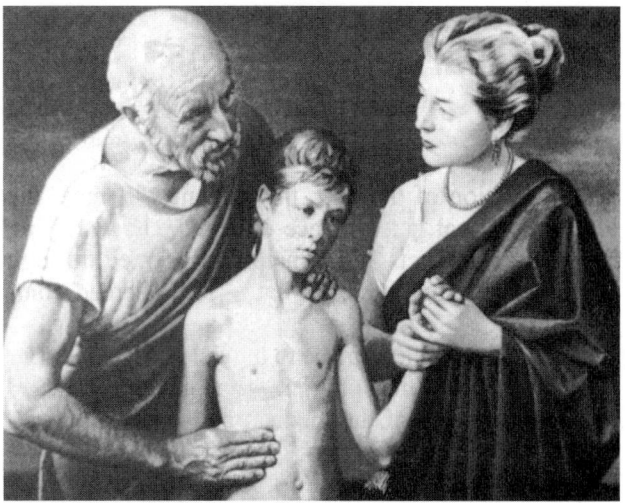

Figure 3-3   Hippocrates examining a child.

why his name surfaces above all other Greek physicians, for some were surely just as prominent. His writings, however, have contributed much to today's medical culture. Hippocrates is remembered by many for his well-known Hippocratic Oath, which established guidelines for a physician's practice of medicine. While few physicians swear to this oath today when they embark on their medical career, it is still recognized for its validity and wisdom. There are various translations of the Hippocratic Oath, although all communicate the same fundamental message.

It would be impossible to identify all the other individuals who made significant contributions to medicine in this text. There are several of note, however, who are mentioned in Table 3-1.

TABLE 3-1 INDIVIDUALS OF NOTE IN THE HISTORY OF MEDICINE	
Moses c. 1205 B.C.	Advocate of health rules in Hebrew religion
Hippocrates c. 460–c. 377 B.C.	Greek physician; "father of medicine"
Andreas Vesalius A.D. 1514–1564	Brussels physician; wrote first anatomical studies
Anton van Leeuwenhoek 1632–1723	Dutch lens grinder; discovered lens magnification
John Hunter 1728–1793	Founder of scientific surgery
Edward Jenner 1749–1823	Developed smallpox vaccine
Rene Laennec 1781–1826	Invented the stethoscope
W. T. G. Morton 1819–1868	Massachusetts physician; introduced ether as anesthetic
Florence Nightingale 1820–1910	Founder of modern nursing
Elizabeth Blackwell 1821–1910	First female physician in America
Clara Barton 1821–1912	Started American Red Cross in 1881
Louis Pasteur 1822–1895	"Father of bacteriology"
Joseph Lister 1827–1912	Laid the groundwork on asepsis
Elizabeth G. Anderson 1836–1917	First female physician in Britain
Robert Koch 1843–1910	Bacteriologist; developed culture-plate method
Wilhelm Roentgen 1845–1923	Discovered X rays (roentgenograms)
Sir Alexander Fleming 1881–1955	Discovered penicillin in 1928

THE OATH OF HIPPOCRATES

I swear by Apollo Physician and Aesculapius and Hygeia and Panacea and all the gods and goddesses, making them my witnesses, that I will fulfill according to my ability and judgment this oath and this covenant:

To hold him who has taught me this art as equal to my parents and to live my life in partnership with him, and if he is in need of money to give him a share of mine, and to regard his offspring as equal to my brothers in male lineage and to teach them this art—if they desire to learn it—without fee and covenant; to give a share of precepts and oral instruction and all the other learning to my sons and to the sons of him who has instructed me and to pupils who have signed the covenant and have taken an oath according to the medical law, but to no one else.

I will apply dietetic measures for the benefit of the sick according to my ability and judgment; I will keep them from harm and injustice.

I will neither give a deadly drug to anybody if asked for it nor will I make a suggestion to this effect. Similarly, I will not give to a woman an abortive remedy. In purity and holiness I will guard my life and my art.

I will not use the knife, not even on sufferers from stone, but will withdraw in favor of such men as are engaged in this work.

Whatever houses I may visit, I will come for the benefit of the sick, remaining free of all intentional injustice, of all mischief, and in particular of sexual relations with both female and male persons, be they free or slaves.

NEW FRONTIERS IN MEDICINE

There has been phenomenal growth in medicine in the past two decades. Only a few advances are mentioned here. Much better imaging leading to much better diagnosis is now available. Where exploratory surgery might have been performed in the past to determine a diagnosis, noninvasive ultrasound, CT scans, and MRIs assist in diagnosis now. People who have worn glasses or contact lenses for many years are turning to eye laser surgery and implantable lenses.

Recently surgeons performed the first successful human larynx transplant. Consider the implications of an AIDS saliva test that creates a needle-free way to test for HIV. Needleless injections are now possible. There is a flu prevention inhaler and an osteoporosis pill.

Experimentation with aromatherapy reveals that some aromas actually improve brain function. Research has shown that individuals suffering from dementia often respond favorably to the odor of freshly roasted coffee and bread baking. Inhaling the scents of green apple, banana, and peppermint stimulates positive feelings. It is thought that with aromatherapy we will soon accelerate learning and speed up rehabilitation for people who have had a stroke.

Who can possibly predict what the future will bring in medicine?

SUMMARY

Medicine's history leaves us with a rich heritage and a sound basis for the future of health care. Medical history continues to be in the making today. For example, research in gene manipulation has the potential benefit of being able to reverse the progression of many debilitating diseases. One day we will look upon medical discoveries of this decade and be impressed by how much further medicine has advanced.

REVIEW QUESTIONS

Multiple Choice

1. A pharmacopoeia is:
   a. a book describing drugs and their preparation
   b. an ancient religious rite used in medicine
   c. a source of magic
   d. used only by twentieth-century physicians

2. In later cultures, women were typically allowed to use their health care skills to:
   a. cure everyone in society
   b. care only for women and to assist in childbirth
   c. become physicians
   d. care only for the elderly

3. An accurate sketch of the spinal vertebrae was created during the Renaissance by:
   a. Leonardo da Vinci
   b. Michelangelo
   c. early Christian monks
   d. Louis Pasteur
4. Hippocrates is considered by many to be:
   a. the founder of scientific surgery
   b. the inventor of the smallpox vaccine
   c. the father of medicine
   d. the father of preventive medicine
5. The first woman physician in the United States was:
   a. Florence Nightingale
   b. Clara Barton
   c. Elizabeth Anderson
   d. Elizabeth Blackwell

Critical Thinking

1. With a group of peers, identify the effects of culture on today's medicine.
2. How does the role of a medical specialist today compare to the role of a medical specialist in the past? Consider both similarities and dissimilarities.
3. You are a male physician on call in your hospital's emergency room when a woman, five months pregnant, is brought in. She is hemorrhaging. Her husband shuns you and demands a female physician. You quickly realize this couple is Muslim. Role play this scenario with a classmate. How can you solve the dilemma? Consider the possibility that your only female physician is out of the country on vacation.
4. You are the medical assistant. Your physician has just prescribed analgesics for a young Oriental woman suffering from migraine headaches. You overhear the young woman arguing with her mother who thinks that she should see a Chinese acupuncturist. What, if anything, would you do?
5. Discuss with a peer the role of women in medicine today. What difficulties, if any, might a female physician face today? Compare today's difficulties to those of female health care practitioners 100 years ago.
6. Write a one-page report on one significant person who contributed greatly to medicine.

WEB ACTIVITIES

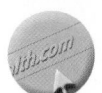

The World Wide Web is an ideal place to seek evidence of new and emerging technologies in medicine. One such avenue is "Medical Breakthroughs" reported by Ivanhoe Broadcast News, Inc. Identify at least two or three recent discoveries you find particularly interesting from your research on the Web.

REFERENCES/BIBLIOGRAPHY

Keir, L., Wise, B. A., & Krebs, C. (1998). *Medical assisting: Administrative and clinical competencies* (4th ed.). Albany, NY: Delmar.

Kinn, M. E., & Woods, M. A. (1999). *The medical assistant: Administrative and clinical* (8th ed.). Philadelphia: W. B. Saunders.

Lewis, M. A., & Tamparo, C. D. (1998). *Medical law, ethics, and bioethics for ambulatory care* (4th ed.). Philadelphia: F. A. Davis.

Lyons, A. S., & Petrucelli, J. R., II (1978). *Medicine: An illustrated history.* New York: Harry N. Abrams, Inc.

Taber's cyclopedic medical dictionary (18th ed.) (1997). Philadelphia: F. A. Davis.

Warden, C. D. (1986). *Health care in the 1980s from a consumer's perspective.* Unpublished doctoral dissertation, Union Graduate School, Seattle, WA.

THE THERAPEUTIC APPROACH

THERAPEUTIC COMMUNICATION SKILLS

KEY TERMS

Active Listening
Bias
Body Language
Buffer Words
Closed Questions
Clustering
Communication Cycle
Compensation
Congruency
Decode
Defense Mechanism
Denial
Displacement
Encoding
Facial Expressions
Feedback
Gestures/Mannerisms
Hierarchy of Needs
Indirect Statements
Interview Techniques
Introjection
Kinesics
Masking
Modes of Communication
Open-Ended Questions
Perception
Position
Posture
Prejudice
Projection
Rationalization
Regression
Repression

(continues)

OUTLINE

Importance of Communication
Cultural Influence on Therapeutic Communication
Biases and Prejudices
The Communication Cycle
The Sender
The Message
The Receiver
Feedback
Listening Skills
Verbal Communication
The Five Cs of Communication
Nonverbal Communication
Facial Expression
Territoriality
Posture
Position
Gestures and Mannerisms
Touch

Congruency in Communication
Perception
Maslow's Hierarchy of Needs
Technology and Communication
Roadblocks to Therapeutic Communication
Defense Mechanisms
Introjection
Denial
Compensation
Regression
Repression
Sublimation
Projection
Displacement
Rationalization
Interview Techniques
Telephone Techniques

OBJECTIVES

The student should strive to meet the following performance objectives and demonstrate an understanding of the facts and principles presented in this chapter through written and oral communication.

1. Define the key terms as presented in the glossary.
2. Identify the importance of communication.
3. Recall at least four influences on therapeutic communication related to culture, and describe four common biases/prejudices in today's society.
4. List and define the four basic elements of the communication cycle.
5. Identify the four modes or channels of communication most pertinent in our everyday exchange.

(continues)

KEY TERMS
(continued)

OBJECTIVES *(continued)*

6. Discuss the importance of active listening in therapeutic communication.
7. Differentiate the terms verbal and nonverbal communication.
8. Analyze the five Cs of communication, and describe their effectiveness in the communication cycle.
9. Demonstrate the following body language or nonverbal communication behaviors: facial expressions, territoriality, position, posture, gestures/mannerisms, touch.
10. Identify and explain congruency in communication.
11. Discuss the use of Maslow's hierarchy of needs in therapeutic communication.
12. Discuss communication modification for electronically transmitted messages.
13. Recall eight significant roadblocks to therapeutic communication.
14. List and describe seven common defense mechanisms.
15. Discuss the possible impact on therapeutic communication that the unequal relationship between physician and patient might have.
16. Compare/contrast closed questions, open-ended questions, and indirect statements.
17. List four tools or considerations when communicating on the telephone.
18. Demonstrate the correct way to speak into the mouthpiece of a telephone by answering an incoming call and closing a telephone conversation.

ROLE DELINEATION COMPONENTS

GENERAL (TRANSDISCIPLINARY)

Communication Skills

- **Treat all patients with compassion and empathy**
- **Recognize and respect cultural diversity**
- **Adapt communications to individual's ability to understand**
- **Use effective and correct verbal and written communications**
- **Use medical terminology appropriately**
- **Use professional telephone technique**

(continues)

SCENARIO

In the two-doctor office of Doctors Lewis and King, four medical assistants constantly interact with patients, allaying their concerns, scheduling their appointments, instructing them on medications, and helping them understand their insurance coverage. On any given day, office manager Marilyn Johnson, CMA, is greeting patients warmly as they arrive for their appointments. Some patients, like Anna and Joseph Ortiz, are new to the practice. Marilyn's warm manner puts them at ease. Other patients, like Martin Gordon, who has prostate cancer, may be depressed and anxious. Marilyn tries to create an environment where they feel free to share their concerns and anxieties.

While Marilyn is busy with patients, administrative medical assistant Ellen Armstrong is on the telephone, scheduling appointments, answering patient questions, and making decisions about what calls need priority attention. Ellen projects a warm, courteous presence over the telephone; she maintains her composure, even when faced with difficult calls and tries always to ask the right questions of callers in a nonthreatening manner.

- Recognize and respond to verbal and nonverbal communications
- Receive, organize, prioritize, and transmit information
- Serve as a liaison
- Promote the practice through positive public relations

INTRODUCTION

Of all the tasks and skills required of the medical assistant in the ambulatory care setting, none is quite so important as communication. Communication is the very foundation for every action taken by health care professionals in the care of their patients. Because medical assistants are often the liaison between patient and physician, it is critical to be aware of all the complexities of the communication process.

Every day, Marilyn and Ellen and the two clinical medical assistants at the offices of Doctors Lewis and King face many communication challenges. This chapter will describe effective communication principles, apply those principles to face-to-face communication as well as telephone communication, and describe the basic roadblocks to communication. The key word to all communication in the medical setting is *therapeutic*. In all conversation with patients, the more therapeutic the conversation, the more satisfied the patient will be with the care provided.

IMPORTANCE OF COMMUNICATION

Communication in the health setting is the foundation for all patient care and is of the utmost importance. The majority of this communication in the ambulatory care setting will be therapeutic—it will utilize specific and well-defined professional skills. Patients' satisfaction with their medical care is as much related to the effectiveness of the communication between themselves and their chosen health care provider as it is to the actual care itself.

A patient choosing a physician wants a clear understanding of the physician's professional and technical skills as well as the physician's ability to communicate. The patient may question family members and friends regarding their personal physician's professional manner and communication skills. Questions often asked include: "Will your doctor talk with me so that I understand what is being said?" "Will your doctor listen to what I have to say?" "Can I talk to your doctor honestly and openly?"

When communication is therapeutic, patients feel validated and respected. **Therapeutic communication** skills create a feeling of comfort for patients even when difficult or unpleasant information must be exchanged.

CULTURAL INFLUENCE ON THERAPEUTIC COMMUNICATION

 For true therapeutic communication to take place, the influence of culture must be considered. Cultural influences include one's ethnic heritage, geographic location and background, genetics, age, gender, economics, educational experiences, life experiences, and value systems.

Any or all of these influences may exhibit themselves when health care is sought by patients. A patient's ethnic heritage may indicate a slant toward the Eastern influence in medicine as opposed to the traditional Western style more commonly taught and practiced in the United States today. Geographic location and background may reveal that a person is more comfortable with a family physician in a very small clinic than one in a large metropolitan multispecialty practice.

Age and gender are factors with a strong influence on communication. How and when do you communicate with a young child? What do you communicate to that child? How do you impress upon an elderly gentleman who has taken little medications throughout his lifetime that he now must take his pill every day? In a culture where the husband is the authority, how does the doctor discuss with the female patient the inadvisability of another pregnancy at this time?

Language barriers will prevent therapeutic communication if great care is not taken. If an interpreter is necessary, it is important to remember to speak directly to the patient, not the interpreter. If English is the second language or a heavy accent is involved, speaking clearly and slowly (not loudly) can greatly enhance communication. It must always be emphasized, however, that the lack of clear and understandable language does *not* imply lack of intelligence.

The influence of economics may reveal a discomfort if the office staff and patients have a different perception

39

about how billing is managed and when and how payment is expected. A discussion of billing and payment procedures at the first office visit or before a major procedure will be beneficial to all concerned parties.

Educational and life experiences will, in part, determine how patients react to their care. Patients with family members being treated for a chronic illness will have more knowledge and understanding of that illness in their own lives. Individuals who have already suffered a great deal of loss and grief in their lives may handle the information of a life-threatening illness more easily than someone who has experienced little grief.

BIASES AND PREJUDICES

Personal preferences, biases, and prejudices will enter into many physician-patient relationships. Such biases affect the types of communication possible. When individuals are not aware of their biases or prejudices, hostile attitudes may prevail.

For therapeutic communication to take place, biases must be examined, a person's comfort level with each bias determined, and measures taken to ensure that a hostile attitude is not present. **Bias** is defined as a slant toward a particular belief. **Prejudice** is defined as an opinion or judgment that is formed before all the facts are known; prejudice is a preconceived and unfavorable concept. Common biases and prejudices in today's society include:

1. A preference for Western style medicine
2. Choosing physicians according to gender
3. Prejudice related to a person's sexual preference
4. Discrimination based on race or religion
5. Hostile attitudes toward people with different value systems than one's own
6. A belief that people who cannot afford health care should receive less care than someone who can pay for full services

 Medical assistants must recognize such biases and prejudices so that their own culture with its biases does not prevent them from responding therapeutically in communications with patients. Such recognition requires being aware of the differences among human beings and willingly accepting the uniqueness of each person.

THE COMMUNICATION CYCLE

All communication, whether social or therapeutic, involves two or more individuals participating in an exchange of information. The **communication cycle** involves sending and receiving messages even when unconsciously aware of them.

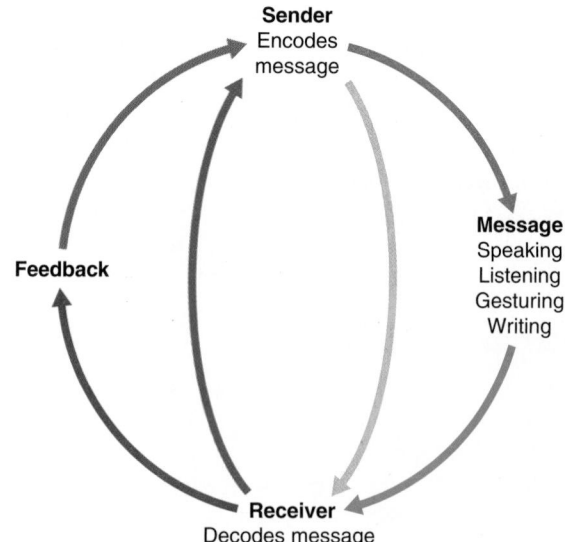

Figure 4-1   The communication cycle and channels of communication.

Four basic elements are included in the communication cycle. They are (1) the sender, (2) the message and a channel or mode of communication, (3) the receiver, and (4) feedback (Figure 4-1).

The Sender

The sender begins the communication cycle by **encoding** or creating the message to be sent. This is an important step, and much care should be taken in formulating the message. Before creating the message, the sender must observe the receiver to determine the complexity of the words to be used within the message, the receiver's ability to interpret the message, and the best channel by which to send the message.

The Message

The message is the content being communicated. The message must be understood clearly by the receiver. Various levels of complexity in communication are used depending upon the ability of the receiver to recognize and understand the words contained within the message. Children do not have the vocabulary base nor the cognitive skills to communicate and understand the same as adults. The health of the receiver also must be considered. A patient who is stressed or in pain may find it difficult to concentrate on the message. If the patient is of a different nationality and/or culture from the sender, verbal communication may require special skill. When visual or hearing acuity is impaired, another challenge must be surmounted.

The four **modes of communication**, also called channels of communication, most pertinent in our everyday exchange include (1) speaking, (2) listening, (3) gestures or body language, and (4) writing. These modes or channels are affected by our physical and mental development, our culture, education and life experiences, our impressions from models and mentors, and in general by how we feel and accept ourselves as individuals. Each mode or channel of communication has its appropriateness and must be considered when formulating the message.

The Receiver

The receiver is the recipient of the sender's message. The receiver must decode, or interpret, the meaning of the message. The primary sensory skill used in verbal communication is listening. It is hard work to concentrate and listen. When decoding the message, the receiver must be aware that not only the spoken words, but the tone and pitch of the voice and the speed at which the words are spoken carry meaning and must be evaluated.

Feedback

Feedback takes place after the receiver has decoded the message sent by the sender. Feedback is the receiver's way of ensuring that the message that is understood is the same as the message that was sent. Feedback also provides an opportunity for the receiver to clarify any misunderstanding regarding the original message and to ask for additional information.

LISTENING SKILLS

A vital part of feedback in the communication cycle is listening. A good listener is alert to all aspects of the communication cycle—the verbal and nonverbal message as well as verification of the message through appropriate feedback.

Active listening is one method used in therapeutic communication. In this technique, the received message is sent back to the sender, worded a little differently, for verification from the sender.

Sender: "How can I possibly pay this fee when I have no insurance?"
Receiver: "You're worried about paying your bill?"

The preceding example illustrates how the receiver is able to validate the sender's concerns at the same time the message is checked for accuracy. The door is then left open for a therapeutic response such as:

Sender: "Our bookkeeper will be glad to work out a payment plan with you that will fit your resources."

VERBAL COMMUNICATION

Verbal communication takes place when the message is spoken. However, one must keep in mind the fact that unless the words have meaning, and unless the sender and the receiver apply the same meaning to the spoken words, verbal communication may be misunderstood. If, for example, you overhear a conversation in a language foreign to you, you are indeed a witness to verbal communication, but you may not understand the message. To have any meaning, the spoken word must be understood by all parties of the communication (Tamparo & Lindh, 2000).

The Five Cs of Communication

In their book *Professional Development,* Mary Wilkes and C. Bruce Crosswait (1991) identified the five Cs of Communication in business. They are (1) complete, (2) clear, (3) concise, (4) courteous, and (5) cohesive. These five Cs apply equally well in health care professions.

Complete. The message must be complete, with all the necessary information given. The medical assistant cannot expect the patient to be compliant if all the instructions are not given and understood.

Clear. The information given in the message must also be clear. The use of eye contact enhances clarity. Health care professionals must be able to articulate by using good diction and by enunciating each word distinctly. The patient must be allowed time to process the message and verify its meaning. The message must also be heard to promote understanding.

Concise. A concise message is one that does not include any unnecessary information. It should be brief and to the point (Figure 4-2). Patients must not be overloaded with technical terms that may not be understood or that tend to distract them by diverting their attention away from the balance of the message.

Patient Teaching Tip

When patients speak a different language or when English is their second language, you may need to urge them to communicate nonverbally; you can encourage them to do so by using appropriate, nonthreatening gestures. Sometimes, it may be important to communicate verbally with a family member to gain specific information. Be sure not to violate any confidentiality of the patient, however.

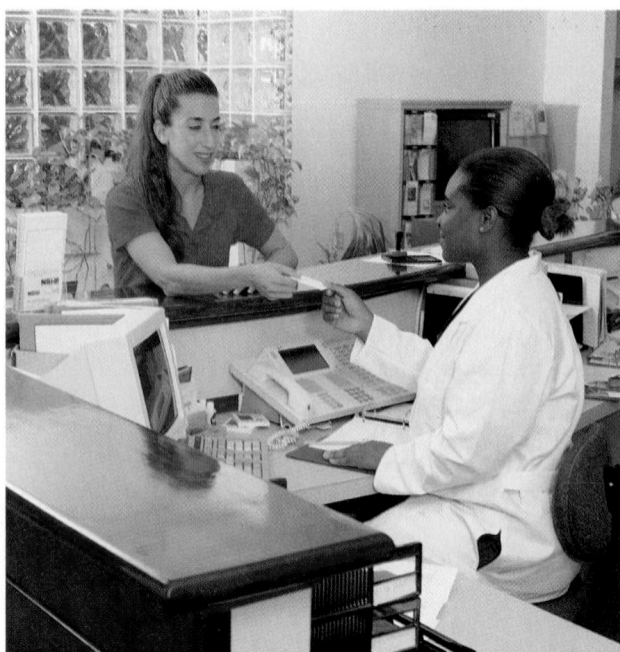

Figure 4-2   To say to the patient after greeting her by name, "I've completed an appointment card to remind you of your next appointment, Tuesday at 2:00 P.M." is an example of a concise message, brief and to the point.

Courteous. Courtesy is important in all aspects of communication. It only takes a moment to acknowledge a patient with a smile or by name. Knocking on the exam room door before entering validates the patient's right to privacy and builds self-esteem.

When a patient must be placed on hold on the telephone, thank the patient for waiting. Try not to keep the patient waiting too long if you must find information.

Remember to be courteous to colleagues in the office. Good working relationships and professionalism are always enhanced by simple courtesy.

Cohesive. A cohesive message is organized and logical in its progression. The cohesive message does not ramble and does not jump from one subject to another. The

Patient Teaching Tip

Sensitive medical assistants will encourage patients to verbalize their concerns. The ability to ask questions in a nonprobing way and to elicit patient response is an important function in any ambulatory care setting, for it is critical to know a patient's history, current medications, and other relevant data.

patient should be able to follow the message easily. The medical assistant should always allow time to summarize detailed messages and utilize responding skills to verify that the patient fully understands the message.

When communicating within the health professions, keep in mind the following:

1. Good communication skills are necessary in establishing rapport with patients.
2. Patients feel respected and validated when called by their full name, such as Mary O'Keefe or Mrs. O'Keefe.
3. Patients should be encouraged to verbalize their feelings.
4. Give technical information to patients in a manner that they can understand.
5. Allow patients to make practical application to their personal health needs.

NONVERBAL COMMUNICATION

Verbal communication alone is not always adequate in conveying the message being sent. In most instances, more than one mode or channel of communication is employed. Nonverbal communication, often referred to as **body language,** includes the unconscious body movements, gestures, and facial expressions that accompany speech. The study of body language is known as **kinesics** (Figure 4-3).

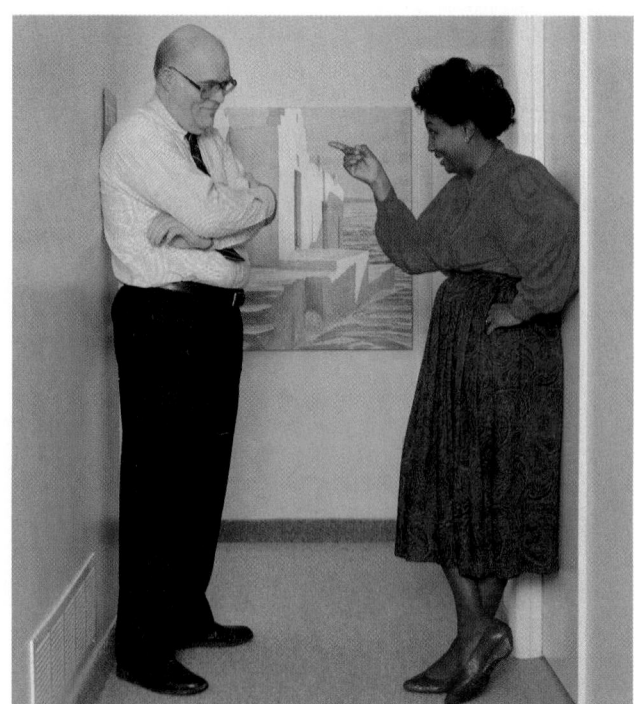

Figure 4-3   Body language can communicate more than spoken words.

Nonverbal communication is the language we learn first. It is learned seemingly automatically when infants learn to return a smile or respond to touches on the cheek. Much of our body language is a learned behavior and is greatly influenced by the primary caregivers and the culture in which we are raised.

Feelings and emotions are communicated most often through nonverbal means. The body expresses its true repressed feelings using body language. Most of the negative messages we communicate are also expressed nonverbally and usually are unintentional. Experts tell us that 70 percent of communication is nonverbal. The tone of voice communicates 23 percent of the message—only 7 percent of the message is actually communicated by the spoken word (Wilkes & Crosswait, 1991).

Facial Expression

Facial expression is considered one of the most important and observed nonverbal communicators. Each facet or aspect of the anatomy of the face sends a nonverbal message.

Often expressions of joy and happiness or sorrow and grief are reflected through the eyes. The anatomy of the eyes does not change, but the movements of the structures surrounding the eyes enhance or magnify the message being communicated.

Children are told it is not polite to stare at people. It is acceptable to stare at animals in the zoo or art objects in the museum, but not at humans. Staring is dehumanizing and is often interpreted as an invasion of privacy.

The medical assistant must learn not to stare when patients present with ailments that make them "look" different. Patients such as these are individuals who have needs and who perhaps feel pain, discomfort, and have decreased self-esteem and value. These feelings will only be amplified if the medical assistant and other health professionals are unable to "see" them as humans. A lack of eye contact may also be viewed as avoidance or disinterest in being involved.

The movements of the eyebrow indicate many nonverbal cues as well. Surprise, puzzlement, worry, amusement, and questioning are often nonverbal messages reflected by the position of the eyebrow. Wrinkling of the forehead sends similar messages.

 Cultural influences affect customs and different forms of facial expressions. In many Latin and Asian countries, it is unacceptable to look adults in the eye so people from these cultures often stare at the floor. This expression may be misinterpreted and misunderstood. Many persons of Eastern cultures communicate nonverbally differently from persons of Western cultures. These differences also may lead to confusion and misunderstanding.

Territoriality

Territoriality is the distance at which we feel comfortable with others while communicating. In the classroom, for example, students claim their territory the first day of class. The area is well-defined by using books and papers or by placing the arm, hand, or chair on boundary lines. When another invades the territory, a shift in body position or the use of eye contact sends the message "This is my area." Individuals may feel threatened when others invade their personal space without permission. Some examples of comfortable personal space follow:

- Intimate
  touching to 6 inches
- Personal
  1½ to 4 feet
- Social
  4 to 12 feet
- Public
  12 to 15 feet

As with facial expressions, territoriality or personal space will be handled differently by various cultures. For example, there is no word for privacy in the Japanese language. Population numbers require crowding together publicly as well as privately. Public crowding is often viewed as a sign of warmth and pleasant intimacy in Japan. In the private home, several generations may live together; however, each considers this space to be his own and resents intrusion into it.

Arabs like to touch their companions, to feel and to smell them. To deny a friend your breath is to be ashamed. When two Arabs talk to each other, they look each other in the eyes with great intensity.

The medical assistant may perform many invasive tasks during the course of an office visit. Examples include taking vital signs or giving injections, both of which require touching the patient. It is beneficial to explain procedures that invade another's space before beginning the procedure so that it will not be perceived as threatening. This helps to empower the patient by involving the patient in the decision-making process and builds a sense of trust in the medical assistant.

Posture

Like territoriality, posture is important to allied health care professionals. Posture relates to the position of the body or parts of the body. It is the manner in which we carry ourselves, or pose in situations. We tend to tighten up in threatening or unknown situations and relax in nonthreatening environments. Those who study kinesics feel a posture involves at least half the body and that the position can last for nearly five minutes.

When the patient is seated with the arms and legs crossed, the message of closure or being opinionated may be relayed. On the other hand, sitting in a chair relaxed with the hands clasped behind the head indicates an attitude of being open to suggestions. Slumped shoulders may signal depression, discouragement, or in some cases even pain.

Position

Position, the physical stance of two individuals while communicating, is a key factor to consider while communicating with the patient. Most physician-patient relationships utilize the face-to-face communication arrangement. When speaking with a patient, the physician or medical assistant will want to maintain a close but comfortable position enabling observation of all cues being sent, both verbal and nonverbal (Figure 4-4).

Standing over a patient can convey a message of superiority, and too much distance between the two parties may be interpreted as avoidance or being exclusive. Generally, leaning toward the patient expresses warmth, caring, interest, acceptance, and trust. Moving away from the patient may be interpreted as dislike, disinterest, boredom, indifference, suspicion, or impatience.

Whenever possible, it is best to have a chair in the examination room and to have the patient seated comfortably there to begin the communication cycle. The medical assistant or physician can sit on a stool that can easily be moved toward the patient. This arrangement aids the patient in feeling valued, listened to, and cared for as a fellow human being.

Gestures and Mannerisms

Most of us use **gestures and mannerisms** when we "talk" with our hands. This form of body language may be useful in enhancing the spoken word by emphasizing ideas, thus creating and holding the attention of others.

Touch

Touch is a powerful tool that communicates what cannot be expressed in words. Its appropriateness in the patient/health professional relationship has well-defined boundaries and requires the use of good judgment on the part of the professional. Infants who are not touched, cuddled, and loved do not grow and develop as those who receive these reassuring gestures. The touch that communicates caring, sincerity, understanding, and reassurance is usually welcomed and considered to be a therapeutic response. Most patients will understand and accept the touching behavior as it relates to the medical setting; however, we

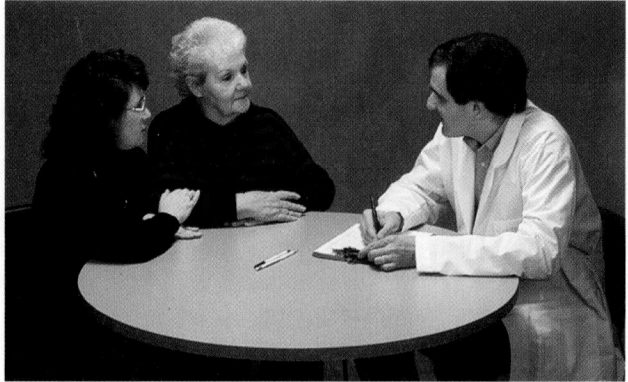

Figure 4-4 Positive posture and position encourage therapeutic communication.

must remember that not all patients are comfortable with touch. Whenever the patient is not comfortable with touch, ask permission and create as safe and reassuring an environment as possible.

CONGRUENCY IN COMMUNICATION

There are some keys to successful communication to employ for communication to be effective. There must be **congruency** between the verbal and nonverbal communication. The two messages must agree; you cannot shake your head NO while saying YES verbally. This response sends a mixed message, and in most cases, the nonverbal messages will be accepted as the intended message.

It is also important to remember that most nonverbal messages are sent in groups of various forms of body language. The grouping of nonverbal messages into statements or conclusions is known as **clustering**. **Masking** involves an attempt to conceal or repress the true feeling

SPOTLIGHT ON AAMA ESSENTIALS THROUGH CAAHEP

- Respect your patient's cultural diversity, and adapt your skills to meeting the patient's needs.
- Remember that body language can often convey feelings not otherwise expressed through verbal communication.
- Consider that a patient may use defense mechanisms to mask true feelings.

or message. The perceptive professional will be aware of all these messages.

Perception

Perception as it relates to communication is the conscious awareness of one's own feelings and the feelings of others (Fast, 1970). To be most useful and therapeutic as health professionals, we must first explore our own feelings and appreciate and accept ourselves.

Learning to use perception involves the ability to sense another's attitudes, moods, and feelings. It takes practice and experience to develop and use this skill effectively. Being attentive to other professionals and observing their use of perception will yield insight into its usefulness and provide an example to emulate. A word of caution— the use of perception may easily be misinterpreted, especially when going with your feeling or assessment of what is happening regarding the patient. Always follow perceived assessments with verbal validation before assuming your perception of the circumstance is correct.

Nonverbal communication is easily misinterpreted. Careful observation for congruency between verbal and nonverbal communication, and clustering nonverbal cues being sent into nonverbal statements will strengthen the ability to interpret the message accurately.

Maslow's Hierarchy of Needs

Abraham Maslow is considered the founder of humanistic psychology and is most well known for his hierarchy of needs (Figure 4-5) (Miliken, 1998).

If you can understand this hierarchy, you can assess a patient's needs. If the most basic of needs are not met, it is highly unlikely that a patient can be successful with any

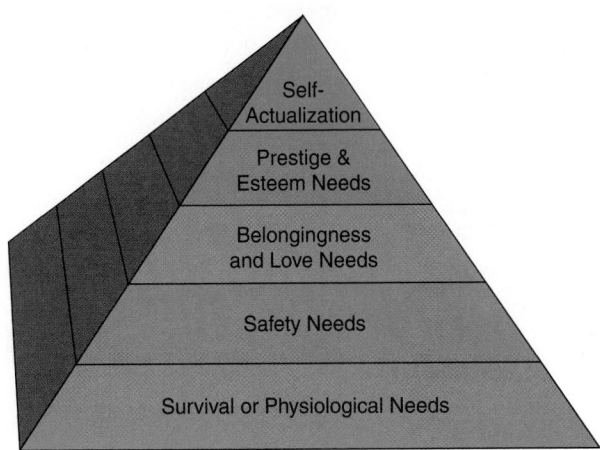

Figure 4-5   Maslow's hierarchy of needs.

treatment protocol. Keeping this hierarchy in mind will help facilitate therapeutic communication.

TECHNOLOGY AND COMMUNICATION

Face-to-face communication is the mode of choice in most physician offices today. However, technological devices are becoming more and more accepted as a means of communication. Technology-mediated communication and a greater reliance on cyberspace technology will greatly affect communication in the twenty-first century. Examples of new technologies in medical offices include fax machines, telecommunication conferences, e-mail, and laptop computers linked to a network of computers that communicate with satellite offices in another part of the community or even in another country.

Do these new communication methods change the communication cycle? There is still a message, a sender, a receiver, and feedback. What changes is the way in which the message is encoded and decoded. The content of the message will be examined for credibility rather than one's dress, eye contact, facial expression, vocal inflection, and posture. Technology does not convey emotions nearly as well as face-to-face or even telephone conversations. Another factor to consider is that your composed message may not look like what your reader sees. The software and hardware that you use for composing, sending, sorting, downloading, and reading may be completely different from what your recipient uses. Modifications to the format may change the intended emphasis or meaning of the message.

There are several advantages for the use of e-mail rather than postal mail (commonly referred to as "snail mail"). E-mail is less expensive and faster than mailing a letter. Because the turnaround time can be so fast, e-mail is more conversational than traditional paper-based media. An e-mail transmission is less intrusive than a telephone call and less bother than a fax. When one uses e-mail transmissions, differences in location and time zone are less of a problem. See Chapter 15 for additional information regarding e-mail.

ROADBLOCKS TO THERAPEUTIC COMMUNICATION

Being sensitive to patients' unique personalities and needs will enable the health care professional to avoid roadblocks to communication (Table 4-1).

It must be the concern of each health care professional to facilitate communication by encouraging and enabling patients to express themselves honestly without

TABLE 4-1 ROADBLOCKS TO COMMUNICATION	
Roadblock	**Example**
Reassuring clichés	"Don't worry, Mr. McKay, about not having a job; you'll find another one really soon."
Moralizing/lecturing	"If you were smart, Mrs. Johnson, you'd lose fifty pounds and you wouldn't have such a problem with your diabetes and hypertension."
Requiring explanations	"Why would you not want to have chemotherapy, Mr. Gordon? Seeing your wife die of cancer should surely make you want to seek treatment."
Ridiculing/shaming	"Ha, ha, Mr. Gordon! It's not *prostrate*—it's prostate cancer."
Defending/contradicting	"Mr. Marshal, I assure you the physician is *very busy.* He will not see you until he has finished with his other patients."
Shifting subjects	"Yes, Mrs. Jover, your work is very interesting, but I must ask you to sign this permission form to test for HIV."
Criticizing	"Mrs. O'Keefe, why in the world would you stay with an abusive husband?"
Threatening	"There is no way you will get rid of this cough if you do not stop smoking, Mr. Fowler."

fear. Roadblocks close communication and prevent quality care of the total person.

DEFENSE MECHANISMS

Defense mechanisms are used often by individuals and may further block the communication cycle. The use of defense mechanisms may be the result of individuals feeling threatened, ashamed, or guilty. In this situation, patients tend to respond defensively to protect themselves. Defense mechanisms are used unconsciously by all individuals at one time or another. They allow individuals to gain composure and/or control in a situation. They can become harmful when they prevent patients from facing problems through to a satisfactory solution. Recognizing common defense mechanisms enables individuals to communicate effectively.

Introjection

Introjection is the identification with another person or with some object. The patient assumes the supposed feelings and/or characteristics of the other personality or object.

Denial

Denial (rejection of or refusal to acknowledge information) is often found in the health care setting. When patient Abigail Johnson does not comply with her diet, she is denying the consequences that might occur as a result.

Compensation

Compensation is the overemphasizing of characteristics to make up for a real or imagined failure or handicap.

Regression

Regression is moving back to a former stage to escape conflict or fear. When three-year-old Chris is faced with another baby in the family, he may feel left out, unwanted, and demand to be nursed or to have a bottle like the baby.

Repression

Repression is temporary amnesia—being unable to cope with the overwhelming situation by temporarily forgetting. When Mary O'Keefe confronts her husband about his hostile attitude, he is likely to deny her allegation because he has repressed his frustration and anger at not having a satisfactory job.

Sublimation

Sublimation is an example of redirecting a socially unacceptable impulse into one that is socially acceptable. If John O'Keefe could release his anger and frustration by playing handball, he would not be so hostile in other settings.

Projection

Projection is the act of placing one's own feelings upon another. Juanita Hansen, who is suspected of child abuse, accuses the medical assistant of being unduly rough with her son.

Displacement

Displacement occurs when individuals displace their negative feelings onto something or someone with no significance to the situation. Cele Little is agitated when Dr. Woo tells her that her hearing is seriously impaired and suggests going to an audiologist for a hearing aid. She yells at her sister, Dottie, about being so clumsy and falling and injuring her back.

Rationalization

Rationalization is the act of justification, usually illogically, that one uses to keep from facing the truth of the situation. Leo McKay rationalizes that his stomach pains are the result of his lousy cooking and have nothing to do with the stress he may be feeling as the result of being laid off his job.

Recognizing defense mechanisms and understanding how best to communicate to get beyond the defense mechanisms to the truth is an art. It takes practice and patience. Medical assistants must be observant, always looking for the nonverbal cues while listening closely to the verbal message. Being present in the moment and giving each patient your full attention will enable you to communicate therapeutically.

INTERVIEW TECHNIQUES

All health professionals must be adept at **interview techniques**—knowing how to encourage the best communication between themselves and the patient. It is important to remember that an unequal relationship exists between the health professional and the patient. The health professional, whether it be the physician or the medical assistant, is in the power position and has a great deal of control over the patient. Therefore, it is important to equalize the relationship as much as possible. That is the reason why some professionals use the term *client* rather than *patient*.

Early in the interview, the patient must feel comfortable enough to risk being honest with the health professional. The health professional must build an atmosphere of trust by showing concern for the patient. A gentle touch and a warm, caring facial expression may be all that is necessary. Always be honest and genuine in your responses to patients. Be sympathetic and empathic and create an environment that is free of hypocrisy.

When the medical assistant is interviewing the patient for the chief complaint, it is important to listen with a "third" ear. Listen to what the patient is not saying but is apt to exhibit through nonverbal communication.

You might choose to share your observation of the nonverbal message with the patient, thus encouraging the patient to verbalize more freely. When feelings are shared, validate and acknowledge those feelings through such statements as "I understand your distress." You can verify the communication by reflecting or paraphrasing what the patient has said.

You will be asking **closed questions** during the interview. Closed questions can be answered with a simple yes or no.

"Are you still taking your medication?"
"Are you in pain now?"

You will also use **open-ended questions** with the patient. These questions encourage therapeutic communication because the patient is required to verbalize more.

"What kind of help will you have at home during your recovery?"
"How are you coming along on this diet?

Indirect statements will also prove helpful in facilitating therapeutic communication. An indirect statement will elicit a response from a patient without the patient feeling questioned.

"Tell me what you've been doing since you retired."
"I'd like to know more about your exercise program."

TELEPHONE TECHNIQUES

It has often been said that the telephone is the lifeline of the physician's office. Communication over the telephone requires understanding on the part of each communicator (Figure 4-6).

Each medium uses the proper tools to get the job done. Speaking on the telephone is much like a conversation

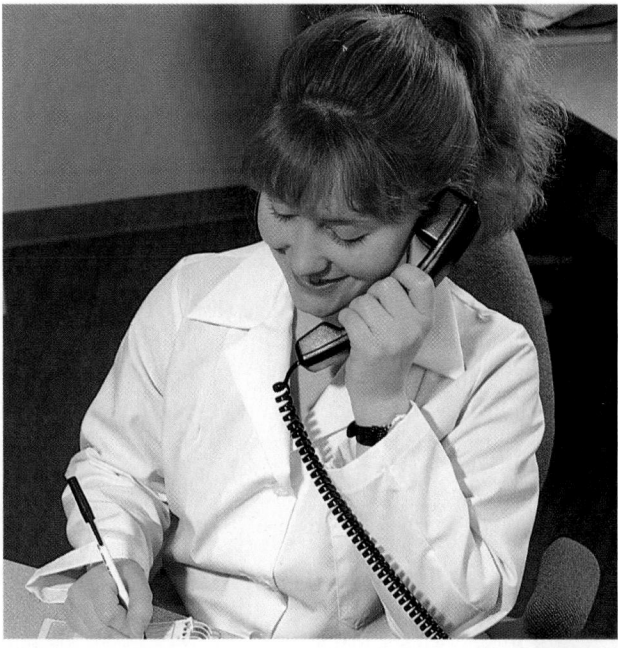

Figure 4-6   When communicating over the telephone, listen with full attention to make certain the message sent and received is correct.

between two blindfolded individuals. The facial expressions cannot be seen, there is no eye contact, and there is no visual feedback. The listener will interpret mood by the tone and pacing of voice and the words spoken. When speaking on the telephone, quick conclusions are drawn. Often, we jump to conclusions, and the communication is misinterpreted.

The old, cold, aloof, formal business greeting comes across like frostbite in the medical office setting. It sounds curt, bored, and uncaring. Think of welcoming a new acquaintance into your home, then practice the same characteristics when speaking on the telephone. Speaking clearly, use words that will be easily understood, and ask questions to verify that the patient has understood the message being conveyed.

Concentrate on enunciating and being understood. If you hear, "What? I didn't understand you. I can't hear you," slow down and speak a little louder with distinct enunciation directly into the mouthpiece. The mouthpiece should be held one to two inches away from the mouth. Project your voice at the mouthpiece and then project another foot further. Your voice is the delivery system for your words and thoughts. Speak with confidence and conviction.

Have you ever called an office and had the firm name clipped off? The name of the office is important. To avoid clipping off the office name, practice using buffer words. Buffer words are expendable; if you clip them off, at least the office name remains intact. Use buffer words before the office name and before you identify yourself. "Good morning, this is Inner City Health Care. This is Walter, how may I help you?" *Good morning* and *this is* are buffer words.

All the techniques for effective face-to-face communication must be more intentionally observed when the communication is over the telephone because you cannot see the person with whom you are speaking. You must listen with full attention to make certain that the message sent and received is correct.

To close a telephone conversation to schedule an appointment, for example, consider the following:

1. Use the patient's name if it can be done without announcing the name to persons in the reception area.
2. Confirm the date and time of the appointment.
3. Identify the physician if there is more than one physician in the office.
4. Give any specific instructions that may be necessary.
5. Say goodbye.

For more information on telephone techniques, see Chapter 12.

SUMMARY

Throughout this text you are reminded of the importance of effective communication techniques. Good communication takes practice. Use the techniques identified in this chapter with your family and with your peers. Watch for roadblocks, be aware of defense mechanisms, and remember the five Cs of communication.

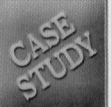

CASE STUDY 4-1

It is a typically active day at the offices of Doctors Lewis and King. Despite the three emergencies in early afternoon and the full schedule of patients, everything is running smoothly with Dr. Lewis and the entire staff responding quickly but thoroughly to patient concerns.

At 4:00 P.M. another emergency patient arrives; at the same time Jim Marshal, an architect in a downtown firm, comes in early for a routine appointment and demands to be seen immediately. Jim, a regular patient, has a history of being difficult and impatient; being a bit arrogant, he tends to put his needs first. However, Dr. Lewis is occupied with another patient. It is critical to treat the patient with the emergency as soon as possible, and Jim is half an hour early.

Joe Guerrero, CMA, the office's administrative and clinical medical assistant, calmly asks Mr. Marshal to please wait until his scheduled appointment time. When he threatens to leave, Joe explains to Mr. Marshal that there are two patients ahead of him but that the doctor will see him at his scheduled appointment time.

continues

CASE STUDY REVIEW

1. What communication roadblocks did medical assistant Joe Guerrero avoid in reacting to Jim Marshal's demands to see the doctor?

2. With another student, role-play the scenario, with one student taking the role of patient and one student the role of the medical assistant. Identify roadblocks to communication imposed by the patient. How is the medical assistant using the five Cs of communication to deal with the situation?

3. Do you think the medical assistant reacted appropriately? What else could he have done? What should he *not* do in this situation?

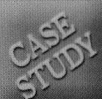

CASE STUDY 4-2

You have learned in this chapter that communication has not been successful until the cycle is complete. Consider the following scenario:

An 82-year-old woman with moderate dementia and a hearing impairment is brought to the surgeon's office for a follow-up appointment after hip replacement surgery. The woman's daughter accompanies her. The goal of the appointment is to make certain the hip is healing nicely and to discuss precautions before the patient returns to her assisted-living apartment. Almost immediately the conversation is directed toward the daughter because it is so much easier to explain to her what should be done.

CASE STUDY REVIEW

1. What might the staff do to help the patient understand the following?
   - Use the walker consistently.
   - Shoes must be leather tennis shoe type or uniform style; consider Velcro closure as opposed to laces that have to be tied.
   - Do not wear pantyhose.
   - You will not be able to walk your dog on a leash.

2. Should the patient be left out of the conversation? Should the daughter be included?

3. In cases such as these, is something other than verbal communication indicated?

REVIEW QUESTIONS

Multiple Choice

1. Culture influences which of the following?
   a. biases and prejudices
   b. ethnic heritage, age, and gender
   c. educational and life experiences and value systems
   d. b and c only

2. In the cycle of communication, encoding means:
   a. deciphering a message
   b. creating the message to be sent
   c. sending the message
   d. receiving the message

3. Body language:
   a. is used to express feelings and emotions
   b. is not as important as verbal communication
   c. only makes up 7 percent of the message
   d. is only used in Eastern cultures

4. A comfortable social space is defined as:
   a. touching to 6 inches
   b. 1½ feet to 4 feet
   c. 12 to 15 feet
   d. 4 to 12 feet

5. A reassuring cliché is:
   a. a way of calming down a patient
   b. a means of rationalizing a decision
   c. a roadblock to communication
   d. always useful in daily communications

6. Redirecting a socially unacceptable impulse into one that is socially acceptable is an example of which of these defense mechanisms?
   a. sublimation
   b. rationalization
   c. projection
   d. displacement

7. When using an open-ended question with a patient, we expect:
   a. a yes or no answer
   b. them to tell us the truth
   c. a response that permits the patient to elaborate
   d. only the right answers
8. Buffer words:
   a. help us get through the day
   b. are meant to soothe a patient's feelings
   c. are expendable words used in answering a telephone call
   d. are important in face-to-face communication

Critical Thinking

1. The 15-year-old girl awaiting a sports physical exam complains that she is overweight and has pimples. What is your therapeutic response?
2. Bill, who is 28 years old, comes for his annual checkup. When reviewing his social data sheet, you discover he is now living in an apartment and has a new phone number. He mumbles to you that his wife left him and won't let him see the kids. What is your verbal therapeutic response?
3. You try to be gentle and gracious with Edith. She is very fragile and difficult to please. While positioning her for an X-ray, she sneers and says, "You are about the roughest person who ever cared for me." What is your therapeutic response?
4. When you report to Herb that his cholesterol is quite high and that the doctor wants to discuss medication and diet, he responds, "That is impossible; you must have made some mistake." What is your therapeutic response?
5. Lenore uses a wheelchair for mobility. When you offer to help her, she says, "Buzz off! I can do this myself." What is your therapeutic response?
6. Leo, age 62, comments on his being laid off, "I simply don't know what I will do with all the extra time on my hands." What is your therapeutic response?
7. Martin says to you, "I wish it would just end," as you schedule him for another series of chemotherapy treatments. What is your therapeutic response?

8. Your physician/employer is leaving for hospital rounds. He must tell the Ward family that their father will never recover. If he does not die within the next thirty-six hours, the physician recommends disconnecting the ventilator. Your physician is close to this family; he has given them care for many years. What is your therapeutic response?

WEB ACTIVITIES

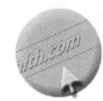

Select three cultures of particular interest to you personally and search the World Wide Web for information regarding these cultures and communication traditions. How might this new information be applied to the physician whose clientele is primarily made up of these cultures? How might this new knowledge benefit a medical assistant employed in this type of setting?

REFERENCES/BIBLIOGRAPHY

Blair, G. M. (January 23, 2000). *Conversation as communication* [On-line]. Available: http://www.ee.ed.ac.uk/~gerard/Management/art7.html

Fast, J. (1970). *Body language*. New York: M. Evans and Company.

Kinn, M. E., & Woods, M. A. (1998). *The medical assistant: Administrative and clinical* (8th ed.). Philadelphia: W. B. Saunders.

Miliken, M. E. (1998). *Understanding human behavior: A guide for health care providers*. Albany, NY: Delmar.

Purtillo, R. (1990). *Health professional/patient interaction*. Philadelphia: W. B. Saunders.

Sherwood, K. D. (January 25, 1999). *A beginner's guide to effective email* [On-line]. Available: http://www.webfoot.com/advice/email.top.html

Taber's cyclopedic medical dictionary. (18th ed.). (1997). Philadelphia: F. A. Davis.

Tamparo, C. D., & Lindh, W. Q. (2000). *Therapeutic communications for health professions*. Albany, NY: Delmar.

Wilkes, M., & Crosswait, C. B. (1991). *Professional development: The dynamics of success*. San Diego: Harcourt Brace Jovanovich.

Chapter

5

COPING SKILLS FOR THE MEDICAL ASSISTANT

KEY TERMS

Burnout
Goal
Inner-Directed People
Long-Range Goals
Outer-Directed People
Parasympathetic Nervous System
Self-Actualization
Short-Range Goals
Stress
Stressors
Sympathetic Nervous System

OUTLINE

What Is Stress?
    Adaptation to Stress
    Coping with Stress
What Is Burnout?
    Burnout in the Workplace
    What to Do If You Are Burned Out
    Preventing Burnout
Goal Setting as a Stress Reliever

OBJECTIVES

The student should strive to meet the following performance objectives and demonstrate an understanding of the facts and principles presented in this chapter through written and oral communication.

1. Define the key terms as presented in the glossary.
2. Differentiate between stress and stressors.
3. Describe Hans Selye's GAS theory.
4. Identify seven approaches to coping with stressors in the ambulatory care setting.
5. Identify three characteristics associated with burnout in the workplace.
6. Identify seven signs or symptoms of burnout.
7. List five aspects of personality that promote burnout.
8. List a minimum of five ways to reduce the risk of burnout.
9. List five considerations when setting a goal.
10. Differentiate between long-range and short-range goals.

ROLE DELINEATION COMPONENTS

GENERAL (TRANSDISCIPLINARY)

Professionalism

- **Project a professional manner and image**
- **Demonstrate initiative and responsibility**
- **Work as a team member**
- **Prioritize and perform multiple tasks**
- **Adapt to change**

SCENARIO

At the office of Doctors Lewis and King, there are four full-time medical assistants who collaborate to make the office run smoothly, both administratively and clinically. One day a month, though, office manager Marilyn Johnson, CMA, is out of town, leaving Ellen Armstrong, the administrative medical assistant, in charge of a busy reception area and an ever-ringing telephone.

On these days, Ellen is particularly careful to organize her work so that things run as they should. She organizes some work the night before, she sets priorities so she is confident that the critical work will get done, and she tries to maintain her calm by taking a short break every couple of hours to review new needs that have come up during the day. While Ellen can't anticipate every emergency, she does try to influence the situation rather than let events control her.

INTRODUCTION

Even in the most well-managed ambulatory care setting, medical assistants and other health providers are likely to feel the effects of stress from time to time. They may be overworked on certain days; they may face difficult patient situations; they may find that the administrative and paperwork load is getting ahead of them.

This chapter helps today's busy, multifaceted medical assistant pinpoint the symptoms of stress and provides ideas for coping with stress as it occurs. The better equipped the medical assistant is to confront and solve the sources of stress, the less likely stressors will become so overwhelming as to lead to burnout on the job. Goal setting, recognizing one's limitations and potentials, setting priorities, and keeping a balanced perspective can work together to reduce stress and enable the medical assistant to take pleasure in working with patients and colleagues.

WHAT IS STRESS?

The body's response to change is termed stress. Stress is the "wear and tear" our bodies experience as we continually adjust to a changing environment. Stress has physical and emotional effects on the body, which create either eustress-positive feelings, or distress-negative feelings. Feeling positive leads to a sense of well being, increased motivation, and awareness of new opportunities and perspectives. Positive stress adds anticipation and excitement to life and is enhancing to our lives. Some stress is beneficial and helps us focus on details, achieve difficult goals, and perform at our best.

Negative feelings, or distress, may result in boredom, frustration, rejection, distrust, anger, and depression. Physical symptoms of distress may include cigarette smoking, obesity, and lack of exercise. It has been estimated that 50 percent of all diseases in the United States have a stress-related origin. Included in these diseases are hypertension, migraine headaches, ulcers, anxiety, allergies and asthma, and some types of cancer and cardiovascular disease (Tecco, 1999).

The demands to change that cause stress are called stressors. Stressors cause the body to go into arousal or alarm and may be anything from fear, worry, threat, or even challenging events. When we experience any type of stress that exceeds what our body can comfortably handle, we are more susceptible to depression and anxiousness. If we become very stressed, the ability to think clearly and objectively may be impaired.

Adaptation to Stress

Hans Selye's General Adaptation Syndrome (GAS) theory proposes that adaptation to stress occurs in four stages, which he defines as alarm, fight-or-flight, exhaustion, and return-to-normal (Figure 5-1).

Alarm. Awareness of perceived stress is recognized by the body during the alarm stage. Pain is a part of this system as it tells us when body tissue is being damaged. A therapeutic response in the ambulatory care setting is to recognize the fact that pain does produce a stress response. The medical assistant who falls behind during the daily rush of scheduling may also experience a slight rise in blood pressure caused by the alarm stage of stress.

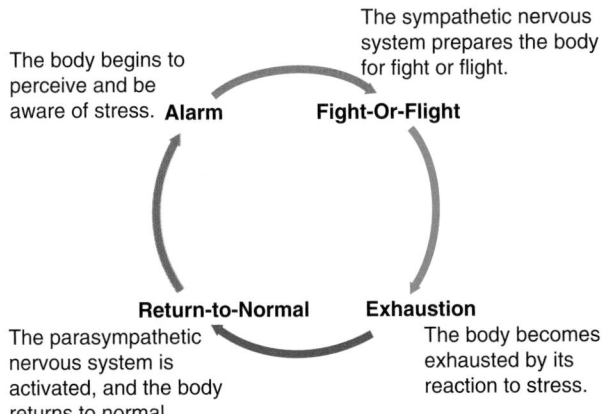

The body begins to perceive and be aware of stress. **Alarm**

The sympathetic nervous system prepares the body for fight or flight. **Fight-Or-Flight**

Return-to-Normal The parasympathetic nervous system is activated, and the body returns to normal.

Exhaustion The body becomes exhausted by its reaction to stress.

Figure 5-1 Hans Selye's General Adaptation Syndrome (GAS) theory proposes that four stages are involved in adapting to stress.

Fight-or-Flight. The **sympathetic nervous system** prepares the body for fight-or-flight. The eyes dilate and the mouth becomes dry. The heart rate is increased, as is the pulse and respirations. Blood vessels in the skin constrict, and blood vessels in the heart and brain dilate. There is decreased motility in the gastrointestinal and genitourinary tracts. All these changes prepare the body for whatever action may need to be taken.

Exhaustion. The body can only stay in the fight-or-flight state for a limited time. If you have ever stretched a rubber band to the maximum and held it there for a period of time, eventually you tired of holding it and released the rubber band. If you were to examine the rubber band after its release, you would find that it has lost some of its elasticity, which can never be regained. The same principle applies to the blood vessels throughout the body. After repeated periods of dilation and relaxation, they become weakened. If you have ever overstretched a rubber band, you know it snaps in two. Blood vessels may burst when they are dilated to an extreme or have developed weakened areas.

Return-to-Normal. During the return-to-normal stage, the **parasympathetic nervous system** is activated, and the body returns to normal. The eyes constrict, salivary glands begin to function, and heart rate, pulse, and respirations decrease. Blood vessels dilate in the skin and constrict in the heart and brain. The gastrointestinal and genitourinary tracts begin to function again (Tamparo & Lindh, 2000).

Each stage in Selye's GAS theory is a mechanism to help protect the body and prepare it to escape from danger. When demands are placed on the body, stress occurs. The way a person reacts to those demands determines the level of stress and whether health is threatened or harmed.

Stress is often considered harmful to health. In reality, stress is essential to one's well-being. The body continually goes through change in the course of a twenty-four-hour period. For example, a quick response while driving to work may be necessary to avoid a collision with another vehicle. During your working hours the telephone rings, the exam rooms are full, and the physician is called to the hospital on an emergency. Immediately the body's stress mode is activated. A moderate to high level of stress for short periods of time enables you to make quick judgments and decisions, to be organized and efficient, and to accomplish tasks within minimal time limits.

When too much stress is experienced or if the stress lasts for a long period of time, it begins to affect the body in a negative way. Often one of the first signs of stress may be a headache caused by an increase in blood pressure. Feeling tired even after plenty of rest may be another signal of stress. If these conditions continue, other vital organs, such as the heart and lungs, for example, may also be affected negatively. Cardiac or respiratory arrest, transient ischemic attack, or fainting may be experienced.

For the medical assistant, new technology, a demanding work load, responding to the needs of people who are ill or hurting, patient diversity, and the continuing need for creative problem solving are examples of the stressors encountered daily in ambulatory care settings.

Coping with Stress

The following suggestions may be helpful in coping with stressors in the work environment.

1. Plan ahead
   - Review the schedule for the next day, and pull charts before leaving the office for the day.
   - Keep an accurate inventory of supplies; order before the last items are used.
   - Read journals and keep current with new technology.
   - Participate in continuing education activities.
2. Arrive early
   - Review the patient charts for the day; notice any special problems or needs.
   - Be sure that each exam room is well-equipped and ready for patients.
3. Personal assessment
   - Get plenty of rest.
   - Exercise and eat balanced meals.
   - Dress appropriately. Clothing or shoes that are too tight cause stress.

4. Laugh
   - Learn to laugh at life's little problems.
   - Laugh at yourself.
   - Establish an appropriate level of humor with other members of the staff.
5. Music, color, light
   - Soft background music has been proven to soothe and promote relaxation.
   - Use color and light to create a calm atmosphere.
6. Breaks
   - Build morning and afternoon breaks into the schedule, even if only five or ten minutes.
   - Close the office during the lunch hour, and if possible, leave the facility.
7. Work smarter, not harder
   - Employ time management techniques for reducing stress by completing one task before moving on to another.
   - Prioritize tasks; when possible do the most difficult task early in the day.
   - Do not procrastinate.
   - Be motivated.
   - Be a team member as well as working well independently.
   - Plan your work, then work your plan.

Incorporating these suggestions for coping with and relieving stress will help you operate efficiently and effectively in the ambulatory care setting. You may begin to experience what Abraham Maslow termed **self-actualization.** During self-actualization, you develop your full potential and experience fulfillment and job satisfaction. See Table 5-1 for some suggestions for relieving tension and stress during your daily work routine.

WHAT IS BURNOUT?

According to New York psychologist Herbert J. Freudenberger, PhD, who coined the term, burnout is a state of

TABLE 5-1 TECHNIQUES FOR REDUCING STRESS AT WORK

- Stretch or change positions.
- Slowly roll your head from side to side and forward and back.
- Slowly rotate your shoulders forward and backward several times.
- Turn away from the computer or close your eyes for several seconds.
- Walk around and deliver charts or lab specimens, and so on.
- Stand or sit tall and take a few deep breaths.
- Meditate for 30 seconds.
- Know your limits and be aware of your body's needs.

fatigue or frustration brought about by a devotion to a cause, a way of life, or a relationship that failed to produce the expected reward (Gehmeyer, 2000). Burnout exhausts one's physical and mental resources, and leaves one feeling angry, helpless, and trapped. The military term for burnout is "battle fatigue." As a medical assistant you are a member of the health care team that battles disease and the ravages of disease on a daily basis.

Burnout does not occur suddenly as does stress. Rather, burnout is a gradual process that occurs slowly over a period of time. Typical signs and symptoms of burnout include:

- Emotional and physical exhaustion
- Anger
- Self-criticism
- Irritability
- Hair-trigger display of emotions
- Impatience
- Negativism
- A sense of being constantly under attack
- Inability to keep even daily frustrations in perspective

Burnout in the Workplace

Burnout happens to people who previously were enthusiastic and bursting with energy and new ideas when first hired on the job or beginning a new experience. When individuals with a high need to achieve do not reach their goals, they are apt to feel angry and frustrated. Failing to recognize these signs as symptoms of burnout, they may throw themselves even more fully into work-related goals. Unless there is some type of revitalization outside of the workplace, burnout occurs.

Three characteristics associated with burnout in the workplace include:

- Role Conflict: When employees have conflicting responsibilities, they feel pulled in many directions. The perfectionist tries to do everything equally well without setting priorities. Fatigue and exhaustion associated with burnout begin to set in after a period of time.

- Role Ambiguity: The employee does not know what is expected and how to accomplish it because there may not be a role model to follow or ask, or established guidelines to follow.

- Role Overload: If the employee cannot say no and continues to accept more responsibility than they can handle, burnout is sure to set in (Gehmeyer, 2000).

What to Do If You Are Burned Out

When you recognize the signs and symptoms of burnout, it is time to do some self-analysis by asking yourself some hard questions. Recall and analyze when you began feeling so tired and unable to relax and enjoy your work. Have you always been a perfectionist? Have you always had a higher need than most of your peers to do a job well? Are you irritable toward coworkers or patients? At what point did you lose your sense of humor? Do you always see work as a chore? Are you so intensely striving to achieve your goals that if you do not succeed you consider yourself a failure? Are you physically and emotionally exhausted?

The next step is to make some changes.

- Make a list of negative words or phrases that you most often use. Now replace the negatives with more neutral words or phrases.

- Create some job diversity for yourself. Drive to work via a different route; enter the building through a different door; change your work routine slightly; change your start time.

- Become creative. Redecorate your area.

- Establish some long- and short-term realistic goals and write them down.

- Take care of yourself; change your eating habits; exercise more; get more sleep.

- Renew friendships; go to lunch with coworkers; laugh with them.

- Implement time management techniques.

- Delegate responsibility to others who are capable.

Table 5-2 will help you assess your risk for burnout.

Preventing Burnout

The best way to treat burnout on the job is to prevent it. This can be accomplished by leaving work-related issues at the office when leaving for the day. Other things you can do to reduce the risk of burnout include:

- Maintain a positive self-esteem and self-image
- Have regular physical examinations
- Take a vacation
- Give up unrealistic goals and expectations
- Develop interests outside of your profession
- Separate work from the rest of your life
- Develop time management techniques
- Develop clear and complete job descriptions for each position in the office

GOAL SETTING AS A STRESS RELIEVER

Do you direct your life or do you allow others to influence and make decisions for you? **Outer-directed people** let events, other people, or environmental factors dictate their behavior. By contrast, **inner-directed people** decide for themselves what they want to do with their lives. Laurence Peter, author of *The Peter Principle*, stated, "If you don't know where you are going, you will end up somewhere else" (Wilkes & Crosswait, 1991).

Discoveries prove that goal-oriented employees are more effective and assertive than colleagues with no goals or future objectives. Recognizing the value of goal planning, many employers arrange planning sessions and/or

TABLE 5-2 ASSESS YOUR RISK FOR BURNOUT		
This simple test, developed by the Center for Professional Well-Being, can help you determine your predisposition to distress in your life. The more questions with a "yes" response, the greater your risk for burnout.	Yes	No
1. Are you highly achievement-oriented?	☐	☐
2. Do you tend to withdraw from offers of support?	☐	☐
3. Do you have difficulty delegating responsibilities to others, including patients?	☐	☐
4. Do you prefer to work alone?	☐	☐
5. Do you avoid discussing problems with others?	☐	☐
6. Do you externalize blame?	☐	☐
7. Are your work relationships asymmetrical; that is, are you always giving?	☐	☐
8. Is your personal identity bound up with your work role or professional identity?	☐	☐
9. Do you often overload yourself and have a difficult time saying no?	☐	☐
10. Is there a lack of opportunities for positive and timely feedback outside of your professional or work role?	☐	☐
11. Do you abide by the laws "don't talk, don't trust, don't feel?"	☐	☐

Musick, J. L. (1997). *How Close Are You to Burnout?* American Academy of Family Physicians. [On-line]. Available: http://www.aafp.org/fpm/970400fm/lead.html

SPOTLIGHT ON AAMA ESSENTIALS THROUGH CAAHEP

- Planning ahead will help the medical assistant deal with stressful situations encountered daily in the ambulatory care setting.

- Maintaining a positive self-esteem and self-image and being able to separate work from the rest of one's life, will help the medical assistant prevent burnout.

- Setting goals and promoting a sense of pride in one's work are two ways the medical assistant can help reduce the stress on the job and cope better with the daily ups and downs of a busy medical practice.

seminars to encourage goal setting as a practical application for coping with stress and/or burnout and to develop career objectives. If this does not happen in your work environment, seek your own seminars for goal setting. Such an activity not only "centers" you in your current employment but helps you clearly picture your future plans and hopes.

What is a **goal**? The dictionary definition of a goal according to *Merriam-Webster's Collegiate Dictionary* is, "the result or achievement toward which effort is directed." To reach a desired goal, a person must implement planning along with a sincere desire to work hard. Skill in goal setting allows the medical assistant to clarify what must be accomplished and to develop a strategic plan to successfully achieve the goal.

A goal must be specific, challenging, realistic, attainable, and measurable. Specific goals are focused and have very precise boundaries. A goal that is challenging creates enthusiasm and interest in achievement. Realistic goals are practical or beneficial for the present and for future self-actualization. An attainable goal refers to the fact that the goal is possible to fulfill. Measurable goals achieve some form of progress or success. By reflecting on the process, one is encouraged to establish additional goals.

Long-range goals are achievements that may take three to five years to accomplish. Long-range goals give direction and definition to our lives and serve to keep us "on track" so to speak. Much discipline, perseverance, determination, and hard work will be expended in accomplishing long-range goals. Some adjustment and readjust-

ment to your goals may be necessary, however. The rewards of goal achievement include satisfaction, pride, a sense of accomplishment, and a job well done.

Short-range goals take apart long-range goals and reassembles the required activities into smaller, more manageable time segments. The time segments may be daily, weekly, monthly, quarterly, or yearly periods.

As a graduate and new employee, one of your long-range goals might be to become the office manager in the ambulatory care setting in which you are currently employed. You may wish to attain this goal within the next three to five years; by breaking it into three longer range goals and a series of short-range goals, you will be able to measure progress and feel a sense of accomplishment. Examples of long- and short-range goals might include:

Long-range goal 1:

To become proficient in all back-office clinical skills during the first year of employment.

Short-range goals necessary to achieve this:

- Practice accuracy and proficiency when performing tasks and skills.

- Practice efficiency by planning ahead for the equipment and supplies needed for each task performed.

- Evaluate your progress on a regular basis, and identify areas that need improvement.

Long-range goal 2:

To add front-office administrative tasks and skills to your routine during the second year of employment.

Short-range goals necessary to achieve this:

- Practice accuracy and proficiency when performing all front-office tasks and skills.

- Practice efficiency by planning ahead for the equipment and supplies needed for each task performed.

- Evaluate your progress on a regular basis, and identify areas that need improvement.

Long-range goal 3:

To begin to focus on office management during the third year of employment.

Short-range goals necessary to achieve this:

- Develop a procedures manual for all back- and front-office tasks and skills.

- Enroll in office management classes.

- Focus on team-building skills.

By year four, you will be ready to move into the office manager position.

Long-range and short-range goals work together to help make changes in our lives. Goals keep life interesting and give us something for which to strive. We can all reach goals successfully with some planning, hard work, discipline, and dedication.

SUMMARY

Stress is very much a part of the medical profession. Each individual working in a medical career experiences consecutive days of demanding, emotionally and physically draining interactions with patients and staff members. This highly technical and ever-changing career requires its professionals to maintain a high level of skill and training and to be familiar with the newest technology.

Goal setting is one approach to reducing stress and burnout and promoting a sense of pride in the workplace, self-actualization, and possible employment promotion. Both long-range and short-range goal planning work together to help make changes in our lives.

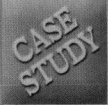

Ellen Armstrong, CMA, is an administrative medical assistant with Doctors Lewis and King. This is her first job. She is just two years out of school, and she is trying to learn everything she can to achieve her long-range goal of becoming office manager at this or some other ambulatory care setting.

Ellen has a great deal in her favor, for she is good with patients, both face-to-face and over the telephone. She is not daunted by the complexity of administrative work her job requires. Ellen knows she has a great deal yet to learn and, although she is a bit intimidated by her, Ellen looks to Marilyn Johnson, CMA, the office manager, for guidance and advice.

CASE STUDY REVIEW

1. How would you advise Ellen to go about achieving her long-term goal of office manager?
2. What are some of the short-term goals Ellen should set? Why are short-term goals important to her success?
3. Besides learning on the job, what else can Ellen do to achieve her goal?

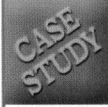

Ellen Armstrong, CMA, has been employed for five years as an administrative medical assistant with Doctors Lewis and King. Ellen is a perfectionist and has pushed herself to achieve many of her short- and long-term goals. The office staff has become aware of the fact that Ellen does not have a sense of humor lately. She seems frustrated and irritable, and is becoming critical of herself and others. Ellen has felt physically and emotionally exhausted, yet she continues to focus on her high standard of job performance; however, work is becoming a chore. At the end of the day if everything has not been completed to her satisfaction, she feels like a failure.

CASE STUDY REVIEW

1. Do you feel Ellen is stressed or experiencing burnout? What do you base your conclusions upon?
2. What might Ellen do to differentiate these two conditions?
3. What changes might Ellen implement to resolve this problem?

REVIEW QUESTIONS

Multiple Choice

1. Which answer is *not* true about stress?
   a. It does not occur suddenly.
   b. It has physical and emotional effects on the body.
   c. It may be positive or negative on its affects on the body.
   d. It is the body's response to change.
2. Hans Selye's GAS theory proposes that adaptation to stress occurs in how many stages?
   a. 2 stages
   b. 3 stages
   c. 4 stages
   d. 5 stages
3. Which is *not* a stage in the General Adaptation Syndrome?
   a. fight-or-flight
   b. exhaustion
   c. burnout
   d. alarm
4. Burnout occurs often if:
   a. a person is aged
   b. the individual works as a health care professional
   c. an individual has certain personality traits
   d. the individual isn't interested in the job
5. Signs and symptoms of burnout include all of the following *except:*
   a. emotional and physical exhaustion
   b. hair-trigger display of emotion
   c. feelings of accomplishment and pride in work
   d. irritability and impatience
6. Working smarter, not harder includes:
   a. taking a sick day now and then, even if you're not sick
   b. prioritizing your tasks and employing time-management techniques
   c. giving as much work to others as possible
   d. making sure others are not taking advantage of you
7. Self-actualization is a term used by:
   a. Laurence Peter
   b. Abraham Maslow
   c. Hans Selye
   d. Harry Levinson
8. Long-range goals are easy to achieve if:
   a. they are not too challenging
   b. they are divided into a series of short-range goals
   c. they don't involve too much hard work
   d. you never change or adjust them

Critical Thinking

1. Discuss a minimum of five methods of dealing positively with stress.
2. Through self-analysis, determine whether you are an outer-directed person or an inner-directed person and what impact this trait may have upon your medical assisting career.
3. List two long-range goals you personally would like to attain within the next five years. Now determine the short-range goals necessary to achieve your long-range goals.
4. Discuss the causes and manifestations of burnout.
5. Discuss the causes of burnout in the workplace and ways in which it may be decreased.

WEB ACTIVITIES

 Search the World Wide Web for additional information on burnout in the workplace. Compile your information into a report for your instructor. Be sure to include a bibliography identifying your web sources.

REFERENCES/BIBLIOGRAPHY

Cooper, J. R. (1993). *The medical reporter: Beware of professional burnout* [On-line]. Available: http://none.coolware.com/health/medical_reporter/burnout.html

drkoop.com. (1998–2000). Wellness: Mental health, stress, ways stress affects individuals. [On-line]. Available: http://www.drkoop.com/wellness/mental_health/stress/page_337_765.asp

Gehmeyr, A. (June 14, 2000). *Burnout* [On-line]. Available: http://155.187.10.12/fun/burnout.html

Gehmeyr, A. (1993). *Prescription for burnout* [On-line]. Available: http://155.187.10.12/fun/burnout.html

Keir, L., Wise, B. A., & Krebs, C. (1998). *Medical assisting: Administrative and clinical competencies* (4th ed.). Albany, NY: Delmar.

Merriam-Webster's collegiate dictionary (10th ed.). (1994). Springfield, MA: Merriam-Webster.

Musick, J. L. (1997). *American Academy of Family Physicians: How close are you to burnout?* [On-line]. Available: http://www.aafp.org/fpm/970400fm/lead.html

Stress management. (2000). [On-line]. Available: http://www.ivf.com/stress.html

Tamparo, C. D., & Lindh, W. Q. (2000). *Therapeutic communications for allied health professions.* Albany, NY: Delmar.

Tecco, A. (1999). *Stress management* [On-line]. Available: http://www.drkoop.com/wellness/prevcenter/stress/stress.asp

Vikesland, G. (1999). *How to prevent burnout and ridding yourself of burnout* [On-line]. Available: http://www.employer-employee.com/Burnout.html

Wilkes, M., & Crosswait, C. B. (1991). *Professional development: The dynamics of success.* San Diego: Harcourt Brace Jovanovich.

THE THERAPEUTIC APPROACH TO THE PATIENT WITH LIFE-THREATENING ILLNESS

KEY TERMS

Acquired Immunodeficiency Syndrome (AIDS)

Culture

Dementia

Durable Power of Attorney for Health Care

Human Immunodeficiency Virus (HIV)

Libido

Living Will

Physician Directive

Psychomotor Retardation

OUTLINE

Life-Threatening Illness
    Cultural Perspective on Life-
    Threatening Illness
**Choices in Life-Threatening
Illness**
**The Range of Psychological
Suffering**

**The Therapeutic Response to the
Patient with AIDS**
**The Challenge for the Medical
Assistant**

OBJECTIVES

The student should strive to meet the following performance objectives and demonstrate an understanding of the facts and principles presented in this chapter through written and oral communication.

1. Define the key terms as presented in the glossary.
2. Describe possible patient perspectives when facing a life-threatening illness.
3. Define "life-threatening" illness.
4. Discuss cultural manifestations of life-threatening illness.
5. Identify the strongest cultural influence in the life of a patient.
6. List at least four choices to be made when facing a life-threatening illness.
7. Briefly describe the use of living wills and physician directives.
8. Discuss the range of psychological suffering that accompanies life-threatening illnesses.
9. Discuss additional concerns/fears when the life-threatening illness is AIDS.
10. Recall a number of challenges faced by the medical assistant when caring for people with life-threatening illnesses.

ROLE DELINEATION COMPONENTS	SCENARIO
GENERAL (TRANSDISCIPLINARY) **Communication Skills** ● **Treat all patients with compassion and empathy** **Legal Concepts** ● **Maintain confidentiality** **Instruction** ● **Instruct individuals according to their needs** ● **Teach methods of health promotion and disease prevention** ● **Locate community resources and disseminate information**	You have seen the medical reports and have agonized with your physician who must tell Suzanne Markis when she comes in today that she has inoperable pancreatic cancer. When she arrives, you treat her as you normally would, making certain she suspects nothing from you. When she emerges from the physician's room, you make certain to meet her, take her arm, and ask if you can call someone for her. You do not present her with a bill or make another appointment at this time. You recognize that anything you say will probably not be remembered, so you focus entirely upon this patient and her immediate needs. In a day or two, as instructed by your physician employer, you will make a phone call to set an appointment for Suzanne and any family members she might want present to visit with your physician so any questions might be answered for them.

INTRODUCTION

Everything learned in Chapter 4 regarding therapeutic communications is heightened and considered more difficult when the patient has a life-threatening illness. If you were told today that your life would probably be shortened because of a serious illness, your perspective would change completely. What was important yesterday may mean little or nothing now. Something that meant nothing to you yesterday suddenly takes on great importance to you now. It is essential for the medical assistant to remember this difference in perspective and what is likely to be important to patients with a life-threatening illness.

It also must be remembered that no two individuals respond to a life-threatening illness in the same way. Some respond with denial and act as if the information had never been shared with them. Others alter their lives radically and drastically change their priorities. Still others quietly continue their lives changing very little outwardly but recognize that their choices may now be limited (Figure 6-1).

LIFE-THREATENING ILLNESS

A life-threatening illness is not easily defined. Some will use the word *terminal*; others refuse to use that word because they believe it removes any hope from the situation. Also, what is life-threatening for one individual may not be for another. For our purposes, life threatening is used to imply a life that in all probability will be shortened because of a serious or debilitating illness or disease. It may be defined as death that is imminent; it may be defined in terms of a serious illness that one will battle for many years but will ultimately shorten his/her life.

Cultural Perspective on Life-Threatening Illness

 Strong cultural manifestations will be seen in the treatment of a life-threatening illness and for anyone facing death. Culture is defined as how we live our lives, how we think, how we speak, and how we behave.

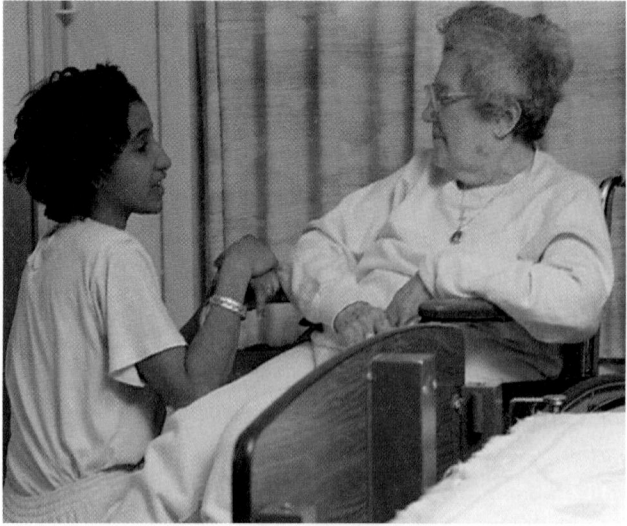

Figure 6-1 Establishing a caring and trusting relationship will help the patient come to terms with a life-threatening illness.

Some cultures prefer that the life-threatening illness not be shared with the patient in the beginning, but with the family who helps to prepare the patient for the inevitable. A few cultures generally do not seek care for an illness until it is quite advanced; this practice can make pain management and treatment more difficult or impossible in some cases. Some cultures surround the person who is ill with great attention, never leaving the person alone. Other cultures view the illness as something that must be removed from the body, perhaps even believing that the individual has been visited upon with this illness due to some past sin or transgression.

In the same manner, pain is viewed. Some cultures believe it is to be endured quietly without complaint; others believe there is to be no pain and family members will go to great lengths to have health care providers relieve the pain. When questioning a patient about the pain level, it must be within a cultural perspective. For example, cultures with an Asian influence are more likely to describe pain in general terms related to the imbalance of the body than in terms of "piercing, intermittent, or throbbing" or on a scale of 1 to 10.

It must also be remembered that the strongest influence in managing any life-threatening illness in the life of the patient is *not* the health care team; it is the family and those closest to the patient. Therefore, great care must be taken to determine and understand the patient's cultural perspective as much as possible, and the patient must be given great respect. Many times the cultural influence may contradict the standard of care preferred by the health care provider. It is better to understand the culture and work within it than to deny it and continually work against the patient's belief system and influence of family.

CHOICES IN LIFE-THREATENING ILLNESS

Many choices are available to a patient with a life-threatening illness, and many decisions are to be made. The urgency of the decisions will depend in part upon possible life expectancy. Sometimes these decisions may seem contrary to recommended medical intervention.

Patients have the right to choose or to refuse treatment in most cases. Some rush into a treatment protocol only to discover later that their choices have brought them pain, disability, and expense far beyond what originally was assumed. While it is the health care professional's goal to heal, if healing is not likely or possible, patients ought not to be "urged" into treatment protocols that are likely to be contrary to their personal wishes for the sake of treatment only.

While health care professionals are less comfortable with death than they are with saving life, there are some issues appropriate to discuss with patients especially when facing life-threatening illness. Those issues include the following:

1. **Living will** or **physician directive** documents may be used in making end-of-life decisions.
2. **Durable power of attorney for health care** allows another to make decisions for the patient when the patient is no longer able to do so.
3. Discussions of pain management and treatment may or may not be a part of a living will document but should be discussed at some point with the patient and/or patient's family.
4. Alternative methods of treatment should be discussed as well as the outcome if no treatment is sought.
5. Finances are to be considered. What will insurance cover (if there is insurance)? Who makes the decisions if managed care is an issue? What family resources can or will be used?
6. Emotional needs of the patient and family members are important. From where does the patient's primary support come? Friends, clergy, other?

It is not the responsibility of the health care professionals treating the individual with life-threatening illness to provide all these services, but a health care professional who raises these issues for patients and families to deal with is more closely in tune with a patient's power in the illness.

While some states were slow to recognize living wills, there is a piece of legislation that is available to all. The federal government passed the

Patient Self-Determination Act in 1991 giving all patients receiving care in institutions receiving payments from medicare and medicaid written information about their right to accept or refuse medical or surgical treatment. The act also requires that patients be given information about their options to create living wills and to appoint someone to act on their behalf in making health care decisions (durable power of attorney for health care). When facing a life-threatening illness, it can be very helpful to have some decisions made about what should be done and who can make decisions if the patient becomes unable to do so.

Any documents of this nature the patient has should be copied in the medical chart that goes with the patient when hospitalized. At any time the patient makes a change in such a document, the old document is to be replaced with the new one.

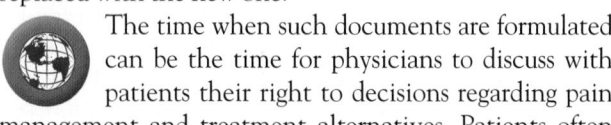 The time when such documents are formulated can be the time for physicians to discuss with patients their right to decisions regarding pain management and treatment alternatives. Patients often fear pain and loss of independence more than anything when facing a life-threatening illness. It is better to have those discussions early in treatment than later when the patient may not be so clear on options. Sometimes treatment alternatives the patient may consider are not within the realm of recognized medical acceptability, but it is better to have that discussion than to ignore the possibility. Remember the earlier statement indicating that the family and friends bring more influence to bear than does the health care professional. If the physician and patient are seen as partners in the patient's care, then the patient may not be so fearful in discussing any nonmedically accepted protocol being considered.

Finances are no one's favorite subjects, especially physicians. However, such a discussion is important. Often patients fear not being able to meet their financial obligations as much as they fear the illness. What methods of payment are there? What does insurance cover? How far will insurance go? What restrictions does any managed care agency hold in a particular illness? Can the medical insurance be cancelled when the patient is no longer able to work or when a life-threatening illness is diagnosed?

Emotional support is vital when dealing with a life-threatening illness. Health care professionals will want to determine where that support comes from for the patient. Should a support group be suggested for the patient and family members? For some patients and families, an individual giving spiritual guidance is seen as a member of the family and a member of the health care team. For others, no spiritual influence is recognized or sought.

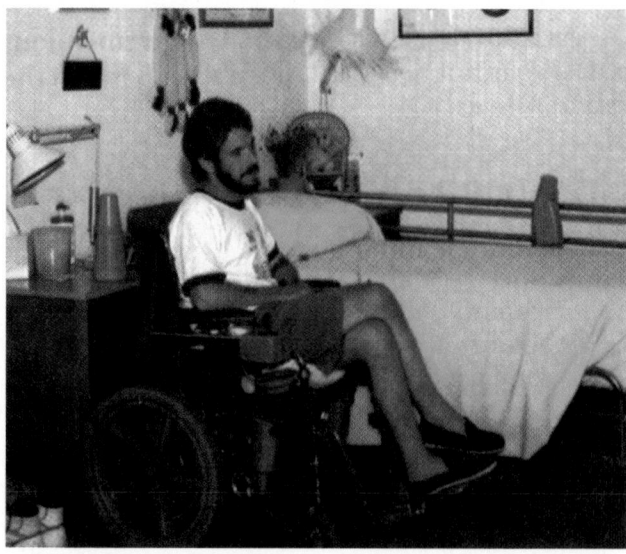

Figure 6-2   Patients living with a serious illness may experience a wide range of emotions.

THE RANGE OF PSYCHOLOGICAL SUFFERING

The range of suffering associated with a life-threatening illness is extensive. Patients feel extreme distress. Anxiety and depression are common. At the time of diagnosis, patients' responses may include denial, numbness, and inability to face the facts. Sadness, hopelessness, helplessness, and withdrawal often are exhibited (Figure 6-2).

The range of psychological suffering leads to physical symptoms, such as tension, tachycardia, agitation, insomnia, anorexia, and panic attacks. The physician may be so intent on treating the physical ramifications of the illness that the psychological suffering is mostly ignored.

THE THERAPEUTIC RESPONSE TO THE PATIENT WITH AIDS

It is not the intention of this chapter to specifically identify the many life-threatening illnesses and their particular needs. However, a few comments about patients testing positive for **human immunodeficiency virus (HIV)** and suffering from **aquired immunodeficiency syndrome (AIDS)** are important.

The discovery of infection with HIV is extremely stressful and is typically accompanied by the fear of developing AIDS. Patients are often preoccupied with illness and the fear of getting other life-threatening diseases. Patients are angry at the disease, at the discrimination that often accompanies it, at the prospect of a lonely, painful death, at the lack of effective treatment, at medical staff, and at themselves.

In many cases, guilt develops about past behavior and lifestyles, or about the possibility of having transmitted the disease to others. When the disease has been contracted through contaminated blood or blood products or by individuals who felt they were protected or safe from the disease, the anger may turn to rage.

Some patients contemplate suicide. Because social and physical assistance are needed, a strong network of friends and family is particularly important. In the case of homosexuals and those addicted to intravenous drugs, however, there are a large number who are estranged from their family's support system. People with AIDS may feel added strain if this is the first knowledge their families have of any high-risk behaviors associated with the transmission of the disease.

Patients with AIDS are apt to suffer central nervous system involvement. Forgetfulness and poor concentration may be followed by **psychomotor retardation** (the slowing of physical and mental responses), decreased alertness, apathy, withdrawal, diminished interest in

> For example, at Inner City Health Care, Dr. Ray Reynolds is known for his compassion and great warmth toward people. On difficult days at the center, this attitude holds him in good stead. Sometimes, he tends to take on the more challenging cases: patients with life-threatening diseases, often young people with AIDS who should be in the prime of their lives.
>
> Clinical medical assistant Wanda Slawson always tries to learn from Dr. Reynolds' example. While she is quieter and not as outgoing as Dr. Reynolds, Wanda always tries to be both courteous and comforting to patients, especially those who are anxious. She makes it a point always to help patients discover a new way to cope with debilitating diseases.

work, and loss of **libido** (sexual drive). Some patients later experience confusion, progressive impairment, and profound **dementia** (progressive impairment of intellectual function).

THE CHALLENGE FOR THE MEDICAL ASSISTANT

As a medical assistant, you face the challenge of caring for people with a life-threatening illness; you must comfort those who face great suffering and death. You will become a source of information for patients and their support members. You must be particularly sensitive and respectful toward individuals who may be viewed as social pariahs. You will have to examine your own beliefs, lifestyle, and biases. You must be comfortable treating all patients, no matter what the illness is or how it was contracted.

As well as assisting your physician or employer in providing the best possible medical care, many nonmedical forms of assistance may be required by patients suffering from a life-threatening illness. You may need to make referrals to community-based agencies or service groups. Health departments, social workers, trained hospice volunteers, and AIDS volunteers may also be helpful to you, your patients, and their families.

The best therapeutic response to the patient with a life-threatening illness will build upon the person's own coping abilities, capitalize on strengths, maintain hope, and show continued human care and concern. Patients may want up-to-date information on their disease, its causes, modes of transmission, treatments available, and sources of care and social support. Be prepared to recommend support groups where patients can discuss their feelings and express their concerns. Treat patients with concern and compassion and assure them everything will be done to provide continuity of care and relief from distress. Patients may be encouraged to call upon clergy for spiritual support.

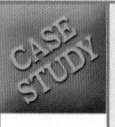

CASE STUDY 6-1

The extended family of Wong Lee is concerned about his illness and his care. Chronic obstructive pulmonary disease (COPD) has ravaged his body. He is on oxygen all the time now. He wants to remain at home to die; his family wants that, too. Yet you are uncertain of how much information to give to members of this expanded family when they call. You wish to protect Mr. Lee's confidentiality.

CASE STUDY REVIEW

1. Are the questions the extended family members raise intended to harm or help Mr. Lee?

2. Is there a durable power of attorney for health care in place?

3. What, if any, of this concern is related to the culture?

4. What can you and your physician-employer suggest to be of help to everyone involved?

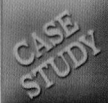

CASE STUDY

6-2

Inner City Health Care, a multi-doctor urgent care center in a large city, has a large roster of patients, some of whom have AIDS. While clinical medical assistant Bruce Goldman tries not to be, sometimes he is wary of patients who he thinks might be homosexual. When patient Bill Swartz was seen for a change in a mole on his calf, Bruce did his best to interact in a professional manner even though he suspected Bill was homosexual. After this patient exchange, medical assistant Bruce Goldman decided it was time to deal with his prejudices against homosexuals and his fear of AIDS and all AIDS patients.

CASE STUDY REVIEW

1. While medical assistant Bruce Goldman may not admit it, he is threatened by AIDS. What should he know about AIDS transmission that may reduce his fears?

2. In the future, Bruce would like to be more open and supportive when he is dealing with an AIDS patient. What are some of the things he can do to help patients?

3. What are some things Bruce can do to reduce wariness regarding patients he feels might be homosexuals?

SUMMARY

Medical assistants must be aware that when caring for people with a life-threatening illness, having even the slightest fear of death can undermine the ability to respond professionally, with empathy and support. If you feel yourself losing the ability to be helpful, it is time to briefly step aside. This does not mean withdrawal from your position or refusal to care for your patients. It means that you do whatever is necessary so that your perspective is not lost. It may mean taking a day off from work to "fill up your soul" and to give your psyche a rest. If the ambulatory care setting has an abundance of patients with life-threatening illnesses, it may require that you spend some time in a support group of your own so that you are better able to cope. Never be afraid to feel sad or weep with your patients. It is better to sense their pain and, at times, feel the pain with them, than it is to be so clinically objective you miss their true needs.

REVIEW QUESTIONS

Multiple Choice

1. When a practice treats patients with AIDS, it is important for medical assistants to:
   a. warn other patients about the dangers of transmission
   b. segregate AIDS patient reception areas from other patient areas
   c. be supportive and free of prejudice
   d. deny any information to patients regarding the seriousness of the illness

2. The Patient Self-Determination Act:
   a. allows a patient to have a choice of physicians
   b. ensures a patient's right to accept or refuse treatment
   c. gives patients the right to formulate advance directives

   d. all of the above
   e. only b and c

3. The strongest influence in a patient with a life-threatening illness is:
   a. the physician
   b. the hospital
   c. the family
   d. the patient

4. Life-threatening illness is defined as:
   a. a life shortened due to serious illness or disease
   b. death that is imminent
   c. serious illness to battle for many years but may shorten life
   d. all of the above

5. Culture may be defined as:
   a. how we live our lives
   b. how we think

c. how we speak and behave

d. all of the above

6. Therapeutic communication with a patient with a life-threatening illness:

a. is no different than communicating with any patient

b. is heightened and considered more difficult

c. is left to nonmedical support staff

d. comes naturally and requires no special skill

7. Cultural influence may in part determine:

a. when/how to involve family members

b. whether spiritual support is sought

c. how the illness and pain associated with it is managed

d. all of the above

8. Durable power of attorney for health care:

a. enables someone other than the patient to make only health care decisions

b. enables someone other than the patient to make any decisions for the patient

c. makes certain that patients' financial responsibilities are met

d. makes certain a patient's wishes are followed

e. only a and d

9. Additional problems people with AIDS may encounter are:

a. loss of family and friends for support

b. being treated as social pariahs in some settings

c. that living wills are not recognized

d. only a and b

10. Effective pain management may depend upon:

a. patient's needs

b. family wishes

c. cultural systems

d. all of the above

e. only a and c

Critical Thinking

1. Research other sections in this text that discuss end-of-life legal documents. Describe additional information you find.

2. Discuss with a friend what cultural influences might affect each of you if you were facing a life-threatening illness. What choices would each of you make?

3. In a paragraph seen only by yourself, describe your greatest fears in caring for patients with AIDS.

4. List common psychological reactions people might have from learning they have a life-threatening illness.

5. Research other sections in this text that discuss AIDS. What additional information do you find beneficial?

6. What steps would you personally take to make certain you do not burn out from caring for persons with a life-threatening illness?

7. List the advantages/disadvantages of the physician directives available.

8. Discuss with a nurse or a nursing student in your school how health care professionals deal with the psychological suffering in persons with a life-threatening illness.

9. Discuss with a classmate your concerns in dealing with patients with a life-threatening illness. Would you choose to work where you seldom lost a patient to a life-threatening illness? If so, what are the reasons?

10. Research the agencies available in your community that can provide support for people and family members facing life-threatening illness.

REFERENCES/BIBLIOGRAPHY

Lewis, M., & Tamparo, C. (1998). *Medical law, ethics, and bioethics for ambulatory care*. Philadelphia: F. A. Davis Company.

Purnell, L., & Paulanka, B. (1998). *Transcultural health care: A culturally competent approach*. Philadelphia: F. A. Davis Company.

Tamparo, C., & Lindh, W. (2000). *Therapeutic communications for health professionals*. Albany, NY: Delmar.

3

RESPONSIBLE MEDICAL PRACTICE

7

LEGAL CONSIDERATIONS

KEY TERMS

Agent
Civil Law
Criminal Law
Defendant
Doctrine
Durable Power of Attorney
Emancipated Minor
Expert Witness
Expressed Contract
Implied Consent
Implied Contract
Incompetence
Informed Consent
Libel
Litigation
Malpractice
Mandate
Minor
Negligence
Noncompliant
Plaintiff
Risk Management
Slander
Statute
Subpoena
Tort

OUTLINE

Civil and Criminal Law
Medical Practice Acts and the
   Medical Assistant's Role
   Patient Rights
The Physician, the Medical
   Assistant, and the Law
Contracts
   Termination of Contracts
Standard of Care and the 4 Ds of
   Negligence
Torts
   Battery
   Defamation of Character
   Invasion of Privacy

Medical Records
   Informed Consent
   Implied Consent
   Consent and Legal Incompetence
   Subpoenas
   Confidentiality
   Statute of Limitations
Public Duties
   Drug Screening
   AIDS
   Abuse
Good Samaritan Law
Physician's Directives
Americans with Disabilities Act
   (ADA)

OBJECTIVES

*The student should strive to meet the following performance objectives and demonstrate
an understanding of the facts and principles presented in this chapter through written and
oral communication.*

1. Define the key terms as presented in the glossary.

2. Compare/contrast civil and criminal law.

3. Define the medical assistant's role in legal issues.

4. Describe the use of contracts in the ambulatory care setting.

5. Discuss the standard of care for health care professionals.

6. Explain the 4 Ds of negligence.

7. Define and give examples of torts.

8. Explain the necessity of informed consent.

9. Describe how to handle subpoenas.

10. Recall the special consideration for patients related to the issues of confidentiality, the statute of limitations, public duties, and AIDS.   *(continues)*

11. Describe procedures to follow in documenting and reporting abuse.
12. Discuss Good Samaritan Laws, physician's directives, and the Americans with Disabilities Act.

ROLE DELINEATION COMPONENTS

GENERAL (TRANSDISCIPLINARY)

Legal Concepts

- **Prepare and maintain medical records**
- **Document accurately**
- **Use appropriate guidelines when releasing information**
- **Follow employer's established policies dealing with the health care contract**
- **Follow federal, state and local legal guidelines**
- **Maintain awareness of federal and state health care legislation and regulations**
- **Comply with risk management and safety procedures**

SCENARIO

At the ambulatory care center of Doctors Lewis and King, a two-doctor family physician office, Dr. Lewis and Dr. King are especially careful about establishing stringent risk management procedures to protect patients from harm and the practice from potential liability.

Dr. King has worked with office manager Marilyn Johnson, CMA, to assemble a policy and procedures manual outlining everything from how telephone calls are answered to how patient medical records are documented and stored. Marilyn, in turn, seeks the input of the other administrative and clinical medical assistants as she frequently updates the manual. To ensure that they are providing the best care for patients while protecting themselves, four times a year the entire staff meets to review office policies, changing them as necessary or incorporating new procedures to meet new situations or legal mandates.

INTRODUCTION

The law as it relates to health care has grown increasingly complex in the past decade. The agendas of federal and state governments include an investigation of quality health care, a desire to control health care costs (while hoping to assure equitable access to health care), and an interest in protecting the patient. A full discussion of health law requires several volumes; therefore, only the laws designated to protect the patient will be identified in this chapter, and emphasis will be placed on the ambulatory care setting.

Being aware of the law and its implications and establishing sound practices and procedures will both safeguard patient rights and protect the health care professional.

CIVIL AND CRIMINAL LAW

The most frequent law exercised in the ambulatory care setting is civil law, or law as it is related to individuals. Restitution awarded when a civil wrong is committed is usually monetary in nature. Criminal law addresses wrongs committed against the welfare and safety of society as a whole; punishment is usually imprisonment or a fine.

If a charge is brought against a physician as the defendant in a civil case, the goal is to reimburse the plaintiff, the person bringing charges (usually a patient), with a monetary amount for suffering, pain, and any loss of wages. For example, a physician who has caused harm to a patient in the course of treatment may be sued in a civil case by the patient for the recovery of time lost from work as well as the pain and suffering that was the result of treatment.

In a criminal case, charges are brought against the defendant by the state with the intent of preventing any further harm to society. For example, a physician practicing medicine without a proper license may be subject to disciplinary action from a professional association and criminal action by the courts.

MEDICAL PRACTICE ACTS AND THE MEDICAL ASSISTANT'S ROLE

Each state has medical practice acts that regulate the practice of medicine with the intent of protecting its citizens from harm. These statutes, or laws, govern licensure, standards of care, professional liability and negligence, confidentiality, and torts. Some states also regulate personnel who may be employed in the ambulatory care setting. For example, some states require that medical assistants be licensed or certified to be able to perform any invasive procedures. Other states require additional training in radiology for the medical assistant to be able to take X rays. Further, some states are so strict in their regulations that medical assistants perform mostly clerical functions. Certainly, medical assistants desiring to utilize their skills must be aware of state regulations and always perform only within the scope of those regulations.

Patient Rights

The Patient's Bill of Rights was developed by the American Hospital Association in 1973 and revised in 1992 to establish more effective patient care and greater satisfaction for patient, physician, and hospital (Figure 7-1). While this Bill of Rights was written with the hospital patient in mind, patients in ambulatory care settings should be accorded the same rights. Although no list of rights can guarantee the kind of treatment patients have a right to expect, medical assistants should make every effort to conduct activities with the concern of the patient in mind.

THE PHYSICIAN, THE MEDICAL ASSISTANT, AND THE LAW

There are a number of ways in which the law governs physicians and their employees. Some of these issues are particularly pertinent to the ambulatory care setting and the medical assistants who work in these health care environments.

CONTRACTS

A contract is a binding agreement between two or more persons. A physician has a legal obligation, or duty, to care for a patient under the principles of contract law. The agreement must be between competent persons to do or not to do something lawful in exchange for a payment.

A contract exists when the patient arrives for treatment and the physician accepts the patient by providing treatment. An example of a valid contract occurs when a patient calls the office or clinic to make an appointment for an annual physical examination. Assuming both physician and patient are competent and that the physician performs the lawful act of the physical examination and the patient pays a fee, all aspects of the contract exist.

There are two types of contracts, expressed and implied. An expressed contract can be written or verbal and will specifically describe what each party in the contract will do. A written contract requires that all necessary aspects of the agreement be in writing. An implied contract is indicated by actions rather than by words. The majority of physician-patient contracts are implied contracts. It is not required that the contract be written to be enforceable as long as all points of the contract exist. An implied contract can exist either by the circumstances of the situation or by the law. When a patient complains of a sore throat and the physician does a throat culture to diagnose and treat the ailment, an implied contract exists by the circumstances. An implied contract by law exists when a patient goes into anaphylactic shock and the physician administers epinephrine to counteract shock symptoms. The law says that the physician did what the patient would have requested had there been an expressed contract.

For a contract to be valid and binding, the parties who enter into it must be competent; therefore, the mentally incompetent, the legally insane, persons under heavy drug or alcohol influences, infants, and some minors cannot enter into a binding contract.

A PATIENT'S BILL OF RIGHTS

First adopted by the American Hospital Association in 1973.

This revision approved by the AHA Board of Trustees on October 21, 1992.

1. The patient has the right to considerate and respectful care.

2. The patient has the right to and is encouraged to obtain from physicians and other direct caregivers relevant, current, and understandable information concerning diagnosis, treatment, and prognosis.

   Except in emergencies when the patient lacks decision-making capacity and the need for treatment is urgent, the patient is entitled to the opportunity to discuss and request information related to the specific procedures and/or treatments, the risks involved, the possible length of recuperation, and the medically reasonable alternatives and their accompanying risks and benefits.

   Patients have the right to know the identity of physicians, nurses, and others involved in their care, as well as when those involved are students, residents, or other trainees. The patient also has the right to know the immediate and long-term financial implications of treatment choices, insofar as they are known.

3. The patient has the right to make decisions about the plan of care prior to and during the course of treatment and to refuse a recommended treatment or plan of care to the extent permitted by law and hospital policy and to be informed of the medical consequences of this action. In case of such refusal, the patient is entitled to other appropriate care and services that the hospital provides or transfer to another hospital. The hospital should notify patients of any policy that might affect patient choice within the institution.

4. The patient has the right to have an advance directive (such as a living will, health care proxy, or durable power of attorney for health care) concerning treatment or designating a surrogate decision maker with the expectation that the hospital will honor the intent of that directive to the extent permitted by law and hospital policy.

   Health care institutions must advise patients of their rights under state law and hospital policy to make informed medical choices, ask if the patient has an advance directive, and include that information in patient records. The patient has the right to timely information about hospital policy that may limit its ability to implement fully a legally valid advance directive.

5. The patient has the right to every consideration of privacy. Case discussion, consultation, examination, and treatment should be conducted so as to protect each patient's privacy.

6. The patient has the right to expect that all communications and records pertaining to his/her care will be treated as confidential by the hospital, except in cases such as suspected abuse and public health hazards when reporting is permitted or required by law. The patient has the right to expect that the hospital will emphasize the confidentiality of this information when it releases it to any other parties entitled to review information in these records.

7. The patient has the right to review the records pertaining to his/her medical care and to have the information explained or interpreted as necessary, except when restricted by law.

8. The patient has the right to expect that, within its capacity and policies, a hospital will make reasonable response to the request of a patient for appropriate and medically indicated care and services. The hospital must provide evaluation, service, and/or referral as indicated by the urgency of the case. When medically appropriate and legally permissible, or when a patient has so requested, a patient may be transferred to another facility. The institution to which the patient is to be transferred must first have accepted the patient for transfer. The patient must also have the benefit of complete information and explanation concerning the need for, risks, benefits, and alternatives to such a transfer.

9. The patient has the right to ask and be informed of the existence of business relationships among the hospital, educational institutions, other health care providers, or payers that may influence the patient's treatment and care.

10. The patient has the right to consent to or decline to participate in proposed research studies or human experimentation affecting care and treatment or requiring direct patient involvement, and to have those studies fully explained prior to consent. A patient who declines to participate in research or experimentation is entitled to the most effective care that the hospital can otherwise provide.

11. The patient has the right to expect reasonable continuity of care when appropriate and to be informed by physicians and other caregivers of available and realistic patient care options when hospital care is no longer appropriate.

12. The patient has the right to be informed of hospital policies and practices that relate to patient care, treatment, and responsibilities. The patient has the right to be informed of available resources for resolving disputes, grievances, and conflicts, such as ethics committees, patient representatives, or other mechanisms available in the institution. The patient has the right to be informed of the hospital's charges for services and available payment methods.

Figure 7-1   A Patient's Bill of Rights. (Reprinted with permission of the American Hospital Association)

Medical assistants are considered **agents** of the physicians they serve and as such must be cautious that their actions and words may become binding on their physicians. For example, to say that the doctor can cure the patient may cause serious legal problems when in fact a cure may not be possible.

Termination of Contracts

A broken contract or breach of contract occurs when one of the parties does not meet contractual obligations. A physician is legally bound to treat a patient until:

- The patient discharges the physician
- The physician formally withdraws from patient care
- The patient no longer needs treatment and is formally discharged by the physician

Patient Discharges Physician. When the patient discharges the physician, the physician should send a letter to the patient to confirm and document the termination of the contract. The notice should be sent by certified mail with return receipt requested. Keep a copy of the letter in the patient's record (Figure 7-2).

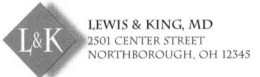

January 6, 20--

CERTIFIED MAIL

Jim Marshal
76 Georgia Avenue
Millerton, TX 43912

Dear Mr. Marshal:

This will confirm our telephone conversation today in which you discharged me as your attending physician in your present illness. In my opinion your condition requires continued medical supervision by a physician. If you have not already done so, I suggest that you employ another physician without delay.

You may be assured that after receiving a written request from you, I will furnish the physician of your choice with information regarding the diagnosis and treatment which you have received from me.

Very truly yours,

Winston Lewis

Winston Lewis, MD
WL:ea

Figure 7-2 Letter confirming physician's discharge by the patient.

Physician Formally Withdraws from the Case. To avoid any charges of abandonment, the physician should formally withdraw from the case as, for example, when the patient becomes **noncompliant** or the physician feels the patient can no longer be served. Again, notice should be sent to the patient by certified mail with return receipt requested and a copy of the notice should be filed in the patient's record (Figures 7-3 and 7-4).

> **Inner City Health Care**
> 222 S. First Avenue
> Carlton, MI 11666
>
> May 9, 20--
>
> CERTIFIED MAIL
>
> Lenny Taylor
> 260 Second Street
> Carlton, MI 11666
>
> Dear Mr. Taylor:
>
> You will recall that we discussed our physician-patient relationship in my office on May 6, 20--.
>
> Your son, George Taylor, and Bruce Goldman, my medical assistant were also present. As you know, the primary difficulty has been your failure to cooperate with the medical plan for your care.
>
> While it is unfortunate that our relationship has reached this stage, I will no longer be able to serve as your physician. I will be available to you on an emergency basis only until June 10, 20--. Meanwhile, you should immediately call or write the Medical Society, 123 Omega Drive, Carlton, MI 11666, Tel. 123-456-7899 and obtain a list of gerontologists. Any delay could jeopardize your health, so please act quickly.
>
> Your physical (and/or mental) problems include: hypertensive heart disease, decreased kidney function, and arteriosclerosis. You could have additional medical problems that may also require professional care. Once you have found a new physician have him or her call my office. I will be happy to discuss your case with the physician assuming your care, and will transfer a written summary of your case to them upon the receipt of a written request from you to do so.
>
> Thank you for your anticipated cooperation and courtesy.
>
> Very truly yours,
>
> *James Whitney*
>
> James Whitney, MD
> JW:kr

Figure 7-3 Letter reiterating "for the record" the physician's decision to withdraw from the case discussed during meeting with patient.

Inner City Health Care
222 S. First Avenue
Carlton, MI 11666

December 5, 20--

CERTIFIED MAIL

Rhoda Au
41 Academy Road
Carlton, MI 11666

Dear Ms. Au:

I find it necessary to inform you that I am withdrawing further professional medical service to you because of your persistent refusal to follow my medical advice and treatment.

Since your condition requires medical attention, I suggest that you place yourself under the care of another physician without delay. If you so desire, I shall be available to attend you for a reasonable time after you have received this letter, but in no event later than January 7, 20--. This should give you sufficient time to select a physician from the many competent practitioners in this area.

You may be assured that, upon receiving your written request, I will make available to the physician of your choice your case history and information regarding the diagnosis and treatment which you have received from me.

Very truly yours,

Mark Woo

Mark Woo, MD
MW:kr

Figure 7-4   Letter notifying patient of physician's withdrawal as attending physician.

The Patient No Longer Needs Treatment.
Unless a formal discharge or withdrawal has occurred, a physician is obligated to care for a patient until the patient's condition no longer requires treatment.

STANDARD OF CARE AND THE 4 DS OF NEGLIGENCE

Physicians, medical assistants, and all health care providers have the responsibility and duty to perform within their scope of training and to always do what any reasonable and prudent health care professional in the same specialty or general field of practice would do. That is what is expected of every physician when a contact is made by a patient. Failure to do what any reasonable and prudent health care professional

would do in the same set of circumstances can be seen as a breach of the standard of care.

Negligence is defined as the failure to exercise the standard of care that a reasonable person would exercise in similar circumstances. Negligence occurs when someone suffers injury because of another's failure to live up to a required duty of care. This is a primary cause of malpractice suits. **Malpractice** is professional negligence. The four elements of negligence, sometimes called the 4 Ds, are:

1. Duty: duty of care
2. Derelict: breach of the duty of care
3. Direct cause: a legally recognizable injury occurs as a result of the breach of duty of care
4. Damage: wrongful activity must have caused the injury or harm that occurred

If an individual has knowledge, skill, or intelligence superior to that of a layperson, that individual's conduct must be consistent with that status. Medical assistants are held to a high standard of care by virtue of their skills, knowledge, and intelligence. As professionals, medical assistants are required to have a standard minimum level of special knowledge and ability. This is what is known as duty of care.

Physicians and members of their staff may be called to testify in court to the standard of care. In such a case, they are usually considered **expert witnesses**. An expert witness is one who has knowledge and experience enough in a field to be able to testify to what is the reasonable and expected standard of care. Expert witnesses are expected to tell what they know to be fact and are best counseled to use lay terms rather than complicated medical language. The goal is for jurors and judges to understand the nature of any medical information shared. Visual aids, charts, and computer simulations are often used to illustrate or clarify testimony given by expert witnesses.

TORTS

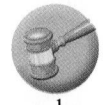 A **tort** is a wrongful act that results in injury to one person by another. Medical assistants may commit a tort that may result in **litigation**. If it can be proven that the injury resulted from the medical assistant (or other health care professional) not meeting the standard of care governing their respective professions, then litigation is a possibility. If, however, the medical assistant (or other health care professional) commits a wrongful act but the patient suffers no injury or harm, then no tort exists. If, for example, the medical assistant changes a wound dressing, breaks sterile technique, and the patient suffers a severely infected wound, the medical assistant has committed a tort and can be held liable, and legal action can be taken. On the other hand, if the med-

ical assistant changes a wound dressing, breaks sterile technique, and the patient's wound does not become infected, no harm has been suffered, and a tort does not exist. If a medical assistant fails to report to the physician a negative result on a blood test that causes the physician to fail to make an early diagnosis of a disease, the assistant's omission of an act has caused a breach in the standard of care.

There are two major classifications of torts, intentional and negligent. Intentional torts are deliberate acts of violation of another's rights. Negligent torts are not deliberate and are the result of omission and commission of an act. Malpractice is the unintentional tort of professional negligence; that is, a professional either failed to act in a reasonable and prudent manner and caused harm to the patient or did what a reasonable and prudent person would not have done and caused harm to a patient.

There are two Latin terms that can be used to describe aspects of negligence. These are known as **doctrines.** *Res ipsa loquitur,* or "the thing speaks for itself," is the term used in cases that involve situations such as a nick made in the bladder when the surgeon is performing a hysterectomy. The negligence is obvious. The other doctrine, *respondeat superior,* "let the master answer," expresses that physicians are responsible for their employees' actions. If a medical assistant violates the standard of care, therein lies the basis for a suit of medical malpractice. For example, the medical assistant used the incorrect solution to clean the patient's wound and the patient sustained injuries to the wound. The physician-employer can be sued under the doctrine of *respondeat superior* because the physician-employer is responsible for the acts of employees committed in the scope of their employment. The medical assistant also can be sued because individuals are responsible for their own actions.

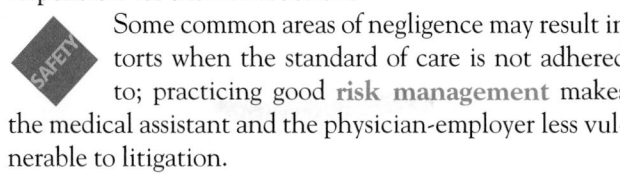 Some common areas of negligence may result in torts when the standard of care is not adhered to; practicing good **risk management** makes the medical assistant and the physician-employer less vulnerable to litigation.

- Protect patients from falling from an examination table, wheelchair, or stretcher.
- Check for faulty electrocautery. Have repair done by qualified technicians.
- Check patient identification by correctly identifying patient before performing a procedure or administering a medication.
- Never leave a patient unattended. If you must leave, pass the responsibility for the patient's care on to another individual.
- Be particularly watchful with patients who have special needs such as the elderly, pediatric patients, and those with physical and emotional disabilities.

- Properly label and identify all specimens. Handle specimens properly.
- Make certain the patient has signed a consent for surgery and other care.
- Follow all policies and procedures established by your employer.
- Do not misrepresent your qualifications.
- Document fully only facts and do not alter medical records.
- Admit any error that may have occurred.

Some specific examples of common torts that can occur in the office or clinic are battery, defamation of character, and invasion of privacy.

Battery

The basis of the tort of battery is unprivileged touching of one person by another. A patient must consent to being touched. When a procedure is to be performed on a patient, the patient must give consent in full knowledge of all the facts. It does not matter whether the procedure that constitutes the battery improves the patient's health. Patients have the right to withdraw consent at any time.

One example of battery is when a medical assistant insists on giving the patient an injection the physician ordered for the patient even though the patient refuses the injection. Another example can be seen when a physician performs additional surgery beyond the original procedure (the surgeon performed a hysterectomy for which consent was given, but is liable for battery for removing an abdominal nevus from the patient's abdomen without consent). It does not matter that the physician does not charge for the additional procedure. It also does not matter if the patient would have given consent if asked in advance.

Defamation of Character

The tort of defamation of character consists of injury to another person's reputation, name, or character through spoken or written words for which damages can be recovered. Two kinds of defamation are **libel** and **slander**. Libel is false and malicious writing about another such as in published materials, pictures, and media. An example can be seen when the medical assistant writes in the patient's record, "Mr. O'Keefe's wife appears to be the cause of his ulcer." A copy of Mr. O'Keefe's records were later sent to a new physician who reviewed the record and saw the remarks quoted by the medical assistant.

Slander is false and malicious spoken words. Slander can be seen in the following comment directed by a patient toward the physician, "Dr. Woo is incompetent. He should have his license revoked." The statement is overheard by the office receptionist and other patients waiting in the reception area.

In order for a tort of defamation of character (either libel or slander) to exist, a third party must see or hear the words and understand their meaning.

Invasion of Privacy

Invasion of privacy is another kind of tort. It includes unauthorized publicity of patient information, medical records being released without the patient's knowledge and permission, and patients receiving unwanted publicity and exposure to public view. For example, if a minor unmarried girl has been examined for possible pregnancy, and the medical assistant telephones the laboratory report to the girl's home and inadvertently gives the results to someone other than the patient, her privacy has been invaded. A second situation exists when persons other than those providing care and performing examinations and procedures (essential or nonessential personnel) are allowed to be present without the patient's consent. Yet another example of the patient's right to privacy being violated is when the patient is asked to walk from the examination room across the hall to a treatment room while wearing only a patient gown in full view of other patients and personnel.

Medical assistants and other health care professionals should:

- Close a door, pull a curtain, or provide a screen when looking at, handling, or examining the patient's body
- Expose only body parts necessary for treatment (drape the patient's body, exposing only that part which is being treated)
- Discuss patients with no one except those individuals involved in the patient's care and then discuss only those aspects that relate to the needs of the patient for care

It is not an invasion of privacy to disclose information required by a court order (**subpoena**) or by statute to protect the public health and welfare, as in the reporting of violent crime.

MEDICAL RECORDS

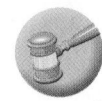

A major responsibility of the physician and the medical assistant is to maintain an accurate and up-to-date record of the patient's care. Whatever style of record is used, the credibility of the medical record will be a key factor in any litigation.

All matters related to a patient's care must be charted, and these charts must be an accurate reflection of actual care rendered and charges made. An act not recorded is generally considered an act not done. Charts that are incomplete or illegible are not easily defensible. Necessary corrections should be made by drawing one line through the error and placing the correction above it with the person's initials and date. All entries should be properly signed and dated, also. Consistency in the medical records becomes a powerful defense for the physician.

Informed Consent

Documentation of **informed consent** becomes an important part of the medical records. Every patient has a right to know and understand any procedure to be performed. The patient is to be told in language easily understood:

1. The nature of any procedure and how it is to be performed
2. Any possible risks involved as well as expected outcomes of the procedure
3. Any other methods of treatment and those risks
4. Risks if no treatment is given

It is the responsibility of the health care provider to make certain the patient understands. If an interpreter is necessary, the physician must procure one.

Often, consent forms will be signed if there is to be a surgical or invasive procedure performed (Figure 7-5). The medical assistant may be asked to witness the patient's

---

CONSENT FOR TREATMENT

Date _____ Time _____

    I authorize the performance of the following procedure(s) _____ on _____ (name of patient) _____ to be performed by _____ (name of physician) _____, MD.

    The following have been explained to _____ by Dr. _____ (name physician) _____.

    Nature of the procedure _____ (describe procedure)
_____.

    For the purpose of _____
_____.

    The possible alternative methods of treatment are
_____.

    The possible consequences of the procedure are
_____.

    The risks involve the possibility of _____
_____.

    The possible complications of this procedure are
_____.

    I have been advised of the serious nature of this procedure and have been further advised that if I desire a more detailed explanation of any of the foregoing or further information about the possible risks or complications, it will be given to me.

    I do not request a more detailed listing and explanation of the above information.

               Signed _____
                                (Patient / Parent / Guardian)

Witnessed by: _____

Figure 7-5   Model formal consent for treatment form.

signature and may be expected to follow through on any of the physician's instructions or explanations but is not expected to explain the procedure to the patient. The signed consent form is kept in the medical chart and a copy is also given to the patient.

Implied Consent

Two circumstances related to consent are worth mentioning at this point. Implied consent occurs when there is a life-threatening emergency or the patient is unconscious or unable to respond. The physician, by law, is allowed to give treatment without a signed consent. Implied consent

occurs in more subtle ways, also. The patient who rolls up a shirt sleeve for the medical assistant to take a blood pressure reading is implying consent to the procedure by the action taken.

Consent and Legal Incompetence

Consent for treatment is not valid if the patient is legally incompetent to give consent. Legal **incompetence** means that a patient is found by a court to be insane, inadequate, or to not be an adult. In such instances, consent must be obtained from a parent, a legal guardian, or the court on behalf of the patient. Consent for treatment may be given only by the natural parent or legal guardian as determined by the court for a **minor** child, typically defined as one under eighteen years of age or the age of majority. An **emancipated minor** is one considered by the courts to be an adult. Emancipated minors may be defined as persons living on their own, who are self-supporting, who may be married, or who are in the military. They can legally give consent for treatment.

    Consent problems may arise when providing care to minors. Consent for medical care such as treatment of sexually transmitted diseases, pregnancy, alcohol or drug abuse, abortion, or birth control pose special problems. Some states allow minors to give their consent in these special situations.

    Questions of ability to give consent related to minors and emancipated minors often must be determined on a case-by-case basis because state statutes vary. Placing a telephone call to the state attorney general's office can help clarify issues, questions, and concerns that involve consent and treatment of minors.

Subpoenas

The medical records may be subpoenaed and/or the physician and health care provider (*subpoena duces tecum*) may be subpoenaed to testify in court. The subpoena is a court order naming a specific date, time, and reason to appear. The staff in the ambulatory care setting usually will have ample time to make certain the record is current and complete prior to its inclusion in court. Out of courtesy, the physician will notify patients whose records have been subpoenaed. If, for any reason, the patient does not want the record released, the physician must call for legal advice on how to respond to the subpoena.

    Certain records, because of their sensitive nature, may require more than a subpoena to be released. These include records related to sexually transmitted diseases, including AIDS and HIV testing, mental health records, substance abuse records, and sexual assault records. For the courts to have access to these records, a court order is required in some states.

Confidentiality

The care taken with subpoenas and court orders for certain information is to assure patients of confidentiality. The information in the medical record, including the information a patient shared with the physician and medical assistant, is private.

No patient information can be given to another (another physician, patient's attorney, insurance company, federal or state agency) without the expressed written consent of the patient. Care must be exercised at all times to ensure that the patient's right to confidentiality is not breached. For example, information given to unauthorized personnel associated with the physician's or clinic's practice in regard to the patient's condition or financial status regarding payment of bills violates the patient's right to confidentiality. Likewise, when discussing issues over the telephone that can be overheard—such as the patient's account being turned over to a collection agency—the patient's right to confidentiality has been violated.

There are certain disclosures of information about a patient's conditions and suspected illnesses that are required by law. Legally required disclosures are necessary when the public needs to know certain information for its safety and welfare. The disclosures supersede the patient's right to privacy and confidentiality. See "Public Duties" in this chapter.

Statute of Limitations

No discussion of medical records is complete without a brief statement regarding the statute of limitations which will, in part, determine how long medical records are kept. Generally speaking, all records should be retained until after the statute has run, usually three to six years. Statutes of limitations most commonly begin at the time a negligent act was committed, when the act was discovered, or when the care of the patient and the patient-physician relationship ended. It is easy to understand why many physicians choose to keep their records indefinitely.

State and federal statutes set maximum time periods during which certain actions can be brought or rights enforced; there is a time limit for individuals to initiate legal action. The statute of limitations varies from one jurisdiction to another and a lawsuit may not be brought after the statute of limitations has run. For example, in the Commonwealth of Massachusetts, the statute of limitations for an act of medical malpractice committed on an adult is three years. If harm to a patient resulted from a medical assistant administering the wrong dose of medication to a patient in Massachusetts, a lawsuit must be brought within three years from the time the medication error was made, with the three years commencing at the time the negligent act was committed.

PUBLIC DUTIES

 Physicians have a duty to the public to report diseases and injuries that jeopardize public health and welfare. Transmittable or contagious diseases and injuries resulting from knife or gunshot are examples; these must be reported to the appropriate authorities. This is done without the patient's consent because it is required by law. When reporting, it is important to do so properly and according to the laws of the state in which one is employed. Knowledge of which illnesses, injuries, and conditions to report, to whom to report, and the appropriate forms to submit is essential. Copies of all information must be kept for the office or clinic.

Other generally required reportables include: births, deaths, childhood immunizations, rape, and abuse toward a child, elder, or domestic partner.

Some states have laws specific to the release of information relative to mental or psychological treatment, human immunodeficiency virus testing, acquired immunodeficiency syndrome diagnosis and treatment, sexually transmitted diseases, and chemical substance abuse.

Local or state health departments can provide lists of diseases and injuries to report and will also provide the appropriate forms.

Drug Screening

States vary in the laws they have regarding the abuse of alcohol and other drugs. In general, employers are allowed to screen an employee for chemical substances if they believe the employee's work performance is being affected by the abuse.

Great controversy surrounds preemployment and random screening for drugs in the workplace. Some states allow widespread random testing of employees. It is important that the worker's right to privacy not be violated. A tort of defamation of character could be claimed against an employer if the results of the testing become known to others.

Get the patient's written consent when asked to collect a specimen for drug screening. Be certain the laboratory that performs the screening is qualified to perform the test. The possibility of liability is great if the ambulatory care setting does not have specific policies and procedures to employ in regard to specimen collection and testing. It should be carefully documented on the patient's record which medical personnel are responsible for the specimen from the time it was collected until the results are known.

The release of patients' records that pertain to chemical substance abuse is protected by federal laws under the Federal Drug Abuse Prevention, Treatment, and Rehabilitation Act. The law prohibits disclosure of information that identifies the patient as a chemical substance abuser. Also, information about the patient's treatment cannot be divulged without the patient's written consent. The records can, however, be released by order of a subpoena to another health care professional during an emergency situation or if the records are to be used for research and program evaluation.

AIDS

The Americans with Disabilities Act of 1990 (ADA) offers protection to persons with AIDS or diseases associated with AIDS. Controversy surrounds the mandatory testing for human immunodeficiency virus (HIV) in medical assistants and other health care professionals and the release of the results to patients who say they have the right to know the HIV status of their caregivers. Health care professionals insist on their right to privacy.

Patients also insist on their privacy. A written informed consent form specific to HIV testing is signed by the patient prior to testing. Laws regarding HIV and AIDS vary from state to state. The best approach regarding release of information regarding the HIV status of a patient is never to disclose this or any confidential patient information.

Abuse

Child abuse, domestic violence, and elder abuse are becoming more common in our society and as a result, patients suffering such abuse may be seen in the ambulatory care setting. In all cases of abuse, medical records hold valuable information if a court procedure ensues. Careful documentation is critical. State laws are fairly specific in mandates to report child abuse, but laws related to elder abuse and domestic violence are not so detailed. In any case, the rights of the victim must be protected.

Child Abuse. The law mandates, or requires, that physicians and health care professionals, teachers, social workers, and certain others who suspect child abuse report the incident to the proper authorities. Confidentiality in the physician-patient relationship does not exist when parents abuse children. If a person has a reason to suspect abuse and reports the abuse to the police and in the case of child abuse to the child protective agency, this individual is protected against liability as a result of making the report. Failure to report could result in criminal or civil penalties. Usually, the Child Protective Unit of the State Department of Social Services is called in to investigate suspected cases of child abuse. Some injuries that are commonly seen in child abuse are bruises, welts, burns, fractures, and head injuries.

If a suspicion of abuse exists, the physician and health care professional should:

- Treat the child's injuries
- Send the child to the hospital for further treatment when necessary
- Inform parents of the diagnosis and that it will be reported to the police and social services agency
- Notify the child protective agency (keep phone number posted)
- Document all information
- Provide court testimony if requested

Elder Abuse. Elder abuse may consist of neglect, physical abuse, punishment, physical restraint, or abandonment. Examples are seen when elders are overmedicated or undermedicated, physically restrained, intimidated by shouting or profanity, sexually abused, neglected or abandoned, or in any other way have their rights and dignity violated. The person reporting the abuse is generally a health care professional, and the reporting agency is most likely one of a social service or welfare nature.

Domestic Violence. Incidents of spousal abuse have escalated since the 1970s. The battered women's syndrome is recognized as a significant problem. The violence of it is a criminal act and failure to report it may be considered a misdemeanor in some states. Victims of domestic violence should be treated as soon as possible after the assault so as to preserve evidence for legal purposes. Community agencies such as rape hot lines are available and the physician may refer the patient for additional services.

GOOD SAMARITAN LAW

Most states have laws regarding the rendering of first aid by health care professionals at the scene of an accident or sudden injury. Good Samaritan laws, although not always clearly written, encourage physicians and health care professionals to provide medical care within the scope of their training without fear of being sued for negligence. In an emergency situation, medical assistants cannot be held liable should an injury result from some form of first aid rendered or from first aid they omitted to render as long as they acted in a reasonable way within the scope of their knowledge. Medical assistants and other health care professionals with skills in cardiopulmonary resuscitation (CPR) who are present when CPR is needed must perform the procedure on the victim or otherwise could be declared negligent. Emergencies that arise in the ambulatory care setting generally are not covered by Good Samaritan laws.

PHYSICIAN'S DIRECTIVES

Medical assistants in the ambulatory care setting will be asked to attach physicians' directives or living wills to patients' charts (Figure 7-6). These directives are legal documents in which patients indicate their wishes in the case of a life-threatening illness or serious injury. Such documents should always accompany the patients to the hospital for any treatment or care. They may be updated from time to time, and the patient can ask to rescind such a document at any time. Medical assistants must remember that these documents reflect the choices of their patients and are to be respected as such.

Another document often seen in the ambulatory care setting is the durable power of attorney for health care or Designation of Health Care Surrogate (Figure 7-7). These documents allow a patient to name another person who is appointed as the official spokesperson for the patient should the patient be unable to speak for herself. The documents may allow another person to manage finances and personal matters or just to make medical decisions. These documents should be recognized and honored.

Every state has different versions of the Living Will and Designation of Health Care Surrogate forms as well as requirements for filling them out. To assure the correct language is used, these forms should be prepared either by an attorney familiar with your state requirements, or by contacting Partnership for Caring, 1035 30th Street NW, Washington, DC 20007, 800-989-9455.

AMERICANS WITH DISABILITIES ACT (ADA)

The federal government established new laws in 1990 to protect physically challenged persons. Barrier-free accommodations are required in public and commercial facilities. The ADA law applies to businesses with at least fifteen employees, but some states have more stringent laws.

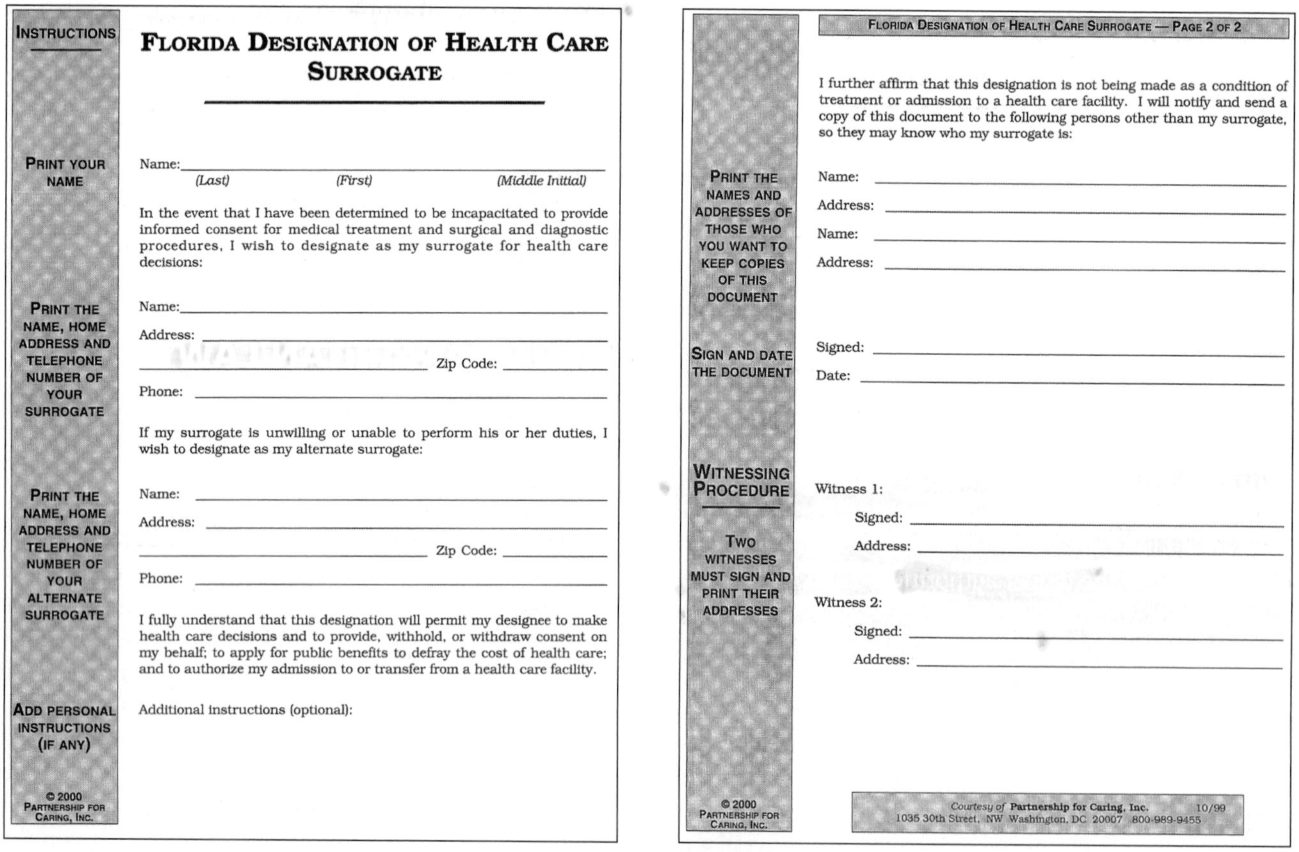

Figure 7-6   Living will declaration. Choice In Dying makes available legally recognized document forms to residents of states that have enacted right-to-die laws. For people in states that have not enacted right-to-die laws, Choice In Dying provides statutory advance directives for each state free of charge, as well as other materials and services relating to end-of-life medical care. (Reprinted by permission of Choice in Dying, 200 Varick Street, New York, NY 10014, 212-366-5540)

INSTRUCTIONS

PRINT THE DATE
PRINT YOUR NAME

PLEASE INITIAL EACH THAT APPLIES

PRINT THE NAME, HOME ADDRESS AND TELEPHONE NUMBER OF YOUR SURROGATE

FLORIDA LIVING WILL

Declaration made this _____ day of _____, _____,
(day)   _(month)_   _(year)_

I, _____, willfully
and voluntarily make known my desire that my dying not be artificially prolonged under the circumstances set forth below, and I do hereby declare that:

If at any time I am incapacitated and
_____ I have a terminal condition, or
_____ I have an end-stage condition, or
_____ I am in a persistent vegetative state

and if my attending or treating physician and another consulting physician have determined that there is no reasonable medical probability of my recovery from such condition, I direct that life-prolonging procedures be withheld or withdrawn when the application of such procedures would serve only to prolong artificially the process of dying, and that I be permitted to die naturally with only the administration of medication or the performance of any medical procedure deemed necessary to provide me with comfort care or to alleviate pain.

It is my intention that this declaration be honored by my family and physician as the final expression of my legal right to refuse medical or surgical treatment and to accept the consequences for such refusal.

In the event that I have been determined to be unable to provide express and informed consent regarding the withholding, withdrawal, or continuation of life-prolonging procedures, I wish to designate, as my surrogate to carry out the provisions of this declaration:

Name: _____
Address: _____
_____ Zip Code: _____
Phone: _____

© 2000 PARTNERSHIP FOR CARING, INC.

FLORIDA LIVING WILL — PAGE 2 OF 2

PRINT NAME, HOME ADDRESS AND TELEPHONE NUMBER OF YOUR ALTERNATE SURROGATE

I wish to designate the following person as my alternate surrogate, to carry out the provisions of this declaration should my surrogate be unwilling or unable to act on my behalf:

Name: _____
Address: _____
_____ Zip Code: _____
Phone: _____

ADD PERSONAL INSTRUCTIONS (IF ANY)

Additional instructions (optional):

I understand the full import of this declaration, and I am emotionally and mentally competent to make this declaration.

SIGN THE DOCUMENT

Signed: _____

WITNESSING PROCEDURE

Witness 1:
Signed: _____
Address: _____

TWO WITNESSES MUST SIGN AND PRINT THEIR ADDRESSES

Witness 2:
Signed: _____
Address: _____

© 2000 PARTNERSHIP FOR CARING, INC.

Courtesy of **Partnership for Caring, Inc.** 6/00
1035 30th Street, NW Washington, DC 20007 800-989-9455

Figure 7-7 **Health care surrogate form.** (Reprinted by permission of Choice in Dying, 200 Varick Street, New York, NY 10014, 212-366-5540)

The ADA allows preemployment physical examinations only after an individual has been offered employment. Medical records of these persons are kept confidential and separate and accessible only to persons who must know what restrictions the patient may bring to a job. Job qualifications and the specific standards for employment must be the same for all applicants. Disabled persons cannot be screened using different standards for employment.

Former drug users and those who are being rehabilitated also are covered by the ADA and cannot be denied employment because of their past history of drug use.

Employers are required to post notices regarding employee and applicant rights and obligations.

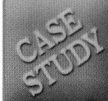

CASE STUDY 7-1

Three weeks ago, Dr. King treated a new patient, Boris Bolski, for lower back pain, which the patient felt was the result of consistent heavy lifting at his job. Medical assistant Joe Guerrero assisted Dr. King during the examination and, today, both Joe and Dr. King were served with subpoenas by Mr. Bolski's attorney. Mr. Bolski is alleging that unsafe conditions at his workplace caused severe strain on his back and he is suing his employer for damages. Dr. King and Joe Guerrero were called as expert witnesses to a civil hearing; Joe, especially, is a bit nervous about this, as he has never been on the witness stand in court and is not sure what is expected of him.

CASE STUDY REVIEW

1. How will Mr. Bolski's medical record help Joe answer questions at the hearing?
2. What information should Joe gather in order to be prepared to testify?
3. As an expert witness, what is Joe expected to communicate to the judge in this case?

SUMMARY

Changing societal values have contributed to an explosion of lawsuits in medical practice. Patients are more aware than ever of their rights, especially those of confidentiality and the right to privacy, consent, and records ownership. They readily seek redress when they perceive their rights to be violated.

A healthy relationship between physicians and patients and between medical assistants and patients, as well as respect for the patient's rights, lowers the likelihood of a lawsuit.

Knowledge of the laws that regulate medical and business practices in your state is necessary in order to be in compliance. Sources of information regarding state and federal laws can be obtained from the state medical society, the physician's liability insurance company, the state medical assistant society, the state attorney general's office, or the public library.

REVIEW QUESTIONS

Multiple Choice

1. The type of contract that most often exists between physician and patient is:
   a. expressed
   b. implied
   c. privileged
   d. civil
2. Which of the following claims of negligence would fit into the category of *res ipsa loquitur?*
   a. improper use of X-ray equipment
   b. failure to use X-ray equipment
   c. incorrect administration of anesthesia
   d. discovery of a surgical instrument inside the patient's body
3. Slander is defamation through:
   a. spoken statements that damage an individual's reputation
   b. written statements that damage a person's reputation
   c. written falsehoods about an individual
   d. a, b, and c
4. Occasionally, a physician will be sued for the negligence of a partner or employee, even though the physician is not guilty of any negligent act. This is done on the basis of the doctrine of:
   a. *res ipsa loquitur*
   b. *respondeat superior*
   c. proximate cause
   d. contract law
5. The standard of care expected of a physician is held by the courts to mean:
   a. on a par with all other physicians engaged in the same medical specialty anywhere
   b. reasonable, attentive, diligent care comparable to other physicians of the same specialty in the same or similar community

   c. the best possible under the circumstances
   d. the same as the national norm
6. Physician's directives:
   a. allow patients to direct how their billing is to be handled
   b. are designed to encourage physicians to render first aid in an emergency
   c. direct physicians based on a patient's wishes in life-threatening circumstances
   d. are not considered legal documents
7. A subpoena:
   a. is a court order requesting data and/or an appearance in court
   b. is sufficient to enforce a release of any type medical record or information
   c. may be ignored without consequences
   d. allows the person being served to select a specific date or time to appear
8. The 4 Ds of negligence are:
   a. duty, danger, damage, and disaster
   b. derelict, direct cause, damage, and danger
   c. danger, direct cause, damage, disaster
   d. duty, derelict, direct cause, damage
9. Emancipated minors:
   a. are considered adults and can consent to treatment
   b. live on their own and are self-supporting
   c. may be married or serve in the military
   d. all of the above
   e. only b and c
10. Torts:
    a. include battery, defamation of character, invasion of privacy
    b. are always intentional in nature
    c. do not require that harm has occurred
    d. do not include malpractice

Critical Thinking

1. Chris is a six-year-old girl whom Dr. King has seen for a broken leg. Chris' parents fail to follow Dr. King's treatment plan for Chris. What, if any, action can Dr. King take? What is the legal term for this situation?

2. Audrey, the medical assistant at Lewis & King MD, has accidentally used an incorrect solution to irrigate a patient's eyes. The patient suffers injuries to both eyes. Can Audrey's error be considered malpractice? Explain your reason.

3. Explain the standard of care as it applies to medical assistants. Give an example.

4. Jaime arrived in the clinic having sustained a serious laceration at his construction site. Dr. Woo ordered Demerol R 100 mg. 1.m - stat which Wanda, the medical assistant, administers. Dr. Woo determines surgery is required. Should a consent form be prepared? If so, by whom, and what should be included?

5. Give two examples of routine office or clinic procedures that might constitute violation of the patient's right to privacy.

6. Discuss the federal law regarding HIV testing, AIDS, and drug screening.

7. What are public duties? Discuss the physician's and medical assistant's obligations in regard to public duties.

8. What is the Good Samaritan Law? What must a medical assistant and any other health care professional remember when giving first aid at the scene of an accident?

9. Describe three types of abuse. Tell what your role and responsibilities are as a medical assistant when Juanita brings her son Henry into the clinic. Henry appears to have bruises on his face and chest.

10. Lenore McDonnell, who uses a wheelchair, has applied for employment in a large bookstore in town. She has not yet been offered the job. She has an appointment today for a preemployment physical examination and tells Audrey, the medical assistant, that the bookstore wants a copy of the results of Dr. Lewis' findings. Discuss the situation in light of the Americans with Disabilities Act.

WEB ACTIVITIES

Research the World Wide Web for the statute of limitations related to claims injuries. What is the time span in your state?

REFERENCES/BIBLIOGRAPHY

Cowdrey, M., & Drew, M. (1995). *Basic law for the allied health professions* (2nd ed.). Sudbury, MA: Jones and Bartlett.

Flight, M. (1998). *Law, liability, and ethics for medical office professionals* (3rd ed.). Albany, NY: Delmar.

Lewis, M. A., & Tamparo, C. D. (1998). *Medical law, ethics, and bioethics for ambulatory care* (4th ed.). Philadelphia: F. A. Davis Company.

McWay, D. A. (1997). *Legal aspects of health information management*. Albany, NY: Delmar.

Chapter 8

ETHICAL CONSIDERATIONS

KEY TERMS

Bioethics
Ethics
Genetic Engineering
Surrogate

OUTLINE

Ethics Defined
Bioethics Defined
Keys to the AAMA Code of Ethics
AMA Ethical Guidelines
    Advertising
    Media Relations
    Confidentiality
    Medical Records
    Professional Fees and Charges
    Professional Rights and Responsi-
        bilities
    Abuse

Bioethical Dilemmas
    Allocation of Scarce Medical
        Resources
    Abortion and Fetal Tissue
        Research
    Genetic Engineering/Manipula-
        tion
    Artificial Insemination/Surrogacy
    Dying and Death
    HIV and AIDS

OBJECTIVES

*The student should strive to meet the following performance objectives and demonstrate
an understanding of the facts and principles presented in this chapter through written and
oral communication.*

1. Define the key terms as presented in the glossary.
2. Identify the two prominent Codes of Ethics.
3. Compare/contrast the AAMA and the AMA Codes of Ethics.
4. Recall the five principles of the AAMA Code of Medical Ethics.
5. Relate the five principles of the AAMA code to patient care in the
   ambulatory care setting.
6. Recall the seven principles or standards of conduct adopted by the AMA.
7. Discuss the guidelines identified in at least six ethical issues presented
   by the *Current Opinions of the Council on Ethical and Judicial Affairs of the
   AMA.*
8. Restate the dilemmas encountered by the following bioethical issues:
   (a) allocation of scarce medical resources; (b) abortion and fetal tissue
   research; (c) genetic engineering/manipulation; (d) artificial insemina-
   tion/surrogacy; (e) dying and death.

**GENERAL
(TRANSDISCIPLINARY)**

Professionalism

- **Adhere to ethical principles**
- **Promote the CMA credential**

Legal Concepts

- **Maintain confidentiality**
- **Prepare and maintain medical records**
- **Use appropriate guidelines when releasing information**

On occasion, ethical dilemmas occur because patients are unsure of the role of the medical assistant. For example, the medical assistants of Inner City Health Care are truly multidisciplinary and have a range of administrative and clinical skills. However, patients sometimes think of them as nurses who have an entirely different set of skills. While most of the medical assistants gently correct patients and make it a point to practice only within their area of expertise, occasionally newer members of the medical assistant staff may feel more "important" when patients regard them as nurses or physicians' assistants.

A few weeks ago, medical assistant Liz Corbin, who is in her early twenties, was taken aback when Walter Seals, the office manager, spoke up about Liz's tendency to let patients assume she was a nurse. While Liz never deliberately intended to mislead patients, she never corrected them about their misconceptions. Walter pointed out that to present a good example of the medical assisting profession, Liz should gently but firmly help patients understand that she was a medical assistant with a specific range of skills that complemented, but did not substitute for, nursing skills.

INTRODUCTION

It is impossible in today's world to function as a medical assistant without an awareness of the impact of ethics and bioethics on health care. Just as an understanding of the law and working within the law is vital information for the medical assistant, it is equally important to understand ethics and bioethics.

From the previous chapter, you have come to realize that there are many circumstances and situations that occur in health care that are guided and directed by state and federal laws. You, personally, are expected to be above reproach in all your actions in this regard. You must also work with your employer and other members of the health care team to assure that each member of the staff functions within the law—protecting both patients and providers.

Ethics plays a huge role in such an endeavor. To function ethically demands that you never function outside the law. Ethics, however, demands something more—ethics calls for honesty, trustworthiness, integrity, confidentiality, and fairness. To function ethically, you must know yourself well and understand weaknesses and any vulnerabilities that might prevent you from acting ethically.

The scenario described above is just one situation in which medical assistants may need to reflect on their actions and be sure that they are acting ethically and within the range of their skills. Medical assistants also need to recognize the warning signs that they, or some other staff member, may be about to breach a code of ethics. Often, this kind of breach occurs when one has, or seeks to have, too much power; when one attempts to take too much authority; and when one has too little knowledge and experience. When a breach seems about to occur, the individuals involved should be encouraged to step back and review their actions and the likely consequences of those actions.

ETHICS DEFINED

Traditionally, **ethics** has been defined in terms of what is right or wrong. For health care professionals, ethics is often defined by a code or creed as seen in the Code of Ethics from the American Association of Medical Assistants (AAMA) or the Principles of Medical Ethics from the American Medical Association (AMA). While these codes, and many others like them, are essential and very helpful, they lose their vitality unless they are understood by individuals who possess a personal and sound moral code or set of values.

Unlike the law, which seldom changes unless challenged and examined in the courts, codes of ethics constantly change and evolve just as personal values and morals change and evolve. Every time values are challenged and examined, a medical assistant's personal ethical codes become stronger, the understanding of others' perceptions becomes clearer, and professionalism is enhanced.

BIOETHICS DEFINED

Bioethics brings the entire focus of ethics into the field of health care and into those ethical issues dealing with life. Never before in the history of medical care has bioethics been such a topic of concern. In the past, most bioethical decisions were made by physicians and esteemed members of the medical and/or legal profession. However, advancing technology giving patients and consumers numerous choices regarding their health care causes each one of us to take an active role in bioethics.

Medical assistants will encounter ethical and bioethical issues across the lifespan. In Figure 8-1, a few issues are identified for contemplation and discussion. Issues of bioethics common to every medical office are the allocation of scarce medical resources, abortion and fetal tissue research, genetic engineering or manipulation, and the many choices surrounding life, dying, and death.

For medical assistants to fully comprehend a discussion of ethics and bioethics, they must be familiar with the Code of Ethics of AAMA (Figure 8-2) and the AMA's Principles of Medical Ethics (Figure 8-3).

A FEW ISSUES FOR CONTEMPLATION AND DISCUSSION

Infants

- In premature, deformed, or severely disabled infants, ethical issues include the decision to provide or withhold treatment. Health care professionals and parents are not always in agreement. Central to this issue, also, is the expense involved in certain treatments and deciding who pays the cost of treatment.
- Vulnerability of infants can lead to issues of negligence, abuse, or rejection. Parents are also vulnerable because they may be unable to cope with the needs of the entire family.

Children

- Children who are ill-fed, housed, educated, and clothed exhibit great needs for preventive, curative, and rehabilitative health care.
- Minors with sexually transmitted diseases can seek treatment without the parents' knowledge. Treatment also must be offered without parental consent to pregnant, infected, or addicted minors.
- Child abuse presents an ethical dilemma, especially when a child confides physical, sexual, or emotional abuse to a health care worker but does not want the information divulged. Health care professionals, as mandated reporters, must report suspected child abuse. Will the child/patient view this as a violation of confidence or suffer dire consequences as a result of the reported abuse?

Adolescents

- Adolescents as young as 13 to 18 years old may seek abortion without parental knowledge or consent. Is this a violation of parents' right to medical information regarding their children? Or should the adolescent, fearful of parental reaction, have the right to decide?
- The adolescent's growing autonomy, need for independence, changing values, and desire for peer acceptance lead to a number of ethical issues that may involve the health care environment. These include the adolescent's decision to be sexually active, to use birth control, to protect against sexually transmitted diseases, and to use drugs and/or alcohol.

Adults

- Many low-income women do not have sufficient access to prenatal care, which has proven to be a cost-saving medical measure that is critical to the health of both mother and infant.
- As employers seek to reduce the cost of health insurance benefit programs, many individuals and families are finding themselves shifted from one insurance program to another, leaving them with little or no continuity of care. Also, in some managed care programs, adults may receive medical services from a number of health care professionals with whom they have no opportunity to establish an ongoing physician-patient relationship.
- Even with a physician's directive or a living will, a dying patient's wishes may not be followed. Technological advances in medicine have created a situation where patients may not be able to exercise a choice in the death issue.

Senior Adults

- Dementia is a common problem that is physically and financially exhausting for the caregiver, who is usually a spouse or adult child. How do caregivers cope with their own needs and the needs of dependent adults? Often, the elderly may reject nursing home placement, and there may be limited funds for such long-term care.
- Elderly patients have the right to maintain dignity and privacy, but their dependency on others may deprive them of these basic rights.
- Physician-assisted suicide for terminally ill patients is a prominent issue in our society, especially when elderly patients sense a total loss of dignity.

Figure 8-1 Ethical issues across the lifespan. (Compiled by Carol Tamparo, CMA-A, PhD, and Marilyn Pooler, RN, CMA-C, MEd)

AAMA CODE OF ETHICS

The Code of Ethics of AAMA shall set forth principles of ethical and moral conduct as they relate to the medical profession and the particular practice of medical assisting.

Members of AAMA dedicated to the conscientious pursuit of their profession, and thus desiring to merit the high regard of the entire medical profession and the respect of the general public which they serve, do pledge themselves to strive always to:

A. render service with full respect for the dignity of humanity;
B. respect confidential information obtained through employment unless legally authorized or required by responsible performance of duty to divulge such information;
C. uphold the honor and high principles of the profession and accept its disciplines;
D. seek to continually improve the knowledge and skills of medical assistants for the benefit of patients and professional colleagues;
E. participate in additional service activities aimed toward improving the health and well-being of the community.

CREED

I believe in the principles and purposes of the Profession of Medical Assisting.
I endeavor to be more effective.
I aspire to render greater service.
I protect the confidence entrusted to me.
I am dedicated to the care and well-being of all people.
I am loyal to my employer.
I am true to the ethics of my profession.
I am strengthened by compassion, courage, and faith.

Figure 8-2 AAMA Code of Ethics and Creed. (Copyright by the American Association of Medical Assistants, Inc. Revised October, 1996)

KEYS TO THE AAMA CODE OF ETHICS

Medical assistants should consider the more salient points in the AAMA code of ethics and ask themselves the following questions:

A. *Render service with full respect for the dignity of humanity.*

- Will I respect every patient even if I do not approve of his or her morals or choices in health care?
- Will I honor each patient's request for information and explain unfamiliar procedures?

PRINCIPLES OF MEDICAL ETHICS: AMERICAN MEDICAL ASSOCIATION

Preamble

The medical profession has long subscribed to a body of ethical statements developed primarily for the benefit of the patient. As a member of this profession, a physician must recognize responsibility not only to patients, but also to society, to other health professionals, and to self. The following Principles adopted by the American Medical Association are not laws, but standards of conduct which define the essentials of honorable behavior for the physician.

I. A physician shall be dedicated to providing competent medical service with compassion and respect for human dignity.
II. A physician shall deal honestly with patients and colleagues, and strive to expose those physicians deficient in character or competence, or who engage in fraud or deception.
III. A physician shall respect the law and also recognize a responsibility to seek changes in those requirements which are contrary to the best interests of the patient.
IV. A physician shall respect the rights of patients, of colleagues, and of other health professionals, and shall safeguard patient confidences within the constraints of the law.
V. A physician shall continue to study, apply, and advance scientific knowledge, make relevant information available to patients, colleagues, and the public, obtain consultation, and use the talents of other health professionals when indicated.
VI. A physician shall, in the provision of appropriate patient care, except in emergencies, be free to choose whom to serve, with whom to associate, and the environment in which to provide medical services.
VII. A physician shall recognize a responsibility to participate in activities contributing to an improved community.

Figure 8-3 American Medical Association Principles of Medical Ethics. (Source: Code of Medical Ethics Current Opinions with Annotations, 2000–2001 Edition, American Medical Association, Copyright 2000)

- Will I give my full attention to acknowledging the needs of every patient?
- Will I be able to accept the indigent, the physically and mentally challenged, the infirm, the physically disfigured, and the persons I simply do not like as equal and valid human beings with an equal right to service?

B. *Respect confidential information obtained through employment unless legally authorized or required by responsible performance of duty to divulge such information.*

- Will I refrain from needless comments to a colleague regarding a patient's problem?
- Will I refrain from discussing my day's encounters with patients with my family and friends?
- Will I always protect a patient's chart and everything in it from unnecessary observation?
- Will I keep patients' names and the circumstances that bring them to my place of employment confidential?

C. *Uphold the honor and high principles of the profession and accept its disciplines.*

- Am I proud of serving as a medical assistant?
- Will I always perform within the scope of my profession, never exceeding the responsibility entrusted to me?
- Will I encourage others to enter the profession and always speak honorably of medical assistants?

D. *Seek to continually improve the knowledge and skills of medical assistants for the benefit of patients and professional colleagues.*

- Will I always be willing to learn new skills, to update my skills, and seek improved methods for assisting the physician in the care of patients?
- Will I keep my certification current and valid?
- Can I always remember that I am a member of a group of broad-based health care professionals and that my goal is to complement rather than to compete with that team?

E. *Participate in additional service activities aimed toward improving the health and well-being of the community.*

- Will I be able to serve in the community where I reside and work to further quality health care?
- Will I promote preventive medicine?
- Will I practice good health care management for myself, being a model for others to follow?

AMA ETHICAL GUIDELINES

The American Medical Association and its nine-member Judicial Council publish a guide for ethical behavior for physicians that is beneficial to medical assistants who act in concert with their physician/employer. The guidelines are based on the Code of Medical Ethics in the publication *Current Opinions of the Council on Ethical and Judicial Affairs of the American Medical Association, 2000.* Information shared here is not meant to be exhaustive; however, physicians and their employees will find it helpful to consider information on the following topics, which was summarized from this publication. The complete guide can be purchased from the AMA in Chicago, IL.

Advertising

Physicians and professional people have traditionally not advertised; however, it is not illegal or unethical to do so if claims made are truthful and not misleading. Advertisements may include credentials of physicians and a description of the practice, kinds of services rendered, and how fees are determined. Managed care agencies may advertise their services and the names of participating physicians. Testimonials from patients are best avoided. Indeed, most physicians discover that word-of-mouth advertisement from patients is the best source of advertisement for their practice.

Media Relations

Physicians and all of their employees are not allowed to discuss a patient's medical condition with any member of the media without the patient's expressed approval. This does not apply to information that is considered "public domain," which includes births, deaths, accidents, and police records. While more hospitals than ambulatory care settings will be involved in media relations, the following is an example of information that is considered public domain and does not require the patient's consent.

"Jaime Carrera, a local construction worker, suffered a severe laceration to the head as a result of an accident at the construction site. He remains hospitalized in good condition."

Confidentiality

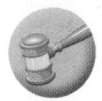

Physicians must not reveal confidential information about patients without their consent unless they are otherwise required to do so by law. Confidentiality must be protected so that patients will feel comfortable and safe in revealing information about themselves that may be important to their health care. The following list contains examples of the kinds of reports that allow or require health professionals to report a confidence.

A patient threatens another person and there is reason to believe that the threat may be carried out.

Certain injuries and illnesses *must* be reported. They include injuries such as knife and gunshot wounds, wounds that may be from suspected child abuse, and communicable diseases such as influenza, AIDS, and sexually transmitted diseases.

Information that may have been subpoenaed for testimony in a court of law.

When in doubt, it is always recommended that a physician have the patient's permission to reveal any confidential information.

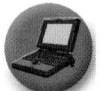
Extra caution must be taken to protect the confidentiality of any patient's data that is kept on a computer database. As few people as possible should have access to the computer data, and only authorized individuals should be permitted to add or alter data. Adequate security precautions must be utilized to protect information stored on a computer.

Medical Records

The medical chart and the information in it are the property of the physician and the patient. No information should be revealed without the patient's consent unless required by law. The record is confidential. Physicians should not refuse to provide a copy of the record to another physician treating the patient so long as proper authorization has been received from the patient. Also, physicians should provide a copy of the record or summary of its contents if a patient requests it. A record cannot be withheld because of an unpaid bill.

Upon a physician's retirement or death, or when a practice is sold, patients should be notified and given ample time to have their records transferred to another physician of their choice.

Professional Fees and Charges

Illegal or excessive fees should not be charged. Fees should be based on those customary to the locale and should reflect the difficulty of services and the quality of performance rendered. Fee splitting (a physician splits the fee with another physician for services rendered with or without the patient's knowledge) in any form is unethical. Physicians may charge for missed appointments (if patients have first been notified of the practice) and may charge for multiple or very complex insurance forms. Physicians and their employees must be diligent to assure that only the services actually rendered are charged or indicated on the insurance claim. Only what is documented in the patient's chart is to be billed.

Professional Rights and Responsibilities

Physicians may choose whom to serve, but may not refuse a patient on the basis of race, color, religion, national origin, or any other illegal discrimination. It is unethical for physicians to deny treatment to HIV-infected individuals on that basis alone if they are qualified to treat the patient's condition. Once a physician takes a case, the patient cannot be neglected nor refused treatment unless official notice is given from the physician to withdraw from the case.

Patients have the right to know their diagnoses, the nature and purpose of their treatment, and to have enough information to be able to make an informed choice about their treatment protocol. Physicians should inform families of a patient's death and not delegate that responsibility to others.

Physicians should expose incompetent, corrupt, dishonest, and unethical conduct by other physicians to the disciplinary board. It is unethical for any physician to treat patients while under the influence of alcohol, controlled substances, or any other chemical that impairs the physician's ability.

Physicians who know they are HIV positive should refrain from any activity that would risk the transmission of the virus to others.

Any activity that might be regarded as a "conflict of interest"(for example, a physician holding stock in a pharmaceutical company and prescribing medications only from that company) should be avoided. Financial interests are not to influence physicians in prescribing medications, devices, or appliances.

Abuse

It is the responsibility of physicians and their employees to report all cases of suspected child abuse, to protect and care for the abused, and to treat the abuser (if known) as a victim also. This is not an

SPOTLIGHT ON AAMA ESSENTIALS THROUGH CAAHEP

- Medical ethics involves providing patients of all socioeconomic backgrounds with quality care.

- Professional and empathetic medical assistants never judge patients whose belief systems differ from their own.

- If a medical assistant suspects that an HIV-seropositive patient is infecting an unsuspecting person, he or she should make every attempt to protect the individual at risk and to encourage the infected person to cease endangering other people.

easy task. Abuse is not easy to witness. While there are very specific laws regarding suspected child abuse, and in most states medical assistants are mandated to report abuse, the laws are vague or nonexistent in elderly and spousal abuse. However, whatever form the abuse takes, it is best to treat all forms of abuse in the same manner by providing a safe environment for those abused and seeking treatment for the abuser and the abused.

BIOETHICAL DILEMMAS

Guidelines for bioethical issues are even harder to define than are guidelines for ethics, because each of the bioethical issues calls upon us to make decisions that directly affect a person's life. In some instances, the bioethical issue requires a choice about who lives and requires a definition of the quality of life. Such dilemmas are difficult, if not impossible, to approach from a neutral point of view even though medical assistants should strive not to impose their own moral values upon patients or coworkers.

Allocation of Scarce Medical Resources

The issue faced daily by health care workers is the allocation of scarce medical resources. Even with the government's attempts at health care reform, medical resources still will not be available to everyone. When the receptionist determines who receives the only available appointment in a day, when patients are turned away because they have no insurance or financial resources to pay for services, when Medicare/Medicaid patients are denied services because of low return from state and federal insurance programs, scarce medical resources are being denied.

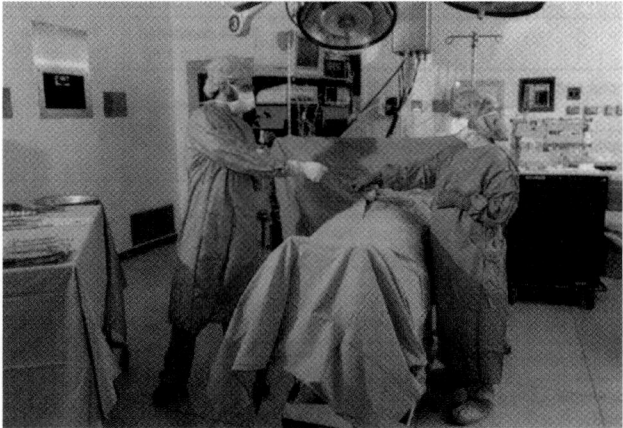

Figure 8-4 Scarce medical resources may limit surgery options for patients whose conditions are not immediately life threatening; some patients may lack insurance and not be able to afford necessary surgical procedures. (Photo courtesy of the U.S. Army)

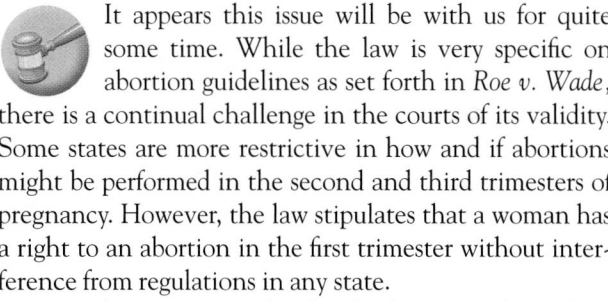

Weightier decisions might include who gets the surgery, a kidney transplant, or the experimental bone marrow transplant, Figure 8-4. These allocations are being made and will continue to require decisions on the part of the health care team. Rationing of health care may become more widespread as managed care operations try to achieve a balance between providing access to care while still curtailing costs.

Decisions made by Congress, health systems agencies, and insurance companies are termed macroallocation of scarce medical resources. Decisions made individually by physicians and members of the health care team at the local level are termed microallocation of scarce resources. No matter what the level, physicians and medical assistants will be involved.

Abortion and Fetal Tissue Research

It appears this issue will be with us for quite some time. While the law is very specific on abortion guidelines as set forth in *Roe v. Wade*, there is a continual challenge in the courts of its validity. Some states are more restrictive in how and if abortions might be performed in the second and third trimesters of pregnancy. However, the law stipulates that a woman has a right to an abortion in the first trimester without interference from regulations in any state.

A physician must decide whether to perform abortions and under what circumstances (within the legal parameters). A physician cannot be forced to perform abortions, nor can any employee be forced to participate or assist the physician to perform an abortion. Employees not wishing to participate in abortions are advised to seek employment where they are not performed.

There are many unanswered ethical questions related to abortion that make it difficult for health care professionals. Should abortion be considered a form of birth control? If not, should birth control be readily available to all who seek it regardless of age? Is it ethical to deny a woman on welfare an abortion while providing one to the woman who either has money for the procedure or whose insurance pays for it? And, of course, the major unanswered question that must be determined by every physician is: when does life begin?

The abortion issue raises another bioethical issue—fetal tissue research and transplantation. Research has shown that transplanted tissue from aborted fetuses can be instrumental in benefiting individuals with serious, life-threatening diseases. This issue is political as well as bioethical, and it changes with each major political shift in our government. If fetal tissue research is allowed, the primary ethical concern is that that fact not be used to encourage women to have abortions; rather, the tissue would be available only after a decision had already been made regarding abortion.

Genetic Engineering/Manipulation

So much is possible today in the area of genetic engineering and more is being discovered daily. Through genetic engineering, we have the potential of identifying genes that predispose individuals to certain illnesses and diseases and manipulating or altering those genes to prevent or lessen the disease or illness. Who among us would not want to be free of certain illnesses? But at what cost? How far do we go in genetic engineering? Would we prefer a society where everyone is healthy and beautiful? If it is determined that a fetus suffers from a serious defect, should abortion be encouraged? If we manipulate the genes prior to implantation, are we playing god? If fertilization takes place *in vitro*, is discarding defective embryos a reasonable and presumed choice?

Artificial Insemination/Surrogacy

For many individuals, artificial insemination is the only means by which they can conceive. Physicians can be called upon to perform artificial insemination for couples, single women, or lesbians who want a child. If artificial insemination is practiced, the AMA recommends the signed consent of each party involved. It is also recommended that physicians practicing AID (Artificial Insemination by Donor), not continually use the same donors for semen, and that meticulous screening be performed prior to the insemination.

Surrogacy is another bioethical issue. Men have been used as **surrogates,** or substitutes, for decades with the practice of artificial insemination, but society has a more difficult time with surrogate mothers than artificial insemination with male donors. Under what circumstances should a surrogate mother be considered? How should the rights of each individual in the exchange be protected? For many of these issues, there is little or no protection or guidance under the law; therefore, physicians and their employees must make decisions on the basis of their own belief systems. The AMA is not supportive of surrogacy as a viable route to parenthood.

Dying and Death

Patients are making more choices regarding their death. We all have the right to direct health care professionals regarding our death in the case of a life-threatening ill-

ness. Through a living will or a physician's directive, we can mandate that life support systems be removed. Sometimes, patients make these decisions before physicians are ready to remove the life support. Other times, physicians can determine when a case is hopeless far quicker than the patient or the patient's family. What should be done then? When a physician is committed to sustaining life, it is very difficult to make decisions to terminate life. In 1994, Oregon voters passed a physician-assisted suicide law. Other states are considering similar laws.

In 1990, Congress passed a bill called the Patient Self-Determination Act, which encourages patients to make living wills and advance directives before life-sustaining measures become necessary. Nearly all states have legislation regarding advance directives.

Choices available to patients who are dying always cause us to ask ourselves what is "quality of life"? While the answer to that question is different for everyone, it is a question often in conflict with today's medical technology that can, in many instances, keep a patient alive much longer than the patient might prefer. The benefits of advanced technology will continue to be weighed against what many consider the right to die with dignity and a minimum of medical intervention.

HIV and AIDS

The general public's fear of AIDS has caused some serious bioethical issues. Patients who may suspect they have come into contact with HIV or AIDS should be tested for the virus. Their confidentiality must be protected as much as possible since persons with AIDS often face loss of employment, medical insurance, and even loss of family and friends. It is unethical to deny treatment to HIV-infected individuals because they test positive for HIV.

While persons with AIDS must be protected, so must the public. Therefore, if physicians suspect that an HIV-seropositive patient is infecting an unsuspecting individual, every attempt should be made to protect the individual at risk. Health professionals must first encourage the infected person to cease endangering any person. Second, if the patient refuses to notify the person at risk or wishes the physician to notify the person, the physician can contact authorities. Many states and cities have Partner Notification Programs that will anonymously notify the patient at risk, keeping the source confidential. The Program informs them that it has been brought to their attention that they are a "person at risk" and provides them with free testing. Third, the physician can notify the person at risk.

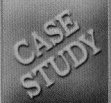

CASE STUDY 8-1

At the end of a busy afternoon, Juanita Hansen, a single mother in her twenties, brings in her son Henry after he fell down a flight of steps. He is badly bruised and crying and also seems to be somewhat fearful of his mother. Medical assistant Liz Corbin recognizes Henry, for his mother brought him in the week before when he fell off his bike. At that time, Liz had assisted Dr. Esposito in examining Henry and both were concerned about the possibility of child abuse, for Henry had been in before for various "accidents." Today, when Liz assists Dr. Esposito once again to examine Henry, it becomes clear that Henry is probably the victim of abuse.

CASE STUDY REVIEW

1. Because Liz and Dr. Esposito strongly suspect that Henry is being repeatedly abused, what are they obligated to do?
2. How can Liz best help Henry to cope with his situation?
3. How can Liz attempt to help Henry's mother come to terms with the fact that she is physically abusing her son?

SUMMARY

As medical technology continues to advance, a greater need for ethical guidelines will be necessary. Physicians and health care professionals at all levels must stay abreast of the issues and carefully consider all aspects prior to any decision making.

Medical assistants must, however, keep the following legal and ethical guidelines in mind: (1) always practice within the law; (2) preserve the patient's confidentiality; (3) maintain meticulous records; (4) obtain informed, written consent; (5) do not judge patients whose belief system differs from yours.

REVIEW QUESTIONS

Multiple Choice

1. Typically, ethics has been defined in terms of:
   a. what is right and wrong
   b. whether an action is legal
   c. the expedient thing to do
   d. professionalism in the workplace
2. Bioethics has to do with:
   a. biological reproduction
   b. the act of artificial insemination
   c. genetic engineering
   d. ethical issues that deal with life and health care
3. The Code of Ethics of AAMA:
   a. is concerned with principles of ethical and moral conduct
   b. defines the duties the medical assistant can perform
   c. is intended for physicians only
   d. applies only to patient rights

4. When a physician or medical assistant suspects child abuse, she should:
   a. give the parent a warning
   b. report it to the proper authorities
   c. not impose her values on the parents
   d. give the child some hints on how to protect against abuse
5. When a patient has HIV:
   a. it is ethical for the physician not to provide treatment
   b. it is unethical for the physician not to provide treatment
   c. other patients should be warned of the possibility of infection
   d. all friends and family members of the patient should be notified
6. A copy of a medical record may be granted to:
   a. a physician the patient is being referred to
   b. a physician's attorney when subpoenaed or released by patient

c. the patient
d. all of the above
e. only a and b

7. A patient's living will or physician's directive:
   a. is a legal document to be kept in the chart
   b. can be changed at any time by the patient
   c. should accompany the patient to the hospital
   d. all of the above
   e. only a and c

8. Your physician employer is considering changing the practice's announcement in the yellow pages of the phone book. Which of the following is not recommended?
   a. Name and specialty of practice
   b. Names and credentials/specialties of participating physicians
   c. Patient testimonials
   d. Managed care participation

9. Which of the following is true?
   a. A physician can choose whom to serve.
   b. A physician may charge for completing multiple and complex insurance claims.
   c. Physicians and their employees cannot be forced to perform abortions.
   d. All of the above
   e. None of the above

10. You are most likely to make ethical decisions correctly when:
    a. you have a clear picture of the situation
    b. you leave emotion out of the decision as much as possible
    c. you understand your weaknesses and vulnerabilities
    d. honesty and integrity are hallmarks of your entire life
    e. all of the above

Critical Thinking

1. In your own words, define ethics and bioethics.
2. List the similarities of and the differences between the AAMA Code of Ethics and the AMA Principles of Medical Ethics.
3. The physician observes another physician put a patient at risk while under the influence of alcohol and does nothing about it. What would constitute ethical behavior?

4. A physician attends a medical seminar related to medical practice every month and charges the seminar fee to the business. Would you consider this ethical or unethical? Why?
5. A physician refuses to accept any more Medicaid patients for medical care. Is this the physician's right? Is it ethical?
6. A medical assistant whispers to the receptionist, "There goes the guy with AIDS." How should the receptionist view this behavior?
7. The services reported on the insurance claim are more complex than those actually rendered. Is this ethical or unethical? State your reasons.
8. The physician refuses to perform a legal abortion. Do you consider this an ethical issue? Why?
9. A physician performs artificial insemination for a lesbian couple; however, the medical assistant refuses to participate or assist the physician. What are the ramifications of the medical assistant's behavior? Do you believe the medical assistant has a right to refuse?
10. Referring to Figure 8-1, select an ethical issue with which you may have had some personal experience. Now, form a small group, with each student leading a discussion on a different issue.

WEB ACTIVITIES

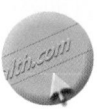 Using the World Wide Web, research particular guidelines to be used for artificial insemination either by donor or by husband. Look under the Current Opinions of the Council on Ethical and Judicial Affairs.

● What are the guidelines for medical records? Why?

● Why is frozen sperm recommended?

REFERENCES/BIBLIOGRAPHY

American Medical Association. (2000). Code of medical ethics. *Current opinions of the council on ethical and judicial affairs, 2000.* Chicago: Author.

Flight, M. (1998). *Law, liability, and ethics for medical office personnel* (3rd ed.). Albany, NY: Delmar.

Lewis, M. A., & Tamparo, C. D., (1998). *Medical law, ethics, and bioethics for ambulatory care* (4th ed.). Philadelphia: F. A. Davis Co.

EMERGENCY PROCEDURES AND FIRST AID

KEY TERMS

Cardiopulmonary Resuscitation (CPR)
Crash Tray or Cart
Crepitation
Emergency Medical Services (EMS)
First Aid
Fracture
Heimlich Maneuver
Hypothermia
Lackluster
Occlusion
Rescue Breathing
Shock
Splint
Sprain
Standard Precautions
Strain
Syncope
Triage
Universal Emergency Medical
   Identification Symbol
Wound

OUTLINE

Recognizing an Emergency
   Responding to an Emergency
   Primary Survey
   Using the 911 or Emergency
      Medical Services System
   Good Samaritan Laws
   Blood, Body Fluids, and Disease
      Transmission
Preparing for an Emergency
   The Medical Crash Tray or Cart
Common Emergencies
   Shock
   Wounds
   Burns

Musculoskeletal Injuries
Heat- and Cold-Related Illnesses
Poisoning
Sudden Illness
Cerebral Vascular Accident
   (CVA)
Heart Attack
**Procedures for Breathing Emer-
gencies and Cardiac Arrest**
   Heimlich Maneuver (Abdominal
      Thrust)
   Rescue Breathing
   Cardiopulmonary Resuscitation
      (CPR)

OBJECTIVES

*The student should strive to meet the following performance objectives and demonstrate
an understanding of the facts and principles presented in this chapter through written and
oral communication.*

1. Define the key terms as presented in the glossary.

2. Learn to recognize, prepare for, and respond to emergencies in the ambulatory care setting.

3. Understand the legal and disease transmission considerations in emergency caregiving.

4. Perform the primary assessment in emergency situations.

5. Identify and care for different types of wounds.

6. Understand the basics of bandage application.

7. Discriminate among first-, second-, and third-degree burns.

8. Assess injuries to muscles, bones, and joints.

9. Describe heat- and cold-related illnesses.   (*continues*)

10. Describe how poisons may enter the body.
11. Recall the eight types of shock.
12. Define a cerebral vascular accident.
13. Describe the signs and symptoms of a heart attack.
14. Demonstrate proficiency in Heimlich maneuver, rescue breathing, and cardiopulmonary resuscitation (CPR).

ROLE DELINEATION COMPONENTS

CLINICAL

Patient Care

- **Adhere to established triage procedures**
- **Recognize and respond to emergencies**
- **Obtain patient history and vital signs**
- **Prepare and maintain examination and treatment areas**
- **Prepare patient for examination, procedures, and treatment**

GENERAL (Transdisciplinary)

Instruction

- **Instruct individuals according to their needs**

SCENARIO

Inner City Health Care, which is located in Carlton, Michigan, has its share of cold, snowy winters and when the temperature drops near freezing, that snow sometimes turns to ice. Last night, as Clinical Medical Assistant Wanda Slawson, CMA, was leaving for the evening, she noticed a woman from an adjacent office slip and fall in the parking lot. Wanda immediately went over to the woman to lend assistance and saw that, in falling, the woman had cut the palm of her hand. Apparently, she had tried to break her fall with her hand only to sustain a large wound that was now bleeding moderately. Fortunately, Wanda knew that one of the physicians was still in the office and she led the woman back to the building, reassuring her all the way. Once in the office, Wanda assisted Susan Rice, the physician, to examine the wound. After determining that sutures were not needed, Dr. Rice and Wanda cleansed the wound, applied a dry, sterile dressing, and covered it with an elastic bandage. The patient was instructed to call her physician first thing in the morning.

INTRODUCTION

While the ambulatory care setting is primarily designed to see patients under nonemergency conditions, occasionally the physician will need to administer emergency care and the medical assistant will be called upon to assist the physician in this care. For the medical assistant who may need to triage or assess the patient's condition, the first and most critical step in responding to an emergency is developing the skill to recognize when emergency measures should be taken.

While some emergencies can be treated in the office, others cannot and the medical assistant must know when to call for outside help. If the emergency occurs in the ambulatory care setting, the physician usually provides immediate care. It is possible, however, that the medical assistant may be the first emergency caregiver should the physician be out of the office. The medical assistant also may be called upon to provide care in an emergency outside of the office environment.

This chapter will acquaint the medical assistant with types of emergency situations that may occur either inside or outside of the office. However, this chapter is merely an introduction to emergency topics and does not substitute for first aid and cardiopulmonary (CPR) instruction taught either through the college curriculum or through the American Red Cross or the American Heart Association. These hands-on classes are vital teaching tools and all medical assistants should take them on a regular basis in order to continually update their skills.

RECOGNIZING AN EMERGENCY

An emergency is considered any instance in which an individual becomes suddenly ill and requires immediate attention. Some common signs that an individual has an emergency include unusual noises, such as yelling, moaning, or crying. A person may appear to be behaving strangely when choking or if having difficulty breathing. To recognize when an emergency exists, it is important to have sharp senses of hearing, sight, and smell and be acutely sensitive to any unusual behaviors.

In the ambulatory care setting, medical assistants will encounter a range of emergency situations requiring first aid techniques. **First aid** is designed to render immediate and temporary emergency care to persons injured or otherwise disabled prior to the arrival of a physician or transport to a hospital or other health care agency.

Emergency situations can include:

- Wounds
- Bleeding
- Burns
- Shock
- Fractures
- Poisoning
- Sudden illnesses such as fainting
- Illnesses related to heat and cold
- Heart attack
- Choking and breathing crises

Some of these will be life-threatening; all will require immediate care. In either case, it is critical to remain calm, to follow the emergency policies and procedures established by the ambulatory care setting, and to be well-versed in first-aid and cardiopulmonary resuscitation techniques.

Responding to an Emergency

Once it has been determined that an emergency exists, it is essential to act quickly. Before making any decisions about how to proceed, it is necessary to assess the nature of the situation. Does it include respiratory or circulatory failure, severe bleeding, burns, poisoning, or severe allergic reaction?

Sometimes, it is possible that more than one type of care must be administered. In this case, it is necessary to **triage** the situation, which is a method of prioritizing treatment. When an individual suffers more than one illness or injury, care must be given according to the severity of the situation. When two or more patients present with emergencies simultaneously, triage also determines which patient is treated first. The main principle of triage states that absence of breath and severe bleeding are immediate life threats. See Table 9-1 for the common ordering of triage situations.

To identify the nature of the emergency and respond effectively, it is critical that the patient be assessed. If the patient is conscious, ask for personal identification and identification of next of kin. Try to obtain information about symptoms being experienced in order to identify the problem. Always check for a **universal emergency medical identification symbol** (Figure 9-1) and accompanying identification card, which will describe any serious or life-threatening health problems of the patient. Quickly observe the patient's general appearance, including skin color and size and dilation of pupils. Check pulse.

TABLE 9-1	EXAMPLES OF TRIAGE SITUATIONS	
First Priority	**Next Priority**	**Least Priority**
Airway and breathing problems	Second-degree burns not on the neck and face	Fractures
Cardiac arrest	Major or multiple fractures	Minor injuries
Severe bleeding that is uncontrolled	Back injuries	Sprains
Head injuries	Severe eye injuries	
Poisoning		
Open chest or abdominal wounds		
Shock		
Second- and third-degree burns		

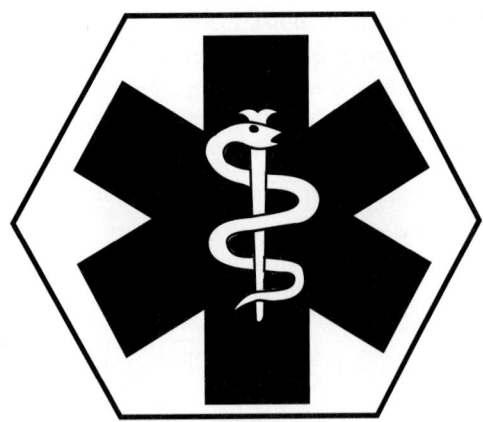

Figure 9-1   The universal emergency medical identification symbol.

Primary Survey

If the patient is unresponsive, it is critical to assess the ABCs, which include:

- Airway (A)
- Breathing (B)
- Circulation (C)

To assess whether the unresponsive patient is breathing and to determine if there is an open airway, place your face close to the patient's face and look, listen, and feel.

Look at the patient's chest and notice whether the chest rises and falls with breathing. Listen for air entering and leaving the nose and mouth and feel for moving air.

If the individual is not breathing, first open the airway by either tilting the head and lifting the chin (Figure 9-2A); or by the jaw-thrust maneuver, which involves placing both thumbs on the patient's cheekbones and index and middle fingers on both sides of the lower jaw (Figure 9-2B). **CAUTION:** Do not attempt to tilt the head and lift the chin when the patient has a head, neck, or spinal cord injury.

If the patient still does not breathe after the airway has been opened, rescue breathing must be performed, which is covered later in this chapter.

To assess circulation, check for the presence of a pulse at the carotid artery on the side of the neck below the ear. If no pulse is present, the patient may be in cardiac arrest and must be given cardiopulmonary resuscitation. CPR techniques are covered in detail later in this chapter.

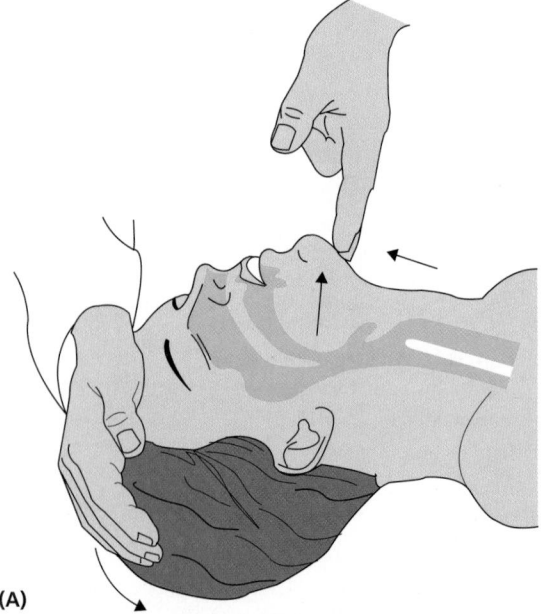

(A)

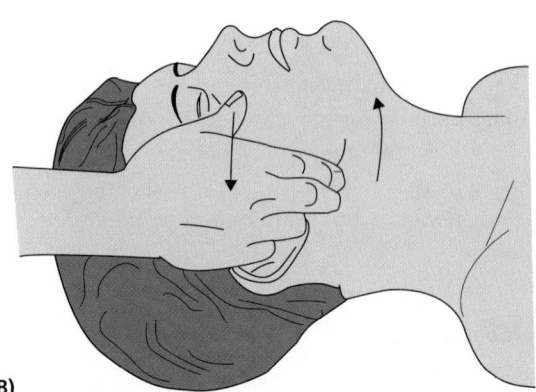

(B)

Figure 9-2   If the individual is not breathing, first open the airway: (A) By tilting the head and lifting the chin or (B) By the jaw-thrust maneuver, which involves placing both thumbs on the patient's cheekbones and index and middle fingers on both sides of the lower jaw.

Using the 911 or Emergency Medical Services System

The **Emergency Medical Services (EMS)** system is a local network of police, fire, and medical personnel who are trained to respond to emergency situations. Other community experts and volunteers also act as resources in an EMS system. In many communities, the network is activated by calling 911. Even when preliminary emergency care is provided by the ambulatory care physician, the patient may still need to be transported or may require follow-up care. It is also possible that the physician may not be equipped to deliver the type of emergency care required, in which case one person should call for EMS help while another stays with the patient until help arrives. Never leave a seriously ill or unconscious patient unattended.

Good Samaritan Laws

When delivering or assisting in delivering emergency care, the medical assistant may be concerned about professional liability. Most states have enacted Good Samaritan laws, which provide some degree of protection to the health care professional who offers first aid.

Most Good Samaritan laws provide some legal protection to those who provide emergency care to ill or injured persons. However, when medical assistants or any other individuals give care during an emergency, they must act as reasonable and prudent individuals and provide care only within the scope of their abilities. Remember that a primary principle of first aid is to prevent further injury.

While Good Samaritan laws give some measure of protection against being sued for giving emergency aid, they generally protect *off-duty* health care professionals. Also, conditions of the law vary from state to state. As part of establishing emergency care guidelines, every ambulatory care setting should understand the explicit and implicit intent of the Good Samaritan Law in its state. See Chapter 7 for more information on legal guidelines.

Blood, Body Fluids, and Disease Transmission

When providing emergency care, medical assistants should always protect themselves and the patient from infectious disease transmission. Serious infectious diseases, such as hepatitis B (HBV) and HIV, which causes AIDS, can be transmitted through blood and body fluids (see Chapter 22 for detailed information).

By establishing and following strict guidelines, the risk of contacting or transmitting an infectious disease while providing emergency care is greatly reduced.

- Always wash hands thoroughly before (if possible) and after every procedure.
- Use protective clothing and other protective equipment during the procedure.
- During the procedure, avoid contact with blood and body fluids, if possible.
- Do not touch nose, mouth, or eyes with gloved hands.
- Carefully handle and safely dispose of soiled gloves and other objects.

Refer to Chapter 22 for more information on standard precautions. **Standard precautions** were issued by the Centers for Disease Control and Prevention (CDC) in 1996 and combine many of the basic principles of universal precautions with techniques known as body substance isolation. These augmented 1996 guidelines represent the standard in infection control and are intended to protect both patients and health care professionals.

PREPARING FOR AN EMERGENCY

Emergencies are unexpected but can and should be anticipated and prepared for in the ambulatory care setting. Being properly prepared assures that the office has the materials and resources needed to respond to emergencies.

An in-office handbook of policies and procedures should be developed and should be familiar to all staff. Telephone numbers for the local emergency medical services (often this is 911) and the poison control center should be posted and kept in an established place so that there is no delay in calling for outside assistance. Materials and supplies should be maintained in proper inventory. All personnel should be trained in the basics of first aid and CPR, so that every staff member can respond to or

---

SPOTLIGHT ON AAMA ESSENTIALS THROUGH CAAHEP

- Treat all patients with compassion and empathy.
- Identifying a patient's cultural needs during an emergency may help to save his or her life.
- Listening to how a patient "feels" is just as important as how the patient appears.

assist the physician in providing care. Proper documentation should be completed after any emergency situation. The office environment itself should be a safe one and as accident-proof as possible. Wipe up spills to avoid falls on a slippery floor, keep corridors clutter-free, and keep medications out of sight. These basic risk management techniques will help medical personnel focus on giving emergency care and also protect the facility from any possible litigation.

The Medical Crash Tray or Cart

Every health care facility should have a **crash tray or cart**, with a carefully controlled inventory of supplies and equipment (Figure 9-3). These first-aid supplies should be kept in an accessible place, and the inventory should be routinely monitored to assure that all supplies are replaced and that all medications are up to date and have not reached their expiration date.

A smaller practice may require only a portable tray for emergency and first-aid supplies; larger urgent care centers may respond more frequently to emergencies and thus may need a cart that can hold a large inventory and variety of supplies. Whether a tray or cart is used, supplies should be customized to the facility and the type of emergencies frequently encountered. Remember that only physicians can order medications or treatment.

Following is a brief list of some common supplies found on most trays and/or carts. Also see Chapter 35 for more information on supplies and medications.

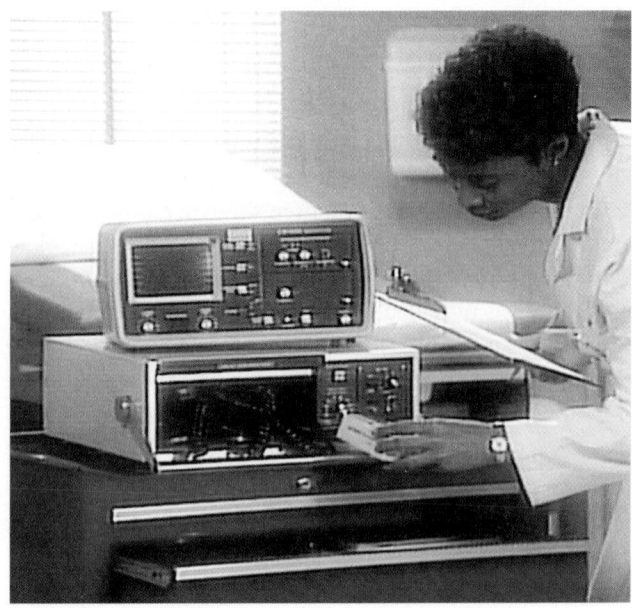

Figure 9-3 Medical crash cart.

General supplies:

- Adhesive and hypoallergenic tape
- Alcohol wipes
- Bandage scissors
- Bandage material
- Blood pressure cuff (standard, pediatric, large)
- Constriction band
- Defibrillator
- Gloves
- Hot/cold packs
- IV tubing
- Needles and syringes for injection
- Orange juice for diabetics (refrigerated)
- Penlight (with extra batteries)
- Personal protective equipment
- Spirits of ammonia
- Sterile dressings
- Stethoscope

Emergency medications:

- Activated charcoal
- Aramine
- Aspirin
- Atropine
- Dextrose
- Diphenhydramine
- Epinephrine
- Glucagon
- Insulin
- Lidocaine
- Nitroglycerin tablets
- Phenobarbital and diazepam (controlled substances; must be kept in a locked cabinet)
- Sodium bicarbonate
- Spirits of ammonia
- Sterile water
- Syrup of ipecac
- Verapamil
- Xylocaine and marcaine

Respiratory supplies:

- Airways of all sizes for nasal and oral use
- Ambu bag™
- Bulb syringe for suction
- Oxygen mask
- Oxygen tank

This list represents just some of the supplies to be found on a well-stocked crash cart or tray. The type and list of supplies should always be overseen by facility physicians and tailored to the emergency demands of the practice. The medical assistant should be familiar with the equipment and medication on the crash cart or tray. Practice "drills" simulating various emergency situations are helpful for preparing staff members for actual emergencies.

COMMON EMERGENCIES

Included in this discussion are shock, wounds, burns, musculoskeletal injuries, heat- and cold-related illnesses, poisoning, sudden illness, cerebral vascular accident, and heart attack.

Shock

When a severe injury occurs, shock is likely to develop. Shock is basically a condition in which the circulatory system is not providing enough blood to all parts of the body, causing the body's organs to fail to function properly.

Shock is always life threatening, and EMS should be activated. The body's attempt to compensate for a massive injury or illness, especially those involving severe bleed-ing, often leads to other problems. During shock several things occur.

- The heart becomes unable to pump blood properly.
- Consequently, the body does not get enough oxygen, which is carried by the blood.
- The body tries to compensate by sending blood to critical organs and reducing the flow of blood to arms, legs, and skin.

Signs and Symptoms of Shock. Learn to recognize the signs and symptoms of shock.

- Patient may be restless or feel irritable.
- Weakness, dizziness, thirst, or nausea may occur.
- Breathing may be shallow and rapid.
- Skin is cool, clammy, and pale.
- Pulse is weak and rapid.
- Blood pressure is low.
- Area around the lips, eyes, and fingernails may turn blue from lack of oxygen.
- The patient may be confused and/or become suddenly unconscious.
- Dilated pupils and lackluster eyes are notable.

Types of Shock. There are eight major types of shock, including respiratory, neurogenic, cardiogenic, hemorrhagic, anaphylactic, metabolic, psychogenic, and septic. See Table 9-2 for a description of each.

TABLE 9-2	EIGHT TYPES OF SHOCK WITH DESCRIPTIONS
Type of Shock	**Description**
Respiratory	Trauma to the respiratory tract (trachea, lungs) which causes a reduction of oxygen and carbon dioxide exchange. Body cells cannot receive enough oxygen.
Neurogenic	Injury or trauma to the nervous system (spinal cord, brain). Nerve impulse to blood vessels impaired. Blood vessels remain dilated and blood pressure drops.
Cardiogenic	Myocardial infarction with damage to heart muscle; heart unable to pump effectively. Inadequate cardiac output. Body cells not receiving enough oxygen.
Hemorrhagic	Severe bleeding or loss of body fluid from trauma, surgery, or dehydration from severe nausea and vomiting. Blood pressure drops, thus blood flow is reduced to cells, tissues, and organs.
Anaphylactic	Results from reaction to substance to which patient is hypersensitive or allergic (allergen extracts, bee sting, medication, food). Outpouring of histamine results in dilation of blood vessels throughout the body, blood pressure drops and blood flow is reduced to cells, tissue, and organs.
Metabolic	Body's homeostasis impaired; acid-base balance disturbed (diabetic coma or insulin shock); body fluids unbalanced.
Psychogenic	Due to overwhelming emotional factors; i.e., fear, anger, grief. Sudden dilation of blood vessels, results in fainting because of lack of blood supply to the brain. In most cases, may not be life-threatening unless it leads to physical trauma as a result of a fall.
Septic	An acute infection, usually systemic, that overwhelms the body (toxic shock syndrome). Poisonous substances accumulate in bloodstream and blood pressure drops impairing blood flow to cells, tissues, and organs.

Treatment for Shock. A person suffering from shock needs immediate medical attention. Call for outside emergency help first, then care for the patient until help arrives. **CAUTION:** Shock requires immediate medical help. Shock is progressive and if not treated immediately, most types are life threatening. Once shock reaches a certain point, it is irreversible.

To care for a patient in shock, follow these procedures.

- Lie the patient down. This minimizes pain and decreases stress on the body.

- Loosen clothing.

- Check for an open airway.

- Control any external bleeding.

- Help the patient maintain normal body temperature. A blanket over and under the patient can help avoid chilling. Do not overheat.

- Reassure the patient.

- Elevate the legs about 12 inches, unless you suspect spinal injuries or broken bones involving the hips or legs.

- Do not give the patient anything to eat or drink.

- Ascertain that outside help has been called and stay with the patient until help arrives.

Wounds

Typically, **wounds** are classified as open wounds or closed wounds. In the closed wound, there is no break in the skin; a bruise, contusion, and hematoma are common closed wounds. An open wound represents a break in the skin and can be classified as an abrasion, avulsion, incision, laceration, or puncture wound.

Closed Wounds. Most closed wounds do not present an emergency situation. If there is pain and swelling, the application of a cold compress can be effective. Protect the patient's skin by placing a cloth beneath the source of cold; apply the compress for 20 minutes, then remove for 20 minutes; continue for 24 hours. Then apply heat 20 minutes on and 20 minutes off for the next 24 hours. A common procedure for treating closed wounds is to RICE it:

- Rest

- Ice

- Compression

- Elevation

Some closed wounds, such as hematomas, can be very dangerous and may cause internal bleeding. If the patient is in severe pain and was subject to an injury caused by high impact, call for help and keep the patient comfortable until the help arrives. Watch for symptoms of shock and monitor vital signs.

Open Wounds. Open wounds can be minor tears in the skin or more serious breaks, but all open wounds represent an opportunity for microorganisms to gain entry and cause an infection. Some major open wounds may involve heavy bleeding, which will need to be controlled, probably by suturing. A tetanus injection is indicated for an open wound if the patient has not had a booster in the past seven to ten years. See Chapter 22 for immunization information.

There are five common types of open wounds.

1. *Abrasions* are a superficial scraping of the epidermis. Because nerve endings are involved, they can be painful. However, they are not usually serious, unless they cover a large area of the body. Administer first aid by cleaning the area carefully with soap and water, apply an antiseptic ointment if prescribed by a physician, and cover with a dressing.
2. In an *avulsion*, the skin is torn off and bleeding is profuse. Avulsion wounds often occur at exposed parts: fingers, toes, ear. First, control bleeding (Procedure 9-1) if necessary. Then clean the wound. If there is a skin flap, reposition it. Apply a dressing, then bandage as necessary. Note that pieces of the body may be torn away. If possible, save the body part, keep moist, and transport with the patient.
3. *Incisions* are wounds that result from a sharp object, such as a knife or piece of glass. Incisions may need sutures. The wound must be cleaned with soap and water and a dressing applied.
4. *Lacerations* tear the body tissue and can be difficult to clean, so care must be taken to avoid infection. If there is not severe bleeding, which in itself is a cleansing mechanism, these wounds may need to be soaked to remove debris. If there is severe bleeding, it must be controlled immediately (Procedure 9-1). Lacerations with severe bleeding are likely to need suturing.
5. *Punctures* pierce and penetrate the skin and may be deep wounds while appearing insignificant. Usually, external bleeding is minimal, but the patient should be assessed for internal bleeding. Because a puncture wound is deep, the risk of infection is great and the patient should be advised to watch for signals of infection, such as pain, swelling, redness, throbbing, and warmth.

Use of Tourniquets in Emergency Care. In the past, tourniquets were regularly used in the field to control hemorrhaging from an extremity when all other attempts to control bleeding were unsuccessful. However, because tourniquet application was meant to completely stop blood flow, many times this complete lack of blood flow resulted in the death of the arm or leg. Often, the affected extremity needed to be amputated.

To remedy this situation, a "constriction band" was substituted for the tourniquet and is now widely used. The constriction band is made of a material similar to that used in the tourniquet. When the band is applied to an extremity to control bleeding, it is applied tightly enough to stem the rapid loss of blood but loosely enough to allow a small amount of blood to continue to flow. A pulse should be felt distally to the constriction band. The use of the constriction band applied in this manner allows a blood supply to the remainder of the extremity unlike the tourniquet, which cuts off all blood flow.

For information on wounds and minor surgery, see Chapter 31.

Dressings and Bandages. When a patient presents with an open wound, after treatment it is critical to dress and bandage it properly to curtail infection. This covering of the wound is accomplished by a series of dressings and bandages.

Typically, dressings are sterile pads placed directly on the wound; they often have nonstick, sterile surfaces, but they are absorbent and will soak up blood and protect the wound from microorganisms. They are often made of a gauze-type material.

Bandages, which are nonsterile, are placed over the dressing. They hold the dressing in place and are made to conform to the area to be covered. Sometimes, as in a Band-Aid, the dressing and bandage are combined. Roller bandages, such as those made of elastic, can be placed over a dressing and used to control bleeding or swelling.

Kling gauze, a type of gauze that stretches and clings as it is applied, and roller bandages, long strips of soft material wound on itself, are other types of bandage materials.

Bandages and their applications can take many shapes and forms, depending on the type of injury and the injury site. In all cases, a bandage must be secure, but not constricting. Avoid too tight or too loose a wrap.

- Spiral bandages are useful for injuries to the arms or legs (Figure 9-4).
- A figure-eight bandage will hold the dressing in place on a wound on the hand or wrist, knee, or ankle (Figure 9-5).
- Fingers, toes, arms, and legs can also be bandaged using a tubular gauze bandage (Figures 9-6, 9-7, and 9-8). Using a cylindrical applicator, a quantity of gauze is stretched over the wound site.
- Commercial arm slings are used to support injured or fractured arms (Figure 9-9). To apply, support the injured arm above and below the injury site while applying the sling.

Burns

Most burns are commonly caused by heat, chemicals, explosions, and electricity. Critical burns can be life threatening, requiring immediate medical care. According to the American Red Cross, critical burns:

- Involve breathing difficulty
- Cover more than one body part
- Involve the head, neck, hands, feet, or genitals

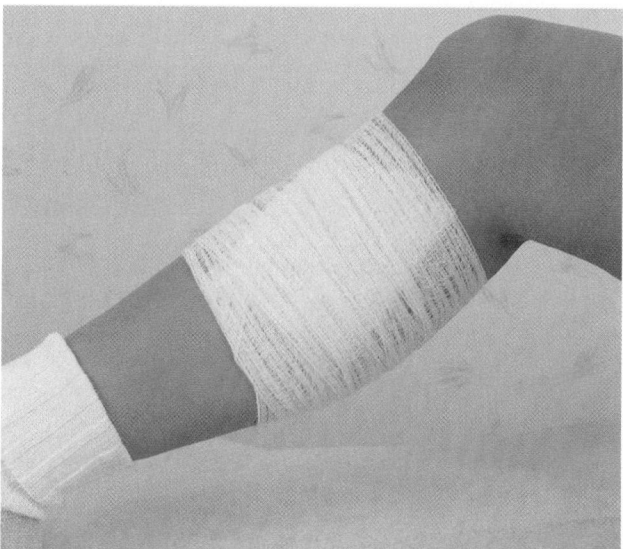

Figure 9-4 The spiral bandage is an option for arm and leg injuries.

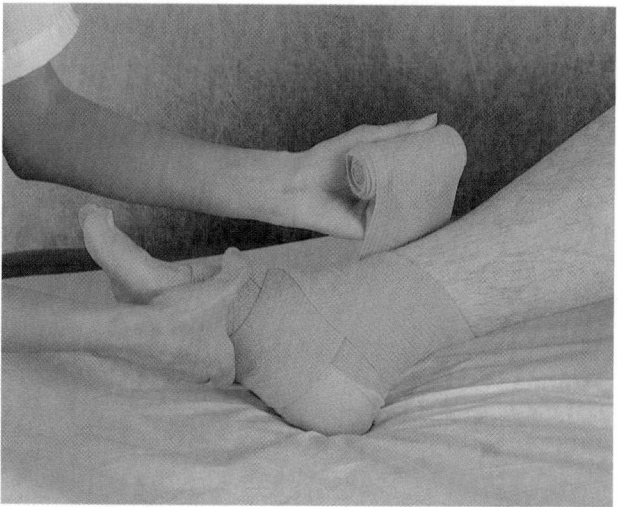

Figure 9-5 An elastic figure-eight bandage holds dressings in place or can be used for immobilization as with an ankle sprain.

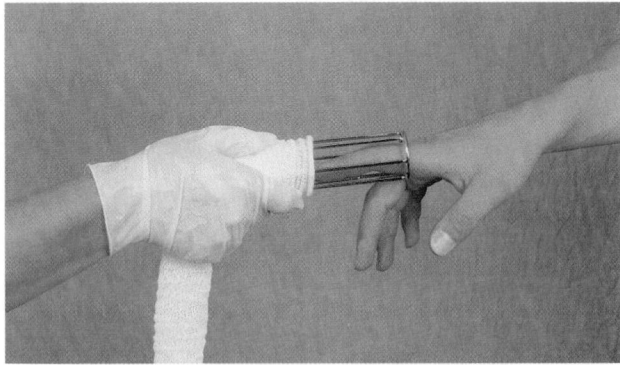

Figure 9-6   There are several types and sizes of tubular gauze applicators, including plastic, solid metal, and metal cage applicators; the metal cage is shown here. All applicators use a seamless elastic gauze bandage (also available in various sizes) that slides over the applicator. The applicator with the gauze then fits over the appendage to be wrapped.

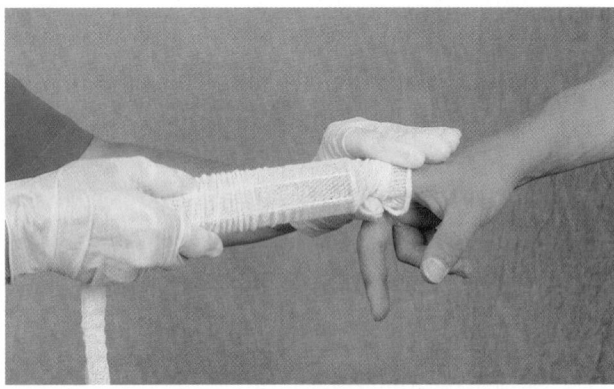

Figure 9-7   The gauze bandage is stretched over the appendage by pulling the applicator away from the base of the appendage. At the same time, the bandage should be held in place at the appendage base with the other hand.

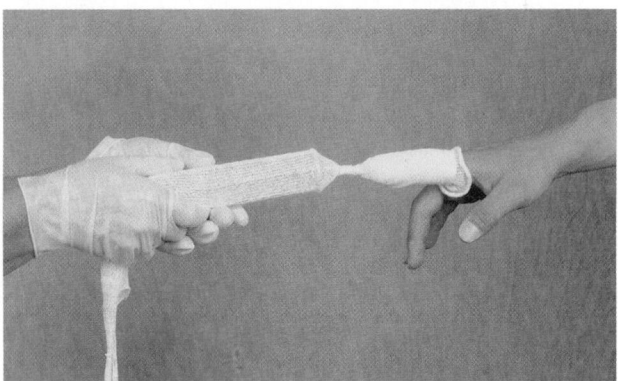

Figure 9-8   Once the applicator has been pulled off the finger, a layer of the bandage will remain on the appendage. To apply another layer, the applicator is again fitted over the finger and a new layer is applied in the same manner as before.

● are any burns to a child or elderly person (other than minor burns)

To distinguish critical from minor burns, it is important to understand the degrees of burns and what they mean.

First-, Second-, and Third-Degree Burns. First-degree burns are superficial burns that involve only the top layer of skin. The skin appears red, feels dry, is warm to the touch, and is painful. First-degree burns usually heal in a week or so with no permanent scarring (Figure 9-10).

In a second-degree burn, the skin is red and blisters are present. The healing process is slower—usually a month—and some scarring may occur. Second-degree burns affect the top layers of the skin, are very painful, and

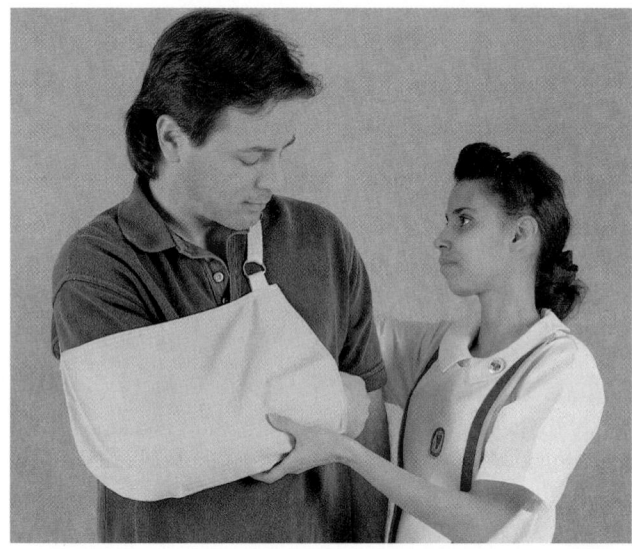

Figure 9-9   A commercial sling is used to support injured or fractured arms.

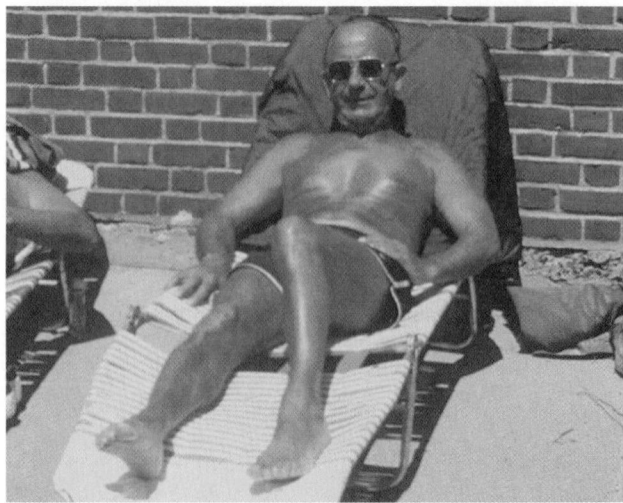

Figure 9-10   First-degree burns involve the top layer of skin. (Courtesy of the Phoenix Society of Burn Survivors, Inc.)

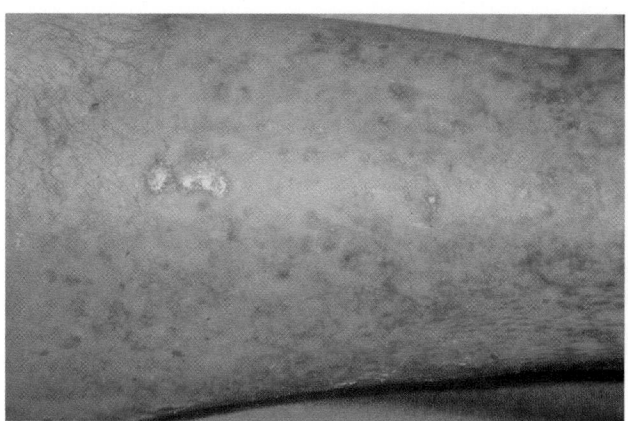

Figure 9-11 Second-degree burns affect the top layers of skin. The healing process is slower and scarring may occur. (Courtesy of the Phoenix Society of Burn Survivors, Inc.)

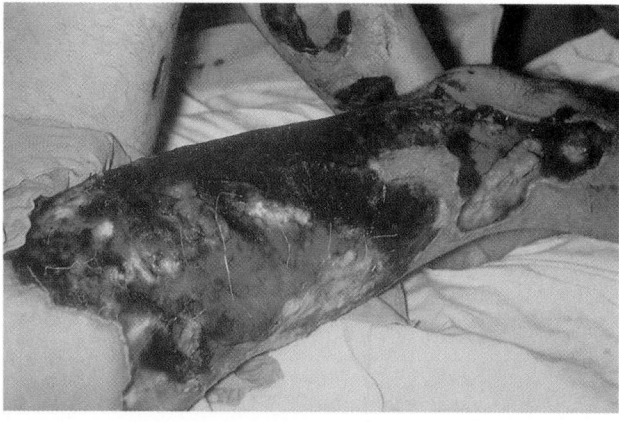

Figure 9-12 Third-degree burns are the most serious, affecting or destroying all layers of skin plus the fat, muscle, bones, and nerves. (Courtesy of the Phoenix Society of Burn Survivors, Inc.)

may take three to four weeks to heal. Some scarring may occur (Figure 9-11).

Third-degree burns are the most serious, affecting or destroying all layers of skin, plus the fat, muscles, bones, and nerves under the skin. These burns look charred or brown. There may be great pain or, if nerve endings are destroyed, the burn may be painless. Victims of third-degree burns must receive immediate medical attention both for the burn and for shock. Of serious concern with a third-degree burn, is the likelihood of infection and the amount of scarring that can result in loss of body function. Skin grafts may be necessary (Figure 9-12).

Figure 9-13 shows the relative penetration level of each degree of burn into the skin and underlying structures.

General Guidelines for Caring for Burns. Treatment for burns depends on the type of agent causing the burn. General treatment strategies for any degree of burn include the following:

- Cool the burn with large amounts of cool normal saline.
- Cover the burn with a sterile dressing if one is available and burn is minor. Otherwise, cover the burn with a sheet or other smooth textured cloth for a burn over a large area of the body.
- Be sure the patient is protected from being either chilled or overheated.

However, it is important to follow these guidelines:

- Do not apply ice or ice water to a burn.
- Do not touch a burn, except with a clean sterile dressing.
- Do not clean a severe burn, break blisters, or use any kind of ointment.
- Do not remove pieces of clothing that may be sticking to the burn.

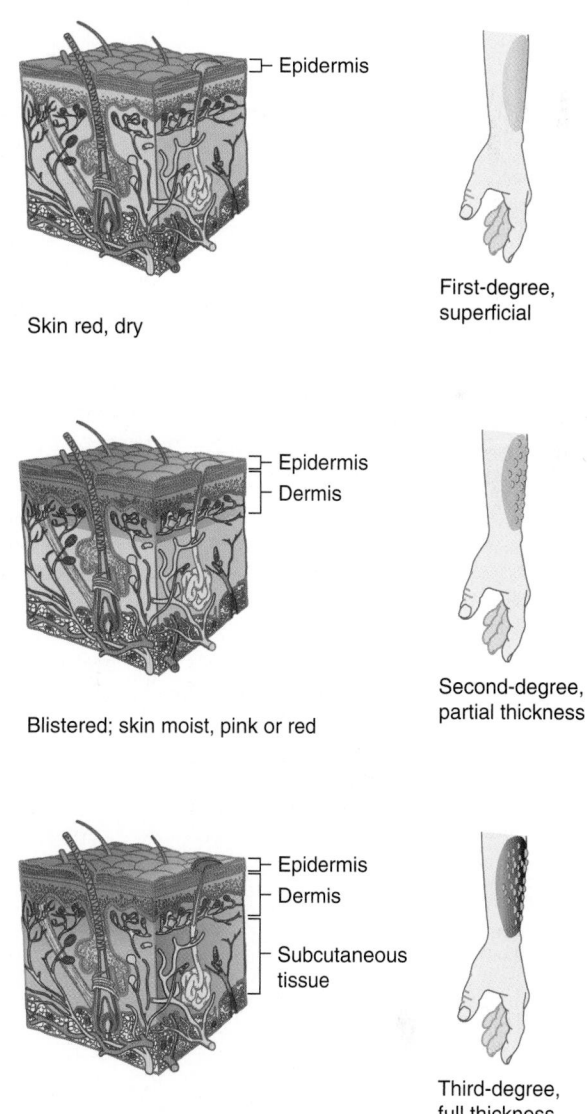

Figure 9-13 Classification of burn injuries.

First Aid for Burns. First aid for burns is outlined in Table 9-3.

Types of Burns. Most burns are caused by heat; however, burns can also be caused by chemicals, electricity, and solar radiation.

Chemical Burns. These can occur in the workplace or even in the home with "ordinary" household chemicals. In order to stop the burning process, the chemical must be removed from the skin. Have someone call an ambulance while you flush the skin or eyes with cool water. Remove any clothing contaminated by the chemicals unless they

TABLE 9-3	FIRST AID FOR BURNS

First-Degree Burn Response Guide

Questions	Responses	Action to Take	Rationale
Is skin reddened without blisters?	YES ⟹	Submerge in cool normal saline 2–5 minutes.	Stops burning process.
NO ⬇			
Does area involve: • hands? • feet? • genitals? • face?	YES ⟹	Patient to come to office.	These are potential danger areas and require evaluation by the physician.
NO ⬇			
Is patient: • elderly? • very young?	YES ⟹	Patient to come to office.	These groups are very susceptible to burn complications.
NO ⬇			
Consult physician.			Physician has final decision whether patient is seen.

Second-Degree Burn Response Guide

Questions	Responses	Action to Take	Rationale
Is skin reddened with blisters or splitting of the skin?	YES ⟹	Submerge in cool normal saline 10–15 minutes if skin is intact. Use compresses if skin is broken. Do not break blisters. Do not use anesthetic creams or sprays.	Stops burning process. If blisters are broken, can allow infection in burn. Creams or spray may slow healing process and increase severity of a burn.
NO ⬇			
Does area involve: • hands? • feet? • genitals? • face?	YES ⟹	Patient to come to office.	These are potentially dangerous areas and require medical attention.
NO ⬇			
Is the area involved larger than a child's hand?	YES ⟹	Patient to come to office.	Burns of this size are very susceptible to complications.
NO ⬇			
Is patient experiencing trouble breathing?	YES ⟹	Patient should go to emergency room.	There may be swelling of the airways because of heat.
NO ⬇			
Consult physician.			Physician has final decision whether patient is seen.

(continues)

TABLE 9-3 (continued)			
Third-Degree Burn Response Guide			
Questions	**Responses**	**Action to Take**	**Rationale**
Is skin gray, black, or charred appearing? Can muscle, fat, or bone be seen in wound?	YES ⇨	Call EMS immediately. Do not ⇨ apply cold; do not remove burnt clothing from burn area.	Life-threatening emergency that requires prompt attention.
NO ⇩			
Is patient experiencing: • pallor • loss of consciousness? • shivering?	YES ⇨	Patient in shock: ⇨ • maintain body temp. • elevate feet if appropriate. • monitor breathing. • call EMS.	Need to control shock due to loss of fluid.
NO ⇩			
Consult physician.			Physician has final decision whether patient is seen.

adhere to the skin. If clothing clings to the skin, it can be cut with scissors. Do not attempt to pull clothing away from burned area.

Electrical Burns. Electrical burns can be caused by power lines, lightning, or faulty electrical equipment in the home or workplace. **It is important to remember never to go near a patient injured by electricity until you are sure the power has been shut off because you could be injured.** If there is a downed line, call the power company and emergency medical services (EMS).

A victim of an electricity burn may be suffering from two burns: one where the power entered the body, and one where it exited. Often, the burns themselves may be minor. Of more serious consequence are the possibilities of shock, breathing difficulties, and other injuries. CPR is often needed here.

Solar Radiation. Most "sunburns," while not advisable nor good for the skin, present minor burns. If the patient has a severe burn, however, he should see a physician who will cover the burn area to reduce infection and protect the patient against chill.

Musculoskeletal Injuries

Most injuries to muscles, bones, and joints are not life threatening, but they are painful and, if not properly treated, can be disabling. Some injuries, such as those to the spinal cord, can be quite serious and can result in paralysis. These injuries are not typically seen in the ambulatory care setting.

Types of Injuries. A **sprain** is an injury to a joint, often an ankle, knee, or wrist, that involves a tearing of the ligaments. Most sprains are minor and heal quickly; others are more severe, include swelling, and may not heal properly if the patient continues to put stress on the sprained joint. Signs of a sprain are rapid swelling, discoloration at the site, and limited function. Many times it is difficult to determine whether the patient has sustained a sprain or a fracture because the degree of pain may not be a true indicator of the patient's injury. As with most closed wounds, treating the injury with the RICE method is beneficial.

A **strain** results from the overuse or stretching of a muscle or group of muscles, as with improper lifting or

Patient Teaching Tip

Some burns can be prevented. Advise patients who insist on sunbathing to protect themselves against harmful rays by using a sunscreen and avoiding the sun between 10 A.M. and 2 P.M.

Patient Teaching Tip

Advise patients not to run should their clothing catch on fire. They should fall to the ground or wrap themselves in a blanket or rug and roll on the ground to extinguish the flames.

moving heavy objects. Applications of ice and heat (as described for treatment of sprains), as well as rest, are indicated for treatment of strains.

Dislocations are painful and involve the separation of a bone from its normal position. These usually occur from the kind of wrenching motion that might result from a fall, automobile accident, or sports injury.

Fractures involve a break in a bone and can be caused by a fall, by a blow, from bone disease, or from sports injuries. There are several types of fractures, but all are classified as either open fractures or closed fractures. An open fracture involves an open wound and is characterized by a protruding bone. In a closed fracture, the skin is not broken. Signs and symptoms that occur with a fracture may include swelling, discoloration, pain, deformity, and immobility of the body part. It is not unusual for patients to tell you that they heard the bone break or that they sensed a grating feeling. Crepitation is the term that describes the grating sensation experienced when bone fragments rub together. Fractures are further defined as follows:

- Incomplete or greenstick: fracture in which the bone has cracked but the break is not all the way through. Frequently seen in children.

- Simple: complete bone break in which there is no involvement with the skin surface.

- Compound: fracture in which the bone protrudes though the skin surface, creating the possibility of infection.

- Impacted: fracture in which the broken ends are jammed into each other.

- Comminuted: more than one fracture line and several bone fragments are present.

- Spiral: fracture that occurs with a severe twisting action, causing the break to wind around the bone.

- Depressed: fracture that occurs with severe head injuries in which a broken piece of skull is driven inward.

- Colles: fracture often caused by falling on an outstretched hand. Involves the distal end of the radius and results in displacement, causing a bulge at the wrist.

See Figure 9-14 for examples of these fractures.

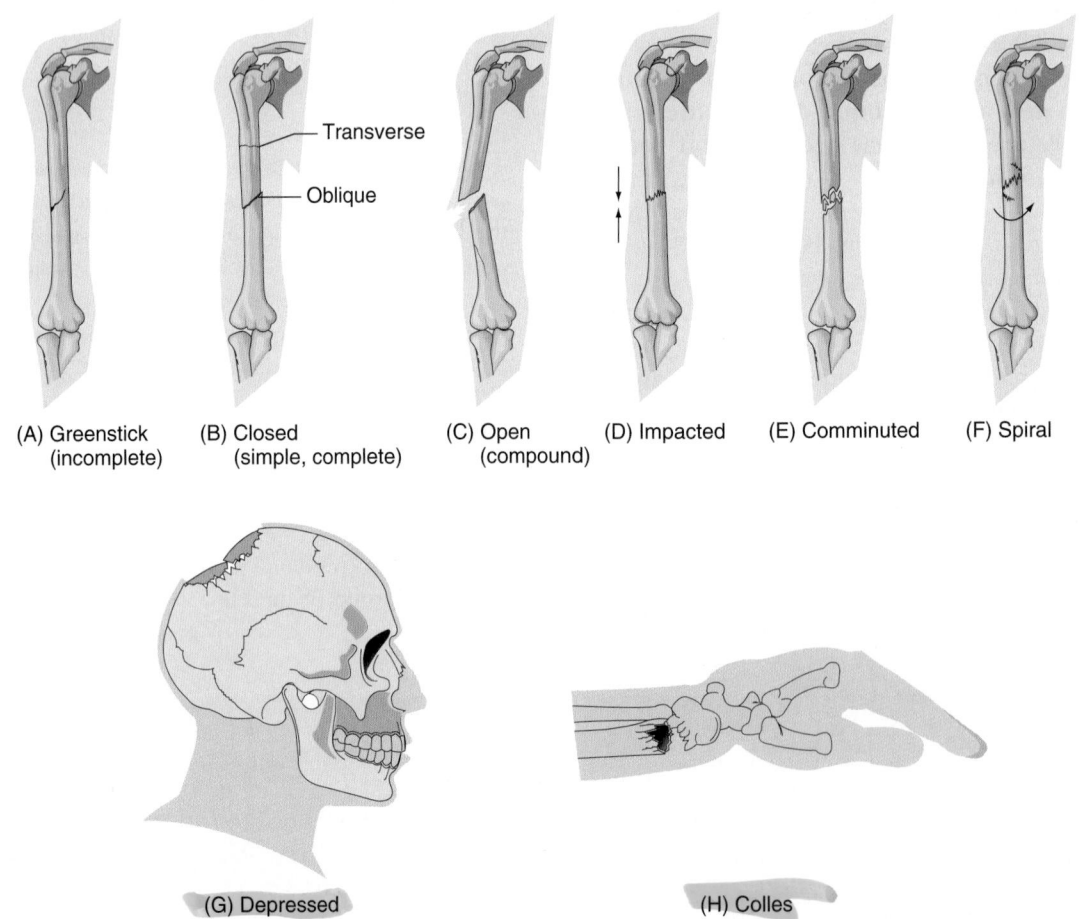

(A) Greenstick (incomplete)   (B) Closed (simple, complete)   (C) Open (compound)   (D) Impacted   (E) Comminuted   (F) Spiral

Transverse
Oblique

(G) Depressed   (H) Colles

Figure 9-14   Types of fractures.

Assessing Injuries to Muscles, Bones, and Joints. Sometimes it is difficult to determine the extent of an injury, especially in closed fractures. There are some assessment techniques to call upon, however, to gauge the seriousness of an injury.

- Note the extent of bruising and swelling.

- Pain is a signal of injury.

- There may be noticeable deformity to the bone or joint.

- Use of the injured area is limited.

- Talk to the patient: what was the cause of the injury? What was the sound or sensation at the time of injury?

Caring for Muscle, Bone, and Joint Injuries. Most injuries to muscles, bones, and joints are treated in a similar way; all require rest, elevation of the injured part, immobilization, and the application of ice to the injury.

After calling for outside care (always check for life-threatening symptoms, such as breathing difficulties, bleeding, or head, neck, or back injuries), it is important to immobilize the injured area if the patient must be moved. EMS personnel employ a variety of **splints** to immobilize bones and joints. See Procedure 9-2 for splinting an arm in the ambulatory care setting.

Heat- and Cold-Related Illnesses

The condition of patients who have been subject to extreme heat and cold can deteriorate very rapidly and either a heat- or cold-related illness can result in death. Individuals especially vulnerable to extreme exposures include the very young and very old; individuals who must work out of doors; and people who may suffer from poor circulation.

Heat-Related Illnesses. Illnesses related to heat, in increasing degree of severity, include heat cramps, heat exhaustion, and heat stroke. Heat cramps, the least serious, involve cramping in the legs and abdomen due to excessive body exposure or exercise in hot weather. Heat cramps should be considered a signal to stop, slow down, rest in a cool place, and drink plenty of water. Salt tablets should not be taken. The individual should lightly stretch the muscles. Heat cramps can progress to heat exhaustion or heat stroke, both more serious conditions.

Heat exhaustion, often experienced by people who work or exercise in extreme heat, is a more serious reaction and is signaled by exhaustion, cold and clammy skin, profuse sweating, headache, and general weakness. The individual should come out of the heat immediately, apply cool, wet towels, and slowly drink cool water. The physician will advise the patient not to resume activity in the heat.

Heat stroke is the least common, but the most dangerous of heat-related illnesses and requires immediate medical attention. Heat stroke is characterized by red, dry, hot skin, an abnormal, weak pulse, and breathing that is shallow and fast. In heat stroke, the body systems are extremely taxed. EMS should be alerted; until they arrive, stay with the patient, watch for breathing problems, and attempt to lower body temperature by applying cool, wet towels or sheets.

Cold-Related Illnesses. Exposure to extreme cold for prolonged periods can lead to frostbite or hypothermia.

Frostbite, which typically affects the extremities such as fingers, toes, ears, and nose, involves the freezing of exposed body parts. Symptoms include skin that becomes off-color, that is cold, or that takes on a waxy appearance. Severity can range from the superficial (frostnip) to more penetrating stages, which may require amputation.

Individuals with frostbite need immediate medical attention. To care for frostbitten extremities, warm the area of injury by wrapping clothing or blankets around the affected body part. Be careful in handling the frozen part. It is best to have the patient transported as soon as possible to emergency care. This type of facility is better able to properly rewarm the frozen part, preventing further tissue damage.

Hypothermia is a serious illness in which the body temperature falls to a perilously low level. It can result in death if the individual does not receive care and if the progression of hypothermia is not reversed. Hypothermia occurs when a person falls through the ice or is exposed to cold temperatures, for example, after getting lost in the woods while hiking. Symptoms include shivering, cold skin, and confusion.

After checking for breathing problems and alerting EMS, care for the patient. Make the individual comfortable, provide a source of warmth, such as a blanket, and *gradually* warm the body. If clothing is wet or cold, remove and put on dry clothing. In extreme cases, it may be necessary to provide rescue breathing, which is covered later in this chapter.

Poisoning

Poisons can enter the body in four ways:

- *Ingestion.* Ingested poisons enter the body by swallowing. Swallowed poisons may include medications, plant material, household chemicals, contaminated foods, and drugs.

- *Inhalation.* Poisons are inhaled into the body in poorly ventilated areas where cleaning fluids, paints and chemical cleaners, or carbon monoxide may be present.

- *Absorption.* Poisons absorbed through the skin include plant materials such as poison oak or ivy, lawn care products such as chemical pesticides, and other chemical powders or liquids.

- *Injection.* Drug abuse is the most common cause of injected poisons. The stingers of insects inject poisons into the body and can be extremely dangerous and lead to anaphylactic shock in allergic individuals.

Whenever a patient calls regarding poisoning or there is a suspicion of poisoning, call the local poison control center or the local emergency number and ask for advice. Telephone numbers of the poison control center should be posted in a familiar and accessible place.

The treatment for poisoning will vary according to the source of the poisoning and must be tailored to the specific incident. The physician will have advised staff regarding specific poisoning antidotes. Generally, do not give the patient anything to eat or drink; try to determine what poison the patient was exposed to and, if ingested, how much was taken; if the patient vomits, save some of the vomitus for analysis.

If prescribed by a physician, two medications used to treat poisoning include syrup of ipecac, which can induce vomiting, and activated charcoal, which is used to absorb certain swallowed poisons.

Insect Stings. The medical assistant in the ambulatory care setting is likely to receive a number of calls every summer from patients who have been stung by insects, typically yellow jackets, hornets, honeybees, or wasps. In the nonallergic patient, the sting is likely to result in localized swelling and tenderness and slight redness. The physician will recommend that these localized symptoms be managed with a topical cream and oral antihistamines. Swelling can be significant and cause for serious concern if the sting occurred in a vulnerable area of the body such as the mouth or tongue. Swelling in these locations can be

Patient Teaching Tip

Remind patients who are parents of young children to remove any potential sources of poisoning from their homes or to keep them in locked cabinets. Also advise them to include the nearby poison control center in their list of emergency phone numbers. They should also keep syrup of ipecac and activated charcoal on hand.

Patient Teaching Tip

Advise all patients with known allergic reactions to be particularly careful when working or playing outdoors. Insects are not usually aggressive until their nests are approached; however, often these nests are not easy to detect and an individual may approach one without being aware of its presence. Patients with allergies to insects should always wear shoes out-of-doors, wear light-colored clothing, preferably with long sleeves and pant legs, look before taking a sip from a beverage when outdoors, and inspect lawn areas, shrubbery, and building walls periodically for evidence of stinging insect nests.

frightening and dangerous because it can impair breathing. An antihistamine, administered as soon as possible after the sting, may help to curtail symptoms somewhat. Treatment for insect stings in nonallergic individuals consists of removing the stinger by scraping it off with the edge of something rigid such as a credit card or your fingernail. Tweezers can cause more venom to be dispersed into the patient's body tissues so should not be used. Wash the area with soap and water, apply a cold pack to the site, and watch for an anaphylactic reaction.

The individual who experiences an allergic reaction or hypersensitivity to a sting needs to be seen immediately, for in severe cases a sting may induce an anaphylactic reaction which can lead to death. If allergic, individuals who have been stung are likely to experience symptoms within a half-hour after the incident. Symptoms are generalized throughout the body and may include hives, itching, lightheadedness, and may progress to difficulty breathing, faintness, and eventual loss of consciousness.

For individuals with known allergic reactions, the physician will prescribe epinephrine, which patients should carry with them and self-inject should they not be able to get immediate emergency care. The patient should then seek immediate emergency treatment. For individuals who present at the ambulatory care setting with an apparent allergic reaction to a sting, the physician will prescribe epinephrine. Attempt to allay patient apprehension and monitor vital signs while waiting for EMS personnel to arrive.

Sudden Illness

Sudden illness is, by definition, an unexpected occurrence. While the cause of the illness may be inexplicable, it is important to respond sensibly and responsibly within the parameters of knowledge and resources.

Sudden illnesses include, but are not limited to, fainting, seizures, diabetic reaction, and hemorrhage.

Fainting. Also known as syncope, fainting involves a loss of consciousness, caused by an insufficient supply of blood to the brain. Loss of consciousness may simply be the result of a fainting episode or it may indicate a more serious medical problem such as diabetic coma or shock. A fall during a fainting incident may result in bodily harm.

If a patient in the office or clinic "feels faint," indicated by lightheadedness, weakness, nausea, or unsteadiness, have the individual lie down or sit down with head level with the knees. This may prevent a fainting spell. As a part of office policy, aromatic spirits of ammonia may be administered to revive the patient who faints. **CAUTION:** Hold the crushed ampule of ammonia at least six inches away from the patient's nose and eyes. Move it back and forth since the fumes are very irritating to eyes and mucous membranes.

If a patient faints, gradually lower the patient to a flat surface, loosen any tight clothing, and check breathing and for any life-threatening emergencies. Elevate the legs if there is no back or head injury. If vomiting occurs, place the patient on the side. While fainting is typically not serious in itself, 911 or EMS may need to be called since the problem may be indicative of a more complex medical condition.

Seizures. Seizures or convulsions occur when normal brain functioning is disrupted, which can occur for a variety of reasons including fever, disease such as diabetes, infection, or injury to the brain. Epilepsy is a common cause of convulsions. Involuntary spasms or contractions of muscles characterize seizures.

To the onlooker, seizures look frightening and painful, which may lead inexperienced individuals to try to stop the seizure when they see it occurring in another individual. A patient suffering from a seizure should never be restrained; simply care for the victim of a seizure with compassion and medical understanding. The goal is to protect the patient from self-injury during the episode. Also, do not force anything between the patient's clenched teeth—individuals experiencing seizures cannot "swallow" their tongues.

Most patients will recover from a seizure in a few minutes. During the seizure, protect the patient from injury, cushion the patient's head, and roll the patient to the side if any fluid is in the mouth. After the seizure subsides, calm and comfort the patient.

If a patient is known to regularly have seizures, and the patient's seizure subsides in a matter of minutes, EMS personnel do not need to be summoned. Repeated seizures during the same time frame, however, dictate a call to emergency services, as does any seizure if the patient is diabetic, pregnant, injured, or does not regain consciousness after the incident.

Diabetes. Diabetes is defined by the American Diabetes Society as the "inability of the body to properly convert sugar from food into energy."

Under normal functioning, the body produces a hormone called insulin, which transports sugars into body cells. In some cases, the body does not produce insulin or does not produce enough insulin; this results in diabetes.

Diabetes occurs in two major types:

- Type I, or insulin-dependent diabetes.

- Type II, or noninsulin-dependent diabetes, which usually occurs in adults. In Type II, the body produces insulin in insufficient quantities.

Complications from diabetes, which you may encounter in a medical office or clinic setting, include diabetic coma (acidosis) and insulin shock or reaction. The physician will prescribe either insulin or glucose prior to the patient being transported to the hospital. Both are serious emergencies that require immediate EMS assistance. See Table 9-4 for common causes and symptoms of diabetic coma or insulin shock.

Hemorrhage. The different sources of bleeding determine the seriousness of hemorrhage, or bleeding.

External Bleeding. External bleeding includes capillary, venous, and arterial bleeding. Capillary bleeding, often from cuts and scratches, usually clots without first-aid measures. Bleeding from a vein, which is characterized by dark red blood that flows steadily, needs to be controlled quickly (see Procedure 9-1) to avoid excessive blood loss. Bleeding from an artery produces bright red bleeding that spurts from the wound; this is the most serious type of bleeding and occurs when an artery is punctured or severed. Like venous bleeding, arterial bleeding requires immediate emergency care, for serious loss of blood and profound irreversible shock can quickly ensue.

Epistaxis, or nosebleed, may be the result of breathing dry air for a long period of time; may result from injury or blowing the nose too hard; may be caused by high altitudes; may be caused by hypertension (high blood pressure); or may result from overuse of medications such as aspirin and anticoagulants.

To control nosebleeds, seat the patient, elevate the patient's head, and pinch the nostrils for at least ten minutes. Assist the patient to sit with head tilted forward so blood running down the back of the throat will not be aspirated. If bleeding cannot be controlled, the physician may request that you activate EMS.

TABLE 9-4   CAUSES AND SYMPTOMS OF DIABETIC COMA AND INSULIN SHOCK

Diabetic Coma or Acidosis		Insulin Shock or Reaction	
Causes	Too little insulin, too much to eat, infections, fever, emotional stress	Causes	Too much insulin or oral hypoglycemic drug, too little to eat, an unusual amount of exercise
Symptoms	Skin: Dry and flushed	Symptoms	Skin: Moist and pale
	Behavior: Drowsy		Behavior: Often excited
	Mouth: Dry		Mouth: Drooling
	Thirst: Intense		Thirst: Absent
	Hunger: Absent		Hunger: Present
	Vomiting: Common		Vomiting: Usually absent
	Respiration: Exaggerated, air hungry		Respiration: Normal or shallow
	Breath: Fruity odor of acetone		Breath: Usually normal
	Pulse: Weak and rapid		Pulse: Full and pounding (gives patient feeling of heart pounding)
	Vision: Dim		Vision: Diplopia (double)
	Blood glucose over 200 mg/100 ml		Blood glucose low (40–70 mg/100 ml)
First aid	Keep patient warm	First aid	If conscious, give patient sugar or any food containing sugar (fruit juice, candy, crackers, etc.)
	Obtain medical help immediately		Obtain medical help immediately

Internal Bleeding. Internal bleeding may be minor or serious depending on the cause of the injury. A contusion, or bruise, will result in minor internal bleeding. A sharp blow may induce severe internal bleeding.

Because there is no visible blood flow, it is important to recognize other symptoms of internal bleeding. Symptoms are similar to those of shock and include a rapid, weak pulse, shallow breathing, cold, clammy skin, dilated pupils, dizziness, faintness, thirst, restlessness, and a feeling of anxiety. There may be pain, tenderness, or swelling at the injury site. The abdomen may be board-like.

If internal bleeding is suspected, ask another staff member to call EMS; until they arrive, stay with the patient and take measures to prevent shock. Monitor vital signs.

Cerebral Vascular Accident (CVA)

The common term for a cerebral vascular accident (CVA) is stroke. A stroke is the result of a ruptured blood vessel in the brain; it can also be caused by the occlusion of a blood vessel or by a clot. Both these situations can result in blood spilling over brain cells and depriving them of oxygen, causing them to die. Symptoms of a stroke

Patient Teaching Tip

Advise the patient not to blow the nose for several hours following an epistaxis.

include numbness in face, arm, leg on one side of the body, loss of vision, severe headache, mental confusion, slurred speech, nausea, vomiting, and difficulty in breathing and swallowing. Paralysis may be present. If a patient is suspected of having a stroke, call EMS, loosen tight clothing, lie the patient down and keep her comfortable. Position the patient's head to facilitate flow of secretion from the mouth to avoid choking and maintain an open airway. Do not give anything by mouth and monitor vital signs. Immediate emergency care is critical for all individuals experiencing strokes. If the stroke is caused by a clot that blocks blood flow, a recently released drug may be able to protect the individual from permanent injury. Rapid transport to the hospital is important for treatment to be instituted as soon as possible. Treatment with the clot-dissolving drug must be given within three hours of onset of symptoms.

Heart Attack

Heart attack, also known as myocardial infarction, is usually caused by blockage of one or more of the coronary arteries. Symptoms include tightness of the chest, pain radiating down one or both arms, or pain radiating into the left shoulder and jaw. Other signs include rapid and weak pulse, excessive perspiration, agitation, nausea, and cold, clammy skin.

If you suspect the patient is experiencing a heart attack, contact EMS immediately, loosen tight clothing, and keep the patient comfortable. Prepare to give oxygen and other medications such as aspirin as directed by the physician. Monitor vital signs. If the patient suffers an episode of cardiac fibrillation, cardioversion or defibrillation may be necessary. See Chapter 30. Prepare to begin CPR if necessary.

PROCEDURES FOR BREATHING EMERGENCIES AND CARDIAC ARREST

Breathing or respiratory emergencies occur for a variety of reasons, including choking, shock, allergies, and other illnesses or injuries such as drowning and electrical shock. When an individual stops breathing, artificial breathing must be given quickly, for without a constant supply of oxygen, brain damage or death will occur.

When the breathing problem is accompanied by cardiac arrest, the rescue breathing must be accompanied by chest compressions. This is known as **cardiopulmonary resuscitation (CPR)**. Cardiac emergencies may occur in the medical office due to the large number of patients who have heart disease.

The procedures that follow will help you respond to breathing emergencies in your clinic or office until EMS arrives. The techniques vary for conscious and unconscious individuals, and for adults, children, and infants. These procedures are for review purposes only; it is essential that every medical assistant take first aid and CPR courses and frequent refresher courses.

Heimlich Maneuver (Abdominal Thrust)

A common cause of breathing difficulty results from choking. If an individual signals distress from choking, assist the patient in coughing up the object (Figures 9-15 and 9-16). If the patient cannot cough up the object, and the breathing airway is becoming completely blocked, act immediately. It is apparent that the airway is becoming blocked when the patient cannot cough or speak and the patient uses the universal sign for choking.

Have someone call an ambulance while you perform abdominal thrusts, known as the **Heimlich maneuver**. Patients can be taught to give themselves abdominal thrusts if they are alone and choking (Figure 9-17).

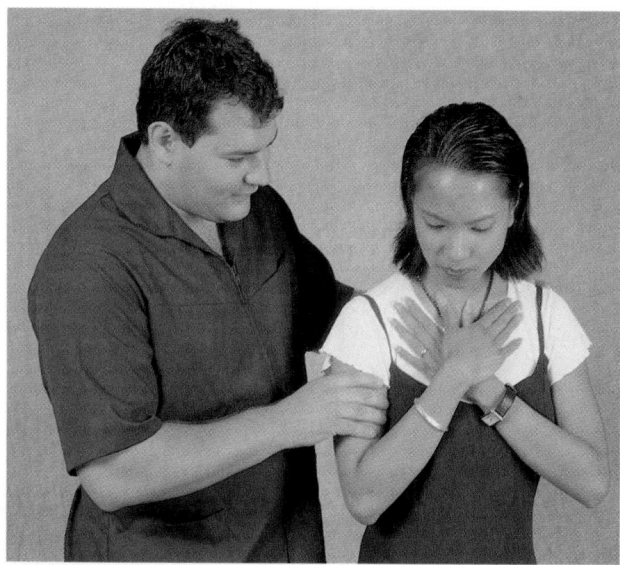

Figure 9-16 Assist the patient in coughing up an object by encouraging continuous coughing.

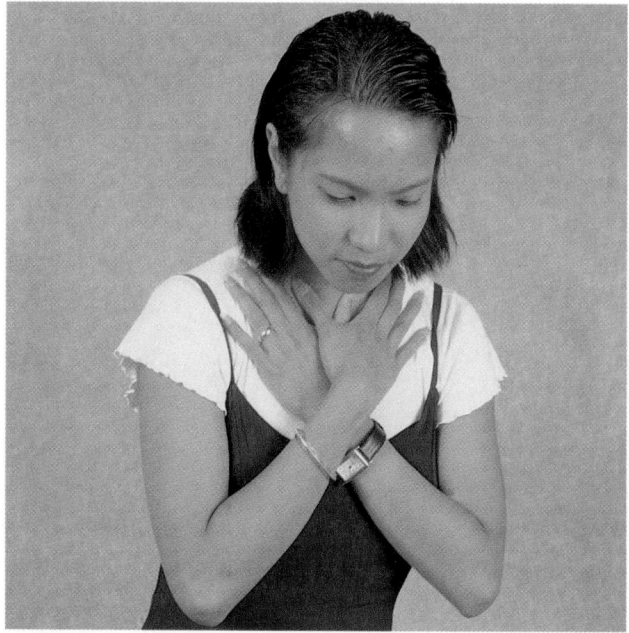

Figure 9-15 Universal sign for choking.

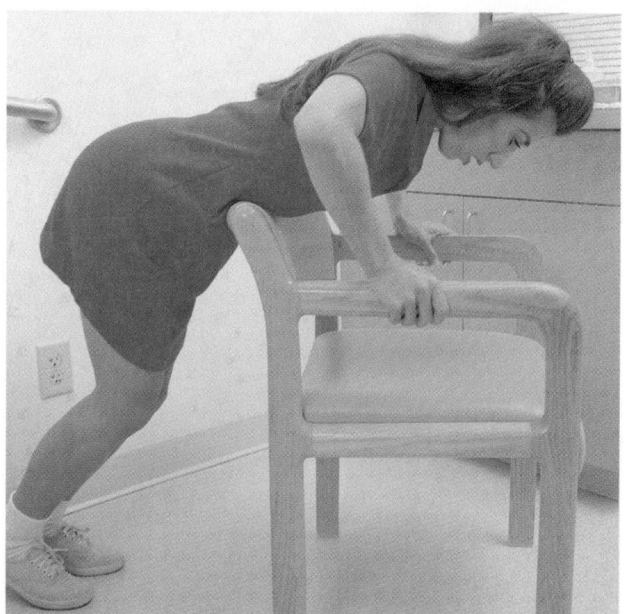

Figure 9-17 If alone, individuals can self-administer the Heimlich maneuver by using the back of a chair or similar hard object.

Procedures 9-3, 9-4, 9-5, 9-6, and 9-7 describe how to perform the Heimlich maneuver for adults, children, and infants.

Rescue Breathing

Individuals in respiratory arrest require immediate emergency care. **Rescue breathing**, previously called mouth-to-mouth resuscitation, provides oxygen to the patient until emergency personnel arrive.

When performing rescue breathing procedures in the ambulatory care setting, it is recommended that resuscitation mouthpieces be used and that direct mouth-to-mouth (i.e., with no personal protective equipment) resuscitation never be used.

Procedures for rescue breathing differ for adults, children, and infants. See Procedures 9-8, 9-9, and 9-10.

Cardiopulmonary Resuscitation (CPR)

The combination of rescue breathing and chest compressions is known as CPR, which stands for cardiopulmonary resuscitation. Alone, CPR cannot save an individual from cardiac arrest—it represents preliminary care until advanced medical help is available to the heart attack victim.

When performing CPR, the rule is that you do not stop until

- another trained person can take over
- EMS arrives and takes over care of the patient
- you are physically exhausted and not able to continue
- the environment becomes unsafe for any reason

Procedure 9-1   Control of Bleeding

STANDARD PRECAUTIONS:

PURPOSE:
To control bleeding caused by an open wound.

EQUIPMENT/SUPPLIES:
Sterile dressings
Sterile gloves
Mask and eye protection
Gown
Biohazard waste container

PROCEDURE STEPS:
1. Wash hands.
2. Put on gloves.
3. Apply eye and mask protection and gown if splashing is likely to occur.
4. Assemble equipment and supplies.
5. Apply dressing and press firmly (Figure 9-18A).
6. Apply pressure bandage over the dressing.
7. If bleeding continues, elevate arm above heart level (Figure 9-18B).
8. If bleeding still continues, press adjacent artery against bone (Figure 9-18C). Notify the physician if bleeding cannot be controlled.

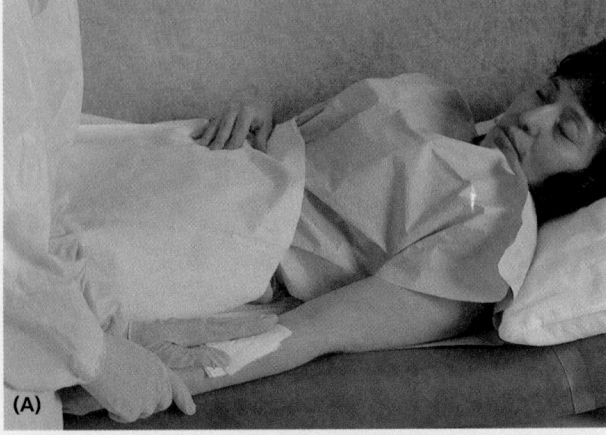
(A)

Figure 9-18   (A) Apply dressing and press firmly.

(continues)

Procedure 9-1 (continued)

9. Dispose of waste in biohazard container.
10. Remove gloves, dispose of in biohazard container.
11. Wash hands.
12. Document procedure.

CAUTION: If bleeding is not controlled, the patient may go into hemorrhagic shock. Be prepared to call EMS immediately.

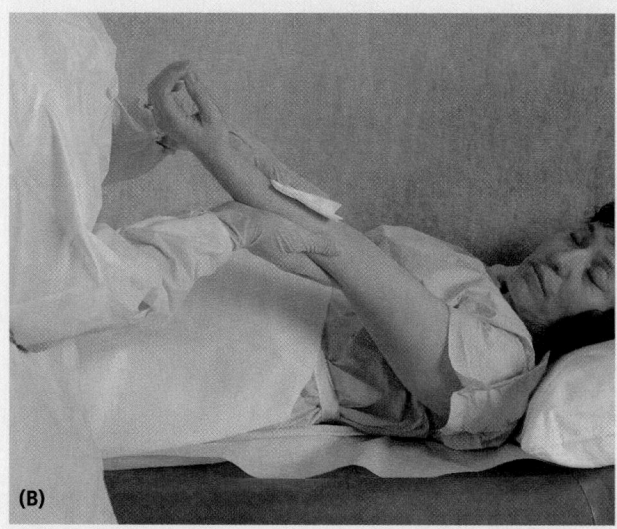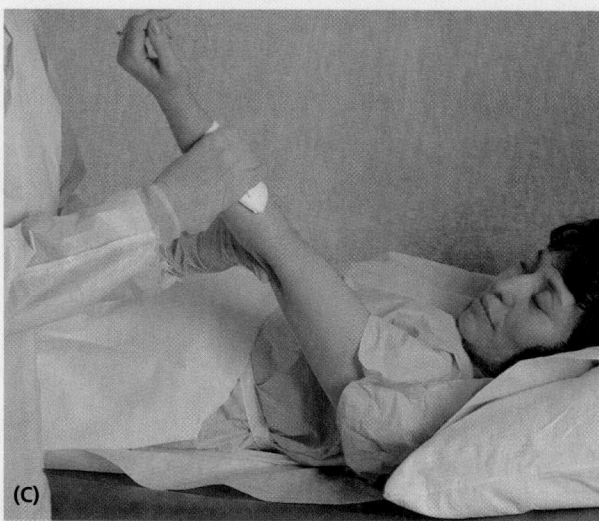

Figure 9-18 (B) Elevate arm above heart level. (C) Press artery against bone.

Procedure 9-2 Applying an Arm Splint

STANDARD PRECAUTIONS:

PURPOSE:

To immobilize the area above and below the injured part of the arm in order to reduce pain and prevent further injury.

EQUIPMENT/SUPPLIES:

Thin piece of rigid board; cardboard can be used if necessary

Gauze roller bandage

PROCEDURE STEPS:

1. Place the padded splint under the injured area.
2. Hold the splint in place with gauze roller bandage.
3. After splinting, check circulation (note color and temperature of skin, check pulse) to ascertain that the splint is not too tightly applied.
4. A sling can now be applied to keep the arm elevated, which increases comfort and reduces swelling.
5. Wash hands.
6. Document the procedure.

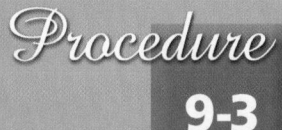

Heimlich Maneuver for a Conscious Adult
9-3

STANDARD PRECAUTIONS:

PURPOSE:
To open up a blocked airway.

EQUIPMENT/SUPPLIES:
None needed

PROCEDURE STEPS:
1. Place the thumb side of your fist against the middle of the abdomen, just above the umbilicus and below the xiphoid process.
2. Grasp your fist with your other hand and give quick upward thrusts (Figure 9-19).
3. Repeat the procedure until the patient coughs up the object. If the person becomes unconscious, perform abdominal thrusts for an unconscious individual (Procedure 9-4).
4. Wash hands.
5. Document the procedure.

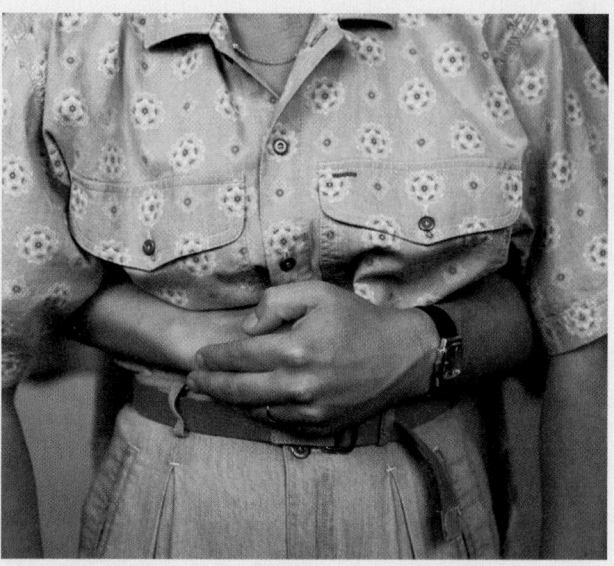

Figure 9-19 Grasp your fist with your other hand and give quick thrusts.

Heimlich Maneuver for an Unconscious Adult or Child
9-4

STANDARD PRECAUTIONS:

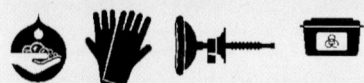

PURPOSE:
To open up a blocked airway.

EQUIPMENT/SUPPLIES:
Gloves
Resuscitation mouthpiece
Biohazard waste container

PROCEDURE STEPS:
1. Have someone call emergency services.
2. Put on gloves if available.
3. Lie person on back. Open victim's mouth and look

for foreign object. Position resuscitation mouthpiece. Tilt back person's head (Figure 9-20A).
4. Give breaths (Figure 9-20B).
5. If air will not go in, retilt head to try to breathe again. If air will not go in, place the heel of your hand against the abdomen above the umbilicus and below the xiphoid process of the sternum (Figure 9-20C).
6. Kneel astride the patient's thighs. Give up to five abdominal thrusts (Figure 9-20D).
7. Lift the jaw and sweep out the mouth (Figure 9-20E).
8. Tilt back the head, lift the chin, and give breaths again. Continue giving breaths and thrusts, and

(continues)

Procedure

9-4 *(continued)*

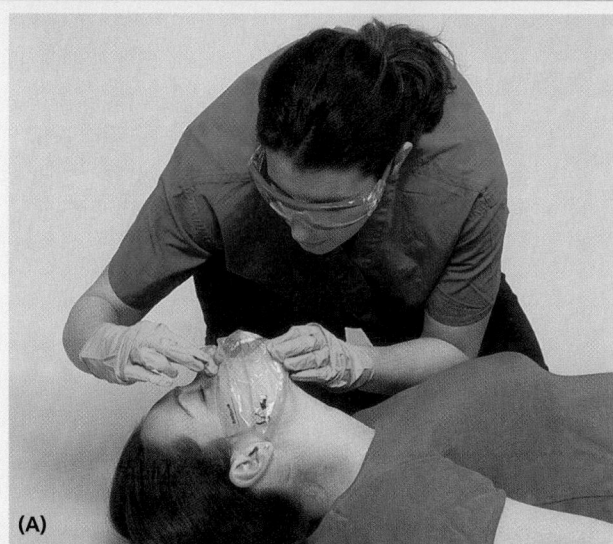

(A)

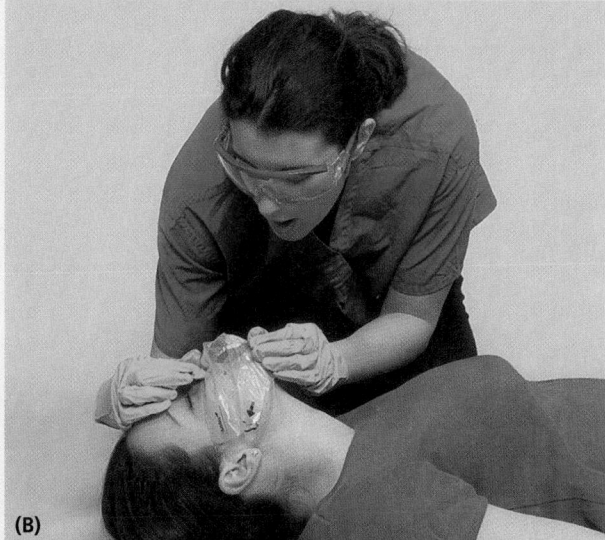

(B)

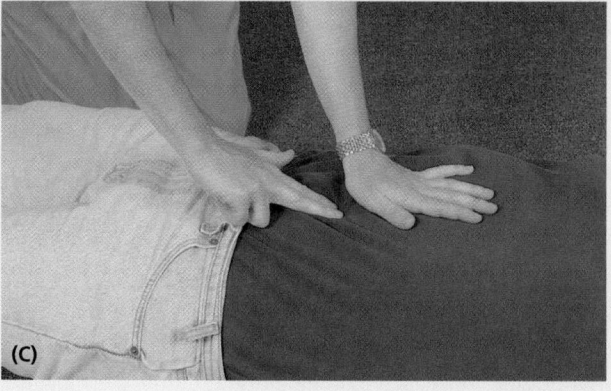

(C)

sweeping the mouth until breaths go in. If the airway is cleared and victim does not begin to breathe on his own, prepare to perform CPR (Procedure 9-11).

9. Dispose of waste in biohazard container.
10. Remove gloves, dispose of in biohazard container, and wash hands.
11. Monitor vital signs.
12. Document the procedure.

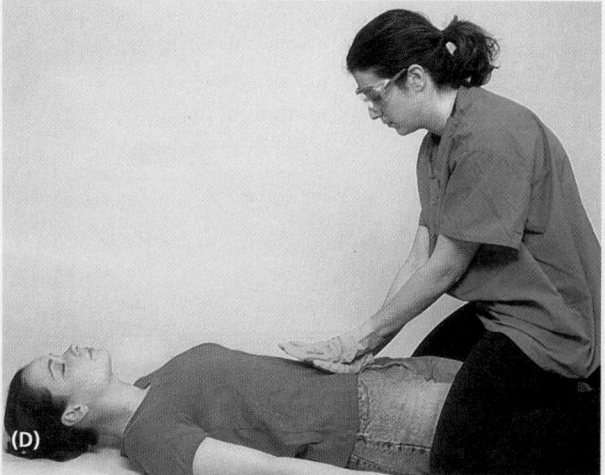

(D)

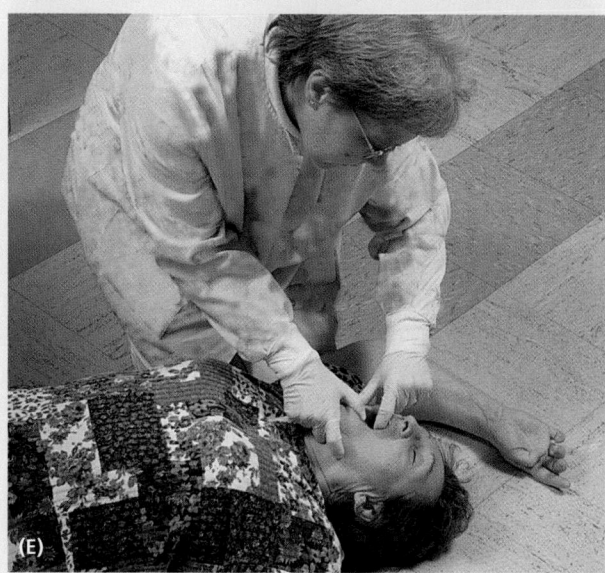

(E)

Figure 9-20 (A) Tilt back head. (B) Give breaths. (C) If air does not go in, place heel of hand against abdomen above the umbilicus and below the xiphoid process of the sternum (2 finger widths or 1½ inches above xiphoid). (D) Give up to five abdominal thrusts. (E) Lift jaw and sweep out mouth.

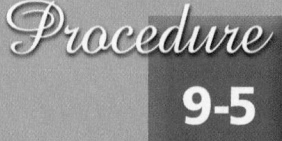

Heimlich Maneuver
for a Conscious Child

9-5

STANDARD PRECAUTIONS:

PURPOSE:
To open up a blocked airway.

EQUIPMENT/SUPPLIES:
None needed

PROCEDURE STEPS:

1. Place the thumb side of your fist against the middle of the child's abdomen, just above the umbilicus and below the xiphoid process (Figure 9-21A).

2. Grasp your fist with your other hand. Give quick upward thrusts (Figure 9-21B). Repeat the procedure until the object is expelled or until the patient loses consciousness (see Heimlich maneuver for unconscious child, Procedure 9-4).

3. Wash hands.

4. Document the procedure.

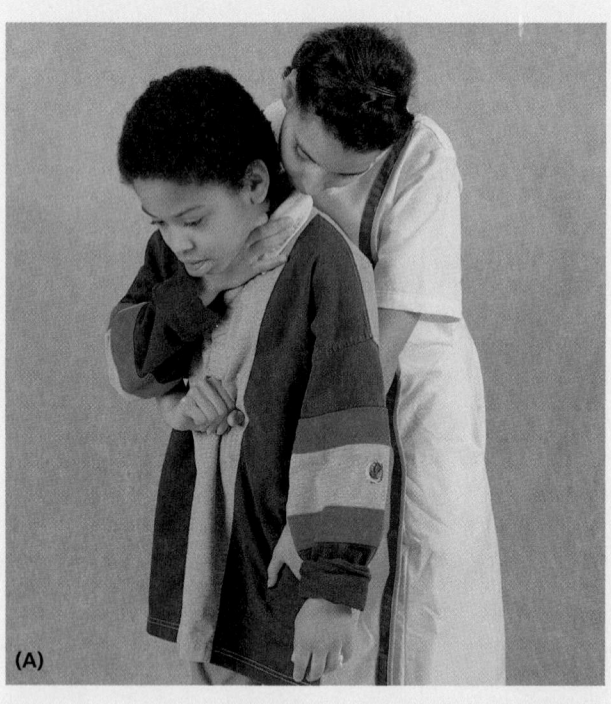

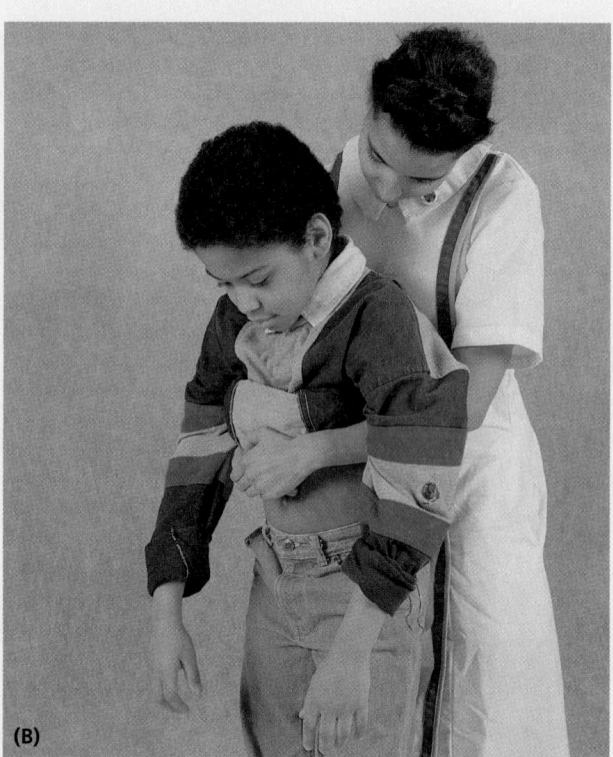

(A)

(B)

Figure 9-21 (A) Place the thumb side of your fist against the middle of the abdomen, just above the umbilicus and below the xiphoid process. (B) Grasp your fist with your other hand and give quick upward thrusts.

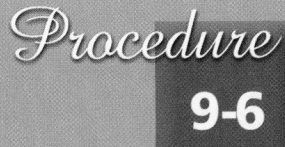

Back Blows and Chest Thrusts for a Conscious Infant Who Is Choking

STANDARD PRECAUTIONS:

PURPOSE:
To open up a blocked airway and assist an infant unable to cough, cry, or breathe.

EQUIPMENT/SUPPLIES:
None needed

PROCEDURE STEPS:

1. With the infant face down on your forearm, give five back blows between the infant's shoulder blades with the heel of your hand (Figure 9-22A).

2. Position the infant face up on your forearm.
3. Give five chest thrusts on about the center of the breastbone (Figure 9-22B).
4. Look in the infant's mouth for the object. Repeat the back blows and chest thrusts and look for object until the infant begins to breathe on own. If the infant becomes unconscious, use back blow and chest thrust techniques for unconscious infants (Procedure 9-7).
5. Wash hands.
6. Document the procedure.

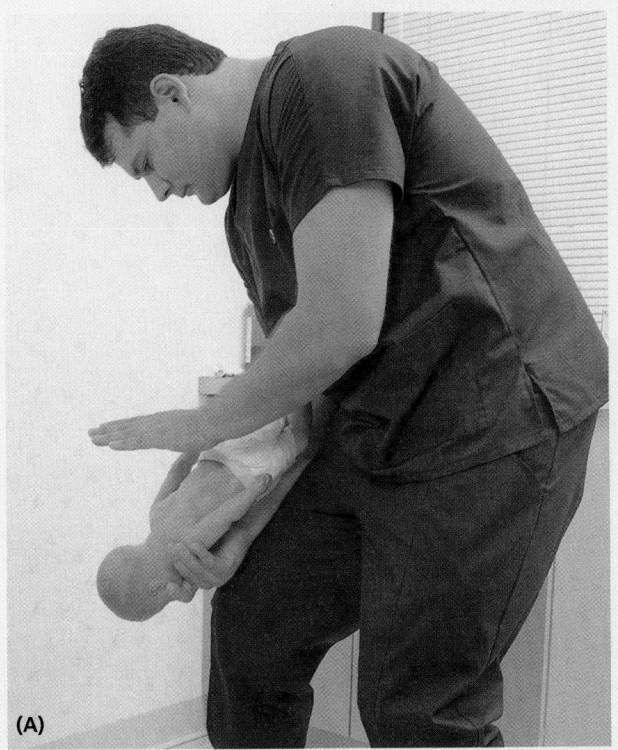

(A)

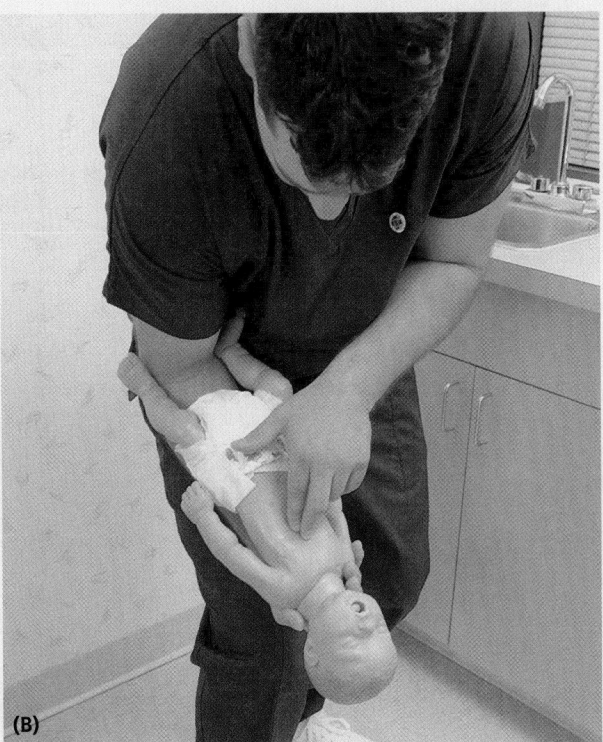

(B)

Figure 9-22 (A) With the infant face down on your forearm, give five back blows. (B) With the infant face up on your forearm, give five chest thrusts.

Procedure 9-7

Back Blows and Chest Thrusts for an Unconscious Infant

STANDARD PRECAUTIONS:

PURPOSE:
To open up a blocked airway.

EQUIPMENT/SUPPLIES:
Gloves
Resuscitation mouthpiece

PROCEDURE STEPS:
1. Have someone call emergency services.
2. Don gloves. Tap the infant gently to check for consciousness.
3. Gently tilt back the infant's head. Do not hyper-extend (Figure 9-23A).
4. Listen and watch for breathing.
5. Apply resuscitation mouthpiece. Give two breaths, covering infant's nose and mouth with your mouth (Figure 9-23B).

6. If air will not go in, retilt head, attempt to give breaths again.
7. If breaths still will not go in, position the infant face down on your forearm.
8. Give five back blows with the heel of your hand between the infant's shoulder blades (Figure 9-23C).
9. Position the infant face up on your forearm.
10. Give five chest thrusts on about the center of the breastbone (Figure 9-23D).
11. Lift jaw and tongue and check for object. If you see the object, sweep it out (Figure 9-23E).
12. Tilt back head and give breaths again.
13. Repeat breaths, back blows, chest thrusts, and checking for object until breaths go in. If the infant does not begin to breath on his own, prepare to perform CPR.
14. Remove gloves. Wash hands.
15. Document the procedure.

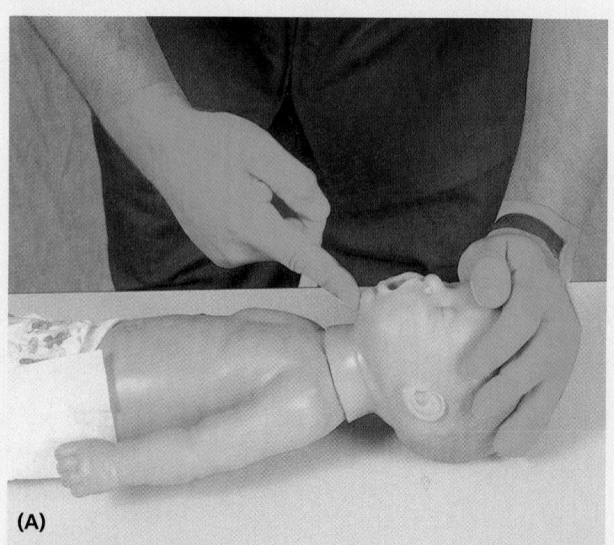

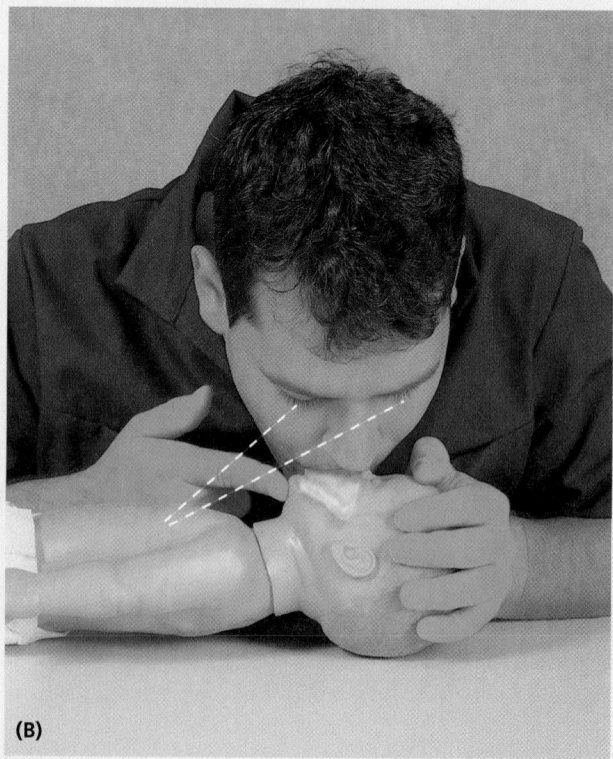

Figure 9-23   (A) Gently tilt back head. (B) Give two breaths, covering the infant's nose and mouth.   *(continues)*

Procedure **9-7** **(continued)**

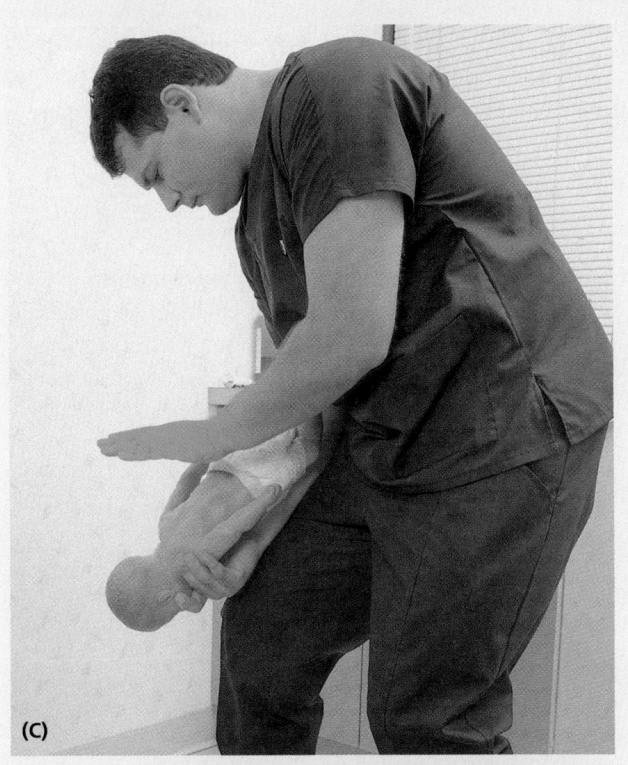

(C)

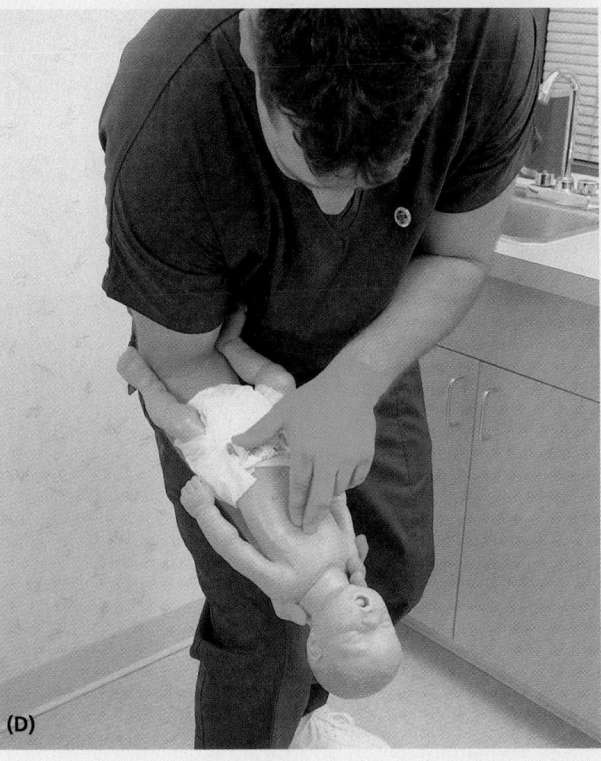

(D)

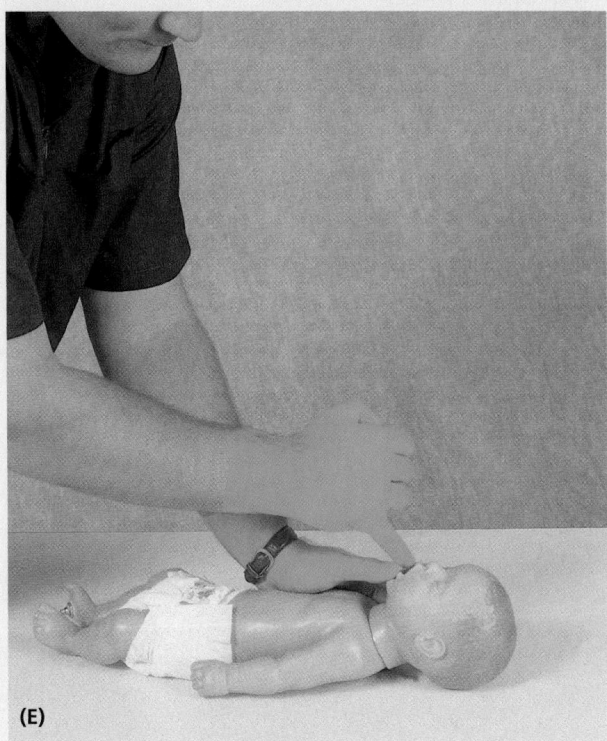

(E)

Figure 9-23 (C) If breaths will not go in, place infant face down on forearm and give five back blows. (D) With infant face up on forearm, give five chest thrusts. (E) Lift jaw and tongue. Check for object and, if seen, sweep out.

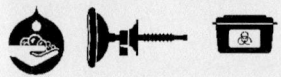

9-8 Rescue Breathing for Adults

STANDARD PRECAUTIONS:

PURPOSE:
To respond to a breathing emergency.

EQUIPMENT/SUPPLIES:
Biohazard waste container
Resuscitation mouthpiece

PROCEDURE STEPS:
1. Have someone call emergency services.
2. Tilt back the head, lift the chin, position resuscitation mouthpiece, and pinch the nose closed (Figure 9-24A).
3. Give two slow breaths. Breathe into patient until the chest gently rises. Turn your face to the side and listen and watch for air to return.
4. Check for pulse on the carotid artery (Figure 9-24B).
5. If pulse is present, but the person is not breathing, give one slow breath every five seconds. Do this for one minute.
6. Recheck pulse and breathing every minute.
7. Continue rescue breathing as long as pulse is present and the person is not breathing. Continue until breathing is restored or another person takes over.
8. Dispose of waste in biohazard container.
9. Wash hands.
10. Document procedure.

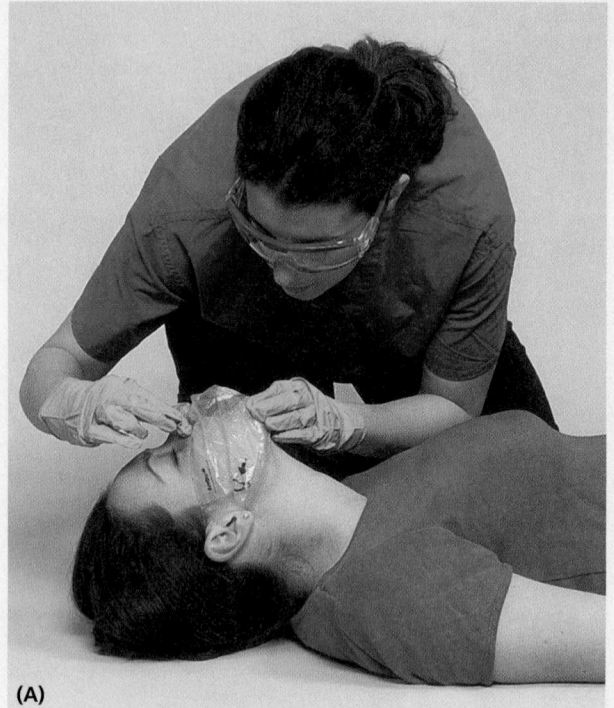

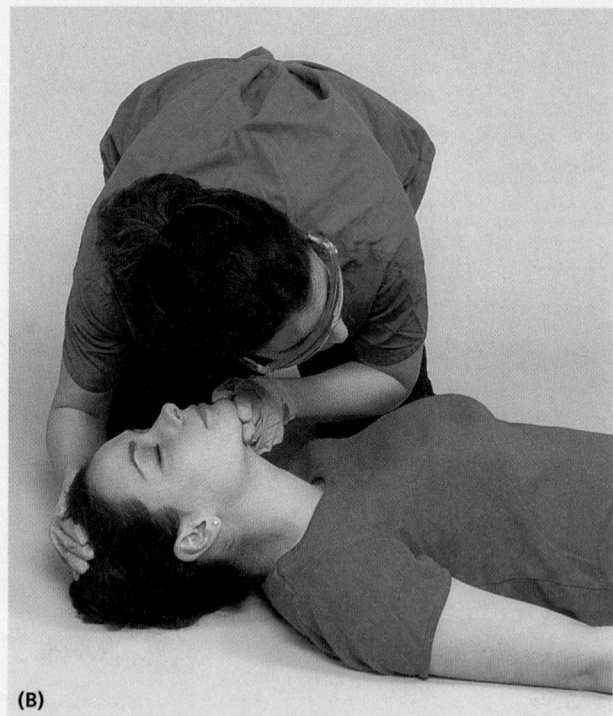

Figure 9-24 (A) Tilt back head, lift chin, position resuscitation mouthpiece, pinch nose closed, and give two short breaths. (B) Check for pulse at the carotid artery.

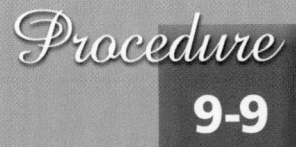

9-9 Rescue Breathing for Children

STANDARD PRECAUTIONS:

PURPOSE:
To respond to a breathing emergency.

EQUIPMENT/SUPPLIES:
Gloves
Resuscitation mouthpiece

PROCEDURE STEPS:
1. Have someone call emergency services.
2. Don gloves.
3. Tilt back the head, lift the chin, position the resuscitation mouthpiece, pinch the nose closed, and give two short breaths (Figure 9-25A). If air does not go in, retilt head and breathe again.
4. Check for a pulse at the carotid artery (Figure 9-25B).
5. If pulse is present, but the child is not breathing, give one slow breath every three seconds. Do this for one minute.
6. Recheck pulse and breathing every minute.
7. Continue rescue breathing as long as pulse is present but the child is not breathing.
8. Remove gloves. Wash hands.
9. Document the procedure.

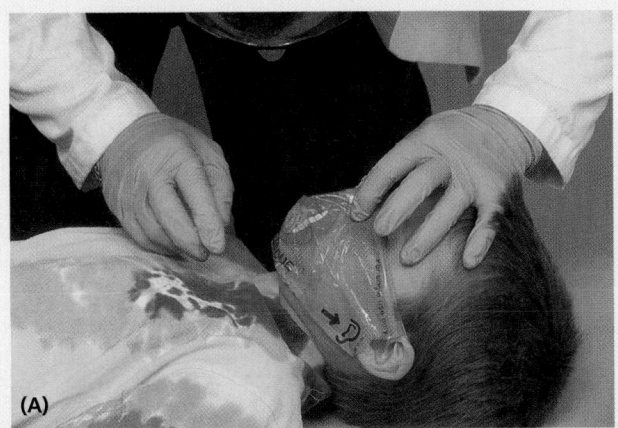

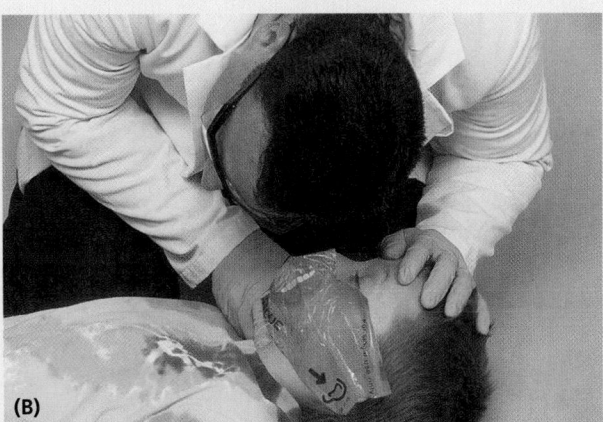

Figure 9-25 (A) Tilt back head, lift chin, position resuscitation mouthpiece, pinch nose closed, and give two short breaths. (B) Check for pulse at the carotid artery.

Procedure

9-10   Rescue Breathing for Infants

STANDARD PRECAUTIONS:

PURPOSE:
To respond to a breathing emergency.

EQUIPMENT/SUPPLIES:
Gloves
Resuscitation mouthpiece

PROCEDURE STEPS:
1. Have someone call emergency services.
2. Don gloves.
3. Tilt back the head (Figure 9-26A).

4. Position resuscitation mouthpiece. Seal your lips tightly around the infant's nose and mouth (Figure 9-26B).
5. Give two slow breaths. Breathe into the infant until the chest rises.
6. Check for a pulse at the brachial artery (Figure 9-26C).
7. If pulse is present, but infant is not breathing, give one slow breath every three seconds. Do this for one minute.
8. Recheck pulse and breathing every minute (Figure 9-26D).
9. Continue rescue breathing as long as pulse is present but the infant is not breathing.
10. Remove gloves. Wash hands.
11. Document the procedure.

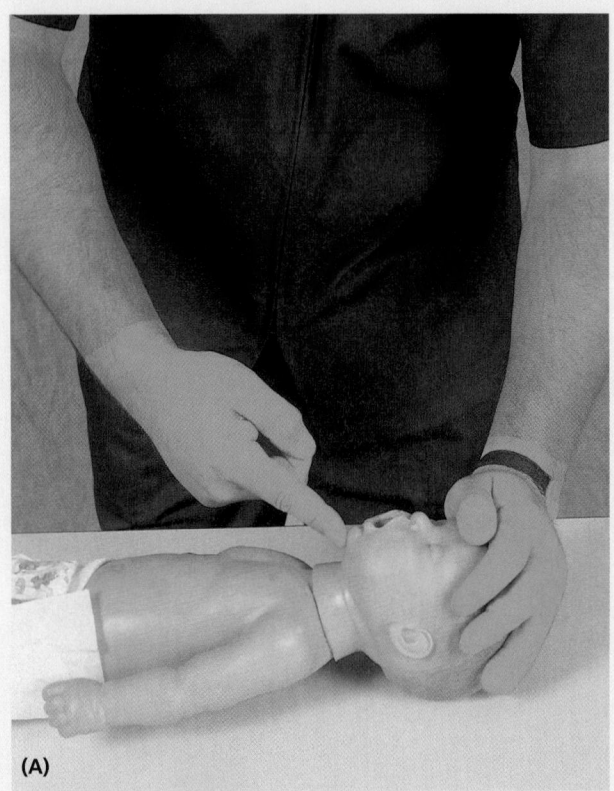

(A)

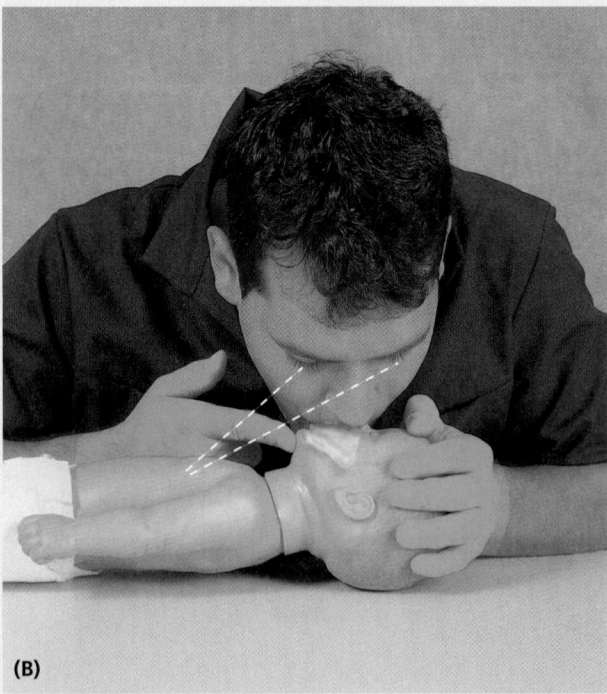

(B)

Figure 9-26   (A) Tilt back head. (B) Position resuscitation mouthpiece. Seal lips around nose and mouth, and give two slow breaths.

(continues)

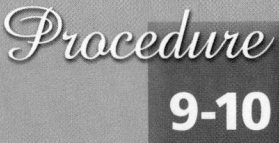

Procedure 9-10 *(continued)*

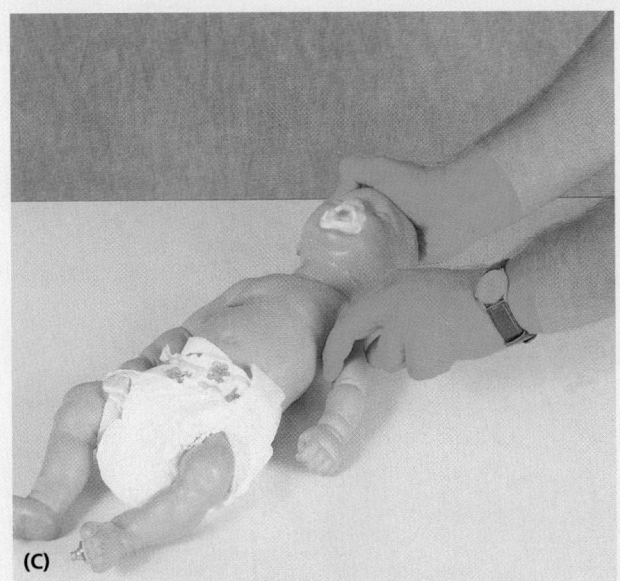

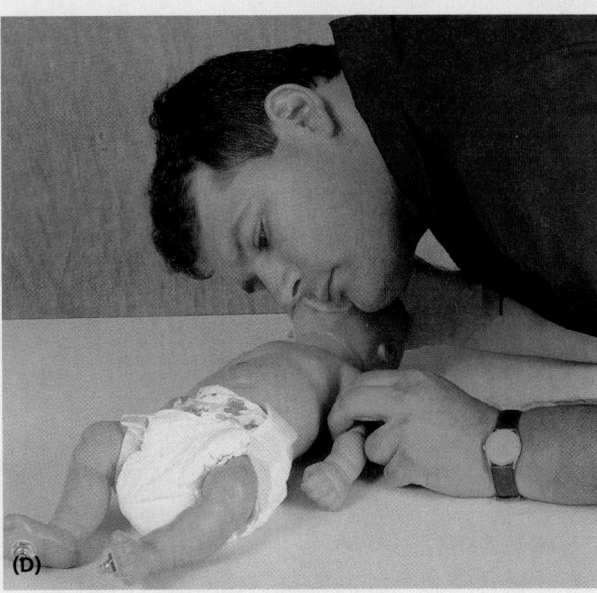

Figure 9-26 (C) Check for pulse at the brachial artery. (D) Recheck pulse and breathing every minute.

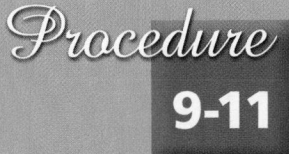

Procedure 9-11 CPR for Adults

STANDARD PRECAUTIONS:

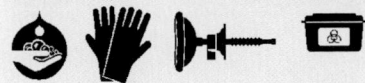

PURPOSE:
To respond to a breathing and cardiac arrest emergency.

EQUIPMENT/SUPPLIES:
Biohazard waste container
Resuscitation mouthpiece
Gloves

PROCEDURE STEPS:
Ask, "Are you OK?" If no response:
1. Have someone call emergency services.
2. Put on gloves if available.
3. Tilt back head and lift chin.

4. Look, listen, and feel for breathing for 10–15 seconds. If the patient is not breathing, keep the airway open, pinch the nose, position the mouthpiece, seal your mouth over the device, and give two breaths through the mouthpiece into the patient's lungs.
5. Check the pulse at the carotid artery for 10 to 15 seconds. If the patient has a pulse, continue rescue breathing. If the patient does not have a pulse, start chest compressions.
6. After locating the area on the abdomen 2 inches above the xiphoid (Figure 9-27A), position your shoulders over your hands and compress the chest about 1½ to 2 inches fifteen times (Figure 9-27B).
7. Give two slow breaths, holding the nose (Figure 9-27C).

(continues)

Procedure

9-11   **(continued)**

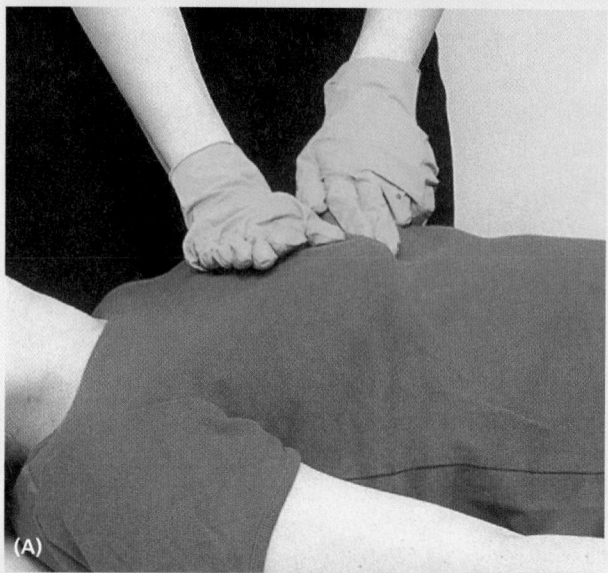

(A)

Figure 9-27   (A) Tilt back head and lift chin. Locate hand on the breastbone two inches above xiphoid process. (B) Position your shoulders over your hands and compress the chest fifteen times. (C) Give two slow breaths, holding nose.

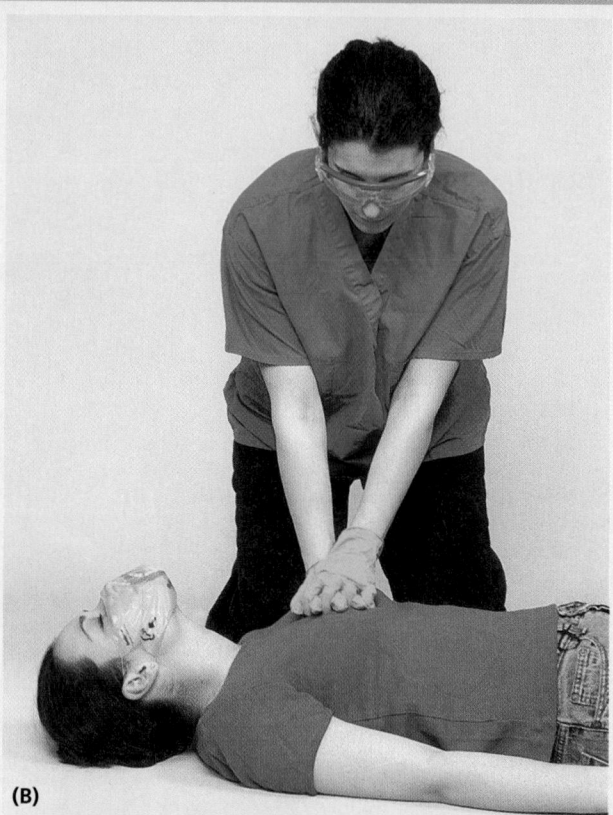

(B)

8. Do three more sets of fifteen compressions and two breaths.
9. Check the pulse and breathing for about 10–15 seconds.
10. If there is no pulse, continue sets of fifteen compressions and two breaths.
11. Dispose of waste in biohazard container.
12. Remove gloves, dispose of in biohazard container, and wash hands.
13. Document the procedure.

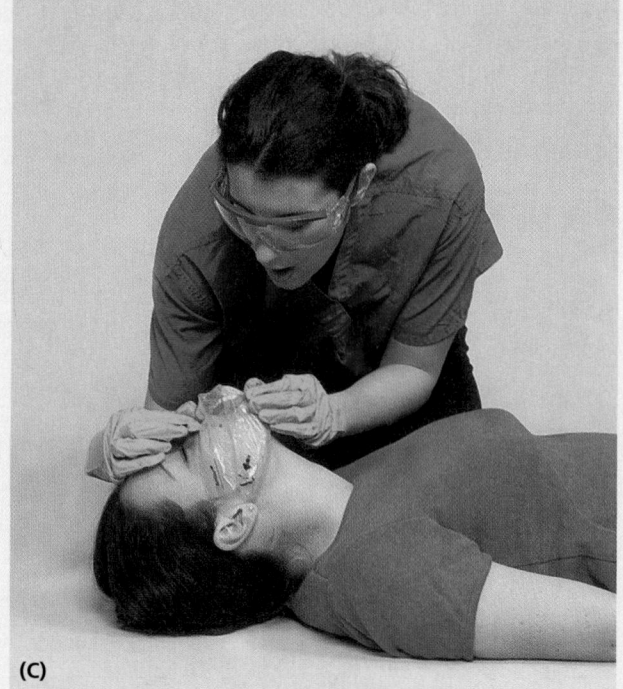

(C)

Procedure

9-12 CPR for Children

STANDARD PRECAUTIONS:

PURPOSE:
To respond to a cardiac arrest emergency.

EQUIPMENT/SUPPLIES:
Gloves
Resuscitation mouthpiece

PROCEDURE STEPS:
1. Put on gloves.
2. Tap child to check consciousness level. Activate EMS.
3. Tilt head, look, listen, and feel for breathing. If there is no breathing, give two slow breaths. Check carotid artery for pulse.
4. Locate one hand on the breastbone and one hand on the forehead to maintain an open airway. Use heel of hand only. Position your shoulders over the child's chest and compress the chest five times (Figure 9-28A).

5. Position resuscitation mouthpiece. Give one slow breath, while pinching the nose (Figure 9-28B).
6. Repeat cycles of five compressions and one breath for about 1 minute.
7. Check the pulse and breathing for about 5–10 seconds (Figure 9-28C).
8. If there is no pulse, continue sets of five compressions and one breath.
9. Recheck the pulse and breathing every few minutes.
10. Remove gloves. Wash hands.
11. Document the procedure.

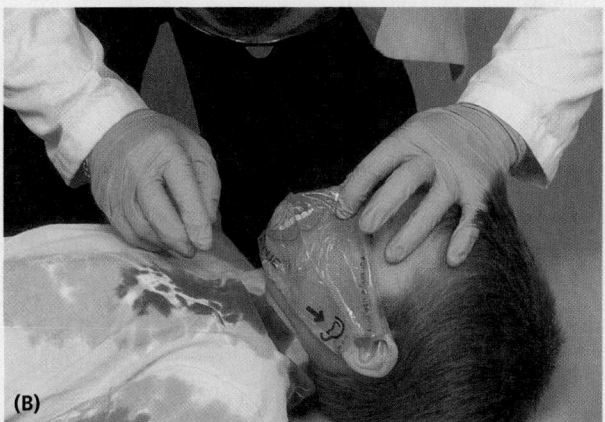

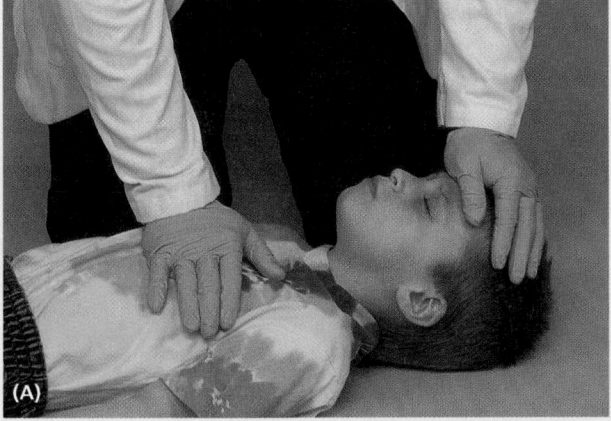

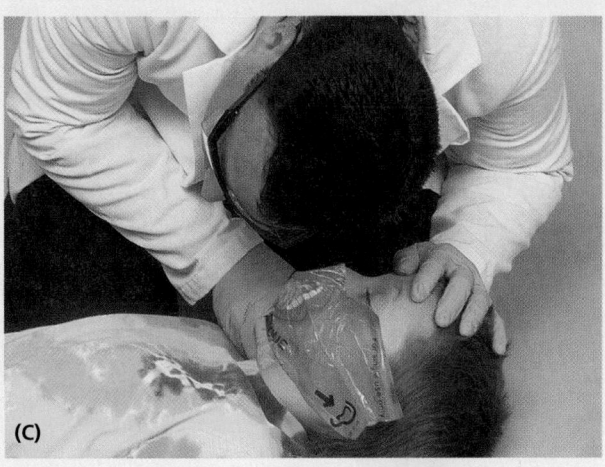

Figure 9-28 (A) Position your shoulders over the child's chest and compress the chest five times. (B) Give one slow breath, holding the nose. (C) Check pulse and breathing for 5 seconds.

Procedure

9-13   CPR for Infants

STANDARD PRECAUTIONS:

PURPOSE:
To respond to a cardiac arrest emergency.

EQUIPMENT/SUPPLIES:
Gloves
Resuscitation mouthpiece

PROCEDURE STEPS:
1. Don gloves.
2. Gently tap the infant to determine consciousness level. Activate EMS.
3. Tilt head. Look, listen, and feel for breathing. If there is no breathing, position resuscitation mouthpiece and give two slow breaths, covering mouth and nose. Check brachial artery for pulse for 5–10 seconds.
4. Find your finger position on the center of the sternum.
5. Compress the infant's chest five times about ½ inch to ¾ inch.
6. Give one slow breath (Figure 9-29A).
7. Repeat cycles of five compressions and one breath for 1 minute.
8. Recheck brachial pulse and breathing for about 5–10 seconds (Figure 9-29B).
9. If there is no pulse, continue cycles of five compressions and one breath.
10. Recheck the pulse and breathing every few minutes.
11. Remove gloves. Wash hands.
12. Document the procedure.

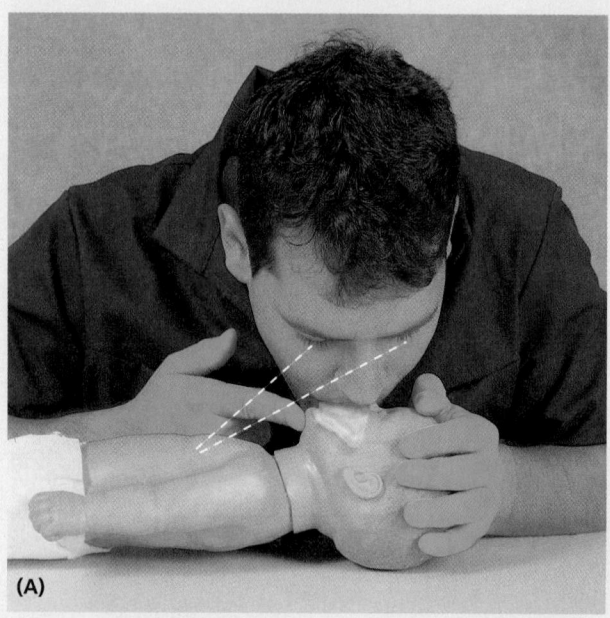
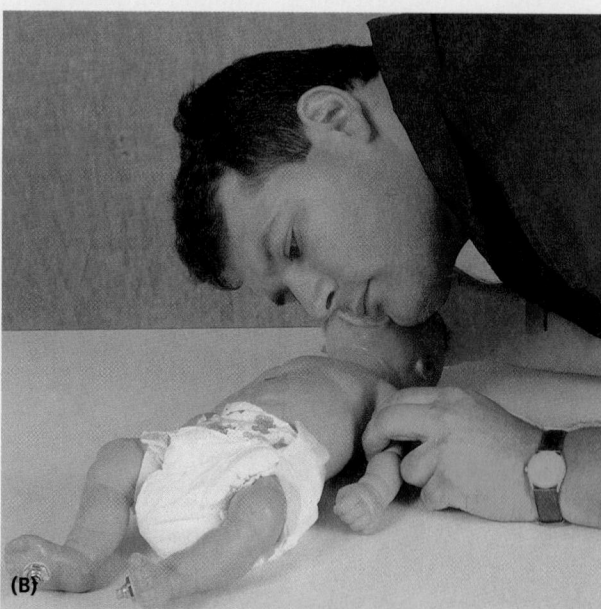

Figure 9-29   (A) Give one slow breath. (B) Recheck brachial pulse and breathing for 5–10 seconds.

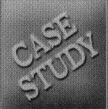

Annette Samuels, a regular patient at Inner City Health Care, is walking her dog one morning, stops to rest on a grassy knoll, and notices a yellow jacket on her arm. She brushes it away, unthinkingly, and then realizes it is stinging her. She receives two more stings and suddenly notices she is at a nest site. Annette is now a half-hour walk from home but not really concerned because she has never had an allergic reaction to a bee sting. However, a few minutes into her walk, her palms become itchy, her ears start to burn, and she feels lightheaded. She is not having difficulty breathing. She is determined to get home and she does, at which point she notices she is covered with hives. She calls Inner City Health Care to ask: should she come in?

CASE STUDY REVIEW

1. Wanda Slawson, CMA, is triaging calls the morning Annette is stung. What questions should she ask Annette?

2. Because Annette obviously is having a hypersensitive or an allergic reaction, she is advised to seek emergency care immediately. What first-aid measures might be taken?

3. What advice about precautions should Wanda give Annette?

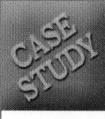

Abigail Johnson has arrived at Inner City Health Care for her scheduled nine o'clock appointment. As she checks in with Bruce Goldman, the medical assistant, she complains of feeling nauseated, having some pressure in her chest, and being short of breath.

CASE STUDY REVIEW

1. What immediate actions should Bruce take to respond to Mrs. Johnson's complaints?

2. What equipment/supplies/medications should be ready and available for Dr. Lewis?

3. Because of the possibility of myocardial infarction, what action would Dr. Lewis direct Bruce to take after Mrs. Johnson has been stabilized?

4. What patient education can Bruce employ in this situation?

SUMMARY

While many of the emergencies covered in this chapter may never be seen by the medical assistant in the ambulatory care setting, it is nonetheless important to develop a broad base of information about the various types of potential emergency situations. This knowledge gives the medical assistant the confidence and the preparation to manage the emergencies that do occur with speed, accuracy, and understanding until outside emergency help arrives. Staff will need to assess their response to emergencies on a continual basis. Was protocol followed? Were there difficulties in the delivery of care? Were staff and equipment prepared and ready to deal with these potentially life-threatening situations? Staff meetings should be held to discuss these and other questions that may have arisen and to allow staff the opportunity to talk about any fears or concerns they might have. It must be stressed that this chapter is at best an introduction to the topic of emergency procedures and first aid; it is highly recommended that all medical assistants in all ambulatory care settings, whether large or small, enroll in either a Red Cross or American Heart Association first aid and CPR program and take refresher courses at least every two years to update skills.

REVIEW QUESTIONS

Multiple Choice

1. Good Samaritan laws:
   a. are designed to protect the public
   b. only protect non-health-care professionals
   c. require that all individuals providing assistance act within the scope of their knowledge and training
   d. only protect health care professionals on the job
2. First-degree burns:
   a. are the most serious and penetrate all layers of skin
   b. affect only the top layer of skin
   c. often leave scar tissue
   d. usually take more than a month to heal
3. A fracture in which the bone protrudes through the skin is called:
   a. greenstick fracture
   b. compound fracture
   c. depressed fracture
   d. comminuted fracture
4. To control a nosebleed, it is important to:
   a. have the patient lie down
   b. tilt the patient's head back
   c. tilt the patient's head forward
   d. call 911 immediately
5. Another name for a heart attack is:
   a. cerebral vascular accident
   b. cardiac arrest
   c. angina pectoris
   d. myocardial infarction

Critical Thinking

1. Discuss the Good Samaritan law and define its purpose and the extent of its protection.
2. Recall what ABC stands for and describe actions that may need to be taken when doing a primary survey of a patient in distress.
3. Define the purpose of a crash cart or tray and compile a list of the major supplies and medications it should contain.
4. Describe shock and tell how and why it is important to prevent a patient from going into shock.
5. Recall three types of bandages and give examples of their use.
6. Describe the difference between first-, second-, and third-degree burns.
7. Recall and describe the four ways that poisons may enter the body.

8. What is hemorrhaging and what kinds of bleeding may the medical assistant encounter? What are the symptoms of each?
9. Explain when and why Heimlich maneuver, rescue breathing, and CPR techniques are performed.
10. What courses should every medical assistant take at least every two years and why?

WEB ACTIVITIES

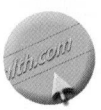

1. Search the web for sites and resources on the Emergency Medical Services (EMS) System. Are there any cities or towns within 100 miles of your place of residence that do not use the EMS System?
2. What sites can you recommend to patients and their families who are looking for first aid information about diabetes and heart attack?
3. What organizations could you use to search for information that deal with first aid for convulsions?
4. Search the web for information regarding first aid for insect stings.
5. What sites are available for information about poisonings?

REFERENCES/BIBLIOGRAPHY

American Red Cross. (1993). *Community first aid & safety*. St. Louis, MO: Mosby-Year Book, Inc.

Bonewit-West, K. (2000). *Clinical procedures for medical assistants* (5th ed.). Philadelphia: W. B. Saunders.

Frew, M. A., Frew, D., & Lane, K. (1995). *Comprehensive medical assisting, competencies for administrative and clinical practice* (3rd ed.). Philadelphia: F. A. Davis.

Keir, L., Wise, B. A., & Krebs, C. (1998). *Medical assisting: Administrative and clinical competencies* (4th ed.). Albany, NY: Delmar.

Kinn, M. E., & Woods, M. A. (1999). *The medical assistant: Administrative and clinical competencies* (8th ed.). Philadelphia: W. B. Saunders.

Prickett-Ramutkowski, B., Barrie A., Keller, C., Dazarow, L., Abel, C. (1999). *Medical assisting: A patient-centered approach to administrative and clinical competencies* (1st ed.). Princeton: Glencoe/McGraw Hill.

Taber's cyclopedic medical dictionary (18th ed.). (1997). Philadelphia: F. A. Davis.

Tuttle-Yoder, J., & Fraser-Nobbe, S. (1996). *STAT! Medical office emergency manual*. Albany, NY: Delmar.

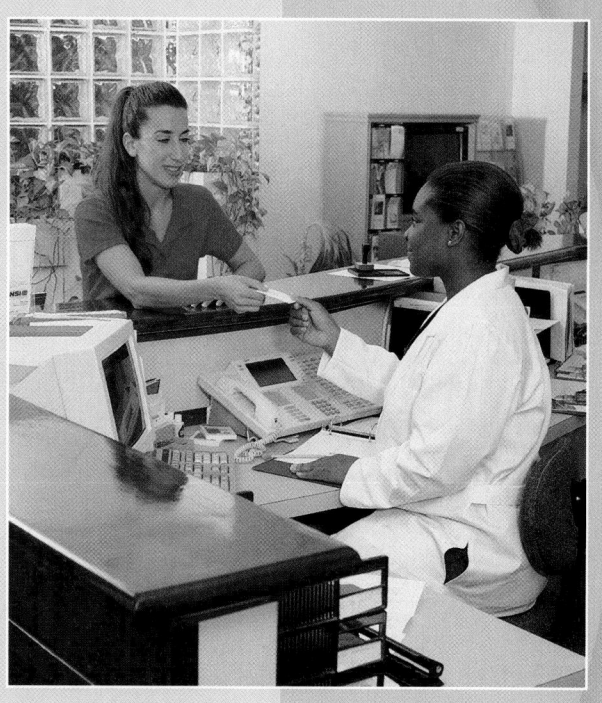

ADMINISTRATIVE
PROCEDURES

INTEGRATED ADMINISTRATIVE PROCEDURES

Chapter

10

CREATING THE FACILITY ENVIRONMENT

OBJECTIVES

The student should strive to meet the following performance objectives and demonstrate an understanding of the facts and principles presented in this chapter through written and oral communication.

1. Define the key terms as presented in the glossary.
2. Describe a comfortable and pleasing reception area.
3. List at least six physical characteristics that may leave patients with an inaccurate impression of the medical facility.
4. Discuss how to ensure a patient's privacy.
5. Describe the role of color in the office environment.
6. Review the purpose of the Americans with Disabilities Act.
7. Discuss the importance of the physical office environment to the patient's care.
8. Identify the important personality characteristics the medical receptionist should possess.
9. Describe the procedure to use when an unexpected delay causes patients to wait for the physician.
10. List at least three tasks to perform upon opening and closing the facility.

GENERAL (TRANSDISCIPLINARY)

Professionalism
- Project a professional manner and image

Legal Concepts
- Maintain and dispose of regulated substances in compliance with government guidelines
- Comply with established risk management and safety procedures

Operational Functions
- Evaluate and recommend equipment and supplies

SCENARIO

The design of any ambulatory setting often evolves as the needs of the office and patients change. In the office of Doctors Lewis and King, which is a two-doctor family practice, the environment has always been warm and welcoming, which is particularly important because the physicians see many children. However, the office was initially designed in the early 1980s, before the Americans with Disabilities Act was passed by the United States Congress.

Once this Act was passed in 1990, the office manager, Marilyn Johnson, CMA, was very aware of the need to comply with its mandates. In addition, Doctors Lewis and King wanted to make all their patients—including those with disabilities—as comfortable as possible. Working with a local architect, Marilyn was able to incorporate changes into the practice's existing space: a ramp was added outside, doorways were widened to provide wheelchair access, and new Braille signage was installed outside for the visually impaired patients. While the changes were not without expense, the staff of Doctors Lewis and King willingly complied with the ADA not only because it is law but because it gave more access to more patients.

INTRODUCTION

The environment of the medical office or clinic contributes almost as much to a patient's well-being as does the medical attention given by the physician and medical assistants. The physical environment can foster a feeling that embraces and welcomes patients or causes them to feel alienated and intimidated.

Interior designers and experts in space planning are advising all individuals involved in designing clinics, medical offices, and hospitals that patient comfort must be considered as important as the facility's functional utility and ease of maintenance. The Americans with Disabilities Act (ADA) also must be taken into account when creating any medical office environment, and provisions must be made to accommodate patients who are physically challenged.

The creation of a health care facility involves many variables. Some are concrete elements, such as lighting, color choice, and furniture arrangement. Yet others are intangible and are expressed in a receptionist's greeting and attitude toward patients. Together, these elements make an ambulatory setting the kind of environment where patients will feel comfortable and secure.

THE RECEPTION AREA

A reception area is just that—a place of reception; it should never be thought of as the waiting room. This is the area that can make the patient feel welcome, secure, and comfortable. Adequate and comfortable seating affords patients room to have their own space.

 Proper seating placement also respects cultural biases. For example, some Americans do not like to be touched by strangers. Middle Eastern and Latin cultures, by contrast, encourage closeness and touching, and individuals from these cultures may cluster themselves close together in the reception area (Figure 10-1).

Current magazines that are appropriate to the clinic clientele, plants, and other features such as a professionally maintained built-in aquarium will help set a welcoming tone. The fabric and texture of draperies, upholstery, and carpet should be pleasing, comfortable, and easy to maintain. It is helpful if there is a place for patients to hang heavy coats or wet umbrellas.

Many physicians provide educational materials for patients in the reception area. For example, new parents always appreciate pamphlets related to raising children. It is also appropriate to have available in the reception area a patient information brochure that describes the services of the office, the function of medical staff members, measures to take in case of an emergency, and other issues that patients may need to consider. See Chapter 45 for more information on developing brochures for patient use.

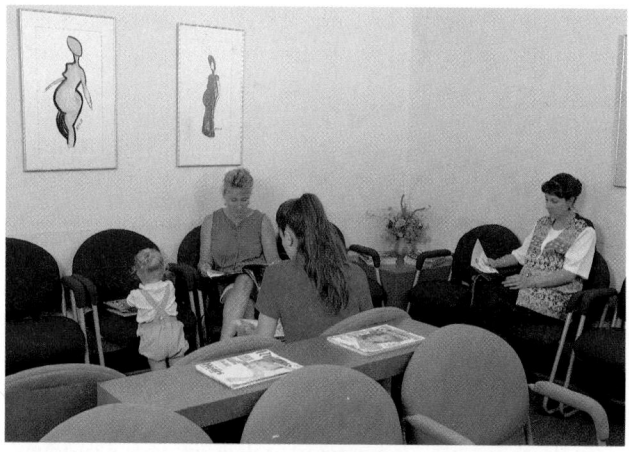

Figure 10-1   An inviting and pleasant reception area has seating arranged so that patients are comfortable sitting together or away from other patients.

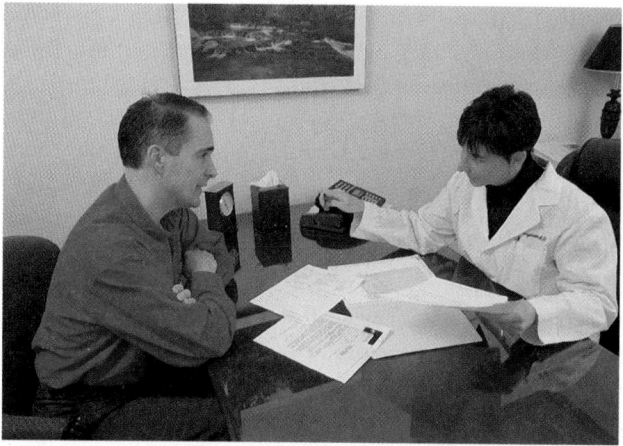

Figure 10-2   Patients should be afforded as much dignity and empowerment as possible. Many patients may feel more comfortable discussing conditions, procedures, or treatments in the physician's office rather than in the examination room.

OFFICE DESIGN AND ENVIRONMENT

Even when the office or clinic is housed in an older building not originally constructed as a medical facility, there is much that can be done to create an environment that enhances patient comfort. Remember to see things from the patient's point of view. If the facility is a labyrinth of corridors where patients can easily get turned around, make certain that directions are clear. Be sure that examination rooms are not made more frightening by an assortment of exposed medical equipment and strange-looking dials, hoses, and nozzles. Be alert to odors that are often distasteful to patients even if the odors are from necessary antiseptics.

A reception window or desk should not make the patient feel closed off from the receptionist; it should provide privacy for the receptionist while allowing a full view of the reception area. A poorly illuminated room may suggest that the physician is trying to hide something—poor housekeeping, dust-encrusted baseboards, soiled carpets, or faded draperies. Lighting can be soft and inviting while providing proper illumination.

Some rooms in the facility, by their very nature, cause patients to feel intimidated. Consider the patient who is naked on an examination table except for a paper or cloth gown interacting with the physician who is fully clothed and wearing a white lab coat and comfortably seated at a counter desk. Consider also the patient who is about to have a sigmoidoscopy and must be placed on a special examination table tilted into the knee-chest position. Both these situations place the patient at an unequal level with the physician for discussion and negotiation. The goal in medical care should be to empower the patient with as much control as possible (Figure 10-2).

Privacy is always important to patients. Provide space for them to hang their clothes and undergarments out of view. A mirror is especially helpful when dressing. Always ask if a patient needs help in disrobing, and always knock before entering a room. Remember, too, that privacy implies that the patient's conversation cannot be overheard in any other part of the facility.

Color can do much to establish an inviting environment. Greens and blues are good in areas that require quiet and extended concentration. Cool colors cause individuals to underestimate time and make heavier items seem lighter, objects smaller, and rooms larger. Warm colors with high illumination cause increased alertness and an outward orientation. The aged will have difficulty distinguishing pastels because of failing eyesight. Strongly contrasting patterns and extremely bright colors can be overwhelming, and even intimidating or threatening in their effect.

Accessories and artwork can easily add a special touch to a facility. While fresh flowers might be a nice touch, fresh flowers harbor microorganisms, and some patients may be allergic to them. There is the tendency to use living plants in the medical facility, but some silk plants and flowers also may be appropriate. It would be worth the investment to have a professional designer look through the facility to make suggestions regarding color, artwork, and the general environment of the office.

Americans with Disabilities Act

Accessibility, or making facilities and equipment available to all users, is a major consideration when creating the health care environment. The Americans with Disabilities Act (ADA) was passed by the United States Congress in 1990. The purpose of this act is to provide a clear and comprehensive national mandate to end discrimination against individuals with disabilities and to bring them into the economic and social mainstream of life. In addition to accessibility regulations, this act also provides employment protection for persons with disabilities. ADA applies to businesses with fifteen or more employees; however, some states may have stricter legislation. Even before ADA became legislation, most health care facilities attempted to make their premises barrier-free and accessible to patients with special needs. While many ambulatory care settings will have less than fifteen employees, accessibility for all patients in all settings is very important.

A professional designer can provide advice on how the facility must be accessible to persons who are physically challenged. For example, all doors and hallways must accommodate a wheelchair. There must be a bathroom facility available for handicapped individuals. Signage in Braille accommodates patients with visual disabilities. Elevators must be provided if the facility is on more than one level. Be alert also, to patients whose impairment is not obvious—individuals with impaired hearing or vision and individuals whose infirmity (temporary or permanent) may prevent them from doing certain physical activities.

THE RECEPTIONIST'S ROLE

The receptionist is the person on the health care team who must always keep a positive "We can help you" attitude, have a smile for each patient, and a genuine "I care about you" personality. This individual, who often is a medical assistant with other duties as well, must be able to perform telephone triage, retrieve records, greet patients, present a bill, make appointments, and log data into the computer all the while remembering that the patient's

comfort is of primary concern. The receptionist must genuinely like people and not be upset when they are grumpy, irritable, or depressed and worried about an illness. The receptionist is the person who sets the social climate for the interchange between the patient and the physician and the rest of the staff, Figure 10-3.

Patients who are very ill should not have to wait in the reception area but should be shown to an examination room away from other patients. The receptionist or medical assistant may also have to entertain children who may be intent on disrupting patients. This is especially necessary if the parent seems unconcerned about keeping youngsters under control, Figure 10-4.

If there are unexpected delays in the physician's schedule, be certain to notify patients of the delay tactfully and graciously and offer them the alternative of making other arrangements. Keep in mind that the patient's time is as valuable as the physician's.

OPENING THE FACILITY

When the facility is opened in the morning, everything should be in readiness. The receptionist or administrative medical assistant, who arrives at least twenty minutes before the first patient, will make a visual check of each room to be certain it is prepared and ready for the day.

Rooms should be of a comfortable temperature, well-organized, pleasantly illuminated, and spotless. All necessary supplies and equipment should be checked for readiness. At all times, patient comfort and safety should be paramount. Patient charts for the day should be retrieved if not done so the prior evening. The receptionist will also check the answering service or machine for any telephone messages.

An effective way to check a room's readiness is to place yourself in the room as a patient. Ask yourself how

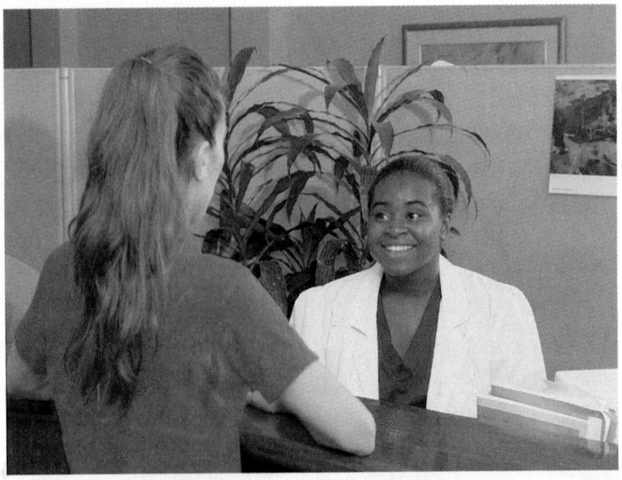

Figure 10-3 A friendly greeting from the medical assistant who is serving as receptionist is reassuring to most patients.

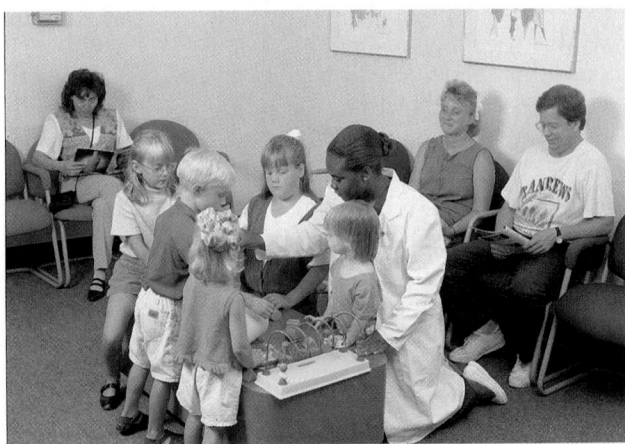

Figure 10-4 The receptionist or medical assistant may need to entertain children while parents are in the examination room or physician's office.

you feel about being there, what mood the surroundings create for you, and whether you would feel welcome and comfortable as a patient.

CLOSING THE FACILITY

At the close of the day, each room should be checked to make certain all equipment is shut down and doors and windows are secured. Be sure that all materials of a sensitive nature are under lock and key. (This is not easily accomplished in facilities that use open-shelf filing, however.) Any drugs identified in the Controlled Substances Act list of narcotics and non-narcotics must be in a locked and secure cabinet and should also be checked when leaving the office. Any petty cash kept on the premises must be locked in a safe container.

It is best, also, to put each room and area in readiness for the next day.

 Local law enforcement officers can advise you on appropriate indoor and outdoor lighting as well as any other security measures to make both during and after office hours.

Always contact the answering service to notify them that the office is closed and where and how the medical staff can be reached in an emergency.

SPOTLIGHT ON AAMA ESSENTIALS THROUGH CAAHEP

- A friendly greeting, a pleasant smile, and a professional attitude, always help to reassure most patients coming into the office.

- Creating an environment that is inviting, pleasant, and arranged in a comfortable manner helps patients feel at ease when coming into the office either for the first time or as a returning patient.

- Affording patients as much dignity and empowerment as possible helps them to feel more comfortable when discussing their medical condition.

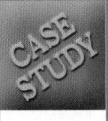

CASE STUDY 10-1

Even though she appears collected on the outside, Abigail Johnson, age somewhere in the seventies, is really quite nervous about having her annual physical. Clinical medical assistant Audrey Jones senses her patient's underlying tension and wants to do what she can to get Abigail to relax. She knows that the patient suffers from hypertension and may be feeling guilty about going off the strict diet that was designed to manage both her high-blood pressure and her diabetes. At this moment, Audrey is helping Abigail get ready to see Dr. King, her physician. She does not want to intrude on her patient's privacy but does want her to relax a bit.

CASE STUDY REVIEW

1. What are some of the actions Audrey can take to ensure her patient's privacy?

2. In what ways can the physical environment itself become a calming influence for the patient, Abigail?

3. How will Audrey's sympathetic attitude affect her patient?

SUMMARY

Keep in mind that the environment in which patient care is given must promote health rather than aggravate illness and feed anxiety. The environment must be clean, fresh, cheerful, and nonthreatening with contemporary furnishings, appropriate colors, proper lighting, and soothing textures.

Even if patients are not consciously aware of the message they are getting from the office design and environment, they are subconsciously receiving it. The office environment reveals things that might subconsciously undermine a patient's confidence in the physician and the health care team.

REVIEW QUESTIONS

Multiple Choice

1. Which of the following is appropriate for the reception area of an ambulatory care setting?
   a. heavily scented flowers
   b. medical journals with colored pictures
   c. dim lighting
   d. live or silk plants
2. One of the goals in treating patients is:
   a. to give them as much control as possible
   b. to see them as quickly as possible
   c. to disregard their desire for privacy
   d. to be sure they arrive on time for their appointment
3. One design element to avoid in a medical office is:
   a. a mirror for dressing
   b. the colors green and blue
   c. strongly contrasting patterns
   d. accessories and artwork
4. The Americans with Disabilities Act is mostly concerned with:
   a. segregating individuals according to type of disability
   b. providing access and opportunity for physically challenged individuals
   c. only the work environment
   d. getting economic benefits for physically challenged people
5. In any medical office, the receptionist's key responsibility is to:
   a. not keep the physician waiting
   b. make sure all plants are watered
   c. greet patients in a friendly, warm manner
   d. be efficient, even if it means ignoring patient requests
6. Making a visual check of each examination room is a function of:
   a. only the physician
   b. opening the office
   c. closing the office
   d. b and c above
7. The American with Disabilities Act applies to businesses with ___ employees:
   a. 10
   b. 5
   c. 15
   d. one or more
8. Children in the reception area:
   a. should sit still and be quiet
   b. may need to be entertained by the receptionist
   c. are not the responsibility of the office staff
   d. should be able to go into the examination room with a parent

Critical Thinking

1. What would an interior designer or space planner do to create a pleasant atmosphere for patients in a medical office? If there is an interior design program in your school, consult with their students on planning a medical office environment.
2. Describe the most pleasant office you have seen. What made it stand out? In what ways was it special? What were your first impressions?
3. Recall your physician's office. Is it accessible to all patients? If not, what would you do to make it accessible to all patients?
4. As the administrative medical assistant employed in a busy ambulatory setting, how will you keep your personality pleasant, warm, and genuinely friendly and caring even on days when you are having your own personal difficulties?
5. With a fellow student, role-play a situation in which a very frustrated and angry patient must be calmed by the medical receptionist. Assume the patient is angry because of a long wait in the reception area.
6. Discuss what you might do to entertain children aged 4 and 6 while their mother is in the examination room.
7. If you felt the facility in which you are employed could benefit from the services of an interior designer either for minor adjustments or a major remodel, what suggestions would you make to your physician employer to convince him/her of the benefits of such a suggestion?

WEB ACTIVITIES

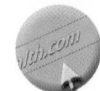 Using the World Wide Web, search for sites identifying companies whose specialty it is to create pleasant interior environments for medical office clinics. Start with the words "interior design and medical facilities." Identify what you are able to locate. What about the pictures displayed is pleasing to you? Why?

REFERENCES/BIBLIOGRAPHY

Keir, L., Wise, B. A., & Krebs, C. (1998). *Medical assisting: Administrative and clinical competencies* (4th ed.). Albany, NY: Delmar.

Kinn, M. E., & Woods, M. A. (1999). *The medical assistant: Administrative and clinical* (8th ed.). Philadelphia: W. B. Saunders.

COMPUTERS IN THE AMBULATORY CARE SETTING

KEY TERMS

Algorithm
Antivirus Program
Application Software
Benchmark
Bit
Byte
Central Processing Unit (CPU)
Data Input Device
Data Output Device
Data Storage Device
Data Storage Memory
Database Management Software
Documentation
Ergonomics
Field
Firewall
Floppy Disk
Footer
Gigabyte
Graphics Software
Hacker
Hard Disk
Hardware
Header
Information Retrieval System
Internet
Jaz® Drive
Macro
Mainframe Computer
Megabyte
Merge Operation
Microcomputer
Minicomputer
Motherboard   (*continues*)

OUTLINE

Types of Computers
Components of a Computer
  System
  Hardware
  Power Outage, Electrical Surge,
    and Static Discharge Protection
    Devices
  Software
  Documentation

Common Software Applications
  in the Medical Office
  Word Processing
  Graphics
  Spreadsheets
  Databases
  Virus Protection
Patient Confidentiality in the
  Computerized Medical Office
Computerizing the Medical Office
The Safe Use of Computers

OBJECTIVES

The student should strive to meet the following performance objectives and demonstrate an understanding of the facts and principles presented in this chapter through written and oral communication.

1. Define the key terms as presented in the glossary.
2. Recall ten examples of what computers can do to improve efficiency in the ambulatory care setting.
3. Describe the six points that must be considered when moving from a manual to a computerized system.
4. Identify the four main types of computers.
5. Define a computer system and identify its components.
6. Explain the difference between system and application software.
7. Differentiate between the five major categories of application software.
8. Explain how database management concepts might be used in an ambulatory care setting.
9. Discuss patient confidentiality and guidelines for maintaining confidentiality.
10. Explain why ergonomics is important, and recall at least six guidelines for setting up a computer workstation.

KEY TERMS (*continued*)

Network Interface
Optical Disk
Orphan
Password
Patch
Personal Computer (PC)

Random Access Memory (RAM)
Read-only memory (ROM)
Record
Server
Software
Sort

Spreadsheet Software
Supercomputer
System Software
Widow
Word Processing Software
Zip® Drive

ROLE DELINEATION COMPONENTS

GENERAL (TRANSDISCIPLINARY)

Legal Concepts

- Maintain confidentiality
- Prepare and maintain medical records
- Use appropriate guidelines when releasing information
- Comply with established risk management and safety procedures
- Develop and maintain personnel, policy, and procedure manuals (advanced)

Operational Functions

- Evaluate and recommend equipment and supplies
- Apply computer techniques to support office operations

SCENARIO

Inner City Health Care, an urgent care center in a large urban area, recently made the transition from a manual to a computerized system. It was a change long overdue, and it required a great deal of fact-finding and research before office manager Walter Seals could convince the center's physicians to purchase a network of computers for the five-physician center.

Once he persuaded his employers of the computer's potential value to the center, Walter, an administrative medical assistant, proceeded very carefully. He spoke with other ambulatory care settings that were already computerized, to establish **benchmarks**, or comparisons. He selected a computer vendor who was familiar with the software needs of a medical office. He made sure all staff would receive training in the use of the computer. Finally, he selected a two-week period when the office was routinely closed for summer vacation to have the computer system installed and operational.

INTRODUCTION

In a little more than a decade, computers have revolutionized the world of health care. Computers assist in performing sensitive surgeries, diagnosing illnesses, and developing patient treatment strategies. In addition to these dramatic clinical applications, computers have changed the nature of the ambulatory care setting from an administrative point of view, streamlining critical tasks such as patient data collection, correspondence, reports, and insurance claim filing.

Yet, by itself, the computer cannot make a medical practice function more smoothly. Talented medical assistants, who understand the uses and potential of the computer, are the key behind an effective computerized office.

Computers are no longer a luxury in the ambulatory care setting; they have become an essential way of doing business. The medical assistant in most ambulatory care settings must be computer literate. In addition, the medical assistant also must be aware of procedures to prevent compromise of confidential medical records.

TYPES OF COMPUTERS

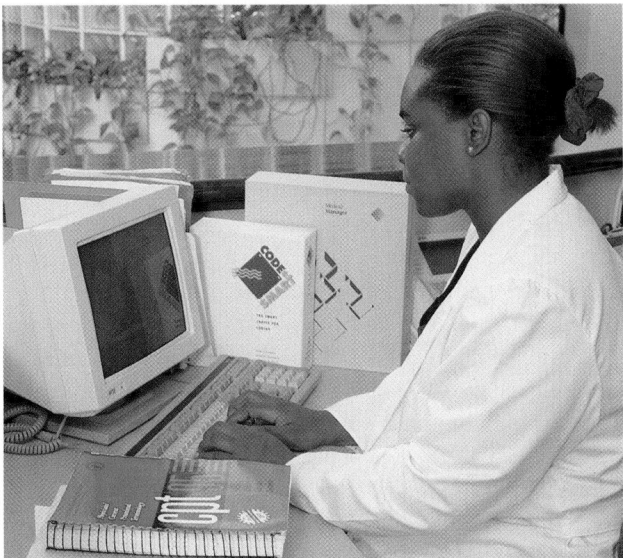

Although the medical assistant will be primarily concerned with the uses of the minicomputer and the microcomputer, commonly known as the personal computer, it is helpful to understand the capabilities of the four major types of computers.

Supercomputers, the fastest and the most powerful computers, are used in medical research to combat cancer and to trace the genetic components for birth defects. They are the most expensive and complex of computers. Relatively few of these systems are up and running. Supercomputer technology is still under development but holds great promise for the advancement of sophisticated medical interventions.

Mainframe computers, the next largest in size and processing ability, are used for large volumes of repetitive calculations. With their high processing speeds, mainframes are invaluable for large governmental provider service programs like Medicaid and Medicare.

Minicomputers, grouped between mainframes and microcomputers in terms of size, speed, and capacity, process data in health care facilities in a variety of ways, including patient account processing, insurance claim processing, and statistical analysis of research data. Minicomputers handle large amounts of processing and challenge the capabilities of older mainframe systems (Figure 11-1).

Microcomputers are the most widely used type of computer in today's health care facility. The smallest of the four types of computers, microcomputers range in size

Figure 11-1 Minicomputers allow different operators to use the same application at the same time. There is no data storage unit (disk or drive) at the operator's station, only a keyboard and monitor.

from easily transportable systems such as handheld, laptop, or notebook systems, to the more common desktop or **personal computer (PC)** (Figure 11-2).

The medical assistant will work with the computer on a daily basis in many different ways. Microcomputers may be used in a medical practice to schedule appointments, maintain patient accounts, and process insurance claims. Handheld micros may be used to input patient information during examination.

COMPONENTS OF A COMPUTER SYSTEM

A system is an assembly of parts that function together to perform a particular task. A computer system consists of hardware, software, and documentation of the installation.

Hardware

The components of a computer system you can see and touch are referred to as **hardware**. Hardware consists of the central processing unit (CPU), data input devices, and data output devices. Each of these items is made up of many subcomponents. However, we will only concern ourselves with the primary function and unique technology employed to perform that function.

Central Processing Unit. The **central processing unit (CPU)** of a computer is the brain of the system. It carries out instructions defined by the program software on the data input and sends the result to the selected output device. The actual heart of the CPU is a silicon microchip approximately 3 inches square with sometimes hundreds of connections to other electronic components. The circuitry printed on the microchip contains logic **algorithms** for performing functions such as addition, subtraction, and multiplication. (Word processing example: The operator presses the letter *a* on the keyboard or data input device. The input device sends the numeric symbol for *a* to the CPU. The CPU then combines this input and whether the shift or caps key was pushed with data previously input when the word processing program was set up and sends the output to memory and to the monitor for you to view the letter A.)

Data Input Devices. **Data input devices** convert hard copy, motion, temperature, position, and other analog signals into digital input for use by a computer. The most common data input devices are the keyboard and mouse. Other input devices are electronic tablets with pointers, pens, airbrush tools, scanners, touch screens, and a host of electronic clinical instruments that can directly

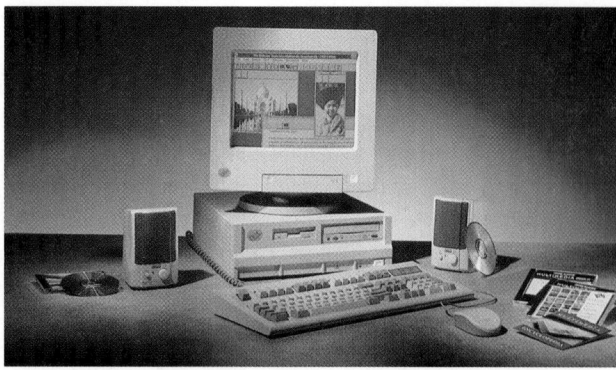

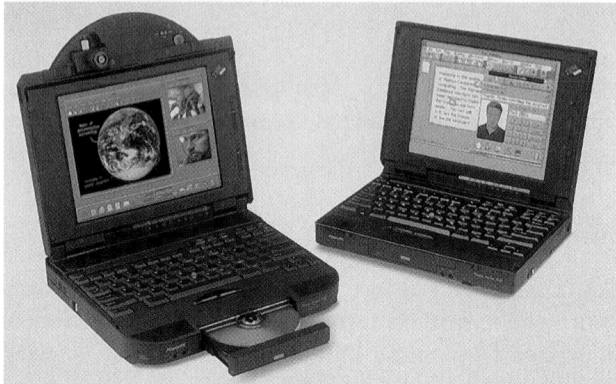

Figure 11-2 Microcomputers come in a variety of sizes and types: (Top) Traditional desktop personal computer. (Bottom) Versatile laptop and Thinkpad models. (Courtesy of International Business Machines Corporation)

record patient laboratory data into a patient's file as either a printed or an electronic record.

Data Output Devices. Data output devices are the user's eyes, showing how the program has manipulated the input data. The most common data output device is the monitor or screen, which provides real-time feedback of what is taking place with input data. It is used interactively by most operators to make in-process changes to format of data output and to correct input errors. Printers, plotters, and facsimile (fax) machines are output devices that provide hard copy for filing, mailing, or transmission to remote locations. Use of a fax machine or connection to the Internet requires a modem to interface between the computer and a telephone line or cable. Modems can be internal to the computer case or external in the form of an add-on device connected by a cable or plug-in slot on the computer case. Modems operate at different speeds of data transfer, and the fastest device compatible with the telephone, cable system, or Internet provider should be utilized. **CAUTION:** Fax transmission of sensitive data requires special protocols to ensure that unauthorized persons do not receive it. Data storage devices also function

as output devices to electronically store output for future manipulation or transmission. The same caution should apply when transmitting output electronically as with electronic fax machine transmission of output or data. See the section on Patient Confidentiality in the Computerized Medical Office.

Data Storage Devices. Data storage devices are devices capable of permanently or temporarily storing digital data. Data storage device capacity is often referred to as memory. Along with computer speed, this area of the computer has seen the greatest improvement, with capability doubling every few years or less. Computers used by most of us today have no functional limitation for memory, with portable memory cartridges providing unlimited memory expansion.

Data storage devices consist of **read-only memory (ROM)**, **random access memory (RAM)**, and **data storage memory**. The computer manufacturer permanently writes data or instructions into the memory on ROM chips, which are installed directly onto the **motherboard**. They contain instructions for operations such as booting the computer when the power is turned on. RAM memory is also in the form of chips and is part of the motherboard. It provides the computer with registers in which to store in-process data. RAM memory is erased or "lost" when the computer is turned off or experiences a power failure. RAM memory is important to the user, in that too small a RAM capacity will cause the computer to run slowly and sometimes not run some software programs. Data storage memory is permanent in that it is not erased when the computer is turned off and can be either read-only or random access. Read-only data storage memory is used to store application programs for loading onto the computer. The following paragraphs describe several devices for providing data storage.

Hard disks are nonportable storage devices, usually installed directly into the computer cabinet that contains the CPU. A hard disk is a read-write device, and the memory is permanent except if the device experiences mechanical failure. Because of the failure potential of these devices, it is considered good practice to back up frequently the stored data by making a copy of files on a portable data storage device. The frequency for data backup is dependent on rate at which data is entered into your system, and upon how long original records are maintained. Original records should never be destroyed until the stored data is backed up.

Floppy disks are portable memory storage devices that can be readily removed and transported. The most common floppies are 3.5 inches square and hold about 1.4 **megabytes** of data, although minicomputers use larger disks that hold correspondingly more data.

Zip® drives and Jaz® drives are found on many new computers. They are slightly thicker than a floppy disk but hold between 100 and 2,000 megabytes of data. They are portable and interchangeable from one computer to another.

Optical disks are portable memory storage devices that can be of the read-only or read-write type. The read-only devices are basically a compact disk commonly used to record digital music and are used to store computer programs for loading onto your computer or to store catalogs, maps, and charts or similar data-intensive applications. The storage capacities of optical disks run into the **giga-byte** range.

Servers are not true data storage devices. They usually contain or are connected to massive hard drives, but in many networked systems they become the storage devices for the user workstations. Servers may be located remote from workstations or even on the Internet. When servers are used, special protocols must be employed to protect confidentiality of records. See the section on Patient Confidentiality in the Computerized Medical Office.

Power Outage, Electrical Surge, and Static Discharge Protection Devices

Protection devices must be an integral part of a medical office computer system. Computer systems should have an uninterruptible power supply, usually a battery backup, to prevent power outages from shutting down the system or destroying data. The power supply should also have a surge protection capability to prevent voltage surges on the utility line from damaging computer components. Static electricity can also be highly damaging to computers by transferring thousands of volts of electrical charge to components that are damaged by only a few hundred volts. This is the type of charge we all experience during dry weather when we get a shock from touching a grounded object and draw a spark. Nylon stockings, synthetic clothing, and walking on a synthetic fiber carpet all create static charges. To prevent damage from static discharges, grounding mats are required at all workstations.

Software

Software, frequently referred to as a computer program, can be thought of as a set of instructions that a computer follows to control computer hardware and to process data. System software and application software are both required by a computer to accomplish its tasks.

System software, frequently just called the operating system, tells the computer hardware what to do and when to do it. Some of the modern systems operate with a graphic interface that utilizes graphic symbols for input to the system and is much more user friendly than systems requiring alphanumeric inputs. Microsoft Windows® and Macintosh systems are probably the best known of the graphic interface operating systems.

Application software performs a specific data processing function. Word processing, accounting, scheduling, and insurance coding are examples of application software functions. Application software must be compatible with the operating system and the computer system hardware. The label on the application package usually defines the minimum system properties for the program to function as designed and in a fashion acceptable to the user. It is usually better to have a system, which has a slightly faster speed, greater RAM capacity, and more memory than required by the program.

Documentation

Computer system documentation consists of the manuals and documents that define how programs operate. Documentation tells how to execute specific functions and gives the specifications for specific hardware, such as the frequency of the internal clock, RAM, and hard disk available memory. Although it is more likely provided on an optical disk that originally provided the specific program, documentation can be in printed format.

Updates to program documentation are increasingly made available on the web site of the company providing the program, along with patches for glitches discovered in the basic program. Third party documents defining how to use application software are becoming increasingly popular and are frequently more user-friendly than documentation from the software supplier. All documentation, including licenses, recovery software, and program disks that come with the computer system, add-on hardware, and software should be maintained in a safe location for the life of the equipment and software and then disposed of when the system or software is phased out of use.

COMMON SOFTWARE APPLICATIONS IN THE MEDICAL OFFICE

In a medical environment, application software can be used either for general or specialized purposes (Figure 11-3). When applications are needed to fulfill specific purposes, customized software might be used. Custom software can be purchased as a prewritten application designed for a specific industry (such as The Medical Manager® software for the medical field, Figure 11-4), or it can be written to meet the needs of a single organization.

Scheduling

Appointment scheduling
Follow-up scheduling
Patient recall lists
Patient reminders

Word processing

Articles
Consultation reports
Correspondence
Labels and addressing
Medical transcription
Memos
Thank you letters
Welcome-to-practice letters

Clinical

Access to national data banks
CME (continuing medical education) programs
Drug interaction and allergy checks
Medical records
Patient education brochures
Prescription writing
Protocols, diagnosis, and treatment
Research
Retrieving medical research from on-line sites
Treatment plans

Accounting

Accounts payable
Cash report
Cash register

Charge slips
Check writing
Cross-posting in multiphysician practices
Daily log
Deposit slip
General ledger
Income and expense statement
Monthly statements to patients
Payroll
Profit and loss statements
Retirement plan accounting
W-2 forms

Billing, collecting, and insurance

Accounts receivable
Aging accounts receivable
Billing forms
Collection letters
Electronic transmission of claims
Insurance claim processing
Patient billing

Practice management

Employee vacation and sick-time records
Hospital lists and charges
Inventories and drug supplies
Ordering drugs and supplies
Patient profiles by age, diagnosis, and so on
Practice profiles by diagnosis, procedure, service
Production reports by physicians
Referrals

Figure 11-3   The computer has great value for the ambulatory care setting.

While custom software can be very expensive, it is valuable because it has many special features developed especially for medical offices (Figure 11-5).

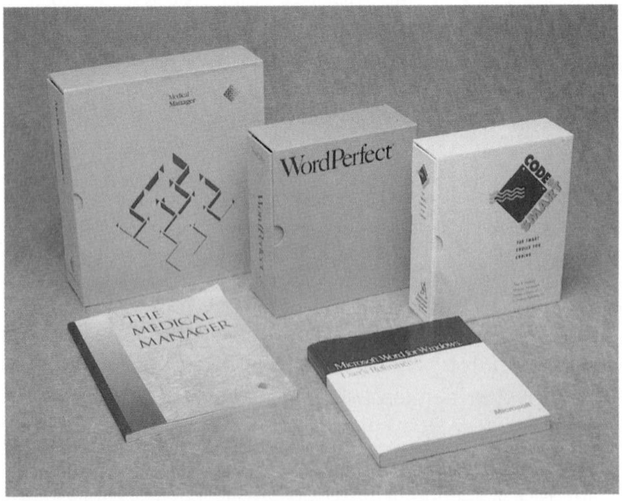

Figure 11-4   Examples of popular application software and documentation packages common to many medical offices.

General-purpose software useful in the ambulatory care setting includes word processing, graphics, spreadsheet, database, and on-line communications programs.

Word Processing

Word processing is largely concerned with the production of textual material. Documents created using **word processing software** may include standard reports, medical transcription, memos, business letters, and articles.

Word processing software allows the medical assistant to produce a document needed quickly and easily; the advantages of word processing over typewriting are considerable, for corrections are easily made and material can be cut or copied and pasted from one file to another.

Common Word Processing Features

- Block operations allow the user to highlight and move "blocks" of text to another position within the document. Text can be copied, appended, deleted, moved, and added to another document. It can be changed

- Provides immediate access to patient records, insurance information and eligibility, office notes, and reports
- Procedure entry routines capture information necessary for any type of claim or HMO report
- Electronic communications include ability to request, receive, and transfer information electronically. An example of this is electronic insurance claim filing
- Advanced billing features may include:
  - Capability for maintaining enrollment lists, automatically calculating co-pay amounts, and monitoring benefit limits for managed care
  - Capability for government reporting such as Worker's Compensation documents
  - Collection tracking system for patient bills and insurance claims
- Automates the scheduling of patient appointments, cancellations, and recalls
- Electronic medical records can store, organize, and present data on various aspects of a patient's medical history on demand
- Automated reporting allows practice to predefine reports and billing jobs to be printed automatically and even unattended

Figure 11-5   Some medical management software capabilities.

from lowercase to all caps, the font or typestyle can be altered, and it can be made italic or boldface.

- Page formatting can create a variety of looks for the printed page. Text can be right and left justified, centered, or aligned on the left with a ragged right. Other page format features include pagination, the placement of numbers on the page, **widow** and **orphan** control (where paragraphs end or begin on the page), and the use of **headers** and **footers** that mark each page of the document in some consistent way.

- Spell check is a feature of most word processing programs. Medical spell checkers can be added to most word processing programs and can be used to check medical terminology in word processed documents or transcribed medical reports. See also the transcription section in Chapter 16. While spell checkers are useful tools, they are not a replacement for proofreading.

- **Macros** are keystrokes that have been saved separately so that the saved keystrokes may be inserted into any document. Macros are useful for increasing productivity when working with repetitive types of

SIX OPERATIONS FUNDAMENTAL TO OPERATING SOFTWARE

1. File creation.
When alphanumeric or numeric data are entered, the information is stored in primary memory (RAM) and made available to the user for viewing on a monitor.

2. Formatting.
Formatting a file, depending on the software, usually refers to the arrangement of information so that its appearance is concise and easy to read. For word processing files, this process entails setting margins, line spacing, tab settings, and other variations. For a spreadsheet file, the process may involve choices about the size of the columns, the placement of headings over columns, and the placement of headings.

3. Editing.
Once a file has been created and formatted, modifications may be made to the original file. Spelling corrections can be made and formatting changes can be implemented. Sections of the document may be cut and pasted.

4. Saving.
If the file is to be retained permanently, it must be saved to a secondary storage medium. When working on any document, it is advisable to use the save command frequently; power interruptions and other events may cause the file to be deleted.

5. Printing.
A hard copy (printed page) is created when the file is complete and all changes have been made. Text viewed on the monitor is called a soft copy.

6. Retrieval.
Saved files may be retrieved from storage at any time. Accessing them is a process known as retrieval.

materials. For example, a letterhead used on every business letter could easily be saved in a macro format and used repeatedly.

- **Merge operations** are also time savers when working with repetitive material. Merges are often used on the individualized form letter. Ambulatory care settings may use merge operations in mailing patient education memos.

- **Sorting** refers to rearrangements of information. Sorts can be performed on alphanumeric (letters and numerals) or numeric (numerals) data. Frequently, sorts are used to arrange labels for mailings by zip code.

● Importing and exporting data allow users to carry a text file into another applications program. Moving data from one program to another can be cumbersome, time consuming, and frustrating without the ability to import (bring in) and export (send out) easily and efficiently.

● Multicolumn output is the arrangement of text on a page in two or more columns for documents such as newsletters and patient education brochures. See Chapter 45 for techniques on developing patient information brochures.

● Desktop publishing refers to the ability to combine text and graphics into documents and produce them in a high-quality format, usually with the use of an inkjet or laser printer. Word processing packages vary greatly in their ability to provide all the options necessary for effective desktop publishing environments.

Graphics

Pictorial representations help to summarize and highlight important ideas and assist professionals in communicating material effectively. **Graphics software** transforms numeric information into line graphs, pie charts, or bar graphs (Figure 11-6). These graphic representations summarize trends in an easy-to-read format.

Graphics programs often allow the medical assistant to import files from spreadsheet or database applications, so that data from these files can be summarized graphically and displayed on screen. Drawing applications also provide a means of creating and developing custom artwork for patient brochures and newsletters.

When more than one application is grouped together and made available in a single prewritten, prepackaged format, the application is said to be integrated. Popular integrated packages include Microsoft Works and Lotus Works.

Spreadsheets

Spreadsheet software "crunches" or calculates numbers. These programs act as electronic calculators, performing mathematical calculations and recalculations. These calculations occur so quickly and accurately that financial and other types of numeric data can be summarized and analyzed in ways that used to be difficult and time consuming. In fact, the introduction of spreadsheets began what we know now as the computer revolution.

Spreadsheets take the form of a worksheet, much like an accountant's columnar pad. The worksheet consists of empty rows and columns. Each row and each column is labeled, either numerically or alphabetically, to give

entries a title. The intersection of row and column has a unique location, identified by the coordinates of the row and column, for example, D5 or AA7760. This intersection is called the cell location or cell address.

Common features found in most spreadsheet packages include the ability to format numbers. Values can be displayed in decimal format, in a currency format with a dollar sign, or as a percent sign (%). Labels can be formatted to be left justified over a column of cells, right justified over a column of cells, or centered over the column.

Spreadsheets are useful for expense sheets, tax reporting, and other financial reporting. Medical billing packages are usually based on spreadsheet software.

Databases

Databases serve to organize large quantities of related data into useful forms. **Database management software** is frequently used to handle employee information, manage inventory systems, record number of patient visits, and manage other patient information. Databases also are used in information retrieval services, which provide access to on-line sites.

Database Management Systems. Databases or database management systems (DBMS) are built from the concept of data organization. Data is organized from its most simple component, the bit, to the most complex data structure, the database. **Bits** are the smallest unit of data that the computer can process. **Bytes**, the equivalent of characters (a, b, 1, 2, @, #, and so on), are made up of codes of bits. Each byte that can be input from a keyboard can be translated into a unique code. These codes make up what is referred to as machine language, the language the computer works with in order to process data.

Bytes are combined together to make fields. **Fields** are pieces of information or data elements. Examples of fields include first names, last names, and disease categories like hypertension or obesity. Fields are pieces of information that we collect about individual entities. These entities are known as **records**, and most of the time entities represent individuals.

Databases can be quite complex, based on sophisticated mathematical models. One of the most flexible models for the database is the relational model. Because of its flexibility, it has been used with microcomputer systems and is becoming more popular with the use of minicomputers and mainframes.

Structuring or Defining the Database. The first step in working with a database is the creation of the database structure itself.

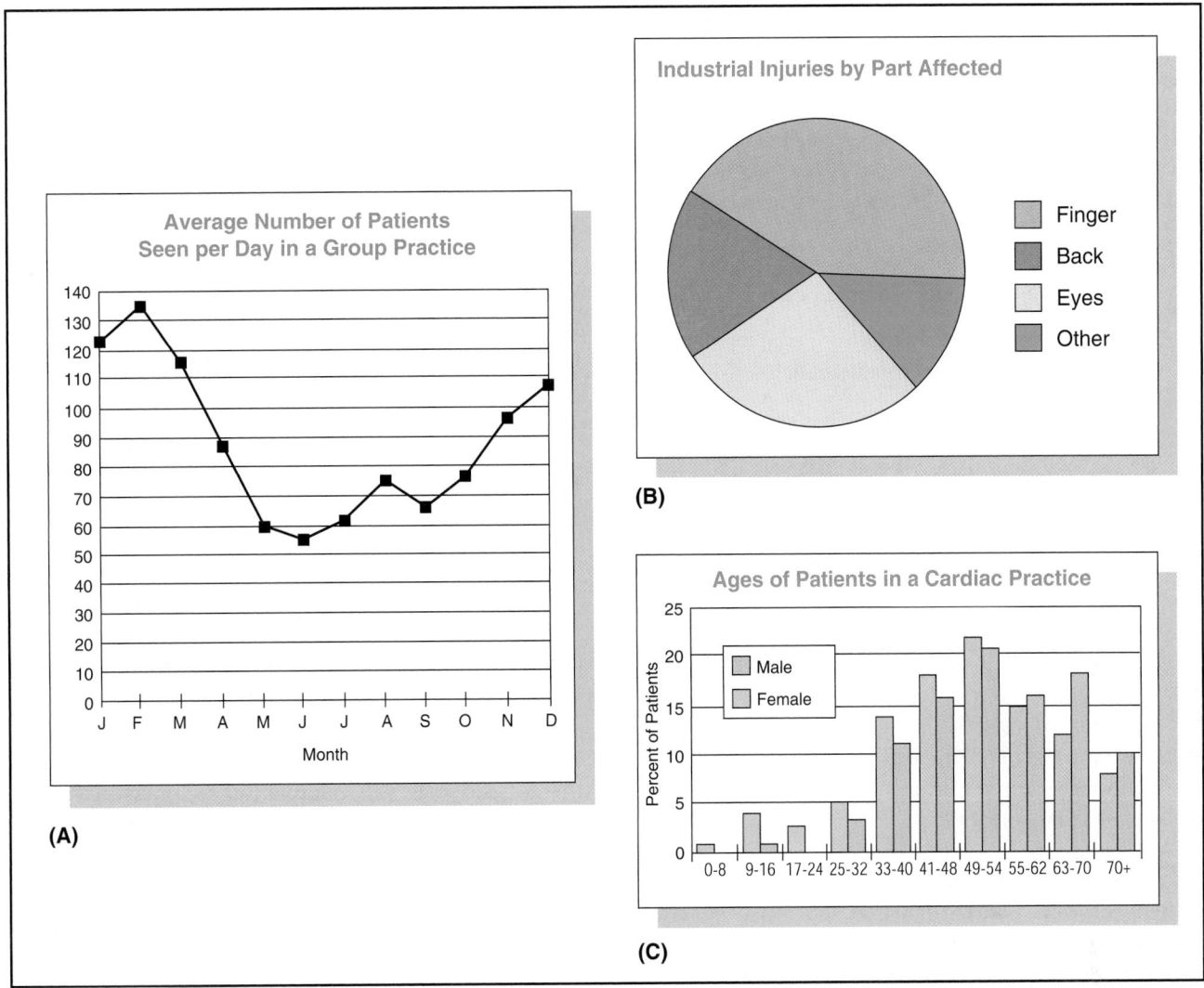

Figure 11-6 Graphs and charts are excellent for presenting information that can be interpreted at a glance: (A) Line graph. (B) Pie chart. (C) Bar graph.

Creating an imaginary patient database for a medical practice will be helpful for illustrative purposes. Consider a two-physician practice with 1,000 patients. The office maintains information on all its patients, including general identifying information, accounting information, and medical records.

A database is needed that will maintain the general identifying information. Minimally, the fields necessary for the database would need:

- Patient name
- Patient address
- Work phone
- Home phone
- Patient insurance

Other fields might also be included such as:

- Gender
- Social Security number
- Date of birth
- Occupation
- Place of employment

These headings provide the basic structure for the database.

The variables involved in health care databases are numerous and might include identification of the patient, identification of the insurance carrier or carriers, type of insurance, limits in plan benefits, diagnosis and procedure codes, and information concerning the primary care physician.

With the influence of managed care, databases that identify patient insurance variables become increasingly important. These databases might include the identification numbers of insurance policies and the insurance carriers or managed care operations that provide coverage for the patient. In developing this database, it is important to consider the following questions:

- Is the patient insured?

- Is there more than one insurance policy?

- Who is the insurer? Does this insurance supplement governmental forms of insurance such as Medicare or Medicaid?

- Does the patient's insurance require co-payments or deductibles?

- What will be covered by which insurance policy?

- Does the patient assign (turn over) benefits directly to the provider?

- Is the patient covered through Worker's Compensation?

Once established, databases can provide invaluable information in very little time. The key is to know what information you need readily available and then structure a database to that objective.

Information Retrieval Systems. Database management software (DBMS) can be adapted to a variety of medical settings. In addition to DBMS's capability of processing patient data, databases are used within the health care environment as information retrieval systems. Through the Internet, it is possible to connect electronically with information retrieval systems to reference topics in health sciences literature. Most medical libraries and many hospitals have the capacity to use the MEDLARS (Medical Literature Analysis and Retrieval Systems) literature database. This database, through the National Library of Medicine, allows researchers to conduct literature reviews on any of their twenty on-line bibliographies.

Information systems that complete biomedical journal searches are also becoming available on a subscription service basis to individual purchasers for use on their microcomputers. One on-line service is Medline; it contains more than six million references on journal articles relevant to health care professionals.

Information retrieval systems are also available for patient use. Cancer treatment protocols, descriptions of treatment regimens, and prognosis information by diagnostic category are now available to individuals who wish to gather information on cancer diagnoses and treatment

options. These information retrieval systems should not be used for complete medical care but are a resource to patients who are frequently bewildered by treatment choices.

Virus Protection

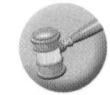

Protecting your computer from viruses, especially when patient records are on the system, is especially important. No office should download information from the Internet or even accept files from other computer systems without having a virus protection software (e.g., Norton Antivirus).

PATIENT CONFIDENTIALITY IN THE COMPUTERIZED MEDICAL OFFICE

The computer and other electronic transmission media are powerful tools, but they are equally powerful in their potential to jeopardize patient confidentiality. A record or test result faxed to a location where the fax is not contained in a secured area can be read by anyone coming past. A fax also can be accidentally sent to the wrong phone, possibly the office fax of the patient since this information is commonly in the patient record. Records sent over the Internet to an external location can be intercepted by a hacker and posted on the web for all to see. These are just a few of the possible scenarios that can occur if protocols are not in place to ensure maintenance of confidentiality.

The starting point for a meaningful information security system is a comprehensive security policy that is understood and supported by staff and employees. All staff and vendors having access to the computer system should be educated on the security policy and should be asked to sign a contract affirming that they will adhere to the policy before they are given access to confidential data.

The next essential step is to ensure that computer literate personnel are employed to set up and structure databases. Protocols should be established defining who can access and modify databases, providing identification, dating, and authentication mechanisms for those changes and additions. Procedures should be in place to ensure that people other than the intended recipient cannot accidentally read misdirected files, and that sufficient firewalls or precautions are taken to prevent people from hacking into the system through Internet or network interfaces. Antivirus programs should be part of the system to prevent loss of the database and/or the unintentional dissemination of files.

Passwords incorporating employee personal identification numbers (PIN) or passwords that are employee-specific are quite successful in controlling access to files and providing an authentication mechanism. Locating fax machines in restricted access areas under the supervision of people with access to all sensitive data can control faxes. Both the sender and the recipient can make sending files on the Internet secure by the use of encryption programs. Development of a firewall to allow outside computers to access your computer while restricting access to your databases is essentially impossible. The U.S. government, with unlimited facilities, hasn't been able to develop a foolproof system, so other approaches are required for an office of limited resources. Probably the best approach is not to allow outside computers access to your database computers, and to communicate to an outside network or Internet using a dedicated computer. Files to be transferred would be loaded into the dedicated computer using one of the portable data storage devices. This would also limit damage in the event a virus invaded your system.

The American Medical Association (AMA) supports the adoption of standards to protect individual confidential information. Figure 11-7 summarizes AMA Policy E5-07, "Confidentiality—Computers," issued prior to April 1977 and updated in 1994 and 1998. Sample security policy guidelines, employee and vendor training, and confidentiality statements have been developed by the Computer-Based Patient Records Institute (CPRI). Their web site is www.cpri-host.org. They are located at 4915 St. Elmo Avenue, Suite 401, Bethesda, MD 20814.

COMPUTERIZING THE MEDICAL OFFICE

While the computerization of an ambulatory care setting may seem like a daunting process, the task is made more manageable if problems are anticipated beforehand. While computerization can simplify cumbersome tasks, and ultimately lead to greater productivity, initially staff members may experience some frustration until they become proficient in the use and language of computers.

When computerizing a medical office, it is important to know what to expect, to understand the uses and limits of computers, and to organize the transition thoroughly, with proper attention to these details:

1. *Know what the office needs in a computer system.* To be useful, a computer system must serve the needs of the facility. Make a list of why you want the computer: it might include word processing, insurance claim filing, and managing a database. You also might want on-line and e-mail capabilities.
2. *Network by talking to other people in the medical industry.* It is advisable to ask questions of other ambulatory care centers that have been through the

---

SPOTLIGHT ON AAMA ESSENTIALS THROUGH CAAHEP

● When computerizing the medical office, asking for input from members of the staff will ultimately make implementation of the system a much more positive experience for all involved.

● Being willing to help others to learn new skills and tackle new office tools, such as the computer, helps to promote adaptability and eventually helps you get ahead in your career.

● A medical assistant who is familiar with computers and how they can be used in the ambulatory care setting can help others understand their usefulness, and thus, help lessen the stress caused by learning something new.

---

manual-to-computerization process. Ask them what computer hardware they prefer, what software applications they advise for different functions, and what problems they encountered during their transition.

3. *Work with a trusted, knowledgeable vendor.* It is important to establish a relationship with a computer vendor who understands not only computers but the needs of a medical office. Reliable vendors should be able to advise you of the best system and software and help you anticipate and allow for future needs as the medical practice grows.
4. *Involve all staff members.* If staff members are not familiar with the use of computers, they may feel threatened and, initially, think that using a computer is more time consuming than doing a task manually. The transition takes time and training. Organize staff training sessions, either on- or off-site, so that all employees are familiar with the basics of computer operation.
5. *Install the operation during a down period.* The installation of a computer network can be very disruptive to patients and the office environment. If possible, schedule the installation during a down period, such as over a long holiday when the office is closed, or at least after office hours.
6. *Allow adequate time for start-up.* Initially, much data from existing records will have to be entered. This is an onerous and time-consuming task, but one that

AMA COMPUTER CONFIDENTIALITY GUIDELINES

The utmost effort and care must be taken to protect the confidentiality of all medical records, including computerized medical records.

The guidelines below are offered to assist physicians and computer service organizations in maintaining the confidentiality of information in medical records when that information is stored in computerized data bases:

(1) Confidential medical information should be entered into the computer-based patient record only by authorized personnel. Additions to the record should be time and date stamped, and the person making the additions should be identified in the record.

(2) The patient and physician should be advised about the existence of computerized data bases in which medical information concerning the patient is stored. Such information should be communicated to the physician and patient prior to the physician's release of the medical information to the entity or entities maintaining the computer data bases. All individuals and organizations with some form of access to the computerized data bases, and the level of access permitted, should be specifically identified in advance. Full disclosure of this information to the patient is necessary in obtaining informed consent to treatment. Patient data should be assigned a security level appropriate for the data's degree of sensitivity, which should be used to control who has access to the information.

(3) The physician and patient should be notified of the distribution of all reports reflecting identifiable patient data prior to distribution of the reports by the computer facility. There should be approval by the patient and notification of the physician prior to the release of patient-identifiable clinical and administrative data to individuals or organizations external to the medical care environment. Such information should not be released without the express permission of the patient.

(4) The dissemination of confidential medical data should be limited to only those individuals or agencies with a bona fide use for the data. Only the data necessary for the bona fide use should be released. Patient identifiers should be omitted when appropriate. Release of confidential medical information from the data base should be confined to the specific purpose for which the information is requested and limited to the specific time frame requested. All such organizations or individuals should be advised that authorized release of data to them does not authorize their further release of the data to additional individuals or organizations, or subsequent use of the data for other purposes.

(5) Procedures for adding to or changing data on the computerized data base should indicate individuals authorized to make changes, time periods in which changes take place, and those individuals who will be informed about changes in the data from the medical records.

(6) Procedures for purging the computerized data base of archaic or inaccurate data should be established and the patient and physician should be notified before and after the data has been purged. There should be no mixing of a physician's computerized patient records with those of other computer service bureau clients. In addition, procedures should be developed to protect against inadvertent mixing of individual reports or segments thereof.

(7) The computerized medical data base should be on-line to the computer terminal only when authorized computer programs requiring the medical data are being used. Individuals and organizations external to the clinical facility should not be provided on-line access to a computerized data base containing identifiable data from medical records concerning patients. Access to the computerized data base should be controlled through security measures such as passwords, encryption (encoding) of information, and scannable badges or other user identification.

(8) Back-up systems and other mechanisms should be in place to prevent data loss and downtime as a result of hardware or software failure.

(9) Security:

(a) Stringent security procedures should be in place to prevent unauthorized access to computer-based patient records. Personnel audit procedures should be developed to establish a record in the event of unauthorized disclosure of medical data. Terminated or former employees in the data processing environment should have no access to data from the medical records concerning patients.

(b) Upon termination of computer services for a physician, those computer files maintained for the physician should be physically turned over to the physician. They may be destroyed (erased) only if it is established that the physician has another copy (in some form). In the event of file erasure, the computer service bureau should verify in writing to the physician that the erasure has taken place. (IV)

Issued prior to April 1977.
Updated June 1994 and June 1998.

Figure 11-7 Computer confidentiality guidelines. (Source: *Code of Medical Ethics Current Opinions with Annotations,* 1994 Edition, American Medical Association, copyright © 1998) must be done with great accuracy. Do not expect the computer system to be 100 percent operational immediately. Allow time for medical records and other data to be entered and for staff to build confidence in their computer skills.

THE SAFE USE OF COMPUTERS

In any environment where computers are routinely used, the concept of ergonomics must be considered. **Ergonomics** is the study of work environments; the purpose of the study is to effectively design work areas that both increase productivity and ensure worker safety and satisfaction.

 Safety issues are of concern in computer environments because of documented adverse health effects. For example, low-level radiation has been correlated with increased incidence of miscarriages

in women and increased incidence of leukemia. Other health and safety concerns relate to a category of problems classified as repetitive strain injuries. One of the most frequently encountered is carpal tunnel syndrome, which can be caused by excessive wrist strain. This syndrome is quite painful for the individual and may require surgical intervention for correction. Other health problems associated with routine computer use include increased stress, fatigue, eyestrain, and headaches.

To minimize the occurrence of health problems, computer equipment needs to be chosen, set up, and used properly so the medical assistant is protected from injury, strain, and discomfort (Table 11-1).

Posture is also critical in preventing injury. Figure 11-8 is a diagram of a recommended sitting posture for computer users developed by Gary Karp, Ergonomics Consultant of Onsight Technology Education Services of San Francisco, California.

TABLE 11-1 PREVENTING COMPUTER INJURY

General Prevention Methods	Workstation Setup	
☐ Maintain good health with proper diet, sleep, and exercise.	**Chair**	☐ Chair back slightly reclined to carry body weight.
☐ Balance lifestyle—work, social, spiritual.		☐ Provide lumbar support to lower back.
☐ Learn principles of ergonomics and the potential causes of injury.		☐ Optimize back height to conform to shape of back.
☐ Do stretching exercises for hands, arms, shoulders and neck.		☐ Provide support to upper back—especially for those who sit for long periods.
☐ Learn breathing and relaxation methods.		☐ Thighs in optimal contact with seat pan, no contact behind knees.
☐ Take ten-second "micro-breaks" several times each hour.		☐ Thighs above knees without sense of sliding out of seat.
☐ Don't continue intense computer work when fatigued.		☐ Feet in firm contact with floor (use foot rest only if necessary).
☐ Mix tasks to allow breaks from computing and the chance to get up and move around.		☐ Armrests—if used—set so shoulders stay relaxed and arms are free to move.
☐ Manage time to avoid unnecessary crises and times of stress.	**Monitor**	☐ Ensure sufficient training in adjustment controls.
☐ Keep temperature comfortable.		☐ Top of screen just below eye level.
☐ Keep arms warm with long sleeves, sweaters, etc. Consider fingerless gloves.		☐ Position close enough to allow sitting back in chair with head relaxed.
☐ Promote a relaxed working atmosphere to reduce stress.		☐ Center in front of body to prevent turning trunk or head.
☐ Minimize loud noises, distracting sound in work environment.		☐ Set optimal contrast and brightness.
☐ Streamline office processes and production systems to reduce stress.		☐ Position to prevent glare from windows, light fixtures.
☐ Don't allow jobs to be typically overloaded or over-specialized.	**Keyboard**	☐ Keep clean of dust and smudges.
☐ Don't maintain "flattened" posture of hands when not actually keying.		☐ Position so that wrists are straight, shoulders are relaxed, arms at side.
☐ Reduce impact on fingers at the keyboards.		☐ Use "feet" of keyboard only if wrists are straighter.
☐ Look away from monitor when waiting for printing, files opening, etc. Allow eyes to focus on distance or close them to rest.		☐ Do not allow wrists to be in contact with edge of desk or hard surfaces.
		☐ Use wrist rest only if needed and comfortable.

(continues)

TABLE 11-1 *(continued)*

General Prevention Methods	Workstation Setup

General Prevention Methods

☐ Learn the computer and software properly to avoid frustration and stress.

☐ Take advantage of shortcuts, automated features, and efficiency utilities.

☐ Pay attention to your body. Do not ignore pain!

Workstation Setup

☐ Center in front of body to avoid twisting or bending wrists.

☐ Move hands and arms rather than stretching fingers or bending the wrist.

Miscellaneous

☐ Consider trackball, programmable mouse, or other alternative inputs.

☐ Headset telephone for people who talk while keying or writing.

☐ Keep oft-used objects close to avoid long reaches.

☐ Use document holders to prevent craning neck looking down to desk.

(Reprinted with permission from Gary Karp, Ergonomics Consultant, Onsight Technology Education Services, San Francisco, CA)

Sitting Diagram

This is the general diagram of the recommended sitting posture for computer users. Keep in mind that fixed postures contribute to the risk of cumulative trauma injury. Variety of posture is crucial, as is the habit of standing up often. The body needs movement. Nothing counts more than comfort, and this illustration is simply a tool to understand what is happening in your body at the computer. Keep these principles in mind as you develop a repertoire of comfortable postures to use throughout the workday, knowing that slumped and leaning postures demand more work from the body leading to early fatigue.

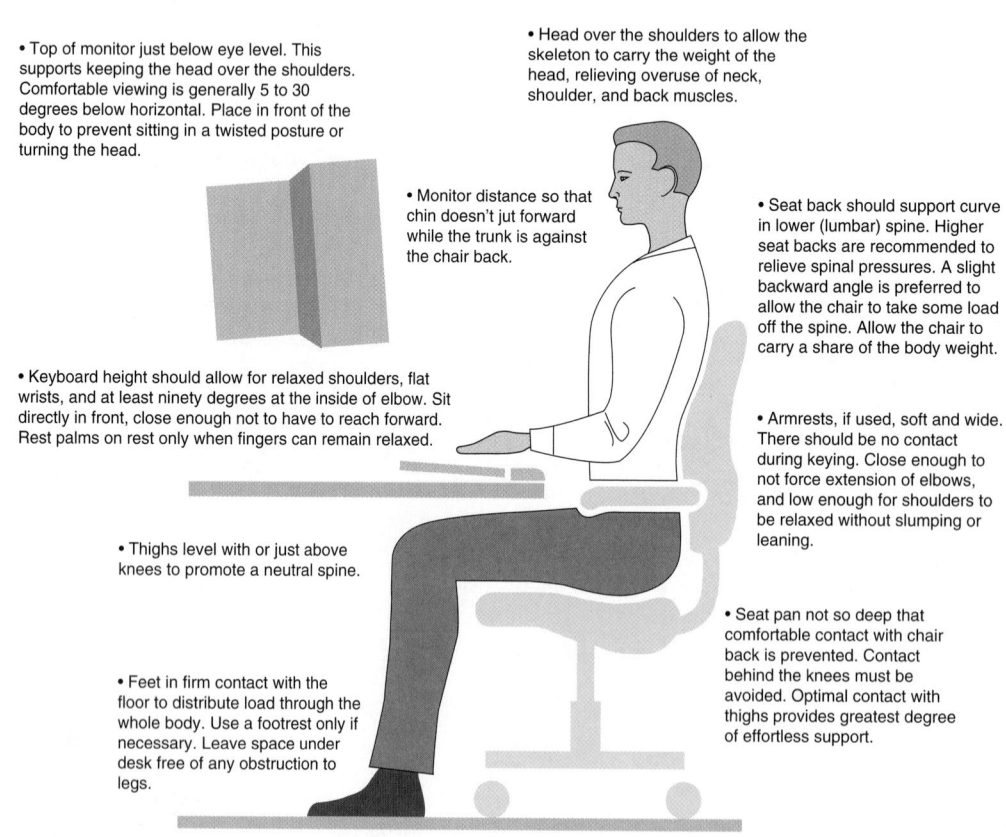

• Top of monitor just below eye level. This supports keeping the head over the shoulders. Comfortable viewing is generally 5 to 30 degrees below horizontal. Place in front of the body to prevent sitting in a twisted posture or turning the head.

• Monitor distance so that chin doesn't jut forward while the trunk is against the chair back.

• Head over the shoulders to allow the skeleton to carry the weight of the head, relieving overuse of neck, shoulder, and back muscles.

• Seat back should support curve in lower (lumbar) spine. Higher seat backs are recommended to relieve spinal pressures. A slight backward angle is preferred to allow the chair to take some load off the spine. Allow the chair to carry a share of the body weight.

• Keyboard height should allow for relaxed shoulders, flat wrists, and at least ninety degrees at the inside of elbow. Sit directly in front, close enough not to have to reach forward. Rest palms on rest only when fingers can remain relaxed.

• Armrests, if used, soft and wide. There should be no contact during keying. Close enough to not force extension of elbows, and low enough for shoulders to be relaxed without slumping or leaning.

• Thighs level with or just above knees to promote a neutral spine.

• Seat pan not so deep that comfortable contact with chair back is prevented. Contact behind the knees must be avoided. Optimal contact with thighs provides greatest degree of effortless support.

• Feet in firm contact with the floor to distribute load through the whole body. Use a footrest only if necessary. Leave space under desk free of any obstruction to legs.

Figure 11-8 Recommended computer operator position. (Courtesy of Gary Karp, Ergonomics Consultant, Onsight Technology Education Services, San Francisco, CA)

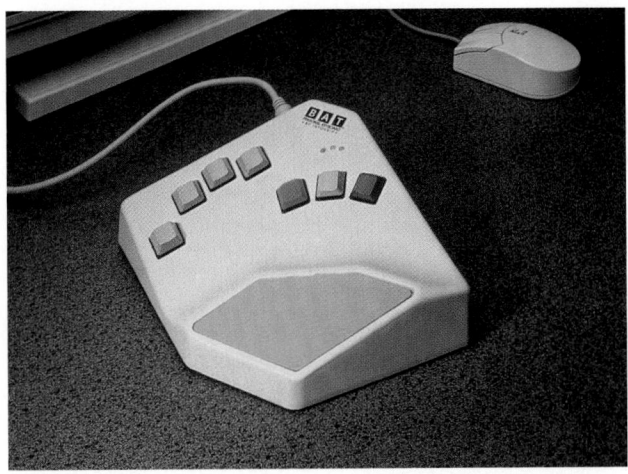 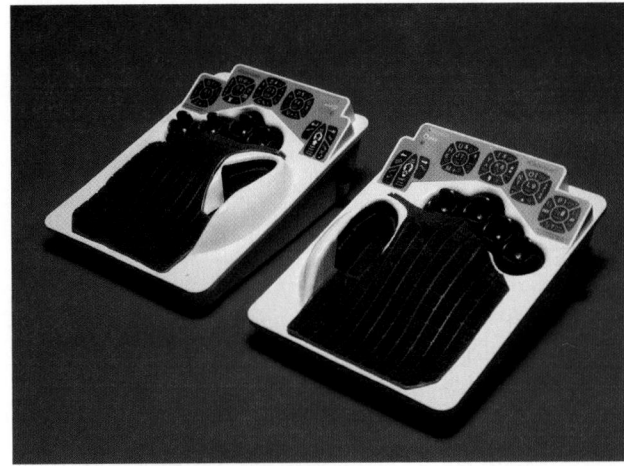

Figure 11-9 A variety of alternative keyboards is available: (Left) The BAT keyboard (Courtesy of Infogrip, Inc.). (Right) Datahand (Courtesy of Industrial Innovations).

Other considerations include using alternative keyboards to reduce wrist strain (Figure 11-9), using screen glare protectors to deflect and reduce monitor glare, positioning monitors appropriately for the individual, and using chairs that offer comfortable lower back support to reduce fatigue. Medical assistants should organize their work so they take frequent breaks away from the computer. These recommendations do not represent a complete ergonomic solution as many other issues specific to the environment would need to be evaluated especially for those medical assistants who may be at computer terminals for most of the workday.

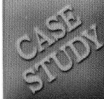

Once medical assistant Walter Seals received the go-ahead to order a computer system for Inner City Health Care, he immediately consulted a professional for advice on how to set up the workstations. As a health care professional, Walter firmly believes in preventive care and he wanted to ensure that staff members, especially those who might be using the computer extensively, did not develop some of the health problems associated with routine or prolonged computer use.

11-1

CASE STUDY REVIEW

1. Imagine that you are helping Walter design a typical computer workstation. Make a list of how chair, monitor, and keyboard should be positioned. Sketch your diagram for a safe and effective workstation.

2. In addition to a proper workstation setup, what are other measures Walter should consider to ensure staff safety?

3. One of the center's medical assistants is reluctant to use the computer, not because of safety issues but because she feels intimidated by the process. How should Walter help her overcome her timidity of the computer?

Walter Seals, a CMA employed by Inner City Health Care, has been given approval to computerize the office. Walter is also concerned about confidentiality issues involved with a computerized medical office.

11-2

CASE STUDY REVIEW

1. Identify the areas where confidentiality is most likely to be jeopardized.

2. Suggest possible solutions to protect confidentiality in each of these areas.

3. Write a one-page summary, and submit it to your instructor.

SUMMARY

As the capabilities for networking and communications between computer systems continue to develop, the potential for increasingly sophisticated uses of computer systems is becoming a reality. We are entering the age of global computing where information is available almost as quickly as it is requested. As these changes occur, the role of the medical assistant will reflect the growing reliance of the medical practice upon the capabilities of computers.

It will become the responsibility of all medical assistants to be information managers, taking advantage of the wealth of resources available by computer that can enhance patient care.

Physicians will require assistance in retrieving information from medical databases that support diagnosis; office staff may need assistance in locating, accessing, and working with applications software.

The medical assistant's professional responsibilities will become even more challenging as computers become indispensable to the ambulatory care setting.

REVIEW QUESTIONS

Multiple Choice

1. Microcomputers:
   a. are the fastest and most powerful computers
   b. handle large amounts of processing and challenge the capabilities of older mainframe systems
   c. are widely used in today's health care facility
   d. are very expensive and complex
2. The CPU:
   a. is the brain of the computer system
   b. consists of electronic tablets with pointers, scanners, and touch screens
   c. is often referred to as memory
   d. frequently is referred to as a computer program
3. Documentation:
   a. performs a specific data processing function
   b. is a set of instructions that a computer follows to control computer hardware and to process data
   c. frequently is called the operating system
   d. consists of the manuals and documents that define how programs operate
4. Spreadsheets are used primarily in:
   a. document production
   b. financial analysis
   c. communications
   d. information retrieval
5. Formatting a document refers to:
   a. setting margins, tabs, and line spacing
   b. macro operations
   c. exporting features
   d. all of the above
6. Fields:
   a. are a collection of bytes
   b. can be logical, alphanumeric, numeric, memo, or date
   c. represent pieces of information or data categories
   d. all of the above

7. Importing and exporting data:
   a. save time when working with repetitive material
   b. allow users to carry a text file into another application program
   c. are keystrokes that have been saved separately so that the saved keystrokes may be inserted into any document
   d. allow the user to highlight and move blocks of text to another position within the document
8. Database management software may be used for all of the following *except:*
   a. employee information
   b. manage inventory systems
   c. tax and other financial reporting
   d. record the number of patient visits
9. All of the following apply to bytes *except:*
   a. they are the smallest unit of data a computer can process
   b. they are the equivalent of characters
   c. each byte that can be input from a keyboard can be translated into a unique code
   d. the above code is referred to as machine language
10. When going from a manual to a computerized medical office, it is important to do all of the following *except:*
    a. know what the office needs in a computer system
    b. install the operation during a down period
    c. work with a trusted, knowledgeable vendor
    d. expect the computer system to be 100% operational immediately

Critical Thinking

1. Assume you work in an ambulatory care setting that operates on a manual system. Make a wish list of every function you would have a computer perform for the office.

2. The same office is now going to make the transition to a computerized system. What steps would you take to make the transition as smooth as possible?

3. Recall the four main types of computers and describe a situation in which each would be used.

4. What are the four components of a computer system? Discuss each component and its function.

5. If you were to create a file, what six functions would you perform in the process?

6. What are the major categories of applications software? What operations do they perform?

7. Your physician/employer has asked you to research a particular medical topic on the computer. How do you proceed?

8. Discuss the importance of patient confidentiality in medical computing. What measures could you take to ensure patient confidentiality?

9. Describe the study of ergonomics and give ten suggestions for preventing computer injury.

WEB ACTIVITIES

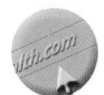 Go to a software provider's web site, such as www.microsoft.com, and list the name and purpose of each patch available for various system and application software programs.

REFERENCES/BIBLIOGRAPHY

American Medical Association. (2000). E-5.07 confidentiality: Computers. [On-line]. Available: http://www.ama-assn.org

Computer-based Patient Record Institute. *Advancing electronic information systems for health care*. [On-line]. Available: http://www.cpri-host.org

Humphrey, D. D. (1996). *Contemporary medical office procedures* (2nd ed.). Albany, NY: Delmar.

Karp, G. (1996). *Preventing computer injury*. Adapted from paper presented at the Association of American Medical Transcriptionists, Baltimore, MD.

Kinn, M. E., & Woods, M. A. (1999). *The medical assistant: Administrative and clinical* (8th ed.). Philadelphia: W. B. Saunders Company.

Chapter

12

TELEPHONE TECHNIQUES

OBJECTIVES

*The student should strive to meet the following performance objectives and demonstrate
an understanding of the facts and principles presented in this chapter through written and
oral communication.*

1. Define the key terms as presented in the glossary.

2. Describe four useful rules for using proper telephone technique.

3. State at least five common telephone courtesies.

4. Discuss proper screening techniques.

5. Outline the proper procedure for answering incoming calls.

6. Describe the information every message should contain.

7. Name at least three calls the medical assistant can take, and state the
   reasons why. Name three calls the medical assistant should refer to the
   physician, and state the reasons why.

(continues)

8. Recall six questions that should be asked during telephone triage.

9. Elaborate on how calls from angry individuals should be handled in a professional manner, and give three steps to take when this type of call is received.

10. Outline the proper procedure for placing outgoing calls.

11. Discuss telephone documentation.

12. Identify ways to ensure patient confidentiality when using the telephone.

13. Recall four examples of telephone technology, and describe their functions.

ROLE DELINEATION COMPONENTS

ADMINISTRATIVE
Administrative Procedures

- Perform basic clerical functions
- Schedule, coordinate and monitor appointments
- Schedule inpatient/outpatient admissions and procedures
- Understand and adhere to managed care policies and procedures

CLINICAL
Patient Care

- Adhere to established triage procedures
- Recognize and respond to emergencies

GENERAL (TRANSDISCIPLINARY)
Professionalism

- Project a professional manner and image
- Adhere to ethical principles
- Demonstrate initiative and responsibility
- Work as a team member
- Prioritize and perform multiple tasks

(continues)

SCENARIO

At a busy two-doctor family physician's office like Doctors Lewis and King, the telephone lines are rarely quiet. Yet, administrative medical assistant Ellen Armstrong has learned to maintain her composure when she is responsible for managing incoming calls. Ellen has in her favor a naturally warm telephone manner, but she has had to cultivate other traits so that she can represent the practice in a professional manner, help patients and other callers feel at ease, and efficiently screen or refer calls as necessary.

This is Ellen's first job since receiving her medical assisting certification, and initially she felt unable to properly screen calls. She was not sure when to refer them to the physician; she did not know when she should record a message. With some advice from Marilyn, the office manager, Ellen devised a simple system to keep herself and her thoughts organized throughout a hectic day of telephone communications. Every day before office hours, she gathers the materials she needs, including the appropriate message pad, a list of information needed to set a patient appointment, and any information she needs on prescription refills for patients. With these few measures, Ellen feels organized and prepared and thus able to focus her attention on interacting with the caller.

INTRODUCTION

As in many office settings, the telephone is the lifeline of the ambulatory care setting. By means of telephone communication, which can also include fax and e-mail transmissions, patient appointments are scheduled, referrals made, critical information related, and the practice personality conveyed.

Medical assistants, more multiskilled than ever, have a wealth of knowledge to bring to their telephone communications. Over the telephone, they will welcome new patients, reassure current patients, collaborate with other organizations on patient care, and calmly and efficiently deal with emergencies. They will need to draw on their vast resource of administrative and clinical knowledge; they will also need to cultivate a telephone personality that is warm and accessible while also being efficient and organized.

In this chapter, medical assistants will come to understand the principles basic to successful telephone communications, whether initiating or answering calls; learn the extent and limits of their authority as medical assistants; discover how to prepare themselves for making or receiving calls; and be introduced to telephone systems and new technologies.

BASIC TELEPHONE TECHNIQUES

The majority of patients seen in ambulatory care settings initiate their first contact with the office through the telephone. Medical assistants responsible for answering the telephone may be the first contact most people have with the practice. First impressions tend to be lasting ones, so both tone of voice and message content are important as communicators.

To create a positive impression, try to answer the telephone at the end of the first ring and always by the third ring. If your office has more than one incoming line and more than one telephone, it may be necessary to interrupt a conversation to answer another call. Some guidelines to follow in that instance include:

- Excuse yourself to the first caller by saying, "Excuse me, another line is ringing. May I put you on hold for a moment?"
- When the first caller has given permission to be put on hold, answer the second call. Ascertain who is calling, and determine if it is an emergency. If it is not an emergency, ask if you may put the person on hold or return the call when you have completed the first call.
- Return to the first caller, and thank the person for holding.

Telephone Personality

First impressions are usually conveyed through verbal and nonverbal communication. (Refer to Chapter 4 for a review of these communication modes.) In telephone communications, however, personality and attitudes are conveyed only through the tone in which words are spoken and the words themselves. Remember, callers are not an interruption of your work but the reason for your job. Even in a large practice, it is rare that someone just answers the telephone and has no other duties. No matter what other duties are pressing, the primary responsibility of every employee in a physician's office is patient care; everything else is secondary. Whoever answers incoming calls should be prepared to give the caller complete attention.

Use a voice that is pleasant and well **modulated** (one that varies in pitch and intensity) and conveys interest in the callers' needs. Hold the handpiece correctly, about 1 to 2 inches away from the mouth, and project your voice *at* the mouthpiece not *over* it.

Volume, enunciation, pronunciation, and speed all have a profound effect on how you sound to the person on the other end of the line.

- Volume should be the same as when speaking conversationally.
- **Enunciation** implies speaking your words clearly and **articulating** carefully.
- **Pronunciation** involves saying the words correctly.
- Speed should be at a normal rate, neither too fast nor too slow.
- **Posture**, the way the body is carried, also affects the voice. If slumped in a chair, the **diaphragm** (the muscle separating the abdominal and thoracic

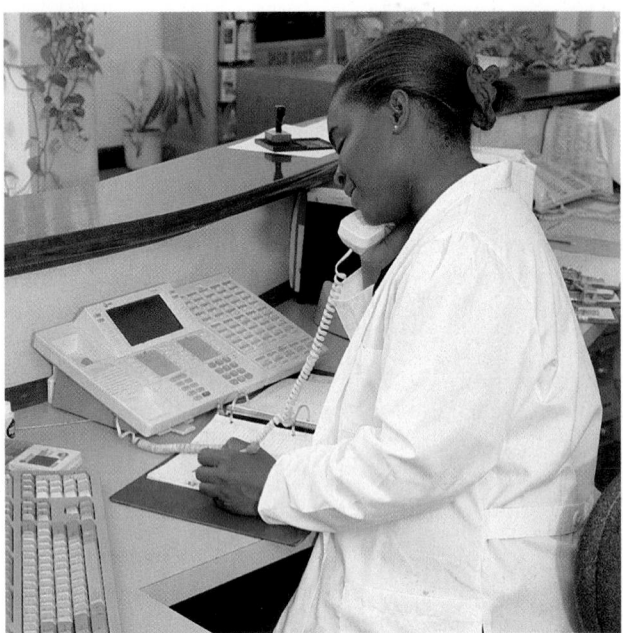

Figure 12-1   Practice proper posture and attitude when using a telephone in a professional setting.

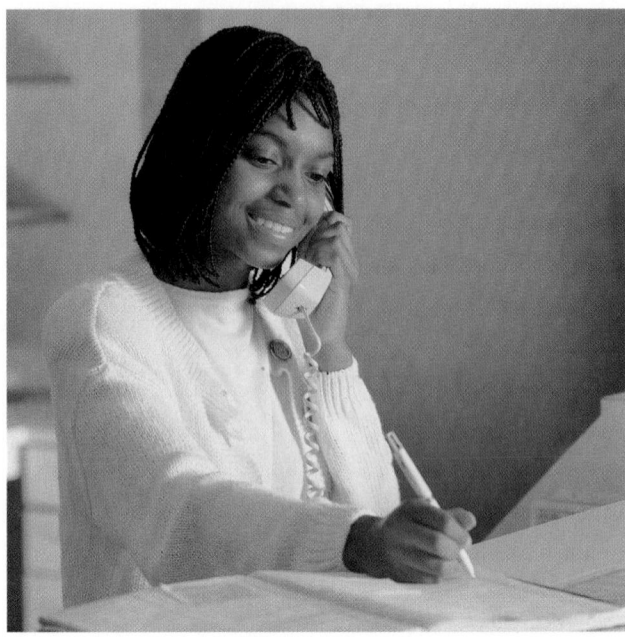

Figure 12-2   Tone of voice is able to put people at ease in a telephone conversation. People can hear an unpleasant mood, just as they can hear a warm smile.

cavities) is compressed and breathing may be restricted. This posture can make an individual sound tired and tense. Additionally, posture affects mood. Sitting up straight creates a professional and alert mood that comes across in the voice (Figure 12-1).

Being organized and prepared in advance for each telephone call enables the medical assistant to respond to each caller as if there is nothing else to do. By taking a breath before answering the telephone and putting a smile on one's lips, a pleasant vocal impression can be delivered to the caller.

Medical assistants who enjoy their work and want to be of assistance to patients communicate enthusiasm. Enthusiasm conveys interest to the caller and projects a sincere, caring attitude that can be "heard" over the telephone (Figure 12-2).

Though some callers will be upset, frightened, or even angry, the medical assistant must always be patient and in control. Some calls may be life-threatening emergencies; medical assistants need to remain calm to be of help to the caller, remembering their professional role as health care providers.

Medical assistants can concentrate on improving telephone communications by setting up a small tape recorder next to the telephone and setting it to record for an hour or two each day. At the end of the day, recorded calls will present an accurate representation of volume, articulation, and tone of voice. After using the tape as a self-improvement exercise, be sure to erase all messages in order to respect the confidentiality of callers.

Telephone Etiquette

Telephone etiquette, as with all good manners, simply involves treating others with consideration. Medical assistants have chosen a profession in which care and concern for others are paramount, so it is especially important to keep the patient's feelings in the forefront at all times. Basic telephone courtesies should be kept in mind when answering any professional call.

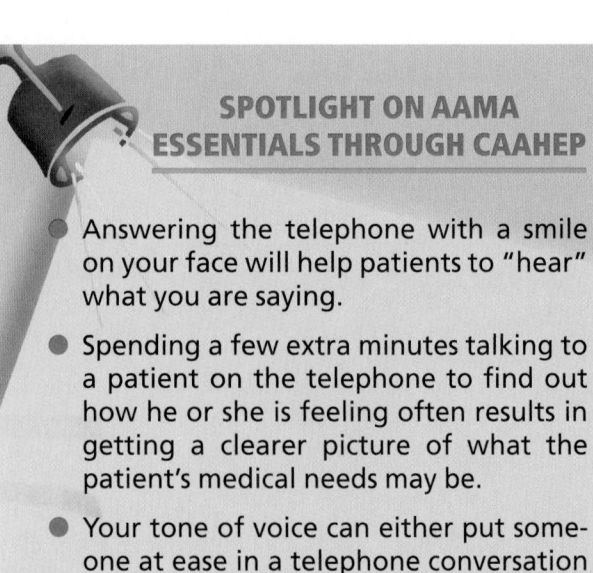

SPOTLIGHT ON AAMA ESSENTIALS THROUGH CAAHEP

- Answering the telephone with a smile on your face will help patients to "hear" what you are saying.

- Spending a few extra minutes talking to a patient on the telephone to find out how he or she is feeling often results in getting a clearer picture of what the patient's medical needs may be.

- Your tone of voice can either put someone at ease in a telephone conversation or cause the person to become angry and put off.

ANSWERING INCOMING CALLS

Most calls received in an ambulatory care setting are from patients or prospective patients, though many are from other physicians or medical facilities. The remainder will be from family members, salespeople, and miscellaneous others. Personal calls should not be permitted in the medical office as they busy lines intended for business. Most physicians will tolerate occasional emergency calls from family members.

Preparing to Take Calls

Before answering incoming calls or making outgoing calls, medical assistants should devise a simple system to keep organized throughout the hectic day of telephone communications. Collect pertinent materials, such as a message pad, information regarding scheduling of patients and prescription refills, internal and outside referral forms, listing of frequently used telephone numbers and extensions, and several sharpened pencils and working pens.

Answering Calls

When answering incoming calls, the name of the facility should be clearly identified and with whom the caller is speaking. The name of the office is very important, as the caller wants to know the correct number has been reached. To avoid clipping off the office name, practice using **buffer words**. Buffer words are expendable words and may consist of introductory words, phrases, or statements. They allow a caller an opportunity to collect their thoughts and focus on what is being said.

Obtain the caller's full name and correct spelling, and ask if this is an emergency call. Determine how you can be of assistance, and complete the call efficiently by following all established office protocols. (Refer to Procedure 12-1.)

Screening Calls

One of the medical assistant's responsibilities will be to **screen** incoming calls. The purpose of screening is twofold: 1) to be sure the caller talks to the person who

---

TELEPHONE COURTESIES

- Always use callers' names and titles (for example, Mrs. O'Keefe or Dr. King) during the course of a conversation when confidentiality is assured; this shows interest in them as individuals.
- Do not use technical terms if simpler ones will convey the information adequately. Using professional jargon, or terminology, is an easy trap to fall into since this terminology is used daily with coworkers. Jargon only confuses people outside the profession; the goal in communication is mutual understanding, not obfuscation, which confuses people.
- Do not use slang or nonstandard terms in a business setting. Slang terms may have entirely different meanings to individuals from another generation or cultural background. Use of slang is not professional and tends to indicate a poor vocabulary range or lack of education. However, patients may use slang in their communications. It is important not to be offended by slang terms; also, be certain that patients who use slang understand any common medical terminology you may use.
- The "hold" button on the telephone is probably the most misused piece of equipment in the practice; always use it sparingly.
  Never put a caller on hold until you know who is calling and why. Never place an urgent or emergency call on hold. Never put a caller on hold without asking for and receiving permission to do so.

- No call should be left unattended for more than 20 to 30 seconds. If it is necessary to keep calls waiting longer, go back to the caller and give the option of continuing to hold or receiving a call back in a few minutes.
- When it is necessary to get additional information and call back later, let the person know when to expect the call. If for some reason the information is not available when the time for the call back arrives, call anyway to let the person know when to expect another call.
- When taking a message for someone in the office, give the caller an idea of when to expect a return call. If the person will be out of the office for an extended period, see if someone else can help or if the caller would rather wait to hear from that specific individual.
- Pay attention to what the person is saying and *how* they sound. Do not interrupt or finish sentences for slow talkers. The caller may have difficulty putting some things into words, but give the person a chance to explain the problem or question. Listen with empathy for the caller. Also listen to what the tone of voice expresses.
- Never talk to someone in the office while on an open line. This is confusing to the caller, and confidential information could inadvertently be overheard.
- Do not attempt to work on other things while talking on the telephone.
- Never eat or chew gum when talking on the telephone. This impedes enunciation and is distracting to the caller.
- Say "goodbye" when closing the call, and allow the caller to hang up first.

will be most helpful (this is not necessarily the person asked for); and 2) to ensure the physician's time with calls is efficiently managed.

Most people who call an ambulatory care setting will ask to speak to the doctor. Patients calling for appointments or with billing problems or insurance questions will frequently ask to speak to Dr. King, assuming she is the person in charge and therefore should answer any question or solve any problem. In most practices, this is not the case. Medical assistants and other administrative employees are equipped to deal with front-office functions; usually, physicians are not involved in these procedures and sometimes may not be aware of administrative routines.

Proper Screening Techniques. Screening is usually a simple process of asking the caller's name and the reason for the call. There are situations, however, that will require tactful persistence to get the information needed to properly direct the caller. Sometimes callers hesitate to give information because the questions are of a confidential and possibly even embarrassing nature.

Occasionally a caller flatly refuses to give any information or will just say, "I'm a friend." If it is a patient who refuses to give information after gentle prodding, respect the patient's privacy and take a message. If you do not know who the caller is and you are unable to get any information, take the message and give it to the physician. Frequently this type of caller is a salesperson. (Physicians are prime targets for all types of sales pitches.) If the physician does not know the person, he or she can decide whether to return the call. In any event, do not argue with the caller. Be polite and professional at all times.

Transferring a Call

During the screening process, calls may mistakenly be directed to someone who is unable to assist the caller adequately. This call will need to be transferred to someone with more expertise in a particular area. Guidelines that ensure successful transfer of calls include:

- Get the caller's full name, telephone number, and any other situation-associated information before attempting to transfer the call.

- Determine who would be the best person to assist with this situation.

- Ask if you may place the caller on hold while you collect any pertinent data and make a call to see that the person best suited to assist is available.

- Return to the caller, thank for holding, and give the name and extension of the person to whom you will be transferring the call.

- Follow your telephone system's procedure for transferring the call.

- Followup to be sure the call transferred correctly.

Taking a Message

When taking messages, it is advisable to use a standard telephone message pad with a carbon that allows the office to maintain a record of all incoming calls (Figure 12-3). The information that should be recorded for *every* message includes:

1. Date and time call is received
2. Who the call is for
3. Caller's name and telephone number
4. When the caller can be reached
5. Nature and urgency of the call
6. Action to be taken (e.g., will call back, returned your call, please call back)
7. Message, if any
8. Your name or initials (in case there are questions)

Be sure to repeat the information back to the caller to verify that you have heard and copied it correctly. When taking a message, give callers an approximate time when they might expect to receive a call back. ("Dr. King will be returning calls between 4:30 and 5:00." "Ellen is out of the office today, but I'll ask her to call you before 10 A.M. tomorrow.")

Always attach a message from a patient to the patient's chart before placing the message on the physician's desk. The physician cannot discuss the patient's condition or answer questions without this information.

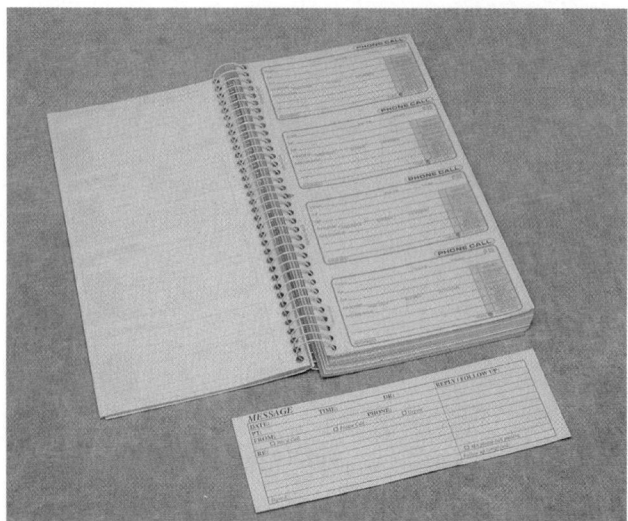

Figure 12-3 Message pads with a carbon allow the office to maintain a written record of all incoming calls.

Ending the Call

Ending the telephone call is as important as answering the call promptly. Bring the conversation to a courteous closure, and repeat any pertinent information back to the caller. ("Your appointment is scheduled for Friday, January 12, at 9 A.M. with Doctor King.") Pause just a moment to see if the caller has any additional questions. If not, say "Goodbye." Never use slang terms such as *bye bye, see you later,* or *so long.* They do not reflect a positive professional image. You should always stay on the line until the caller hangs up. They might think of something else they wanted to ask or verify, and staying on the line gives the caller the opportunity to verbalize a thought rather than have to call back. Figure 12-4 summarizes four rules of proper telephone technique.

TYPES OF CALLS THE MEDICAL ASSISTANT CAN TAKE

Keep in mind that, no matter how experienced, the medical assistant has definite limitations of authority and knowledge. The vast majority of calls can be handled by the knowledgeable medical assistant, but there are situations that only the physician should manage simply because the physician ultimately is responsible for what happens in the practice.

1. Established patients: When an established patient calls to set up an appointment, record the patient's name, daytime telephone number, and the reason for the appointment.
2. New patients: Require the same information as the established patient plus some additional information, including:

   - Address
   - Age/birthdate
   - Employer
   - Insurance carrier or HMO
   - Name of insured (self, spouse, or parent)
   - Name of referral source

   This information serves as a source for the establishment of the chart and may lead to a discussion regarding payment of fees. The information should be entered into the appointment book for both new and established patients. See Chapter 13 for more information on patient scheduling.
3. Scheduling appointments: A major portion of telephone communications will be spent scheduling patient appointments. See Chapter 13 for detailed information on patient scheduling and rescheduling.
4. Scheduling patient tests: Scheduling tests for patients can involve a great deal of coordination, for

often appointment times need to involve physician, patient, and the facility where a test may be conducted.
5. Patients' billing questions: Billing questions can be involved and complex and medical assistants should be prepared to answer questions by retrieving information on the patient's insurance and billing status.
6. Insurance information: Calls will come from patients about insurance as well as from insurance carriers and HMOs with questions about patients or their treatment. If the call is from an insurance company or HMO, be sure there is a signed "Release of Information" in the patient's chart before giving information.

Rule 1. Callers are not an interruption of your work, but the reason for your job.
Even in a large practice, it is rare that someone just answers the telephone and has no other duties. No matter what other duties are pressing, the primary responsibility of every employee in a physician's office is patient care; everything else is secondary. Whoever answers incoming calls should be prepared to give the caller complete attention.

Rule 2. Always attach a message for the physician from a patient to the chart before putting it on the physician's desk; the physician cannot discuss the patient's condition or answer questions without that information.
The information that should be recorded for every message will include: date and time the call is received; who the call is for; the caller's name and number; when the caller can be reached; and the nature and urgency of the call; and initials of person writing the message.

Rule 3. When you take a message, give callers an approximate time when to expect to receive a call back.
For example, "Dr. King will be returning calls between 4:30 and 5:00." "Ellen is out of the office today, but I'll ask her to call you before 10 A.M. tomorrow." This basic courtesy respects the caller's time.

Rule 4. Complete patient confidentiality is an ethical and legal obligation.
One of the most important issues in a medical setting is patient confidentiality. No information about patients should be discussed outside the office, even with family or friends, or with other patients. Violations of confidentiality leave the practice vulnerable to lawsuits. More importantly, violations of confidentiality erode patient trust. See Chapters 7 and 8 for more information on legal and ethical issues.

Figure 12-4 A summary of useful rules for the medical assistant to follow for using proper telephone technique.

7. Requests for prescription refills: If a patient or family member is requesting that a prescription be refilled, medical assistants may take the call. However, they may not authorize a refill or tell the patient that a prescription will be refilled without the physician's approval. Most offices ask that the patient call their refill requests into the pharmacy; the pharmacy then calls the physician's office for approval. Messages taken on these calls should be attached to the patient's chart and given to the physician for review and for permission to refill. When the physician approves the refill, the pharmacy may be called with an approval.

8. Receiving routine progress reports: Frequently physicians will ask patients to report on their progress. *If the patient is doing well,* it is acceptable for you to take that information on a message form to be given to the physician.

9. General information about the practice: People may call requesting information about hours, location, financial policies, or areas of practice.

10. Salespeople: The medical office will have policies regarding the scheduling of pharmaceutical representatives.

TYPES OF CALLS REFERRED TO THE PHYSICIAN

1. Requests for test results: Only the physician should give this information. A seemingly simple report may frighten or confuse the patient; at the very least it will probably generate questions that medical assistants are not qualified to answer. Many physicians allow medical assistants to report on satisfactory test results.

2. Medical emergencies: There should be standard procedures for dealing with emergencies. The physician, when present, should be interrupted and notified of all emergency calls.

3. Medical questions: Medical assistants may not give medical advice without risking practicing without a license.

4. Other physicians: When other physicians call, always ask if they need to speak to the physician on staff immediately or if they would like a call back. Be sure to ask if the call is regarding a current patient; if so, pull the chart.

5. Patients who refuse information: If a patient will not provide information about a problem, take a message for the physician to call them back. Some patients are not comfortable discussing physical problems with anyone except the physician; they have a right to that privacy.

6. Complaints: In a medical office, all patient complaints should be viewed as potential malpractice suits. A patient with complaints about the office or the quality of care is best referred to the physician.

7. Poor progress reports: If a patient calls to report that a treatment regimen is not working, the information should be given to the physician immediately. Changes in the treatment or medication may need to be made or the patient may need to be seen right away. This is a medical judgment that medical assistants are not qualified to make.

8. Requests for patient information from a third party: Unless there is a signed release, patient information may not be given to anyone. Any such requests (other than from the patient's insurance carrier or HMO) must be referred to the physician.

9. Requests for referrals: (unless the physician has given the front office a list of specialists to use).

10. Requests for medication: (other than standard refills).

SPECIAL CONSIDERATION CALLS

Working in an ambulatory care setting brings the medical assistant into contact with emergencies, angry callers, and people of all ages, ethnic backgrounds, and educational levels. As a professional, your goal is to treat every individual with courtesy and respect regardless of age, race, creed, or national origin.

Referring Calls

Calls will often need to be referred to someone else in or out of the office—the physician, bookkeeper, insurance clerk, a hospital, laboratory, or other facility.

Internal Referrals. If it is necessary to transfer a caller to someone else in your office:

- Tell the caller to whom you are transferring the call and why.

- Call the party to whom you are transferring the call and tell them the caller's name and reason for the call in as much detail as the caller has provided.

See the example of internal referral.

External Referrals. If it is necessary to refer the caller to someone outside the office, such as to a laboratory or another physician, be sure to tell the caller:

- Why they should speak to someone else

- The telephone number to call (be sure to include the extension and area code, if necessary)

- Who, specifically, to speak with at that number

- What information to have ready when they make the call

- When to call

● If your office should be called back after the call is made

See the example of external referral.

Emergency Calls

Triage is the act of evaluating the urgency of a medical situation and prioritizing treatment. Keep in mind that most patients, when ill or injured or if a family member is ill or injured, feel the situation requires immediate medical attention. Triage is one of the most important functions for the person answering the telephone. Triage takes skill and experience. Do not be afraid to ask questions of other professionals in the office. To determine if a call is truly a medical emergency, keep a list of questions near the telephone to assist in evaluating the situation. Standard triage questions can determine the nature of an emergency. Not all questions are appropriate to every call; suitable questions depend on the nature of the situation. (Refer to Procedure 12-2.)

EXAMPLE: INTERNAL REFERRAL

Mrs. O'Keefe is calling about her account and asks specific questions regarding some tests done on her husband. You do not have access to the information she needs since Marilyn Johnson handles the bookkeeping and financial arrangements for the office.

Poor Technique

Medical Assistant: Oh, I don't do bills, hang on. *Dials Marilyn's extension.*
Medical Assistant: Marilyn, line 3 is for you." *Medical assistant hangs up. Marilyn picks up the telephone unprepared and has to put Mrs. O'Keefe on hold while she looks for the records. Once Marilyn has the records, Mrs. O'Keefe has to explain again why she is calling.*

Correct Technique

Medical Assistant: Mrs. O'Keefe, I would be happy to help you, but Marilyn has all the financial records in her office and is more knowledgeable about your account and better able to help you. If you would like to speak with Marilyn I can transfer you to her office." *When Mrs. O'Keefe acknowledges that she is willing to be transferred, you would then call Marilyn.*
Medical Assistant: Marilyn, I have Mary O'Keefe on the line and she wants to know why there are charges for three different blood tests on John's statement. Could you take the call? *This gives Marilyn the opportunity to pull the O'Keefe's ledger before she answers the phone. When Marilyn does answer, she can say,* "Hello, Mrs. O'Keefe, I have the information regarding John's lab charges in front of me. The receptionist tells me you have some questions about the charges for three blood tests on this last statement . . ." *Marilyn can then explain the reason for the charges.*

EXAMPLE: EXTERNAL REFERRAL

Herb Fowler needs to have a glucose tolerance test done at the laboratory next door and make an appointment in your office for one week after the test is done.

Poor Technique

Medical Assistant: Mr. Fowler, you need to call Johnston Labs to arrange for those tests. We'll see you after the tests are done.

Correct Technique

Medical Assistant: Mr. Fowler, Dr. King has ordered a glucose tolerance test for you with Johnston Laboratory in Suite 516 of this building. Since you are working, we felt it would be better to have you call them yourself to make the appointment. If you have a paper and pencil, I'll give you the information you need.

The lab is open from 6:30 A.M. to 7 P.M. Monday through Friday. The phone number is 555-1234 and you should ask for Susan at Ext. 23; she makes the appointments. She will need your name, address, phone number, age, social security number, the name and address of your insurance company, and your insurance ID and Plan numbers.

After you make your appointment with Susan, please call me so we can make an appointment for you here for one week later. Dr. King will have your test results by then and will want to go over them with you at that time.

Do you have any questions or do you need any of the information repeated? Fine, I'll speak to you after you talk to Susan and we'll set up your appointment with Dr. King.

- What happened?

- Who is the patient? (Ask name and age.)

- Is the patient breathing?

- Is there bleeding? How much? From where?

- Is the patient conscious?

- What is the patient's temperature?

- If the patient ingested something:

  – What did the patient take?

  – How much?

  – Are there poison or overdose instructions on the bottle?

Triage does not only pertain to emergency calls. Triage techniques can also help determine when a patient with symptoms should be seen. By asking the caller questions such as:

- How long have you had the symptoms?

- Is there any fever?

- Are you taking any medications?

This information helps determine whether an appointment should be scheduled immediately or if it can wait a few days.

 The practice should periodically review procedures for handling emergency calls. If an office situation involves a great deal of telephone triage, the staff should enroll in an advanced Red Cross first-aid course. This will enable all participants to more accurately give emergency instructions or to handle these calls if there is no physician in the office at that moment. Remember, Good Samaritan laws only protect persons rendering aid *within the areas of their training and expertise.* All ambulatory settings should also post a list of numbers to be used in case of emergencies, such as the poison control telephone number. See also Chapter 9 for more information on triage.

Angry Callers

Medical assistants will probably have occasion to speak with callers who are angry or upset. Though these calls may eventually need to be referred to the office manager or the physician, medical assistants need techniques for managing problem calls.

The first priority is to diffuse the situation. This cannot be accomplished if you become angry or upset. As a professional, it is important to remain calm and in control at all times. Like most skills, diffusing a difficult situation becomes easier with practice. See Procedure 12-2.

Elderly Callers

There are several issues that may arise when dealing with elderly patients: impaired hearing, confusion, and an inability to understand procedures or technical information.

Do not assume that all elderly people are senile or hard of hearing. This is a dangerous pitfall into which many people stumble.

If the individual has a hearing impairment, speak more slowly, more clearly, and a little louder than normal. Do not shout. If uncertain that the person has heard everything, ask if there are any questions or ask the person to repeat information back to you.

If the person has difficulty understanding you, simplify the information, ask frequently if there are any questions, and try to explain in simple, concrete terms. At times, if it is difficult to communicate with an elderly patient, someone from the patient's family should be given certain information. Discuss this option with the office manager or physician first.

English as a Second Language Callers

 In any ambulatory care setting, it is possible to have contact with many patients whose primary language is not English.

It is extremely helpful to have at least one person in the office who is bilingual, particularly in an area such as the Southwest where many people speak a language other than English. For the non-bilingual medical assistant, certain techniques may help when communicating with all but totally non-English speaking patients.

- A patient who does not *speak* fluent English may still *understand* as well as anyone. Do not assume that individuals with strong accents cannot understand you.

- Speak at a normal volume; raising the voice does not increase the other person's ability to comprehend.

- If the other person has difficulty understanding, speak more slowly. Avoid complicated words when simple ones will express the meaning just as well.

- Ask the person if clarification is needed. Be willing to review the information again.

- Be patient.

If these techniques are not successful, it is the responsibility of your physician-employer to provide an interpreter (who may or may not be a member of the patient's family) if necessary.

PLACING OUTGOING CALLS

When making calls for the medical office, whether to patients, health care facilities, or other physicians, know what information is needed and have it at hand before making the calls.

For example:

- If arranging for a patient to receive care at another facility, have the patient's chart and insurance information. Determine physician instructions as to the diagnosis and type of care (specific tests, x-rays, and so on) that need to be ordered.

- If calling insurance companies for claim follow-up, gather copies of all claim forms in question so you can answer specific questions regarding each claim.

- If scheduling meetings or outside appointments for office physicians, have their schedules in front of you.

Arrange to make outgoing calls from a telephone in a location that is not distracting. If the calls concern patients (whether bills, insurance, or care), it is mandatory that the calls be made from a telephone where you cannot be overheard by other patients or people in the reception area.

Always choose a time when calls can be made without interruption. Arrange for someone else to cover incoming calls during this period and to take messages on any calls that you need to handle personally.

It is best to establish a routine for making various types of outgoing calls. Most offices call the next day's patients to confirm appointments near the end of each day. Collection and insurance calls, as well as pharmacy callbacks, are usually done either before the office is open for patients in the morning, during the period from noon to 2 P.M. when the office is closed for lunch, or after the last patient has been seen.

Procedure 12-3 summarizes guidelines for placing outgoing calls.

PLACING LONG DISTANCE CALLS

Placing Calls

Most long-distance calls medical assistants make are likely to be direct dialing calls; that is, calls placed without the help of an operator. To direct dial a local long-distance call, which is a call within the area code but out of the local calling area, dial 1 plus the telephone number; in some parts of the country, it is no longer necessary to dial 1 before the seven-digit telephone number.

For long-distance calls out of the area code, dial 1 plus area code plus number. Nationwide area codes are usually listed in your telephone directory before alphabetical entries. When giving another party the medical office number, always include the area code.

When it is necessary to make an operator-assisted call, dial 0 plus area code plus number. Operator-assisted calls, many of which are automated, include collect calls, person-to-person calls, and occasionally credit card calls.

Time Zones

When making a long-distance call out of the area code, it is likely that a time zone change may occur (Figure 12-5). When scheduling the day's calls, it is important to keep in

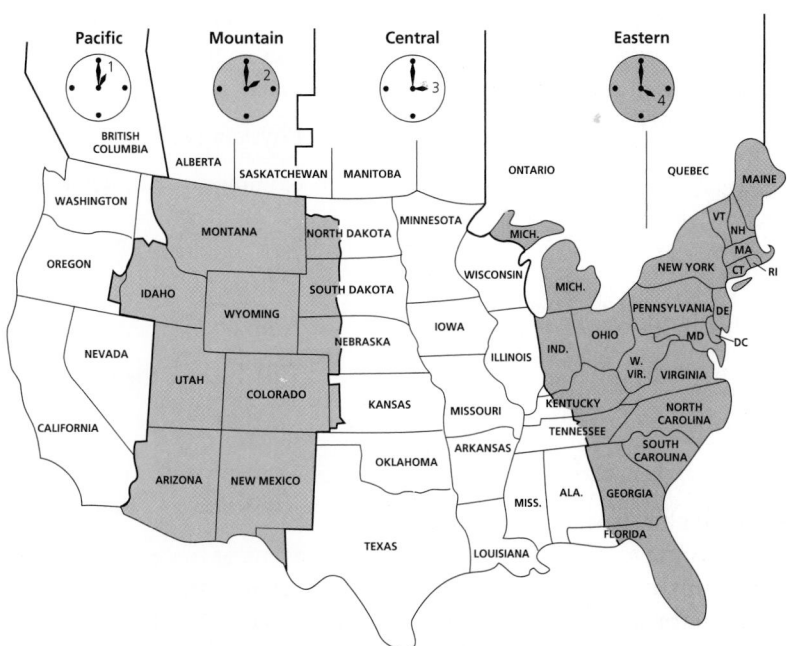

Figure 12-5 Time zone map.

mind the location of the call and plan accordingly. Time zones include Pacific, Mountain, Central, and Eastern times and usually span a three-hour difference. If it is noon in New York, it is 11 A.M. in Illinois, 10 A.M. in Arizona, and 9 A.M. in Washington state.

Long-Distance Carriers

Many companies, some well-known, others new to the market, are competing for long-distance business. Judging the offers and services of long-distance companies can be a complex task, but a wise choice can save an ambulatory care setting hundreds of dollars a year or more in telephone charges. It is important to analyze the medical office long-distance requirements and then make comparisons among several long-distance companies. Company representatives are usually more than willing to discuss their services in light of specific needs to help you comparison shop.

TELEPHONE DOCUMENTATION

Requests for medical information over the telephone should be discouraged. A physician or facility that needs the information to treat the patient usually places an emergency request. A "call-back" verification procedure should be implemented for this type of request. Request the caller's name and telephone number, and state that you will call back with the necessary information. Then call back to verify the identity of the caller, and provide or fax the information. It is important to follow this procedure during routine telephone interchanges that take place between facilities/provider offices and labs seeking test results or consult findings.

All telephone requests should be documented either in a log reserved for that purpose or in the patient's medical record. Documentation includes the following:

- Date of the request
- Name of the requestor
- The information requested
- Patient's name (and patient number)
- Name of the treating physician
- The information released
- To whom the call was referred (if applicable)

When a patient telephones the office to request prescription refills, is displeased with medical treatment, or expresses some form of a complaint, documentation of the call should always be recorded in the medical chart.

USING TELEPHONE DIRECTORIES

The medical assistant should have on hand in the office a variety of telephone directories and be skilled in their use. The telephone directory contains an organized, accurate, and complete listing of the name, address, zip code, and area code with telephone number for most individuals with telephone service. Often, the pages within the directory are color-coded; residences listed on white pages, business numbers on blue, and advertisements on yellow pages. The front pages of many directories contain other very useful information such as:

- Information regarding emergency and nonemergency numbers.
- The Internet guide makes it easy to get on-line.
- Information guide and consumer tips provide a variety of free facts and answers about the things you want to buy and the services you need.
- Community pages provide attractions, events, and the general-interest information unique to a particular area. Often, maps are provided on these pages.
- Phone service pages answer questions you may have regarding your phone service.
- Government pages contain information about county, state, tribal, and federal government office as well as information regarding public schools and voter registration information.
- An index makes finding what you need easy.

Many metropolitan medical centers and hospitals produce another type of directory. These directories list important telephone numbers specific to that facility. Examples of information available within these directories include:

- Physician referral information
- Community education services
- Nurse counseling service/nurse line
- Main hospital/facility telephone number
- Automated operator
- TTY line for the hearing impaired
- Medical center departments
- Medical staff including department and photo of physicians and their names with credentials

Some of these publications list physicians no longer maintaining their active/associate privileges at the facility. Often a map of the facility is included within the front or back pages. The large facilities also may produce supplements to maintain current information.

LEGAL AND ETHICAL CONSIDERATIONS

One of the most important issues in the medical setting is patient **confidentiality**, or right to privacy. Respecting the confidentiality of all patient information is a legal and **ethical** obligation. No information about patients is to be discussed outside the office, with family or friends, or with other patients. Violations of confidentiality leave you and your physician open to lawsuits. More importantly, they are violations of patient trust.

When calling patients, whether to discuss treatment or finances, do so with respect for the patient's privacy at all times. The front desk is certainly not the place to make collection calls when other patients are in the reception room. Either make calls from another location or choose a time when other patients cannot overhear you. Always be aware of the surroundings and who may be able to overhear conversations.

There are many situations when individuals will call the office to discuss a patient. Parents, spouses, grandparents, other relatives, significant others, employers, and friends often will have questions about a patient's condition or finances. Usually these people are asking questions out of genuine concern and a desire to help. The information they request may seem harmless, but discussing anything about a patient can turn into an ethical and legal issue.

See examples on this page.

To ensure patient confidentiality and practice sensible risk management, never discuss a patient with:

- The patient's spouse or family, without specific permission
- The patient's employer
- Insurance carriers, HMOs, or attorneys without a signed release
- Credit bureau/collection agency (reporting a patient to a credit bureau or collection agency is a violation of confidentiality)
- Other patients
- People outside the office (friends, family, acquaintances)

When necessary for medical or administrative reasons, you can discuss a patient with:

- Members of the office staff as necessary to the patient's care
- The patient's insurance carrier or HMO, if you have a signed release
- The patient's attorney (usually in accident or Worker's Compensation cases), if you have a signed release
- The patient's parent or legal guardian, except concerning issues of birth control, abortion, or sexually transmitted disease (check the laws in each state regarding minors' right to privacy)
- Another health care provider (physician, lab, or hospital) that is providing care to the patient under orders from the patient's physician
- Referring physician's office

TELEPHONE TECHNOLOGY

Though much of this chapter has been dedicated to the interpersonal nature of telephone communications, astute medical assistants will also investigate and become knowledgeable about the technology of telephone communications.

Ongoing advances in telecommunications have had a tremendous impact on how the staff of a medical office communicates both within the office and with patients, hospitals, and others outside the office. These advances include telephone systems with automated routing units (ARUs); electronic transmissions (fax and e-mail); cellular telephones; and paging systems.

EXAMPLES: LEGAL AND ETHICAL

Situation 1

A medical assistant called the home of a patient inquiring about the delinquent status of his account. The patient was not home, but his wife answered the phone. The medical assistant discussed the situation with the patient's wife, who wanted to know what the charges were for. Upon checking the file, it was discovered the patient had been tested for a sexually transmitted disease.

Situation 2

A patient's employer calls to find out "how Boris is doing and when he can come back to work. We really miss that guy!" The medical assistant, who just saw Boris in the reception area yesterday, responds without thinking, "Oh, he seems to be doing great, I'll bet you'll have him back in a few days." If he had checked the patient chart, he might have seen that Boris was filing a disability claim as well as a negligence suit against the employer for unsafe working conditions. He might also have seen that Boris is still in physical therapy and on pain medication or that he may have permanent problems as a result of the accident.

Automated Routing Units

Many hospitals and larger ambulatory care settings have automated routing unit (ARU) telephone systems to manage heavy telephone traffic. The system answers the call and a recorded voice identifies departments or services the caller can access by pressing a specified number on the Touch-Tone telephone. If callers indicate they are having a medical emergency, the system can be programmed to immediately route calls to the medical assistant. This saves patients with immediate medical problems from waiting during busy telephone times.

Some automated telephone systems have electronic mailboxes so the caller can leave a message if the person they are calling is unavailable. In many ARU systems, selecting any of the numbered choices often gives the caller a second, third, or fourth menu of choices. If the caller does not select an option, the ARU will usually switch the call automatically to a "live" operator.

A disadvantage with ARU systems is that the recorded voice may be difficult to hear, especially for elderly or hearing-impaired patients. Many patients may not understand the recorded options. Offices with an ARU system should provide an information sheet to all patients explaining their options when calling the office and how to get through to the office quickly in an emergency.

Answering Services and Machines

One responsibility of the office manager/medical assistant is to ensure that patient calls are answered after office hours, both on evenings and weekends. While in smaller ambulatory care settings it may not be possible to have staff on telephone duty twenty-four hours a day, nonetheless calls must be answered and messages taken. Answering services—typically staffed by a live operator—and answering machines are two methods of taking calls after hours.

Many ambulatory care centers favor answering services because a live operator is reassuring to patients and other callers. These services also can provide flexibility in routing calls and locating the physician for emergencies. Typically, fees for answering services are by the month or by the number of calls.

Answering machines are convenient but perhaps less reassuring for the caller. The machine must be checked frequently for messages should an emergency occur. Sometimes, the message may leave a telephone number where the physician can be reached, but this system is likely to be cumbersome, for too many nonemergency calls may be directed to the physician. If an answering machine is used, the message often contains a number, other than the physician's, that callers can use for emergencies. That call is answered by a live operator who then screens and refers the call appropriately.

Facsimile (Fax) Machines

Fax machines are more and more common in the ambulatory care setting as they are used to send reports, referrals, insurance approvals, and informal correspondence. A fax is a facsimile transmission sent over telephone lines from one fax machine to another or from a modem to a fax machine. A fax document may contain data like typed characters, photographs, or line art.

While fax machines are a great timesaver for the ambulatory care setting, confidentiality is a critical issue for fax machines are typically located in centralized areas where documents may be seen by unauthorized personnel. Before sending any document, be sure it will not violate confidentiality, have permission to transmit it by fax, and attach a cover sheet that stipulates the information is for the intended recipient only. Review fax machine information contained in Chapter 16.

Electronic Mail

Electronic mail (e-mail) is the process of sending, receiving, storing, and forwarding messages in digital form through telephone lines. E-mail can save time and money. Instead of having to make personal or telephone contact, the sender can leave a message in an electronic mailbox via a computer where it can be retrieved by the receiver at a convenient time. Insurance inquiries lend themselves to this type of communication system. If a response is required, it can often be returned by the same system. If it is not retrieved within a certain amount of time, some electronic mail systems either send a printed copy of the message or delete the message from the system.

Another advantage of e-mail is flexibility. When computers are networked, electronic mail can substitute for the interoffice memo with one staff member composing information on the computer screen to be automatically transmitted to all members of a medical facility. Any message stored can be brought up on a computer screen and saved to a disk or printed.

It is possible to subscribe to an on-line computer information service that incorporates an e-mail system and communicate with any other users on the system around the world. Medical assistants, medical transcriptionists, medical billing services, and others subscribe to these services to network information to each other. These services also feature bulletin boards (electronic method of exchanging information publicly). Some of these computer information services are known as America On-Line, CompuServe, and Prodigy. Review the electronic mail section found in Chapter 16.

Cellular Service

Since the 1980s cellular telephones have become very popular and are now available and used in all populated areas of the country. Cellular communication offers convenience and flexible communication. The telephones themselves are available in many models and sizes and some can even fit in the palm of the hand. Many physicians have car and/or portable phones allowing immediate verbal contact with their office or hospital staff. 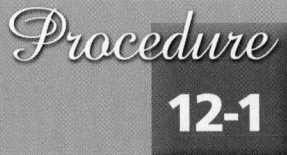 Cellular signals are not secure, which means that other people may be able to listen to the conversations with certain scanning radios. Therefore, staff and physicians should be very careful not to use patients' full names or reveal any confidential information over the cellular phone. Cellular phone usage is much more expensive than using traditional telephone lines, so calls should be kept brief and to the point.

Paging Systems

Another telecommunication option available is the use of pagers or "beepers." Hospitals have used paging systems for many years both inside the hospital and for physicians on call. Several types of paging systems are available, and many physicians now use the same type of pagers available to individual consumers. Some paging system options include:

1. Voice alerts. The voice message is automatically heard by the person being paged. Not only does the person being paged hear the message but anyone in the vicinity will hear it as well.
2. Beep alerts. The pager emits a beeping sound or silent vibration that notifies the person being paged to call one designated phone number to obtain the message.

3. Digital message display.
   a. Alphanumeric display: displays the message on a digital screen. The message can include an entire typed message via a computer modem or through an operator who will input the message and transmit it to the receiver. The receiver can scroll through the text message and save or delete messages as needed.
   b. Numeric display: displays the callback telephone number on small screen. The number displayed is selected by the person initiating the page.

Pagers are not as convenient as cellular phones because they allow only one-way communication; cellular phones allow automatic two-way communication between caller and receiver. However, pagers are less expensive to use and typically have a set monthly charge while cellular phone bills include a monthly rate plus charges for each minute of phone use, whether the call is made or received by the user.

DOCUMENTATION

In the log reserved for telephone documentation, the following entry could be made based on Case Study 12-2.

07/16/--   Claussen-Mason Laboratories requested previous laboratory findings from Qwik Lab in Nashville, Tennessee, for Juanita Hansen, patient number 306-30-7840. Juanita is a patient of Dr. King. The information was released to Janet Bailey, employee of Claussen-Mason Laboratories as directed by Dr. King. W. Slason 7/16/--.

Procedure 12-1   Answering Incoming Calls

PURPOSE:
To answer telephone calls professionally, acquiring all necessary information from the caller, documenting it correctly, and properly acting on it.

EQUIPMENT/SUPPLIES:
Telephone
Message pad
Appointment calendar
Pen or pencil

PROCEDURE STEPS:
1. Be prepared. Have materials such as a message pad, notepad, appointment calendar, sharpened pencils, and working pens nearby. RATIONALE: Being ready for calls conveys professionalism and lets the caller know you are prepared to assist.
2. Answer the telephone promptly. The phone should not ring more than three times before it is answered. RATIONALE: Callers may become annoyed and hang up if a call is not answered within a reasonable time.

(continues)

Procedure

12-1   *(continued)*

3. Answer the call with the preferred office greeting, speaking directly into the mouthpiece. The mouthpiece should be 1 to 2 inches away from the mouth. For example, "Good morning. Doctors Lewis and King. Ellen speaking." RATIONALE: Take a breath before answering the phone, put a smile on your lips, and use a pleasant tone of voice to convey a warm greeting. Holding the phone correctly and speaking directly into the mouthpiece aid the caller in hearing your message clearly.

4. Ask the name of the caller as quickly as possible, and determine if this is an emergency call. RATIONALE: Using the caller's name personalizes the call and acknowledges that you heard the name correctly. If this is an emergency call, follow emergency protocols.

5. Focus on the call. Concentrate on dealing with the call, and put aside other work. RATIONALE: This gives the caller a sense that you are listening attentively, and information will be transmitted correctly. You are less apt to have to ask the caller to repeat information or to record it incorrectly.

6. Repeat information back to the caller. RATIONALE: This technique confirms facts are complete and accurate. The caller also has opportunity to hear the message and confirm that it is accurate or may wish to modify the message meaning for clarity.

7. When using a multiline telephone as shown in Figure 12-6, it is helpful to keep a notepad by the telephone. When you answer the phone and have the caller's name, jot the name, which line the caller is on, and some quick notes about the content of the call. RATIONALE: Using this simple technique avoids problems if another line rings and you must put the first person on hold. No matter how many incoming lines there are, you will not forget who is on which line or what the call is about.

8. Ask if the caller has any other questions. RATIONALE: This saves you and the caller time. It is frustrating to have to place a second call because you forgot to ask something. It also ties up the telephone lines.

9. End the call courteously. Say "thank you" and "goodbye" (not "bye-bye"). RATIONALE: Saying goodbye conveys professionalism and leaves the caller with a positive image of the office.

10. Let the caller hang up before you disconnect. RATIONALE: Often callers think of questions just as they are ready to hang up. It is more time efficient to handle the question immediately rather than have the caller have to return a call.

11. Document information, and record any future actions necessary. RATIONALE: This procedure is necessary for legal reasons. Remember, a deed not documented is a deed undone in a court of law.

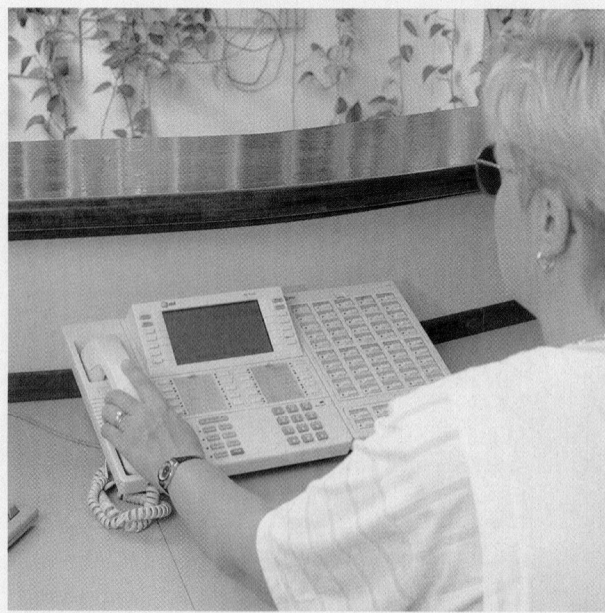

Figure 12-6   An example of a multiline telephone system.

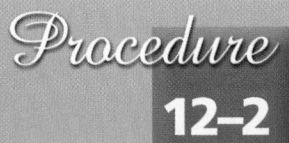

12–2   Handling Problem Calls

PURPOSE:
To handle calls in a positive and professional manner while providing necessary comfort, empathy, and information to the caller to resolve the problem.

EQUIPMENT/SUPPLIES:
Telephone
Message pad
Pen or pencil

PROCEDURE STEPS:

1. Remain calm and avoid becoming upset with an angry caller. Let the caller say what needs to be said without interruption (unless it is a medical emergency requiring immediate action). RATIONALE: This permits the caller to express concerns without having to repeat information or to forget something important.

2. Lower your voice both in pitch and volume. RATIONALE: This technique has a calming effect on an angry caller.

3. Listen to what the caller is upset about. Paraphrase information for verification that you have understood the problem. RATIONALE: This technique lets the caller know you are truly listening and have understood the problem.

4. Use the words "I understand" and show that you are interested in hearing the caller's concerns. RATIONALE: This does not necessarily mean you agree with the caller but that you are willing to empathize and at least accept that, from a particular point of view, there is a reason to be upset.

5. Do not take the call personally. RATIONALE: It is the situation that made the caller angry; you have not done so.

6. Offer assistance. RATIONALE: Ask what you can do to help, and then follow through.

7. Document the call accurately and properly. RATIONALE: Complete documentation promotes risk management and prevents lengthy litigation experiences.

8. When dealing with a frightened or hysterical caller, speak in a soothing voice; use a slower, lower tone than normal. RATIONALE: This often has a calming effect on the caller.

9. If the call is an emergency, begin triage procedures as needed. RATIONALE: Have a list of triage questions at hand to refer to or instruct the caller to dial 9-1-1. Be sure you have the name and telephone number for followup.

10. Always have the caller repeat instructions. RATIONALE: People who are upset may not hear or comprehend much of what is said. Your instructions may deal with an emergency situation, so it is important they are clearly understood.

11. Finalize and follow through on action to be taken, whether it is to confirm emergency medical personnel are on the scene or scheduling an emergency appointment. RATIONALE: Ensure quality patient care.

12. Always report problem calls to the physician or office manager at once. RATIONALE: This will ensure appropriate action is taken, and it is important for risk management purposes.

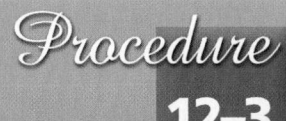

Procedure

12–3   Placing Outgoing Calls

PURPOSE:
To place calls efficiently and effectively.

EQUIPMENT/SUPPLIES:
Notepad
Pen or pencil
All materials specifically applicable to the call

PROCEDURE STEPS:

1. Preplan the call by preparing all materials in front of you prior to making the call; for example, gather telephone number, chart, financial information, or appointment book. Also, have notes of questions you have or information you need to relay. RATIONALE: This technique uses time efficiently and conveys professionalism.

2. Make calls from a location and telephone that will not be disrupted with noise and distractions.

RATIONALE: This type of location permits you to concentrate on the call without distractions or interruptions.

3. Try to schedule specific times of the day for calls; for example, early morning before patients arrive, midday, or after the last patient has been seen. Be aware of the time zone you are calling, so you do not disturb people at inappropriate times. RATIONALE: Return calls to outside labs or consulting physicians may be done early in the morning before patients arrive and offices become busy with patient loads. Midday may be an appropriate time to call in prescription refills or reminders of appointments.

4. Use appropriate language and tone following proper telephone techniques. RATIONALE: Ensure that your message is conveyed clearly and understood accurately.

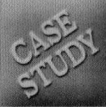

12-1

Audrey Jones, the young clinical medical assistant at Doctors Lewis and King, was on telephone duty on a busy Thursday afternoon. This was only the third or fourth time Audrey was responsible for answering incoming calls, but her energy and quick judgment saw her through some difficult situations when all the lines were ringing at the same time. Audrey just received a call; a young man is calling about his mother, a patient of Dr. Lewis, who is having trouble breathing.

CASE STUDY REVIEW

1. What are the critical questions Audrey should ask the young man to triage the situation?
2. How will Audrey's training and background in Red Cross first aid help her assess the situation?
3. If Audrey needs to give medical information over the telephone, what limits should she respect?

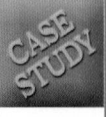

12-2

Wanda Slawson, Clinical Medical Assistant at Inner City Health Care, receives a telephone call from Claussen-Mason Laboratories requesting medical information about patient Juanita Hansen. Wanda is told by lab personnel that the information is needed to perform the tests scheduled by Dr. King. Wanda is not familiar with this request and asks if she can check the chart and return a call to the lab (call-back verification procedure).

CASE STUDY REVIEW

1. What information will Wanda need from Claussen-Mason Laboratories?
2. What is the purpose of the call-back verification procedure?
3. After the verification has been established, what should Wanda do?

SUMMARY

Proper telephone techniques require the medical assistant to have excellent communication and listening skills. The ability to convey warmth and reassurance is vital to patient relationships. Efficiency and organization are also key elements in effectively managing the variety of telephone calls answered and placed in the ambulatory care setting. Medical assistants responsible for incoming and outgoing calls need to be able to perform telephone triage, screen calls, take messages, and refer calls professionally and efficiently.

Medical assistants also need to be aware of telephone technology in order to choose and productively use the office's telephone systems. An understanding of technology can result in savings of both time and money for the efficient ambulatory care setting.

REVIEW QUESTIONS

Multiple Choice

1. Positive first impressions are conveyed over the telephone by:
   a. using the hold button sparingly
   b. being authoritative with the caller
   c. not permitting the caller too much leeway to speak
   d. working while talking on the telephone
2. Basic telephone techniques involve:
   a. volume, enunciation, pronunciation, and control of speed
   b. being assertive with the caller
   c. not spending too much time talking
   d. referring all calls to the physician
3. Buffer words:
   a. are necessary for clarity
   b. confuse the caller
   c. are used to avoid clipping off the office name
   d. are not considered introductory words, phrases, or statements
4. Guidelines that ensure successful transfer of calls include all of the following *except*:
   a. determine who would be the best person to assist
   b. follow your telephone system's procedure for transferring the call
   c. followup to be sure the call transferred correctly
   d. getting the caller's name and telephone number is not necessary
5. Medical assistants should refer calls to the physician when:
   a. an appointment needs to be scheduled
   b. a patient has a billing question
   c. a salesperson is planning a call
   d. a patient requests test results
6. Triage:
   a. is the act of evaluating the urgency of a medical situation and prioritizing treatment
   b. is expressing oneself clearly and distinctly
   c. uses expendable words while answering the telephone
   d. is the ability to be objectively aware of and have insight into others' feelings, emotions, and behaviors
7. In handling a problem call, the medical assistant should:
   a. take it personally
   b. listen calmly to the upset person
   c. become upset to identify with the patient
   d. ask emotionally charged questions to calm down the patient
8. The "call-back" verification procedure:
   a. should never be documented
   b. should always be documented
   c. should sometimes be documented
   d. is not appropriate in the ambulatory office setting
9. ARU telephone systems:
   a. transmit over telephone lines via modem
   b. involve transmissions sent from one fax machine to another
   c. use a recorded voice that identifies departments or services the caller can access by pressing a specified number
   d. process messages in digital form through telephone lines
10. Pagers or beepers are:
    a. useful for calling back patients
    b. old technology
    c. capable only of one-way transmission
    d. now replaced by fax machines

Critical Thinking

1. When is it acceptable to put a caller on hold?
2. What can you do to improve your sound on the telephone?
3. List six types of calls that must be referred to the physician.

4. Why should complaints be referred to the physician or office manager instead of managed by the staff?
5. What is triage?
6. List six questions you might ask to evaluate the urgency of a call.
7. What are the eight elements necessary to a proper telephone message?
8. When taking a message for someone, what information do you always give the caller?
9. When giving the physician a message from or about a patient, what should always be attached?
10. Describe how to properly transfer a call to someone else in your office.
11. How would you handle an angry caller?
12. If an individual is hearing impaired, what three changes do you make in the way you speak to them?

WEB ACTIVITIES

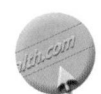 Using the World Wide Web, search for current information relative to legal and ethical considerations when using the telephone in the ambulatory care setting. Compile your information into a one-page report, and list your URL addresses for your instructor.

REFERENCES/BIBLIOGRAPHY

Hosley, J. B., Jones, S. A., & Molle-Matthews, E. A. (1997). *Lippincott's textbook for medical assistants*. Philadelphia: Lippincott, Williams, and Wilkins.

Humphrey, D. D. (1996). *Contemporary medical office procedures* (2nd ed.). Albany, NY: Delmar.

Kinn, M. E., & Woods, M. A. (1999). *The administrative medical assistant* (4th ed.). Philadelphia: W. B. Saunders Company.

Saunders, J., & McGee, R. R. A. (1996). *Patient confidentiality*. Salt Lake City, UT: Medicode, Inc.

Chapter

13

PATIENT SCHEDULING

KEY TERMS

Clustering
Double Booking
Established Patient
Matrix
Modified Wave
New Patient
No-Show
Open Hours
Practice-Based
Slack Time
Stream
Triage
Wave

OUTLINE

OBJECTIVES

The student should strive to meet the following performance objectives and demonstrate an understanding of the facts and principles presented in this chapter through written and oral communication.

1. Define the key terms as presented in the glossary.

2. Review six of the major scheduling systems.

3. Describe the six considerations in scheduling appointments.

4. Explain the importance of triage in scheduling patient appointments.

5. Review proper cancellation procedures and explain the legal necessity of documenting cancellations.

6. Recall three types of reminder systems. *(continues)*

7. Choose an appropriate appointment scheduling tool and describe its advantages.

8. Establish a matrix for a new year and a new practice.

9. Prepare a daily appointment sheet. Describe how it differs from a daily worksheet.

10. Describe the purpose and content of a patient informational brochure.

ROLE DELINEATION COMPONENTS

ADMINISTRATIVE

Administrative Procedures

- Schedule, coordinate, and monitor appointments
- Schedule inpatient/outpatient admissions and procedures

CLINICAL

Patient Care

- Adhere to established triage procedures

GENERAL (TRANSDISCIPLINARY)

Communication Skills

- Receive, organize, prioritize and transmit information
- Serve as liaison
- Promote the practice through positive public relations

Legal Concepts

- Document accurately

Instruction

- Explain office policies and procedures

Operational Functions

- Apply computer techniques to support office operations

SCENARIO

At Inner City Health Care, medical assistant Walter Seals is responsible for efficient patient flow. Because Inner City is an urgent care center, patients are seen as walk-in appointments, on a first-come, first-served basis unless there is an emergency situation. Inner City also operates specialty care clinics, and these clinics require scheduled appointments. Walter has found that the clustering system is most efficient for these specialized care clinics, with certain days dedicated to certain procedures.

Because of the high volume of patients and the need to coordinate multiple physician schedules, Walter's job is not an easy one. However, Inner City is computerized, so paperwork is easy to generate as appointments are made, canceled, or rescheduled. And while Walter manages a smooth patient flow, he makes it a point to remain flexible to accommodate patient needs and keep stress to a minimum.

INTRODUCTION

While patient appointment scheduling may seem like a routine function, a smooth patient flow often determines the success of a day in the ambulatory care setting. A variety of administrative skills are utilized in the performance of this vital office function. By effectively scheduling patients to fit a particular practice, it is possible to make profitable use of physician and staff time.

In addition, efficient patient flow is satisfying to the patient. A common patient complaint is the time spent waiting in the reception area. Most patients appreciate an office that recognizes the value of patients' time. Accordingly, these patients do not hesitate to advertise their experience (good or bad) to friends and families—a fact of great significance to any medical office.

In addition to the required administrative skills, medical assistants involved in scheduling patients must put into practice their interpersonal and communication skills. Scheduling an appointment may be the first contact patients have with the medical office. They remember and value the treatment they receive from the time of first contact. The personality of the ambulatory care setting is always reflected in the treatment and respect accorded to patients.

TAILORING THE SCHEDULING SYSTEM

The schedule of each medical office will determine the best method for scheduling appointments. A surgeon's office will have a much different flow of patients than a pediatrician's office. The key is to customize the system to best accommodate the practice. Primary goals in determining this should include:

- a smooth flow of patients with a minimal amount of waiting time for the patients
- flexibility to accommodate acutely ill, STAT (or emergency) appointments, work-ins, cancellations, and no-shows

TYPES OF SCHEDULING SYSTEMS

There are a number of methods for patient scheduling. The best method for a practice is the one that effects good patient flow and proper utilization of staff and physical facilities.

Open Hours

In open hours scheduling patients are seen throughout a particular time frame; e.g., 9:00 A.M. to 11:00 A.M. or 1:00 P.M. to 3:00 P.M. Patients sign in and are seen on a first-come, first-served basis. Emergency rooms and many clinics frequently choose this method as they are able, by their nature, to maintain a steady flow of patients.

Double Booking

With the double-booking method, two or more patients are given a particular appointment time. This method is limited to a practice where patients can be attended to more than one at a time. For instance, Maria Jover and Jim Marshal are both given a 9:30 A.M. appointment. Ms. Jover requires a complete checkup including lab tests, vitals, and so on. Mr. Marshal is being seen for suture removal. While the physician's staff conducts the lab tests on Ms. Jover, the physician can be seeing Mr. Marshal. Obviously, this method requires a precise accounting for time and rooms and adequate staff. A good rule to remember is that if patients are consistently having to wait for staff to attend to them, double booking is not a wise choice of method.

Clustering

The clustering method utilizes the concept used in production line work, namely that performing only one step or process allows for efficient processing. In the ambulatory care setting, patients with similar problems are booked consecutively. Obstetricians and pediatricians commonly choose this method. A block of time, either hours or days of the week, is set aside for particular types of cases. For instance, an obstetrician might see only third trimester patients on Mondays and Fridays and gynecology patients on Tuesdays and Thursdays. A pediatrician's office might be organized for immunizations on Tuesday mornings and well-baby checkups on Monday and Friday afternoons.

Wave

Wave scheduling is another method that can be used effectively in medical facilities that have several procedure rooms and adequate personnel to staff them. Using the wave scheduling system, patients are scheduled in the first half hour of each hour. This method takes into account the fact that there will be no-shows and late arrivals. It can also accommodate work-in appointments. However, it does require personnel who are able to triage patient problems precisely when establishing the appointments.

Modified Wave

This is a variation of the wave method where patients are scheduled in "waves." In the modified wave method, two or three patients are scheduled at the beginning of each hour, followed by single appointments every 10 to 20 minutes the rest of the hour.

A variation of this method assesses major and minor problems (Figure 13-1). Major time-consuming problems are seen at the beginning of the hour; e.g., new patients. Minor problems are seen from 20 minutes past the hour to half past the hour; e.g., follow-ups, bandage changes, and other minor procedures, and walk-ins; e.g., a child with a 103° temperature, are accommodated at the end of the hour. Again, good triaging will determine the success of this method.

With both the clustering and wave methods, empty or unscheduled periods can be used for dictation or the processing of paperwork.

Stream

Stream scheduling is perhaps the best known and most widely used scheduling system. When this system works as it should, there is a steady stream of patients at set appointment times throughout the workday; e.g., 30-minute appointment at 9:00 A.M.; 15-minute appointment at 9:30 A.M.; 15-minute appointment at 9:45 A.M. Each patient is assigned a specific time. This can best be

TIME	TYPE OF APPOINTMENT
8:15	Major
8:20	Minor
8:50	Work-in
9:00	Major
9:20	Minor
9:50	Work-in
10:00	Major
10:25	Minor
10:40	Work-in
11:00	Major
11:25	Minor
11:45	Minor

Figure 13-1 Modified wave variation. Major problems are scheduled at the beginning of the hour, minor problems scheduled 20 to 30 minutes past the hour, and work-ins toward the end of the hour.

accomplished by establishing time guidelines for particular types of appointments such as 60 minutes for returns, 15 minutes for immunizations, and 30 minutes for a hearing test.

Practice-Based

As discussed earlier in this chapter, some ambulatory care settings find it necessary to develop a system unique to their patient load. In these customized systems (practice-based), the practice determines the schedule. An orthopedist might schedule cast removals on Mondays and Fridays using double booking and stream scheduling for new patients with each patient having a 60-minute appointment. A group of vascular surgeons might employ both a double-booking and a modified-wave system. They might double book patients for short rechecks and quick procedures, while using the modified wave for patients with pre- and postoperative checks and long specialty procedures.

There are many variations on these basic scheduling systems. Some offices use double booking for quick follow-ups and clustering for all new patients. Other facilities use

open hours for most patients but 15-minute interval appointments for follow-ups. Another system of double booking is to schedule follow-up calls in a two-column book while scheduling new patients for half-hour appointments. The medical assistant responsible for appointment scheduling will use the system that enables the ambulatory care setting to function smoothly and efficiently.

ANALYZING PATIENT FLOW

When setting up a new practice or reviewing current scheduling practice, a simple analysis can maximize an office's scheduling practices. This entails looking at appointment times, patient arrival times, the actual time a patient is seen, and the time a visit is completed. A simple grid chart can be produced for a given period of time; e.g., one to two weeks (Figure 13-2). In addition, chart the number of no-shows and cancellations.

This analysis should provide a clear picture of patient flow and whether office personnel are being utilized efficiently. The data will assist in estimating how many patients to schedule and realistic time frames for particular problems or procedures. If the physician is scheduling return patients every 15 minutes yet the analysis shows these visits average 24 minutes, the scheduling method needs adjustment. This may mean either allowing 25 minutes for follow-up visits or building in slack time, or unscheduled time, where no appointments are made.

Develop a simple list of commonly scheduled visits with time estimates for each. This procedural sheet will be particularly useful when training new employees or when temporary help is utilized for scheduling (Figure 13-3).

PATIENT FLOW ANALYSIS

February 2, 20—

Patient Name	Length of Appt.	Appt. Time	Dr. King Time Seen	Time Out
Martin Gordon	15	10:20	10:22	10:45
Jason Jover	45	11:20	11:20	12:30
Nora Fowler	30	1:00	1:25	1:45
Jim Marshal	15	1:30	1:50	2:10
Herb Fowler	60	2:45	2:15	3:25

Figure 13-2 Patient flow analysis helps a practice determine realistic time frames for appointments.

TYPICAL SCHEDULING TIMES FOR INTERNAL MEDICINE PRACTICE

New patients . . . . 30 minutes
Patients for consultation . . . . 45 minutes
Patients requiring complete
   physical examinations . . . . 45 minutes
All other patients (minor illnesses,
   routine checkups, etc.) . . . . 15 minutes

Figure 13-3   Most practices will have a list of typical visits with time estimates.

Waiting Time

One of the most frequently voiced frustrations with physicians' offices is excessive waiting time. Obviously, emergencies and other unexpected interruptions cannot be anticipated. However, there are certain measures one can take when attempting to keep the schedule on target. If patients are kept waiting, it is a better strategy to explain the reason for the delay and give patients an estimate of how long the delay will be. *Never* ignore the delay hoping patients will not notice; this, in fact, seems to increase perceived waiting time. Find ways to make patients comfortable while they wait; e.g., providing an appropriate choice of reading materials (or in the case of children, activities). If a delay can be anticipated, e.g., the physician was called away for a delivery or surgery, attempt to contact patients before they leave home to reschedule the appointments.

If the delay is likely to be a half hour or longer, provide patients with options:

1. Offer patients the opportunity to run an errand, having them return at a specified time.
2. Offer to reschedule appointments for another day or later in the day.

In any case, remember that good customer relations dictate your willingness to acknowledge the inconvenience to the patients and attempt to provide an acceptable solution. Remember also that some patients simply will not appreciate any efforts to apologize for a delay, in which case you must continue to act professionally toward them.

Flexibility

One principal above all else in scheduling is be *flexible*. Policies should be established to ensure effective patient flow; however, it is more important to meet the needs of patients. At times, patients cannot be scheduled accord-

ing to the structured appointment times, and the medical assistant will need to decide how to best accommodate their needs.

In every ambulatory care setting, emergency patients must be seen. This situation can be handled in a variety of ways. After determining through triage that it is an emergency, the patient is most often told to come into the office and will be seen as soon as possible. (See Triage Calls in this chapter.) Some offices refer patients to the emergency room, thus minimizing disruption to other patients. Other offices let scheduled patients know of the emergency and offer them the opportunity of rescheduling or waiting until the emergency patient has been seen. A built-in slack time of 30 minutes in the morning and 30 minutes in the afternoon can provide some flexibility in last-minute scheduling.

LEGAL ISSUES

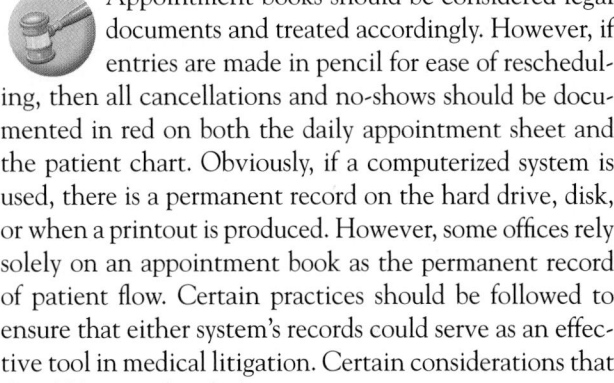 Appointment books should be considered legal documents and treated accordingly. However, if entries are made in pencil for ease of rescheduling, then all cancellations and no-shows should be documented in red on both the daily appointment sheet and the patient chart. Obviously, if a computerized system is used, there is a permanent record on the hard drive, disk, or when a printout is produced. However, some offices rely solely on an appointment book as the permanent record of patient flow. Certain practices should be followed to ensure that either system's records could serve as an effective tool in medical litigation. Certain considerations that should be noted include:

1. The Internal Revenue Service (IRS) can legally demand records from the beginning of a practice. While they generally do not go back more than three to five years, compared to other documents required for legal purposes, the space required for patient records seems minimal compared to the value these permanent records might have to IRS or litigation proceedings.
2. Many facilities make it a practice to keep appointment books in pencil because of the ease of making changes in the schedule. If this is the practice, ensure that there is a typewritten daily appointment sheet as a permanent legal record of each day's appointments.

Remember that anyone looking into a practice will be looking at the record of documentation. Taking the time to accurately and consistently document all aspects of patient care makes a statement about the physicians in the practice and their staff and reflects positively on the presumed quality of patient care.

INTERPERSONAL SKILLS

Scheduling appointments requires interpersonal skills. Medical assistants convey a great deal to patients through attitude and actions. A hurried or disinterested manner communicates that the patient is not a priority. Because patients are often distraught or anxious when making appointments, it is extremely important to reduce rather than increase anxiety. Also, the medical assistant scheduling appointments may be the first contact a patient has with the office; patients do not easily forget rude or insensitive staff. A hurried, disinterested manner toward patients is more often the basis for legal action than is a negligent act.

The patient should always be made to feel worthy of attention. If scheduling a patient in the office and the phone rings, answer the call but excuse yourself first. Ask the caller to please hold for a moment. If on the telephone scheduling a patient and another patient walks in, acknowledge with a nod or signal that you will be right there—never let the person feel ignored. Today patients have a variety of options for health care and tend to be much more consumer-conscious of the treatment they receive.

GUIDELINES FOR SCHEDULING APPOINTMENTS

Whether completed by manual methods or computer technology, the process of scheduling appointments for patients and other visitors to the ambulatory care setting involves a number of variables, including (1) the urgency of the need for an appointment; (2) whether the appointment has a referral from another physician, (3) recording methods for new and established patients; (4) implementation of check-in, cancellation, and rescheduling policies; (5) use of reminder systems; and (6) accommodating visits from medical supply and pharmaceutical company representatives.

Recently, the *Wall Street Journal* reported on physicians in some health maintenance organizations who are paid by a salary rather than by patient visit, experimenting with group scheduling. The group visits may be set up around patients with specific chronic ailments such as diabetes, hypertension, or geriatric complaints. While not yet widely accepted, it is one alternative to keep costs down while maintaining patient/physician relationships in providing health care.

Triage Calls

Urgent calls will need to be triaged, or assessed, before they can be scheduled. In other words, the office personnel making the appointment will need to determine the actual urgency of that call and determine how the patient can best be scheduled. This requires a combination of both communication skills and medical knowledge.

Appropriate questions need to be asked to determine the actual urgency. Is the patient in immediate need of medical assistance? Is there any bleeding? Are there chest pains? The medical assistant needs to determine if this is a life-threatening matter or if the problem is "urgent" in the patient's eyes but not an emergency.

In triaging, also obtain information that will assist in determining the urgent nature of the call. How long have the symptoms/complaint been present? If there is bleeding or discharge, where is the origin? How profuse is it? If it is pain, how intense is it? Is it localized? Precise information will assist the physician in determining the critical or noncritical nature of the call.

In triaging the patient's urgency of care, be tactful in questioning and avoid making the patient feel that the need is insignificant. If questioning indicates this is a medical emergency, follow office policy for having the patient seen (whether it be an emergency appointment or referral to the emergency room). If it is determined that the situation is not an emergency, work the patient into the schedule as the situation warrants and time allows. Be sure to leave the patient with the understanding that you have done your best to address the situation. For more information on triage, see Chapters 9 and 12.

Referral Appointments

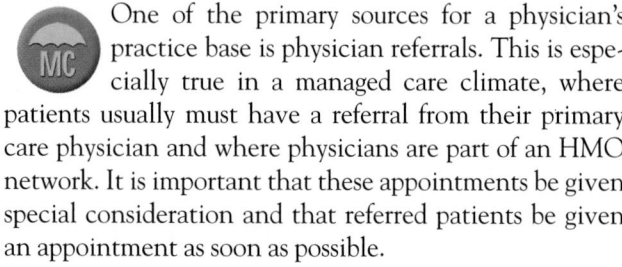

One of the primary sources for a physician's practice base is physician referrals. This is especially true in a managed care climate, where patients usually must have a referral from their primary care physician and where physicians are part of an HMO network. It is important that these appointments be given special consideration and that referred patients be given an appointment as soon as possible.

Adequate information needs to be obtained to determine the urgency of scheduling. If the referring physician or office staff calls directly, the situation can be triaged at that time. However, if the referred patient calls, it is best to obtain necessary records and/or information from the referring physician to determine the urgency and appropriateness of an appointment. This can be done by obtaining general information from the patient and then scheduling an appointment after the physician's office is contacted for complete information regarding the patient's condition. Be polite and assure the patient of an appointment as soon as the referring physician is contacted.

Recording Information

Patients can be sensitive to the amount of information they are required to provide to make an initial appointment. Keep the information as simple as possible and obtain only essential information. It should be tailored to fit the practice; e.g., an obstetrician and a pediatrician will have very different questions for the first-time patient.

Generally, these basic items should be obtained from a **new patient**, someone being seen for the first time in the office:

1. The patient's full legal name (with the correct spelling)
2. A daytime telephone number
3. The chief complaint or reason for the visit
4. The referring physician, if relevant.
   Repeat this information back to the patient to assure accuracy.

 Some offices today, particularly those with computerized scheduling and billing, will require a few additional items:

1. Date of birth
2. Type of insurance
3. Insurance number

The critical determination is whether the information is essential to the first contact or whether it could be obtained at the time of the visit.

An **established patient**, someone who has already been seen in the office, should require only:

1. Full legal name
2. Chief complaint or reason for the visit
3. A daytime telephone number

When the information is recorded, print it legibly and accurately in a manual system, and check for accuracy in the same manner when using a computer system for scheduling. Record the appointment as soon as it is made—never rely on memory.

When scheduling an appointment time, ask the patient what day and time would be most convenient for them and then make the appointment for the first available time stated. If possible, provide the patient with a choice of possible appointment times. Finally, confirm that the patient clearly understands the date and time of the appointment; be sure to repeat the date and time to ensure that both of you have recorded the same information. Spell the patient's name back if confidentiality is assured. If the patient is making the appointment in person, provide them with an appointment card (Figure 13-4).

Scheduling an appointment for the office's available times for a parent who works outside the home, serves in a carpool, and is a coach for the gymnastics or swim team can require a great deal of patience. If the patient requests a particular appointment and this is not possible, courteously offer an explanation.

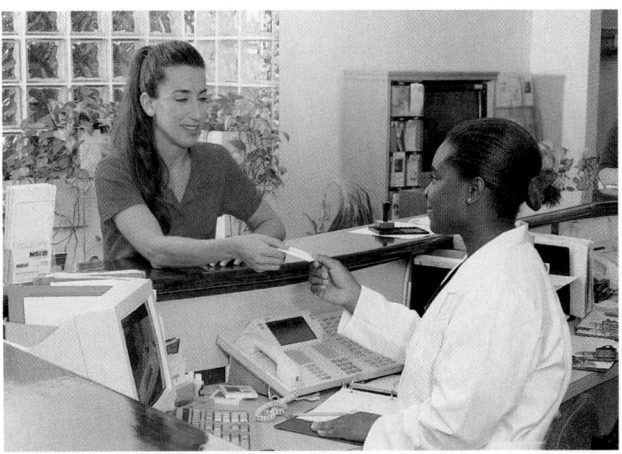

Figure 13-4 Provide patients with appointment cards neatly printed with the date and time of their next appointment.

Computer Scheduling

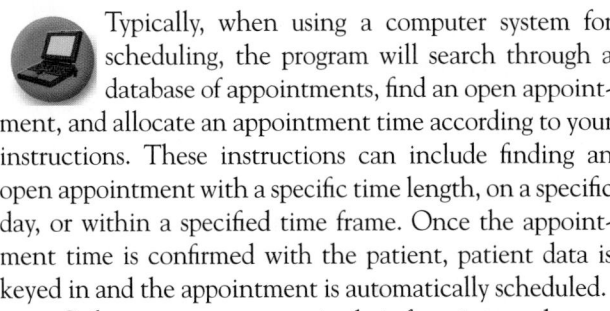 Typically, when using a computer system for scheduling, the program will search through a database of appointments, find an open appointment, and allocate an appointment time according to your instructions. These instructions can include finding an open appointment with a specific time length, on a specific day, or within a specified time frame. Once the appointment time is confirmed with the patient, patient data is keyed in and the appointment is automatically scheduled.

Software programs vary in their functions and capabilities; it is always advisable to network with other ambulatory care settings to discover their program likes and dislikes before choosing and purchasing scheduling software.

Patient Check-In

Records of patient appointments serve a legal purpose. Establishing a procedure for checking in appointments simplifies tracking of the arrival of patients. (See Procedure 13-1.) This is particularly true in multiphysician settings or offices where a number of staff are attending to patients before, or instead of, seeing the physician.

There are offices where patients are required to sign a check-in list.

A word of caution here. The patient's right to privacy requires that patients do not see the names of other patients. Patients may be reluctant to sign in on such a list and it is within their legal rights to refuse. It is a better policy for the office staff to check the patients off on a list (Figure 13-5). When a patient checks in, a red √ or other appropriate mark should be used in the appointment book.

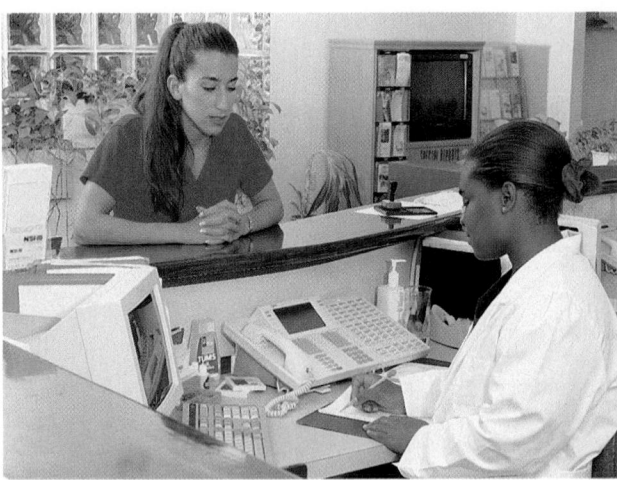

Figure 13-5 The medical assistant/receptionist should be able to see patients as they enter the office. Patients may sign themselves in, or preferably check in with the medical assistant who will keep the patient check-in list current.

Patient Cancellation and Appointment Changes

When using pencil on a manual appointment book system, a permanent record of no-shows should be designated on the appointment sheet with a red **X**. Cancellations should be marked through on the appointment sheet with a single red line (Figure 13-6). Computer scheduling will provide an area to indicate no-shows and cancellations also. No-shows and cancellations should always be noted in the patient's individual chart. Again, it is imperative that the physician's care of the patient be thoroughly documented. Should a patient develop complications and claim the physician was unavailable, the daily appointment sheet and chart should document the patient's failure to show.

Many offices have established firm policies for multiple no-shows and/or cancellations. The general rule is that after three no-shows and/or cancellations in a row, the physician will review the records. In order for the physician to adequately treat a patient, the patient's cooperation is necessary. A no-show pattern may indicate that the patient is not truly committed to assisting in treatment. If a patient routinely cancels or does not show, the physician will write a letter terminating services and explaining why the physician is discontinuing care. This should be sent by certified mail, return receipt requested, to ensure that the patient received the notice. See Chapter 9 for more information on termination of services and Chapter 15 for information on certified mail. Procedure 13-2 outlines the proper cancellation procedures.

		Dr. King	Dr. Lewis
7	00		
	15		
	30		
	45		
8	00	Hospital	
	15		Surgery
	30	Rounds	
	45		
9	00	Abigail Johnson - Black	Lenore
	15	Diabetes Check/466-2964	McDonell
	30	Marge O'Keefe/CPE/296-7234	
	45		
10	00		Joseph Ortiz/New Pt/462--1121
	15		
	30	Nora Fowler/Back Pain/466-2234	Maria Tover/Stomach Problems/292-2104
	45		
11	00	Jim Marshal/CPE/763-2067	Maria Tover/Stomach Problems/292-2104
	15		
	30	Partners	Partners
	45		
12	00		
	15		
	30		
	45		
		Lunch Meeting	Lunch Meeting
1	00	Matt. Hanes/Consultation/763-3284	Boris Bolski/New Pt./466-8156

MONDAY, NOVEMBER 23

Figure 13-6 Multiphysicians' office where physicians' commitments and no-shows are marked with a red "X" and cancellations are marked with a single red line. Other offices may have slightly different systems for tracking appointments, but in all offices all no-shows and cancellations should be marked in the patient's record.

Computer Cancellations

While software programs differ, cancellations are typically performed by deleting the patient's name from the time slot: if the appointment is to be rescheduled, the name is then keyed in to the appropriate time. The first time opens for other appointments.

When canceling appointments by computer, be certain that the program maintains a list of canceled appointments including patient name, date, and time. This documentation is necessary for legal purposes; also record canceled appointments on the patient chart.

Reminder Systems

Studies have shown that reminding patients of appointments results in a higher rate of fulfilled appointments. There are three ways of reminding patients of appointments. Appointment cards are the most obvious and perhaps the most widely used method. However, the card may be tucked in a wallet and forgotten. Many offices call patients in the afternoon to remind them of an appointment the next day. This can be particularly effective in this day and age with voice mail and message machines.

Patient Teaching Tip

Encourage patients to participate in their health care by keeping appointments or by notifying the ambulatory care setting that they need to reschedule. Some cancellations are unavoidable but gentle reminders and a two-way physician/patient relationship encourage responsible patient behavior.

However, remember that this is confidential information and should never be left on such a recording device without the patient's express permission to do so. (When initially seeing the patient, obtain a number where a personal message could be left.) Finally, reminders can be mailed. This would be most appropriate for patients who come on a regular basis; e.g., once every six months.

Scheduling Representatives

Every medical office needs to schedule time with representatives of pharmaceutical and medical supply companies. These representatives can provide a valuable service to physicians and patients and with clear guidelines regarding when and how often representatives can visit, a working partnership can develop. Most physicians set aside a specific time during the week to meet with these representatives; generally a time allotment of 15 to 20 minutes is sufficient for these appointments.

SCHEDULING MATERIALS

Whether using a manual system for scheduling patients or a computer system, a thorough understanding of the manual system is helpful in understanding the whole process of patient scheduling. Materials needed for scheduling should be customized to the ambulatory care setting. For instance, a smaller practice may prefer a manual method involving appointment books; a large urgent care-type setting may use a computer program for patient scheduling. Increasingly, all appointment scheduling is done by computers. No matter what materials and which methods are used, the proper tools will enable patient scheduling to be a smoothly functioning, easily documented process.

Appointment Books

An appointment book appropriate to the medical practice is essential to any ambulatory care setting. Each office has unique needs in its physical facilities and staff. This applies to the appointment book as well. In addition to the physical arrangement of the date pages, there are various combinations of time allotments. Some books have major headings for hours with minor spaces for 15-minute intervals. Others have 10-minute intervals, and others only hour intervals.

Appointment Sheets

Another vital tool in efficient patient flow is a daily appointment sheet, which provides a permanent record for both legal risk management and quality management purposes. Figure 13-7 is a sample of a daily appointment sheet.

DAILY APPOINTMENT SHEET

Thursday, August 21

9:15	Chris O'Keefe	30 minutes	Immunizations
9:30	Jim Marshal	15 minutes	Blood pressure check
10:00	Martin Gordon	60 minutes	PE/lab work
11:00	Nora Fowler	30 minutes	URI
2:00	Maria Jover	30 minutes	Suspicious rash
4:00	Joseph Ortiz	30 minutes	Choking problems

Figure 13-7   Daily appointment sheet.

DAILY WORKSHEET

Thursday, August 21

8:00	Hospital Rounds		
9:15	Chris O'Keefe	30 minutes	Immunizations
9:30	Jim Marshal	15 minutes	Blood pressure check
10:00	Martin Gordon	60 minutes	PE/lab work
11:00	Nora Fowler	30 minutes	URI
11:30	Lunch break		
12:30	Dentist Appointment, Dr. Schleuter		
2:00	Maria Jover	30 minutes	Suspicious rash
2:45	Meet with drug rep regarding new beta-blocker agents		
4:00	Joseph Ortiz	30 minutes	Choking problems

Figure 13-8   Daily worksheet.

Using the daily appointment sheet, it is easy to check off shows, no-shows, and cancellations. If the sheet is double-spaced, walk-ins can easily be written in (in ink). For quality management purposes, check-in times can be indicated as well as check-out times. Perhaps more importantly, the daily appointment sheet assists the physician and staff and enables them to see the total scheme of the day's patient flow. If a physician works between two clinics or a hospital and office, it is helpful to have available a pocket-sized edition of the daily appointment sheet for easy referral. This is a simple task with today's reduction feature on many photocopiers—reduce the schedule and secure onto a 3 × 5 index card.

Daily Worksheets

Some offices may also use daily worksheets that include not only patient appointments but also other physician commitments such as meetings and visits from pharmaceutical representatives. This is helpful in scheduling work-in and emergency appointments, as an empty section of time on a sheet with only patient appointments may in fact be booked for another purpose. Figure 13-8 is a sample of a daily worksheet.

Computer Equipment

Although computers greatly simplify the scheduling process, the same guidelines as those required in a handwritten system will need to be employed. Obvious advantages are that appointments can be quickly changed and a daily list of appointments generated. There is also an easily accessible source of vital information on a patient without having to pull the chart.

There are a number of software programs specially designed for scheduling of appointments, such as *The Medical Manager*, published by Delmar Publishers. Many of them can be customized for individual office needs.

Appointment Cards

In addition to the appointment book, offices should have available appointment cards. Studies show that fewer patients report at the wrong time or forget appointments when provided with an appointment card (Figure 13-9).

ESTABLISHING AN APPOINTMENT BOOK

After selecting the type of appointment book that is most appropriate, the book must be readied for scheduling of patients.

Procedure 13-3 outlines the key steps in establishing the appointment matrix. Once these steps have been followed and information recorded, the appointment book is ready for patient scheduling. If done properly, the appointment book will serve as a valuable tool in effecting good patient flow and promoting satisfied clientele.

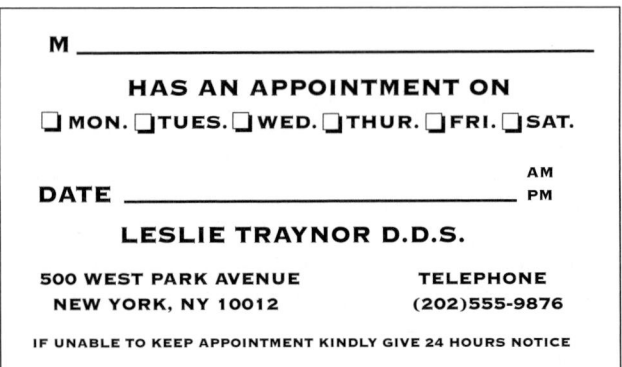

M _____

HAS AN APPOINTMENT ON

☐ MON. ☐ TUES. ☐ WED. ☐ THUR. ☐ FRI. ☐ SAT.

DATE _____ AM PM

LESLIE TRAYNOR D.D.S.

500 WEST PARK AVENUE   **TELEPHONE**
NEW YORK, NY 10012   **(202)555-9876**

IF UNABLE TO KEEP APPOINTMENT KINDLY GIVE 24 HOURS NOTICE

Figure 13-9   Sample appointment card.

Inner City Health Care

Meeting Families' Total Health Care Needs

Commitment to Patient Care

Our staff is committed to providing our patients with the best in medical care. We view your medical care as a team effort—providing you with qualified medical staff while encouraging you to be active participants in your total care. This brochure is designed to help you understand how our practice can best serve you. You are a very important part of our practice and we welcome your questions and comments.

Professional Staff

We are pleased to service the metropolitan area with a well-trained staff of physicians and support staff. Our team of physicians is available to meet your medical needs, assisted by our registered nurses, and certified medical assistants, lab technicians, and radiology technicians. Our urgent care clinic is an alternative to expensive emergency room visits and is open Monday through Saturday.

Services

We provide your family with complete medical facilities through our on-site diagnostic services, including X rays and clinical laboratory. In addition, we are located within five minutes of the local hospital should more extensive services be required. Our **triage line** is available 24 hours a day to assist in assessing problems.

Scheduling

To better serve you, we utilize different methods of scheduling your visits.

In our **Urgent Care Center**, no appointments are necessary. Patients will be seen on a first-come first-served basis, but patients with an urgent need for care will be attended to first. We do, however, request that you call the office first to let us know you are coming. The Urgent Care Center is best suited for problems that arise unexpectedly (fevers, flus, fractures, etc.).

Our **Clinics** require scheduled appointments. General medical appointments are made every day during regular hours. We make every attempt to see you as close to your scheduled appointment time as possible. Our **specialty clinics** utilize a clustering system so that we reserve certain days and times for particular types of appointments. These are as follows.

Orthopedics—Cast removals,
Mon/Wed 9 AM - 3 PM
Tues/Fri 11 AM - 7 PM
Obstetrics
Mon/Wed 9 AM - 2 PM   Friday 1 - 7 PM
Gynecology—Tues and Thurs, 9-7
Pre-Surgery—Mon-Fri, 9 AM - noon
Vascular Lab—Tues and Thurs, 1-7 PM

Cancellations

We request you provide 24 hours notice of an appointment cancellation. You will be billed $20 if you fail to show without notifying our office at least one hour in advance.

Payment Plans

To assist you in obtaining proper medical care and minimizing your concerns for cost, we have established several methods of payment. We directly bill Blue Cross/Blue Shield, HMO Michigan, Shield Care, Care Michigan, and Medicare/Medicaid. Our **billing coordinator**, Karen Ritter, CMA, will be happy to assist you in setting up payment plans if you do not have insurance coverage. In addition, we accept pre-approved credit card payments.

For More Information

Our staff is here to assist you with questions and concerns you may have. Please refer to the following phone numbers for quicker service with specific needs:

Billing
Karen Ritter, CMA, 555-7155, ext. 4

Insurance Preauthorization
Jane O'Hara, CMA, 555-7155, ext. 12

Lab Results
555-7155, ext. 22

Appointment Scheduling
555-7158

Triage Line
555-7159

Clinic #1
Office Hours: Monday-Thursday, 9-7
                      Closed Friday
Clinic #2
Office Hours: Monday, Wednesday, and
                      Friday, 10-7, Saturday, 10-3
                      Closed Tuesday and Thursday
Dr. Brown's Hours:
   Clinic #1—Monday-Thursday, 9-2
   Clinic #2—Monday & Wednesday, 2-7
                      Friday, noon-7, Saturday, 9-4
Dr. Rice's Hours:
   Clinic #1—Monday-Thursday, 2-7
   Clinic #2—Monday & Wednesday, 10-2,
                      Friday, 10-12
Urgent Care Center
Office Hours: Monday-Friday, 9-8
                      Saturday, 9-2
Dr. George's Hours:
   Monday & Wednesday, 9-5
   Friday & Saturday, 9-2 every other week
Dr. Woo's Hours:
   Monday and Wednesday, 1-8
   Friday & Saturday, 9-2 every other week
Dr. Reynolds' Hours:
   Tuesday, 1-8, Wednesday, 9-1, Thursday, 9-2,
   Friday, 9-2
Dr. Esposito's Hours:
   Monday, 9-8, Tuesday, noon-8, Wednesday, 4-8,
   Thursday, 11-8, Friday, 3-8, Saturday, 9-2
Dr. Whitney's Hours:
   Tuesday, 9-8. Thursday & Friday, 11-8,
   Saturday, 9-2

Figure 13-10   Informational brochure.

INFORMATIONAL BROCHURE

Informed patients make better clients. This is as true with scheduling as it is with procedural changes. A simple brochure on scheduling practices can elicit the cooperation of patients and reduce the time spent with explanations when efforts are required for other duties. See sample brochure in Figure 13-10.

In the facility brochure, list office hours. If a clustering system is used, explain to patients what this involves and why they may not be able to get an appointment for the particular day they desire. Provide simple instructions on what information is required by the medical office to make an appointment. Explain policies regarding cancellations and no-shows. In a tactful manner, emphasize to patients that their cooperation in observing scheduled times and cancellation procedures helps your office serve them better. For more information on developing patient brochures, see Chapter 44.

Procedure 13-1 Checking in Patients

PURPOSE:
To ensure the patient is given prompt and proper care; to meet legal safeguards for documentation.

EQUIPMENT/SUPPLIES:
Patient chart
Required forms
Check-in list and/or appointment book

PROCEDURE STEPS:
1. The evening before or prior to opening the ambulatory care setting, prepare a list of patients to be seen and assemble the charts.
2. Check charts to see that everything is up to date.
3. When patients arrive, immediately acknowledge their presence. If you cannot assist them right away, acknowledge their presence, and then thank them for waiting.
4. Check the patient in, reviewing vital information such as address, telephone number, insurance, and reason for visit. **Be certain to protect the patient's privacy by reviewing this information where doing so cannot be overheard by others.**
5. Use a pen to check the patient's name off in the appointment book and/or day sheet if one is used for the permanent record.
6. Politely ask the patient to be seated and indicate the appropriate wait time, if any.
7. Following office procedures, place the chart where it will be used to route the patient to an appropriate location for the visit.

Procedure 13-2 Cancellation Procedures

PURPOSE:
To protect the physician from legal complications; to free up care time for other patients; to assure quality patient care.

EQUIPMENT/SUPPLIES:
Appointment sheet
Pen (red)
Patient chart

(continues)

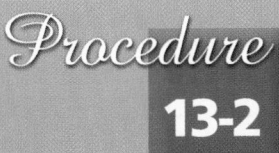

Procedure 13-2 (continued)

PROCEDURE STEPS:

Develop a system so it is evident to staff making appointments that, due to cancellations, time is now open to schedule other appointments. Indicate on the appointment sheet all appointments that were changed, canceled, or failed to show by:

1. *Changes:* Note changes in the appointment sheet margin and directly in the patient's chart and indicate the new appointment time.

2. *Cancellations:* These should be noted also on both the appointment sheet and the patient chart. Draw a single red line through canceled appointments. Be sure to date and initial notations in the patient chart.

3. *No-shows:* These should be noted in both the appointment book and the patient chart. Be sure to date and initial notations in the chart. No-shows can be indicated with a red **X** on the appointment sheet.

Procedure 13-3 Establishing the Appointment Matrix

PURPOSE:

To have a current and accurate record of appointment times available for scheduling patient visits.

EQUIPMENT/SUPPLIES:

Appointment book
Physician's schedule
Staff schedule
Office calendar

PROCEDURE STEPS:

1. Block off times in the appointment book when patients are not to be scheduled by marking a large "X" through these time slots. This establishes the matrix. Ideally the whole year can be mapped out to avoid scheduling patients when the physician has other commitments or when the office is closed.

2. Write in all vacations, holidays, and other office closures as soon as they are known. It may be helpful to indicate absences that might affect patient scheduling; e.g., the vascular lab tech is gone April 20–23 so no Dopplers will be scheduled.

3. Write in all physician meetings, hospital rounds, appointments, conferences, vacations, and other prescheduled physician commitments. If the physician has routine items, such as a Medical Society meeting that is always held on the first Thursday of the month at 7:00 P.M. or daily hospital rounds at 8:00 A.M., write these in.

4. If the office has a scheduling system for certain examinations or procedures; e.g., all cast removals are done in the morning before 10:30 A.M., these can be color-coded with highlighters. This way it is easily and quickly evident where particular types of appointments are available to be scheduled.

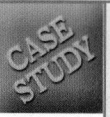

CASE STUDY

13-1

Rhoda Au has persistently canceled her appointments at Inner City Health Care; while she always reschedules, she has canceled the last four appointments. Today, she did not call to cancel nor did she show up for her fifth appointment. Walter Seals, CMA, who is responsible for scheduling and patient flow, is concerned that Rhoda is canceling because she is afraid to come in for some reason. Rhoda has been a patient for a few years now, and she was always responsible about keeping her appointments.

CASE STUDY REVIEW

1. From the point of view of the urgent care center, why should Walter be concerned that Rhoda is canceling appointments? What action might be taken?
2. From the patient point of view, why should Walter be concerned?
3. How should Walter record these cancellations and no-shows if using a manual method of scheduling? If using a computer program?

SUMMARY

Today's ambulatory care setting needs to function efficiently to provide quality care, ensure adequate patient flow, and maintain positive patient relationships. Proper scheduling of patients and other visitors is key to an efficient operation, and the well-organized medical assistant will design a system that meets with both physician and patient satisfaction.

There are at least six common methods of scheduling; ambulatory care settings should use the one that is most appropriate to their patient population, practice areas, and physician preferences. Scheduling methods can and should be customized to the setting, for this usually provides the most adaptable, workable system.

Patient scheduling tools, too, vary and can be tailored to facility needs. While all ambulatory care settings must carefully document appointments, cancellations, and no-shows, they may do so by either manual methods or computer technology. Whichever method is chosen, the goal is to use that tool wisely and consistently in all scheduling activities.

REVIEW QUESTIONS

Multiple Choice

1. Appointment books should always be:
   a. recorded only in pencil
   b. recorded only in red ink
   c. left out on the front desk where patients enter
   d. a current and accurate record and saved as documentation
2. Triaging:
   a. involves taking only emergencies
   b. is assessing the urgency of a call and need for appointment
   c. means sorting appointments by specialized procedure
   d. is only performed by physicians
3. Representatives from medical supply and drug companies:
   a. should only be seen as a last resort
   b. should not be scheduled, but seen only if the physician has time
   c. can provide a valuable service and should be scheduled for short visits
   d. have complex information to communicate and need one-hour appointments
4. The double-booking method:
   a. gives two or more patients the same appointment time
   b. keeps patients waiting unnecessarily
   c. is never the system of choice
   d. is purely for the physician's convenience
5. The stream method:
   a. gives patients appointments as they walk in
   b. schedules appointments at set times throughout the workday
   c. only works in one-physican offices
   d. refers to streamlining paperwork for each appointment
6. Daily appointment sheets:
   a. indicate when physicians and staff take lunch
   b. provide a permanent record for legal risk management and quality management

c. are available only in computerized patient scheduling
d. both a and b

7. Analyzing patient flow:
   a. can maximize an office's scheduling practice
   b. often reveals why patient flow is not efficient
   c. may indicate a change in pattern for patient scheduling
   d. all of the above

8. One principal above all else to be observed in scheduling is:
   a. always schedule in ink
   b. schedule for the patient's convenience
   c. be flexible
   d. referral patients are first

9. If a patient must wait for an appointment:
   a. it is best to say nothing about the delay
   b. explain the delay and offer options when possible
   c. find ways to make the patient comfortable
   d. both b and c

Critical Thinking

1. Discuss the rationale and the procedure to follow for a canceled appointment and a no-show appointment.
2. Describe the following appointment systems: Stream; cluster; modified wave. Give examples of each.
3. Why is there no one best system of scheduling?

Form small discussion groups and develop solutions to the following problems by (1) defining the problem, (2) describing the appropriate steps if required, and (3) developing a possible solution.

4. Lenore McDonnell has called to cancel her appointment for the third consecutive time. (Background: Her last blood pressure reading in the office was 195/115, and there is a known history of stroke in her family.)
5. Dr. Lewis is running an hour behind schedule. It is now 1:00 P.M. He is just seeing a return patient. He has two new patients scheduled and has a surgery scheduled for 2:00 P.M. (Background: Return patients require 30 minutes and new patients 60 minutes.)
6. Your urology office has been using a double-booking system. Through tracking the patient flow, you find that patients are having to wait consistently half an hour or longer. (Background: There is one medical assistant and two examination rooms.)

7. You are using the modified-wave system. You have three appointments scheduled for 10:00 A.M., one for 10:50 A.M., and three for 11:00 A.M. The office closes at 11:30 for lunch so Dr. King can speak at a hospital luncheon. A patient calls and insists to be seen on an emergency basis. (Background: Dr. King's partner is unavailable to cover for her.)
8. Two patients are scheduled to be seen at 11:30. It is now 11:50 and Dr. Whitney has indicated that he will not be through with his current patient for another 20 minutes. (Background: Both patients waiting to see Dr. Whitney are for nonemergency problems.)

For the following situations, briefly explain which type of appointment book and scheduling system you would choose and why.

9. A four-physician practice has only two physicians seeing patients at any one time. There are three medical assistants sharing front and back office duties for all of the physicians.
10. An obstetrics practice specializes in problem pregnancies. There is one front and one back office medical assistant.

WEB ACTIVITIES

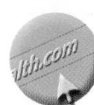

Research the World Wide Web for information related to the types of appointment books and/or computer software that might be appropriate to the ambulatory care setting for patient scheduling. What features might you especially want to have?

REFERENCES/BIBLIOGRAPHY

Fordney, M. T., & Follis, J. J. (1998). *Administrative medical assisting* (4th ed.). Albany, NY: Delmar.

Humphrey, D. D. (1996). *Contemporary medical office procedures* (2nd ed.). Albany, NY: Delmar.

Martinez, B. (2000, August 21). Now it's mass medicine. *The Wall Street Journal*, p. B1.

Montone, D. (1997). *Power building in scheduling*. Philadelphia: W. B. Saunders Co.

Chapter 14

MEDICAL RECORDS MANAGEMENT

KEY TERMS

Accession Record
Caption
Coding
Color Coding
Consecutive or Serial Filing
Cross-Reference
Cut
Guides
Identification Label
Indexing
Inspect
Key Unit
Nonconsecutive Filing
Out Guide
Problem-Oriented Medical Record (POMR)
Purging
Release Mark
Shingling
SOAP
Source-Oriented Medical Record (SOMR)
Tickler File
Unit

OUTLINE

The Importance of Accurate Medical Records
Equipment and Supplies
   Vertical Files
   Open-Shelf Lateral Files
   Movable File Units
   File Folders
   Identification Labels
   Guides and Positions
   Out Guides
Basic Rules for Filing
   Indexing Units
   Filing Patient Charts
   Filing Identical Names
   Filing Business and Organizational Records
Steps for Filing Medical Documentation in Patient Files
   Inspect
   Index
   Code
   Sort
   File

Filing Techniques and Common Filing Systems
   Color Coding
   Alphabetic Filing
   Numeric Filing
   Subject Filing
   Choosing a Filing System
Filing Procedures
   Cross-Referencing
   Tickler Files
   Release Marks
   Check-Out System
   Locating Missing Files or Data
   Filing Chart Data
   Retention and Purging
Correspondence
   Incoming Correspondence
   Outgoing Correspondence
   Filing Procedures for Correspondence
Computer Applications
   Databases
   Archival Storage
   Transfer of Data
   Confidentiality

OBJECTIVES

The student should strive to meet the following performance objectives and demonstrate an understanding of the facts and principles presented in this chapter through written and oral communication.

1. Define the key terms as presented in the glossary.
2. State the reasons for accurately maintaining ambulatory care office files.

(continues)

3. Recall eight common supplies used in medical records management.
4. Name ten of the twenty rules described under Basic Rules for Filing.
5. Describe the five steps commonly used when filing any documentation.
6. State three advantages and three disadvantages of the alphabetic filing system.
7. Name the two other filing systems most often used in the ambulatory care setting.
8. Analyze the purpose of cross-referencing.
9. Recall four common documents filed in the patient's medical record.
10. Describe computer databases and their usefulness to the ambulatory care setting.

ROLE DELINEATION COMPONENTS

ADMINISTRATIVE

Administrative Procedures

● **Perform basic clerical functions**

GENERAL (TRANSDISCIPLINARY)

Legal Concepts

● **Maintain confidentiality**

● **Prepare and maintain medical records**

● **Document accurately**

Operational Functions

● **Apply computer techniques to support office operations**

SCENARIO

Consider a situation that might arise at the multiphysician Inner City Health Care. Patient Juanita Hansen was seen on Tuesday morning by Dr. Whitney for acute stomach pain. She was given a thorough examination and sent for appropriate testing that afternoon. She was then scheduled to return to Inner City on Friday to see Dr. Whitney.

After she was seen Tuesday morning, Juanita received an upper and lower GI series; the results were then sent to Dr. Whitney's office. However, because Karen Ritter, the medical assistant, could not locate Juanita's chart to file the test results, she just set them aside. Friday arrived and Juanita came back to Inner City for her appointment, anxious to know the results of her tests. Dr. Whitney found Juanita's chart, which was inadvertently left on his stack of dictation, and realized the patient's test results had not been filed.

This left Dr. Whitney with a very anxious patient. Karen Ritter is off today so the physician checks with the other medical assistants on duty. They have no knowledge of the test results. Two acts—not replacing the file and not promptly filing Juanita's test results—cause undue stress for the physician, medical assistants, and the patient.

INTRODUCTION

With the vast number of medical records that must be maintained in the ambulatory care setting today, accurate filing of patient charts is the only method by which a facility can efficiently track information vital to patient care. Current medical litigation requires every health care facility to have an efficient filing system and staff who are experienced in using and maintaining medical records.

Medical assistants are often vitally involved in developing filing systems and maintaining accurate tracking of patient records.

Physicians provide the best care for patients when all pertinent data is readily accessible. The medical assistant in charge of filing and retrieving records must file information accurately and retrieve the file efficiently.

THE IMPORTANCE OF ACCURATE MEDICAL RECORDS

Accurate medical records are essential to patient care in any ambulatory care setting. Patient files are critical to the facility's smooth functioning and are important when referring the patient to outside specialists with whom the facility may need to coordinate care. Each treating physician must be aware of tests, procedures, and diagnoses. Maintaining a conscientious record of patient care is also absolutely essential in controlling the costs of medical care.

Medical records management is also important due to the legal issues that every medical office and health care professional must face today. The standard in court is that if there is no written record of a temperature, a visit, a history or physical, a lab report, and so forth, it did not happen. To be prepared in the event of medical litigation, all medical treatment must be documented. No matter how competently a physician has performed treatment, if a written record cannot prove how and what was done, there is no basis for a defense in a court of law.

EQUIPMENT AND SUPPLIES

There are three primary types of file cabinets used in medical offices. These include vertical, lateral, and movable file cabinets.

Vertical Files

Vertical files are cabinets that have pull-out drawers where files are stored (Figure 14-1). Files are retrieved by

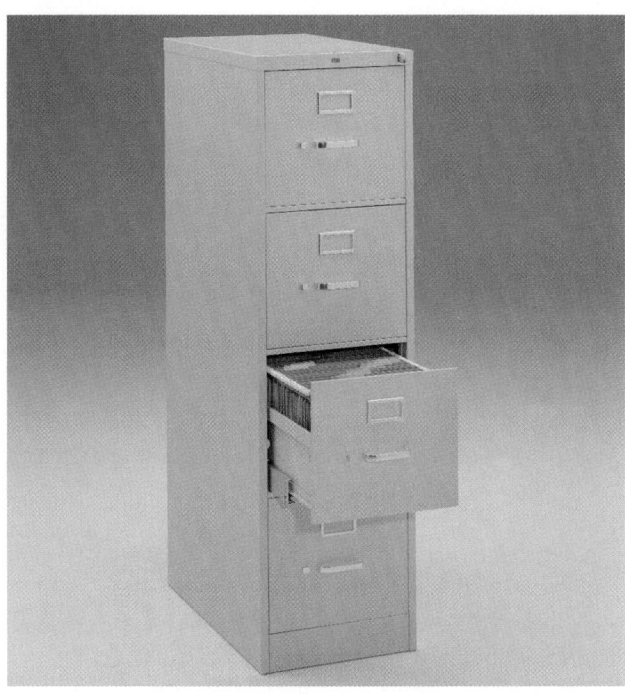

Figure 14-1   Vertical file cabinet. (Courtesy HON® Company)

lifting the appropriate file up and out. These may be used for business records and documents.

Open-Shelf Lateral Files

These are open file cabinets that make quick retrieval of files possible (Figure 14-2). The records are retrieved by pulling them out laterally from the shelf. They are used most often with color-coded filing systems where visual inspection makes it possible to ensure files are kept in the proper order.

Movable File Units

Movable file units allow easy access to large record systems and require less space than vertical or lateral files. These units may be electrically powered to move on floor

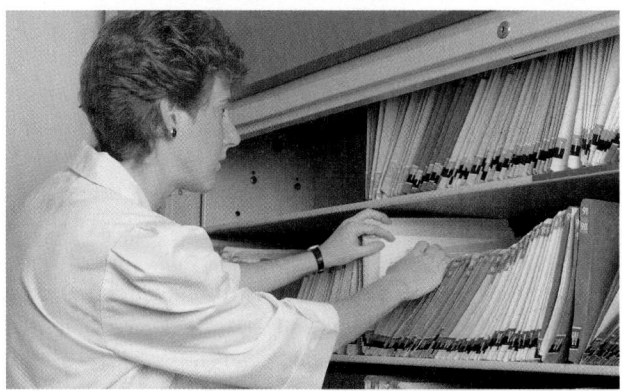

Figure 14-2   Open-shelf lateral file cabinet.

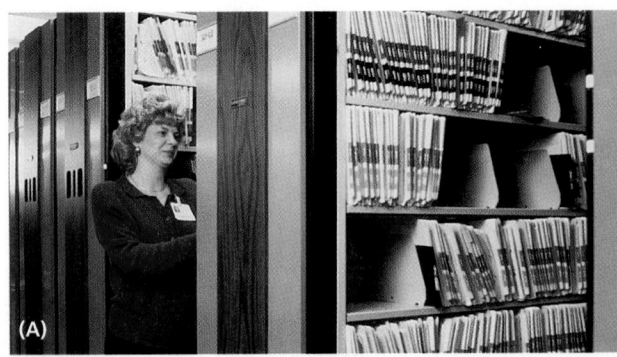

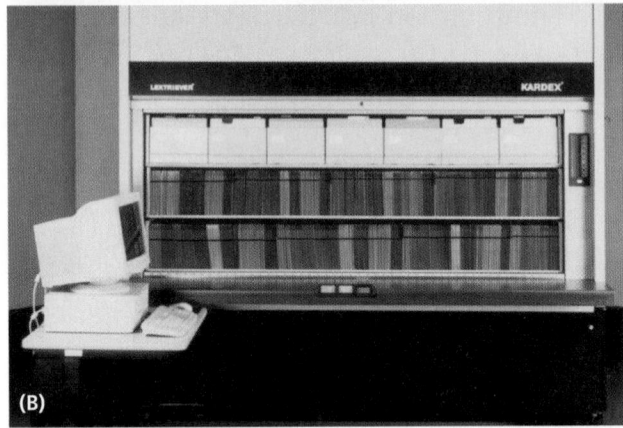

Figure 14-3 Movable file units: (A) Kompakt movable shelving; (B) Lektriever vertical carousel with computer unit. (Courtesy of KARDEX Systems, Inc., Marietta, OH)

tracks or may be physically moved with an easy-to-turn handle mechanism. The movable shelving unit shown in Figure 14-3A is electrically powered to open aisles for accessing files or to close aisles when those files do not need to be accessed. There are also movable file storage units that will automatically travel on a computer-controlled carousel track moving files around until the required section reaches the operator, Figure 14-3B.

File Folders

File folders are designed for different types of labels. Extending along the top edge (the edge that will be visible when filing) are tabs that are cut in varying sizes and positions to allow for different methods of labeling. Figure 14-4 shows the types of cuts, or tabs, found on file folders.

Identification Labels

A variety of labels are used to display the information required to select the correct name or number designation for a particular file. The identification label is adhered either along the top of the file folder (top tab) in vertical file cabinets or along the side of the file folder (side tab) in lateral file cabinets.

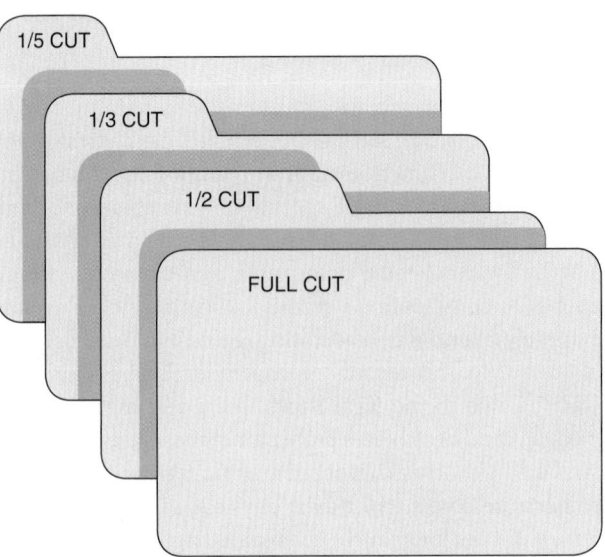

Figure 14-4 Types of cuts, or tabs, on file folders.

Guides and Positions

Guides are used to separate file folders. Guides are somewhat larger than file folders and are of heavier stock. Guides are described by the position of the tab, designated according to its location. For instance, a tab located at the far left would be in the first position, the next one to the right would be in the second position, and so forth. If using third-cut file folders, there are three positions of guides; if using fifth-cut file folders, there are five positions.

Captions. Captions are used to identify major sections of file folders by more manageable subunits (AA–AC, A, B, Office Supplies). Captions are marked on the tabs of the guides (Figure 14-5). These are denoted as single caption and double caption.

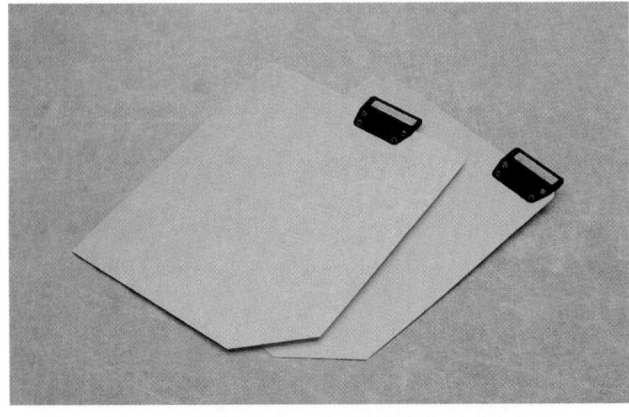

Figure 14-5 Guides separating file folders into subsections. Captions such as A, B, C (single captions) or Ab–Be, Co–Dy (double captions) are placed on the tabs of the guides to identify the sections.

● **Single captions** contain just one letter, number, or unit:
  – A, B, C, D
  – Adams, Smith, Jones

● **Double captions** contain a double notation to denote a range of files:
  – Ab–Be, Co–Dy, Ho–Le
  – Appleston–Bertram, Cody–Devoe

Out Guides

Out guides or out sheets are a device to help in tracking charts. An out guide is a cardboard or plastic/paper sheet kept in place of the patient chart when charts are removed from the filing storage (Figure 14-6).

BASIC RULES FOR FILING

Regardless of the type of filing system used, alphabetizing is the key to organizing files and charts. It is easily recognizable that Adams would be filed before Benson, as A comes before B. In what order, though, are Winston Adams and Winston Alexandar Adams filed? What about Joseph Lee Masters, III and Joseph Lee Masters, Jr.? Is Northwest Diagnostic filed before or after North West Diagnostic? It is necessary to know more than just the alphabetic order of the letters A to Z. Thus, certain indexing rules have been developed to facilitate the alphabetic process in maintaining files in the medical office.

Indexing Units

There must be an organized method of identifying and separating items to be filed into small subunits. This is accomplished with the use of what we call indexing units. A unit identifies each part of a name. In this process each unit is identified according to unit 1 (the key unit), unit 2, unit 3, and so forth, with each segment of the filing

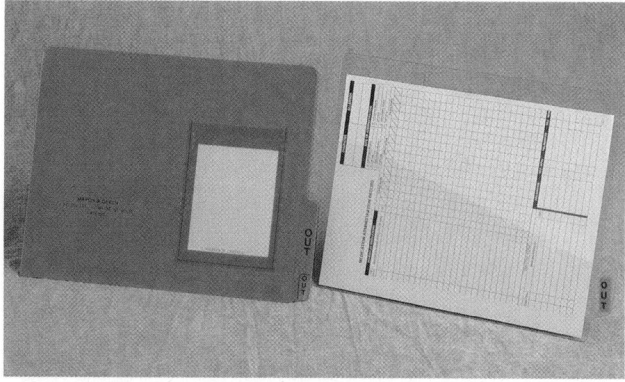

Figure 14-6 An out guide indicating the name of the person who has possession of the file should always be put in place of a patient's record when it is removed from the file.

label identified. This process can be applied to individual names, organizations, or clinics. Accepted filing rules describe how to assign unit numbers to each element.

Example. Annette Barbara Samuels

Unit 1	Samuels
Unit 2	Annette
Unit 3	Barbara

When working in a medical setting with patient charts the patient's legal name is always used for the chart rather than a nickname or abbreviation. If the office has a practice of calling patients by preferred names, a note of name preferences and nicknames may be noted on the chart. However, the filing label should use the proper name.

Example. The following items to be filed would be assigned units as illustrated:

	Units Assigned		
	1	**2**	**3**
Cole Blanche Little	Little	Cole	Blanche
Wayne Lee Elder	Elder	Wayne	Lee
Kelso Medical Supply	Kelso	Medical	Supply
GT Pharmacy	GT	Pharmacy	

Filing Patient Charts

Rule 1. The names of individuals are assigned indexing units respectively: last name (surname), first name, middle and succeeding names.

	Units Assigned		
	1	**2**	**3**
Jaime Renae Carrera	Carrera	Jaime	Renae
Lee Allen Au	Au	Lee	Allen
Bill Hugo Schwartz	Schwartz	Bill	Hugo
Dottie Marie Tate	Tate	Dottie	Marie

Rule 2. Foreign language prefixes are indexed as one unit with the unit that follows. Spacing, punctuation, and capitalization are ignored. Such prefixes include *d, da, de, de la, del, des, di, du, el, fitz, l, la, las, le, les, lu, m, mac, mc, o, saint, sainte, san, santa, sao, st, te, ten, ter, van, van de, van der, and von der* (*st, sainte,* and *saint* are indexed as written).

	Units Assigned		
	1	**2**	**3**
Gerald Steven St. Simon	Stsimon	Gerald	Steven
Carol Louise del Rio	Delrio	Carol	Louise
Richard Saint Louis	Saint	Louis	Richard

Rule 3. Titles are considered as separate indexing units. If the title appears with first and last names, the title is considered to be the last indexing unit. When dealing with patient charts, the first name always accompanies the title and last name.

Units Assigned

	1	2	3	4
Dr. Marlene Elaine Smith	Smith	Marlene	Elaine	Dr
Prof. Marcia Tai Lewis	Lewis	Marcia	Tai	Prof

Rule 4. Names that are hyphenated are considered as one unit.

Units Assigned

	1	2	3
Adele Marie Johnson-Smith	Johnsonsmith	Adele	Marie
Ray Steven Reynolds-Martin	Reynoldsmartin	Ray	Steven

Rule 5. When indexing names of married women, the name is indexed by the legal name. Remember that patient charts are legal documents, making this practice necessary (see cross-referencing to use husband's name).

Units Assigned

	1	2	3	4
Amy Sue Sung (Mrs. John)	Sung	Amy	Sue	Mrs John
Tami Jo Strizver (Mrs. Todd)	Strizver	Tami	Jo	Mrs Todd

Rule 6. Seniority units are indexed as the last indexing unit.

Units Assigned

	1	2	3	4
James Edward Brown Jr.	Brown	James	Edward	Jr
Manuel Louis Garcia III	Garcia	Manuel	Louis	III

Rule 7. Seniority units are filed in numerical order from first to last.

	Matthew Earl Wallesz, Jr.
BEFORE	Matthew Earl Wallesz, Sr.
	Patrick James O'Neill, Jr.
BEFORE	Patrick James O'Neill, Sr.
	Virgil James Garcia, I
BEFORE	Virgil James Garcia, II
	Alex Curtis Jordan, I
BEFORE	Alex Curtis Jordan, II

Rule 8. Numeric units are broken down such that numeric seniority terms are filed before alphabetic terms.

	Edward Lee Kletka, IV
BEFORE	Edward Lee Kletka, Jr.
	George Lee Curtis, II
BEFORE	George Lee Curtis, Sr.

Filing Identical Names

When names are identical, the address may be used to order files. The address is indexed by:

> First: . . . . .City
> SECOND . . . . .STATE
> *Third* . . . .*Street Name*
> **Fourth:** . . . .**Address #**

Therefore, the following Acme Drug Supply files would be arranged from first to last as follows:

1. Acme Drug Supply, **839** *Kentucky Boulevard,* <u>Crawford</u>, MISSOURI
2. Acme Drug Supply, **683** *Wildflower Avenue,* <u>Fairbanks</u>, ALASKA
3. Acme Drug Supply, **1539** *Wildflower Avenue,* <u>Fairbanks</u>, ALASKA
4. Acme Drug Supply, **742** *Terminal Street West,* <u>Fairbanks</u>, ARIZONA
5. Acme Drug Supply, **731** *Terminal Street East,* <u>New York</u>, NEW YORK

Although this is the official indexing rule, most medical offices prefer alternative methods for filing identical charts. The primary consideration here is that patient addresses often change frequently. Therefore, preferred methods include date of birth or social security number.

Filing Business and Organizational Records

When indexing businesses and organizations, the rules learned under filing individual names (Rules 1–8) will be used when individual names appear as part of the filing units. Rules for business and organizational records (Rules 9–20) do not apply to the filing of patient charts. However, they are used when filing business correspondence related to the running of the office, including correspondence for business equipment, maintenance contracts, medical equipment, and delivery services.

Rule 9. The order assignment of units for indexing businesses/organizations is as written.

	Units Assigned		
	1	2	3
Ace Bandage Supplies	Ace	Bandage	Supplies
Kent Memorial Hospital	Kent	Memorial	Hospital

Rule 10. When *the* is the first unit of a business-organization, it is indexed as the last unit. The same would be true of *in, at,* and other prepositions and articles or words that do not provide a clearly identifiable key unit.

	Units Assigned		
	1	2	3
The Office Assistants	Office	Assistants	The
The Medical Specialists	Medical	Specialists	The

Rule 11. Symbols such as &, ¢, $, #, and % are indexed as units, spelled out as words.

	Units Assigned			
	1	2	3	4
Lawless & Krakoa, Attorneys	Lawless	and	Krakoa	Attorneys
# One Secretarial Service	Number	One	Secretarial	Service

Rule 12. When indexing the $ sign before a number, the first unit is the number.

	Units Assigned			
	1	2	3	4
$1 Quick Fax	1	Dollar	Quick	Fax
$5 Florists	5	Dollar	Florists	

Rule 13. When punctuation marks are included as part of the indexing units, they are disregarded. Punctuation marks include: ." ' : ; - ! ? ( ).

	Units Assigned			
	1	2	3	4
L. L. Transcription	L	L	Transcription	
M. E. Medical Equipment	M	E	Medical	Equipment

Rule 14. When indexing numbers, the numbers are indexed as written.

	Units Assigned		
	1	2	3
Rx 2-Go	Rx	2go	
Number Two Florists	Number	Two	Florists

Rule 15. When indexing figures, the numbers are written as figures. *NOTE: d, nd, rd, st,* and *th* are ignored when indexing.

	Units Assigned			
	1	2	3	4
2nd Hand Office Supplies	2	Hand	Office	Supplies
1st Rate Secretaries	1	Rate	Secretaries	

Rule 16. When indexing numbers, if the number is written as a single word, it is indexed as a single unit.

	Units Assigned		
	1	2	3
Flowers 4 You	Flowers	4	You

Rule 17. When indexing numbers, if the number is written with a word, it is indexed as one unit with the word.

	Units Assigned	
	1	2
Flowers 4U	Flowers	4U

Rule 18. When indexing hyphenated numbers, they are indexed only by the number before the hyphen.

	Units Assigned		
	1	2	3
8–4 Temporary Help*	8	Temporary	Help

*If there happened to be an "8–4 Temporary Help" and an "8–5 Temporary Help," then the second number could be used.

Rule 19. When indexing alpha characters and numeric characters, the numeric characters are always filed before alpha characters.

NAME	ORDER	FILE SECTION
18th Street Pharmacy	First	Before any alphabetic sections—numeric*
72nd Avenue Clinic	Second	Before any alphabetic section (72 follows 18)—numeric
Eighteenth Street Pharmacy	Third	The letter "E" section

*The files could be set up with one file for all numeric designations followed by "A" to "Z" files/sections.

Rule 20. When indexing words that can be compound or two single words, the "as written" rule applies.

	North West Rehabilitation
filed before	
	Northwest Rehabilitation

STEPS FOR FILING MEDICAL DOCUMENTATION IN PATIENT FILES

Before a discussion of the common filing systems, it is helpful to review procedural steps that accurately and efficiently process data sheets, laboratory requests, dictation, and so forth from the time they are generated to the time the file is returned to the medical records section. Efficiently following these steps will save considerable time in the ambulatory care setting.

Inspect

Carefully inspect the report to identify the patient, subject, or file to whom the information belongs. Remove clips and staples. Make certain the information is complete.

Index

Use the indexing process to determine how the chart would be located, properly identifying indexing units and their order.

Code

Coding is the process of marking data to indicate how information is to be filed. If using a system other than a strict alphabetic system, determine the proper coding (numbers, Tab-Alpha, or other) for the chart so it can be retrieved. Otherwise, identify the indexed units by underlining or highlighting. This makes refiling more effective and assures that the item will always be filed in the same place. If a cross-reference is required, identify the cross-reference by double underlining and placing an "X" nearby. This chapter includes detailed information on coding and cross-reference.

Sort

If there are a number of reports/documents to be filed, sort them into units according to the captions on the charts. This will eliminate wasted time in working back and forth through the alphabet or numbers.

File

The papers are placed in the proper charts and the charts returned to their proper place in the medical records section. Be alert to the labels and refile any information or charts that have been misfiled.

FILING TECHNIQUES AND COMMON FILING SYSTEMS

There are three major filing systems commonly used in the ambulatory care setting: alphabetic, numeric, and subject filing. The alphabet is intrinsic to all methods, and the basic rules for filing covered previously are used in all systems.

Color coding is used a high percentage of the time in all three systems to minimize filing errors. Another system, geographic, is seldom used in the ambulatory care setting unless there are multiple offices. Even then, a form of color coding may be used.

Color Coding

Color coding is a technique often used in the three major filing systems. Color-coding methods most widely employed in medical facilities are Tab-Alpha® by Tab Products, Inc., Alpha-Z® by The Smead Manufacturing Company, and other variations of color coding methods. By working with these systems medical assistants will understand the principles behind the color-coding and be able to apply these principles to variations in any ambulatory care setting.

Color coding makes retrieval of files more efficient with the use of visible color differences that facilitate easier maintenance of the files. Color-coding filing systems utilize an alphabetic system in that after they are coded by color that designation is used to order the files alphabetically.

Tab-Alpha System. This system is designed primarily for filing systems that use vertical files where all individual charts are clearly visible in one unit.

Each alphabetic letter is assigned a different color. Each folder has a color-coded label. Only full-cut folders are used:

- Colored labels are applied over the edge of the full cut for the first two letters of the key indexing unit (Winston Paul Lewis: WI).

- A third white label is placed over the tab edge, which contains all of the indexing units (Winston Paul Lewis).

- In addition, some offices utilize a color-coded label to indicate the last year the patient was seen. This makes an efficient method for easily identifying active and inactive files.

- Any additional labels; e.g., allergies, last year seen, or industrial claim, are attached to the chart according to the office procedure.

Alpha-Z System. This particular system is designed for use with either open lateral files or vertical drawer files (Figure 14-7A). Alphabetic letters are utilized as the primary guides. Breakdowns of alphabetic combinations are added as determined by the needs of a particular facility.

A combination of thirteen colors is utilized in the Alpha-Z system with white letters on a solid colored background for the first half of the alphabet and white letters on a colored background with white stripes for the second half of the alphabet (Figure 14-7B).

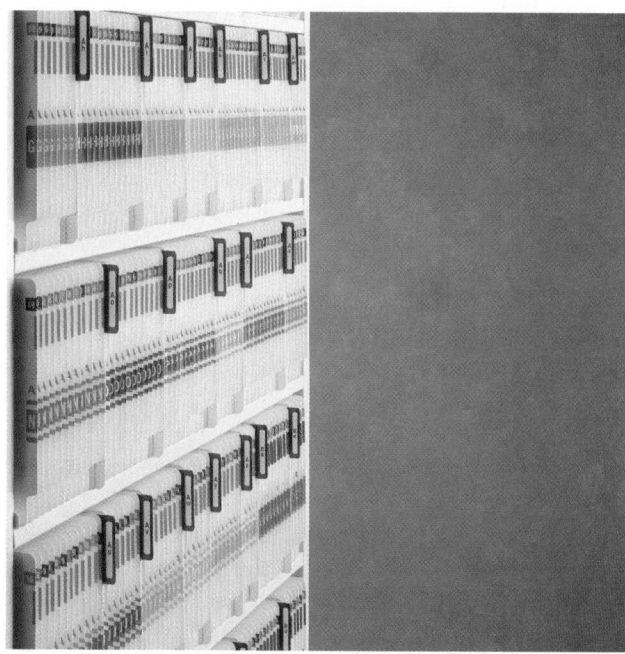

Figure 14-7A Alpha-Z Color-Coding Filing System uses open lateral shelving unit with color-coded files. (Courtesy Smead Manufacturing Company)

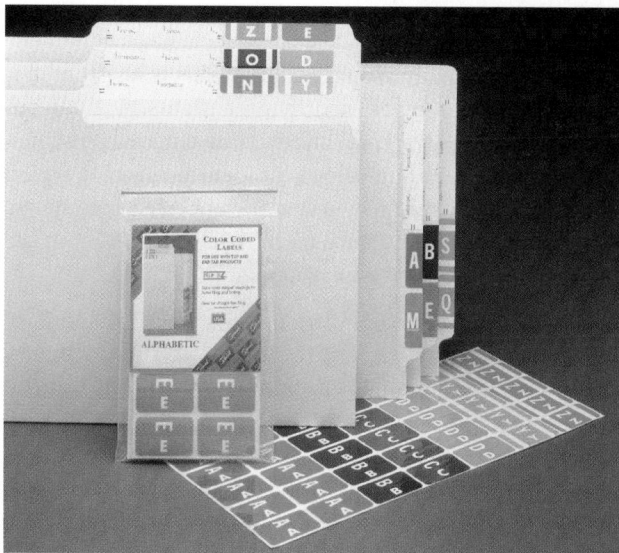

Figure 14-7B Alpha-Z Color-Coded Labels shown on top- and side-cut files.

The thirteen colors utilized are shown in Table 14-1. Folders have three labels:

- The first label contains the typed name, a color block, and the letter of the alphabet for the first letter of the first indexing unit:

  Winston, Lewis Paul YELLOW "W"

- The second and third labels are color-coded to correspond to the second and third letters of the first unit:

  "I" on pink background and "N" on red striped background

Customized Color-Coding Systems. Many offices utilize color systems to meet specific needs.

TABLE 14-1	THIRTEEN COLORS ARE USED IN THE ALPHA-Z SYSTEM	
White Letter Colored Background	**White Letter Striped Colored Background**	**Color**
A	N	Red
B	O	Dark Blue
C	P	Dark Green
D	Q	Light Blue
E	R	Purple
F	S	Orange
G	T	Gray
H	U	Dark Brown
I	V	Pink
J	W	Yellow
K	X	Light Brown
L	Y	Lavender
M	Z	Light Green

Colored File Folders by First Name. One method color-codes the first letter of the first name. The folders then are filed alphabetically by last name.

Example. *A* is assigned red folders; *M* is assigned green folders; *S* is assigned blue folders

Michael Taylor	Green Folder
Annette Samuels	Red Folder
Susan Boyer	Blue Folder

Many small medical offices utilize this system and find it quite effective. In the multiphysician urgent care center, this would be quite time-consuming when locating files for patients of all physicians.

Color File Folders by Last Name. Another method utilizing this system assigns colored folders according to the first letter of the last name. The folders are then filed alphabetically.

Example. *S* is assigned pink folders; *B* is assigned gray folders.

Bill Schwartz	Pink Folder
Corey Boyer	Gray Folder

This system makes it easy to spot folders that have been misfiled under an incorrect first letter but does not break it down further for misfilings within the first-letter guides.

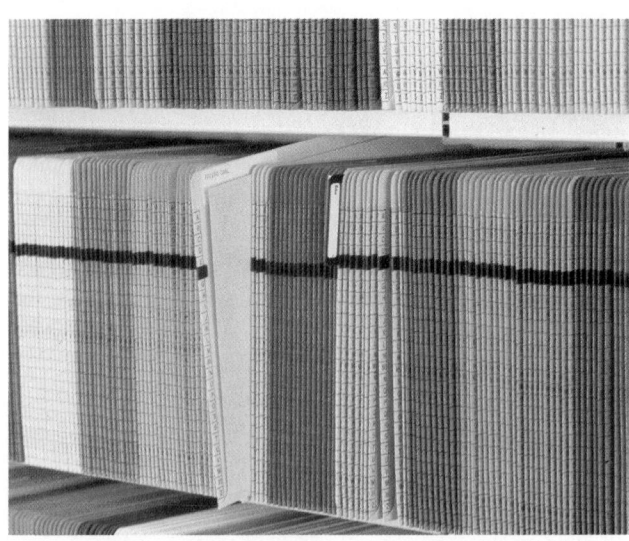

Figure 14-9   Colorscan Color-Coded Filing System. Yellow file selected for "Carl"; "F" side tab selected for "Friend." (Courtesy of KARDEX System, Inc., Marietta, OH)

Colorscan System. The Colorscan Color-Coded Filing System by *KARDEX Systems, Inc.*, assigns color folders based on ten color groups (Figure 14-8). The color folder is assigned to a specific record based on the first letter of the second unit (usually patient's first name). Figure 14-9 shows that the yellow color file was selected because of the "C" in Carl. The files are further segmented by side tabs assigned to the first letter of the first unit (usually last name). In Figure 14-9, the side tab is assigned to the letter "F" for the patient's last name "Friend." All color folders would be used behind each alphabetic guide. If a record has only one unit, the first letter determines both position and color.

This system makes it easy to spot folders that have been misfiled under the incorrect first or second unit.

Physician Coding. In large clinics this is a system that many practices use for identifying patients by their primary care physician. Each physician is assigned a particular color of folder. This allows for identification of folders that have been misfiled under the incorrect physician. The folders themselves are filed under either the alphabetic or numeric system for each particular physician.

Example. Edith Leonard is a patient of Dr. Rice who has been assigned pink folders. Her chart is pink and is found under the "L's" as an alphabetic system is used.

Color-Coded Numbers. This system is utilized in a numeric filing system and operates in the same way as alphabetic systems. Numbers from 0 to 9 are color coded. The appropriate colored numbers are then placed on the tabs of the patient's folder.

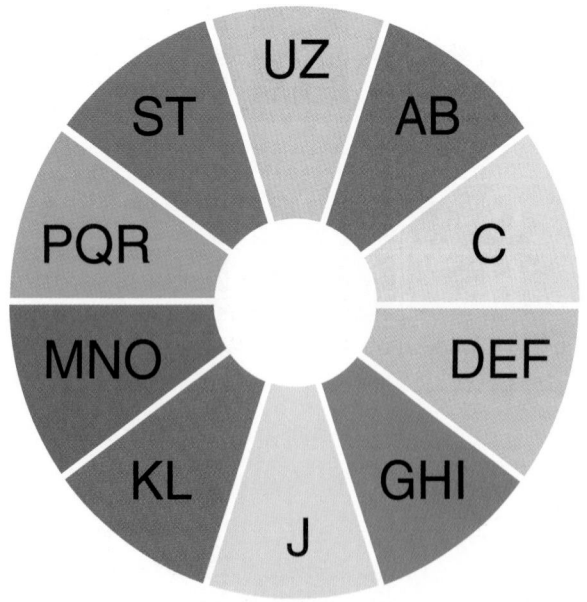

Figure 14-8   Colorscan Color-Coded Filing System Color Wheel. (Courtesy of KARDEX System, Inc., Marietta, OH)

Alphabetic Filing

Strict alphabetic filing is one of the simplest filing methods, as files are strictly maintained by assigning a label to each file. The first letter of that label (e.g., Jones, Invoices, Pharmacies) is then used to alphabetize the files from A to Z. When a limited number of files is accessed, this is a very acceptable method of maintaining records.

Numeric Filing

Numeric filing is organized by number rather than by letter. A key benefit of numeric filing is that it preserves patient confidentiality since the individual's name is not obviously apparent on the file folder.

Numeric filing systems are either consecutive (serial) or nonconsecutive.

Consecutive or Serial.
The consecutive or serial filing method is commonly used in handling invoices, sales orders, and requisitions. Each record is numbered and filed in ascending order.

Example.   576 93 or 57693

Unit 1	5
Unit 2	7
Unit 3	6
Unit 4	9
Unit 5	3

Nonconsecutive.
The nonconsecutive filing system uses groups of two, three, or four or more digits; e.g., social security numbers or telephone numbers. Numbers are grouped and arranged in ascending order using the digits to the far right or the terminal digits. Each group of numbers is considered a unit (one number). To file the terminal digit files in numerical order, begin with strictly the terminal digit unit.

Example.   2108 23 879

Unit 1	879
Unit 2	23
Unit 3	2108

Components of Numeric Filing.
There are four essential components that are used with a numeric system, whether it is a manual or computerized system.

Serially Numbered Dividers with Guides. Consecutive numeric guides (5, 10, etc.; 50, 100, etc.) separate the individual file folders into smaller groups of files.

Miscellaneous (General) Numeric File Section. This is reserved for records that have not been assigned numbers. Patients should automatically be assigned a number on the first visit. However, there are occasions where patients cannot be assigned a number initially. The miscellaneous section is generally in front of all the numeric folders for ease of locating items. Files in the miscellaneous section are filed alphabetically by patient name. This is the best place for the miscellaneous file(s) for two reasons:

1. They do not have to be moved each time a numbered file is added to the back of the order.
2. In a large system of files, retrieval from the front is quick and easy.

Alphabetic Card File. This alphabetic file is necessary as a source to locate files or records.

A card contains name, address, and file number (or an M if located in the miscellaneous section); any cross-reference is here rather than in the numeric files.

The alphabetic card file and accession record in a manual system would be equivalent to the computerized record of the patient and whatever number is assigned to them in that computer record. If using a computerized system, the program generally will automatically cross-reference the number with the alphabetic list that was generated with the initial entry. If laboratory data come into the office on Leo M. McKay, there would need to be a method to know where to locate his chart to file the report; i.e., the alphabetic listing.

With a manual system, the alphabetic file is kept in an index card fashion. This file needs to contain the complete name and address (and any other information denoted by the office policy; e.g., insurance and emergency numbers).

Noted with this information there needs to be either an M for miscellaneous (for those items not assigned a number) or an assigned number (Figure 14-10 A and B).

If a cross-reference is required, prepare a cross-reference card and include an X next to the file number (or M) to indicate this is the cross-reference card and not the primary location (Figure 14-10C).

Accession Record. The accession record is a journal (or computer listing) where numbers are preassigned. Each new item to be assigned is written on the line next to the number (Figure 14-11). Each new entry for which a chart will be created must be assigned a number. A computerized system would have an accession record in its memory bank.

See Procedure 14-1 for numeric filing steps.

Subject Filing

There are many reasons why material would be filed using a system of subjects in a medical office. If physicians are doing research, they might wish to index research according to diseases. Subject files are convenient for locating

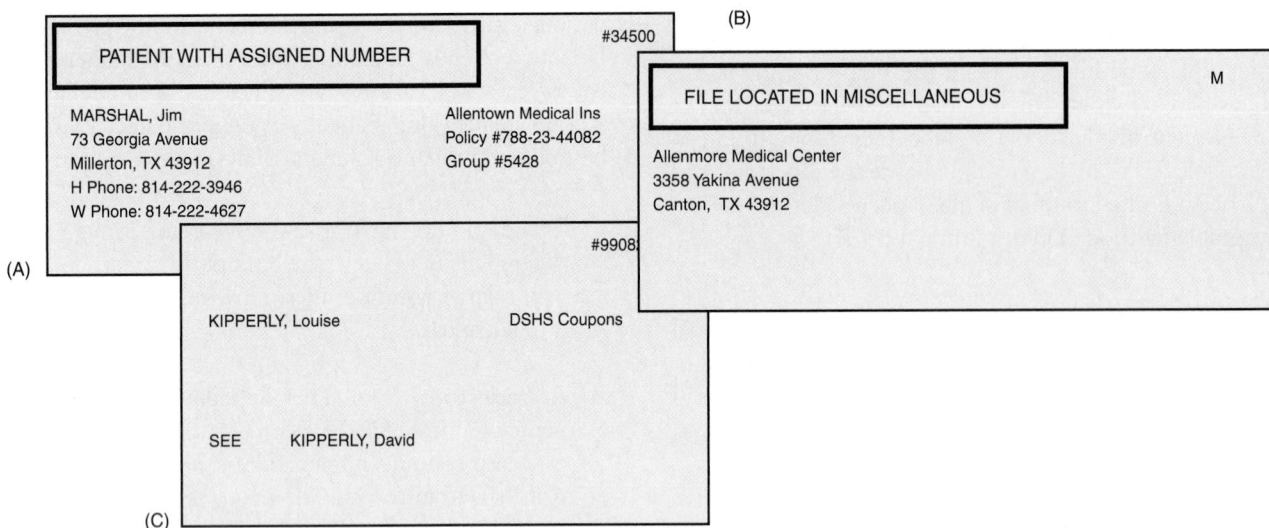

Figure 14-10 Card files used in a numeric filing system: (A) Patient with an assigned number. (B) Patient record has not had a number assigned and is located in miscellaneous section. (C) Cross-reference card.

frequently used services or for filing reference materials for patient needs. Insurance company information also might be filed by subject.

When using a subject filing system, scan the material to determine the subject or theme. As with color-coding and numeric filing, an alphabetic file is necessary. This can be either a subject list or an index card file listing the subjects. Also, as with numeric filing, all cross-reference cards are done only with alphabetic file listings.

Within the folders, material can be arranged either alphabetically or chronologically; keep in mind the objective for maintaining the particular files. For instance, if using subject indexing for research projects physicians

have conducted, identify the subject category, and then in the material, code an item for reference to that specific material. See Procedure 14-2 for subject filing steps.

Choosing a Filing System

To select a filing system, each office must decide what the primary objectives are with respect to storage of patient files, business records, and research files within the office. How will the charts be used primarily? Is there information that will need to be tracked by others not familiar with the records? It is often the case that more than one filing system will be utilized, such as alphabetic filing for patient charts, a numeric system for research subjects, and a subject system for miscellaneous correspondence (Table 14-2).

The number of documents to be filed seems to be one primary determinant in selecting an alphabetic or numeric system. Alphabetic filing is quite manageable when dealing with a relatively small number of patients. However, when the number of patients increases to several hundred or more, a numeric system becomes much more practical because there are an infinite set of numbers available. With the numeric system there is only one of each assigned designation. However, with an alphabetic system, there are a number of common names (e.g., Smith, Jones, Adams, and Johnson) that can have many

ACCESSION LOG BOOK

#	File Name
800	CARRERA, Jaime
801	AU, Rhoda
802	TREMONT Drug Supply
803	
804	
805	
806	
807	

Figure 14-11 Accession record or log sequentially lists numbers to be used to assign to numeric records. The next number available in this system is 803.

TABLE 14-2	ALPHABETIC OR NUMERIC FILING SYSTEM CONSIDERATIONS

1. Consider the type, purpose, and use of the information.
2. Take into account the number of files or records.
3. Recognize the need for confidentiality.

multiples requiring additional sorting to narrow the search for the correct chart. In addition, with multiple charts of the same last name, the chances for misfiling increases. With the current trend in health care toward larger ambulatory care settings, there is likely to be an increase in the use of numeric filing over alphabetic filing. Confidentiality is another reason to select a numeric filing system. Confidentiality of charts is maintained more easily with numeric files as there is no visible name on the outside of the chart. Additionally, numerically referenced records can be utilized in research activities where random sampling and anonymity are required.

FILING PROCEDURES

By adhering to some common principles in medical records management, any filing system will be more effective and enable the medical assistant to store, identify, retrieve, and maintain medical records efficiently.

Cross-Referencing

In running an efficient medical office files must be stored for quick and accurate retrieval. If there is any doubt as to where a particular file would be located, cross-reference the file. Many offices fail to take the extra time it requires to do this. However, with the growing number of foreign names, hyphenated names, and stepfamilies, it is well worth the effort. When the office receives a letter and a release of information form inquiring about medical facts on Mr. David Kipperly's four stepchildren who were involved in an accident, how will these files be located? If they are cross-referenced under the stepfather's name, this will be a relatively easy procedure. However, if the medical assistant is unfamiliar with the family (as in a larger urgent care center with a large volume of patients), this may become a time-consuming job. Another scenario might involve insurance information on Janet Morgan. A search of the records does not produce a file for any Janet Morgan. The reason for this is that Janet Morgan is married and her chart has been filed under Janet Hill-Morgan. Time spent cross-referencing contributes to a more efficient method of retrieving information.

A cross-referencing system does not need to be elaborate. It is quite sufficient to use inserts with labels attached that are inserted in the appropriate place in the storage units. For instance, a plain piece of cardboard, rather than a file or chart, could be inserted for "Janet Morgan." This insert would simply have a label directing one to the location of the primary file.

The proper steps for cross-referencing along with several examples where cross-referencing might be used follow.

Steps for Cross-Referencing

1. Identify the primary filing label.
2. Make a proper file to be used as the primary location for all medical records.
3. Identify one (or more) alternatives where one might find the file.
4. For the alternative filings, make a cross-reference sheet, card, or dummy chart that lists the primary reference and refers back to the location of the primary file.

Example. The patient, Jaime Renae Carrera, has made it known to the office that most of the correspondence received will refer to the name Renny Carrera as this is his preference. The SEE reference will identify where the primary file is located.

PRIMARY FILE:	Carrera, Jaime Renae
X-REFERENCE FILE:	Carrera, Renny
	SEE Carrera, Jamie Renae

Rule 1. Married Women. The primary file would be the patient's legal name with the cross-reference being listed under her husband's name.

PRIMARY FILE:	Au, Rhoda A. (Mrs.)
	Lee Au
X-REFERENCE FILE:	Au, Mrs. Lee
	SEE Au, Rhoda A. (Mrs.)

Rule 2. Foreign Names. The primary file would be located under the patient's legal name. It is important therefore that you identify the first, middle, and surname (last name) when the patient comes for the first visit. Unless people are familiar with a particular group of names, the first, middle, and surnames are often confused with one another. Again, your experience will teach you which cross-references should be set up.

PRIMARY FILE:	Sing, Yange Teah
X-REFERENCE FILE:	Yange, Sing Teah
	SEE Sing, Yange Teah
X-REFERENCE FILE:	Teah, Yange Sing
	SEE Sing, Yange Teah

Rule 3. Hyphenated Names. With the proliferation of hyphenated names, it is common for materials to be listed under different combinations of the hyphenated name. For instance, a married woman may have records under her maiden name, her husband's surname,

and her hyphenated name. Therefore, it is necessary to make two cross-references.

PRIMARY FILE:	Krenshaw-Skiple, Rose Marie
X-REFERENCE FILE:	Skiple, Rose Marie
	SEE Krenshaw-Skiple, Rose Marie
X-REFERENCE FILE:	Krenshaw, Rose Marie
	SEE Krenshaw-Skiple, Rose Marie

Rule 4. **Multiple Listings.** A great deal of correspondence is received with multiple listings of names. At times the medical office may receive correspondence from only one of the involved parties. Rather than keep a separate file for each, maintain a primary file as listed on the letter and then cross-reference file(s) for the individual names.

PRIMARY FILE:	Olsen, Piper, and Dillard Associates
X-REFERENCE FILE:	Piper, Richard C., M.D.
	SEE Olsen, Piper, and Dillard Associates
X-REFERENCE FILE:	Olsen, Francis William, M.D.
	SEE Olsen, Piper, and Dillard Associates
X-REFERENCE FILE:	Dillard, Thomas E., M.D.
	SEE Olsen, Piper, and Dillard Associates

Tickler Files

Sticky notes and writing notes on the calendar are popular methods of reminding office personnel to follow up with some required action. However, a well-organized, efficient office will maintain what is known as a tickler file, a method that serves as a reminder that some action needs to be taken at a date in the future.

Many computer systems today have provision for establishing ticklers on files. However, a standard practice of using index cards for tickler files is easy to maintain (Figure 14-12).

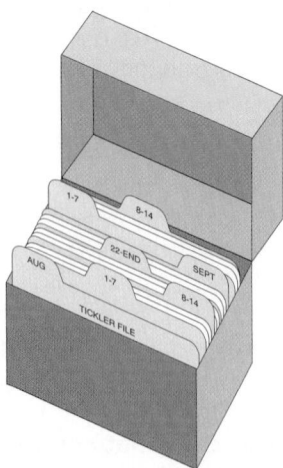

Figure 14-12 Tickler files should be reviewed daily or weekly to follow up on activities and actions that must be taken.

The tickler card should contain the following information:

- Patient name
- Tickler date (when action should be taken)
- Required action (e.g., schedule surgery or mail reminder)
- Additional relevant information (telephone number)

If action is to be taken with a patient or on behalf of the patient; e.g., scheduling a hospital admittance or sending a reminder of a checkup visit, place the information on the tickler card as soon as possible so this task is not forgotten.

When filing records, be sure to look for such words as "on _____ date we will," "pending action," or "follow-up," indicating that some course of action needs to be taken.

Release Marks

It is a good practice to use some type of release mark on every item that is filed (date stamp, initials, check mark). Ideally the physician should initial the document after it has been read. Then, if action is required by the medical assistant, a release mark is in a consistently identified place on every document. If no action is required after the physician has signed or initialed it, place a release mark on the document. A release mark on every piece of correspondence serves as an excellent quality control measure.

Check-Out System

Many offices have developed dummy charts or cardboard files labeled "out sheets" or "out guides." Most of these guides are identified by an OUT label or metal holder, but they could be assigned a particular color; the key is that they stand out as different from the primary folders.

On the out guide there should be at the least:

- A record of when the chart was removed
- Where the chart can be located

Other information that is useful to note includes:

- Expected date of return
- Actual date the chart was returned
- Signature of the personnel checking out the record.
- Notation on what section of the chart file was borrowed, such as a lab report or specialty examination.

Some clinics prefer to have *temporary folders* rather than just an out guide. There are also out guides with pockets to file data in the absence of a chart. This allows for data storage on a temporary basis until the primary file is returned. The data can then be filed permanently when the primary folder is returned. If these folders are of a different color or have a different type of tab/label, they can be spotted easily so the staff can track the temporary files to be sure they do not become permanent folders.

Locating Missing Files or Data

Misfiling can occur for a number of reasons. When this situation occurs, a specific procedure must be established to conduct a search for the missing information. By systematically searching, the missing data usually can be located. This systematic search can be aided by making a mental note of the particular items that commonly are misplaced; i.e., thin-paper lab reports, small lab slips, look-alike names such as "Ward" filed under "Wart" or "Adam" filed under "Adams." Make a note of what was misfiled and where the information was located to more easily locate similar items in the future.

To locate missing pieces of information when the correct file is located but not the particular item within that file:

- Check all of the items within the file.
- Check other files with similar labels.

To locate missing files:

- Check the folders filed before and after the proper location of the misplaced file.
- Look at folders with similar labels.
- Check the physician's desk, desk tray, and other office personnel.
- If using a color-coding system, look for folders with the same color-coding as the misplaced file.
- If using a numeric system, look for possible transposition of combinations of numbers.
- Check for transposition of first and last names.
- Check for alternative spellings of names or look-alike names.

Misplaced files can be very frustrating and time-consuming to locate. The best strategy is to check files for the proper filing order whenever returning or retrieving a file folder. When removing a file to answer a question, leave the file following it sticking out slightly to make its return easy and correct. Most importantly, when finished with a record, refile it immediately.

Filing Chart Data

Types of Reports. The patient's chart is the key source of information relating to treatment. There are a number of reports kept in the chart, all serving to provide a total picture of patient care. Following are the most common documents that will be part of the patient's medical record:

Clinical Notes. These include documentation such as the medical history, the physical examination, and the follow-up notes. They track the patient's course of treatment.

Correspondence. This varies from office to office. Some offices file all types of correspondence together. Other offices file correspondence about the patient's treatment with the clinical notes.

Laboratory Reports. Included in this section are X-ray reports, CT scans, ultrasound reports, blood work, urinalysis, EEGs, ECGs, physical therapy-related reports, and pathology reports—information related to clinical data that assess the patient's condition.

Miscellaneous. This category includes insurance-related papers, requests for transfer of medical records, and personal notes from/to patients. In general, miscellaneous would encompass matters not related to direct treatment.

Methods of Arranging Charts. Just as the choice of a filing system is important to the efficient use of files, so too is the arrangement of materials within the charts. Again, the choice of method must be in accordance with how the information needs to be accessed and utilized for each individual office. No one method is correct.

Problem-Oriented Medical Record (POMR). The problem-oriented medical record (POMR) type of record-keeping uses a sheet, generally on the inside cover or other prominent location, which lists vital identification data, immunizations, allergies, medications, and problems. The problems are identified by a number that corresponds to the charting relevant to that problem number; i.e., bronchitis #1; broken wrist #2; and so forth. If the patient returns in nine months with recurring bronchitis, the same number (#1) is used.

The patient chart is then further built by adding a numbered and titled page for each problem the patient experiences; e.g., bronchitis #1; broken wrist #2.

Each problem is then followed with the SOAP approach for all progress notes:

S   Subjective impressions
O   Objective clinical evidence
A   Assessment or diagnosis
P   Plans for further studies, treatment, or management

This process makes the chart easier to review and helps in follow-up of all the patient's medical needs (Figure

```
                    OUTLINE FORMAT PROGRESS NOTES
              Patient Name    Yvette Garcia
  Prob.              S    O    A    P
  No. or
  Letter   DATE  Subjective Objective Assess  Plans                    Page ___4___
    5    9/6/01  Patient complains of two days of severe high epigasitric pain and burning.
                 radiating through the back. Pain accentuated after eating.

                         On examination there is extreme guarding
                         and tenderness, high epigastric region
                         no rebound. Bowel sounds normal. BP 110/70

                              R/O gastric ulcer, pylorospasm

                                   To have upper gastrointestinal series.
                                   Start on Ametidine 300 mg g. i. d.
                                   Eliminate coffee, alcohol & aspirin
                                   Return two days.
```

Figure 14-13 Example of POMR progress notes. (Courtesy of Bibbero Systems, Inc., Petaluma, CA)

14-13). The SOAP approach also allows medical personnel to be aware of the patient's current medications. Starting and resolution dates for each problem also are noted on the tracking sheet.

Internists, family practitioners, and pediatricians use the POMR system more commonly than do specialists because they see their patients for a variety of problems over a long span of time.

Source-Oriented Medical Record (SOMR). The source-oriented medical record (SOMR) groups information according to its source; for example, from laboratories, examinations, physician notes, consulting physicians, and other sources. Many offices use this method as it makes different types of information quickly accessible. A fastener-folder is used that contains several partitions with their own fasteners. This allows for a separate section for lab reports, pathology, progress notes, physical examinations, and correspondence to be filed chronologically within each section. In the SOMR system, many physicians will use the SOAP method to record their chart notes.

Strict Chronological Arrangement. Using this method, data are filed strictly with the most recently charted materials to the top of the folder. For instance, a patient is followed from 1963 to 1986. To locate information recorded in 1973, it would be necessary to flip through the chart until the material for the year 1973 was located. This method makes it difficult for a physician or medical assistant to quickly assess a patient's clinical picture.

Shingling. This method is generally used to file laboratory reports. Many of these reports are smaller than the standard size sheets of paper. Shingling ensures that medical personnel have quick access to the most recent data. In addition, it keeps small pieces of paper from being misplaced or lost within the medical record. Simply put, the sheets of paper are "shingled" either up or across the page, the most recent report placed on top of the previous one (Figure 14-14).

Retention and Purging

As information accumulates, it is necessary to maintain files by the process known as purging. Purging can involve several forms of action.

Record purging. This process requires sorting through records and removing those not in active use. Each facility should establish a standard policy for control and processing of records.

States have different time requirements for retention of various types of records. See Table 14-3 for general guidelines. As a way of controlling risk and practicing responsible risk management, many facilities are choosing to maintain large inactive files rather than destroy records. Some keep them on optical disks or microfiche as discussed later in this chapter. Check with the Medical Practice Act in your state to determine record-keeping requirements.

Active Files. Active files include records that need to be readily accessible for retrieval of information.

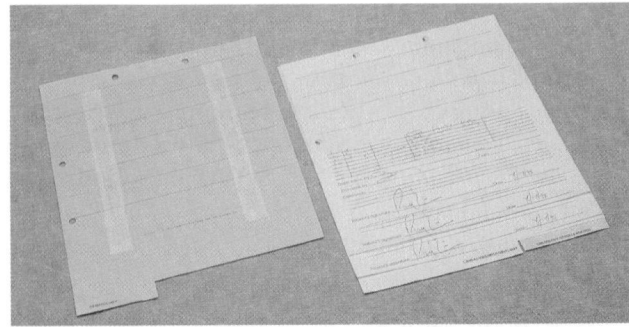

Figure 14-14 Shingled lab reports: (Left) shingling base form with sticky tape for attaching lab forms; (Right) shingled lab forms attached to base.

TABLE 14-3 RECORDS FOR RETENTION

Patient Index Files

These include appointment books or daily appointment sheets. They are kept for an indefinite period of time. They may be required for litigation and/or research.

Case Histories

The length of storage depends on state requirements and individual practice requirements. Product liability cases have deemed long-term storage of these records necessary (20+ years). The records of minors must be retained at least until the age of majority. The statute of limitations is a deciding factor as well.

If records are to be destroyed due to death of physician or closure of a practice, the following procedure is required: Each patient should be notified of the circumstances and given the opportunity to have his or her records forwarded to another physician. After notification, the records must be retained for a "reasonable" period of time (determined by state regulations). A period of three to six months is generally determined to be a "reasonable" period of time. The records must be destroyed by burning or shredding to protect confidentiality.

Personal/Professional Records

Professional licenses should be stored permanently in a secure location.

Office Equipment Records

These records are generally kept until the warranties and/or depreciation are no longer valid. They should be kept in an easily accessible location if under maintenance contract.

Insurance Records

Professional liability policies are kept permanently. Other policies are kept in active files while in force.

Financial Records

Bank records are kept in active files for up to three years and then placed in inactive storage. Tax records must be retained permanently.

Laboratory and X-ray Data

Originals should be retained permanently with the patient's case history.

Inactive Files. Inactive files consist of records that need to be retained for possible retrieval of information. Files not currently being accessed for information would thus become inactive. Often the type of practice will dictate the relevant time period when files are determined to be inactive (generally two to three years).

Closed Files. Closed files are those that are no longer required. Again, patient files are retained for significantly longer periods of time due to litigation and research considerations.

CORRESPONDENCE

Most ambulatory care settings process a considerable amount of correspondence not directly related to patient care. Such items include employment applications, letters from/to pharmaceutical representatives, advertisements for medical supplies, magazine subscription information, and letters to/from other physicians on a variety of subjects. This correspondence is processed using alphabetic filing rules. However, an additional step is necessary to determine whether the correspondence is incoming or outgoing. The correspondence must be filed under some aspect that will be distinctly identifiable; i.e., what idea, subject, name would most likely be thought of if someone wanted to retrieve that correspondence or file additional relevant correspondence.

Incoming Correspondence

This is defined as correspondence received *into* the office from an outside source. This type of correspondence is filed under the most important name—that is, the most likely name were someone to retrieve the correspondence. The key place to look for filing information is the letterhead name or the patient or item referenced in the letter.

Outgoing Correspondence

Correspondence sent *out* of the medical office is considered outgoing correspondence. The key place to inspect here is the inside address or the patient or item referenced in the letter. Again, remember to identify the most probable place to locate the copy of this correspondence should it be needed for future use.

Filing Procedures for Correspondence

Once it is determined whether correspondence is incoming or outgoing, follow the basic rules for filing. In addition:

- Remove paper clips and staple items together.
- Inspect to see if the item is ready to be filed; i.e., any appropriate action has been taken. If not, take care of copies, enclosures, and place note in the tickler file for future action before proceeding with the indexing.
- On incoming correspondence, be sure the letterhead is related to the letter.

Example: A personal letter written by a patient on hotel stationery—index the signature on the letter.

Example: When both the company name and the signature are important, index the company name. A letter from Preston

Industries written by the company president—index Preston Industries, not the president's name, which may change.

Example: If there is no letterhead and you have determined the material is not relevant to a patient, index the name on the signature line. A letter received from Carlton Fiske, RPT, advising your office of services his firm has to offer your patients—index Fiske.

- On outgoing correspondence, look at the inside address and the reference line.

Example: A letter to the District Court regarding Karen Ritter, an employee who is summoned to jury duty—index Karen Ritter rather than District Court.

Example: If the correspondence is relevant to a patient, index the patient's name. A letter RE: Wayne Elder—index under Elder.

Example: If the correspondence is not relevant to a patient, look to the inside address for the indexing information. A letter inquiring about cost estimates for redecorating the office reception room—index the firm in the inside address.

Example: When the inside address is relevant and contains both a company name and a person's name, index the company name. (This avoids the problem of personnel changes.) Cross-referencing would be done under the individual name. A letter to Marvin Fairchild, President of Brandex Pharmaceuticals—index Brandex Pharmaceuticals with a cross-reference for Morgan Fairchild, President, SEE Brandex Pharmaceuticals.

Example: If the letter is personal, the name of the person to whom the letter is written would be used for indexing purposes. Dr. Whitney writes a letter to Dr. Lewis, one of his colleagues, asking if he plans to attend an upcoming conference—index Dr. Lewis.

- On incoming or outgoing correspondence, code the indexing units of the designated label. If the correspondence is being cross-referenced, be sure to note the cross-referencing unit and place the X in a visible place. You may find that the body of the letter contains an important name or subject.

- Create a miscellaneous folder for items that do not have enough in number (office policy will dictate this number, which can be from two to four pieces) to warrant an individual folder. Items in the miscellaneous folder are filed alphabetically first and then identical items are filed with the most recent piece on top. An individual folder is then created when enough pieces accumulate on a particular item.

COMPUTER APPLICATIONS

While the majority of patient charts are still maintained manually, computers are playing an ever-increasing role in the management of records in the ambulatory care setting. Even offices that do not do a great deal of medical records management by computer find the basic database application of great assistance.

Databases

Databases are exceedingly useful in a number of ways. A database is a tool for storing information in a form that allows easy retrieval of information related to a specific topic or element. Maintaining a list of patients with telephone numbers, addresses, family members, and insurance policies is perhaps the simplest use of a database. However, from this can spring a wealth of other information with which the medical office can form other databases; e.g., to retrieve information about patients in a particular locality, patients who are on a particular drug in the event of a drug recall, and general mailing lists for address labels that can be sorted by zip code, state, city, or patient name (Figure 14-15).

Any number of software programs are available to create databases. The steps involved are simple:

1. Design a form by designing the items of interest (called fields) such as patient name, address, date of birth, and sex.
2. Enter the data into each of these fields.
3. Name the database and save the file on the computer for future use.

Simple databases do not require an extensive knowledge of computers to be utilized effectively for routine office applications.

Biomedical, Clinical, and Other Databases. Because technology is changing so rapidly, physicians must stay up to date on medical and health developments.

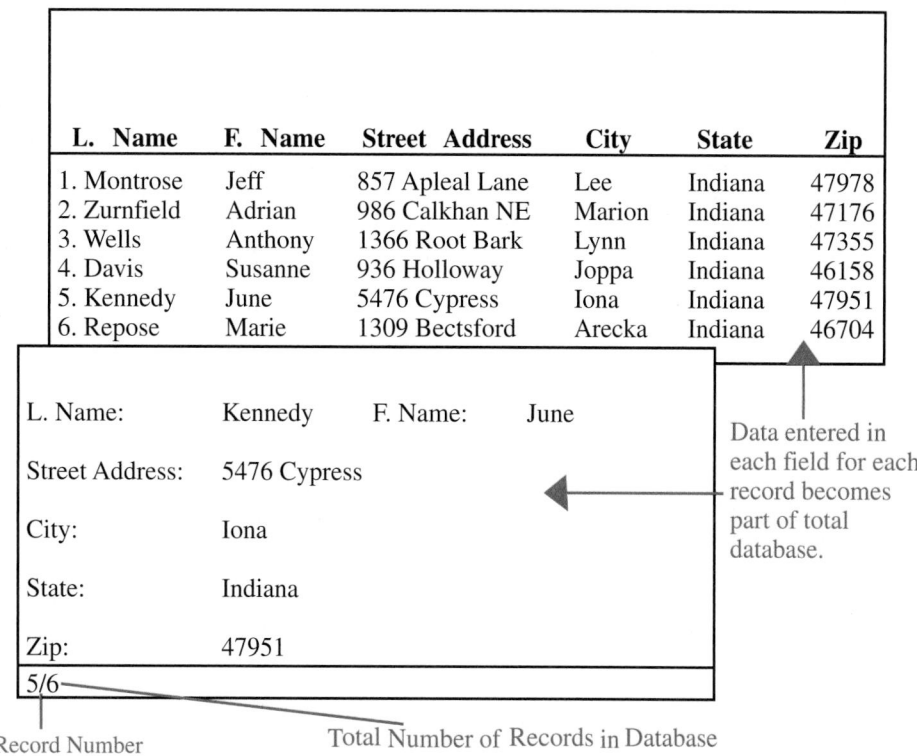

	L. Name	F. Name	Street Address	City	State	Zip
1.	Montrose	Jeff	857 Apleal Lane	Lee	Indiana	47978
2.	Zurnfield	Adrian	986 Calkhan NE	Marion	Indiana	47176
3.	Wells	Anthony	1366 Root Bark	Lynn	Indiana	47355
4.	Davis	Susanne	936 Holloway	Joppa	Indiana	46158
5.	Kennedy	June	5476 Cypress	Iona	Indiana	47951
6.	Repose	Marie	1309 Bectsford	Arecka	Indiana	46704

L. Name: Kennedy   F. Name: June

Street Address: 5476 Cypress

City: Iona

State: Indiana

Zip: 47951

5/6

Record Number   Total Number of Records in Database

Data entered in each field for each record becomes part of total database.

Figure 14-15 Patient information can be entered into a database once and then recalled to update, change, review, or manipulate order as needed.

A biomedical database, essentially a library of health information that can be accessed by a personal computer and modem, allows a physician to search available literature for a topic or combination of topics.

Medical assistants may be assigned the task of researching available databases before the physician subscribes to a particular database service or to search for specific pieces of information the physician requires. If so, look for a database that gives information from around the world. A good biomedical database should index at least 4,000 journals, including foreign journals.

Clinical databases are another aid in researching questions about drugs or chemicals. These databases index drugs and their interactions, poisons and their antidotes, emergency illnesses and their treatments, as well as scores of other clinically related topics. An ambulatory care setting seeking a service of this type should contact the local medical association, the American Medical Association, or a major vendor of medical software for names and addresses of the most widely used clinical database services. Poisindex™, Drugdex™, Emergindex™, and Identidex™ are typical information services. Each is offered by Micromex, Inc., in conjunction with the Rocky Mountain Poison and Drug Center and the University of Colorado.

Hospitals routinely use databases such as Med-Line, Cumulative Index for Nursing and Allied Health

Literature (CINAHL), GENONE (genetic information), and Micromedics. Users access these databases through networks such as Prodigy, CompuServe, Dialog, and Internet.

Nonmedical databases such as Nexus, which might occasionally be used in large medical offices, provide information on just about every imaginable subject, from travel schedules to financial information, art history, and physics.

Electronic databases work in the same way as magazine subscription services. A subscriber selects a particular database service, then pays a monthly fee. In addition, the subscriber pays long-distance telephone charges for the amount of time on-line each month with the database service.

Archival Storage

Most physicians preserve patient medical records for at least the life of their practice. This obviously is a space-consuming prospect, particularly in today's large practices. Computers are helping to solve this dilemma through a process similar to microfiche and microfilm. Records can be copied with a laser beam onto what are called optical disks. This method not only eliminates the bulky storage problems encountered with traditional records but records can be retrieved and viewed almost instantaneously on a computer screen.

Transfer of Data

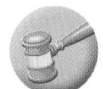 Computers are also streamlining transfer of records from one office or medical facility to another. Faxing is an everyday part of the medical office. Gone are the days when it took a physician's office days to obtain information vital to treating a patient. Within minutes, a patient's entire medical record can be sent via a facsimile from one office to another. Refer to Chapter 12. Offices that are networked can also exchange information via e-mail (electronic mail) or computer modem (see Chapter 12). This requires a software program that allows one computer to communicate with another, sending information via the electronic network or telephone rather than via the post office. Scanners (optical character recognition) are devices that allow information to be converted to an image on the computer screen. For instance, a patient's entire medical record can be "scanned" by running this device over the pages; it is then recreated as a computer file just as it was in paper form.

Confidentiality

Maintaining confidentiality is a major issue in utilizing the computer and on-line devices for storage and transfer of medical information. Key considerations are:

- Maintaining confidentiality with transmission of data. A cover sheet that advises the receiver of the confidential nature of the material, instructions for return to the medical office if received in error, and a telephone number where you (the sender) can be advised of a transmission error are critical.

- Precautions must be taken that the fax or computer receiving the information is in a location where the information will be accessed only by appropriate personnel.

- When using the computer to store and transfer data, consider how many personnel have access to that information. Security measures should be in place to limit access to only those with a legitimate reason for accessing the information. Refer to Chapters 12 and 15 for legal considerations when electronically transmitting patient information.

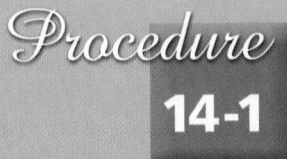

Procedure 14-1   Steps for Manual Filing with a Numeric System

PURPOSE:
To demonstrate an understanding of the principles of the numeric filing system.

EQUIPMENT/SUPPLIES:
Documents to be filed
Dividers with guides
Miscellaneous numeric file section
Alphabetic card file and cards
Accession journal if needed

PROCEDURE STEPS:
1. Inspect and index.
2. Code for filing units. Check the alphabetic card file for each piece to see if the card has already been prepared.
3. Write the number in the upper right-hand corner if the piece has been assigned a number.
4. If no number is assigned (i.e., it has an M for miscellaneous), check the miscellaneous file. If a miscellaneous item is ready to be assigned a number, make a card and note the number in the right-hand corner of the card file, cross out the M, and make a chart file.
5. If there is no card, make up an alphabetic card including a complete name and address, and then write either M or assign a number.
6. Cross-reference if necessary and file the card properly. You are then ready to file the document in the appropriate file folder/chart.
7. File in ascending order.

Procedure 14-2 Steps for Manual Filing with a Subject Filing System

PURPOSE:
To demonstrate an understanding of the principles of the subject filing system.

EQUIPMENT/SUPPLIES:
Documents to be filed by subject
Subject index list or index card file listing subjects
Alphabetic card file and cards

PROCEDURE STEPS:
1. Review the item to find the subject.
2. Match the subject of the item with an appropriate category on the subject index list.
3. If the item contains information that may pertain to more than one subject, decide on the proper cross-reference.
4. If the subject title is written on the material, underline it.
5. If the subject title is not written on the item, write it clearly in the upper right-hand corner and underline (_____) it.
6. Use a wavy (⌇) line for cross-referencing and an X as with alphabetic and numeric filing.
7. Underline the first indexing unit of the coded units.

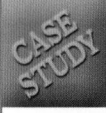

CASE STUDY 14-1

Karen Ritter, administrative medical assistant at Inner City Health Care, has been chiefly responsible for managing this urgent care center's medical records. However, since Karen is only part-time, the office manager feels she needs to delegate some of the responsibility of maintaining all office files to Liz Corbin, a medical assistant who also works part-time. Karen knows the system well and had a hand in designing an effective numeric filing method that both ensures patient confidentiality while meeting the needs of Inner City with its large volume of patients. Now she is trying to orient Liz, who has little experience of the filing system, to the intricacies of medical records management.

CASE STUDY REVIEW

1. What is a good starting point for Liz Corbin's education in medical records management?
2. What are the basic procedures for filing any piece of documentation that Liz needs to learn?
3. Under the direction of the office manager, Inner City is gradually shifting to a computerized system for all operations. Eventually, patient files will be computerized. What can Karen and Liz do to prepare for this eventuality?

SUMMARY

Records management plays an ever-increasing role in the ambulatory care setting today. With the need for thorough and proper documentation, a majority of interaction on the patient's behalf is concerned with proper information processing. It is imperative that medical records be managed efficiently and that the medical assistant possess the skills required for sorting, filing, retrieving, and maintaining information effectively.

A key aspect of managing patient records is selecting a filing system that achieves the goals of information access and storage. Once an alphabetic, numeric, or subject filing system is chosen, patient charts must be assembled and maintained accurately. Technology and computer applications will play a more prominent and varied role in the organization and utilization of files in the medical office.

REVIEW QUESTIONS

Multiple Choice

1. Maintaining order in files by separating active from inactive files is:
   a. indexing
   b. coding
   c. purging
   d. alphabetizing
2. A system used as a reminder of action to be taken on a certain date is called:
   a. accession log
   b. tickler file
   c. release mark
   d. purging system
3. To maintain an accurate filing system, select from the following list the tool used to ensure that records are tracked when borrowed:
   a. release mark
   b. out guide
   c. alphabetic card file
   d. cross-reference file
4. The correct indexing from first to last for assigning units to the name John Porter O'Keefe II would be:
   a. O'Keefe John Porter II
   b. John Porter O'Keefe II
   c. II O'Keefe John Porter
   d. the "II" would be disregarded
5. Of the four systems of filing, the best for every ambulatory care setting is:
   a. the numeric system
   b. the color-coding system
   c. the one that is customized to the needs of the office
   d. the alphabetic system
6. Three main primary types of file cabinets used in medical offices are:
   a. vertical, horizontal, and movable
   b. vertical, open-shelf lateral, and movable file units
   c. vertical, horizontal, and lateral
   d. none of the above
7. Out guides:
   a. are used when the staff is out of the office
   b. are devices to help track charts
   c. may be cardboard or plastic/paper sheets kept in place of a patient's chart
   d. both b and c
8. The first indexing unit for Jayne Carol Warden-Bloomberg is:
   a. Carol
   b. Jayne
   c. Warden
   d. Wardenbloomberg
9. When identical names are being indexed, which system is preferred in medical offices:
   a. index street address next
   b. index using a social security number
   c. index by city
   d. index by state
10. The preferred order for steps in filing medical documentation is:
    a. code, index, sort, inspect, file
    b. inspect, code, index, sort, file
    c. sort, inspect, index, code, file
    d. inspect, index, code, sort, file

Critical Thinking

1. Discuss the importance of maintaining accurate records with regard to the two key issues involving the management of a patient's medical records identified in the text.
2. Discuss briefly two considerations for choosing a filing system for a particular medical office.
3. Briefly outline the differences between the Alpha-Z and the Tab-Alpha color-coding systems.
4. Discuss the significance of the alphabetic card file in a numeric filing system.
5. Provide an example of a subject for subject filing and define five divisions for using this system for a physician working in communicable diseases.
6. Determine the correct filing order for the following pharmaceutical companies from first to last:
   a. Ledsoe-Watson Pharmaceuticals, 789 North Fifth Street, Beckwood, Alabama
   b. Ledsoe-Watson Pharmaceuticals, 345 Ninth Avenue, Little Rock, Arkansas
   c. Ledsoe-Watsen Pharmaceuticals, 893 North Eighth Street, Minneapolis, Minnesota
   d. Ledsoe-Watson Pharmaceuticals, 621 Tenth Street, Shreveport, Louisiana
7. If a chart cannot be located, discuss strategies for locating the missing file.
8. Review the use and capabilities of the computer in regard to medical records management.
9. Properly index and cross-reference (if necessary) your own name. Using the Alpha-Z system, color code your name. Color code your name using the Colorscan Color-Coded Filing System.
10. Research the Statute of Limitations in your state for medical records to determine how long a medical record should be kept. The statute will also tell you what "triggers" activity on a medical file that might dictate it be kept longer than normally indicated.

11. When determining the type of equipment to purchase for storage of medical records, identify a minimum of three indicators to keep in mind.
12. It has been said that filing records is the easiest task the medical assistant will perform; yet it is often the most difficult. What reasons can you give for this statement?

WEB ACTIVITIES

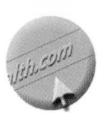

Research the World Wide Web for information that relates to how patient records can be kept confidential in an age of electronic transfer of data. From this information determine what steps you might take to assure patients of their privacy.

REFERENCES/BIBLIOGRAPHY

Fordney, M. T., & Follis, J. J. (1998). *Administrative medical assisting* (4th ed.). Albany, NY: Delmar.

Humphrey, D. D. (1996). *Contemporary medical office procedures* (2nd ed.). Albany, NY: Delmar.

Johnson, J. (1994). *Basic filing procedures for health information management*. Albany, NY: Delmar.

Kalles, N. F., & Johnson, M. M. (1992). *Records management* (5th ed.). Cincinnati: South-Western Publishing Co.

Montone, D. (1998). *Power building in documentation*. Philadelphia, PA: W. B. Saunders Company.

Seare, J. G. (1996). *Medical documentation*. Salt Lake City, UT: Medicode.

WRITTEN COMMUNICATIONS

KEY TERMS

Agenda
Blind Copy
Bond Paper
Clinical E-Mail
Database
E-Mail
Form Letter
Full Block Letter
Keyed
Memorandum (Memo)
Minutes
Modified Block Letter, Indented
Modified Block Letter, Standard
Optical Character Reader (OCR)
Portfolio
Proofread
Simplified Letter
Uniform Resource Locators (URLs)
Watermark
ZIP+4

OUTLINE

Composing Correspondence
    Writing Tips
    Spelling
    Proofreading
Components of a Business Letter
    Date Line
    Inside Address
    Salutation
    Subject Line
    Body of Letter
    Complimentary Closing
    Keyed Signature
    Reference Initials
    Enclosure Notation
    Carbon Copy Notation
    Postscripts
    Continuation Page Heading
Letter Styles
    Full Block
    Modified Block
    Simplified

Supplies for Written
    Communication
    Letterhead
    Second Sheets
    Envelopes
Other Types of Correspondence
    Memoranda
    Meeting Agendas
    Meeting Minutes
Processing Incoming and
    Outgoing Mail
    Incoming Mail and Shipments
    Outgoing Mail and Shipments
    Postal Classes
    Formats for Efficient Processing
    International Mail
Technologies
    Facsimile (Fax)
    Electronic Mail (E-mail)
Legal and Ethical Issues

OBJECTIVES

The student should strive to meet the following performance objectives and demonstrate an understanding of the facts and principles presented in this chapter through written and oral communication.

1. Define the key terms as presented in the glossary.
2. Describe the impact of written communication in the ambulatory care setting.
3. Identify the role of the medical assistant in producing written communications.
4. List the four major letter styles. *(continues)*

5. Compose and key letters using appropriate components of a business letter.

6. Identify various types of form letters that may be written by the medical assistant.

7. Proofread a letter for grammar, spelling, and content.

8. Use proper proofreading marks to correct a document.

9. Describe the various classifications of mail and determine when each class should be used.

10. Address envelopes to satisfy postal regulations.

11. Describe the use of new communication technology in the ambulatory care setting and discuss appropriate confidentiality issues.

ROLE DELINEATION COMPONENTS

ADMINISTRATIVE
Administrative Procedures
- **Perform basic clerical functions**
- **Understand and adhere to managed care policies and procedures**

GENERAL (TRANSDISCIPLINARY)
Communication Skills
- **Adapt communications to individual's ability to understand**
- **Use effective and correct verbal and written communications**
- **Recognize and respond to verbal and nonverbal communications**
- **Use medical terminology appropriately**
- **Receive, organize, prioritize, and transmit information**
- **Promote the practice through positive public relations**

Legal Concepts
- **Maintain confidentiality**
- **Use appropriate guidelines when releasing information**

(continues)

SCENARIO

When they are produced with care, written communications can be a time-consuming part of the administrative medical assistant's day. This is why Marilyn Johnson, CMA, the office manager at Doctors Lewis & King, has compiled a style manual for the two-physician practice. Marilyn is clearly aware that professional looking and sounding letters send a message to all recipients. Yet, she wants to make correspondence writing and producing as efficient as possible, and her style manual provides an easy-to-use resource for anyone in the office responsible for composing or sending written documents.

In her style manual, Marilyn has included examples of the "house" letter format, which is a block style; a list of commonly used medical terms for easy spelling reference; answers to common questions staff have in regard to word usage; proofreader's marks; proper addressing procedures for envelopes and packages, depending on whether they are being sent by United States mail or by an alternative delivery method; and a quick list of the best ways to send various types of correspondence. Marilyn has also included a list of "Do Nots" in order to help her staff avoid mistakes in their written communications.

INTRODUCTION

One of the key responsibilities of the administrative medical assistant is written communication. All written material produced by the ambulatory care setting is critical, for it reflects positively or negatively on the professionalism of the office. Letters to patients, to referring physicians, to other health care organizations, and even interoffice correspondence should be thoughtfully composed, carefully produced according to the style selected by the office manager, and mailed and delivered in a way that is both time- and cost-efficient.

Written correspondence is important in conveying a professional image of the ambulatory care setting and impacts public relations either positively or negatively. It must also be remembered that written documents provide a permanent or legal record in the event of any litigation and thus must be carefully and accurately worded.

ROLE DELINEATION COMPONENTS (*continued*)

● Participate in the development and maintenance of personnel, policy, and procedure manuals

Operational Functions

● Evaluate and recommend equipment and supplies

● Apply computer techniques to support office operations

In most ambulatory care settings, medical assistants will be responsible for creating many forms of written communications. Examples of these forms of communications include:

● Various types of letters, such as letters to order supplies and equipment, letters replying to various types of inquiries, collection letters, promotional letters

● Memoranda or interoffice communications

● Referrals, consultation, and surgical report letters

● E-mail and fax correspondence

● Written instructions for patients

● Meeting agendas and minutes

● Travel itineraries

● Promotional brochures

COMPOSING CORRESPONDENCE

The medical assistant must always remember that the quality of the correspondence reflects the standards of the medical office. It is important to also remember that there is a difference between social correspondence and business correspondence. Social correspondence tends to be lengthy and personal in nature while business correspondence should be clear, concise, courteous, and accurate. It is best to keep business letters to one page in length whenever possible.

Writing Tips

Rosemary Fruehling, a writer and lecturer, states, "Business writing is good when it achieves the purpose the author intended." Practice and careful attention to detail are required to write effective business letters. Writing tips for consideration include:

● Follow the style and format determined by your physician/employer. Physicians often prefer a professional, formal style of letter composition.

● Think about key points to be addressed in the letter and organize them before beginning composition. The first paragraph should state the reason for writing and focus the reader's attention.

● Establish a tone of voice. Be personable and cordial in tone while remaining professional.

● Use only language that the reader will understand.

● Most sentences should be short and contain only one idea or thought.

Spelling

It is important that all correspondence contains no misspelled or incorrectly used words. When in doubt always look the word up in a dictionary (Table 15-1). When checking spelling in a dictionary, develop the habit of reading the definition as well. This will help you imprint the correct spelling and meaning of the word.

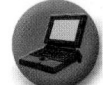 Be careful about relying on the spell check function of your computer; many medical words are not formatted into the computer. The computer also does not recognize if you have used the wrong word, only that the word is spelled incorrectly. For example the words *to*, *too*, and *two* may all be spelled correctly but may be misused within the sentence structure.

TABLE 15-1	FREQUENTLY MISSPELLED WORDS
abscess	ischemia
aneurysm	larynx
arrhythmia	malaise
calcaneus	ophthalmology
cirrhosis	palliative
clavicle	parenteral
curettage	pharynx
hemorrhage	pneumonia
hemorrhoids	psychiatrist
homeostasis	pyrexia
humerus	rheumatic
ischium	roentgenology
ilium	sphygmomanometer
ileum	staphylococcus

TABLE 15-2   FREQUENTLY MISUSED WORDS

advice	advise	
affect	effect	
capital	capitol	
coarse	course	
coma	comma	
command	commend	
complement	compliment	
comprehensible	comprehensive	
council	counsel	
conscience	conscious	
deposition	disposition	
device	devise	
elicit	illicit	
eligible	illegible	
elude	allude	
ensure	insure	assure
explicit	implicit	
farther	further	
heal	heel	
hear	here	
hole	whole	
knew	new	
know	no	
lean	lien	
patience	patient	
personal	personnel	
plain	plane	
precede	proceed	
principal	principle	
right	write	
stationary	stationery	
taught	taut	
their	there	they are
to	too	two
vain	vein	
weak	week	
weather	whether	
you	your	you are

It may be helpful to develop a list of frequently misused words in an alphabetized notebook, card index, or in a special file on your computer (Table 15-2). Several computer word processing software packages contain English/medical spell check features. A new word that is not currently identified in the spell check or medical check package may be added to the program.

SPOTLIGHT ON AAMA ESSENTIALS THROUGH CAAHEP

- A well-written, clear, and concise communication, free from errors, personifies a positive and professional attitude.

- High standards of professionalism and good judgment must always be maintained when dealing with patients and their medical histories.

- It is important to remember that a non-threatening tone of correspondence is more apt to promote the profession than one that is harsh and negative in nature.

Proofreading

Prior to presenting any correspondence to the physician for signature or mailing, the document should be **proofread**. Proofreading is the process of reading the document and checking for accuracy. Accuracy involves checking to be sure that the correct grammar, spelling, punctuation, and capitalization have been used and that the message is clear and concise and presented in a logical organization.

Proofreading marks most commonly used are shown in Figure 15-1. Standard proofreading marks used to indicate corrections hasten the editing process. Some proofreading tips that may be useful include:

- Proofread each document twice; once on the screen checking for obvious errors and then as a hardcopy to be sure everything is accurate and makes sense.

- Prepare the document, set it aside, and proofread a third time later. Inaccuracies or errors may "jump" out after a period of time.

- Do not proofread when tired.

- If the document is long, proofread in several short intervals.

- Read a long document to another person and have him or her check sentence structure and content accuracy.

- Use a card or ruler as a guide to maintain your place within the document.

- Use a piece of colored clear plastic over the document to rest your eyes. This is especially helpful when proofing a long document.

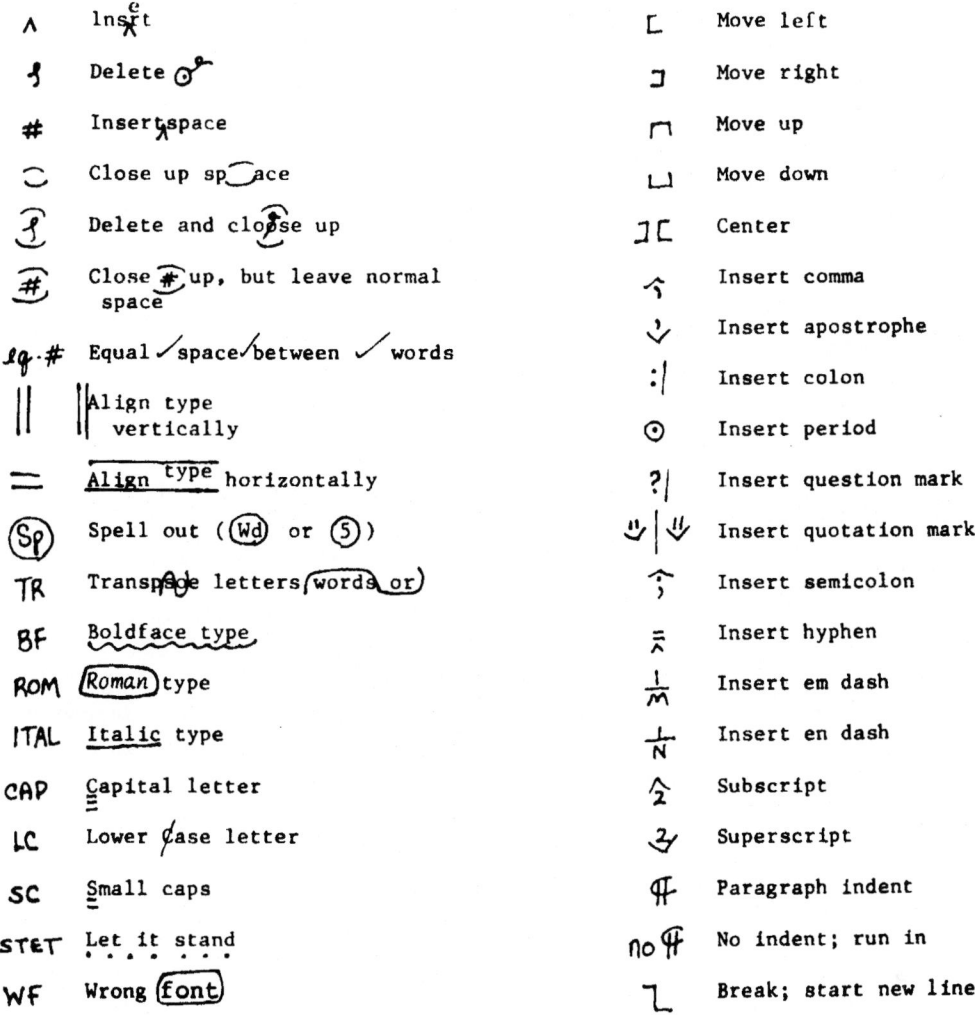

Figure 15-1 Common proofreader's marks.

COMPONENTS OF A BUSINESS LETTER

The following sections of this chapter describe the components of most business letters. (See Procedure 15-1, Preparing and Composing Business Correspondence Using All Components.)

Date Line

The date is usually **keyed** on line 15 or two to three lines below the letterhead. Keying is when data is input by keystrokes on a computer. The date should be completely written out as January 15, 20__ rather than 1/15/20__. (If military style is used, the format would be 01 JAN __.)

Inside Address

The inside address is keyed flush with the left margin. This address may be two, three, or four lines. Some rural areas only require two lines. If the letter is addressed to a physician, the credentials appear after the name. Do not type Dr. John Jones, MD. (Both Dr. and MD are titles; use one or the other.)

Salutation

The salutation is keyed flush with the left margin on the second line below the inside address. A colon follows the salutation. The formal salutation should refer to the receiver of the letter using title and last name; e.g., "Dear Mr. Marshal:". If the receiver and sender know each other well, the receiver's first name may be used, e.g., "Dear Jim:".

Subject Line

If used, the subject line is keyed on the second line below the salutation starting at the left margin. This may begin flush with the left margin, indented five spaces, or centered.

The patient's name or subject (meeting and/or topic) may be used on the subject line.

Body of Letter

The body of the letter should begin on the second line below the salutation unless a subject line is used that precedes two lines above the body. The body format will depend upon the style of letter used. Paragraphs will begin flush with the left margin in full block letter style, or they may be indented five spaces when using the modified block letter style.

Complimentary Closing

The complimentary closure begins on the second line below the body of the letter. The closure depends upon the formality of the letter. Only the first letter of the first word of the complimentary closure is upper case.

The style used in the complimentary closure should correspond with the salutation.

Letter Style	Complimentary Closing
Formal	Respectfully yours or Respectfully
General	Very truly yours or Truly yours or Sincerely or Sincerely yours
Informal (Used when reader and writer are on first name basis.)	Regards or Best wishes

Keyed Signature

A keyed signature is a professional courtesy to the reader. Often a letter is received in which the signature of the sender is not legible. The keyed signature should be at least four lines below the complimentary closing. This space may be lengthened to six lines if you are keying a short letter.

Reference Initials

The keyed signature may be the only initials used if the same person composed and signed the letter. If reference initials are used, the name of the individual composing the letter should be in uppercase letters with the medical assistant's initials keyed in lowercase letters.

Example.
WL:jg or WL/jg

Enclosure Notation

The enclosure indication can be either one or two lines below the keyed reference initials.

The number of enclosures may be indicated by several methods:

- Enclosures
- Enc.
- 1 Enc.
- 2 Enclosures
- Enclosures (2)

Some enclosures should be identified specifically, i.e., check for $84.

Enclosures also may be sent under separate cover. If this method is used, state that the enclosure is under separate cover. It may be written as Enclosure under separate cover: Sarah Jones's medical record.

Carbon Copy Notation

If copies of the letter are to be sent to other parties, the copy notation "cc" should be one or two lines below the reference initials. Although the practice of making a carbon copy is obsolete, the abbreviation of "cc" is still acceptable. The notation "cc" or "pc" (photocopy) should be followed by the name of the person receiving the copy. When more than one person is to receive a copy of the original letter, key cc: by the first name. Align the other names under the first person identified alphabetically or by rank.

Example.

cc:	John Smith, MD
	Joseph Brown, MD

A blind copy notation "bcc:" may be used to send copies of the letter to individuals without the recipient's knowledge. This message is only keyed on the copy of the individual receiving the blind copy. The use of blind carbon copies has decreased and in some practices is no longer used.

Postscripts

Postscripts (abbreviated as P.S.) may be used to:

1. Express an afterthought
2. Identify a thought that has been intentionally deleted from the body of the letter
3. Make a strong significant point

Postscripts are keyed two spaces below reference initials and enclosures.

Continuation Page Heading

There are two methods used to begin the continuation page heading. There should be at least one inch space at the top of each continuing page of the letter. Plain paper matching the color, weight, size, and quality of the letterhead should be used. The following are examples of appropriate continuation page headings.

Example.

(one inch from top of page)
Jeremy Brown, MD   -2-   May 4, 20__
or
Jeremy Brown, MD
Page 2
May 4, 20__

See Table 15-3 and Figure 15-2 for guidelines in letter placement.

LETTER STYLES

The administrative medical assistant may be responsible for creating a variety of letters that support the needs of the ambulatory care facility. One efficient approach to letter composition is to create a **portfolio** or **database** of frequently used **form letters**. Individualize letters by using the current date and the receiver's name and mailing address. When a form letter is carefully composed and produced, it may not be perceived as a form letter by the recipient.

With the physician/employer's permission, the medical assistant may sign certain letters, including most form letters. Form letters that may be written by the medical assistant include:

- Letters to thank referring physicians
- Letters emphasizing to patients criteria for care as directed by the physician
- Letters announcing new insurance or HMOs accepted

- Letters to order supplies or subscriptions
- Letters acknowledging speaking engagements
- Letters to announce vacation schedules or other office closures
- Letters to announce new staff
- Letters to remind patients of payment due or notification of collection procedures

Letters prepared for the physician's signature should be placed with an addressed envelope on the physician's desk for review and signature. Place the envelope flap over the letter and attach with a paper clip. Also include with the letter any enclosures for the physician's approval.

Four major styles of letters are utilized by medical and professional offices. These are:

1. Full block
2. Modified block, standard
3. Modified block, indented
4. Simplified

Full Block

The **full block letter** is most time-efficient for the ambulatory care setting because the medical assistant does not have to use excessive motion to tab indentions or to place

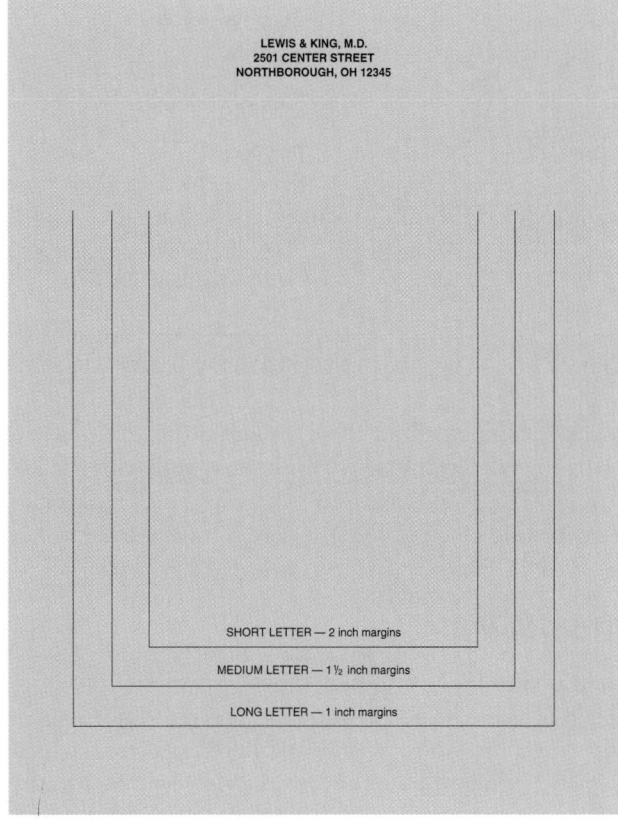

Figure 15-2   Spacing of letter.

TABLE 15-3   GUIDELINES IN LETTER PLACEMENT
The following guidelines are helpful in preventing errors in placement.
1. An imaginary picture frame should surround the letter. Margins may be one inch, one and one-half inch, or two inches (Figure 15-2).
2. The last line of the letter should end no less than one inch from the bottom of the page.
3. Do not divide the last word on a page.
4. A minimum of three lines should be keyed on the second page of a letter. When dividing a paragraph at the bottom of a page, keep a minimum of two lines on the bottom of the page and two lines at the top of the next page.
5. If using a computer to prepare letters, it is easy to make adjustments in order to create a professional letter.
6. Single-space within paragraphs.
7. Double-space between paragraphs.

LEWIS & KING, MD
2501 CENTER STREET
NORTHBOROUGH, OH 12345

NORTHBOROUGH
FAMILY MEDICAL GROUP

Date Line

January 12, 20__   (approximately 15th line)

Inside Address

Jeremy Brown, MD   (approximately 20th line)
111 S Main
Blossom, UT 10283-1120
    (double-space)

Salutation

Dear Dr. Brown:
    (double-space)

Subject Line

Blossom Medical Society Meeting
    (double-space)

Thank you for inviting me to speak at the Blossom Medical Society Meeting June 15, 20__. As requested, my topic will describe the use of the MRI in assisting physicians to make a more accurate diagnosis without resorting to invasive procedures. The exact title of my speech will be sent by next Friday.
    (double-space)

Please have your office manager send information regarding the number of participants expected, time of meeting, location, and any other details that will assist me in preparing my speech.

I will write or call if I have any additional questions.
    (double-space)

Complimentary Closing

Yours truly,

Winston Lewis, MD   (4–5 line spaces)

Keyed Signature

Winston Lewis, MD
    (double-space)

Reference Initials

WL:jg
    (double-space)

Enclosure Notation

Enclosure: Handout on MRI

Figure 15-3   Sample full block style letter; all elements start at the left margin.

address, complimentary close, or keyed signature. When using the full block style, all lines begin flush with the left margin. This style is suggested when desiring a contemporary-looking efficient letter. Figure 15-3 illustrates a full block style letter.

Modified Block

In the **standard modified block** style letter, all lines begin at the left margin with the exception of the date line, complimentary closure, and keyed signature, which usually begin at the center position or a few spaces to the right of center. Figure 15-4 illustrates a modified block style letter without indention.

The assistant may choose to use the **indented modified block** style letter. In this format, paragraphs may be indented five spaces. Figure 15-5 illustrates a modified block style letter with indented paragraphs.

Simplified

The **simplified letter** style omits the salutation and complimentary closure. All lines are **keyed** (input by keystroke) flush with the left margin. The subject line is keyed in capitals three lines below the inside address. The body of the letter begins three lines below the subject line. The signature line is keyed in all capital letters four lines below the body of the letter. The Administrative Manage-

LEWIS & KING, MD
2501 CENTER STREET
NORTHBOROUGH, OH 12345

L&K

NORTHBOROUGH
FAMILY MEDICAL GROUP

January 12, 20___ (approximately 15th line)

(approximately 20th line)

Jeremy Brown, MD
111 S Main
Blossom, UT 10283-1120

Dear Dr. Brown:

Blossom Medical Society Meeting

Thank you for inviting me to speak at the Blossom Medical Society Meeting June 15, 20___. As requested, my topic will describe the use of the MRI in assisting physicians to make a more accurate diagnosis without resorting to invasive procedures. The exact title of my speech will be sent by next Friday.

Please have your office manager send information regarding the number of participants expected, time of meeting, location, and any other details that will assist me in preparing my speech.

I will write or call if I have any additional questions.

Yours truly,

Winston Lewis, MD

Winston Lewis, MD

WL:jg

Enclosure: Handout on MRI

Figure 15-4 Sample standard modified block style letter; all elements start at left margin except date, complimentary closing, and keyed signature.

LEWIS & KING, MD
2501 CENTER STREET
NORTHBOROUGH, OH 12345

L&K

NORTHBOROUGH
FAMILY MEDICAL GROUP

January 12, 20___ (approximately 15th line)

Jeremy Brown, MD (approximately 20th line)
111 S Main
Blossom, UT 10283-1120

Dear Dr. Brown:

Blossom Medical Society Meeting

Thank you for inviting me to speak at the Blossom Medical Society Meeting June 15, 20___. As requested, my topic will describe the use of the MRI in assisting physicians to make a more accurate diagnosis without resorting to invasive procedures. The exact title of my speech will be sent by next Friday.

Please have your office manager send information regarding the number of participants expected, time of meeting, location, and any other details that will assist me in preparing my speech.

I will write or call if I have any additional questions.

Yours truly,

Winston Lewis, MD

Winston Lewis, MD

WL:jg

Enclosure: Handout on MRI

Figure 15-5 Sample modified block style letter with indented paragraphs; this format is the same as the standard modified except that the subject line and paragraphs are also indented.

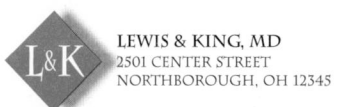

January 12, 20___   (approximately 15th line)

Jeremy Brown, MD   (approximately 20th line)
111 S Main
Blossom, UT 10283-1120

(triple-space)

BLOSSOM MEDICAL SOCIETY MEETING

(triple-space)

Thank you for inviting me to speak at the Blossom Medical Society
Meeting June 15, 20___. As requested, my topic will describe the use of
the MRI in assisting physicians to make a more accurate diagnosis
without resorting to invasive procedures. The exact title of my speech
will be sent by next Friday.

Please have your office manager send information regarding the number of participants expected, time of meeting, location, and any other
details that will assist me in preparing my speech.

I will write or call if I have any additional questions.

Winston Lewis, MD   (4 line spaces)

WINSTON LEWIS, MD

WL:jg

Enclosure: Handout on MRI

Figure 15-6   The simplified style letter has no salutation or complimentary closing. The subject line and keyed signature are all upper case.

ment Society recommends this style of letter. However, in medical offices this style is most often employed when sending a form letter. Figure 15-6 illustrates a simplified style letter.

SUPPLIES FOR WRITTEN COMMUNICATION

The paper should be **bond**, of good quality, and at least 20–24 pound stock with a watermark. A **watermark** is legible when paper is held to the light. Choose a shade of white, cream, or grey.

Although colored paper may be more eye-catching, it does not display a professional image. Also be sure that the paper stock is compatible with printers used in the ambulatory care center.

Letterhead

The letterhead style and design is usually chosen by the physician(s) and may include a specially designed logo for the practice. The physician/practice name, street address and/or post office box number, city, state and zip code, and telephone number with area code are usually printed on the letterhead. Many offices also add their fax number and e-mail address. Letterhead information may be placed at either side or in the center of the paper.

Second Sheets

When an order is placed for letterhead, the medical assistant should order additional plain paper of the same stock as the letterhead to be used for second page sheets. The number of sheets will vary from office to office. If physicians normally dictate long letters, this must be taken into consideration when ordering quantities.

Envelopes

The stock and quality of the envelopes should match the stationery used in the office. With the use of **ZIP+4** and City State Files, mail is processed more efficiently and effectively. The address should be standardized so it contains all delivery address elements. The correct name, city, state and ZIP+4 codes must be used.

Example:

JEREMY BROWN MD
1111 S MAIN
BLOSSOM UT 10283-1120

If Dr. Brown uses a post office box for the delivery of his mail, that address should be used. The postal service delivers to the last line before the city, state, and zip code.

Example:

JEREMY BROWN MD
PO BOX 1453
BLOSSOM UT 10283-1120

Place the intended delivery address on the line immediately above the city, state, and ZIP+4 code. The other address may be placed on a separate line above the delivery line.

Example:

JEREMY BROWN MD
1111 S MAIN
PO BOX 1453
BLOSSOM UT 10283-1120

This letter would be received at the post office box, not the street address.

General Standards for Addressing Envelopes.
For successful processing by **optical character readers (OCRs)**, the United States Postal Services suggests that the address on letter mail needs to be machine-printed, with a uniform left margin. It should be formatted in a manner that allows an OCR to recognize the information and find a match in its address files.

Optical character readers are used by the post office to scan an address. This scanner reads the zip code on the bottom line and prints a bar code in the lower right corner of the envelope.

Envelopes that are handwritten cannot be read by the OCR. Envelopes with handwritten addresses are "spit-out" by the automatic mail sorter. These letters must wait for more costly and slower manual sorting.

New encoding facilities have been established at various sites in the United States. A picture of the handwritten address is taken by a high-speed camera. This picture is transmitted by telephone line to the encoding center. The operators translate the handwritten address into an electric bar code. This code is printed on the envelope, which allows for automatic sorting.

The United States Postal Service publishes several pamphlets and booklets that describe the format to be used when sending any mail. Check with the postal service regarding the latest publications. Service and deliverability will be improved if these standards are used.

To conform to standards, eliminate all punctuation in the envelope address with the exception of a hyphen in the ZIP+4 code. Leave a minimum of one space between the city name and two character state abbreviations and the ZIP+4 code. The OCR can read a combination of uppercase and lowercase characters in addresses but prefers all uppercase characters. See Procedure 15-2.

Dark ink on a light background using uppercase letters is the suggested method in preparing a keyed address. There should be a uniform left margin on all lines of the address. An imaginary rectangle which extends $\frac{5}{8}$ inch to $2\frac{3}{4}$ inches from the bottom of the envelope with one inch on each side should contain the address. The lower right edge should be kept free of any marks. This area will contain the bar code whether it is preapplied or printed by an OCR. The bar code area is $\frac{5}{8}$ inch from the bottom and $4\frac{1}{2}$ inches from the right side of the envelope.

Types of Envelopes.
Number 6¾ and number 10 are the envelopes most often used. A window envelope may also be used, especially when mailing statements.

Number	Size
6¾	6½″ long × 3⅝″ wide
10	9½″ long × 4⅛″ wide
7	7½″ long × 3⅞″ wide

The address on the statement need only be keyed once. The entire address is capitalized with no punctuation. Only one space should be used between the state abbreviation and the zip code. When this statement is folded with the address in view, it may be inserted into a window envelope. Make certain that the entire address is visible through the window. To prepare envelopes for mailing, lay all envelopes facing upward in a row with the flaps displayed. Moisten all the envelopes with a sponge. With the dominant hand, seal the flap and with the non-dominant hand, push the envelope aside while the next flap is closed. This method will speed the process. Procedure 15-3 illustrates letter folding and placement of envelopes for moistening prior to closure.

OTHER TYPES OF CORRESPONDENCE

Other specialized types of correspondence the medical assistant may be involved in preparing include memoranda, meeting agendas and meeting minutes, and travel itineraries.

Memoranda

A type of interoffice correspondence is the **memorandum** or **memo** for short. The use of memos permits messages to be sent quickly and without labor intensive preparation. The memo format may already be preformatted on your computer software. If not, it is easy to design your own memo format.

The side margins should be set for 1 inch. Begin to key the memo heading 2 inches from the top of the page (line 13). The heading includes the words *date, to, from,* and *subject,* which should be emboldened and capitalized. The words should each be keyed on a separate line with a double space between each word. By setting a tab stop 10 spaces in from the left margin, you will be able to tab to each entry and clear the headings to add the appropriate information. Triple space after the entry for the subject heading.

The body of the memo may begin at the left margin or may be set 10 spaces in so that the text starts directly beneath the typed headings. No salutation is required in a memo. Figure 15-7 provides a sample memo.

Meeting Agendas

Most meetings operate by following *Robert's Rules of Order, Newly Revised,* as their parliamentary authority. The outlined order of business is as follows:

- Reading and approval of the minutes
- Reports of officers, boards, and standing committees
- Reports of special committees (ad hoc)
- Special orders
- Unfinished business and general orders
- New business
- Date and time of next scheduled meeting

The **agenda** lists the specific items that the group plans to discuss at the meeting under each of the above-mentioned divisions. The medical assistant preparing the agenda must determine the topics that are to be discussed. Copies of the agenda should be sent to each group member before the meeting date and extra copies should be taken to the meeting for those who may have misplaced or forgotten to bring the agenda with them to the meeting. Figure 15-8 provides a sample meeting agenda.

DATE: August 25, 2001 (key heading 2 inches from top of page, line 13)

TO: Staff of Doctors Lewis & King (embolden and capitalize headings and double space between them)

FROM: Walter Seals, Office Manager

SUBJECT: Vacation Schedule (triple space after the subject)

Doctors Lewis & King will be on vacation January 1–15. Please do not schedule appointments during that time for either doctor. Office personnel should report to work as usual. During this two-week period, we will be preparing for the annual audit.

Figure 15-7   Sample memorandum.

AGENDA
STAFF MEETING
Tuesday, September 1, 2001
Location–Conference Room

Reading and approval of last months' minutes
Reports
     Risk Management Committee
     Personnel
Unfinished business
     Purchase of new X-ray machine
New business
     Doctors Lewis & King vacation January 1–15
     Annual Audit
Date and time for next meeting
Adjournment

Figure 15-8   Sample meeting agenda.

Meeting Minutes

A written record of what transpired during a meeting is called the **minutes**. The minutes should record what business actions were taken during the meeting, who made each motion and what it was, who seconded the motion, any pertinent discussion, and whether the motion was passed or not.

The first paragraph of the minutes should contain the following information:

- Kind of meeting (regular, special, emergency)
- Name of the group or association
- Date, time, and place of the meeting
- Who officiated at the meeting and names of members present and absent
- If the previous meeting minutes were read and approved

The body of the minutes should include a paragraph discussing each subject matter or each item listed on the agenda. All motions should be recorded including the exact wording of the motion, the name of the person making the motion, the person seconding the motion, and if the motion passed or failed. If the meeting had a guest speaker, the speaker's name and title and the subject of the presentation may be included in the minutes.

The last paragraph should contain the next meeting date, time, and place, and the time of adjournment for this meeting. The person recording the minutes should sign them, and a copy of all minutes should be maintained in a notebook designated for that purpose. Corporations are required to have regular meetings with recorded minutes for legal purposes. Figure 15-9 provides a sample of recorded minutes.

STAFF MEETING MINUTES

The monthly staff meeting of Doctors Lewis & King was held Tuesday, September 1, 2001, in the conference room. The meeting was called to order by Walter Seals, Office Manager. Those members present included: Dr. Lewis, Dr. King, Marilyn Johnson, Ellen Armstrong, Jane O'Hara, Wanda Slawson, and Bruce Goldman.

The previous meeting's minutes were read and approved as published.

Marilyn Johnson, CMA heading the Risk Management Committee reported that a thorough walk through of the clinic had taken place to assess for safety issues. It was determined that the pull cords on the blinds could pose a potential hazard to small children. Marilyn made a motion that the blinds be upgraded with new vinyl louvered blinds with the plastic rod-type louver adjuster. Wanda Slawson seconded the motion. After discussion, a unanimous vote was cast to replace the blinds at the earliest time possible.

Walter Seals, Human Resource Manager, announced that he would be posting an opening for a CMA to work in the lab. All staff personnel were asked to share information about this opening with professionals who might be interested in working with Doctors Lewis & King.

Discussion was presented by Doctors Lewis & King regarding the purchase of a new X-ray machine. A committee consisting of Wanda Slawson, Bruce Goldman, and Marilyn Johnson was appointed to investigate the specific needs of the clinic and to locate appropriate vendors. They will present their findings at the next scheduled staff meeting.

New Business items include the fact that Doctors Lewis & King will be on vacation January 1–15, 2002. We are asked to not schedule appointments during that time.

Walter Seals discussed preparations for the annual audit during the vacation period of Doctors Lewis & King. He will provide a schedule and timeline at the next staff meeting.

The next scheduled meeting will be October 3 at 12:30 p.m. in the conference room.

The meeting adjourned at 1:45 p.m.

Ellen Armstrong

Figure 15-9   Sample meeting minutes.

PROCESSING INCOMING AND OUTGOING MAIL

The management of written communications also involves developing procedures for sorting, distributing, and otherwise processing incoming mail. It also includes posting and shipping outgoing items by the most cost- and time-effective method.

Incoming Mail and Shipments

All mail should be sorted by type prior to opening. Incoming mail includes telegrams, faxes, certified or registered letters, personal letters, e-mail, checks from patients, insurance forms, invoices, medical journals, newspapers, magazines for the reception area, and advertisements regarding equipment and supplies.

Once it is categorized, incoming mail is directed to the appropriate personnel in the office. Checks from patients and invoices may be distributed to the bookkeeper, insurance forms to the insurance clerk, medical journals and advertisements can be placed on the physician's desk, and magazines and newspapers can be placed in the reception area. Personal or confidential letters should not be opened unless the medical assistant has been given this responsibility by the physician or office manager.

Use a letter opener to open all mail before taking out the contents and reading the document. After removing the contents:

- Stamp the date it was received in the office.

- If the address is not included on the letter, write the address on the letter, as identified on the envelope or on the bank check (if patient is making a payment).

- When a colored reply envelope is sent with the statement to the patient, payments returned in these envelopes can speed the sorting process.

- Look into the envelope to make certain that all contents have been removed.

- Attach the letter to the envelope with a paper clip, preferably on the left side.

Reply promptly to all requests, answering letters according to date of arrival; emergency situations need to be managed immediately.

Outgoing Mail and Shipments

Before placing postage on outgoing mail, weigh the item to be mailed, using a manual or electronic scale. A manual scale will read ounces. The assistant will then affix the appropriate postage, either stamps or postal meter. An electronic scale will automatically display the correct postage. If your office has a postal meter, this should be used to expedite mail. Metered mail does not have to be canceled or postmarked at the post office.

A postage meter is leased or purchased from a manufacturing company recommended by the postal service. However, the postage meter must be taken to the post office to purchase postage. The meter is locked for the amount of postage purchased. Ambulatory care centers that send a large volume of mail may purchase a postage meter.

See Procedure 15-4 for preparing outgoing mail.

Postal Classes

Check with the local post office to determine anticipated delivery turnaround to specific destinations. Common postal classes include:

1. *First-class mail.* Correspondence and statements are usually sent first class. All single-piece letters weighing less than 11 ounces are included in first-class mail. A postal card may be sent via this method if the card is not larger than 4¼ inches by 6 inches. The card may not be smaller than 3½ inches by 5 inches. If the recipient has moved, first-class mail may be forwarded at no additional cost.

2. *Priority mail.* Mail weighing more than 11 ounces and up to 70 pounds may be sent via priority mail. Check your postal service for current cost. The fee is based on weight and destination. Use the free priority mail stickers available from your local post office.

3. *Second-class mail.* Only newspapers and periodicals that have been authorized second-class privileges are sent by this manner.

4. *Third-class mail (bulk mail).* Circulars, books, catalogs, and other printed material and merchandise weighing less than 16 ounces can be sent via this method. Regular and special bulk rates are available only to authorized mailers. A minimum of 200 pieces of mail is required to utilize the bulk rate, and an annual fee must be paid to send via this classification. All mail must be sent from one post office.

5. *Fourth-class mail (parcel post).* Fourth-class mail must weigh more than 16 ounces (1 pound) and not more than 70 pounds.

6. *Certified mail.* This service provides proof that a letter has been received. For example, if a physician dismisses a patient from the practice due to noncompliance of orders, a letter should be sent by certified mail, return receipt requested. When the receipt of acceptance of the letter is returned to the office, make certain that this receipt is filed in the patient's medical record. This provides legal protection for the physician. Other examples of mail that should be certified include birth certificates, marriage licenses, and deeds to property.

7. *Registered mail.* When an item has an intrinsic (real) value it should be sent via registered mail. Receipts are provided to identify the individual who accepted this mail. The sender declares a value on the item. A signature is required prior to delivery being made. Examples of items that should be sent by registered mail include clothing and jewelry.

8. *Express mail.* This service is available seven days per week for mailing items up to 70 pounds and 108 inches in combined length and girth. Express mail may be sent for noon delivery on the next day between major business markets.

Formats for Efficient Processing

Certified, registered, and special delivery markings should be placed below the stamp or approximately nine lines from the right top edge of the envelope. "Personal" or "confidential" notation should be keyed in all caps three lines below the return address. Adherence to other regulations will ensure accurate, timely delivery.

ZIP+4. ZIP+4 consists of the basic five ZIP code digits followed by a hyphen and four additional digits. The use of ZIP+4 will expedite the delivery of mail. If the envelope has been prepared properly to be read through OCR, the digits will be converted to a bar code. This piece of mail then goes to the bar code sorter which rapidly sorts for the final destination.

Abbreviations. When addressing mail, use the abbreviations for states and United States possessions (Figure 15-10) and official postal service abbreviations for street suffixes, directionals, and locators (Figure 15-11).

International Mail

Classes of international mail include letters and letter packages, postcards and postal cards, aerogrammes, printed matter, direct sacks of printed matter, matter for the blind, small packets, and parcel post. Special services such as insurance, recorded delivery, registered mail, restricted delivery, return receipt, special delivery, COD mail, and certified mail are also available. For the most current information on rates and services, inquire at the local postal service.

TECHNOLOGIES

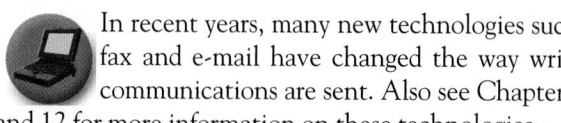

In recent years, many new technologies such as fax and e-mail have changed the way written communications are sent. Also see Chapters 11 and 12 for more information on these technologies.

Facsimile (Fax)

A facsimile, or fax, is the transmission of a written document through a telephone line using a fax machine both at the sender's and receiver's end. A fax can be sent as easily as putting the document in the machine similar to the way a document is put in a copy machine and dialing the receiving telephone number. See Procedure 15-5. There are

AL	Alabama	NE	Nebraska
AK	Alaska	NV	Nevada
AS	American Samoa	NH	New Hampshire
AZ	Arizona	NJ	New Jersey
AR	Arkansas	NM	New Mexico
CA	California	NY	New York
CO	Colorado	NC	North Carolina
CT	Connecticut	ND	North Dakota
DE	Delaware	MP	No. Mariana Islands
DC	Dist. of Columbia	OH	Ohio
FL	Florida	OK	Oklahoma
GA	Georgia	OR	Oregon
GU	Guam	PA	Pennsylvania
HI	Hawaii	PR	Puerto Rico
ID	Idaho	RI	Rhode Island
IL	Illinois	SC	South Carolina
IN	Indiana	SD	South Dakota
IA	Iowa	TN	Tennessee
KS	Kansas	TX	Texas
KY	Kentucky	TT	Trust Territory
LA	Louisiana	UT	Utah
ME	Maine	VT	Vermont
MD	Maryland	VI	Virgin Islands, U.S.
MA	Massachusetts	VA	Virginia
MI	Michigan	WA	Washington
MN	Minnesota	WV	West Virginia
MS	Mississippi	WI	Wisconsin
MO	Missouri	WY	Wyoming
MT	Montana		

Figure 15-10 Abbreviations for states, territories, and District of Columbia. (Courtesy United States Postal Service)

AVE	Avenue	PL	Place
BLVD	Boulevard	RD	Road
CT	Court	STA	Station
CTR	Center	ST	Street
CIR	Circle	TPKE	Turnpike
DR	Drive	VLY	Valley
EXPY	Expressway		
HTS	Heights	APT	Apartment
HWY	Highway	RM	Room
IS	Island	STE	Suite
JCT	Junction	PLZ	Plaza
LK	Lake		
LN	Lane	N	North
MTN	Mountain	E	East
PKY	Parkway	S	South
		W	West

Figure 15-11 Abbreviations for street suffixes, directionals, and locators. (Courtesy United States Postal Service)

TABLE 15-4	ADVANTAGES OF THE FAX
Speed	The document is transmitted immediately or within minutes of sending.
Cost	Cost of a fax is the approximate cost of the telephone call. For long-distance faxes, this can be many times less than the cost of an overnight service.
Patient Care	Patient care could be enhanced, especially in emergency situations where the receiver may need to make decisions based on information in the document.
Legality	The receiver has the "hard copy" document versus relying on verbal information if the information is needed immediately.

several advantages to using the fax machine over traditional postal or carrier services. These advantages are listed in Table 15-4.

There are other issues involved in using the fax, especially when sending patient information. Figure 15-12

provides insight on several legal and confidentiality issues that should be considered before sending any communications via the fax. See Chapter 11 for additional guidelines related to fax use.

Electronic Mail (E-Mail)

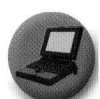

Medical information previously communicated via mail, telephone, or fax may now be sent from computer to computer using **e-mail**. Just as business communication requires proper use of written language, so does e-mail.

Composing e-mail is similar to composing any written communication. Just as a letter or memo has a particular format, the e-mail transmission should also follow a format style. The subject line should be brief and clearly identify the content of the e-mail body.

If your message is in response to another piece of e-mail, your e-mail software will probably preface the subject line with *Re:* (for regarding). If your e-mail software

---

DON'T FAX YOUR WAY INTO A LAWSUIT

One of the cornerstones of the doctor/patient relationship is professional confidentiality. But quality care often depends on sharing patient information, swiftly and accurately, with other medical professionals.

About the fastest and most accurate way to transmit medical information is by fax. But faxed records can all too easily fall into the wrong person's hands.

In this lawsuit-driven age, all of us know why we must never fax confidential records, but in our convenience-driven culture, we also know that confidential records are being faxed every day, all across America. So the question becomes: How can we keep faxed records as confidential as mailed, messengered, or verbally-summarized-over-the-phone records?

The answer is to set up a *Fax Security System*, as follows:

Fax Security System

1. Make sure you have an Authorization To Release Records form, dated and signed by the patient or legal guardian, before you fax any information (just as you'd make sure you had a signed release if you wanted to send records any other way).
2. Never fax financial information. You can justify (in court) the faxing of medical information on the basis of medical necessity; but you cannot justify (anywhere) the faxing of financial data that the patient deems confidential.
3. Before you fax, ask yourself: "Is this really necessary? Or are we better off mailing or messengering these records?"
4. After you answer yourself, ask your office manager: "Will you sign an approval to fax these records? You will? I'll do

it right away. You won't? Thanks for taking the decision off my back."
5. Only fax to telecopiers located in physician offices, nursing stations, or other secure areas. Do *not* fax to machines in mail rooms, office lobbies, or other open areas unless they are secured with passwords. When in doubt about the machine's exact location, "Hold your fax 'til you see the whites of their thermal paper."
6. Use a cover sheet that contains the warning: "The following material is strictly confidential; all persons are advised that they may be prosecuted under federal and state law for sharing this information with unauthorized individuals."
7. If your fax has a display showing the phone number being faxed to, make sure the displayed number corresponds to the number you want to fax to.
8. After faxing, call the faxee and confirm that the fax was received. If not, use your "recall" to find the last number dialed (your manual should show you how). Fax an urgent alert to that number and ask "all persons of goodwill to immediately and effectively destroy all documents received in the previous transmission."

Photocopy this Fax Security System and post it right above your fax machine. Make sure every staff member reads and understands it.

Oh? You say you can't be bothered with all this "security stuff"? That's all right; there's a much easier item to post for practices that aren't all that security-conscious: Your lawyer's telephone number.

Figure 15-12 Don't fax your way into a lawsuit. (Copyright © 1994 The Doctor's Office. Reprinted with permission.)

does not do this, it would be polite to key in "RE:". If your message is time critical, starting with "URGENT" is appropriate. If you are referring to previous e-mail, you should explicitly quote that document to provide context.

If your message is being addressed to several parties, list the e-mail addresses in "bcc" which stands for **blind copies**. This procedure protects the privacy of your audience. "Cc" permits all recipients to view the full list of addresses. It is a good practice to put your own e-mail address at the top of the list, as a quality check, so you can see what everyone else is receiving and/or maintain a copy for the file.

The body of the message should contain short and clear sentences. In trying to be brief and to the point, however, it is important to not leave out important facts or information. Remember also that some e-mail software only understands plain text. Italics, bold, and color changes should be used sparingly. Some software will also recognize **URLs (Uniform Resource Locators,** or web site addresses) in the text and make them "live." Since different software recognizes different parts of the address, if you include a URL in your e-mail, it is much safer to use the entire address, including the initial http://.

The advantages of using e-mail as a means of communication include:

- Asynchronous communication—both parties need not be available at the same time for communication to take place
- Physicians and patients can prepare, leave, read, and respond to messages at times that are convenient
- Can be used to automate certain tasks such as sending out appointment reminders or reports of lab results
- Creates a documentation trail of interactions between physician and patient
- Some patients may be more forthcoming using e-mail than in face-to-face discussion

The disadvantages of e-mail communications include:

- Lack of real-time interaction and feedback
- Lack of body language or vocal inflection, which may lead to misunderstanding
- Reimbursement for the time spent responding to patient messages and receipt of messages from non-patients may not be defined
- May not be suitable for time-sensitive material since determination of when the message will be delivered or read can not be assessed

LEGAL AND ETHICAL ISSUES

Written communication, no matter what form is used, must take into consideration legal and ethical issues. A

 copy of all written communication should be maintained in the patient chart or in office files should it be needed at a later date.

It is important to include e-mail in your office's confidentiality policy. Confidentiality issues must be considered if the ambulatory care office sends or receives **clinical e-mail** from a computer that can be used by more than one person. Many offices use a privacy disclaimer to establish boundaries and ground rules for e-mail messages. The following is an example of such a disclaimer:

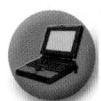 This message is a privileged and confidential clinical communication intended solely for the person to whom it is addressed. If you are not the intended recipient, please be advised that any dissemination, copying, or distribution of this message is strictly prohibited. If you received this message in error, please forward it back to the sender.

Clinical e-mail to or from patients should be treated the same as telephone messages or letters. That means that they should be printed out and filed in the chart. It is important to remember to file both the initial message and any reply.

Before your office begins to use clinical e-mail, a written agreement of understanding should be designed for signature by the patients. In addition to obtaining the patient's permission for you to use clinical e-mail, key elements to include in such an agreement may include:

- E-mail will be exchanged with established patients only.
- E-mail from the patient will include the patient's full name and number.
- The physician is not responsible for e-mail that is not received or responded to in a timely manner.
- E-mail may not be private and confidential.
- E-mail may be read by others, intercepted, or misaddressed.
- E-mail will be filed in the chart.
- E-mail will not be permanently stored on the computer system.
- Urgent issues need to be handled by telephone or in person.

Examples of appropriate uses of e-mail in the ambulatory care setting include:

- Appointment requests
- Prescription refill requests
- Reminder notices
- Insurance or billing questions
- Managed care referrals

Procedure 15-1

Preparing and Composing Business Correspondence Using All Components

PURPOSE:
Prepare and compose a rough draft and final-copy letter using appropriate language and letter style to convey a clear and accurate message to the recipient.

EQUIPMENT/SUPPLIES:
Computer or word processor and printer; or typewriter
Printed letterhead and plain second sheet
Dictionary
Thesaurus
Medical dictionary
Style manual

PROCEDURE STEPS:

1. Organize key points to be addressed in a logical sequence. RATIONALE: To assist in writing an effective letter.

2. Compose a rough draft of the letter. With time and experience, these outlining steps may be eliminated before drafting the letter. RATIONALE: Business correspondence should be clear, concise, courteous, and accurate. A draft letter aids in checking that the letter is logical and achieves the intended purpose.

3. Use language that is easily understood. State the reason for the letter in the first paragraph and encourage action in the last paragraph. RATIONALE: For communication to take place, both parties must understand the message. The letter must be written so that the recipient understands the language and responds appropriately.

4. Read the draft for obvious errors in grammar, spelling, and punctuation. Use the appropriate reference material (dictionary, style manual, and so on) to check any inaccuracies. Read again for content; is the message accurate, logical, and organized appropriately? Lay the letter aside and read it a third time at a later time. RATIONALE: Reading several times allows you to concentrate on different elements of the letter. Errors may "jump" out when reading the third time.

5. Choose the letter format that is customary to the ambulatory care setting. RATIONALE: The letter style should be efficient to prepare and professional in appearance and content in order to represent the physician/employer in a professional manner.

6. Begin keying the letter, referring to the chosen format. Key the date on line 15 or two to three lines below the letterhead. The date should be completely written out; i.e., January 15, 20__, rather than 1/15/__. RATIONALE: Using the component parts of a business letter ensures that the letter is professional in appearance and represents the physician/employer in a professional manner.

7. Key the recipient's name and address flush with the left margin beginning on line 20. RATIONALE: Using the component parts of a business letter ensures that the letter is professional in appearance and represents the physician/employer in a professional manner.

8. On the second line below the recipient's address, key the salutation flush with the left margin. Follow the salutation with a colon unless you are using open punctuation. RATIONALE: Using the component parts of a business letter ensures that the letter is professional in appearance and represents the physician/employer in a professional manner.

9. Key the subject of the letter on the second line below the salutation flush with the left margin, if the subject line is being used. RATIONALE: Using the component parts of a business letter ensures that the letter is professional in appearance and represents the physician/employer in a professional manner.

10. Begin the body of the letter on the second line below the salutation or subject line. The body format will depend upon the style of letter used. For example, if the full block format is used, paragraphs will begin flush with the left margin. Single-space within paragraphs; double-space between paragraphs. RATIONALE: Using the component parts of a business letter ensures that the letter is professional in appearance and represents the physician/employer in a professional manner.

11. Key the complimentary closure on the second line below the body of the letter. Capitalize only the first letter of the first word of the complimentary closure; e.g., Respectfully yours. RATIONALE: Using the component parts of a business

(continues)

Procedure 15-1 *(continued)*

letter ensures that the letter is professional in appearance and represents the physician/employer in a professional manner.

12. Key the signature four to six lines below the complimentary closing. RATIONALE: This ensures that the recipient will be able to determine who sent the letter.

13. If reference initials are used, key the initials two lines below the keyed signature; e.g., WL: jg. RATIONALE: Using the component parts of a business letter ensures that the letter is professional in appearance and represents the physician/employer in a professional manner.

14. Key the enclosure or carbon copy notation one or two lines below the reference initials. RATIONALE: Using the component parts of a business letter ensures that the letter is professional in appearance and represents the physician/employer in a professional manner.

15. Proofread the document and make corrections as necessary. RATIONALE: All information contained in the letter must be accurate and written in a clear and concise manner with logical organization. The grammar, spelling, punctuation, and capitalization must be correct to ensure a professional appearance and represent the physician/employer in a positive manner.

16. Prepare the envelope. Place the envelope flap over the letter and attach it with a paper clip. RATIONALE: Prepare the envelope using United States Postal regulations to ensure delivery in a timely manner. Proofread to be sure the address is accurate to ensure deliverability. By placing the envelope flap over the letter and attaching it with a paper clip the two will not become separated.

17. Place the letter on the physician's desk for review and signature. RATIONALE: The physician's signature signifies the letter is accurate, sends the intended message, and represents the office in a professional manner.

Procedure 15-2 Addressing Envelopes According to United States Postal Regulations

PURPOSE:
To address envelopes according to United States Postal Service regulations to ensure timely delivery.

EQUIPMENT/SUPPLIES:
Computer or word processor and printer with envelope tray; or typewriter
Envelopes
United States Postal Service Publication 221, *Addressing for Success*

PROCEDURE STEPS:

1. Insert the envelope in the typewriter or select the envelope format from the software program. When using a word processor or computer, labels may be used rather than printing directly on the envelope. The label is then adhered to the envelope. RATIONALE: United States Postal regulations suggest that the address on letter mail should be machine-printed, with a uniform left margin.

2. Visualize an imaginary rectangle on the envelope. The rectangle extends ⅝ inch to 2¾ inches from the bottom of the envelope, with 1 inch on each side. The address is placed within this rectangle (Figure 15-13). RATIONALE: United States Postal regulations suggest that the address on letter mail should be machine-printed, with a uniform left margin.

(continues)

Procedure

15-2   *(continued)*

3. Key the address in uppercase letters. Be sure to maintain a uniform left margin on all lines. Eliminate all punctuation in the address except the hyphen in the ZIP+4 code. Leave a minimum of one space between the city name and the two-character state abbreviation and the ZIP+4 code. RATIONALE: A scanner reads the Zip code on the bottom line and prints a bar code in the lower right corner of the envelope. The OCR prefers all uppercase characters.

4. If you are not using preprinted envelopes, key the return address in uppercase letters in the upper left corner of the envelope. Include the name on the first line, address on the second line, and city, state, and ZIP+4 code on the third line. RATIONALE: The return address should be printed in the upper left corner of the envelope should the letter need to be returned to the sender for any reason.

5. Proofread the envelope, make corrections as necessary. RATIONALE: When all information is correct, processing will take place efficiently and correctly.

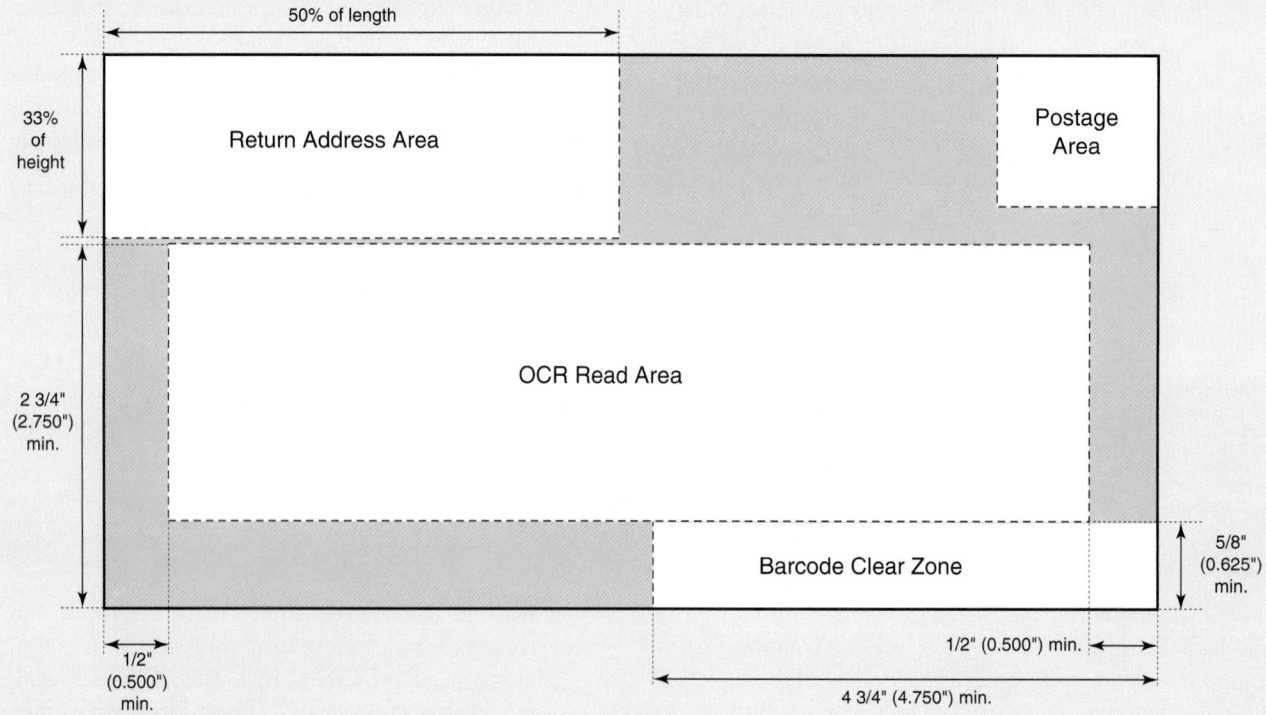

Figure 15-13   Designated zones for accurate reading of envelopes by optical character reader (OCR), the U.S. Postal Service's computerized scanner. (Courtesy United States Postal Service)

Procedure 15-3 Folding Letters for Standard Envelopes

PURPOSE:
To fold and insert letters into envelopes so that the letters fit properly in the envelopes.

EQUIPMENT/SUPPLIES:
Letters to be mailed
Number 6¾ envelope
Number 10 envelope
Window envelope

PROCEDURE STEPS:
1. To fit a standard-size letter into a number 6¾ envelope, fold the letter up from the bottom, leaving ¼ inch to ½ inch at the top, and crease it. Then fold the letter from the right edge about one-third the width of the letter. Fold the left edge over to within ¼ inch to ½ inch of the right-edge crease. Insert the left creased edge first into the envelope (Figure 15-14A). RATIONALE: Ensures a proper fit of the letter into the envelope with a minimum of folds. The last crease made enters the envelope first. This enables the recipient to begin to read the letter with minimum effort.

2. To fit a standard-size letter into a number 10 envelope, fold the letter up about one-third the length of the sheet and crease it. Then fold the top of the letter down to within ¼ inch to ½ inch of the bottom crease, and crease the top. Insert the top creased edge first into the envelop (Figure 15-14B). RATIONALE: Ensures a proper fit of the letter into the envelope with a minimum of folds. The last crease made enters the envelope first. This enables the recipient to begin to read the letter with minimum effort.

3. To fit a standard-size letter into a window envelope, turn the letter over and fold the top of the letter up about one-third the length of the page

(continues)

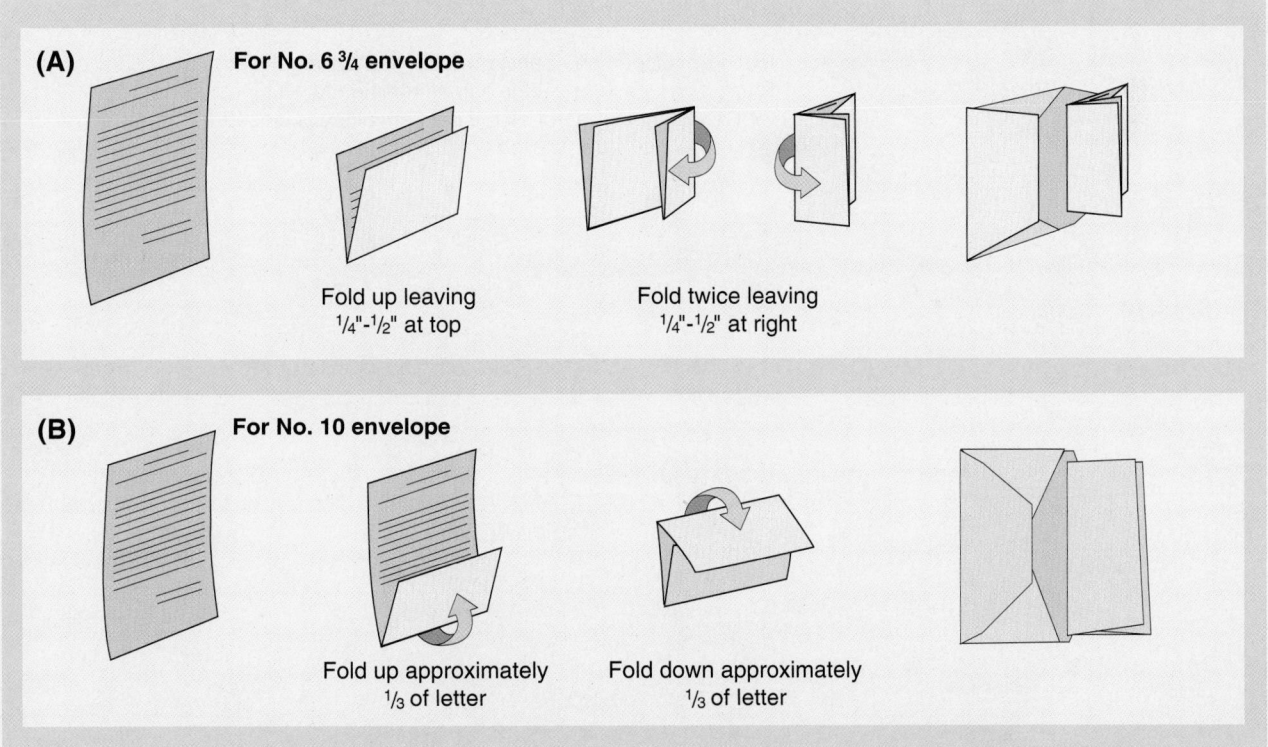

(A) For No. 6 ¾ envelope

Fold up leaving
¼"-½" at top

Fold twice leaving
¼"-½" at right

(B) For No. 10 envelope

Fold up approximately
⅓ of letter

Fold down approximately
⅓ of letter

Figure 15-14 Proper letter folding procedures for various envelope types (A–C) and bulk placement of envelopes for moistening prior to closure (D).

Procedure

15-3   *(continued)*

so that the address is facing you. Then fold the bottom of the letter back to the first crease. Insert the letter into the envelope bottom first (Figure 15-14C). You should be able to read the entire address through the window. RATIONALE: Ensures that the entire address can be read through the window envelope and be delivered correctly.

4. Place envelopes as shown in Figure 15-14D to moisten prior to sealing. RATIONALE: Efficient method of sealing multiple letters for mailing.

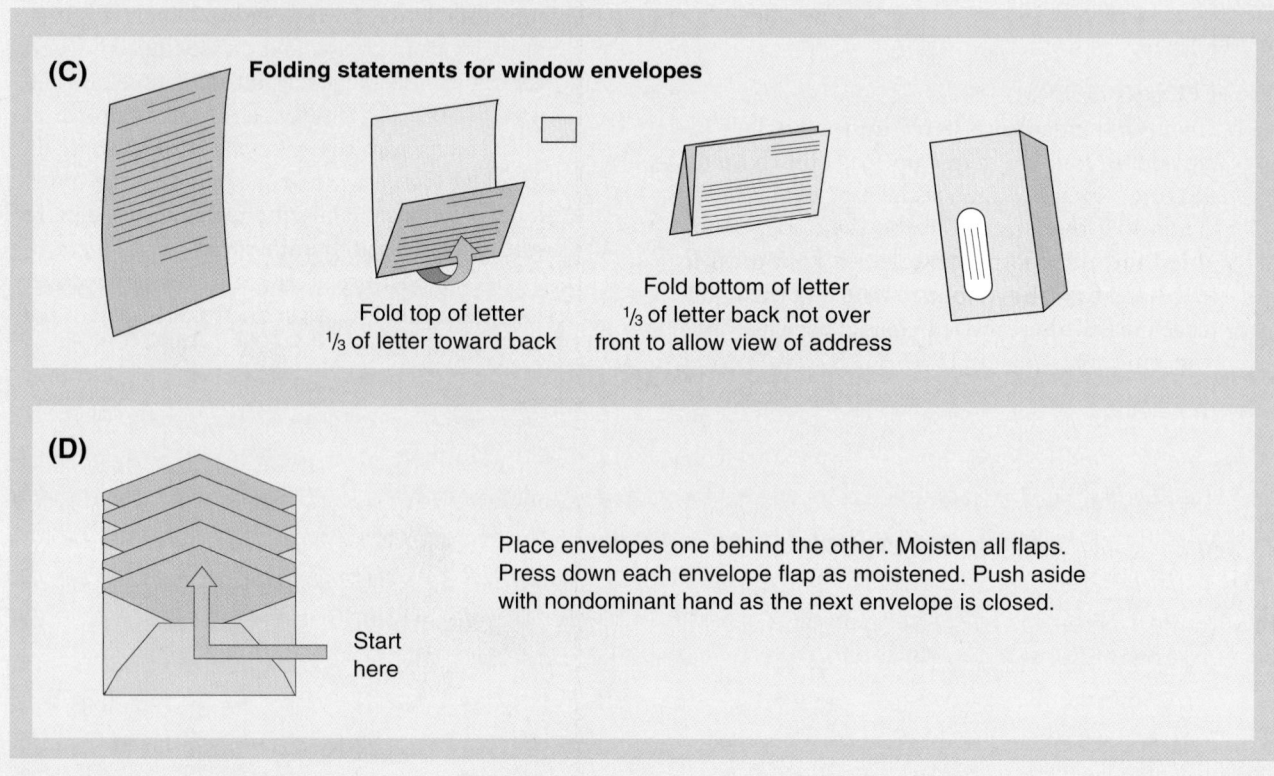

(C)   **Folding statements for window envelopes**

Fold top of letter
⅓ of letter toward back

Fold bottom of letter
⅓ of letter back not over
front to allow view of address

(D)

Start
here

Place envelopes one behind the other. Moisten all flaps. Press down each envelope flap as moistened. Push aside with nondominant hand as the next envelope is closed.

Figure 15-14   *(continued)*

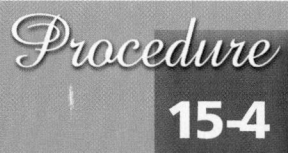

Procedure 15-4 — Preparing Outgoing Mail According to United States Postal Regulations

PURPOSE:
To prepare outgoing mail for expeditious delivery.

EQUIPMENT/SUPPLIES:
Manual or electronic scale
Postage meter or stamps
Envelope or package to be mailed

PROCEDURE STEPS:

1. Sort the mail according to postal class. For example, all single-piece letters that weigh less than 11 ounces are included in first-class mail. Correspondence and statements are sent in this classification. RATIONALE: Sorting by postal class expedites processing at the Post Office.
2. Using the manual or electronic scale, weigh the item to be mailed. If you are using a manual scale, read the weight in ounces and compute the amount of postage due. If you are using an electronic scale, the correct postage will be displayed on the scale. RATIONALE: Correct postage on each postal item is essential to ensure faster delivery service.
3. Using a postal meter or stamps, affix the appropriate postage to the piece to be mailed. Use of a postal meter expedites delivery of mail because metered mail does not have to be canceled or postmarked at the post office. RATIONALE: Correct postage on each postal item is essential to ensure faster delivery service.
4. Place the prepared mail in the area of the office designated for outgoing mail or deliver the mail to the post office according to office policy. RATIONALE: Ensures that all mail going out is centrally located and that the postal worker can pick up outgoing and deliver incoming mail efficiently.

Procedure 15-5 — Preparing, Sending, and Receiving a Fax

PURPOSE:
To send and receive information quickly and accurately by fax (facsimile).

EQUIPMENT/SUPPLIES:
Fax machine
Telephone

PROCEDURE STEPS:

To send a fax:

1. Prepare a cover sheet or use a preprinted cover sheet for the document to be faxed. Include the names of the sender and receiver, the number of pages being sent and whether this includes the cover sheet, and a short message if necessary. RATIONALE: A cover sheet aids in the correct delivery of a fax to the designated person. It also provides a disclaimer should the fax be received in error and what to do if it is misdelivered.

CAUTION: Fax machines may be located in areas where unauthorized personnel may see confidential material. Always include a notice of confidentiality on the cover sheet and always ask the receiver for permission to fax a confidential document.

2. Place the document face down in the fax machine, similar to the way a document is put into a copy machine. RATIONALE: Ensures that content will be read for transmission.
3. Dial the telephone or dedicated fax number of the receiver. If your fax machine has a display showing the number being faxed to, check to be sure the number you dialed is correct. Then press start. RATIONALE: Verify number to be sure fax is being transmitted to correct phone.

(continues)

Procedure
15-5   *(continued)*

4. After the document passes through the fax machine, press the button requesting a receipt. Some fax machines automatically issue a report. RATIONALE: A receipt is your documentation of the date, time, and where the fax was sent.

5. Remove the document from the machine and, when necessary, call the recipient to be sure the fax was received. RATIONALE: Maintains confidentiality and verifies fax was received by intended recipient.

To receive a fax:

6. Be sure that the fax machine is turned on and that the telephone line to the machine is not being used. Most offices will have dedicated fax lines. RATIONALE: Enables you to receive a fax.

7. Remove the document from the machine after it is received and immediately deliver it to the addressee. RATIONALE: Maintains confidentiality and enables recipient to take action immediately if necessary.

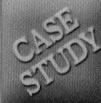

CASE STUDY 15-1

When she was assembling the style manual for all written communications generated by the office of Doctors Lewis & King, office manager Marilyn Johnson wanted it to be as comprehensive as possible. Therefore, she gathered research over a period of months, noting problems the office had experienced in written communications, such as letters going out without the physician's signature; she became very familiar with proofreading devices that would ensure letter-perfect correspondence; and she developed source materials on the different classes of mail and the services of the United States Post Office.

CASE STUDY REVIEW

1. Marilyn is ready to outline the manual. Review the chapter information and create an outline indicating major topic headings for the Lewis & King style manual.

2. Because a few of the medical assistants are not comfortable with composing, what writing tips can Marilyn include to make them more confident?

3. Marilyn wants all letters to look alike. What information should she include to educate the manual users about the components of a standard letter?

CASE STUDY 15-2

Doctors Lewis & King are considering adopting the use of clinical e-mail since many of their patients have home computers and use e-mail in their day-to-day communications. Office manager Marilyn Johnson is concerned about maintaining patient confidentiality and appropriate use of clinical e-mail. She has decided to develop a written agreement of understanding and plans to ask each patient to sign the agreement before transmission of any clinical e-mail is instituted. Marilyn also feels a privacy disclaimer could be of legal value to the office.

CASE STUDY REVIEW

1. Marilyn is developing the agreement of understanding. What are some key elements that should be included in the agreement?

2. Responding to patients using e-mail correspondence is different than social communication. What are some guidelines for e-mail correspondence that will be helpful to remember?

3. List several advantages and disadvantages to using e-mail in the ambulatory health care setting.

SUMMARY

Communication is vital in any ambulatory care setting, and the proper management of written communications ensures both a professional image and an efficient operation. Because of our ability to write letters, send reports, transcribe physician notes, and otherwise communicate with others, the quality of patient care is enhanced, for communication is at the core of much patient treatment.

As well as becoming knowledgeable about the techniques of written communication, it is important for the medical assistant to become comfortable with the act of composition and writing. Proper techniques in letter formatting and proofreading ensures quality control and the maintenance of high administrative standards. Ease in writing and communicating on paper ensures that information is accurate, reliable, and capable of being held up in a court of law if this becomes necessary.

The administrative medical assistant must be skilled in the use of technologies and understand and follow confidentiality and legal policies and procedures.

REVIEW QUESTIONS

Multiple Choice

1. When proofreading a letter, you should:
   a. never read it against the document
   b. proof it on the computer screen
   c. read long documents a section at a time
   d. always finish the job no matter how tired you may be
2. Form letters should be used:
   a. for all patients
   b. for all referring physicians
   c. only for pharmaceutical salespeople
   d. with individualized addressing when possible
3. Of the four major letter styles, which is the most contemporary?
   a. full block
   b. modified block, standard
   c. modified block, indented
   d. simplified
4. Form letters may be written for each of the following except:
   a. letters containing laboratory and/or diagnostic results
   b. letters announcing new insurance or HMOs accepted
   c. letters to announce new staff
   d. letters to order supplies or subscriptions
5. The subject line is keyed:
   a. on line 15 or two to three lines below the letterhead
   b. on the second line below the inside address
   c. four lines below the complimentary closing
   d. on the second line below the salutation

6. When keying a second page, all of the following apply except:
   a. always use a second-page heading
   b. when dividing a paragraph at the bottom of a page, keep one line on the bottom of the page and one line at the top of the next page
   c. a minimum of three lines should be keyed on the second page of a letter
   d. never use a letterhead page as a second page
7. After removing the contents from incoming mail, what should you do?
   a. stamp the date it was received in the office
   b. look in the envelope to make certain that all contents have been removed
   c. if the address is not included on the letter, write it on the letter as it appeared on the envelope
   d. all of the above
8. In the ambulatory care setting, the postal class likely to be used most frequently is:
   a. express
   b. first class
   c. bulk rate
   d. second class
9. The body of an e-mail communication should:
   a. contain short and clear sentences
   b. be written in italic, bold, and color for emphasis
   c. be brief and to the point but contain all pertinent information
   d. answers a and c only
10. To establish boundaries and ground rules for e-mail messages, many offices are developing:
    a. privacy disclaimers
    b. written agreements of understanding
    c. itineraries
    d. agendas

Critical Thinking

1. Recall the five writing tips for more effective communication. Now write a letter using these points.
2. With a group of students, organize a spelling bee of commonly used medical words. Include some of the words that are often misspelled.
3. Identify the four major letter styles. Compose and key a letter using each of these styles.
4. List the component parts of any business letter. Give a brief description of the placement of each component part.
5. State at least eight of the guidelines of letter composition.
6. Use those guidelines to revise a letter. Work from an existing draft that needs corrections, then rewrite, rekey, and proofread the revised letter.
7. In a small group, exchange the original and revised letters produced in number 6. Make comments on how (and whether) the letters are improved.
8. Address an envelope with all address elements in proper format for expeditious handling by the United States Postal Service.
9. Prepare a document with a cover sheet for faxing. Before you fax the document, however, recall the eight points from Figure 15-16. Does your document meet these guidelines?
10. Discuss legal and ethical issues regarding the use of clinical e-mail.

WEB ACTIVITIES

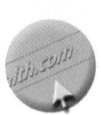 Use the Internet to research additional information pertaining to confidentiality and legal issues related to faxing medical records or electronic mail to transmit medical information. Follow instructor's instructions on completing and turning in your results.

DOCUMENTATION

Clinically related e-mail to or from patients should be treated the same way as telephone messages or letters. That means they should be printed out and filed in the chart.

From:	Elizabeth J. Parker
Sent:	Tuesday, July 20, 20__ 8:55 AM
To:	Dr. King [King@doctor.com]
Subject:	Prescription refill

Please call in a prescription refill for my thyroid medication. The pharmacy is Inner City Pharmacy and the phone number is 890-271-2600. The prescription number is RX6437350 and I have enough pills for three days.

REFERENCES/BIBLIOGRAPHY

Humphrey, D. D. (1996) *Contemporary medical office procedures* (2nd ed.). Albany, NY: Delmar.

Kinn, M. E., & Woods, M. A. (1999). *The medical assistant: Administrative and clinical* (8th ed.). Philadelphia: W. B. Saunders.

Pearce, F. (1999). *Business netiquette international.* [On-line]. Available: *http://www.bspage.com/inetiq/Netiq.html*

Physicians Insurance 2000. March/April 2000. *Physician's risk management update.* (Vol. XI, No. 2.) Author.

Robert, H. M., III, Evans, W. J., Honemann, D. H., Balch, T. J. (2000). *Robert's Rules of Order Newly Revised* (10th ed.). Cambridge, MA: Perseus Publishing.

Sherwood, K. D. (1998). *A beginner's guide to effective e-mail.* [On-line]. Available: *http://www.webfoot.com/advice/email.top.html.*

Tessier, C. (1995). *The AAMT book of style for medical transcription.* American Association for Medical Transcription.

United States Postal Service. (1995). *Addressing for Success* (Pub. 221). Washington, DC: Author.

Virtual mail center not your ordinary sort. (1995, October 16). *Tulsa Daily World.*

Chapter

16

TRANSCRIPTION

KEY TERMS

American Association for Medical
  Transcription (AAMT)
Breach of Confidentiality
Certified Medical Transcriptionist (CMT)
Chart Notes
Chief Complaint (CC)
Confidentiality
Confidentiality Agreement
Consultation Report
Continuing Education (CE)
Continuous Speech Recognition (CSR)
Digital Dictation
Editing
Flag
Freelance MTs
History of the Present Illness (HPI)
History and Physical Examination
  (H&P) Report
Home-Based MTs
Index Counter
Joint Commission on Accreditation of
  Healthcare Organizations (JCAHO)
Medical Transcriptionist (MT)
Medical Transcriptionist Certification
  Program (MTCP)
Privileged
Progress Notes
Proofreading
Quality Assurance (QA)
Recertification
Review of Systems (ROS)
Risk Management
Split Keyboard
STAT
Transcriber
Wrist Rest

OUTLINE

**History of the American
  Association for Medical
  Transcription**
  AAMT Membership
**The Medical Transcriptionist's
  Career**
  Attributes of the Medical
    Transcriptionist
  Job Description
  Employment Opportunities
  Certification for Medical
    Transcriptionists
Transcription Tools
  Equipment
  Ergonomics
  Facsimile Machines
  Photocopy Machines
Transcription Guidelines

**Proofreading and Making
  Corrections**
  Proofreading Skills
  Where Errors Occur
  Editing
  Making Corrections
Medical Reports
  Chart Notes and Progress Notes
  History and Physical Examination
    Reports
  Consultation Reports
  Correspondence
Turnaround Time
Ethical and Legal Issues
  Confidentiality
  Risk Management
New Technology
  Continuous Speech Recognition
  Integrating Digital Photographs
    into Medical Transcription

OBJECTIVES

*The student should strive to meet the following performance objectives and demonstrate
an understanding of the facts and principles presented in this chapter through written and
oral communication.*

1. Define the key terms as presented in the glossary.

2. Briefly describe the history of medical transcription.

3. List a minimum of ten benefits of membership in AAMT.

4. Describe the two major categories of attributes of the medical
   transcriptionist.

5. Compare and contrast the various types of work environments for the
   medical transcriptionist. *(continues)*

6. Describe the certification and recertification process for the medical transcriptionist.
7. List important considerations when setting up a workstation ergonomically.
8. Describe the process of flagging and its significance.
9. Discuss the proper ways to make corrections within medical record transcription.
10. Differentiate between chart notes, history and physical examination reports, consultation reports, and medical correspondence.
11. Describe turnaround time and its importance.
12. Discuss ethical and legal issues as they apply to medical transcription.

ROLE DELINEATION COMPONENTS

ADMINISTRATIVE
Administrative Procedures
- **Perform basic clerical functions**

GENERAL (TRANSDISCIPLINARY)
Legal Concepts
- **Document accurately**

SCENARIO

Inner City Health Care, a multispecialty clinic, employs two full-time medical transcriptionists. Marilyn Johnson, CMA, is the office manager and has former training and experience as a medical transcriptionist. This experience provides her with the basic understanding necessary to manage the medical transcription and medical records department of the clinic. Marilyn has involved the transcriptionists in the ergonomic set up of workstations and in the selection of state-of-the-art equipment and latest reference resources to create a safe work environment and one that encourages quality documents in a timely manner.

INTRODUCTION

In early times, when only a few people could read and write, scribes copied and interpreted the spoken word. Often the scribes transcribed legal and sacred orations into written documents that became the principles and rules by which society was governed. The word *transcription* is composed of two word elements: *trans* and *scriba*. *Trans* is a prefix meaning across, beyond, through, or so as to change. *Scriba* means official writer. Translated, transcription means to change the spoken word to a written record.

Ancient cave writings testify to the beginning of patient care documentation. Hieroglyphics changed to papyrus and parchment using berries to produce ink, to paper using typewriters, and most recently to computer-generated medical records. Until the twentieth century, physicians were both providers of medical care and scribes maintaining their own records. With the standardization of medical data for research purposes after 1900, medical stenographers replaced physician scribes by taking their dictation in shorthand. The career of medical transcription came into being with the development of dictation equipment during World War I. Today medical transcriptionists use computers to transmit patient records electronically to distant locations. Future technology includes incorporating digital images into medical records and the use of continuous voice recognition systems.

HISTORY OF THE AMERICAN ASSOCIATION FOR MEDICAL TRANSCRIPTION

The American Association for Medical Transcription (AAMT) began in 1978 as a nonprofit organization incorporated in California. One of the greatest desires of AAMT's founders was that medical transcriptionists (MTs) be appropriately recognized for the important contribution they make in health care. As a direct result of AAMT's continued efforts to promote the profession, medical transcription is a respected profession, with practitioners recognized as medical language specialists.

The definition of a medical transcriptionist according to the *AAMT Model Job Description* is "a medical language specialist who interprets and transcribes dictation by physicians and other healthcare professionals regarding patient assessment, workup, therapeutic procedures, clinical course, diagnosis, prognosis, etc., in order to document patient care and facilitate delivery of healthcare services." (AAMT, 1990)

For someone seeking education and training, advertisements for medical transcription education programs appear in many places. Here are four ways to evaluate the advertising:

1. The advertising should accurately represent the profession as a medical language specialty requiring a substantial educational investment.
2. When describing a home-based transcription business opportunity, the advertising should indicate the need for additional training in accounting procedures and management protocols for operating a business.
3. A reference source for the income should be cited within the advertising if potential income is discussed.
4. If certification is referenced, it should clearly state that a certificate will be granted upon completion of the educational course. Certification, or the recognized professional credential of certified medical transcriptionist (CMT), can be obtained only through successful completion of both parts of the core certification exam administered by the Medical Transcriptionist Certification Commission (MTCC) at AAMT.

At the present time AAMT does not accredit or approve educational programs. A complete checklist for the evaluation of medical transcription schools and education programs is included on AAMT's web site: http://www.aamt.org.

AAMT Membership

AAMT offers individual membership for professional development, and corporate or institutional membership for visibility and promotion. Other types of membership include practitioner, associate, and student. Student membership is available to any person who is not working as a transcriptionist and is verified as being enrolled in a nine-month or two-semester (defined as 15 to 18 weeks) medical transcription program that includes a student-instructor relationship. Student application requirements include (1) obtain a signed letter from your instructor on school letterhead, indicating enrollment date and length of the program and (2) enclose the letter with an AAMT membership application and your annual payment of $50.

Membership benefits include:

- One-year subscription to *Journal of the American Association for Medical Transcription* (JAAMT)
- *AAMT Desk Companion* (updated annually)
- Information on state-of-the-art technology
- Networking opportunities
- Continuing education
- Access to professional assistance
- Membership help desk (e-mail, fax, or toll-free)
- Discounts on AAMT programs, products, and services
- Professional development opportunities
- Peer recognition
- Pride of accomplishment
- Insurance programs available: errors and omissions, group life and income disability insurance, and equipment insurance
- Optional benefits (from outside companies): discounted travel services and car rental, and no-fee credit card

THE MEDICAL TRANSCRIPTIONIST'S CAREER

Medical transcription is a prosperous industry that offers the educated and experienced transcriptionist opportunities for employment around the world. Diverse work settings and a variety of specialty areas and complexity levels make medical transcription an engaging occupation. The MT career continues to evolve, offering the opportunity for continued learning experiences, rewards in excellent salary packages, and self-actualization. The following paragraphs describe the attributes of a transcriptionist, job description, employment opportunities, and certification.

Attributes of the Medical Transcriptionist

The attributes of the medical transcriptionist may be broken into two major categories: personal attributes and acquired skills developed specific to the career itself. These two categories are key elements to being successful as an MT.

Personal attributes include the love of words. It is not uncommon to find medical transcriptionists working on crossword puzzles and involved with various word games. They have an innate ability to listen closely to what others say and the skill for hearing and understanding different accents and languages. They enjoy detective work and are curious; if terminology is new to them, they use references to research and learn more. MTs are self-disciplined, detail-oriented, independent, and are usually perfectionists. They are dedicated to professional development and enthusiastically committed to learning. They are not afraid to ask questions. They have a genuine caring attitude and an interest in patient care from a medical record point of view. MTs possess integrity and understand the importance and legal implications of medical confidentiality.

Medical transcriptionists must have excellent keyboarding skills. Entry-level positions may require 60 words per minute, while experienced MTs may transcribe more than 80 words per minute. Today's MT must be able to operate a variety of software programs efficiently and maintain continued learning as new programs are developed. Excellent language skills and above-average spelling skills are mandatory. It is recognized that the MT must understand the anatomy and physiology of the human body, have knowledge of surgical terms, equipment, instruments and anesthesia, and directional and body plane terms. A background in common laboratory tests, radiology techniques and terms, drug names and their uses, both brand and generic, common signs and symptoms of diseases and treatment modalities is also required.

New technology, breakthroughs in medicine, and new medications are recognized daily as researchers explore ways in which to treat disease and to produce longevity. MTs must remain current with new medical developments to maintain their professionalism.

Job Description

The *AAMT Model Job Description* is a practical, useful compilation of the basic job responsibilities of a medical transcriptionist. It is designed to assist human resource managers, department managers, supervisors, and others in recruiting, supervising, and evaluating individuals in medical transcription positions. It is also useful for prospective medical transcriptionists as a checklist for employment readiness. The complete *AAMT Model Job Description* may be downloaded from the following web address: http://www.aamt.org/model.htm.

Employment Opportunities

Medical transcriptionists may seek employment in a variety of settings—hospitals, multispecialty clinics, solo physician practices, transcription services, home-based offices, research facilities, radiology clinics, pathology laboratories, tumor boards or registries, law offices, and/or veterinary hospitals. MTs may work as employees, supervisors, managers, or teachers, or may be self-employed or freelancers.

Hospitals, multispeciality clinics, and solo physician practices generally offer competitive salary and benefit packages. Payment for professional membership and/or registration fees for continuing education opportunities may also be included in the benefit package. Some offices will also include money to purchase reference materials. A wide range of dictation types, including a variety of medical specialties, dictator styles and dialects, and a vast degree of complexities are transcribed in these facilities. State-of-the-art equipment is often available, and opportunities for advancement into supervisory positions may be a possibility. A stable work schedule and job security are experienced for those who perform to their standard and have a positive work ethic.

The disadvantages of working in hospital and multispeciality clinics are the inflexible work schedule, low wages, facility politics, and the prospects of a supervisor who is unfamiliar with the needs of transcriptionists. The impacts of managed care and its associated cost-cutting efforts lead more of these facilities to out-source their medical transcription.

Transcription service employees often enjoy competitive pay rates. They transcribe a variety of accounts (physician offices, specialty offices, and so on), so there is a vast difference in the complexity and length of the documents. The work environment is usually quite comfortable and flexible scheduling is a primary advantage. Disadvantages may include the absence of immediate feedback concerning questions regarding dictation and compensation. Often in these types of settings compensation is based on production. If there is a lack of tapes available for transcription, or if the MT experiences an off-day, it will be reflected in the paycheck.

Transcription services often employ **home-based MTs** who transcribe exclusively for those employers. The employer may provide the equipment and the MT works directly under the supervision of the employer. The disadvantages of a home-based business include the fact that larger facilities frequently out-source dictation that is difficult because of the specialty or has been dictated by a foreign-speaking physician. It has been estimated that seven out of ten dictating physicians are foreign-born today. If you do not have an ear and an aptitude for dialects, it may be impossible to service these accounts and maintain a livable wage.

The entrepreneurial MT may opt to establish a freelance business. **Freelance MTs** function as independent contractors. Often they transcribe hospital overflow. The advantages of freelance are a sense of accomplishment and independence, and opportunity to work flexible hours. If you have been employed specifically for medical offices, clinics, or other specialties and feel well qualified, it is best to concentrate your independent transcription work within your field of expertise. Generally, independents are paid by production—by the line, page, or character count. Your earnings will probably be excellent *if* you are highly productive, transcribe accurately, and remain focused on building the business. The disadvantages of freelance include having to handle all areas of a business including bookkeeping, pickup of dictation and delivery of completed work, and finding other MTs to cover during illness, vacation or overload periods. Another disadvantage is the unpredictable income; income is dependent on someone else's need. Some freelance MTs feel isolated and never free to get away from their work.

Insurance companies and law offices also may employ MTs. In these environments the MT analyzes discrepancies in health records and translates medical language in a chart into lay language for attorneys. Other opportunities for MTs include teaching within hospitals, community colleges, or vocational/technical schools, preparing manuscripts for research documentation, or authoring textbooks for MTs.

Certification for Medical Transcriptionists

A qualified MT, described as one with a minimum of two years' experience in performing medical transcription in a variety of medical and surgical specialties, may apply for the certification examination through the Medical Transcriptionist Certification Commission (MTCC). The MTCC is the credentialing program of the AAMT. MTCC offers a voluntary two-part certification exam to individuals who wish to become certified medical transcriptionists (CMTs).

The purpose of MTCC's core examination is to assess core knowledge and skills needed to practice medical transcription. This is accomplished by demonstrating competence to interpret and transcribe routine patient care documentation in a wide variety of work settings and across a broad range of specialty areas.

Part I of the test is written. It includes 120 multiple-choice questions (only 100 of which are scored) in six major content areas:

1. Medical terminology, 30%
2. English language and use, 25%
3. Anatomy and physiology, 20%
4. Disease processes, 15%
5. Health care record, 5%
6. Professional development, 5%

The test is given electronically on touch-screen computers with a time allocation of three hours. No reference materials are permitted while testing. The test is available year-round at testing centers across the United States. For details about exam content and instructions on scheduling an exam, request the MTCC *Candidate Handbook* from AAMT's web site: http://www.aamt.org/certinfo.htm. Anyone who feels ready to take the exam after self-assessing skills and knowledge based on the content outline may apply. The cost is $150, and test results are available immediately. A passing score of 85 (not a percentage) is required.

Part II of the test is practical. About 15 minutes of dictation representing a variety of report types and specialties must be transcribed, proofread, and printed within two hours. Reference materials, notes, spellcheckers, and abbreviation expanders are permitted. The examination sites and an appropriate proctor to administer the examination are chosen by the candidate. The third weekend in February, June, and October, and a choice of Thursday evening, or Friday or Saturday morning test administration are test options.

Individuals who have passed Part I within the previous two years are eligible for Part II of the test. Products from MTCC and AAMT are available to help assess readiness and supply information regarding the application/registration process. Application/registration materials must

SPOTLIGHT ON AAMA ESSENTIALS THROUGH CAAHEP

- When transcribing medical records, maintain confidentiality and never discuss the contents of the medical record with the patient.

- Encouraging the physician to explain the contents of the transcribed medical record to the patient helps to alleviate the patient's confusion and distress about what has been said in the record.

- Respect for the medical information being transcribed into the patient's medical record is just as important as maintaining confidentiality and providing good patient care.

be postmarked seven weeks before exam dates. Results are available within ten weeks and a passing score of 85 (not a percentage) is required. The cost is $150.

Recertification is through **continuing education (CE)** activities. The purpose of recertification is to maintain competency in the field of medical transcription and must be done every 3 years. Recertification is accomplished by accruing at least 30 CE credits (at least 20 of which must be in the medical science category) over a 3-year cycle. The recertification fee is $60 or $45 by early-bird deadline. CE guidelines for CMTs are updated annually and provide details about credit-worthy activities and recertification procedures.

CMTs are not required to be members of AAMT, but membership is encouraged because of the opportunities and benefits that result from professional commitment and involvement. For additional information regarding certification, check AAMT's web site: http://www.aamt.org/certinfo.htm.

TRANSCRIPTION TOOLS

Machine transcription came into its own in the 1950s replacing written shorthand as a method of recording physician notes. Carbon paper and manual typewriters produced the required copies for record management. A few years later analog dictation and electronic typewriters came into use. During the end of the 1960s, self-correcting typewriters were the newest technology. Word processors evolved during the 1970s making production and storage of reports possible in an electronic environment. Cassette tapes were the dictation medium of choice in hospitals and physician offices for years. Personal computers with word-processing software were developed in the 1980s. Magnetic tape was still the most common method of recording dictation; however, transcribing machines were improved. In the 1990s, **digital dictation**—dictation recorded directly into computers and managed by computers—was developed. Digital dictation can be transferred over telephone lines via computer modems, transcribed live, re-recorded for later transcription, and even transferred by waveform audio format (WAV) file. Using file transfer protocol (FTP), encrypted WAV files can be transferred between computers that are connected via the Internet, eliminating long-distance costs involved with telephone transfers.

Equipment

The **transcriber** is a device that makes it possible to transform voice recordings into a transcript or printed documents. **Index counters** measure the length of dictation on a cassette. The index counter is useful to scan cassettes or to find the correct dictation location. The auto playback/auto rewind feature allows you to replay a word or a phrase. Some repeat at the beginning is helpful to ensure that you have not missed any words. The speaker button permits you to listen to dictation out loud or to play the tape for someone. The eject button opens the cassette door. The speed control feature allows you to increase or decrease the speed at which the words are spoken. If the speed is decreased too much, the words will become distorted and difficult to recognize. A normal speaking rate is suggested for the best results. The volume control feature permits you to increase or decrease the volume to compensate for dictators having a soft or loud voice. The tone feature is similar to the treble/bass feature in your car radio. It mutes or accentuates consonants for nasal tones or a stuttering style of dictation. Finally, the erase feature allows you to clear or erase the tape once you have completed the transcription.

Earphones plug into the transcriber and allow you to hear what has been dictated. Earphones should be cleaned with rubbing alcohol after each using. Use a cotton swab to reach into small areas.

Standard cassette transcribers play standard audio tapes. When inserting the cassette, be sure the side you want to play is top side up. There are also microcassette and minicassette transcribers. You will need to use the correct audio tape size when using these transcribers.

The foot pedal frees your hands to use the keyboard. Pushing the foot pedal causes the transcriber to play, and releasing the pedal stops the transcriber. In most cases, the center of the foot pedal is the position to press for play; fast forward is on the left; and rewind is on the right. Study the foot pedal manual to learn how to use your particular model correctly.

Ergonomics

Working at a computer for long periods of time can produce sore muscles, headaches, eyestrain, tension, and fatigue. Carpal tunnel syndrome is soreness, tenderness, and weakness of the muscles of the thumb caused by pressure on the median nerve at the point at which it goes through the carpal tunnel of the wrist. If conservative therapy fails, surgical relief of tension is required. Wearing softFLEX Computer Gloves™ may relieve wrist resting syndrome, which is the true cause of carpal tunnel syndrome symptoms in most keyboard users. The gloves are biomedically engineered and developed by a hand surgeon. They are said to be comfortable and effective, and work without restricting hand motion.

Careful thought should be taken when setting up your workstation, and an emphasis on developing specific habits to prevent injury should be instituted. Take short, frequent breaks and focus on distant objects to relieve eye strain. Wear tinted glasses to reduce glare from the screen.

Arrange the monitor so that it is away from windows; or use drapes, blinds, or an antiglare screen. Adjust the contrast and brightness levels to satisfy eye comfort level. Select a screen color that is restful to your eyes. Practice blinking as it has been documented that computer workers blink at one-fifth the normal rate while they are watching the screen. This causes dry, scratchy eyes.

Prevent ear infections by keeping earphones clean and not allowing others to use them. As much as possible, work in a relatively quiet area.

Keyboards are being redesigned to decrease carpal tunnel syndrome and other repetitive motion injuries. The **split keyboard** is slanted to accommodate the natural position of the hands as opposed to a straight, flat keyboard that does not support the wrists. **Wrist rests** may be purchased for use with the straight, flat keyboard for wrist support. These two devices may also alleviate back pain caused by tensing the muscles around the shoulders. Taking frequent breaks and exercising are recommended for preventative measures.

Adjust the workstation for your individual body. Raise or lower the chair and provide support for the lower back with a lumbar cushion, a rolled up towel, or a small, thin, firm pillow. Use a footrest if you are short-legged. Adjust the table or desk height if possible. Time spent setting up a comfortable, personalized workstation will pay in productivity and decreased health risks. See Chapter 11 for additional ergonomic information.

Facsimile Machines

Facsimile (fax) machines are used in the medical community today to transmit various documents within the facility, to distant communities, and internationally. It is important to note that fax machines print on plain, thin paper or thermally treated paper. Exposure to sunlight quickly fades the printed material, and some paper does not produce clear images. A photocopy of important documents using bond paper will preserve the contents. It is a courtesy to send a hard copy of any important faxed document. Review Chapters 11 and 15 for additional information regarding fax machine use and confidentiality in the medical setting.

Photocopy Machines

Medical offices use photocopy machines in a variety of ways on a daily basis. A photocopy machine should be selected that will satisfy the office needs, produce copies that closely resemble the original, represent the office professionally, and be relatively maintenance free. When disposing of unwanted or extra copies, remember confidentiality. Many offices shred unwanted pages to protect confidentiality and prevent litigation issues.

TRANSCRIPTION GUIDELINES

Punctuation creates more problems than any other aspect of document preparation for the transcriptionist. Authorities disagree with one another, and on occasion there may be more than one correct way to punctuate a sentence. Basic capitalization rules should be followed in medical transcription. The purpose of capitalizing a word is to give it emphasis, distinction, authority, or importance.

The MT must have a clear understanding of when a number should be keyed as a figure, keyed in spelled-out form, or keyed as a roman numeral. Knowledge of the use of symbols and abbreviations commonly found in medical documents is also contradictory.

Guidelines for these specifics may be found in AAMT's *Book of Style*. Your instructor will provide you with additional instructions regarding the actual rules that apply to the transcription of documents.

PROOFREADING AND MAKING CORRECTIONS

Proofreading is the process of checking a document for spelling, sentence structure, punctuation, capitalization, style and format, accuracy, and sense. While transcribing the document, it is a good idea to proofread as you look at the screen and key the information. Many software programs identify spelling and grammar errors making it easy to locate and make corrections as you go.

Proofreading Skills

Proofreading is easier said than done. It has been proven that errors are more often missed while proofreading on the computer screen than proofing a printed copy. The beginning MT should first proof for accuracy by listening to the dictation again while reading the transcribed document. A second reading should be done to identify any misspelled words, incorrect grammar usage, punctuation errors, and inconsistencies in style and format. When time permits, the document should be read a third time after it has been set aside for a period. Errors often "jump out" after being away from the document for awhile.

Transcription departments and services often employ **quality assurance (QA)** reviewers. These individuals check a percentage of each MT's work against dictation. Quality assurance measures documents to be sure they are accurate, complete, consistent in health care documentation, and prepared in a timely manner. Every reasonable effort should be made to resolve inconsistencies, inaccuracies, risk management issues, and other problems.

Where Errors Occur

Examples of where errors occur within dictation include incomplete and run-on sentences, subjects and verbs that do not agree, and dictated spelling and/or punctuation that is incorrect. These types of errors are easily corrected without changing the dictator's style or meaning.

Sound-alike words are another area in which errors may occur. Examples of sound-alike words include ilium/ileum, right/write, site/cite, and aural/oral. Be aware of your personal errors and take steps to avoid them.

Editing

Editing is the process of reviewing the transcribed document for accuracy and clarity. It is important to remember that you must not change the dictator's style or meaning when editing. If the MT encounters a term that cannot be interpreted or something new that cannot be referenced, they should ask other MTs or QA personnel. If the question cannot be resolved, the document should be flagged to alert the dictator something needs to be corrected or resolved. The flagged message may indicate the doctor was cut off, what the term sounds like, or the message is incomprehensible. Provide as much information as you can to assist the dictator in recalling the dictated area in question.

Flagging procedures vary from one facility to another. In large facilities, flagged documents may be referred to QA personnel. The notation may be incorporated into the computerized document using a color code approach with a flag message. The correct information can then be added to the document and the color coding removed. In-house flagging may simply consist of a sticky note or a preprinted flag attachment.

Up-to-date reference materials, adequate equipment, adequate dictating methods and equipment, continuing education, an ergonomically and psychologically safe work environment, and supervision by qualified MTs are essential conditions for successful QA in medical transcription.

Making Corrections

Errors that are made while keying the document should be corrected before the document is printed. Errors that are found in handwritten chart notes are corrected by drawing a single line through the error. The correction is made either just above or just below the error, and if space is available add your initials and the date. Identify the location of correct information as a cross-reference when possible. This procedure gives credibility to the record. Entries into the medical record should always be made using black ink. Black ink is considered more permanent and produces clear, dark writing that photocopies better when necessary.

When errors are found on self-adhesive typing strips, make the corrections as if the document had been handwritten. If the strip is not legible, or if it looks too messy once the corrections have been made, rekey a new strip and place it below the original. Be sure to identify it as "corrected for keying errors." The physician should sign the original and the corrected copy.

MEDICAL REPORTS

Physicians employed in all types of medical specialties including oral surgeons, dentists, and veterinarians dictate numerous types of medical reports. The transcribed medical report is a legal document and is formatted in a variety of styles similar to business correspondence. Medical reports frequently dictated by ambulatory care facilities include:

- Chart or progress notes
- History and physical examination reports
- Consultation reports
- Correspondence

Hospitals and large medical centers dictate numerous medical reports including:

- History and physical examination reports
- Consultations
- Operative reports
- Discharge summaries

Physicians employed in specialty departments within hospitals dictate specialized medical reports. Examples may include:

- Pathology reports
- Radiology reports
- Autopsy reports
- Psychiatric reports
- Medicolegal reports

Medical records become part of the patient's permanent medical record and are vital to continued patient care. Other physicians, attorneys, insurance companies, or the court may review the medical records in part, or entirety. Therefore, the medical record must be neat, accurate and complete. *Neat* refers to a medical record that is legible and assembled to permit easy access to information as needed. *Accurate* means that the dictation has been transcribed as dictated, and *complete* indicates that the document has been dated correctly and signed or initialed by the dictator. If the medical record is subpoenaed for evidence in court, the signed or initialed document indicates that the content was true and correct at the time it was written.

Complete documentation of medical records is also important for payment and/or reimbursement of services for which the physician expects to be paid. The billing and diagnosis codes reported on the health insurance claim form must be supported by the documentation contained with the medical record.

Chart Notes and Progress Notes

Chart notes are also known as progress notes or follow-up notes. They may be formal (keyed) or informal (handwritten) notes taken by physicians when they meet with or examine a patient in the office, clinic, ambulatory care center, or hospital setting. Chart notes are a concise description of the patient's present problem, the physician's physical findings, and the treatment plan. Laboratory test results may also be included within the chart note. Figure 16-1 is a sample chart/progress note.

History and Physical Examination Reports

The history and physical examination (H&P) report includes information relating to the patient's main reason for encounter. The report is divided into two sections. The first is the history, which includes the chief complaint (CC), a description of symptoms, problems, or conditions that brought the patient to the office; history of the present illness (HPI), a chronological description of the development of the patient's illness; past medical and surgical history; family history; and social history. The second section is the review of systems (ROS), an inquiry about the system directly related to the problems identified in the HPI. The physician determines the extent of the examination performed and documented based on the problems presented. The findings of the actual physical examination make up the documentation for the physical examination section of the report.

Consultation Reports

When one physician requests the services of another physician in the care and treatment of a patient, a consultation report is generated. The information may be disseminated in the form of a report or within the body of a letter. The contents of the consultation report/letter usually contain all of the elements of an H&P with a focused history of the patient's illness and the body system directly related to the consultant's area of specialty. The consultant also includes within the report/letter the findings, supporting laboratory data, diagnosis, and suggested course of treatment. Figure 16-2 is a sample consultation.

Correspondence

It is important for the MT to remember that medical correspondence also is considered medical documents and must be transcribed with the same care as any other medical record would. Review Chapter 15 for information regarding various styles and formats for business correspondence. Figure 16-3 is a sample of medical correspondence.

TURNAROUND TIME

Specific time limits are often established for completion of medical reports. Turnaround time is a term used to indicate the specific time period in which a document is expected to be completed from the time it is received by the transcriptionist until it is back for the physician to sign and made a part of the permanent medical record. Examples include:

> STAT: means immediately. Used frequently with radiology, pathology, and laboratory reports. These reports should be reported within 12 hours or less.
>
> Current: H&Ps, consultations, and operative reports. These reports should be turned around within 24 hours.

```
1/4/20__                                    HANSEN, HENRY

RV following treatment for fx of the left wrist. The cast was removed
last week. The skin texture and turgor are returning to normal. Range
of motion has increased with physical therapy, and strength is slightly
improved at -4/5. PLAN: Continue whirlpool and ROM exercises. RV 4 weeks.
                                                          AE/rf
```

Figure 16-1   Sample chart/progress note.

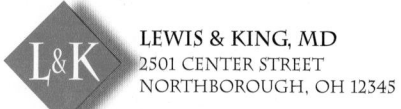

LEWIS & KING, MD
2501 CENTER STREET
NORTHBOROUGH, OH 12345

NORTHBOROUGH
FAMILY MEDICAL GROUP

January 4, 20____

Margaret Holly, MD
Metroma Medical Center
900 Union Street, Suite 208
Metroma, MI 11666

RE: MARY O'KEEFE

Dear Dr. Holly:

Thank you for referring Mary O'Keefe to our clinic. She presented
today stating that she recently relocated to Clinton with her husband
and children to be closer to her parents. Mary has been experiencing
symptoms suggestive of pregnancy and is here for evaluation. Over the
past three weeks, she has noticed increased tenderness of her breasts,
fatigue, and a feeling of being bloated. A home pregnancy test was
positive.

Her past medical history is positive for the usual childhood diseases
and the births of two children, following normal pregnancies. She has a
negative past surgical history.

She has no allergies to medications and takes Tylenol for occasional
headaches. She is married and has two children, ages 3 years and 12
months. She is employed part-time in an insurance office. She does not
smoke or drink.

The family history is noncontributory.

On review of systems, her complaints are limited to those described
above. She has had no nausea or vomiting, and no change in bowel habits.
She has no dizziness, no fevers, and no urinary symptoms.

Physical examination revealed a 32-year-old white female in no acute
distress. HEENT normocephalic, atraumatic. PERRLA, EOMI. The thyroid
was not enlarged, and there was no cervical adenopathy. The lungs were
clear. The heart had a regular rate and rhythm. The abdomen was soft
and nontender. Bowel sounds were normal. The extremities revealed trace
ankle edema. The neurological examination was within normal limits.
Pelvic examination confirmed a gravid uterus, compatible with a very
early pregnancy.

An abdominal ultrasound has been ordered and a beta HCG was drawn.

I believe Mary is pregnant and I will put her on our OB regimen starting
with monthly visits. Thank you for your kind referral.

Sincerely,

Elizabeth M. King, MD

EMK/lmb

Figure 16-2   Sample consultation.

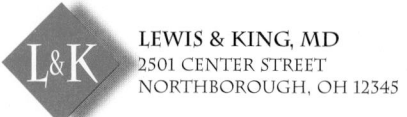

LEWIS & KING, MD
2501 CENTER STREET
NORTHBOROUGH, OH 12345

NORTHBOROUGH
FAMILY MEDICAL GROUP

January 4, 20___

Susan Smith, Coordinator
Special Project Division
American Drug Company
90058 Northover Road
Welfond, PA 44578

Dear Ms. Smith:

It is my understanding that your department oversees the Aid for
Patients program, which provides Glucogenasin for indigent patients.
I am interested in learning more about this.

I have a 74-year-old female patient who would be greatly helped by this
medication. She suffers with hypertension, adult onset diabetes mellitus,
and moderate angina. Medication compliance has been a problem; however,
we feel that this new drug, with its q.d. dosage, will be easy for her
to deal with.

Any information you could forward would be appreciated.

Yours truly,

Winston Lewis, MD

WL/bk

Figure 16-3 Sample medical correspondence.

Old: Discharge summaries and emergency department notes. These reports should be turned around within 72 hours.

ETHICAL AND LEGAL ISSUES

You will remember from Chapter 8 that ethics are not laws but rather standards of conduct. These standards vary from state to state so you will want to research your specific state's standards. The AAMT adopted a Code of Ethics for professional MTs and CMTs who are employed in hospital settings and/or are self-employed. Health Professions Institution in Modesto, California, has established Medical Transcription Industry Alliance Code of Ethics and Standards for MTs employed by transcription services.

The **Joint Commission on Accreditation of Healthcare Organizations (JCAHO)** is a commission established to improve the quality of care and services offered in health care settings through a voluntary accreditation process. Their accreditation standards are published in the *Accreditation Manual for Hospitals* (AMH). Legal aspects of the medical record applicable to the MT are not addressed by AMH; however, standards are given pertaining to medical record format. The MT is responsible only for the accuracy of the transcribed medical report and for seeing that it remains confidential.

The JCAHO requires that each hospital submit a list of abbreviations and symbols along with their meaning for approval. The approved abbreviations and symbols are the only ones that may be used by the MT for a specific hospital. Each hospital's approved list will vary, so it is important for the MT to review the list before beginning work.

The date the material was dictated, not the date it was transcribed, is the date used on a document. This is extremely important because statements within the document could reference this date. In case of litigation in which the document was entered as evidence, the physician's credibility could be questioned if dates are inconsistent.

The physician dictating the document must sign the report. If the physician is away from the office after dictating a report, and the report is urgent, the MT has two options. The MT may opt to sign the physician's name with the MT's initials after it, or to send a photocopy of the report and state that a signed original will be forwarded upon the physician's return.

Confidentiality

Confidentiality means treating the patient's medical information as private and not for publication. The patient has a right to privacy, and as such medical infor-

mation is **privileged**. Privileged information may only be communicated with the patient's permission or by court order. The MT must learn to follow the motto: *What you see here and what you hear here, must stay here when you leave here*.

The institution of **confidentiality agreements** has been established in many transcription businesses today. A signed confidentiality agreement signifies that the MT is committed to keep all patient information confidential. A **breach of confidentiality**, the unauthorized release of confidential information, is one of the few areas in which the MT can be held liable.

Risk Management

The AAMT explains **risk management** as follows: "Healthcare institution activities that identify, evaluate, reduce, and prevent the risk of injury and loss to patients, visitors, staff, and the institution itself" (1990). Medical transcriptionists are vital in this area because of their commitment to quality and their awareness of dictated data that may indicate risk management problems. The MT should immediately report this information to the appropriate designated personnel. Appropriate personnel may include the risk management manager, the office manager, a supervisor, or your employer's attorney. The MT falls under the jurisdiction of *respondeat superior,* meaning "let the master answer." In actuality, this means that the physician/dictator is liable in certain cases for the wrongful acts of the MT.

NEW TECHNOLOGY

Technology is continually changing especially in the areas involving computerized systems. The following items are areas of new technology that hold promise of significant impacts on the MT.

Continuous Speech Recognition (CSR)

Continuous Speech Recognition (CSR) is the process of direct conversion of spoken documentation into a written text (electronic) version using a computer equipped with voice recognition software. Some proponents of this advance in technology wrongly predict that when perfected, CSR will spell transcription's demise. Nothing could be further from the truth for the foreseeable future. CSR, once it is perfected, will constitute one of the most significant advances in the history of patient care delivery; but it will not replace the MT. It will, however, have a significant impact on the productivity of the MT.

CSR is currently not refined to the point where it is sufficiently accurate to be used without the MT acting as the quality control interface. The rate at which CSR software is being improved will continue to accelerate; however, it has been predicted that 10 to 20 percent of all clinical processes and records of health care delivered will never be fully converted using CSR due to complex rapidly changing vocabularies.

Accents, pronunciation, grammar, and other aspects of the clinician's personal style are difficult and costly for the CSR software to address. The MT adjusts to accents, dictation speed, and individualized pronunciations to overcome difficulties without requiring the clinician to change habits.

In most specialties it is desirable to standardize the content of patient records and ensure that critical information is included. The MT normally performs this function by cutting and pasting sections together to maintain a standardized format, and filling in gaps in sentences and information to preserve meaning without altering clinical information. CSR technologies cannot be expected to restructure reports and emphasize critical information in the foreseeable future.

CSR will become an important tool of the MT, not a replacement. It will increase productivity, and reduce the time between dictation of the oral patient record and availability of the electronic record for use by others in the health care network.

Integrating Digital Photographs into Medical Transcription

A new trend in transcription is the integration of digital images directly into the transcribed record. The response to inputting digital images (photographs, scans, and x-rays) has been very positive from both the local health care community as well as patients themselves. This is attributed to easier understanding of a picture by patients and more precise presentation using both pictures and written text to medical professionals.

The tools required for integrating digital images into word processing is already available to most MTs in their current Microsoft Word® or Corel WordPerfect® software packages. They only have to obtain a disk containing digital images from their physician/employer. If the transcribed record is included in the computer-based electronic record, also known as the electronic chart, digital images can be attached allowing other clinicians to view, enlarge, and manipulate the images at will.

DOCUMENTATION

right Marilyn Johnson 9/12/01 See entry dated 8/28/01
CXR shows perihilar infiltrate.

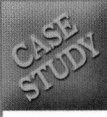

Erin Saunders is a recent graduate from a reputable junior college offering a two-year program in medical transcription. Erin was an excellent student and graduated at the top of her class. She is investigating types of employment opportunities available and has put her resume together. Erin's long-range goal is to become a CMT.

16-1

CASE STUDY REVIEW

1. List the types of work environments available for MTs and briefly describe the transcription with which each would be involved.
2. Review the CMT test content and determine which work environments would best prepare Erin for the examination. Provide the rationale for your decision.

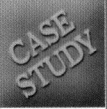

At the offices of Doctors Lewis and King, the medical transcriptionist has just completed the following content in a document: "This patient developed a persistent lesion on the inner aspect of the left upper lip. This lesion was at the junction of the vermilion and mucous membrane. A punch biopsy was obtained of this 1 cm lesion and was read as a probable verrucous squamous cell carcinoma of the lower lip."

16-2

CASE STUDY REVIEW

1. What inconsistencies, if any do you find within this document?
2. What should the MT do to verify inconsistencies and/or inaccuracies?
3. How should these inconsistencies and/or inaccuracies be corrected?

SUMMARY

Medical transcription is a vital part of patient health care. Without appropriate medical documentation it is impossible to provide quality health care, to bill insurance carriers properly to ensure physicians are reimbursed for services rendered, and to support and protect the physician should records be subpoenaed. The MT must keep all patient information strictly confidential and may be asked to sign a confidentiality agreement. A breach of confidentiality is one of the few areas in which the MT can be held liable.

Professional MTs often become CMTs and recertify every three years. A current credential indicates the active involvement in continuing education activities that keep the transcriptionist knowledgeable of new technologies, techniques, procedures, and drugs being used. Medical transcriptionists will continue to be medical language specialists. Their role and job description may change, however, with the innovation and use of new technology.

REVIEW QUESTIONS

Multiple Choice

1. AAMT student membership is available to:
   a. anyone working as an MT who has completed training
   b. anyone not working as an MT and currently enrolled in a two-year program
   c. anyone not working as an MT and currently enrolled in a nine-month or two-semester student-instructor related course
   d. anyone not working as an MT and currently enrolled in a correspondence course
2. Acquired skills developed specific to MTs include:
   a. minimum keyboarding speed of 60 words per minute
   b. love of words
   c. ability to listen and understand different accents and languages
   d. self-disciplined, detail-oriented, and independent
3. The MT who is employed by a transcription service but works from the home is known as a(n):
   a. home-based MT
   b. freelance MT
   c. associate MT
   d. self-employed MT
4. The credentialing program of AAMT is known as the:
   a. JCAHO
   b. AAMA
   c. MTCC
   d. CSR
5. Examples of ergonomics include all of the following *except:*
   a. split keyboards
   b. lumbar cushions
   c. footrests
   d. straight, flat keyboards
6. Quality assurance measures documents for all of the following *except:*
   a. line length of document
   b. accuracy and completeness
   c. consistency in health care documentation
   d. timely preparation
7. MTs with a question that cannot be resolved should:
   a. guess at what is being dictated
   b. edit the document and exclude what cannot be understood
   c. flag the document
   d. refuse to transcribe documents for that physician
8. Types of documents transcribed in ambulatory care settings include all of the following *except:*
   a. chart notes
   b. HPI
   c. H&Ps
   d. consultation reports
9. Turnaround time for most laboratory reports should be:
   a. STAT
   b. current
   c. within 12 hours
   d. both a and b
10. Continuous speech recognition:
    a. cannot restructure reports and emphasize critical information
    b. involves the integration of digital images into the transcribed document
    c. operates on the premise that a picture is worth a thousand words
    d. is available with MS Word® and Corel WordPerfect® software packages

Critical Thinking

1. List the personal attributes and acquired skills specific to the medical transcription career, and discuss why these are important.
2. Read through the section on employment opportunities again. Now use the World Wide Web for additional research and develop a work environment in which you personally would feel comfortable as an employee. Discuss with classmates your discoveries, and explain why you arrived at them.
3. Design a workstation on paper, and list a minimum of 10 ergonomic considerations.
4. Discuss the meaning of QA and its implications on insurance billing.
5. Identify possible legal issues that could arise if medical records are not corrected appropriately.
6. Discuss the importance of turnaround time and its legal implications.
7. Discuss the requirements of JCAHO and the use of abbreviations within medical records.

WEB ACTIVITIES

Using the World Wide Web, locate the AAMT web site, and search through the web pages to locate the *Medical Transcriptionist's Bill of Rights*. Download this item. Discuss it with a classmate, or follow your instructor's directions related to this activity.

REFERENCES/BIBLIOGRAPHY

American Association for Medical Transcription. (1990). *AAMT Model Job Description: Medical Transcriptionist*. Modesto, CA: author.

American Association for Medical Transcription. *A medical transcriptionist's bill of rights* [On-line]. Available: http://www.aamt.org/billorts.htm

American Association for Medical Transcription. *MTCC Disciplinary Policy and Procedures* [On-line]. Available: http://www.aamt.org/certcode.htm

American Association for Medical Transcription. *Student membership* [On-line]. Available: http://www.aamt.org/stu.htm

Burns, L., & Maloney, F. (1997). *Medical transcription and terminology: An integrated approach*. Albany, NY: Delmar.

Diehl, M. O., & Fordney, M. T. (1997). *Medical keyboarding, typing, and transcribing techniques and procedures* (4th ed). Philadelphia: W. B. Saunders Company.

Ettinger, B., & Ettinger, A. G. (1997). *Medical transcription*. St. Paul, MN: Paradigm Publishing, Inc.

Kinn, M. E., & Woods, M. A. (1999). *The medical assistant: Administrative and clinical* (8th ed). Philadelphia: W. B. Saunders Company.

The medical transcription workbook (1999). Modesto, CA: Health Professions Institute.

Shaha, S. (1999). The future of transcription with continuous speech recognition. *Journal of the American Association for Medical Transcription, 18*(6), 12–14.

Tessier, C. (1995). *AAMT Book of Style for Medical Transcription*. Modesto, CA: author.

Tossey, K. L. (1998). The integration of digital photographs into medical transcription. *Journal of the American Association for Medical Transcription, 17*(6), 19–21.

MANAGING FACILITY FINANCES

DAILY FINANCIAL PRACTICES

KEY TERMS

Accounts Payable
Accounts Receivable
Adjustments
Balance
Cashier's Check
Certified Check
Charges
Charge Slip
Credit
Currency
Day Sheet
Disbursement
Ledger
Money Market Account
Notary
Payee
Pegboard System
Petty Cash
Petty Cash Voucher
Posting
ROA
Superbill
Traveler's Check
Usual, Customary, and Reasonable
  (UCR)
Voucher Check
Write-It-Once System

OUTLINE

Determining Patient Fees
Usual, Reasonable, and Customary
  Fees
Discussion of Fees
Adjustment of Fees
Credit Arrangements
Payment Planning
The Bookkeeping Function
Managing Patient Accounts
The Importance of Good Working
  Habits
The Pegboard System
Computerized Systems
Banking Procedures
Types of Accounts
Types of Checks

Deposits
Accepting Checks
Lost or Stolen Checks
Writing and Recording Checks
Reconciling a Bank Statement
**Purchasing Supplies and
Equipment**
Preparing a Purchase Order
Verifying Goods Received
Preparing the Invoice for Payment
Petty Cash
Establishing a Petty Cash Fund
Tracking, Balancing, and
  Replenishing Petty Cash

OBJECTIVES

*The student should strive to meet the following performance objectives and demonstrate
an understanding of the facts and principles presented in this chapter through written and
oral communication.*

1. Define the key terms as presented in the glossary.
2. Understand the importance of communication in regard to establishing
   patient fees.
3. Develop a knowledge of various credit arrangements for patient fees.
4. Differentiate between manual and computerized bookkeeping systems.
5. State the advantages of the pegboard system.
6. State the advantages of computerized systems.
7. Demonstrate a knowledge of banking procedures, including types of
   accounts and services.
8. Show proficiency in preparing bank deposits, writing checks, recording
   checks, and reconciling accounts. *(continues)*

9. Explain the process of purchasing equipment and supplies for the ambulatory care setting.

10. Demonstrate proficiency in establishing and maintaining a petty cash system.

ROLE DELINEATION COMPONENTS

ADMINISTRATIVE

Administrative Procedures

- **Perform basic clerical functions**

Practice Finances

- **Apply bookkeeping principles**
- **Document and maintain accounting and banking records**
- **Manage accounts receivable**
- **Manage accounts payable**
- l **Develop and maintain fee schedules (advanced)**

GENERAL (TRANSDISCIPLINARY)

Legal Conceps

- **Document accurately**

SCENARIO

At the offices of Doctors Lewis & King, many different types of patients are seen: most have some kind of insurance, either a traditional plan or an HMO-type plan, some are on Medicare, a few on Medicaid, and occasionally a patient does not have any insurance or any financial resources to pay for treatment. Whoever schedules the first patient appointment also opens a frank but courteous discussion with the patient about physician fees and the patient's anticipated method of payment. Initiating this discussion of fees at the beginning of the physician-patient relationship keeps patients informed of their responsibility for payment and helps the medical assistants at Doctors Lewis & King make any necessary credit arrangements with the patient before treatment begins.

INTRODUCTION

Ambulatory care settings are primarily designed to serve the patient. However, without sound financial practices, patient care will suffer and the office will not thrive and grow. The health care industry has become more complex in recent years with the explosion of managed care. The impact of managed care has been tremendous and it affects not only the way patients receive treatment but the manner in which the ambulatory care center is administered from a financial point of view.

Of course, this discussion of fees is only a small part of the ambulatory care setting's daily financial practices. Selecting an appropriate bookkeeping method, taking responsibility for banking, managing the purchase of supplies, and establishing a petty cash system are all vital to the smooth functioning of today's ambulatory care setting.

DETERMINING PATIENT FEES

In today's managed care climate, ambulatory care settings have many different arrangements with insurance carriers and with their patients. Often, the office or urgent care center will have a contract with HMO-type insurance carriers in which they agree to a specific fee for certain procedures. In this instance, the physicians of the center are usually known as participating providers. In some plans, the patient pays what is known as a copay amount for each visit. In other situations, the patient is liable for a certain percentage of the fee. This is usually known as coinsurance. Ambulatory care centers may also accept Medicare and Medicaid patients, usually for a predetermined fee.

The situations for payment are numerous and varied, and subsequent chapters in this unit will examine them in greater detail. Of critical importance at the onset of the patient relationship, however, is that both patient and physician have an understanding of their fiscal responsibility to each other. The patient must also be made aware of any fees imposed for missed appointments, telephone consultation, and other charges the patient may not anticipate. It is not unethical to charge for these, but it is not recommended without prior notification to the patient. Insurance carriers will not reimburse missed appointment charges. If the office plans to implement charges, they need to have a signed waiver from the patient. The waiver explains that you have notified the patient in advance that these charges will be added to their account.

Usual, Customary, and Reasonable Fees

A fee schedule often used by Medicare and some insurance carriers is referred to as usual, reasonable, and customary fees. Usual refers to the fee typically charged by a physician for certain procedures; customary is based on the average charge for a specific procedure by all physicians practicing the same specialty in a defined geographic region; and reasonable refers to the midrange of fees charged for this procedure. Also see Chapter 18.

Discussion of Fees

The manner in which billing is done and fees established will vary depending on the type of medical facility, the needs of the practice, and the professional services rendered. Years ago, personnel in medical facilities would typically ask patients at the end of their visits if they would like to pay then or be billed later. It is now customary and in some offices mandatory to request payment at the time of service. Today, the fee for the visit is simply stated, and if a person does not have cash or a check, the option of credit card payment is often provided. If a patient is a member of an HMO, and the ambulatory care setting is a member of that HMO, then the patient is typically responsible only for any established copay amount.

Inherent to the total billing process (see Chapter 20) is the necessity of initially establishing a fee schedule and informing patients of charges and exactly what portion of the bill they are expected to pay. Ideally, the patient should be told the approximate cost of the procedures at the start of treatment. For Medicare and Medicaid patients, this must be in writing and should indicate the type of procedure(s), the total responsibility of the patient, and the reason why this is the patient's responsibility. This form is officially known by Medicare as an Advanced Beneficiary Notification, or by Medicaid as a waiver. These forms are the only legal means an office has to collect payment on charges not allowed by Medicare or Medicaid. Charges for some daily routine visits may be submitted to the insurance carrier, and the office may not know what portion is covered until information is received from the carrier. The facility may accept numerous insurance plans and participation in these plans determines the amount that the patient owes. Many misunderstandings will be prevented and subsequent collection of delinquent accounts expedited when the office staff is well informed about insurance reimbursement and carefully explains fees to the patients.

Adjustment of Fees

If an office accepts assignment with Medicare and Medicaid, they are mandated to charge every patient the same amount for similar services rendered. If an office extends a professional courtesy, it is considered insurance fraud. The office would then be billing insurance an increased rate than what they charge others. More specifically, deductibles are to be collected from the patient; this is part of their premium expectation. Unless you follow government guidelines for establishing when a patient is financially unable to pay their portion of the bill, you cannot give discounts to patients for cash payments.

Adjustments may be made for patients with limited income. For example, if a patient had been going to the ambulatory care center for many years, but recently lost a job or ran into unfortunate financial circumstances, the physician may "write off" a portion of the bill. This sum will be written off against the physician's income, and the patient will not have to pay any amount or will pay a reduced amount according to what is affordable. This courtesy usually applies to only existing patients and is not offered to new patients.

Adjustments also may occur with Medicare, Medicaid, Blue Shield, and private health insurance patients. Physicians who accept assignment in these programs agree to accept as payment in full what the insurer allows. For instance, a fee of $150 may be charged, but $95 is accepted as payment in full by the provider. The remainder of the bill, $55, is written off so that the patient is not responsible for this remainder of the fee.

Medical assistants must be aware, however, of the pitfalls of adjusting or reducing fees. It is difficult to accept all hardship cases and still remain a viable practice. It is always a helpful resource to patients who cannot pay to be given the names and telephone numbers of local health care clinics that may be able to accept them as patients on a sliding scale or no-fee basis.

CREDIT ARRANGEMENTS

If the patient will need to pay a substantial out-of-pocket amount, it is helpful to make the patient aware of this and discuss different credit arrangements that can be made. Many ambulatory care settings will work out installment payments, usually without finance charges, to spread the cost of services over a pre-agreed period of time. This eases the financial burden on the patient and also makes it more likely that the office will be able to collect monies due.

Payment Planning

Medical assistants can help patients plan for anticipated medical expenses (having a baby, surgery, extensive therapy). When patient and physician know in advance that there will be costly medical expenses, the medical assistant should review the patient's insurance coverage. It is also helpful to prepare an estimate sheet, which will give the patient an idea of the cost of the medical services for the planned treatment. The estimate may also include the cost of anesthetist, consultants, and hospital charges.

More recently, ambulatory care settings have begun to accept credit cards as a means of payment. It must be remembered that this is strictly for the convenience of the patient. According to the AMA Code of Ethics, physicians should not increase their charges for patients who wish to use credit cards nor encourage patients to use credit cards. Physicians, therefore, may offer the service, but not actively encourage its use.

The one advantage to the ambulatory care setting that accepts credit cards is that monies for fees charged are usually available within 24 hours or so. Also, the physician is relieved of the responsibility of collection. However, credit card companies do assess a fee for every charge made, which the ambulatory care center must pay.

When a patient decides to use a credit card, it is extremely important that confidentiality be maintained to the fullest extent possible. When writing a description of the services on the credit card receipt, the medical assistant should be as vague as possible to preserve patient confidentiality. For example, medical services versus STD testing.

THE BOOKKEEPING FUNCTION

Daily financial management in the ambulatory care setting is most important to the functioning of the office as it

SPOTLIGHT ON AAMA ESSENTIALS THROUGH CAAHEP

- Portraying a positive attitude when dealing with the patient regarding his or her financial obligations will help the patient maintain a positive relationship with all members of the health care practice.

- Positive communication between members of the staff responsible for daily financial practices and those responsible for caring for the patient's needs is paramount to the efficiency of a smooth-running and financially stable practice.

- Members of the staff responsible for the practice's daily financial duties must maintain a high level of integrity and honesty; the physician-employer must be able to depend upon them for his or her livelihood and for the livelihood of those employed at the practice.

directly affects overall accounting and bookkeeping procedures. Accounting generates financial information for the ambulatory care setting and is defined as a system of monitoring the financial status of a facility and the specific results of its activities. Accounting provides financial information for decision making. (See Chapter 21.) Bookkeeping, the actual daily recording of the accounts or transactions of the business, is the major part of this accounting process. This chapter deals with daily bookkeeping (or recording) functions necessary to manage the income and expenses of an ambulatory care setting.

Managing Patient Accounts

All businesses must keep careful records of income and expenses for tax and legal purposes. One aspect of this recordkeeping in a medical practice is maintaining patient accounts. Since few patients are able to pay in full each time they are seen by the physician, it is necessary to maintain account records for each individual or family as opposed to simply keeping a record of cash received as is done in many other types of business. The money owed to the office by patients is known as **accounts receivable**, and must be carefully monitored to assure that the physician is paid for services provided and that patients are properly credited for payments made.

There are various ways to track patients' balances. In this chapter we will discuss the two most common methods:

- The **pegboard** system (also known as the **write-it-once** method)

- Computerized systems

Though many practices are fully automated, all except the newest ones probably started with some sort of manual system (generally pegboard). Converting from manual to computerized record-keeping is initially expensive, requires thorough retraining of staff, and takes a great deal of time at the beginning. However, it offers great versatility and reduces the need to record and re-record entries.

However, it is necessary for a well-prepared medical assistant to be fully versed in both bookkeeping systems.

The Importance of Good Working Habits

In managing the day-to-day finances of the ambulatory care setting, always observe two guidelines:

1. Always work with care and accuracy; it is extremely easy to transpose numbers (i.e., writing 23 instead of 32) or make other posting errors. A moment of carelessness can result in hours spent trying to find the mistake.
2. The work must be kept current or it may become an overwhelming chore.

Also, develop these habits:

- Form your numerals and letters carefully with good penmanship.
- Use a consistent ink color.
- Align your columns.
- Be careful when carrying decimal points.
- Double-check your math.
- If a mistake is found, neatly cross out the incorrect figure and write the correct figure above it.

The Pegboard System

A complete pegboard or write-it-once system consists of day sheets, ledger cards, charge slips, and receipt forms. The forms are designed to work together to simplify the task and to avoid costly and embarrassing mistakes in patient accounts. All forms will have matching columns

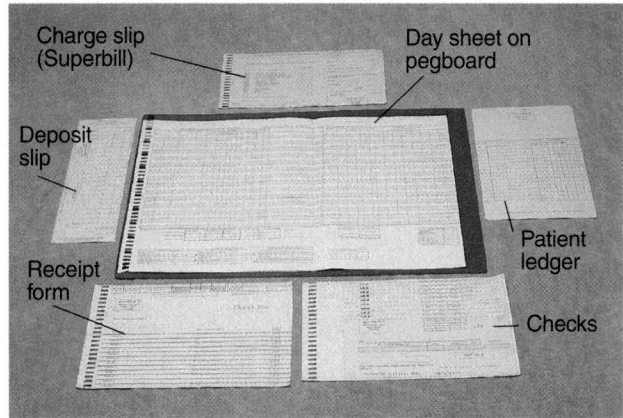

Figure 17-1 An example of the pegboard system and possible overlays.

that align and are held in place on the pegboard when the system is in use (Figure 17-1). The forms are generally carboned or on NCR© paper (no carbon required), which permits entering of **charges**, credits or **adjustments**, or **posting**, onto the day sheet, charge slip, or receipt and the patient's ledger card simultaneously. Some major advantages of the pegboard system include:

- The system is efficient and timesaving—by only having to enter information once, it is impossible to enter incorrect information on one of the forms due to copying errors or errors of omission. (This can also be a major disadvantage when an error made and entered appears on *all* forms.)

- The **day sheet** provides complete and up-to-date information about accounts receivable status at a glance.

- A pegboard system is relatively inexpensive.

Several companies produce pegboard systems, all with slight variations. Though the information and method of use are the same, it is not usually possible to "mix and match" forms from different companies since even a slight difference in column width or location will make the forms incompatible.

Day Sheets. The day sheet is used to list or post each day's charges, payments, credits, and adjustments: the daily financial transactions. This is an important part of the overall bookkeeping process, so legibility and absolute accuracy are critical. At the close of each business day, the day sheet will be balanced to provide a complete picture of all patient financial activity for that day. Those balances carried over from day to day will provide the accumulated data needed for month-end closing.

The day sheet consists of five sections (Figure 17-2), the first three of which are used when posting transactions

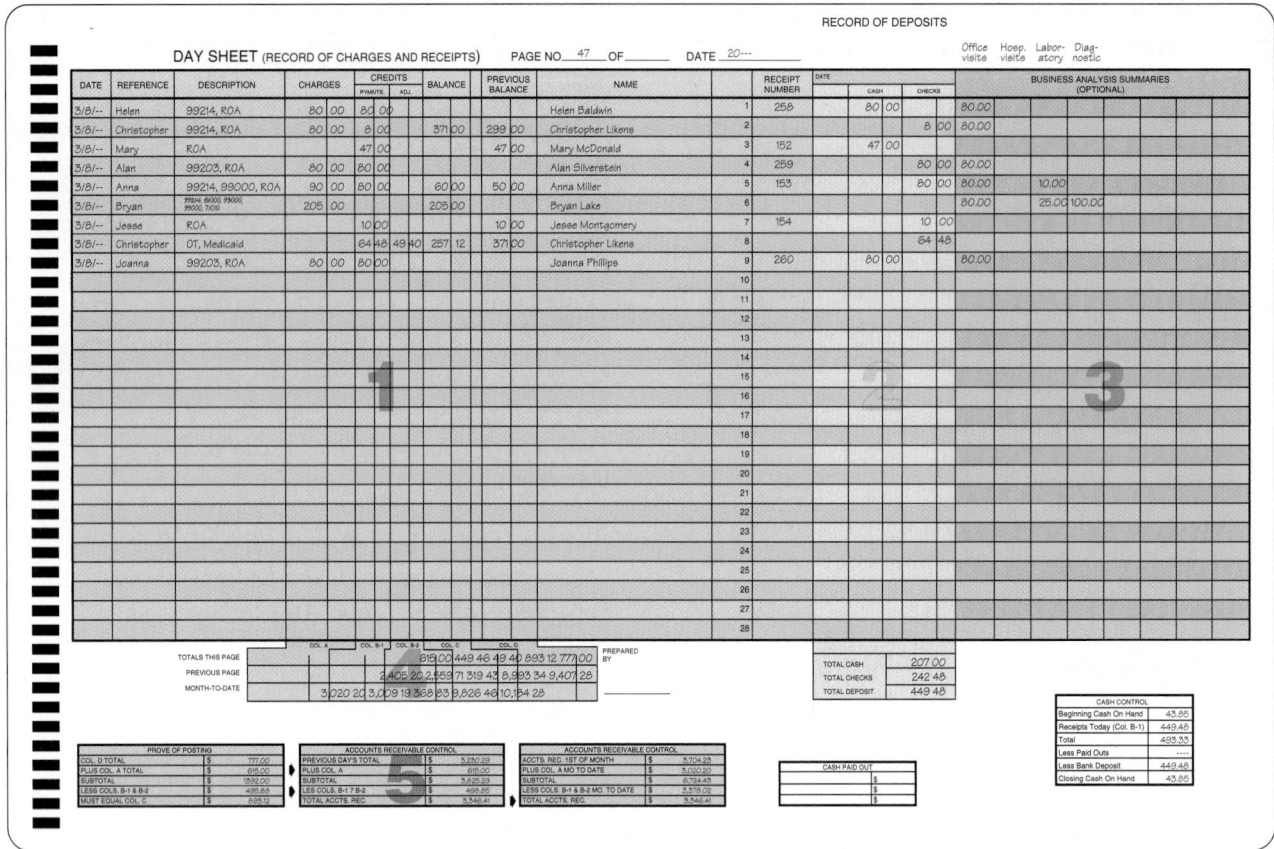

Figure 17-2   Pegboard day sheet with major sections.

and the last two of which are for balancing, proof of posting, accounts receivable control, and accounts receivable proof.

- *Section 1* is where individual transactions are posted, using the ledger card and charge slips, or receipt forms. The information here includes the date, patient name, description of transaction or service, charges, credits, and previous and current balances. This is the write-it-once portion of the day sheet.

- *Section 2* is the deposit portion (some companies make this part detachable to be used as an actual deposit slip). If a transaction includes a payment, the payment amount will be listed under the appropriate right-hand column showing method of payment after the ledger portion is posted.

- *Section 3* is for business analysis. These columns might be used for recording payments or charges to be credited to different physicians or they are often used as a breakdown for types of service (i.e., office examination, hospital visit, surgery, and so on). The use of this area will vary from practice to practice.

- *Section 4* is where transactions are totaled and balanced at the end of the day. (See Procedure 17-5 later in the chapter.)

- *Section 5* is used to verify the daily balances and to balance and track cumulative accounts receivable figures. The total accounts receivable figure shows how much is owed to the practice by all patients to date, allowing the physician or administrator to see the total outstanding balance at a glance without having to add hundreds of individual balances.

Ledger Cards. It is, of course, necessary to maintain a record of services provided and charges and payments for each individual seen in the office or hospital. This is accomplished by creating a separate **ledger** for each patient household. In order to easily keep track of patient accounts, there should be a responsible party for each family whose name and address will appear in the mailing window at the top of the ledger card (Figure 17-3). In a case where both spouses are employed and each is covered by employer-provided insurance, there may be more than one responsible party. It is also possible to have more than one responsible party for a household if one child is from a

STATEMENT

LEWIS & KING MD, PC
2501 CENTER STREET
NORTHBOROUGH, OH
(312) 824-6925

DATE	REFERENCE	DESCRIPTION	CHARGES	CREDITS		BALANCE

BALANCE FORWARD ➔

RB40BC-2

PLEASE PAY LAST AMOUNT IN BALANCE COLUMN

THIS IS A COPY OF YOUR ACCOUNT AS IT APPEARS ON OUR RECORDS

(A)

TELEPHONE	SPOUSE NAME	DATE OF BIRTH	SOC. SEC. NO.	DRIVERS LIC. NO.

EMPLOYER: CITY - STATE - PHONE | SPOUSE EMPLOYER: CITY - STATE - PHONE

NAME - ADDRESS - PHONE OF NEAREST RELATIVE | OTHER PROF. SERVICE USED: CITY - STATE - PHONE

CREDIT/INSURANCE INFORMATION

OWN ☐ RENT ☐

COMMENTS

USE LEAD PENCIL - FELT TIP MARKER - TYPEWRITER

(B)

Figure 17-3 Patient ledger card: (A) Front of ledger. (B) Back of ledger.

spouse's prior marriage and the responsible party is the noncustodial parent. Services or payments for any other members of the family seen in the office or hospital will be entered on the same ledger and the patient's first name (or coded number) will be written in the space provided (reference space columns). If the office is doing insurance billing or receiving insurance payments, it is extremely important that charges and credits be applied to the correct family member, so never omit this step when making entries.

The columns on the front of the ledger card will show the date of activity, name of patient, a clear description of type of activity, amount of charge or credit, adjustments (if any), and the family's total balance due.

The back of the ledger card in Figure 17-3 includes all pertinent patient and insurance information needed for collection purposes.

The ledger is placed under the charge slip or receipt, directly on the day sheet, and aligned prior to posting. *Never* post any patient entry without the patient's ledger in place. This prevents recording information on the day

sheet and thus omitting it inadvertently from the patient's ledger.

Charge Slips and Receipts. The charge slip (or superbill) shown in Figures 17-1 and 17-4 is a three-part form that:

1. Provides patients with a record of account activity for the day
2. May eliminate the need for separate insurance forms
3. Provides the office with a copy of that day's services, which will be filed in the individual's chart

Charge slips can be ordered to fit the practice. Information on the charge slip includes not only the amount of the day's transaction, but procedure codes and diagnosis codes (see Chapter 19) that satisfy the requirements for most insurance companies to reimburse the patient or physician. When the slips are ordered, the office will indicate the most common services provided, which will be printed on the form with the applicable procedure codes

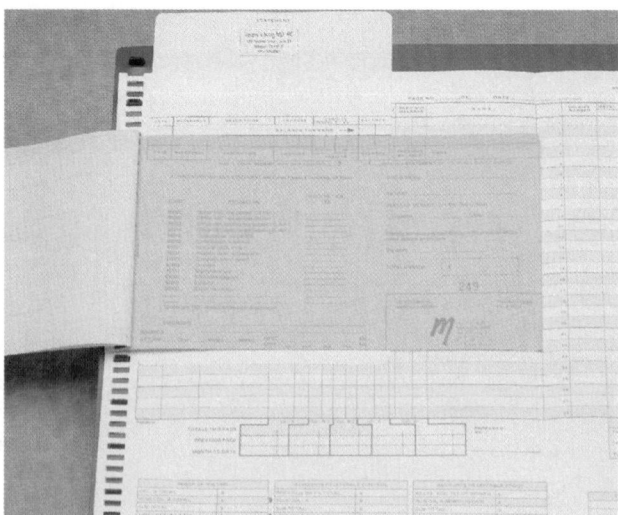

Figure 17-4 Pegboard with day sheet, ledger card, and charge slip.

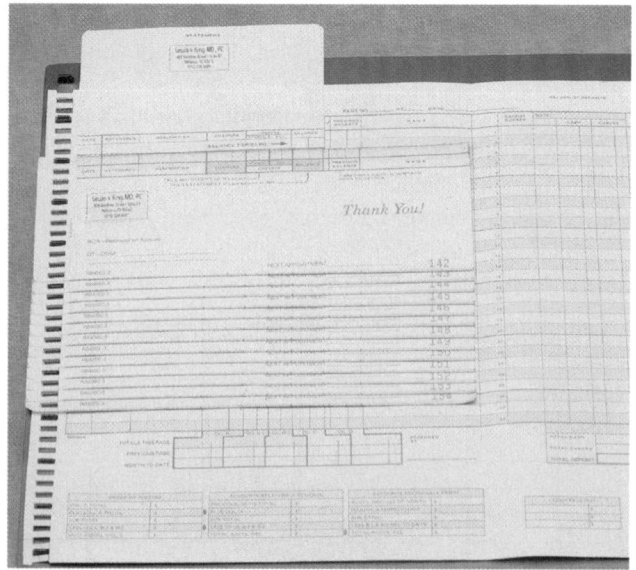

Figure 17-5 Pegboard with day sheet, ledger card, and receipt.

(and some blank lines for infrequently used procedures). After seeing the patient, the physician places a check mark beside the services rendered. In addition, there is an area for the diagnosis code to be filled in by the physician at the same time. The charge slip is printed with the name, address, and telephone number of the practice.

Unlike charge slips, the receipt forms (Figures 17-1 and 17-5) used for payments on account are not customized other than to have the name, address, and telephone number of the practice preprinted. The receipt form is only used when someone makes a payment on account and no services are rendered that day. There is only one copy of this form, which is given to the patient after the payment is recorded. Like many charge slips, the receipt form may include a space to write in the date of the patient's next appointment. It is not necessary to keep any other record of the transaction, since it is entered on the day sheet and ledger card at the time the receipt is filled out using the write-it-once procedures.

Recording Information: Charges, Credits, and Adjustments.
Procedures 17-1, 17-2, 17-3, and 17-4 provide step-by-step details on posting and recording activities.

Adjustments.
These are entries made to change the patient's balance but do not represent charges or payments. The adjustment column is a **credit** column, and therefore entries here normally reduce the balance due. When making an adjustment intended to increase the balance, a negative entry (in parentheses) is made to show that you will reverse the function when you balance (add instead of subtract the amount).

As noted earlier in this chapter, adjustments are frequently made to show a reduction in fee for service granted by the physician, a write-off to the account if the physician has agreed to accept insurance as payment in full, or to correct an error in posting. For example, Edith Leonard had surgery for which the physician agreed to reduce his fee by half of the balance remaining after insurance has paid. At the time of the surgery a charge of $2,500 was entered on her ledger and the day sheet. Today payment is received from her insurance company in the amount of $2,000, which would normally leave a balance of $500. However, since the physician agreed to write off half of that amount ($250), you would enter $250 in the adjustment column when posting the insurance payment. Since the adjustment column is a credit column, this amount, along with the payment received, is subtracted from the previous balance to arrive at the new balance of $250.

Balancing Day Sheets.
In any bookkeeping function balancing is done to be certain all entries are correct. Day sheets are always balanced at the end of each workday. Occasionally, in a busy practice, more than one day sheet will be required to record all of the transactions for a full day. If that happens, **balance** each day sheet as if it were the end of the day and carry the standard information forward to the next sheet just as if it were a new day. The day sheet will have a place to enter the page number if more than one page is needed for posting transactions for a single day (i.e., Page 1 of 2). Be sure to number and date all pages.

Most medical assistants will be entering an established practice, where there is a financial history and previous accounts receivable balance and work with the first and second day sheets of a new month. This means that there will be a figure on the line of "Accounts Receivable

Control" and the "Accounts Receivable Proof" boxes showing the accounts receivable balance from the end of the preceding month. Since the first day sheet being balanced is for the first working day of the month, the column boxes marked "Previous Page" will all contain a zero that can be entered at the same time as the information carried forward at the beginning of the day. See Procedure 17-5 for steps in balancing day sheets. NOTE: When balancing any financial information, always use a calculator with the print function turned on to create a tape of the calculations. These tapes will be an invaluable timesaver if the initial balance is incorrect and you need to search for mistakes.

Month-End. When the last day sheet for the month has been balanced, it is then necessary to verify that the month-end figures on the day sheet agree with patients' ledgers. Though this may be a time-consuming process, it will find mistakes before they grow into major accounting or collection problems.

Reconciling the month-end sheet to the patient ledgers is accomplished by adding all the open balances on the ledger cards and verifying that the total agrees with the end-of-month accounts receivable balance on the last day sheet of the month. When these figures agree, the accounts receivable balance is correct.

By following these procedures of "checks and balances," it is likely that all monies have been properly credited to patient accounts and deposited and that all charges shown as outstanding on the day sheet agree with the outstanding balances of the individual patient accounts. If a payment is somehow misplaced, the deposits will not agree with the credits or with the patient ledgers and it will be known immediately that money is missing. Not only does this catch errors, it also eliminates the possibility of undetected theft of funds, for when a mistake is caught immediately, the payer can stop payment on the missing check or credit card slip and a new payment can be made.

Computerized Systems

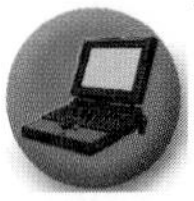

With increasing numbers of medical facilities turning to computers for word processing, patient records, and bookkeeping, there is an ever-increasing number of medical practice software packages on the market. These ready-made systems are available for both single or dual physician offices and large group practices. Often, a consultant is hired to design a customized program, though this is far more expensive than purchasing mass-produced software. When selecting and using any computer bookkeeping software:

- Be sure the system will meet not only current needs but future needs as well (some packages can be expanded to grow with the practice).
- The hardware (computer system) must be powerful enough to run the program.
- To use the automated system, it is necessary to understand the workings of the manual procedures on which the computerized accounting is based.

Computerized Patient Accounts. A software management program offers many advantages in managing patient accounts. The program automatically creates a charge slip at the time of each patient's visit. After the physician's examination, the program calculates the charges for the monthly billing statement (Figure 17-6). The management program also creates and updates the

LEWIS & KING, MD
2501 CENTER STREET
NORTHBOROUGH, OH 12345

STATEMENT DATE 08/29/--
PATIENT NUMBER 113
PREVIOUS BALANCE $0.00

OFFICE PHONE: (404) 555-0078

DATE	CODE	DESCRIPTION	AMOUNT
02/12/--	00000	BALANCE FORWARD	23.00
02/16/--	71020	CHEST X RAY, 2 VIEWS	40.00
03/14/--	81000	URINALYSIS	20.00
04/22/--	85022	CBC	12.50
06/13/--	99221	INIT. HOSP. EXAM, EXTENSIVE	75.00
07/05/--	93040	RHYTHM STRIP	—
07/26/--	93000	ELECTROCARDIOGRAM	52.00
08/29/--	PMT	PERSONAL CHECK	-93.65 CR
		BALANCE DUE	$128.85

OFFICE CLOSED SEPTEMBER 5TH.
NEW CHARGES HAVE BEEN SENT
TO YOUR INSURANCE CARRIER(S).

STATEMENT DATE 08/29/--

CURRENT	0.00
OVER 30-DAYS:	52.00
OVER 60-DAYS:	75.00
OVER 90-DAYS:	1.85
BALANCE DUE	$128.85

THANK YOU FOR YOUR PAYMENT.

113

MARTIN GORDON
107 KNOWLEDGE DRIVE
NORTHBOROUGH, OH 12345

Figure 17-6 Computerized patient bill.

```
                              PATIENT LEDGER
                              ==============


      Patient #218              O'KEEFE, MARY              Date:    06/24/--
                                43 KINGSBORO AVENUE
                                NORTHBOROUGH, OH 12345     PHONE: (404) 555-6123


               Insured #1                        Insured #2

               SAME                              O'KEEFE, JOHN
                                                 43 KINGSBORO AVENUE
                                                 NORTHBOROUGH, OH 12345

      Insurance #1:  PRUDENTIAL       Policy #:  987654321    Group #:  987700
      Insurance #2:  BLUE CROSS       Policy #:  321654907    Group #:  123456987

      ================================================================================

      01/26/--     59400      TOTAL OBSTETRICAL CARE                    1200.00
      01/26/--     99202      INTERMEDIATE EXAM, NEW PT.                  30.00
      01/26/--     88150      PAPANICOLAOU SMEAR                          18.50
      01/26/--     PMT           DEPOSIT OB CARE                        -250.00
      02/18/--     PMT           Insur. Pmt.   01/26/-- 90015            -20.00
      02/18/--     ADJ           Adj. Cat. #1  01/26/-- 90015            -10.00
      02/25/--     85022      CBC                                         12.50
      02/25/--     99212      LIMITED EXAM, ESTAB. PT.                    15.00
      02/25/--     PMT           Cash Pmt.    01/26/-- 94000             -75.00
      04/26/--     85022      CBC                                         12.50
      04/26/--     99212      LIMITED EXAM, ESTAB. PT.                    15.00
      04/26/--     76805      DIAGNOSTIC ULTRASOUND                       55.00
      04/26/--     88150      PAPANICOLAOU SMEAR                          18.50
                                                                     ---------
                              Balance for MARY O'KEEFE                $1,022.00
```

Figure 17-7   Computerized patient ledger card.

ledger card, adds new names to the list of patients and to the daily log, and transfers data to produce insurance forms, statements, a list of checks received each day, and deposit slips. In addition, the program automatically ages accounts at each billing cycle and creates billing statements. As a result, when patient accounts are computerized, practice collections usually increase.

Computerized Patient Ledger. The computerized patient ledger contains personal information about each patient, including the name, address, and telephone number, the person responsible for payment, and all insurance carriers (Figure 17-7). The ledger also lists all previous office visits and the procedures, procedure codes, charges, payments, and adjustments for each visit. Most account management software can be customized to meet the special needs of the individual ambulatory care setting.

As information is entered from the charge slips, the computer automatically updates the ledger by adding a description of each procedure and procedure code and each diagnosis and diagnosis code (see Chapter 19 for coding information). It automatically posts the charges and calculates the balance after credits and adjustments are entered.

Although the ability to view a patient's account is fairly accessible, once charges and/or payments have been entered they are not easily removed or changed. This is important as it ensures that monies are not removed from receivables credited to a previous month. This procedure would cause the practice year-end balance to be off.

As useful and efficient as a computerized bookkeeping system can be, it is important to recognize that an inadequate manual system will not get better once computerized. Also, it takes far more time than predicted to move to a computerized system, train personnel, and enter patient data. A manual and computer system may need to run concurrently for several months.

BANKING PROCEDURES

Understanding banking accounts and services, making deposits, writing checks, and reconciling accounts are all a part of daily financial practices. While many banking services are similar from one bank to another, it is a good idea for the medical assistant in charge of maintaining daily accounts to investigate the banking resources of the local community. In an effort to secure new business, many banks compete for customers by offering special services that can be of utility to the ambulatory care setting.

Types of Accounts

Checking and savings accounts are the two primary types of accounts.

Checking Accounts. The checking account is the primary account type the medical assistant will use in the ambulatory care setting. Stated simply, a checking account allows the depositor to write checks against money placed in the account. Today, there are many variations on checking accounts; in the event that the medical assistant is responsible for establishing a new account, it is worthwhile to investigate features of different checking accounts both within the same bank and at competing banks.

Some features that may differ include:

- Interest paid
- Monthly fees
- Per check fees
- Automated teller machine (ATM) access and fees
- Initial deposit and balance requirements
- Fees for checks
- Special services extended free of charge such as notary, cashier's checks, traveler's checks, balance reconciliation, and services designed expressly for small businesses.

When selecting an account, do not only choose the account with the lowest fees. Also consider convenience, the relationship possible with a given bank, number of bank locations, and other factors.

Savings Accounts. Savings accounts were initially distinguished from checking accounts because they paid interest on the money deposited. However, many checking accounts also pay interest now as well. In either case, the interest is usually minimal on accounts that give immediate access to the deposit. Some money market savings accounts pay a higher rate of interest, although they require a higher initial deposit and maintenance of a higher balance, usually around $2500. Access to the account is limited; often the depositor is permitted to write three checks a month on the account. Savings accounts are useful when money is not needed on demand or when putting monies aside for long-term goals.

Types of Checks

For the most part, the ambulatory care setting will use a standard business check. However, for special purposes, it is useful to understand the other check types available:

- A cashier's check is often used when a check must be guaranteed for the amount in which it is written. Because a cashier's check is the bank's own check drawn against the bank's accounts, the recipient has the assurance that the check will clear.

Cashier's checks are obtained at the bank by paying the bank representative cash or sometimes a personal check for the amount of the cashier's check.

- A certified check is the depositor's own check which the bank has "certified" with a date and signature to indicate that the check is good for the amount in which it is written.

- Money orders are available from banks and the United States Postal Service. They are purchased with cash and are used in ways similar to cashier's checks.

- A voucher check is a type of check with a stub attached to it which can be used to indicate invoice dates, services provided, and so on. Many payroll checks are written on voucher checks; the voucher check is also frequently used in the ambulatory care setting for accounts payable.

- Traveler's checks are available in most banks and are convenient and safer to use than cash when traveling. They are written in specific denominations ($10, $20, $50) and require a signature when purchased and when used.

Deposits

Deposits are usually made daily since they serve as another proof of posting and because it is unwise to leave large sums of money in the office overnight. The office should have a rubber endorsement stamp from the bank; use it to immediately imprint the back of all checks received directly from patients and in the mail. Before depositing them, be sure all checks are stamped.

Because the endorsement transfers rights to whoever holds the check, it is important to take certain precautions. A blank endorsement consists of a signature only (whether in pen or with a stamp) and presents a danger in that, if the check is lost or stolen, someone else could endorse the check below the signature and cash it. A restrictive endorsement should be used on all checks received in the ambulatory care setting. Restrictive endorsements include the signature as well as the words "for deposit only" or "pay to the order of (include the name of bank and account number. Additionally, all possible payees' names should be listed under the company name, with the practice address)." This restricts the use of the check should it be lost or stolen.

Most business accounts use a deposit slip similar to the one in Figure 17-8. They are always filled out in duplicate—one copy to accompany the deposit, one to be retained for office records. As shown, these deposit slips are longer than those generally used for personal accounts and have room for more entries and more information. If

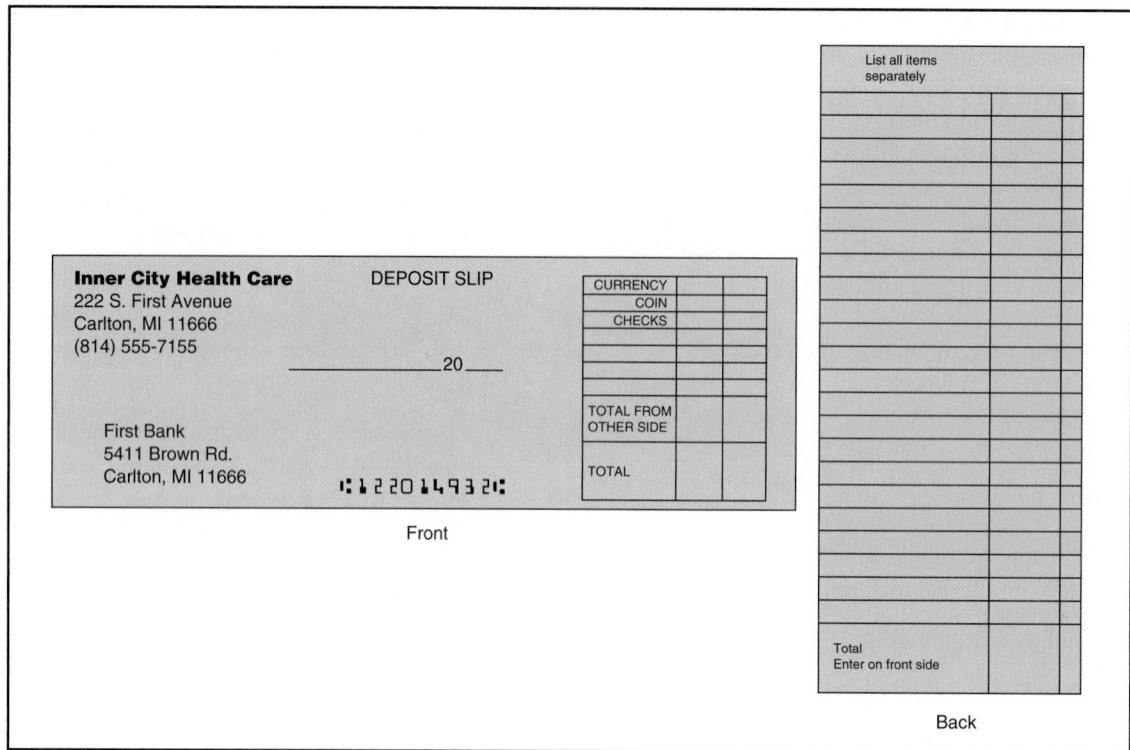

Figure 17-8   Sample deposit slip.

your day sheet has a built-in duplicate deposit slip, it will have been completed during posting (see Day Sheets in this chapter).

Procedure 17-6 outlines the steps in preparing a deposit.

Accepting Checks

When accepting checks from patients and other individuals, take a few minutes to inspect the check; this may eliminate checks returned from the bank for various reasons:

- Inspect the check for correct date, amount, and signature.

- Do not accept a third-party check (a check written to the patient from another person or company) unless it is from the insurance carrier.

- If a deposited check is returned marked "insufficient funds," call the bank that returned it and verify availability of funds. If funds are available, immediately redeposit the check for processing. If the check is returned again, add any fees the bank may charge your office to the patient's account. Be sure to adjust the checking account balance accordingly. Follow office procedure for notifying the patient that the check was returned.

Lost or Stolen Checks

In the event that a check is missing and is thought to be lost or stolen, report this to your bank immediately. In some cases, you may be advised to stop payment to prevent unauthorized cashing of the check. In other situations, the bank may place a warning on the account, advising bank representatives to be especially careful about checking signatures to detect any attempt at a forged signature.

Writing and Recording Checks

Part of daily financial practices includes writing checks to pay bills (**accounts payable**), refunds of overpayment, and replenishment of petty cash. It is important that checks be typed or written legibly to avoid bank errors. Checks should be dated and must include the name of the **payee** and the amount of payment entered both in figures and in words. It is also advisable to complete the "memo" line on the check indicating what the check is for or, in some cases, an account number and/or invoice number for reference purposes. Most medical practices use computerized accounting software packages such as Quickbooks™ or Quickbooks Pro™. These software packages enable you to write checks and keep a running register. They also have the ability to run payroll with tax tables automatically loaded.

CHAPTER 17 *Daily Financial Practices* **269**

In addition, business checking accounts need to make reference to the **disbursement** of the funds. Disbursement accounts are numbered accounts that break all expenditures into categories (i.e., salaries, rent, supplies) in the general ledger. At the end of the year, the accounts in this ledger will provide the figures for all tax-deductible expense. When the accountant completes the tax form for the practice, the information from the disbursement accounts is then easily transferred to the tax forms.

Before preparing the actual check, complete the check stub, which is the only record of payments made from the account. The stub should include the same information entered on the check as well as the disbursement account name or number for the accountant. Remember, it is critical for tax purposes that each check stub contain disbursement information so the bookkeeper can post the information to the correct accounts in the general ledger.

When the checks have been prepared, verify that the check amounts agree with the amounts written on the stubs, then subtract those amounts from the checkbook balance (Figure 17-9).

Rules for Writing Checks. Follow these few rules to assure that checks are properly written and recorded:

- Check that the numerical and written amounts agree.

- Check that everything is spelled correctly.

- Determine that the check has been signed by an individual with signature privileges.

- Follow office procedure for having the physician or office manager approve all expenditures and/or sign all outgoing checks.

- Check that it is payable to the correct payee and that the current date is used.

Reconciling a Bank Statement

Each month the bank will send a statement for the checking account (Figure 17-10). The statement will show the account balance according to the bank's records, a listing of all checks that have cleared the bank, deposits received by the bank, and any service charges deducted from the account. It is necessary to reconcile the entries in the checkbook against this statement to be sure there are no errors either in the checkbook or in the bank's records. Your bank statement is another means of ensuring that the accounts receivable is accurate for the previous month. If you use an accounting software package, this will also have a computerized option for reconciling.

Procedure 17-7 details the steps involved in reconciling the statement.

PURCHASING SUPPLIES AND EQUIPMENT

It is important to ensure proper control over purchasing of supplies and equipment for several reasons:

1. To avoid purchase of unnecessary items
2. To avoid duplication of items purchased
3. To prevent employees from ordering items for personal use
4. To provide a system for payment of only those items properly ordered and received

In order to accomplish these things, the first rule of purchasing should be that nothing is ordered or paid for without a purchase order or purchase order number. A copy of the purchase order is sent to the supplier and a copy is retained by the office for verification of shipment and payment of invoice.

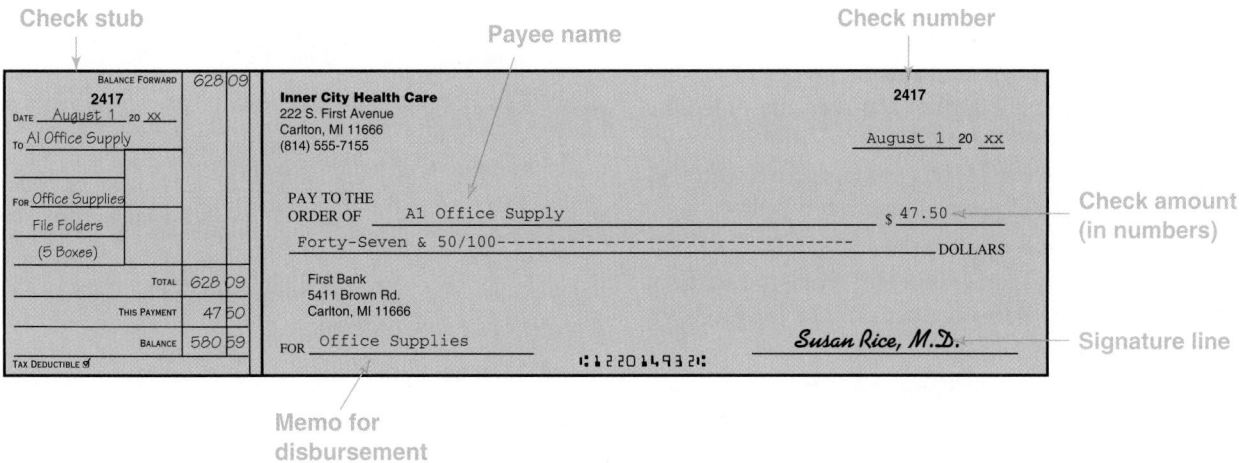

Figure 17-9 Sample of a properly completed check and check stub.

Summary of Account Balance			Closing Date 1/15/02		
Account # 1257-164013			Ending Balance $8,347.62		
Beginning Balance		$7,152.18			
Total Deposits and Additions		$8,643.86			
Total Withdrawals		$7,433.21			
Service Charge		$ 15.24			
Number	Date	Amount	Number	Date	Amount
201	12/18/01	173.82	234	1/4/02	96.31
223*	12/18/01	44.12	235	1/4/02	73.48
224	12/20/01	586.00	236	1/6/02	325.40
225	12/21/01	24.15	237	1/7/02	40.00
226	12/22/01	33.90	238	1/8/02	66.77
228*	12/23/01	1250.00	241*	1/9/02	15.55
229	12/24/01	11.75	242	1/10/02	12.45
230	12/24/01	19.02	243	1/10/02	4441.25
231	1/2/02	43.80	244	1/10/02	64.55
232	1/3/02	39.00			
233	1/4/02	71.50			

*Denotes gap in check sequence

Date	Deposit Amount	Date	Deposit Amount
18-Dec	361.75	4-Jan	825.00
19-Dec	586.00	5-Jan	1286.71
20-Dec	918.21	7-Jan	608.00
21-Dec	201.00	8-Jan	811.15
2-Jan	475.00	9-Jan	1092.68
3-Jan	1478.36		

Front

1. Enter Ending Balance from the front of this statement
$ 8,347.62

2. Enter deposits not shown on this statement
$ 3,162.50

3. Subtotal (add 1 & 2)
$ 11,510.12

4. List outstanding checks or other withdrawals here

Check #	Amount
222	37.89
227	161.15
239	11.50
240	92.12
245	835.17
246	21.75
247	586.00

5. Total outstanding checks
$ 1,745.58

Balance (subtract #5 from #3)
$ 9,764.54
This should equal your checkbook balance

Back

Figure 17-10 Sample bank statement.

Preparing a Purchase Order

Purchase order forms are available from office supply companies or can be ordered from a printer and customized to the needs of the ambulatory care setting. Figure 17-11 shows a typical purchase order form properly completed, which will be reveiwed section by section.

The purchase order form can vary greatly; some have more or less information. The form shown in Figure 17-11 contains the usual information required. The important thing is that the purchase order is used consistently.

- *Purchase order number.* A preprinted number that is used on invoices and statements from the supplier and on the check used to pay the invoice. It is also important for tracking the status of the order. In smaller practices, the purchase order number may simply be the name of the person ordering with the date the order was placed immediately following.

- *Bill to address.* Generally used when items are to be shipped to an address different from the address where the supplier will send the bill for goods or services.

- *Ship to address.* When items are to be sent by supplier; this must always be completed.

- *Vendor information.* Name and address of supplier where purchase order is to be sent.

- *Req. By.* States which individual or department has requested the item(s).

- *Buyer.* States the individual in the office who is authorized to issue a purchase order.

- *Terms.* Agreement between buyer and seller as to when payment is due.

- *QTY.* Quantity of item being ordered (number of units).

- *Item.* Vendor's catalogue part or item number.

- *Units.* How the item is sold—individually (ea.), by the box, case, or dozen. Many suppliers will not split units (i.e., sell less than a full case).

- *Description.* Brief description of item (helps as a cross-check for vendor in the event that an item number is entered incorrectly).

- *Unit Price.* How much *one* unit (ea., box, case, dozen) costs.

- *Total.* Cost of one unit multiplied by the number of units being ordered.

- *Subtotal.* Sum of the "Total" column.

- *Tax.* Sales tax required by the state.

- *Freight.* How much the customer must pay to have the order delivered (not always applicable).

PURCHASE ORDER

NO. 1742

Bill To:	Ship To:	Vendor:
Inner City Health Care 222 S. First Avenue Carlton, MI 11666 (814) 555-7155	**Inner City Health Care** 222 S. First Avenue Carlton, MI 11666 (814) 555-7155	**AZ Medical Supply** 4721 E. Camelback Rd. Phoenix, AZ 85252 (602) 555-3246

REQ BY	BUYER	TERMS
Karen Ritter	Walter Seals	Net 30

QTY	ITEM	UNITS	DESCRIPTION	UNIT PR	TOTAL
10	427A	Box	Surgical Gloves - Sz 7	6.75	67.50
1	327DC	Case	2" gauze pads	42.75	42.75
5	1943C	Box	Tongue Depressors	4.00	20.00
15	7433	Ea	Examination Table paper (roll)	5.75	86.25
				SUBTOTAL	216.50
				TAX	14.07
				FREIGHT	Prepaid
				BAL DUE	230.57

Figure 17-11 Purchase order form.

● *Bal. Due.* The sum of the subtotal, tax, and freight charges—this is how much the office will be billed.

Verifying Goods Received

Proper purchasing procedure does not stop with the completion and mailing of the purchase order. When goods are received, it is necessary to verify that the correct items and quantities were shipped by the vendor. All packages include a packing slip either on the inside of the box or attached to the outside. This packing slip should be attached to the office copy of the purchase order that is later attached to the invoice. Sometimes this packing slip serves as the original invoice as well.

As each item is unpacked, the item number and quantity received are checked against the office copy of the purchase order. If any discrepancies are noted between what has been received and what was ordered, they should be indicated on the office copy of the purchase order and the vendor should be contacted immediately and arrange-ments made to ship any missing items or provide return procedures for any incorrect or overshipped items.

Preparing the Invoice for Payment

When an invoice is received from the vendor (it may be included in the shipment or mailed later), it is necessary to confirm that charges are correct for the items ordered and the shipment received.

The invoice should be compared to the original purchase order to verify quantities, unit prices, and other charges. If there are discrepancies, contact the vendor's accounts receivable department to have the errors corrected before you send payment.

Once the invoice and purchase order are reconciled, the purchase order number is noted on the invoice (if not already printed there by the vendor) and the invoice is marked as "OK to pay." The invoice is then forwarded to the accounts payable department in the office for payment.

PETTY CASH

Petty cash is money kept in the office for minor, routine, or unexpected expenses such as postage-due mail or coffee supplies and cash back for patients paying their co-payments. Keeping this cash on hand eliminates the necessity of the physician or office manager having to sign checks for such items. Petty cash is not used to pay bills or make large routine purchases.

The amount of cash on hand for this purpose is small, usually $75 to $100, and is usually kept in small denominations such as ones and fives and only a few tens. However, records must be as carefully maintained as for any other financial transactions and balanced weekly.

Establishing a Petty Cash Fund

If your office does not already have a petty cash fund or if you are in a new practice and one has not yet been established, the physician or office manager will need to decide how much the fund should be and write a check to "Cash" for that amount.

Tracking, Balancing, and Replenishing Petty Cash

Tracking. Keep a supply of **petty cash vouchers** on hand for tracking how petty cash was used (Figure 17-12). When money is taken from petty cash, a voucher must always be completed and the receipt from the purchase attached. Vouchers and receipts are kept in the petty cash box with the money until the fund is replenished.

PETTY CASH VOUCHER

Amount: $16.98   December 18, 20__

For: Coffee filters, coffee, creamer, sugar

Account: Office supplies

Approved By: Received By:

Jane O'Hara   Karen Ritter

Figure 17-12   Petty cash voucher.

Balancing and Replenishing. When the fund gets low, write another check to "Cash" to bring it back up to the original amount. To determine the amount of the check, it is necessary to first balance the account. After the account is balanced, list how funds were spent in such a way that the bookkeeper can disburse the check properly.

Procedure 17-8 outlines the steps involved in balancing a petty cash account.

DOCUMENTATION

Financial and ongoing billing records should not be maintained in the patient's chart. Keep financial information separate from medical information to ensure that the physician's care is not influenced by the patient's ability to pay.

Procedure

17-1   Preparation for Posting a Day Sheet

PURPOSE:
To ensure that the medical assistant in charge of recording patient transactions prepares the day sheet before patients arrive.

EQUIPMENT/SUPPLIES:
Pegboard
Quantity of new charge slips and receipt forms
New day sheet
Ledger cards of patients scheduled for the day

PROCEDURE STEPS:

1. At the start of the day, a new day sheet and strip of charge slips are placed on the pegboard. RATIONALE: Prepares the day sheet for a new day's transactions.
2. Information at the top of the day sheet (date and page number) is filled in. RATIONALE: Establishes the sequential order of the business' daily financial record throughout the year.

(continues)

Procedure
17-1 (*continued*)

3. Balances forwarded from the previous sheet are carefully entered in Section 4, "Previous Page" columns A–D and the "Previous Day's Total" and "Accts. Rec. 1st of Month" in the Accounts Receivable Control and Accounts Receivable Proof boxes. Now the day sheet is ready to use. RATIONALE: Provides information for the month-end closing.
4. The ledger cards for all scheduled patients are pulled from the storage file and kept at the front desk in the order in which patients will be seen. RATIONALE: Ensures efficiency when patients arrive for their appointment.
5. A strip of receipt forms is kept at hand in case someone comes into the office to make payment on account. RATIONALE: Allows efficient use of time when patient makes a payment on their account.

Procedure
17-2 Recording Charges and Payments Requiring a Charge Slip (Patient Visits)

PURPOSE:
To record information pertaining to a patient's visit to the physician on the patient's ledger and the day sheet and to provide a charge slip for insurance billing.

EQUIPMENT/SUPPLIES:
Patient ledger card
Day sheet
New charge slip

PROCEDURE STEPS:
When a patient comes in for an appointment:
1. Place the ledger under the next charge slip and turn back the first two pages of the slip. RATIONALE: Takes complete advantage of the write-it-once system.
2. Write the date, responsible party's name and the patient's name (often entered in the "Reference" column), and any previous balance on the charge slip in the spaces provided. The information automatically transfers to the ledger through the carbon strip on the last page of the charge slip and to the day sheet through the NCR© paper. RATIONALE: Documents appropriate information.

3. Remove the charge slip from the pegboard and clip it to the front of the patient's chart to be given to the physician. RATIONALE: Allows physician to indicate appropriate procedure and diagnosis codes.
4. When the physician has completed treatment or examination, the spaces for procedures will be checked, the diagnosis filled in, and the physician will sign the bottom of the form. The form is then given to the patient to carry to the receptionist. RATIONALE: Physician marks the appropriate codes and signs the charge slip indicating it is correct.

When the patient returns the form to the front desk:
1. Enter the charge next to each procedure and write in the total on the front of the slip. RATIONALE: Completes the form.
2. Replace the charge slip on the pegboard, carefully lined up with the patient's name on the day sheet, and insert the ledger card under the last page of the charge slip. CAUTION: Be sure to align the *first blank line* of the ledger with the entry strip on the charge slip. RATIONALE: Uses the write-it-once system to record charges and any payment on the ledger card.

(*continues*)

Procedure 17-2 *(continued)*

3. Turn back the first two pages of the charge slip and enter the total charge and any payment the patient makes in the correct columns. RATIONALE: Uses the write-it-once system to record charges and any payment on the ledger card.

4. To arrive at the final balance, simply look at the day sheet at the column that shows previous balance, add the day's charge, and subtract payment made. RATIONALE: Provides the final balance on the day sheet.

Most day sheets have additional columns to the right of the charge slip. Information recorded here usually includes:

1. Receipt number (if your system uses numbered charge slips and receipts). RATIONALE: May be used to trace charges or payments related to specific patient transactions.

2. The method of payment (columns are provided for cash, by check, or credit card payments). RATIONALE: Provides a current record of cash, checks, or credit card totals after each entry.

3. Business analysis to be used as outlined by office procedure. RATIONALE: Business analyses require specific records as designed by the office. CAUTION: Be sure to complete the posting of each transaction all the way to the far right and on the same line of the day sheet as instructed by office procedure.

4. When posting is complete, keep the first copy of the charge slip for filing in the patient's chart, keep second copy for submission for insurance reimbursement, and give third copy to the patient. RATIONALE: Ensures a record is distributed to all parties involved.

Procedure 17-3 Receiving a Payment on Account Requiring a Receipt

PURPOSE:
To record a payment on the day sheet and patient's ledger card and to provide a receipt to the patient.

EQUIPMENT/SUPPLIES:
Day sheet
Patient ledger card
New receipt form

PROCEDURE STEPS:
When someone comes into the office to make a payment:

1. Receipt forms are placed on the pegboard in place of the charge slips. RATIONALE: A receipt documents the payment.

2. The patient's ledger is pulled and placed under the receipt form with the *first blank line* of the ledger under the carbon strip. RATIONALE: Takes advantage of the write-it-once system.

3. The following information is then entered along the top of the receipt: date, reference, description, payment amount, previous balance. RATIONALE: Ensures correct patient is referenced and credited the correct amount.

4. The new balance is calculated by subtracting the payment amount from the previous balance. RATIONALE: Indicates the new balance.

5. The receipt is given to the person making payment. RATIONALE: Proof of payment.

NOTE: No copy of the receipt is needed for the office since the information has been recorded on both the patient's ledger and the day sheet.

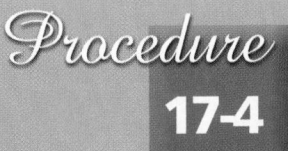

Recording Payments Received Through the Mail

17-4

PURPOSE:

To record payments received in the mail on the day sheet and patient ledger card. Payments received through the mail include payments from patients and from insurance companies on the patients' behalf. Both payments are handled in the same manner.

EQUIPMENT/SUPPLIES:

Day sheet
Patient ledger cards

PROCEDURE STEPS:

If a patient mails in a payment or if payment is sent by an insurance company:

1. Pull the appropriate ledger card and place it directly on the day sheet. RATIONALE: Utilizes the write-it-once system.
2. Temporarily remove the strip of charge slips from the pegboard. RATIONALE: Charge slip is not needed when recording a mail payment;

patient should never send cash and would have canceled check or money order receipt.

3. Enter the patient's previous balance on the day sheet (your ledger card does not extend to this column). RATIONALE: Indicates previous balance since ledger card does not extend to the column.
4. Post directly onto the ledger card the date, reference (patient name), description*, and payment amount. RATIONALE: Provides accurate information, including differentiating ROA and ROA ins.
5. Calculate the new balance as you did with personal payments. RATIONALE: Provides the new balance.

NOTE: No receipt forms or charge slips are used when posting payments received through the mail.

*ROA = Received on Account
*ROA Ins = Received on Account from insurance company

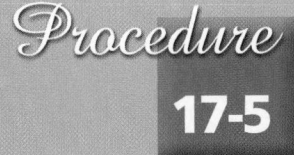

Balancing Day Sheets

17-5

PURPOSE:

To verify that all entries to the day sheet are correct and that the totals balance.

EQUIPMENT/SUPPLIES:

Day sheet
Calculator

PROCEDURE STEPS:

1. *Column Totals.* The first step in balancing a day sheet is to total columns A, B_1, B_2, C, and D and enter the total for each column in the boxes marked "Totals This Page." The column totals are then added to the figures entered in the "Previous Page" column boxes to arrive at

the "Month to Date" totals which provide the total charges, credits, and so forth entered from the first working day of the month to the present. RATIONALE: Establishes column totals.

2. *Proof of Posting.* This box is used to verify that entries have been made correctly and that the column totals are accurate. *All figures entered here are taken from the "Totals This Page" column boxes.*

   a. Enter today's column D total which shows the sum of all the previous balances entered when the transactions were posted.
   b. Added to this is the column A total of all charges for that day to arrive at a subtotal and enter the amount where indicated in the box.

(continues)

Procedure

17-5 *(continued)*

c. Since columns B_1 and B_2 are both credit columns which reduce balances, they are added together, entered in the box labeled "Less Cols B_1 and B_2," and the total of credits is subtracted from the subtotal. If all entries and addition are correct in the posting area, the result should equal the amount in column C and the transactions for that day are balanced. RATIONALE: Verifies entries have been made correctly and that the totals are accurate.

Overview: When an individual transaction is entered, the patient's previous balance (D) is added to the charges for the day (A). If there are any payments or adjustments made at that time, they are entered in the B columns and subtracted from the A + D amount to achieve the new balance (C). Since each transaction is actually D + A − B = C, the column totals of D + A − B will always equal the C total.

$$
\begin{array}{ccccccc}
D & & A & & B & & C \\
10 & + & 5 & - & 2 & = & 13 \\
2 & + & 7 & - & 1 & = & 8 \\
\hline
\textbf{Column Totals} \quad 12 & + & 12 & - & 3 & = & 21
\end{array}
$$

3. *Accounts Receivable (A/R) Control.* This box simply adds the previous day's Accounts Receivable balance to the current day's totals to include the current day's business and arrive at the new A/R total.
   a. The column A and column B totals are carried straight across from the Proof of Posting box to the corresponding blanks in the A/R Control box.
   b. Add the amount already entered in the Previous Day's Total space to the Column A amount to arrive at a subtotal.
   c. Subtract the amount carried over from the "Less Columns B_1 and B_2" box to find the new Accounts Receivable amount. RATIONALE: Determines new accounts receivable balance.
4. *Accounts Receivable Proof* verifies, or proves, the A/R balance in the A/R Control box. *The figure entered on the first line of this box will not change during a calendar month* as it shows how much the A/R balance was on the first working day of the month. *All other figures entered will be taken from the "Month-To-Date" column boxes.*

a. Enter the amount from column A (month-to-date) where shown.
b. Add the column A amount to the "A/R 1st of Month" figure and enter the sum in the subtotal space.
c. Enter the B_1 and B_2 month-to-date amounts and subtract from the subtotal. This amount goes in the Total Accounts Receivable space.

If all posting and addition are correct, the Total Accounts Receivable amounts in the A/R Control and A/R Proof boxes will match and the day is balanced. RATIONALE: Verifies the accounts receivable balance in the accounts receivable control box.

5. *Deposit verification* involves totaling the columns in Section 2 and entering the sum of the columns in the space marked "Total Deposit."

NOTE: The total deposit and the total of payments received in column B_1 should match. RATIONALE: Verifies deposit total.

6. *Business Analysis Summary.* If this section is used, total each column in the summary section.

NOTE: If the Business Analysis Summary is used to break out charges by type or by physician, the sum of the columns should equal today's column A total. If it is used to credit payments to different physicians, the sum of the columns will equal today's payment column. RATIONALE: The total deposit and the total of payments received in column B_1 should match to prove totals.

7. *After the Day Sheet is Balanced,* there is one step remaining: the transfer of balances.
   a. Take out a new day sheet for the next day.
   b. Transfer the "Month-To-Date" column totals to the "Previous Page" columns boxes on the new sheet.
   c. Enter the Total Accounts Receivable amount from the last day sheet in the "Previous Day's Total" space of the A/R Control box on the new day sheet.
   d. Enter the Accounts Receivable 1st of Month Amount in the A/R Proof box on the new sheet. RATIONALE: Transfers balances to prepare a new day sheet for the next day's activities.

The new day sheet is now ready for posting.

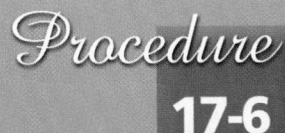

17-6   Preparing a Deposit

PURPOSE:
To create a deposit slip for the day's receipts.

EQUIPMENT/SUPPLIES:
New deposit slip
Check endorsement stamp
Calculator
Cash and checks received for the day

PROCEDURE STEPS:

1. Separate all checks from **currency** (paper money). RATIONALE: Each must be entered as a separate total.
2. Count all currency to be deposited and enter the amount in the space provided. Gather bills in order; i.e., fifties, twenties, tens, and so on. RATIONALE: Follows bank procedure.
3. Count all coins to be deposited and enter the amount in the space provided. Coins may need to be wrapped. RATIONALE: Follows bank procedure.
4. On the back of the deposit slip list each check separately. Include the patient name in the left-hand column and enter the amount of the check in the right-hand column. RATIONALE: Follows bank procedure.
5. Total the checks listed and copy the total on the front where it is indicated to place the total from the other side. RATIONALE: Follows bank procedure.
6. The sum of currency, coins, and checks should always equal the total in the "payments" column on that day's day sheet. RATIONALE: Proof of accuracy.
7. Attach the top copy of the deposit slip to the deposit, leaving the carbon on the pad. RATIONALE: Provides the office and bank with record of deposit.
8. Enter the date and amount of the deposit in the space provided on the checkbook stubs. RATIONALE: Keeps checkbook register current with money in account.
9. Add the amount of the deposit to the checkbook balance. RATIONALE: Keeps checkbook register current with money in account.
10. Deposit at the bank, either in person or at the night deposit. In either case, be sure a record of deposit is received (it will be mailed if the night deposit is used). It is not recommended that deposits be made through automated teller machines (ATMs); currency should never be deposited in an ATM. RATIONALE: Proof bank processed the deposit as indicated.

17-7   Reconciling a Bank Statement

PURPOSE:
To verify that the balance listed in the checkbook agrees with the balance shown by the bank.

EQUIPMENT/SUPPLIES:
Checkbook
Bank statement
Calculator

PROCEDURE STEPS:

1. Make sure the balance in the checkbook is current (all deposits and checks entered have been added or subtracted). RATIONALE: Ensures totals are accurate.
2. If there is a service charge listed on the statement, subtract that amount from the last balance listed in the checkbook. RATIONALE: Reconciles current balance.

(continues)

Procedure
17-7   (continued)

3. In the checkbook, check off each check listed on the statement and verify the amount against the check stub. RATIONALE: Verifies accuracy.
4. In the checkbook, check off each deposit listed on the statement. RATIONALE: Verifies accuracy.
5. The back of the statement contains a worksheet to be used for balancing.
6. Copy the ending balance from the front of the statement to the area indicated on the back.
7. Go through the check stubs and list on the back of the statement in the area provided any checks that have not cleared and any deposits that were not shown as received on the statement.

8. Total the checks not cleared on the statement worksheet.
9. Total the deposits not credited on the worksheet.
10. Add together the statement balance and the total of deposits not credited.
11. Subtract the total of checks not cleared. This amount should agree with the balance in the checkbook. If so, the checkbook is balanced and the statement should be filed in the appropriate place. RATIONALE: Following procedure steps 5–11 completes verification of accuracy.

Procedure
17-8   Balancing Petty Cash

PURPOSE:
To verify that the amount of petty cash is consistent with the beginning amount less expenditures shown on receipts.

EQUIPMENT/SUPPLIES:
Petty cash box
Vouchers
Calculator

PROCEDURE STEPS:
1. Count the money remaining in the box. RATIONALE: Verifies amount of cash and coin remaining in petty cash.
2. Total the amounts of all vouchers in the petty cash box. RATIONALE: Determines amount of expenditures.
3. Subtract the amount of receipts from the original amount in petty cash. This should equal the amount of cash remaining in the box. RATIO-

NALE: Proves that the amount of expenditures deducted from the beginning amount equals the amount left in the box.
4. When the cash has been balanced against the receipts, write a check *only for the amount that was used.* RATIONALE: Brings dollar amount back to original petty cash amount.

PETTY CASH CHECK DISBURSEMENT:
1. Sort all vouchers by account.
2. On a sheet of paper list the accounts involved.
3. Total vouchers for each account, and record individual totals on the list.
4. Copy this list with its totals on the "memo" portion of the stub for the check written to replenish petty cash.
5. File the list with the vouchers and receipts attached, after noting the check number on the list.

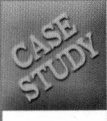

CASE STUDY 17-1

At the offices of Doctors Lewis & King, office manager Marilyn Johnson, CMA, is training a new administrative medical assistant in the practice's bookkeeping functions. The new medical assistant, Joann Crier, is a recent medical assistant graduate. This is her first position since earning her credentials. Joann has a basic interest in bookkeeping but wants Marilyn to instruct her, if possible, in the range of daily financial practices she may eventually be responsible for at Doctors Lewis & King.

CASE STUDY REVIEW

1. Suppose Marilyn were to give Joann a broad overview of every activity involved in Doctors Lewis & King's daily financial practices. What topic areas would she include?

2. Marilyn is very proficient in the pegboard system but knows little about computerized bookkeeping systems. Joann has current information on computer systems because she is a recent graduate; however, she is not really sure of herself with pegboard accounting. How can Marilyn and Joann use their complementary skill areas to help one another?

3. Joann will be helping Marilyn with accounts payable. What does she need to know and what rules should she observe?

SUMMARY

In this chapter we have discussed the daily financial duties in a medical office: patient bookkeeping, working with the checkbook, purchasing supplies and equiment, and petty cash. By becoming proficient in these functions, you will be prepared to handle the day-to-day financial aspects of any ambulatory care setting.

Patient bookkeeping involves not only a responsibility to the physician/employer (you are keeping track of income), but also to the patient to be certain that charges for services rendered are correct and that payments are properly credited. The pegboard system is a comprehensive manual system to post and track this data. Computerized bookkeeping offers advantages of speed, high accuracy, and elimination of some routine tasks.

It is also important to maintain a scrupulous accounts payable system to ensure that bills are paid on time and that payments are properly documented for tax purposes. To accomplish this, checks must be written properly and on time and recorded on the check stubs to effectively track expenditures.

Whether working with a pegboard or computerized system, accuracy is important at all times. To ensure maximum accuracy in all bookkeeping functions, observe a few rules: record all charges and receipts immediately; make deposits of checks and currency the same day they are received; always verify and recheck totals of all deposits and expenditures; stay current with all checking account duties such as account reconciliation; be prompt with all accounts payable.

REVIEW QUESTIONS

Multiple Choice

1. "Usual" refers to:
   a. the fee based on the average charge for a specific procedure by all physicians practicing the same specialty in a defined geographic region
   b. the fee typically charged by a physician for certain procedures
   c. the midrange of fees charged for this procedure
   d. the fee based on the physician's decision

2. The use of credit cards by patients to pay for services in ambulatory care settings is:
   a. never done
   b. highly unethical
   c. sure to compromise the integrity of the office
   d. a credit arrangement that can be used with discretion

3. The first section of the day sheet is used:
   a. to record deposits
   b. for business analysis

c. to post individual transactions

d. to total transactions

4. Good working habits for bookkeeping functions include:
   a. always using pencil
   b. always using red ink
   c. being meticulous about aligning columns
   d. relying on a calculator only

5. When moving from a manual to computerized book-keeping system:
   a. it can be expected to be up and running within a week or so
   b. the manual and computer systems may need to run concurrently for a few months
   c. it is not necessary to understand manual book-keeping systems
   d. accuracy will be assured in the computerized system

6. Charge slips (or superbills):
   a. may be ordered to fit the practice
   b. is a separate ledger for each patient household
   c. lists common services provided, procedural code, and diagnosis code
   d. only a and c are correct

7. Posting is the process:
   a. that increases or decreases patient accounts not due to charges incurred or payments received
   b. that decreases balance due
   c. that records financial transactions into a book-keeping or accounting system
   d. that increases the balance due

8. When accepting checks from patients, all of the following are true *except:*
   a. always accept third-party checks
   b. always inspect the check for correct date
   c. always inspect the check for correct amount in numbers and written portion
   d. always inspect the check for the signature

9. A check with an attached stub for recording information is called a:
   a. certified check
   b. cashier's check
   c. voucher check
   d. money order

10. It is important to ensure proper control over pur-chasing of supplies and equipment for all of the following reasons *except:*
    a. to avoid purchase of unnecessary items
    b. to avoid duplication of items purchased
    c. to permit employees to order items for personal use
    d. to provide a system for payment of only those items properly ordered and received

11. Petty cash:
    a. is usually $25 to $50
    b. is usually $75 to $100

c. usually consists of small denominations

d. only b and c are correct

12. To balance petty cash do all of the following *except:*
    a. count the money remaining and total the amounts of all vouchers
    b. subtract the amount of receipts from the original amount of petty cash
    c. write a check for only the amount that was used (bringing the petty cash back to original amount)
    d. in the checkbook, check off each check listed on the statement and verify the amount against the check stub

Critical Thinking

1. List the three functions of a charge slip. How can charge slips be customized?
2. What is the primary advantage of a pegboard system of bookkeeping? Discuss the forms required for a complete pegboard system.
3. Explain the necessity of maintaining ledger cards.
4. What is the purpose for "running a tape" on the cal-culator whenever you are working on bookkeeping tasks?
5. Describe the five sections of a day sheet and the function of each.
6. What is the procedure for preparing a new day sheet?
7. Explain the difference in procedure between receiv-ing a payment in person versus a payment that has been mailed to the office.
8. Why are bank deposits usually done daily?
9. When should the checkbook be balanced? Why?
10. Explain the purpose of petty cash.

WEB ACTIVITIES

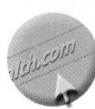 Utilize the World Wide Web to gather informa-tion on several different computerized account-ing programs and compare the advantages and disadvantages of each. Follow your instructor's instructions for additional information regarding this activity.

REFERENCES/BIBLIOGRAPHY

Andress, A. A. (1996). *Manual of medical office management.* Philadelphia: W. B. Saunders Company.

Humphrey, D. D. (1996). *Contemporary medical office procedures* (2nd ed.). Albany, NY: Delmar.

Chapter

18

MEDICAL INSURANCE

KEY TERMS

Assignment of Benefits
Bar Code
Basic Insurance
Beneficiary
Birthday Rule
Capitation
Catchment
Claim
Coinsurance
Coordination of Benefits (COB)
Copayment
Deductible
Diagnosis Code
Diagnosis-Related Groups (DRGs)
Direct Payment
Drug Formulary
Elective Procedures
Envoy
Exclusion
Exclusive Provider Organization (EPO)
Fiscal Intermediary
Health Care Financing Administration (HCFA)
Health Maintenance Organization (HMO)
Integrated Delivery System
International Classification of Diseases, 9th Revision, Clinical Modification (ICD-9-CM)
Major Medical Insurance
Managed Care Organization (MCO)
Medicare Allowable
Medicare Assignment
Medicare Part A
Medicare Part B
Medigap Policy   *(continues)*

OUTLINE

The Evolution of Medical Insurance Coverage
  Changes in Health Insurance Today
  Screening for Insurance
Medical Insurance Terminology
  Terminology Specific to Insurance Policies
  Terminology Specific to Billing Insurance Carriers

Types of Medical Insurance Coverage
  Traditional Insurance
  Managed Care
  Medicare
  Other Types of Coverage
Prospective Payment Systems and Diagnosis-Related Groups
Legal and Ethical Issues

OBJECTIVES

The student should strive to meet the following performance objectives and demonstrate an understanding of the facts and principles presented in this chapter through written and oral communication.

1. Define the key terms as presented in the glossary.

2. Describe the history of medical insurance in this country and its evolution in recent years.

3. Define the terminology necessary to understand and submit medical insurance claims.

4. Recall at least five examples of medical insurance coverage and discuss their differences.

5. Explain the significance of diagnosis-related groups.

6. Describe six primary managed care organization models.

7. Discuss legal and ethical issues related to medical insurance and the physician office.

Nonavailability Statement
Physician-Hospital Organization (PHO)
Preauthorization
Pre-Existing Condition
Preferred Provider

Preferred Provider Organization (PPO)
Primary Care Physician (PCP)
Proof of Eligibility (POE)
Prospective Payment

Resource-Based Relative Value Scale (RBRVS)
Usual, Customary, and Reasonable (UCR)
Utilization Review Organization
Waiting Period

ROLE DELINEATION COMPONENTS

ADMINISTRATIVE

Administrative Procedures

- Understand and apply third-party guidelines
- Obtain reimbursement through accurate claims submission
- Monitor third-party reimbursement
- Understand and adhere to managed care policies and procedures

GENERAL (TRANSDISCIPLINARY)

Legal Concepts

- Document accurately

Instruction

- Explain office policies and procedures

Operational Functions

- Apply computer techniques to support office operations

SCENARIO

At Inner City Health Care, a multidoctor urgent care center in a large city, medical assistant Jane O'Hara, CMA, is responsible for all patient billing procedures. While she delegates much of the responsibility for encoding claim forms to her two assistants, Jane oversees the process. Inner City participates in a number of insurance plans, so Jane must stay abreast of policy changes regarding reimbursement, preauthorizations, and claims filing. She also tries to become acquainted with the conditions of each patient's insurance coverage and helps patients understand their responsibility, if any, for payment. Finally, Jane holds periodic meetings with her assistants to update them; she continually stresses to them the importance of timeliness in filing claims and the need for absolute accuracy in diagnosis and procedure codes, which must always reflect services actually performed.

INTRODUCTION

An understanding of medical insurance and proper coding techniques is absolutely critical to the survival of the ambulatory care setting. In recent years much has changed in medical insurance coverage: more patients are choosing HMO and other managed care options, and even traditional insurance carriers like Blue Cross and Blue Shield are modifying their insurance plans to include some aspect of managed benefits.

In some ways, managed care coverage has simplified the patient's responsibility for payment, but it is more important than ever for the medical assistant to be accurate, timely, and conscientious in both filing insurance claim forms and understanding—and helping the patient understand—the conditions of individual insurance policies.

The increasing complexity of health insurance today means that medical assistants must continually update their base of information. This chapter will provide the groundwork for understanding the role of insurance, its terminology, and its various forms, and will give the medical assistant the confidence to take responsibility for claim filing in the ambulatory care setting.

THE EVOLUTION OF MEDICAL INSURANCE COVERAGE

The first medical insurance contract began in 1929 when a group of Texas teachers made an agreement for each member to pay Baylor University Hospital the amount of $6 a year to cover any of the group for hospitalization up to 21 days if that should become necessary.

Prior to this time, there was no formal medical insurance as we know it today. Then, if someone became ill, the family had to pay hospital, physician, and any related medical bills. If no family members were available to help, or if the family did not have adequate resources to pay these fees, the patient sometimes had to work for years to repay the debt. The physician sometimes gave the patient a reduced bill for office services.

In today's medical insurance, most carriers pay for hospitalization due to illness, accident, or disease. If a patient wishes to undergo an elective procedure (e.g., face-lift or abdominoplasty), most carriers will not pay the costs associated with that procedure. Not all insurance carriers cover the same exposures equally and none of the carriers pays at the same rate. Similarly, not many of the carriers charge the same premiums to policyholders. Some insurance companies cover individuals, families, or employee groups through work or through groups such as American Association of Retired Persons (AARP). Some premiums reflect an insured's past medical history and the company's exposure in covering the person. Premiums may be lower if the insured selects a higher annual deductible. Other premiums represent the rate that a group is able to obtain based on the group's claim history.

Changes in Health Insurance Today

There is much discussion today about changes in the health care insurance industry. Foremost is the idea that health care insurance should be available to all citizens of the United States. At this time, health insurance is usually tied to the employment package that covers the employee, spouse, and dependent children. One problem with work-related coverage is that some part-time employees are not eligible for health insurance and thus often go uninsured. Another problem is if an employee takes a position elsewhere, medical benefits may not transfer equally. If a family member is ill with an ongoing disease like cancer, or diabetes mellitus, the new insurance policy may not cover that disease or condition for at least one year. This is an **exclusion** known as a pre-existing condition. Current changes in the law prevent insurance companies from penalizing a patient with a pre-existing condition.

Another controversial aspect of health insurance is refusal to provide coverage for certain procedures because they are not sufficiently proven to be effective. In the early 1990s, bone marrow transplants were being performed on patients with breast cancer, at that time an experimental treatment for breast cancer. Because most insurance carriers will not extend coverage to experimental treatment, family and friends of patients often gathered for fund-raising drives to ensure that medical costs would be covered.

Screening for Insurance

Until universal coverage becomes a reality, it is the responsibility of the medical assistant to screen all new patients for their insurance. Clear all the insurance hurdles (authorizations, referrals) before giving treatment. If not cleared in advance, these hurdles may be insurmountable when trying to collect for fees for physician services.

Always ask:

- Is the patient covered by insurance?
- Is this procedure covered by the insurance?
- Is the primary care provider performing the procedure?
- Is a referral required? Is an authorization number or authorization code required? Has evidence of qualifying been received?

If the ambulatory care center does not participate in a particular plan and a patient with that plan does not have a referral to the physician, tell the patient in advance that there must be a referral or insurance will not pay. Requesting a referral when scheduling the first appointment should be routine practice and makes the billing process much easier for patient and office.

When screening patients for insurance, it is important to understand the philosophy of the medical office. Some may see patients regardless of ability to pay; responsible medical assistants will investigate all avenues for reimbursement first. Some situations may include the patient who is eligible for Medicaid but has not yet applied, or the patient who has applied for Medicaid but has not yet received notification of qualification.

The medical assistant should investigate and verify that all avenues have been taken to achieve the **proof of eligibility (POE)** that the office will need to receive reimbursement from Medicaid. This may include calling the Medicaid office to verify eligibility, or going on-line and printing a POE directly from the Medicaid system. This electronic data exchange system is called an **envoy**. POE cards are distributed to recipients and are in effect for at least one year. However, the most common avenue to ensure that services will be reimbursed is not to see any patient that does not have proof of Medicaid coverage. Medicaid sends their eligibility statements (medical coupons) to the patient the first day of the month. This coupon guarantees the ambulatory care center payment for the services provided. The majority of offices will not schedule Medicaid patients, unless it is an emergency, before the fifth of each month. This allows ample time for the beneficiary to receive the medical coupon. If the patient presents for their appointment without a medical coupon and proof of eligibility cannot be determined elsewhere, it is common practice to have that patient reschedule the appointment. The exception would be in the instance of an emergency.

Medical assistants with responsibility for billing are one key to a thriving ambulatory care center. Billing the insurance carriers promptly, completing claim forms properly, billing patients as needed, and keeping track of aging accounts will do much to ensure there is a flow of adequate income. In all insurance matters, be available to patients with questions regarding their insurance or accounts, for a friendly attitude helps patients feel positive about the care they receive and establishes a long-term relationship.

There are many hurdles to pass before the idea of universal health care, or coverage for all U.S. citizens, becomes reality. Many people believe that universal coverage will give everyone equal access to health care, regardless of their ability to pay. Others are of the opinion that universal health care will overload the system and result in delayed availability of health care to most people. Which point of view is correct is open to debate.

MEDICAL INSURANCE TERMINOLOGY

Before discussing the types of insurance coverage, one must understand the language used by the insurance industry. The terminology is specific in meaning and has been tested in courts of law to further define its meanings.

Terminology Specific to Insurance Policies

A policy is an agreement between the insurance company and the insured or beneficiary, the person covered under the terms of the policy. The insured person may include as beneficiaries the spouse and dependent minor children and others if related by blood and dependent upon the insured for more than 50 percent of their support. The insurance carrier pays a percentage (coinsurance) of the cost of the services covered under the policy in exchange for a monthly premium or charge. This premium is paid by the insured, the employer, or shared by both.

At the inception or beginning of the policy, the insured is given an identification card, which must be presented before receiving medical treatment (Figure 18-1). This card contains the insured's name, identification number, group number, and any copayment amount or restrictions for treatment. The back of the insurance card contains an address where claims should be submitted and telephone numbers needed to receive prior authorization for treatment.

Deductible. The language of the policy spells out the terms of the coverage. Usually there is an annual **deductible**, or an amount of money that the insured must incur for medical services before the policy begins to pay. This deductible can range from $100 to $1,000 or an even greater amount depending upon the language of the policy. The deductible must be met by medical charges that are incurred after the inception or anniversary date of the policy.

For instance, if Boris Bolski went to the physician on January 22 and incurred $258 in charges but his policy did not go into effect until February 1, none of these charges would apply toward his deductible. If, however, he returned to the doctor on February 3 and incurred another $85, this amount could be applied against his deductible.

Coinsurance. After the application of the deductible to the submitted bills, the insurance policy pays a percentage of the remaining amount. This percentage or coinsurance can vary from 50 percent to 100 percent depending upon the language in a specific policy. Most companies pay 80 percent.

Figure 18-1   Example of a Blue Cross/Blue Shield insurance identification card. (Courtesy of Empire Blue Cross/Blue Shield)

Copayment. Some insurance policies, especially **health maintenance organizations (HMOs)** and other managed care policies, require the patient to make a payment of a specified amount, for instance $5 or $10, at the time of treatment. This is usually done in place of a coinsurance being applied to the claim. This payment must be collected at the time of the office visit. Some policies have both a **copayment** and coinsurance clause.

Pre-Existing Condition. The example of Boris Bolski presents another problem. If a person had an illness, disease, or injury prior to the inception of the insurance whether or not treatment was received, there is a good chance that most insurance policies will not cover any charges related to that specific illness, injury, or disease because it is considered a **pre-existing condition**. Most policies have a specific **waiting period** before coverage is extended to those pre-existing conditions. This waiting period can be a matter of months, years, or the lifetime of the policy. If the person had a previous insurance policy that was not as inclusive as the new policy, often the new policy would still consider this a pre-existing condition and will deny payment until the waiting period is met. However, if the new policy has similar benefits and the person had no lapse in coverage, legally, the company must cover those conditions without applying a pre-existing condition or waiting period to the policy.

Exclusions. Exclusions are an important part of a policy. Some policies exclude **elective procedures** (procedures that are not medically necessary) such as cosmetic surgery, where other policies may allow some elective procedures. Other examples of exclusions might be pre-existing conditions, dental services, chiropractic services, or routine eye examinations. Not every policy has the same exclusions.

Coordination of Benefits. When more than one policy covers an individual, the policy language provides for **coordination of benefits (COB)**. This is determined by the policy language and coordinates payments between the policies so that the final total benefit is not greater than the original charge. Policy language again determines which of the two policies is primary or will pay first.

The employee's policy will pay first for the employee. For instance, if John O'Keefe is covered by an insurance policy where he works and is also covered by his wife's medical coverage, the policy Mr. O'Keefe gets from his employer will pay benefits first for him. The coverage under his spouse's policy will pay second because John is considered a dependent under that policy.

If one policy has coordination of benefits and the other policy does not, the policy *without* coordination of benefits will pay first.

When children of undivorced parents are covered under both parents' policies, often the **birthday rule** will be used to determine which policy is primary. This rule simply states that the policy of the parent with the birthday falling earlier in the year is primary. Thus, if the father's birthday is October 17 and the mother's birthday is May 12, the mother's policy will be primary. The year of the birth date is not relevant.

If the parents share the same birthday, then the policy with the earlier inception date is primary. If John and Mary both have birthdays on July 12, and the policy for John started August 1, 2001, and the policy for Mary started December 1, 2000, Mary's policy would be primary for their dependent children.

For children of divorced parents who are covered under both parents' policies, the policy of the custodial parent is usually primary.

Terminology Specific to Billing Insurance Carriers

There is specific terminology that one must understand when submitting insurance claims for medical benefits. Most ambulatory care settings will bill all appropriate insurance carriers to ascertain that the claim is made and the physician receives payment.

Many policies require **preauthorization** before certain procedures or before a visit can be made to a specialist or even a physical therapist. In these cases, the medical assistant must contact the insurance carrier with all of the diagnosis information and the proposed course of treatment. For instance, in a patient with a diagnosis of cholecystitis, preauthorization requires notification and approval before referring that patient to a surgeon for possible cholecystectomy. If this is not done, the surgery may not be covered.

A **claim** occurs when patients, having received treatment, wish to receive reimbursement under their insurance policies for charges for treatment. The patient (or the center's billing office) sends the claim to the insurance carrier for the amount of the treatment. This is done via a claim form, the most common of which is the HCFA-1500 (12-90) (Figure 18-2). This form was developed by the **Health Care Financing Administration (HCFA)** and is available with or without the **bar code** feature.

The claim form contains all of the identification information that the insurance company will need to process, or analyze, the claim for payment. The patient's name, address, telephone number, and, if they differ, the insured's name, address, and telephone number, social security number, group number, and member number are contained in the upper portion of the claim form. The lower portion of the form includes an area for up to four diagnosis codes, the procedure and visit codes, and the charges for those. Finally, the bottom section of the claim form includes the physician's name, address, telephone number, Internal Revenue Service (IRS) number, and Physician Identification Number (PIN).

All of the diagnoses as well as the visit types and procedures are coded. This coding will be discussed in Chapter 19. The completed claim form is sent to the insurance carrier either by mail, electronically, or through

---

PLEASE DO NOT STAPLE IN THIS AREA

(SAMPLE ONLY - NOT APPROVED FOR USE)

UNDERSTANDING HEALTH INSURANCE CLAIM FORM PICA

1. MEDICARE   MEDICAID   CHAMPUS   CHAMPVA   GROUP HEALTH PLAN   FECA BLK LUNG   OTHER
(Medicare #) (Medicaid #) (Sponsor's SSN) (VA File #) (SSN or ID) (SSN) (ID)

1a. INSURED'S I.D. NUMBER   (FOR PROGRAM IN ITEM 1)

2. PATIENT'S NAME (Last Name, First Name, Middle Initial)

3. PATIENT'S BIRTH DATE   MM   DD   YY   SEX   M   F

4. INSURED'S NAME (Last Name, First Name, Middle Initial)

5. PATIENT'S ADDRESS (No. Street)

6. PATIENT RELATIONSHIP TO INSURED   Self   Spouse   Child   Other

7. INSURED'S ADDRESS (No. Street)

CITY   STATE

8. PATIENT STATUS   Single   Married   Other

CITY   STATE

ZIP CODE   TELEPHONE (Include Area Code) ( )

Employed   Full-Time Student   Part-Time Student

ZIP CODE   TELEPHONE (INCLUDE AREA CODE) ( )

9. OTHER INSURED'S NAME (Last Name, First Name, Middle Initial)

10. IS PATIENT'S CONDITION RELATED TO:

11. INSURED'S POLICY GROUP OR FECA NUMBER

a. OTHER INSURED'S POLICY OR GROUP NUMBER

a. EMPLOYMENT? (CURRENT OR PREVIOUS)   YES   NO

a. INSURED'S DATE OF BIRTH   MM   DD   YY   SEX   M   F

b. OTHER INSURED'S DATE OF BIRTH   MM   DD   YY   SEX   M   F

b. AUTO ACCIDENT?   PLACE (State)   YES   NO

b. EMPLOYER'S NAME OR SCHOOL NAME

c. EMPLOYER'S NAME OR SCHOOL NAME

c. OTHER ACCIDENT?   YES   NO

c. INSURANCE PLAN NAME OR PROGRAM NAME

d. INSURANCE PLAN NAME OR PROGRAM NAME

10d. RESERVED FOR LOCAL USE

d. IS THERE ANOTHER HEALTH BENEFIT PLAN?   YES   NO   If yes, return to and complete item 9 a - d.

READ BACK OF FORM BEFORE COMPLETING & SIGNING THIS FORM

12. PATIENT'S OR AUTHORIZED PERSON'S SIGNATURE I authorize the release of any medical or other information necessary to process this claim. I also request payment of government benefits either to myself or to the party who accepts assignment below

SIGNED   DATE

13. INSURED'S OR AUTHORIZED PERSON'S SIGNATURE I authorize payment of medical benefits to the undersigned physician or supplier for services described below

SIGNED

14. DATE OF CURRENT   ILLNESS (First symptom) OR   INJURY (Accident) OR   PREGNANCY (LMP)   MM   DD   YY

15. IF PATIENT HAS HAD SAME OR SIMILAR ILLNESS GIVE FIRST DATE   MM   DD   YY

16. DATES PATIENT UNABLE TO WORK IN CURRENT OCCUPATION   FROM MM DD YY   TO MM DD YY

17. NAME OF REFERRING PHYSICIAN OR OTHER SOURCE

17a. I.D. NUMBER OF REFERRING PHYSICIAN

18. HOSPITALIZATION DATES RELATED TO CURRENT SERVICES   FROM MM DD YY   TO MM DD YY

19. RESERVED FOR LOCAL USE

20. OUTSIDE LAB?   YES   NO $ CHARGES

21. DIAGNOSIS OR NATURE OF ILLNESS OR INJURY. (RELATE ITEMS 1, 2, 3, OR 4 TO ITEM 24E BY LINE)
1. __   3. __
2. __   4. __

22. MEDICAID RESUBMISSION CODE   ORIGINAL REF. NO.

23. PRIOR AUTHORIZATION NUMBER

24. A DATE(S) OF SERVICE   From MM DD YY   To MM DD YY | B Place of Service | C Type of Service | D PROCEDURES, SERVICES, OR SUPPLIES (Explain Unusual Circumstances) CPT/HCPCS   MODIFIER | E DIAGNOSIS CODE | F $ CHARGES | G DAYS OR UNITS | H EPSDT Family Plan | I EMG | J COB | K RESERVED FOR LOCAL USE

1
2
3
4
5
6

25. FEDERAL TAX I.D. NUMBER   SSN   EIN

26. PATIENT'S ACCOUNT NO.

27. ACCEPT ASSIGNMENT? (For govt. claims, see back)   YES   NO

28. TOTAL CHARGE $

29. AMOUNT PAID $

30. BALANCE DUE $

31. SIGNATURE OF PHYSICIAN OR SUPPLIER INCLUDING DEGREES OR CREDENTIALS (I certify that the statements on the reverse apply to this bill and are made a part thereof.)

SIGNED   DATE

32. NAME AND ADDRESS OF FACILITY WHERE SERVICES WERE RENDERED (if other than home or office)

33. PHYSICIAN'S SUPPLIER'S BILLING NAME, ADDRESS, ZIP CODE & PHONE #

PIN#   GRP#

(SAMPLE ONLY - NOT APPROVED FOR USE)   *PLEASE PRINT OR TYPE*   SAMPLE FORM 1500   SAMPLE FORM 1500 SAMPLE FORM 1500

PATIENT AND INSURED INFORMATION   PHYSICIAN OR SUPPLIER INFORMATION   CARRIER

Figure 18-2   HCFA-1500 claim form (revised 12-90).

a holding system that batches and transmits claims at timed intervals, usually weekly. The most common and expeditious method for submitting claims is electronically. Only a few carriers do not accept electronic billings. This is generally when the HCFA-1500 form will be used. Additionally, the HCFA-1500 would be used when additional documentation will be needed to expedite the claim processing. Depending upon the policy language and the **assignment of benefits**, payment is sent either directly to the physician (known as **direct payment**) or to the patient/insured but payable to both the insured and the physician (known as indirect payment). With Medicaid, payment is made to the insured and the physician must collect from the insured.

TYPES OF MEDICAL INSURANCE COVERAGE

In today's health care environment, medical assistants will need to be aware of the different types of medical insurance policies.

Traditional Insurance

Traditional policies include coverage on a fee-for-service basis. There is usually a deductible and a coinsurance amount. Bills are submitted to the insurance carrier and if the annual deductible has been met, the coinsurance is applied to the difference. Payment is made either to the physician directly or to both the insured and physician.

Usually these policies pay only when there are diagnoses of illness, disease, or injury. Generally, they will not cover examinations to diagnose or to treat fertility problems; only a few carriers cover routine physicals or preventative health care.

Medical insurance policies often defined two types of coverage: basic insurance and major medical insurance. **Basic insurance** covers a specific dollar amount for physician fees, hospital care, surgery, and anesthesia.

Major medical insurance was developed to cover the costs of catastrophic expenses from illness or injury.

Many of the traditional insurance policies require that each policyholder, or insured, choose a **primary care physician (PCP)**, and to coordinate all of their medical care through that primary care physician.

Blue Cross and Blue Shield. While many traditional policies are offered by commercial carriers, the "Blues" are a well-known type of traditional insurance company. The 1929 Baylor University Hospital insurance agreement was the beginning of what we know today as Blue Cross. Over the years it has grown and matured into a nonprofit organization providing basic and major medical coverage. In most parts of the United States, Blue Cross and Blue Shield work in conjunction with each other. Blue Cross normally covers the hospitalization, radiology, and other basic coverages under the health plan. Blue Shield steps in as the major medical portion, picking up physicians' fees, medications, and other charges not covered on the basic portion of the plan. Blue Cross and Blue Shield plans usually have a large network of participating providers. In addition to the traditional Blue Cross and Blue Shield plans, they also offer several HMO-type plans that feature managed benefits and managed care options.

Managed Care

In an attempt to curb medical costs and create efficient use of medical resources, managed care is increasingly used around the country. Some companies require that policyholders seek medical attention only from **preferred providers**. Preferred providers are physicians and other health care professionals who contract with the insurance carrier to provide patient care. This contract states that in return for accepting a discounted fee for services, the insurance carrier will pay the physician directly each month for billings it receives from the physician. This is becoming more common as employers look for ways to reduce insurance costs, employees look for ways to reduce their share of the insurance premium and the cost of medical care, and physicians look for a secure payment situation with a shorter turnaround time.

Managed care organizations (MCOs) have multiplied with concentrations varying widely across the United States. Figure 18-3 illustrates these concentrations. The major principles of MCOs are to offer health insurance programs that ensure cost-effective services by employing case managers or PCPs to save dollars. To accomplish this, MCOs:

- Use PCPs or case managers.

- Utilize preauthorization for medical services, prospective and retrospective view of treatment plans, and significant discharge planning.

- Use specific treatment guidelines for high cost chronic disorders.

- Place emphasis on outpatient care versus hospitalization.

- Use a **drug formulary**, or list of medications that may be prescribed without preapproval.

- Place emphasis on health education and preventive care.

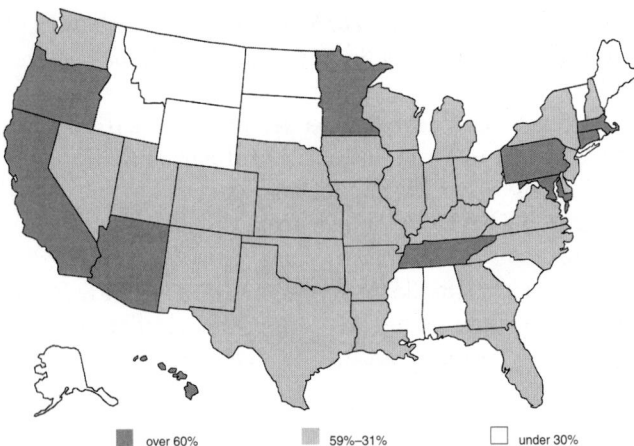

Figure 18-3   National managed care concentrations.
(Source: Rowell, 1998)

Legend: ■ over 60%   ■ 59%–31%   □ under 30%

● Place emphases on patient/family collaboration with health care providers to improve patient's compliance with treatment regimen.

● Utilize selective contracting with all health care providers and institutions involved to achieve discounted rates.

Six primary MCO models operate across the country. They include:

1. Integrated delivery systems
2. Health maintenance organizations
3. Exclusive provider organizations
4. Preferred provider organizations
5. Physician-hospital organizations
6. Utilization review organizations

Integrated delivery systems are groups of affiliated provider sites that operate under single ownership to offer full service/specialty services to their subscribers. The affiliated providers may include physician offices/clinics, hospitals, ambulatory surgery sites, and other ancillary allied health facilities. The patient's health record may be accessed at any affiliated site through a common computerized medical record system.

Health maintenance organizations (HMOs) are another type of managed care facility. In a total departure from the philosophy of the traditional insurance, HMOs cover a large group of people for a monthly premium and a small copayment from the patient at each time of service (usually $5 or $10). Sometimes, physicians are employed by the HMO and are paid according to the number of members enrolled (**capitation**) rather than the number of visits. Two types of HMOs are available: HMOs "with walls" and HMOs "without walls." HMOs "with walls" are facilities that offer all types of services under one roof. For

example, physicians in a variety of specialty areas, x-ray and laboratory departments, physical therapy, and pharmacy facilities are all in one building. HMOs "without walls" establish a network of preferred providers. Each provider may be located in its own building and location. Ideally, members can have all their medical needs met by the HMO. Members cannot see a physician outside the HMO setting unless they pay out-of-pocket for services rendered or only in those instances when the HMO refers the patient outside the HMO, in which case the treating specialist bills the HMO for the treatment and services rendered.

See Table 18-1 for common differences between traditional and managed care policies.

An **exclusive provider organization (EPO)** often requires the provider to work exclusively for the EPO organization. Subscribers receive no benefits if they choose to receive care from a provider who is not associated with the EPO.

A network of physicians and hospitals that have contracted together with insurance companies to provide health care at a discounted fee is known as a **preferred provider organization (PPO)**. Usually, PPOs do not have contracts for laboratory or pharmacy services, but they do offer reduced-rate contracts with specific hospitals. Patients have a greater out-of-pocket fee if they choose to receive health care from a non-PPO. The advantage of a PPO is that the fee-for-service is lower than HMOs; however, the disadvantage is that the premiums, deductibles, and copayments are usually higher than an HMO.

A hospital and selected physicians may form an entrepreneurship known as a **physician-hospital organization (PHO)**. Their primary function is to contract with MCOs to provide health care to their subscribers.

TABLE 18-1	DIFFERENCES BETWEEN TRADITIONAL AND MANAGED CARE POLICIES
Traditional	**Managed Care**
Usually can go outside physician network	Usually must stay inside physician network
Coinsurance	Copay each visit
Annual deductible	No annual deductible
Illness or injury only	Preventive treatment as well as illness and injury
Premium paid monthly to company by employer or subscriber	Premium paid monthly to company by employer or subscriber
MD paid by fee for service	Physician paid by capitation

Utilization review organizations are also known as third-party administrators. They supervise funds set aside to cover medical expenses to employees under self-insured plans. The utilization review organization determines medically necessary treatments, approves/denies payment of health care claims for these services, and completes a retrospective utilization review.

Medicare

In 1965 the United States Congress created Title 18 of the Social Security Act giving all senior citizens (age 65 and above) access to health care coverage. Congress recognized that with advancing age, the likelihood of illness and the need for health care increases. Medicare was created to give continuing medical coverage to senior citizens, most of whom had retired and had only limited, if any, access to health care coverage through their former employers. Many Medicare recipients also buy supplementary insurance policies through private carriers, which are known as **Medigap policies**.

Medicare is administered by the Health Care Financing Administration (HCFA). Claims are handled locally by a **fiscal intermediary**, or insurance carrier that has signed a contract with Medicare to handle all claims for a particular area. Recently, in some areas of the country, Medicare has contracted with managed care companies to administer benefits.

When a physician agrees to accept **Medicare assignment**, **Medicare's allowable** charge is accepted as payment in full for that particular service. Medicare pays 80 percent of that amount and the patient pays the remaining 20 percent. The difference between the physician's charge and the Medicare allowable charge is adjusted or written off by the physician. The benefits to the physician are that Medicare makes a direct payment to the physician, and the fee schedule is 5 percent higher for physicians who accept assignment than for those who do not.

Medicare has two parts: **Medicare Part A** covers hospitalization, home health care, and hospice care. This part has a monetary deductible as well as a limit to the number of days per hospitalization and the number of hospitalizations per year that a person may have. Part A involves just these services, so the hospital or agency responsible bills for the services.

Medicare Part B covers outpatient services including physicians' fees, physical therapy and occupational therapy charges, diagnostic tests, lab tests, radiological studies, ambulance services, and charges for durable medical equipment such as walkers and wheelchairs.

Currently, an annual deductible of $100 must be paid by the patient before Medicare will begin to pay its share of the bills. The rate at which Medicare then reimburses is 80 percent of the Medicare fee schedule for medical care and 100 percent for laboratory fees, which was adopted in 1992 and is based on the **resource-based relative value scale (RBRVS)**. The RBRVS was developed using values for each medical and surgical procedure based on work, practice, and malpractice expenses and factoring for regional differences.

For instance, if a patient goes to the physician for an office visit and the fee is $75, the patient will submit the bill to Medicare through the local Medicare fiscal intermediary to apply against the deductible. At the next visit, the bill is $50. This bill will also be submitted to Medicare. Total bills submitted: $125. Ideally, Medicare will subtract the $100 deductible, apply the 80 percent coinsurance to the amount in excess of the deductible, or $25, and pay $20. The patient would be responsible for the difference (20 percent coinsurance) or $5, plus the $100 deductible.

Example:	
Office visit	$ 75.00
Return visit	+ 50.00
Total Charges	$125.00
Less deductible	−100.00
Subtotal	$ 25.00
Apply 80% coinsurance	× 80%
Insurance Payment	$ 20.00
Patient Owes	$ 5.00

The example shows how the worksheet would look if there were no exclusions or deductions. Medicare, however, as well as many other insurance companies, uses a fee schedule based upon **usual, customary, and reasonable (UCR)** fees. *Usual* refers to the fee that the specific physician charges most of his patients for the same treatment. *Reasonable* refers to the midrange of fees charged for this type of procedure or visit. *Customary* is based on the average charge for a specific procedure by all the physicians practicing the same specialty in a specific geographical location. Also see Chapter 17 for a discussion of fees.

Based on the Medicare fee schedule, Medicare might decide it will only consider $70 of the first bill and $45 of the second bill or a total of $115. From this amount Medicare subtracts $100 (the deductible), which leaves an amount of $15 on which to base payment. Now the 80 percent coinsurance is applied resulting in a payment of $12. The patient is left owing one of the following amounts in addition to the $100 deductible: $3 if the physician accepts Medicare assignment or $13 if the doctor does not accept assignment ($3 plus the $10 disallowed by Medicare).

Example:

	Total Charges	Allowed Charges
Office visit	$ 75.00	$ 70.00
Return visit	+ 50.00	45.00
Total Charges	$125.00	$115.00
Less deductible	−100.00	−100.00
Subtotal	$ 25.00	$ 15.00
Apply 80% coinsurance	× 80%	× 80%
Insurance Payment	$ 20.00	$ 12.00
Patient Owes	$ 5.00	$ 3.00*

*(or $13.00 if physician does not accept assignment)

Other Types of Coverage

In addition to the coverages described, there are other insurance coverages for persons unable to work due to illness or life circumstances (Medicaid), for dependents of persons serving in the Armed Forces (CHAMPUS and CHAMPVA), and for workers who are injured on the job (Workers' Compensation or State Industrial Insurance).

Medicaid. Medicaid was created in 1965 by Congress under Title 19 of the Social Security Act to provide funding for medical care for qualifying persons. It is federally funded but administered through each state's department of human services. People who are on Aid for Families with Dependent Children and Supplemental Security Income (SSI), single women who are pregnant and whose income is at or below the national poverty level, and people who for many reasons due to physical, emotional, or mental difficulties are unable to work may qualify for this program. The recipient is given an identification card which is presented to the medical provider at the time of the office visit. A claim form is then completed and the identification card or a copy of the card is attached to the form and mailed to the administrator's address. Some states have a requirement for a copayment by the recipient at the time of service but collection cannot be enforced.

Many medical practices accept Medicaid but when referring a patient to a specialist or another provider, it is wise to ascertain whether that provider accepts Medicaid patients. A referral form usually must be completed by the

primary care or referring physician prior to the visit with the specialist.

Billings to Medicaid are considered only after all other insurance payments have been made. When a person has both Medicare and Medicaid, charges are submitted first to Medicare and last to Medicaid. Both are federal programs and errors in billing could be construed as fraud, for which there are criminal penalties. It is therefore imperative that all billing practices conform to the legal requirements of these programs.

CHAMPUS and CHAMPVA. Military personnel are covered by the medical personnel in the Armed Services. However, their dependents (spouse and children) often are not able to receive medical care on the base, or in many cases they live outside the catchment area of a 40-mile radius of the assigned base. When these dependents need medical care and no military medical care is easily available to them or they need emergency medical care, they may seek medical care from nonmilitary medical providers without prior authorization. CHAMPUS, the Civilian Health and Medical Program for Uniformed Services, covers the dependents of active duty personnel, retired personnel, dependents of retired personnel, and dependents of personnel who died while on active duty.

CHAMPVA, the Civilian Health and Medical Program of the Veteran's Administration, covers the spouse and unmarried dependent children of a veteran with permanent total disability from a service-related injury and the surviving spouse and children of veterans who died of a service-related disability.

As in all the previous insurance plans, each person covered by CHAMPUS or CHAMPVA will have an identification card showing name, identification number, and program covered. A person cannot be covered by both CHAMPUS and CHAMPVA.

CHAMPUS and CHAMPVA are billed after all other insurance coverages except Medicaid. Preauthorization is required for patients living within a catchment area for treatment. Patients living outside the catchment area do not need preauthorization. Preauthorization is obtained using a nonavailability statement. This form is completed and submitted to the local CHAMPUS office. If treatment is rendered and payment is denied, an appeal process is available to the patient and physician.

Workers' Compensation or State Industrial Insurance. When an on-the-job accident or illness results in injury and/or disability, workers' compensation insurance pays the medical bills and a significant portion of the lost wages if the patient was covered by a workers' compensation policy.

In most states, the employer pays a premium to an insurance carrier for a policy known as Workers' Compensation insurance. This premium is rated upon the number of workers employed and the degree of risk a job entails. A few states provide coverage through a statewide fund, often called State Industrial insurance, which is funded by premiums paid to the state by employers. Again, the premiums are based upon the number of employees and the job risk.

When a claim is made, a workers' compensation claim form is completed and sent to the insurance carrier or to the state fund for reimbursement (Figure 18-4). The injured worker receives no bills, pays no deductible or coinsurance, and is covered 100 percent for medical expenses related specifically to that injury.

Self-Insurance. Many larger companies, nonprofit organizations, and state and county governments choose to self-insure in an attempt to reduce the costs of medical insurance and to gain more control over their finances. In self-insured plans, special accounts are established and, rather than paying premiums to an insurance carrier, the entity makes payments into the plan. Each self-insured plan will differ in its organization and claim filing requirements; if a patient is covered by a self-insured plan, call the plan administrator before scheduling a patient appointment.

PROSPECTIVE PAYMENT SYSTEMS AND DIAGNOSIS-RELATED GROUPS

In an effort to control the costs of hospital care for Medicare patients, in 1983 the Health Care Financing Administration (HCFA) adopted a plan called **diagnosis-related groups (DRGs)**. DRGs, a concept that originated at Yale University, is a method of **prospective payment** in which hospitals are paid a flat fee for Medicare patients. The fee is based on an *average* cost of service, not the *actual* cost of service for a particular patient. With the DRG plan, patients are classified into categories based on principal diagnosis, principal procedure, and discharge status. All patients in the same DRG are predicted to respond in a clinically similar way.

While the DRG system of pricing is typically applied in a hospital setting, the medical assistant in the ambulatory care setting will benefit from an awareness of how this system works. The forty-seven DRG categories are derived from the *International Classification of Diseases, 9th Revision, Clinical Modification* (ICD-9-CM), which contains all standard **diagnosis codes** used to encode a claim form. If responsible for filing any Medicare claim based on the DRG, the medical assistant should note that, like all claim filing, accuracy is essential

and assignment of the correct DRGs helps to ensure maximum financial reimbursement in the processing of medical insurance claims.

LEGAL AND ETHICAL ISSUES

It is critical that the medical assistant be well versed on various insurance plans carried by patients. Explanations regarding insurance submission policies and patient financial responsibilities are often part of the day's work. It is essential that signatures to authorize insurance billing and supply information to insurance carriers be secured. Without the signature, release of information is illegal.

Many Medicare claims are now submitted electronically and private payers in growing numbers are also using electronic claims submission. In a computerized system, everything related to billing and reimbursement is computerized and transmitted electronically. If the office is participating in HCFA's Electronic Data Interchange (EDI), they will be assigned a unique identifier number that constitutes their legal electronic signature. Be cautious with this electronic signature as the office is responsible for any and all claims made with it. The Health Insurance Portability and Accountability Act of 1996 (specifically title II, subtitle F) regulates the security and privacy of transmitted health care information.

INSTRUCTIONS

1. Type answers to All questions and file original with the Workers' Compensation Commission within 72 hours after first treatment.
2. DO NOT FAIL to forward to the Workers' Compensation Commission PROGRESS REPORTS and FINAL REPORT upon discharge of patient.

DO NOT WRITE IN THIS SPACE

WORKERS' COMPENSATION COMMISSION
6 NORTH LIBERTY STREET, BALTIMORE, MD. 21201-3785
SURGEON'S REPORT

WCC CLAIM #

EMPLOYER'S REPORT Yes ☐ No ☐

This is First Report ☐   Progress Report ☐   Final Report ☐

EVERY QUESTION MUST BE ANSWERED AND FORM SIGNED

1. Name of Injured Person: Maureen A. Santega	Soc. Sec. No. 610-98-7432	D.O.B. 7/19/69	Sex M ☐ F ☒

2. Address: (No. and Street) 905 Raymond Lane   (City or Town) Atlanta   (State) GA   (Zip Code) 30385-8893

3. Name and Address of Employer: Majors Concrete Company, 238 Leaf Lane, Atlanta, GA   30342-3329

4. Date of Accident or Onset of Disease: 4/9/__	Hour: A.M. ☒ P.M. ☐	5. Date Disability Began: 4/9/__

6. Patient's Description of Accident or Cause of Disease:
Concrete truck struck and backed over patient's foot while she was pouring concrete at the job site.

7. Medical description of Injury or Disease:
massive bruising to left foot, no broken bones, great deal of pain associated with bruises

8. Will Injury result in:
(a) Permanent defect?   Yes ☐   No ☒   If so, what? ____   (b) Disfigurement   Yes ☐   No ☒

9. Causes, other than injury, contributing to patients condition:
None

10. Is patient suffering from any disease of the heart, lungs, brain, kidneys, blood, vascular system or any other disabling condition not due to this accident?
Give particulars: No

11. Is there any history or evidence present of previous accident or disease? Give particulars:
No

12. Has normal recovery been delayed for any reason? Give particulars:
No

13. Date of first treatment: 4/10/__	Who engaged your services? patient

14. Describe treatment given by you:
Darvon, 100 mg q4h prn for pain

15. Were X-Rays taken: Yes ☐ No ☒	By whom? — (Name and Address)	Date 4/10/__

16. X-Ray Diagnosis:

17. Was patient treated by anyone else? Yes ☐ No ☒	By whom? — (Name and Address)	Date

18. Was patient hospitalized? Yes ☐ No ☒	Name and Address of Hospital	Date of Admission: Date of Discharge:

19. Is further treatment needed? Yes ☐ No ☒	For how long?	20. Patient was ☒ will be ☐ able to resume regular work on: 4/14 Patient was ☐ will be ☐ able to resume light work on:

21. If death ensued give date:	22. Remarks: (Give any information of value not included above)

23. I am a qualified specialist in: orthopedics	I am a duly licensed Physician in the State of: Georgia	I was graduated from Medical School (Name) Emory	Year 1967

Date of this report: 6/21/__   (Signed) *John N. Sparks, M.D.*

8504 Capricorn Drive, Atlanta GA 30312   (404)544-0078
Address: Phone:

(This report must be signed PERSONALLY by Physician)

Figure 18-4   Sample workers' compensation claim form.

DOCUMENTATION

Documentation must support all claims submitted. Failure to document a service translates into nonperformance of that service, from the perspectives of quality patient care, legal safeguards, and reimbursement issues. In other words, a deed not documented is a deed not done.

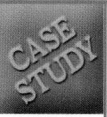

CASE STUDY 18-1

Jane O'Hara, CMA, is responsible for all patient insurance billing procedures. Jane has the following information:

	Total Charges	Allowed Charges
Office visit	$85.00	$80.00
Return visit	$65.00	$55.00

Deductible has not been satisfied.

CASE STUDY REVIEW

1. Calculate the correct billing if the physician accepts assignment.
2. Calculate the correct billing if the physician does not accept assignment.

SUMMARY

An understanding of medical insurance terminology and various types of coverage is vital to a thriving ambulatory care setting. The astute medical assistant will perceive the challenges involved in understanding the role in the management of medical office insurance. The medical assistant must be able to explain insurance procedures to the patient and know how to make contact with appropriate representatives to determine eligibility and coverage questions.

REVIEW QUESTIONS

Multiple Choice

1. The most common avenue to ensure that services will be reimbursed is:
   a. not see any patient that does not have proof of Medicaid coverage
   b. complete an envoy
   c. go on-line and print a proof of eligibility directly from the system
   d. ask the patient if they are covered
2. The most common insurance claim form is the:
   a. UB92 form
   b. ICD-9-CM
   c. HCFA-1500 form
   d. CPT
3. Medicare:
   a. was created by Title 19 of the Social Security Act
   b. was created in 1965
   c. is designed to cover prescriptions
   d. is handled separately by each state

4. If the charge is $150 and the deductible has not been met, Medicare will pay:
   a. $20
   b. $40
   c. $120
   d. 80 percent of UCR after $100 deductible
5. There are _____ primary MCO models operating across the country.
   a. four
   b. three
   c. six
   d. eight
6. EPOs:
   a. often require the provider to work exclusively for that organization
   b. are groups of affiliated provider sites that operate under single ownership
   c. are paid according to capitation
   d. are also known as third-party administrators

7. Medicaid:
   a. was created by Title 19 of the Social Security Act
   b. is designed to cover prescriptions
   c. is handled separately be each state
   d. accommodates only military personnel
8. CHAMPUS:
   a. is a type of HMO
   b. is a type of EPO
   c. is a civilian health and medical program of the Veteran's Administration
   d. stands for Civilian Health and Medical Program for Uniformed Services

Critical Thinking

1. What is the difference between basic insurance and major medical insurance?
2. What is the difference between copayment and coinsurance?
3. Explain the birthday rule and when it is used.
4. What are four insurance considerations to keep in mind when treating a patient?
5. Compare the traditional approach of insurance companies to HMOs.
6. Dr. Lewis accepts Medicare assignment. What does this mean to Dr. Lewis? What does this mean to Abigail Johnson, one of Dr. Lewis' Medicare patients?
7. If a patient lives six miles from an Army hospital, will a preauthorization for treatment be needed by a specialist in the nearby city? Why or why not?

WEB ACTIVITIES

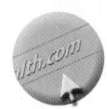

Use the Internet to locate the Intermediary-Carrier Directory for Medicare. Determine the Medicare Part A intermediaries and the Medicare Part B carriers for the state or region in which you live. Follow instructor guidelines to submit your findings.

REFERENCES/BIBLIOGRAPHY

HCFA. (2000). *Medicare Part B basic billing manual*. Noridian Mutual Insurance.

Humphrey, D. D. (1996). *Contemporary medical office procedures* (2nd ed.). Albany, NY: Delmar.

Keir, L., Wise, B. A., & Krebs, C. (1993). *Medical assisting: Administrative and clinical competencies* (3rd ed.). Albany, NY: Delmar.

Kinn, M. E., & Woods, M. A. (1999). *The medical assistant: Administrative and clinical* (8th ed.). Philadelphia: W. B. Saunders Company.

Rowell, J. C. (1998). *Understanding medical insurance* (4th ed.). Albany, NY: Delmar.

Spock, M. (2000). *The coding answer book*. Rockville, MD: Physician Practice Coder.

MEDICAL INSURANCE CODING

KEY TERMS

Breach of Confidentiality

Charge Slip

Claim

Claim Register

Current Procedural Terminology (CPT)

Diagnosis Codes

E Codes

Explanation of Benefits (EOB)

Fraud

HCFA-1500 (12-90)

HCFA Common Procedure Coding System (HCPCS)

Insurance Abuse

International Classification of Diseases, 9th Revision, Clinical Modification (ICD-9-CM)

Point-of-Service (POS) Device

Procedure Codes

Subrogation

Superbill

Uniform Bill (UB92)

V Codes

OUTLINE

OBJECTIVES

The student should strive to meet the following performance objectives and demonstrate an understanding of the facts and principles presented in this chapter through written and oral communication.

1. Understand the process of procedure and diagnosis coding.

2. Code a sample claim form.

3. Explain the difference between the HCFA-1500 and the UB92 forms.

4. Describe the way computers have altered the claims process.

5. Discuss why claims follow-up is important to the ambulatory care setting.

6. Discuss legal and ethical issues related to coding and insurance claims processing.

At Inner City Health Care, a multi-doctor urgent care center in a large city, medical assistant Jane O'Hara, CMA, is responsible for all patient billing procedures. While she delegates much of the responsibility for encoding claim forms to her two assistants, Jane oversees the process. Jane and the assistants must be acquainted with the requirements of each patient's insurance coverage and help patients understand their responsibility—if any—for payment. Finally, Jane holds periodic meetings with her assistants to update them; she continually stresses to them the importance of timeliness in filing claims and the need for absolute accuracy in diagnosis and procedure coding which must always reflect services actually performed and documented within the patient's chart.

INTRODUCTION

Coding is the basis for the information on the claim form. Medical coding is mandatory for the accurate transmission of procedures and diagnosis information between health care providers and various agencies that compile health care statistics and the insurance companies that act as third-party payers for health care services rendered to patients. In order to code accurately, the medical assistant must have a good understanding of medical terminology, especially of those medical specialties found in the ambulatory care setting.

The issue of who owns the medical record, health care provider or patient, has been debated for decades. Generally, it is considered that the health care provider is responsible for maintaining and preserving the patient record, but the patient has a right to access and copy the information contained within the record upon appropriate request. It is extremely important to maintain confidentiality when dealing with physician/patient privilege. Before releasing any information to a third party, a medical release must be obtained from the patient.

INSURANCE CODING SYSTEMS

The process of converting descriptions of diseases, injuries, and procedures into numerical designations is termed coding. **Current Procedural Terminology (CPT)** was developed by the American Medical Association (AMA) to convert commonly accepted, uniform descriptions of medical, surgical, and diagnostic services rendered by health care providers into five-digit numeric codes. The **International Classification of Diseases, 9th Revision, Clinical Modification (ICD-9-CM)** was compiled by the World Health Organization (WHO). It is designed for the classification of patient morbidity (sickness) and mortality (death) information for statistical purposes and for the indexing of hospital records by disease and operation for data storage and retrieval. Medical assistants employed in ambulatory care facilities will use procedure codes and diagnosis codes on a regular basis.

Procedure Coding

Procedure codes for procedures done and for visits of all kinds—office, hospital, nursing facility, home services—is found in *Current Procedural Terminology* (CPT). This volume is updated annually and is divided into seven sections:

1. Evaluation and Management
2. Anesthesia
3. Surgery
4. Radiology, Nuclear Medicine, and Diagnostic Ultrasound
5. Pathology and Laboratory
6. Medicine
7. Index

Evaluation and Management Section. The Evaluation and Management section takes every possible combination of visits into consideration and assigns each its own number. For instance, Mary O'Keefe, a new patient, is seen for a period of 45 minutes during which the physician takes a detailed history, examines the patient, and makes a medical decision of moderate complexity. The CPT code for this visit (99204) is found by looking under office services, new patient, time and service provided. In another instance, Abigail Johnson, an established patient, is seen in the hospital for several days. These visits (99231, 99232, or 99233) would be found under hospital services, subsequent hospital care, and the time and service provided. Codes for any type of evaluation and/or management are found in this section. In many offices the physician will determine the level or charge for visits; however, the medical assistant must be very familiar with all of the codes to make certain that billings are correct and that codes match the physician's documentation.

Anesthesia Section. The Anesthesia section includes all codes for anesthesia required for any procedure. The codes begin with the head and continue down the body to the legs and feet, concluding with anesthesia for radiological procedures. If you want to find the correct code for anesthesia during a total hip replacement, you will find "Anesthesia" in the index, look for "hip" and refer to the codes listed: 01200–01214. When you refer back to the Anesthesia section, you find:

01200	Anesthesia for all closed procedures involving hip joint
01202	Anesthesia for arthroscopic procedures of hip joint
01210	Anesthesia for open procedures involving hip joint; not otherwise specified
01212	hip disarticulation
01214	total hip replacement or revision

As you read through the codes, you see that the correct code is 01214.

Surgery Section. The section on Surgery divides codes according to system. It begins with the skin, subcutaneous and areolar tissues, and continues through subsequent systems ending with ocular and auditory systems. The codes are very specific. For instance, a simple laceration repair is found as:

12001*	Simple repair of superficial wounds of scalp, neck, axillae, external genitalia, trunk and/or extremities (including hands and feet): 2.5 cm or less
12002*	2.6 cm to 7.5 cm
12004*	7.6 cm to 12.5 cm
12005	12.6 cm to 20.0 cm
12006	20.1 cm to 30.0 cm
12007	over 30.0 cm

Thus, the exact length of the laceration and complexity of repair can be found and coded correctly on the claim form. The * signifies a surgical procedure for which a charge is made that does not include pre- or post-operative visits.

Radiology, Nuclear Medicine, and Diagnostic Ultrasound Section. Coding in the Radiology section covers each procedure done and each specific alteration to the procedure. For instance,

75889	Hepatic venography, wedged or free, with hemodynamic evaluation, radiological supervision, and interpretation
75891	Hepatic venography, wedged or free, without hemodynamic evaluation, radiological supervision, and interpretation

Radiological procedures are not often done in the physician's office, although they may be in larger urgent care centers. Occasionally chest X rays are done or, in an orthopedic specialty, many skeletal X rays may be done. More often, though, radiological studies are ordered by the physician through a local facility which bills the insurance company directly, using the diagnosis the physician has provided.

Pathology and Laboratory Section. The Pathology and Laboratory section includes every test and combination of laboratory tests that can be ordered as well as a section on surgical pathology. This latter section includes specimens sent for examination, such as Pap smears, analysis of biopsy tissue from surgical sites, and tissue typing. Following is an example of a laboratory procedure code for hepatitis B and illustrates the complete selection of tests that may be ordered:

87340	Hepatitis B surface antigen (HBsAg)
86704	Hepatitis B core antibody (HBcAb); IgG and IgM
86705	IgM antibody
86706	Hepatitis B surface antibody (HBsAb)
87350	Hepatitis Be antigen (HBeAg)
86707	Hepatitis Be antibody (HBeAb)

The medical assistant should be aware of laboratory codes because when a lab test is ordered, the lab may call to clarify the order. If the coding is correct, the lab should have no questions.

For surgical pathology, the codes are different. The level of examination for the item determines the code. The physician usually determines these levels or the charge for these services.

Medicine Section. The section of the CPT entitled Medicine includes codings for immunizations, injections, dialysis, allergen immunotherapy, and chemotherapy, as well as ophthalmologic, cardiovascular, pulmonary, and neurological procedures, to name a few. As in the earlier sections, there is a comprehensive breakdown of each procedure. Under Cardiography, for example:

93000	Electrocardiogram, routine ECG with at least 12 leads; with interpretation and report
93005	tracing only, without interpretation and report
93010	interpretation and report only

Under Chemotherapy Administration:

96408	Chemotherapy administration, intravenous, push technique
96410	infusion technique, up to one hour
96412+	infusion technique, one to 8 hours, each additional hour
96414	infusion technique, initiation of prolonged infusion (more than 8 hours), requiring the use of a portable or implantable pump

The plus symbol indicates that the procedure is an add-on to a previously described procedure. For example, 96410 would be used to describe the service and the time administered up to one hour. Anything over one hour would use the add-on code of 96412 for each additional hour administration took place.

Index. The final portion of the CPT is a comprehensive index listing every procedure alphabetically. The proper use of the CPT involves looking for the procedure in the index and then checking the number given to determine the precise code.

Each code found in the CPT has five numerical digits. Note that there are no letter codes and no decimal points in these codes. Each five-digit code stands for a specific procedure not duplicated elsewhere.

Modifiers. Occasionally a service or procedure needs to be modified. In that case, there are two-digit numerical modifiers that can be applied to the five-digit code. These modifiers can indicate unusual procedural services (-22), bilateral procedure (-50), multiple procedures (-51), two surgeons (-62), surgical team (-66), or repeat procedure by same physician (-76). When any of these or other modifiers are used and a full five-digit code for the modifier is desired, use 099 before the modifier code. Thus, they become 09922, 09950, 09962, and so on. The modifiers are delineated in the front of each section of the CPT to alert the coder to modifiers available for that section.

If more than one modifier is needed for a procedure, use (-99) before any other modifier. Thus, if a procedure required a modifier of -22 and -51, code -99 before the other modifiers. For instance, "33411 Replacement, aortic valve; with aortic annulus enlargement, noncoronary cusp," becomes 33411-99. This can also be written 33411 and 09999 indicating multiple modifiers.

HCFA Common Procedure Coding System (HCPCS). Medicare uses a supplement to the CPT codes. Level I of the **HCPCS** is the regular CPT system.

Level II is a coding system that uses a five-digit alphanumeric code to clarify procedures. The code begins with a letter from A to V followed by four numbers. An example might be A4550 Surgical trays, A4615 Nasal Cannula, or E0609 Blood Glucose Monitor with special features (voice synthesizers, automatic timers, and so on). Injections are listed under J codes. All of these codes can have an additional two-digit letter modifier. These modifiers can be simply LT for left, RT for right, or even CC to indicate a code change when resubmitting a claim that was previously denied by Medicare. The Level II codes were developed by Medicare for all procedures performed in the medical office in place of CPT codes which may not be specific. For instance, to bill a cyanocobalamin or Vitamin B_{12} injection, the CPT code for an intramuscular injection is used (90782), but a Level II code for the medication (J3420) is also required.

Level III codes are similar to Level II but are assigned by the fiscal intermediary rather than the national administration. These codes use the letter codes W, X, Y, and Z.

Diagnosis Coding

In addition to coding for procedures, a code is required for each diagnosis. **Diagnosis codes** are found in the current International Classification of Diseases, 9th Revision, Clinical Modification or ICD-9-CM, also referred to as ICD-9 or simply ICD. It is expected that in the future there will be a new way of coding diagnoses, known as ICD-10. This will be an alphanumeric code and will take the place of the current ICD-9 system. This is a collection of codes published by the World Health Organization for every disease, illness, condition, injury, and cause of injury known. The codes are found in three volumes, the first two of which depend upon each other for diagnosis coding.

Volumes I and II are used for coding diagnoses in ambulatory care centers and outpatient departments of hospitals; Volume III is used for inpatient procedures. The ICD-9-CM is usually now available in separate versions: one for physician offices and one for hospitals. The physician version has Volume I and II combined into one book, and the hospital version has all three volumes combined in one book.

Volume I, Tabular List, contains all the codes in numerical order. This volume is the second place that is referred to when coding a diagnosis.

Volume II, Alphabetic Index, contains all possible diagnoses, including symptoms, accidents and their causes, and concurrent diagnoses. This volume also contains a table of drugs and chemicals and a list of external causes for injuries. This volume is the first place that is referred to when coding a diagnosis.

Volume III, Procedures: Tabular List and Alphabetic Index, includes procedures used. The procedure codes of the CPT are more commonly used in the United States and are accepted by all the insurance companies. If you are unable to find a correct procedure code in the CPT, Volume III of the ICD-9-CM does contain helpful information. Often there is enough information in this volume to help identify a procedure in the CPT.

In the codes, initials such as NEC and NOS will be encountered. NEC means "not elsewhere classified" and is used only if there is not enough information to find a more specific code. NOS refers to "not otherwise specified." If a more specific diagnosis can be found, do not use a diagnosis with either of these references.

ICD-9-CM codes have a three-digit base with modifiers to that base added *after a decimal point*. For instance,

the code for cellulitis is 682. When looking back to Volume I, the code for 682 is broken down according to various areas of the body. Cellulitis of the leg is 682.6 and includes ankle, hip, knee, and thigh. Cellulitis of the foot is 682.7. Another example is pyelonephritis. Chronic pyelonephritis is 590.0 and acute pyelonephritis is 590.1.

The fifth digit defines the diagnosis even more specifically. In the preceding example, under 590.0 there are two choices: 590.00 without lesion of renal medullary necrosis, or 590.01 with lesion of renal medullary necrosis. If that specific information is known, code the fifth digit.

The fifth digit may also define a location more specifically. As in the example for cellulitis where the fourth digit identified a location, the fifth digit can also define a location. The diagnosis osteomyelitis is found in Volume II as

> Osteomyelitis (general) (infective) (localized) (neonatal) (purulent) (pyogenic) (septic) (staphylococcal) (streptococcal) (suppurative) (with periostitis) 730.2

When found in Volume I, 730.2 reads:

> Unspecified osteomyelitis, osteitis or osteomyelitis NOS, with or without mention of periostitis

There is also noted a requirement of a fifth digit to indicate the location of the disease. Thus, 730.27 is Unspecified osteomyelitis of the ankle or foot.

Some diagnosis codes cannot stand alone. For instance, in Volume II we find "Tuberculosis, kidney" as 016.0 [590.81]. These two codes when checked in Volume I read:

> 016.0 Tuberculosis of kidney
>   Renal tuberculosis
>   (Use additional code to identify manifestation, as:
>   tuberculous: nephropathy (583.81)
>   pyelitis (590.81)
>   pyelonephritis (590.81).)

Looking up 590.81 we find:

> *Pyelitis or pyelonephritis in diseases classified elsewhere*
>   *Code first underlying disease as:* tuberculosis (016.0).

The italics refer to manifestation codes and these must be shown after the underlying disease code. Thus, both codes 016.1 and 590.81 must be used when completing the claim form for this diagnosis.

Injury codes also cannot stand alone. If a patient comes in for treatment of a fractured arm, the first code to be found will be the diagnosis of the injury: 812.21 fracture of the humerus shaft. Upon referring to Volume I, 812.21 states this is a fracture of the shaft of humerus, closed. Since fractures are not usually a disease but rather the result of an injury, the cause of the injury must be coded as well. Again, refer to the back of Volume II under the appendix for **E codes**—Index to External Causes. For this exercise, Jaime Carrera fell from a ladder. Under "Fall, Ladder" the code E881.0 is given. Checking that code in Volume I, E881.0 states Fall from ladder. (E881.1 is fall from scaffold.) It is apparent that diagnosis codes are precise.

It is important to document all information related to an injury. Insurance carriers will often deny an injury **claim** until they have received information that there is no other insurance available to pay the medical charges. Often auto insurance, homeowner liability insurance, or workers' compensation insurance will pay the entire cost of treatment. These policies are primary and the medical insurance policies pay *after* the primary coverage is exhausted. In these situations, make sure the correct insurance company is billed first for the physician's services. If the medical insurance company pays the bill and later discovers there is accident coverage available, the medical insurance company will bring a claim against the accident policy to seek reimbursement of the monies it has paid out. This is called **subrogation**.

Supplementary Health Factors. V Codes are the last main section of Volumes I (numeric) and II (alphabetic). This section contains "Supplementary Classification of Factors Influencing Health Status and Contact with Health Services." These codes reflect exposure to diseases, such as "V01.1 Exposure to tuberculosis." They also reflect potential health hazards to the patient, such as "V16.1 Family history of malignant neoplasm in lung."

Well-child examinations, routine pregnancy examinations and delivery, screening for diseases, or conditions such as "V78.0 Iron deficiency anemia" are also found in this section. Again, just because the code is found in Volume II does not mean coding is complete. It must be checked in Volume I to make certain the code is accurate.

If the diagnosis is Weight gain, Volume II shows: "Weight gain (abnormal) (excessive) 783.1." When 783.1 is checked in Volume I, it reads:

> Abnormal weight gain
> *Excludes*: excessive weight gain in pregnancy (646.1)
> obesity (278.0).

When 278.0 is checked, it states

> Obesity
> *Excludes*: adiposogenital dystrophy (253.8)
> obesity of endocrine origin NOS (259.9).

At this point, the patient's chart must be checked to determine whether the correct code is 278.0, 259.9, or 783.1.

Coding Accuracy. The more accurate the coding on the claim form, the less chance there is for error, the more

quickly the physician is reimbursed, and the better chance that the physician's reimbursement will reflect the actual charge. Many insurance carriers keep a fee profile of each physician's charges. This profile reflects the amount of each charge for each service and can affect the physician's reimbursement for those services.

If an error is made in the coding, the insurance carrier will always downcode. That is, insurance will pay the lesser of the two amounts in question. For instance, Dr. Woo spent 45 minutes with an established patient for a complex medical problem, but instead of billing 99215, the medical assistant billed 99213 which reflects a time of 15 minutes and a problem of low complexity. Even though the diagnosis indicates a complex group of problems, the insurance company will pay according to the physician's fee profile for a 15-minute visit.

Do not guess when coding. The coding that is used becomes a permanent part of the patient's medical record with the insurance carrier. If an incorrect code is used, that coded diagnosis will stay with that patient. This can be a very difficult problem for insureds if they change insurance carriers or if other health problems occur.

Consider a patient with hip pain. She has a history of ovarian cancer for which she has had radiology treatments. The hip pain is thought to be possible metastases from the original cancer site. When ruling out this possibility, the physician indicates the following code for the claim form:

> 198.89 Secondary malignant neoplasm of other specified sites: hip.

When the pain is finally discovered to be arthritis and it is determined that the patient needs a hip replacement, the insurance carrier denies coverage for this operation. Reason: the patient's condition is terminal and the company does not want her to spend her last months having surgery and recovering from surgery when she is already in poor health. And, of course, there is the cost factor to consider in the eyes of the insurance carrier.

Incorrect coding can be a problem with ruling out a diagnosis. For instance, a patient presents many symptoms of peptic ulcer disease. Do not immediately code that patient as having that disease until the diagnosis is confirmed. Instead, code the symptoms. When the tests come back and a specific diagnosis of peptic ulcer can be made, then code the disease as

> 533.70 chronic without mention of hemorrhage or perforation without mention of obstruction.

When coding:

- Be as precise as possible
- Do not guess
- Do not code what is not there

CODING THE CLAIM FORM

In order for the insurance company to understand what is being billed, the claim form is completed by the medical assistant or billing clerk in the ambulatory care setting. The physician completes a charge slip at the time of the visit. This **charge slip** (see Figure 19-1), also known as an encounter form, includes the date of service, the visit or consult code, diagnoses for this visit, procedures done and lab tests ordered, and, if necessary, the date the patient is to return. This information is then translated onto the claim form. In some physician offices, charge slips are referred to as **superbills**.

The **HCFA-1500** is the claim form accepted by most insurance carriers. This form is prepared using words and CPT codes for procedures performed and ICD-9-CM codes for diagnoses. Keep in mind that the codes must correlate; for instance, if a person had an ICD-9-CM diagnosis code of earache, otitis media, or 382.9, and the CPT procedure code indicated was 69090, ear piercing, the insurance company would question the claim and reject it for payment. The person completing the claim form must be *as precise as possible*. If the coding is wrong, the claim will be denied and the physician will not receive pay-

ment. Coding must correlate with the physician's note in the chart; otherwise, fraud is committed.

Coding the claim form is a precise way to communicate with the insurance carrier. Coding indicates the complexity of the visit, the diagnosis for the visit, and the specific procedures performed during the visit. This results in very little confusion, and a minimum of communication is needed between the carrier and the physician's office because all information is contained in the codes.

For instance: Leo McKay, a regular patient, is seen for an extended visit to determine the cause of his abdominal pain. Symptoms include diarrhea, fever, nausea, and anorexia. An abdominal ultrasound is ordered as well as lab tests, and the results are unknown at the time of the insurance billing. The visit lasts 30 minutes and includes a full physical examination and a history of the present illness.

The CPT procedure coding for this visit is 99214, which reflects the examination and time spent with the patient, the history taken of this illness, and a medical decision of moderate complexity.

The ICD-9-CM diagnosis coding for abdominal pain is 789.0, for diarrhea 787.91, for nausea 787.02, and for anorexia 783.0. The claim form is submitted to the insurance carrier with these codes, and even though they are all symptoms, the claim will be paid because the visit and the tests ordered interrelate.

When the test results are known, they show a positive diagnosis of Giardia lamblia. The diagnosis code is changed to 007.1. Any further charges sent to the insurance carrier while Leo McKay is being treated for this problem are coded 007.1. The symptom codes from the first submission are dropped.

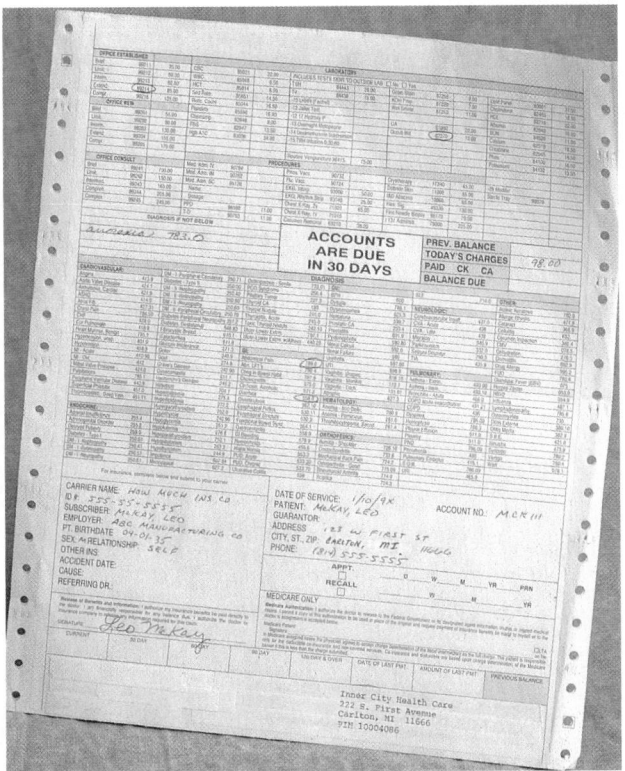

Figure 19-1 Sample charge slip (or superbill), currently known as an encounter form. The physician marks the procedures performed (CPT codes) and the diagnosis (ICD-9-CM codes). There are a variety of charge slip formats available. Note this sample charge slip is different than the charge slips shown in Chapters 17 and 20.

COMPLETING THE HCFA-1500 (12-90)

The HCFA-1500 (12-90) has been adopted by insurance carriers as the only acceptable form on which to submit insurance claims. However, each insurance carrier has its own thoughts on how the form should be completed and no two companies agree entirely on the information required, the boxes checked, and the rationale about what information goes in which boxes.

To illustrate the completion of a claim form, a fictitious insurance carrier will be used. (Insurance carriers change their rules and regulations for submitting claims constantly. One example is Medicare, which changes its requirements several times a year.) In order to avoid out-of-date material, this claim for payment is sent to How Much Insurance Company. Using the example given of Leo McKay in the coding section, the HCFA-1500 in Figure 19-2 shows the properly completed claim form:

Example:

Block 1.	X in "other."
Block 1a.	555-55-5555
Block 2.	McKay, Leo M
Block 3.	04 01 35 X in "M."
Block 4.	McKay, Leo M
Block 5.	123 West First Street Carlton, MI 11666 (814) 983-2831
Block 6.	X in "self."
Block 7.	Same as insured.
Block 8.	X in "single"—no other boxes marked in this block for this claim.
Block 9.	Leave blank. (If the patient has other insurance, that information would go here.)
Block 10.	a. X in "no." b. X in "no." c. X in "no."
Block 11.	1122334 a. Leave blank. b. ABC Manufacturing Company c. How Much Insurance Company d. X in "no."
Block 12.	Needs date and "signature on file" typed in.
Block 13.	Needs "signature on file" typed in.
Block 14.	01 10 xx
Block 15.	In this example, Leo did not have previous symptoms of similar nature, so this will be left blank.
Block 16.	Leave blank.
Block 17.	Leo is a regular patient of Dr. Woo so no referring physician name goes here. If he had been referred to Dr. Woo by another physician, the referring physician's name would go here.
Block 18.	Leave blank.
Block 19.	Leave blank.
Block 20.	X in "yes" since outside labs were ordered in this example.
Block 21.	Use only ICD-9-CM codes here. 1. 789.0 2. 787.91 3. 783.0 4. This can be left blank since there were only three diagnoses. A claim may be submitted using only one diagnosis code if it substantiates the charges.
Block 22.	Leave blank.
Block 23.	Leave blank.
Block 24.	A. 1/10/xx B. 3 (indicates office visit) C. Leave blank. D. 99214 E. 1,2,3 F. 85.00

	G. 1 (indicates one unit) H. Leave blank. I. Leave blank. J. Leave blank. K. Leave blank. (In Medicare, Medicaid, and Workers' Compensation claims, the medical provider's number is entered here.)
Line 2.	A. 1/10/xx B. 3 C. Leave blank. D. 82270 E. 1,2 F. 13.00 G. 1
Block 25.	91-5555555 and X in "EIN."
Block 26.	MCK111
Block 27.	X in "no" unless physician accepts assignment for that plan.
Block 28.	98.00
Block 29.	-0-
Block 30.	98.00
Block 31.	Physician's name, telephone number, date claim sent in.
Block 32.	Leave blank since care provided at Dr. Woo's office
Block 33.	Inner City Health Care 222 South First Avenue Carlton, MI 11666 (PIN#) 10004086

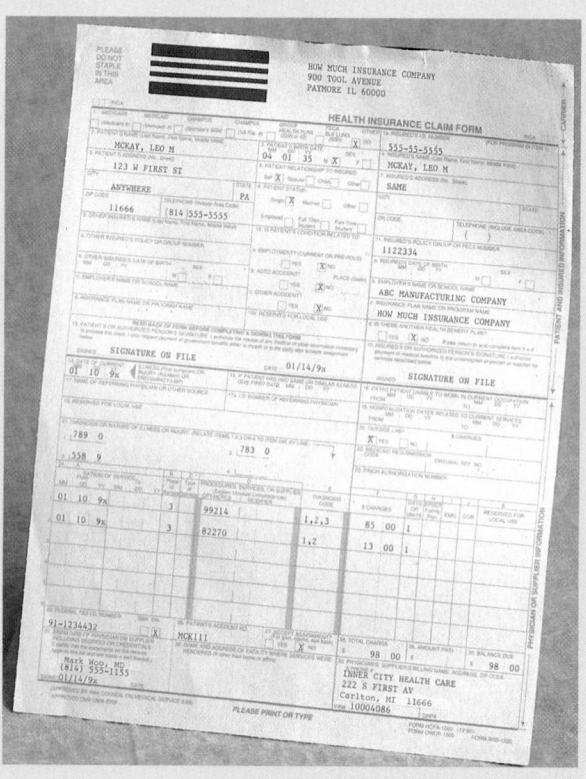

Figure 19-2   Completed HCFA-1500 claim form for Leo McKay.

Remember, many insurance carriers will require some of the boxes to be filled in and others left blank. The billing person for the medical office will need to comply with the current requirements of the insurance carrier that is being billed. There is no right or wrong answer for every insurance carrier. If there is a question about billing, check with that carrier about their requirements.

Although the HCFA-1500 is the most common claim form in the ambulatory care setting, medical assistants who become claims processing specialists in different settings will need to be familiar with the UB92 (Figure 19-3). The **Uniform Bill 92 (UB92)** form was originally developed in the 1970s as a unique form for filing inpatient, home health care, hospice, and long-term

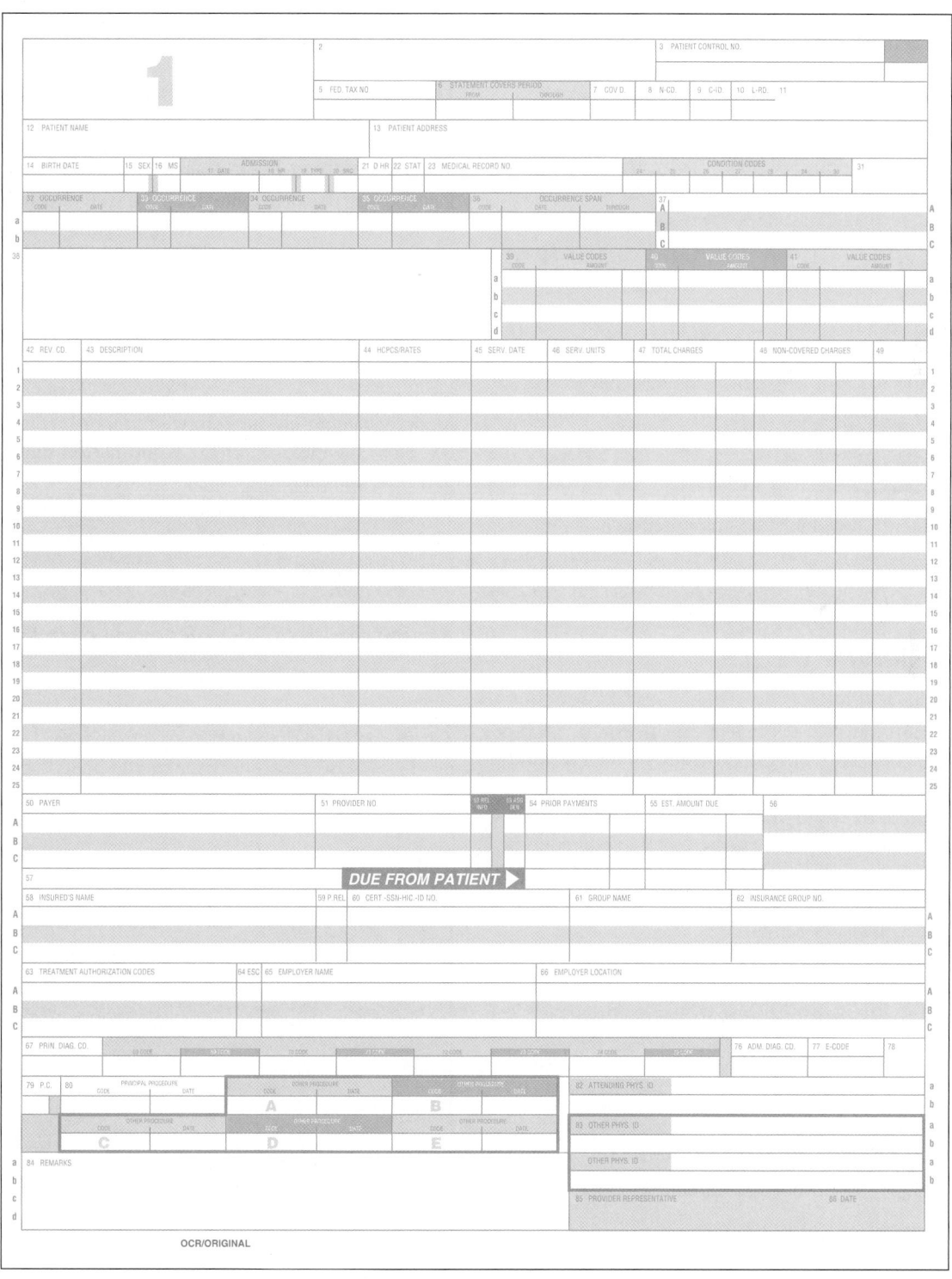

Figure 19-3 UB92 claim form (also known as the HCFA-1450 form).

care benefits under a health plan. It is also known as the HCFA-1450 and may also be referred to as a summary bill.

Although medical assistants in ambulatory care facilities will not typically encounter hospital billing forms such as the UB92, many medical assistants are now finding opportunities as claims processing specialists in hospital, nursing facility, and clinic billing offices. As a claims processing specialist, skills are transferable to anywhere in the United States and interchangeable between provider specialties and insurance carriers. The UB92 claim form is the standard form used for inpatient and outpatient services by acute care hospitals, psychiatric, drug, and alcohol facilities, clinical and laboratory services, walk-in centers, nursing facilities, subacute facilities, home health care agencies, and emergency rooms.

OVERSEEING THE CLAIMS PROCESS

Once the claim form has been coded, a series of events take place: the medical assistant, who may have used a referral number generated by a point-of-service device, enters the claim into the office register of submitted claims; the insurance carrier processes the claim; an explanation of benefits is sent to the insured; and, if necessary, follow-up procedures are instituted if payment is not received from the carrier within a specified time period. We will discuss each of these events in detail.

Point-of-Service Device

A new electronic device now available to some health care providers is a **point-of-service (POS) device**. This device provides immediate and direct access to patient eligibility information and managed care functions through an electronic network connecting the medical office and the health plan's computer.

The POS is a small card-swipe box similar in design and function to a credit card terminal (Figure 19-4). It allows medical office personnel to:

- Record a patient visit
- Check eligibility for patients in the health plan
- Enter referrals for patients in managed care plans
- Verify referral information
- Check authorization status
- Enter inpatient authorization requests
- Enter outpatient authorization requests

After the information is input by the medical assistant, the POS communicates with the health plan's computer

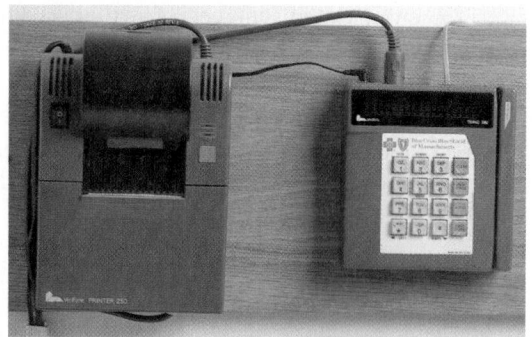

Figure 19-4   Point-of-service (POS) device allows direct communication between medical offices and the health care plan's computer. (Right) To enter information, the patient's insurance card is swiped through the machine or the patient's identification number is entered on the keypad along with specific transaction code numbers. (Left) Responses from the plan's computer are printed directly in the medical office.

system. The computer then returns an acknowledgment to the medical office confirming the transaction or giving an error message code. For example, when visits are recorded accurately, a reference number is generated that is used as the medical office's confirmation that the transaction is complete. Upon successful entry of a referral, a referral number is generated. Specialists may use this number on claims they submit for services they render under the referral.

Maintaining Claim Register or Diary

When claim forms are sent to the appropriate insurance carrier, it is wise and necessary for the medical office personnel to keep a diary or register of submitted claims (Figure 19-5). This **claim register** should include the patient's name, the insured's name if it is different from the patient's name, the dates of service for which the claim is being made, the amount of the claim, and the date the claim is

Date	Patient Name	Insured Name	Insurance Company	Dates Billed	Total Charges	Amount Received
1-18-__	McKay, Leo	—	How Much Ins Co.	1-10-__	98.00	

Figure 19-5   Example of claim register used to track insurance claims.

submitted. When payment is received, date of payment should be entered. When aging and reconciling accounts, the bookkeeper then can check the diary to note where the claim is in the process.

The Insurance Carrier's Role

Upon receipt of the claim form, the claims processor at the insurance carrier checks the codes to make sure that the procedures and accompanying diagnoses agree. The processor then analyzes the information to make certain that:

1. The coverage was in force at the time of treatment
2. The physician has contracted with the insurance carrier
3. There are no exclusions or restrictions on the policy for payment of that diagnosis
4. There are no pre-existing condition restrictions
5. The diagnosis and procedures done are reasonable

The processor also checks to make sure that the billed amount falls within the usual, customary, and reasonable fee that the insurance carrier has developed for that specific procedure.

Explanation of Benefits

Upon completion of the processing of the claim, the insurance company sends an **Explanation of Benefits (EOB)** to the insured. This form includes the dates, charges, amounts applied toward the deductible, amounts not covered either due to an exclusion or excess over the usual, customary, and reasonable charge, and the amount the company is paying for this claim. Some Explanation of Benefits forms even serve as a "bill" or "notice" in that they indicate the amount the insured must forward to the physician for payment in full of the account.

Following Up on Claims

Occasionally, claims may be denied because the claim form was not properly coded. However, if there is no payment from the carrier and no other notification after a period of four to six weeks, it is necessary to follow up on the claim. The claim register will enable the office to keep track of the progress of claims.

To follow up, a toll-free number is provided by most carriers. The necessary information to have before making the call includes a copy of the claim form and the patient's name and insurance identification number. The carrier should be able to give the status of the claim. If payment is delayed, the carrier should be able to give the date when it can be expected. It is possible that payment was sent to the insured, in which case a statement should be sent to the patient. If there is a problem with the claim, the medical assistant may need to investigate the cause of the error and submit a revised claim.

For information on billing and collection procedures, see Chapter 20.

THE COMPUTERIZED CLAIMS PROCESS

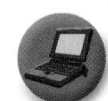 Many ambulatory care settings are coding claim forms on the computer. Most medical software is capable of automatically printing the HCFA-1500 form, which many physician offices and/or billing services will submit electronically from one computer to another. This tends to speed the claims process, although it is still important to take as much care as when manually coding a claim.

Typically, a computer program will receive instructions to print claims forms and to track the forms on a standard schedule. The information for each patient is keyed into the computer; once entered, the information is stored and can be utilized, with revisions as necessary, for future claim forms for that patient. This eliminates some of the tedious typewriting involved in filling out the claim form and ensures greater accuracy since much of the information only needs to be entered once.

LEGAL AND ETHICAL ISSUES

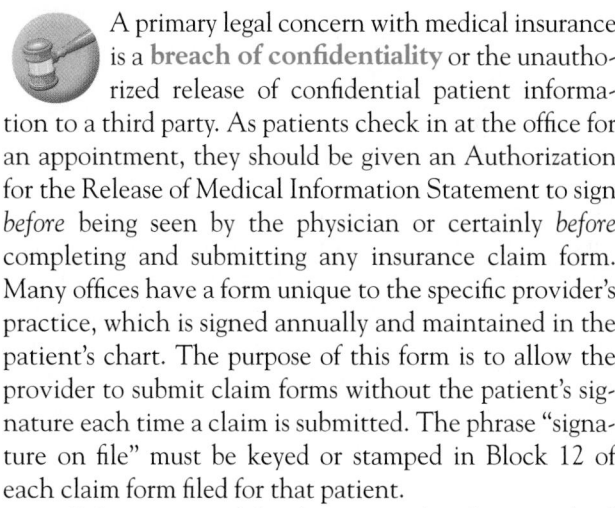 A primary legal concern with medical insurance is a **breach of confidentiality** or the unauthorized release of confidential patient information to a third party. As patients check in at the office for an appointment, they should be given an Authorization for the Release of Medical Information Statement to sign *before* being seen by the physician or certainly *before* completing and submitting any insurance claim form. Many offices have a form unique to the specific provider's practice, which is signed annually and maintained in the patient's chart. The purpose of this form is to allow the provider to submit claim forms without the patient's signature each time a claim is submitted. The phrase "signature on file" must be keyed or stamped in Block 12 of each claim form filed for that patient.

Other types of legal issues related to medical insurance include fraud and insurance abuse. **Fraud** is defined as an intentional deception or misrepresentation that an individual makes, knowing it to be false, which could result in some unauthorized benefit. Examples of fraud in the medical office may include, but are not limited to:

- Using a higher level of service code in order to increase practice revenue
- Billing for services, equipment, or supplies that were not provided or required

● Misrepresenting a patient diagnosis to justify the level of services performed to increase practice revenue

Insurance abuse is defined as incidents or practices of providers, physicians, or suppliers of services and equipment that, while not considered fraudulent, are inconsistent with accepted sound medical, business, or fiscal practices. Examples of insurance abuse in the medical office may include, but are not limited to:

● Overcharging for services, equipment, or supplies

● Submitting claims for items or services that are not medically necessary to treat the patient's condition

● Billing practices that result in payment by a government program when the claim is the legal responsibility of another third-party payer

Coding errors pose another type of legal and ethical issue. The Omnibus Budget Reconciliation Acts of 1986 and 1987 state that physicians can be assessed civil penalties if they "know of or should know that claims filed with Medicare or Medicaid on their behalf are not true and accurate representations of the items or services actually provided." This means that physicians can be held responsible not only for negligent mistakes they make but also for mistakes made in their behalf by their medical assistants completing insurance claim forms. The penalties assessed are usually in the form of a monetary fine and may also involve exclusion from Medicare and Medicaid programs for a period of time.

HEALTHCARE COMPLIANCE

The Office of Inspector General (OIG) issued compliance program guidelines in 2000 to assist physicians in solo or small group practices. These guidelines, consisting of seven steps, are not mandatory but focus on the development of meaningful voluntary compliance programs. They serve as a resource to be considered in addition to other OIG outreach efforts and other federal agency efforts to promote compliance.

Seven Basic Elements of a Voluntary Compliance Program

1. Conduct periodic internal monitoring and auditing.
2. Implement compliance and practice standards by developing written standards and procedures.
3. Designate a compliance officer or contacts to monitor compliance efforts and enforce practice standards.
4. Conduct appropriate training and education on practice standards and procedures.

SPOTLIGHT ON AAMA ESSENTIALS THROUGH CAAHEP

● Establishing a positive relationship with the patient during the first appointment assists the medical assistant in gathering important data and information necessary for coding and billing services at a later time.

● When following insurance and coding procedures, the medical assistant must always maintain a professional attitude and confidentiality when talking to patients regarding their care and treatment.

● The medical assistant responsible for coding procedures must prepare the billing and insurance forms with care and be understanding and positive when discussing the payment schedule with the patient.

---

5. Respond appropriately to detected violations by investigating allegations and disclosing incidents to appropriate government entities.
6. Develop open lines of communication, such as (1) discussions at staff meetings regarding how to avoid erroneous or fraudulent conduct and (2) community bulletin boards, to keep practice employees updated regarding compliance activities.
7. Enforce disciplinary standards through well-publicized guidelines.

Each practice is encouraged to undertake reasonable steps to implement the seven basic elements as best reflects their practice. Advantages of participating in a compliance program include:

● Helps prevent fraudulent or erroneous claims

● Demonstrates the practice is making a good faith effort to submit claims appropriately

● Considered analogous to practicing preventive medicine

Employees have an affirmative, ethical duty to come forward and report fraudulent or erroneous conduct so that it may be corrected. Individuals who fail to detect or report violations of the compliance program may be subject to discipline. Disciplinary actions could include verbal warnings, written reprimands, probation, demotion, temporary suspension, discharge of employment, restitution of damages, and referral for criminal prosecution. Including disciplinary guidelines in training and procedure manuals is sufficient to meet the well-publicized standard.

DOCUMENTATION

An auditor should check claim forms, whether submitted electronically or by hard copy, to see that they are completed correctly. Include all pertinent dates and diagnostic and procedural coding information necessary for insurance payers to generate reimbursement. Auditors will look specifically for any indicators of insurance fraud and abuse.

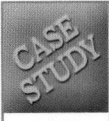
CASE STUDY
19-1

Leo McKay, an established patient at Inner City Health Care, schedules a visit, complaining of nausea and severe abdominal pain. Dr. Mark Woo spends 30 minutes taking a history and doing an examination. He suspects an ulcer and orders lab tests (CBC complete, guaiac, lipid panel, and UA) to be done in the office and sends Mr. McKay for an upper GI series. Mr. McKay returns in 10 days to the test results which show a duodenal ulcer.

CASE STUDY REVIEW

1. What would the proper diagnosis codes be for Mr. McKay?
2. What would the proper procedure codes be for Mr. McKay?
3. In coding the claim form for Mr. McKay's visit, what ethical principle and legal principle should guide the medical assistant?

SUMMARY

Much material has been covered in this chapter. Remember, you can be the person to make the difference in insurance billing. By checking and double-checking your work, you make certain that the physician's time is being billed at the appropriate rate, that all procedures are billed with the proper diagnoses, and that the billing is sent to the correct insurance carrier. It takes much less time to double-check work once

and have it correct *before* it is sent out than to send it out with errors that cause difficulty in the future.

An understanding of medical insurance coverages and coding procedures is vital to a thriving ambulatory care setting. The astute medical assistant will perceive the challenges involved in proper coding techniques and understand their role in the management of the physician's office.

REVIEW QUESTIONS

Multiple Choice

1. CPT codes:
   a. are for diagnosis coding
   b. have five digits and may have two-digit modifiers
   c. have three-digit codes with a decimal point and one to two additional digits
   d. are updated semiannually
2. When coding a diagnosis, go first to:
   a. CPT
   b. Volume I of ICD-9-CM
   c. Volume II of ICD-9-CM
   d. E codes in ICD-9-CM

3. A plus symbol on a CPT code indicates:
   a. unusual procedural services
   b. bilateral procedures
   c. procedure is an add-on to a previously described procedure
   d. repeat procedure by the same physician
4. Level II of HCPCS:
   a. uses a five-digit alphanumeric code to clarify procedures
   b. is the same as the regular CPT system
   c. is assigned by the fiscal intermediary
   d. uses the letter codes W, X, Y, and Z

5. The ICD-9-CM codes:
   a. were developed by the AMA as uniform descriptions of medical, surgical, and diagnostic services
   b. are divided into seven sections
   c. use modifiers
   d. code every disease, illness, condition, injury, and cause of injury known

6. Most insurance carriers accept which claim form?
   a. UB92
   b. HCFA-1500
   c. CPT
   d. HCFA-1450

7. Claim registers are used to:
   a. anticipate claims to be sent to insurance companies for processing
   b. check how many claims are sent to Medicare
   c. monitor claims that have been sent to insurance companies for processing
   d. help in aging accounts

8. Insurance abuse:
   a. is the unauthorized release of confidential patient information to a third party
   b. is an intentional deception or misrepresentation that an individual makes, knowing it to be false, which could result in some unauthorized benefit
   c. refers to incidents or practices of providers, physicians, or suppliers of services and equipment that are inconsistent with accepted sound medical, business, or fiscal practices
   d. is impacted by the Omnibus Budget Reconciliation Acts of 1986 and 1987

Critical Thinking

1. Which claim form is accepted by most insurance companies?
2. Which book is used to code a diagnosis? What is the proper order in using the diagnosis coding book?
3. Which book is used to code office visits and procedures?
4. What are three things to keep in mind when coding a claim?
5. Where should accident-related charges be billed first?

WEB ACTIVITIES

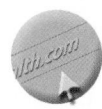

Use the Internet to search for current information on fraud and insurance abuse in Medicare billing. Document your findings following instructor guidelines.

REFERENCES/BIBLIOGRAPHY

American Medical Association (1999). *Current procedural terminology.* Chicago: American Medical Association.

American Medical Association (Oct. 1999). *International classification of diseases, clinical modifications* (2nd ed., 9th rev.). Chicago: American Medical Association.

American Medical Association (1999). *Principles of CPT coding.* Chicago: American Medical Association.

Back, C. J. (2000). *Step-by-step medical coding.* Philadelphia: W. B. Saunders Company.

HCFA (2000). Medicare part B billing manual: Noridian Mutual Insurance.

Humphrey, D. D. (1996). *Contemporary medical office procedures* (2nd ed.). Albany, NY: Delmar.

Keir, L., Wise, B. A., & Krebs, C. (1998). *Medical assisting: Administrative and clinical competencies* (4th ed.). Albany, NY: Delmar.

Kinn, M. E., & Woods, M. A. (1999). *The medical assistant: Administrative and clinical* (8th ed.). Philadelphia: W. B. Saunders Company.

Office of Inspector General, U.S. Department of Health and Human Services. (2000). *Compliance program guide for individual and small group physician practices* [On-line]. Available: http://oig.hhs.gov/modcomp/webcpg.txt

Rizzo, C. D. (2000). *Uniform billing: A guide to claims processing.* Albany, NY: Delmar.

Rowell, J. C. (1998). *Understanding medical insurance* (4th ed.). Albany, NY: Delmar.

Chapter

20

BILLING AND COLLECTIONS

KEY TERMS

Account Aging
Collection Agency
Credit Bureau
Cycle Billing
Fair Debt Collection Practice Act
Monthly Billing
Probate Court
Statute of Limitations
Truth-in-Lending Act

OUTLINE

Billing Procedures
Credit and Collection Policies
Payment at Time of Service
Truth-in-Lending Act
Components of a Complete Statement
    Computerized Statements
Monthly and Cycle Billing
    Monthly Billing
    Cycle Billing
Past-Due Accounts
Collection Process
Aging Accounts
    Computerized Aging

Collection Techniques
    Correspondence to Insurance
      Carriers
    Telephone Collections
    Collection Letters
**Use of an Outside Collection
    Agency**
Use of Small Claims Court
Special Collection Situations
    Bankruptcy
    Estates
    Tracing "Skips"
Statute of Limitations

OBJECTIVES

*The student should strive to meet the following performance objectives and demonstrate
an understanding of the facts and principles presented in this chapter through written and
oral communication.*

1. Define the key terms as presented in the glossary.
2. Analyze the importance of billing and collections to the ambulatory care setting.
3. Describe the advantages of billing at time of service.
4. Recall the components of a complete statement.
5. Differentiate between monthly and cycle billing.
6. Describe the process of sending a series of collection letters.
7. Analyze the importance of correct manner in telephone collections.
8. Explain the process of aging accounts.
9. Recall three special collections problems encountered in the ambulatory care setting.
10. Explain the ramifications of the statute of limitations.

SCENARIO

At Doctors Lewis & King, patient billing is typically done at time of service, and a charge slip noting date, description of charges, and fees is given to the patient upon leaving the office. Office policy states that, if possible, patients should pay their part of the fee, or their copay, at time of service. Marilyn Johnson, the office manager, has found that this is the most efficient way to ensure timely payment and eliminates the need to mail a separate statement. However, the office is flexible and, if the patient cannot pay all or part of the charge at the visit, Marilyn works out a payment schedule that is acceptable to both office and patient.

INTRODUCTION

In the ambulatory care setting, patient billing is a critical administrative function that helps to maintain a healthy, viable practice. Timeliness is essential in billing, for the ambulatory care setting depends on its accounts receivable to pay its bills in a responsible manner. Billing need not be a complex activity, but it must be completely accurate. In offices still using pegboard accounting, billing and collection procedures are done manually, often using the patient's ledger card as the basis for the statement. If the office is computerized, patient bills and collection notices are typically computer generated.

While not all ambulatory care settings expect payment at the time of service, it is certainly common. The best method of patient billing and collections is a method that is customized to the practice and that regards the patient as a consumer who should be respected. Patients appreciate knowing in advance what charges and fees to expect. Many offices include these in their informational brochures or post them in a prominent place in the office.

BILLING PROCEDURES

The ambulatory care setting's cash flow and collection process are dependent on accurate billing techniques. The financial status of the practice is reflected in monthly statements indicating unpaid patient balances, which, if they persist, are reviewed for appropriate action, including referral to a **collection agency**. Copies of all billing forms will be retained in the patient account record.

Timeliness and accuracy have a significant influence upon prompt payment and how soon collection of the patient account will be finalized. In other words, billing performance can be measured by the time it takes to generate and submit a complete statement, that is, a statement with full documentation. If an office is experiencing problems generating patient bills, a billing timeliness analysis worksheet can be constructed to identify internal delays that affect how quickly an account is billed and thus paid. By focusing on inefficiencies in the revenue cycle, processes may be identified that need to be streamlined. For example, the date of service and insurance verification, the date the bill was generated, and the date the bill was submitted to the patient or third party can determine the efficiency of the billing process.

A billing efficiency report is another instrument that may be used to monitor efficiency. This report lists the previous month's billing backlog, which is added to the number of new accounts. The number of processed accounts is then subtracted. The weekly number of accounts that were rebilled also is noted, and the amount of time billing personnel spent on billing accounts is recorded. Production efficiency is calculated from this data. Inherent to this system is the careful monitoring of follow-up bills: whether they were paid, if the insurance was paid, and assessing the patient's responsibility for payment.

CREDIT AND COLLECTION POLICIES

Even uncomplicated patient billing should be done according to credit and collection policies established by the physician employers of the ambulatory care setting. Having a formalized policy makes decision making easier and gives the medical assistant responsible for billing and collections authority to act. For example, some questions the physicians and office manager may want to address include:

- When will payment be due from the patient?

- What kind of payment arrangements can be made if the patient does not pay at time of service?

- Will a collection agency be utilized? Who decides?

- At what point should a patient be reminded of an overdue bill?

- How is that reminder initially managed: by telephone or letter?

- At what point will a patient bill be considered delinquent?

- If exceptions to office policy are to be made, who makes these exceptions?

By answering these and other questions, a straightforward credit and collection policy can be devised that is a guide to both patients and the medical assistant in charge of billing.

Patient Teaching Tip

Patients appreciate knowing their responsibility in terms of payment. Whoever schedules the first appointment with a new patient should diplomatically inform the patient of office policy on payment of fees. If the patient anticipates a problem in paying promptly, a schedule can be worked out that is agreeable to both parties.

PAYMENT AT TIME OF SERVICE

Because the best opportunity for collection is at the time of service, many ambulatory care settings provide the patient with a bill and require payment at that time. This assures prompt collection, eliminates further bookkeeping work, and provides better cash flow for the practice. To accommodate the patient, most offices accept cash, personal checks, and possibly credit cards.

It is important to note that payment at time of service will be adjusted according to the patient's insurance and the terms of that policy. If the patient is a member of an HMO, and the ambulatory care center is a participating provider, it is bound to the terms of that agreement.

It is always helpful to discuss fees with patients when scheduling the first appointment, especially if payment is appreciated at time of service. See also Chapter 17 for a discussion of fees.

TRUTH-IN-LENDING ACT

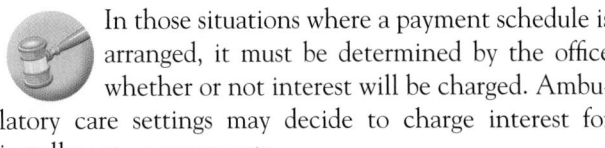 In those situations where a payment schedule is arranged, it must be determined by the office whether or not interest will be charged. Ambulatory care settings may decide to charge interest for installment arrangements.

Medical assistants need to be aware of the conditions of the **Truth-in-Lending Act** (also called the Consumer Credit Protection Act of 1968) which was established to protect consumers by requiring that providers of installment credit state the charges clearly in writing and express the interest as an annual rate. When there is a bilateral agreement between the physician and patient to pay in more than four installments, the physician must disclose finance charges in writing. Even if no finance charges are made, the forms must still be completed.

COMPONENTS OF A COMPLETE STATEMENT

Statements to patients must be professional looking, neat, accurate, and inclusive of all services and charges. If the statement is to be mailed, an enclosed self-addressed envelope is a convenience for many patients and may result in a faster turnaround of payment.

Charge slip (also known as superbill), statement, and insurance reporting information are often combined on one form (Figure 20-1). A well-prepared patient statement should contain not only information for the patient, but information needed to process medical insurance claims as well.

- Patient's name and address

- Patient's insurance identification number

- Insurance carrier

- Date of service

- Description of service

- Accurate procedure (CPT) and diagnosis (ICD-9-CM) codes for insurance processing (see also Chapters 18 and 19)

- Physician's signature

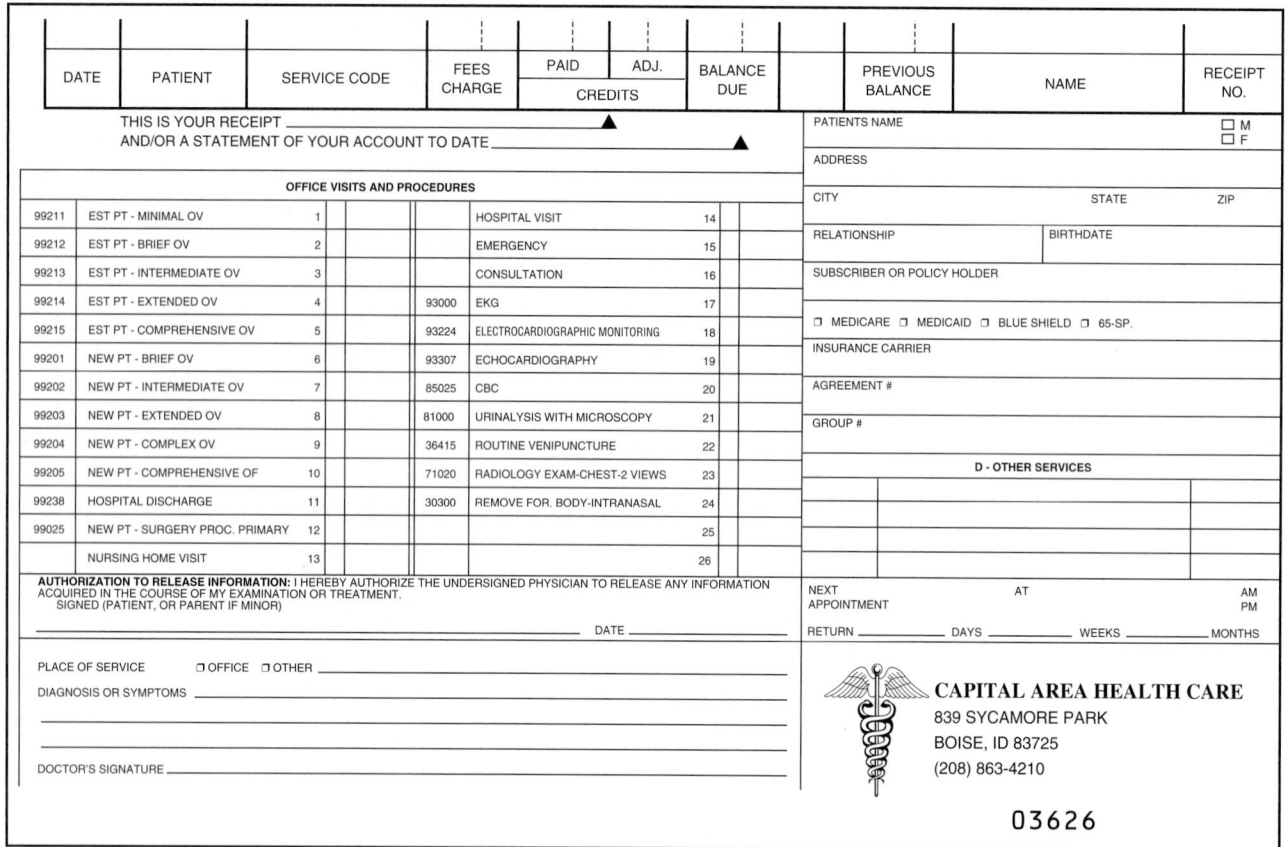

DATE	PATIENT	SERVICE CODE	FEES CHARGE	PAID	ADJ.	BALANCE DUE		PREVIOUS BALANCE	NAME	RECEIPT NO.
				CREDITS						

THIS IS YOUR RECEIPT _____
AND/OR A STATEMENT OF YOUR ACCOUNT TO DATE _____

OFFICE VISITS AND PROCEDURES

99211	EST PT - MINIMAL OV	1				HOSPITAL VISIT	14	
99212	EST PT - BRIEF OV	2				EMERGENCY	15	
99213	EST PT - INTERMEDIATE OV	3				CONSULTATION	16	
99214	EST PT - EXTENDED OV	4		93000		EKG	17	
99215	EST PT - COMPREHENSIVE OV	5		93224		ELECTROCARDIOGRAPHIC MONITORING	18	
99201	NEW PT - BRIEF OV	6		93307		ECHOCARDIOGRAPHY	19	
99202	NEW PT - INTERMEDIATE OV	7		85025		CBC	20	
99203	NEW PT - EXTENDED OV	8		81000		URINALYSIS WITH MICROSCOPY	21	
99204	NEW PT - COMPLEX OV	9		36415		ROUTINE VENIPUNCTURE	22	
99205	NEW PT - COMPREHENSIVE OF	10		71020		RADIOLOGY EXAM-CHEST-2 VIEWS	23	
99238	HOSPITAL DISCHARGE	11		30300		REMOVE FOR. BODY-INTRANASAL	24	
99025	NEW PT - SURGERY PROC. PRIMARY	12					25	
	NURSING HOME VISIT	13					26	

AUTHORIZATION TO RELEASE INFORMATION: I HEREBY AUTHORIZE THE UNDERSIGNED PHYSICIAN TO RELEASE ANY INFORMATION ACQUIRED IN THE COURSE OF MY EXAMINATION OR TREATMENT.
SIGNED (PATIENT, OR PARENT IF MINOR)

_____ DATE _____

PLACE OF SERVICE   ❑ OFFICE ❑ OTHER _____

DIAGNOSIS OR SYMPTOMS _____

DOCTOR'S SIGNATURE _____

PATIENTS NAME   ❑ M
                                                                      ❑ F
ADDRESS
CITY   STATE   ZIP
RELATIONSHIP   BIRTHDATE
SUBSCRIBER OR POLICY HOLDER

❑ MEDICARE ❑ MEDICAID ❑ BLUE SHIELD ❑ 65-SP.
INSURANCE CARRIER
AGREEMENT #
GROUP #

D - OTHER SERVICES

NEXT   AT   AM
APPOINTMENT   PM
RETURN _____ DAYS _____ WEEKS _____ MONTHS

CAPITAL AREA HEALTH CARE
839 SYCAMORE PARK
BOISE, ID 83725
(208) 863-4210

03626

Figure 20-1   Sample charge slip shown is a multipurpose form used to document information for insurance claims as well as to provide the patient with a receipt and documentation of procedures, diagnoses, and fees.

● Ambulatory care center name, address, telephone number, and possibly fax number

Computerized Statements

If the ambulatory care setting uses a computer system of bookkeeping, then statements will be computer generated. Typically, the medical assistant issues instructions to search the patient database for outstanding balances and directs the computer to print statements.

During this process, the computer program will also "age" accounts (see Aging Accounts in this chapter) and print collection letters (already in the database) for over-due accounts.

MONTHLY AND CYCLE BILLING

The billing schedule is often determined by the size of the medical practice. Monthly billing is a system in which all accounts are billed at the same time each month. In a smaller ambulatory care setting, monthly billing may be the most efficient method. Cycle billing staggers bills during the month and is a flexible system for larger practices.

Monthly Billing

In a **monthly billing** system, one or two days are devoted to billing and mailing all statements. Typically, statements should leave the office on the 25th of the month to be received by the first of the month. The major disadvantage of monthly billing is that a medical assistant may neglect other activities during this time-consuming period. To avoid these problems, billing statements may be prepared intermittently over a one- or two-week period and stored until the mailing date. To avoid confusion caused by delays in mailing, a message to "Disregard if payment has already been made" should be printed on the form. Patients become annoyed and the practice appears disorganized if a statement arrives several days after payment has been made.

Cycle Billing

In a **cycle billing** system, all accounts are divided alphabetically into groups, with each group billed at a different time. In this way, office personnel with numerous bills to process each month will be able to handle them in a more efficient manner. Statements are prepared on the same

To cycle bill patient accounts:

1. Divide the alphabet into four sections: A–F, G–L, M–R, S–Z.
2. Prepare statements for patients whose last names begin with A through F on Wednesday and mail them on Thursday of Week 1.
3. Prepare statements for patients whose last names begin with G through L on Wednesday and mail them on Thursday of Week 2.
4. Prepare statements for patients whose last names begin with M through R on Wednesday and mail them on Thursday of Week 3.
5. Prepare statements for patients whose last names begin with S through Z on Wednesday and mail them on Thursday of Week 4.

Figure 20-2 Typical schedule for cycle billing system.

schedule each month. They can be mailed as they are completed, or held and mailed at one time. A typical cycle billing schedule is shown in Figure 20-2. The system can be varied to suit the needs of the individual practice.

PAST-DUE ACCOUNTS

As efficient and effective as the billing process may be, there will still be collections on some accounts. The most common reasons for past due accounts include:

- Inability to pay. People may have financial hardships from time to time.
- Negligence. People may forget to make a payment because they have been away or dealing with a family emergency.
- Unwillingness to pay. When a patient complains about a charge or refuses to pay, it may have nothing to do with finances. Often, they are dissatisfied with the care or treatment they have received. These patients should be referred to the physician or office manager for immediate attention.

COLLECTION PROCESS

The process of collecting delinquent accounts begins with first establishing how much has been owed for how long.

Ideally, collection of accounts receivable should be prompt and conducted in a timely fashion. Management consultants recommend that fees should be collected at the time of service and that a collection ratio of at least 90 percent should be maintained. A collection ratio is a method used to gauge the effectiveness of the ambulatory care setting's billing practices. Typically, the collection

ratio is figured by dividing the total collections by the net charges (gross charges minus adjustments). This yields a percentage, which is the collection ratio.

Another important factor is the accounts receivable ratio, which measures the speed with which outstanding accounts are paid. The desirable ratio is less than two months for collection of accounts receivable. To figure the accounts receivable ratio, divide the current accounts receivable balance by the average monthly gross charges. This yields the typical turnaround for collecting accounts receivable. Also see Chapter 21 for more information on account receivable and collection ratios.

The longer an office puts off attempting to collect delinquent accounts, the less chance there is of receiving payment. Statistics show that the value of the dollar decreases rapidly in the collection process. The more time and energy you put into collections, the less value you receive in return. In other words, you may manage to collect the full amount due, but when you consider the time and expense involved, it may not have been worth the effort and expense. Therefore, the value of the debt to be received following successful collection must be considered when determining how aggressive to be in debt collections. It is evident that as time passes the value of outstanding accounts as well as the percentage that will be collected declines.

AGING ACCOUNTS

Account aging is a method of identifying how long an account is overdue. This means that past due accounts are identified according to the length of time they have been unpaid. When using a pegboard bookkeeping system, color-coded strips are attached to the ledger cards to show the age of an account, or the cards can be stored behind a color-coded divider in a separate file labeled "Unpaid." For example, a red strip might be used for accounts one month overdue, a blue strip for accounts two months overdue, and other colors for additional months overdue. A written code such as "OD3/2/23" should be written on the ledger card to indicate when the overdue notice was mailed, meaning "Overdue notice No. 3 mailed on February 23."

Depending upon the type of patient served, different aging systems are used. In a computerized billing system, the accounts are automatically aged, and the aging schedule or process is shown on the computerized ledger card. A typical aging schedule for a private patient is shown in Figure 20-3.

Computerized Aging

Aging accounts using a computerized system is very simple. Before printing billing statements, the medical assistant keys the appropriate

Charge slip (Superbill) given to patient at time of visit.

1. Itemized statement mailed at end of first month.
2. Itemized statement with overdue notice mailed when account is past due two months.
3. Telephone call reminding patient of overdue account and offering to help arrange a payment schedule.
4. Letter stating, "We have not received payment for your account," when account is past due three months.
5. Letter or telephone call stating, "Your account will be turned over to a collector," if this is the policy of the facility.
6. Certified letter stating (if outside collectors are used), "Your account was turned over to a collection agency." No further telephone calls are necessary, as they might antagonize the patient and leave the medical assistant open to verbal abuse.

Figure 20-3 Sample aging process for a patient with private insurance.

commands to age the accounts. The program can age accounts according to several criteria: for example, by past due balance, zero balance, or credit balance accounts. Accounts can also be aged by government agency category or by insurance carrier. All Medicare or Medicaid accounts might be aged separately from other accounts.

The computer can also generate and print an accounts receivable report showing each overdue account, the balance overdue, and a breakdown showing how long the account is overdue. This breakdown is usually divided into accounts 0 to 30 days overdue, 31 to 60 days overdue, 61 to 90 days overdue, and 90 days or more overdue. Additional reports can be generated from the accounts receivable report. For example, the office staff may wish to reprint a report showing accounts that have been delinquent for more than 90 days or accounts that are delinquent by more than a certain dollar amount.

COLLECTION TECHNIQUES

Ambulatory care settings use both telephone and written communications in their collection techniques. While both have some measure of effectiveness, some practices prefer to call the patient with a past due account before officially initiating collection proceedings. The patient may have misplaced the statement, forgotten a payment, or been away on an extended vacation; a quick telephone call can often resolve the situation without the time and expense involved in collections. Also, the patient appreciates the courtesy and personal approach.

Correspondence to Insurance Carriers

Many patients have some form of medical insurance. Most claim departments of insurance carriers and government agencies employ large numbers of employees who have varying levels of experience. Payment can be delayed because of an overburdened claim department, a form that has been lost in transit, a misfiled form, an inexperienced employee, or numerous other reasons.

The medical assistant should maintain an up-to-date claims register (see Chapter 18) or tickler file and take firm control of the practice's collection procedures to ensure that claims are paid promptly. In offices where the medical assistant files claims for patients, a follow-up collection policy is important to maintain strong cash flow. When carriers do not pay in full or question or deny a claim, the medical assistant will have to determine the nature of the problem and notify the patients.

Telephone Collections

The medical assistant is likely to use the telephone for collection procedures. Telephoning is often an effective measure, for a patient may remember a call more so than a bill received in the mail.

A successful telephone collection call is enhanced by keeping to the facts, being tactful, pleasant, and diplomatic. When making calls to patients regarding past due accounts, there are some things to keep in mind in order to maintain the desired relationship with patients. Always remain courteous and respectful. Do not treat patients with suspicion or threats. Remember, the health profession is dedicated to helping people; avoid antagonizing patients.

Most people do not let their bills become past due on purpose or out of spite. Keep this in mind when making calls. Work with patients to encourage and enable them to pay any fees they owe.

Certain legal rules and ethical guidelines govern telephone collections.

- When making collection calls, callers must identify themselves and ascertain that they are talking to the person who is responsible for the account.
- A collection call could be embarrassing to the patient; therefore it should not be made to the patient's place of employment.
- In most states, a debtor may be contacted only between 8 A.M. and 9 P.M.
- Do not threaten to turn the person over to collection agencies.

Violating these rules makes the caller vulnerable to charges of harassment under the **Fair Debt Collection Practice Act.**

When collecting by telephone, it is helpful to keep complete accurate records of who said what and how much was promised as payment. If, after two weeks nothing has been resolved as a result of the calls, then another course of action, such as retaining the services of a collection agency or **credit bureau**, may be the solution, especially for large sums of money owed.

Collection Letters

Collection letters are sent to encourage patients and third-party carriers to pay overdue balances. After two statements are mailed to patients and the charge slip has brought no response, the ambulatory care setting begins sending collection letters.

Lack of payment from a patient is usually not considered serious until after 60 days. When the patient fails to respond to the charge slip, to the statement, or to a 60-day statement with an "Overdue" remark, a series of collection letters begins. One typical collection letter series is shown in Figure 20-4 A through C.

USE OF AN OUTSIDE COLLECTION AGENCY

Occasionally, the ambulatory care setting may turn over highly delinquent accounts to an outside collection agency. Discretion is always advised here, however, for the expense of collection may not justify the fees to be collected. For unpaid accounts with large balances, however, this is often a viable solution.

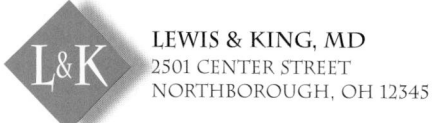

LEWIS & KING, MD
2501 CENTER STREET
NORTHBOROUGH, OH 12345

June 14, 20—

Mr. John O'Keefe
12 Gravers Lane
Northborough, OH 12345

Dear Mr. O'Keefe:

Your account with our office is three months past due, and you have not responded to our previous requests for payment. Please pay your balance of $852 at this time, or contact us with an explanation of why you cannot pay.

Please call me at 312-824-6925 if you have a question about your account. Otherwise, we expect your payment immediately.

Sincerely,

Marilyn Johnson
Office Manager

NORTHBOROUGH
FAMILY MEDICAL GROUP

(A)

Figure 20-4 Sample collection letters: (A) First letter.

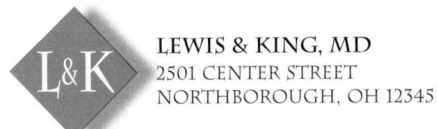

LEWIS & KING, MD
2501 CENTER STREET
NORTHBOROUGH, OH 12345

July 15, 20—

Mr. John O'Keefe
12 Gravers Lane
Northborough, OH 12345

Dear Mr. O'Keefe:

Your son, Chris, was seriously ill in March when he came to Dr. King for treatment. Dr. King was pleased to use her experience and education to treat Chris, and it was in this same spirit of cooperation that we expected you to pay your account within a reasonable amount of time.

Four months have passed and you have still not remitted the $852 outstanding balance on your account. We cannot continue to keep your unpaid account on our books. If you are experiencing financial difficulties, please call the office so we can arrange a payment schedule that is agreeable to both of us.

Sincerely,

Marilyn Johnson
Office Manager

NORTHBOROUGH
FAMILY MEDICAL GROUP

(B)

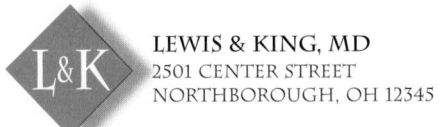

LEWIS & KING, MD
2501 CENTER STREET
NORTHBOROUGH, OH 12345

August 17, 20—

CERTIFIED MAIL

Mr. John O'Keefe
12 Gravers Lane
Northborough, OH 12345

Dear Mr. O'Keefe:

This is our final attempt to collect your account of $852, which is five months past due. You have ignored all our previous letters [or letters and phone calls], so we have no alternative but to turn over your account to a collection company.

Your account is being assigned to Ambler Medical Collection Service, which will pursue whatever legal means is necessary to collect this debt. If you contact me at 312-824-6925 within seven days, we will retrieve your account from the collection service to protect your credit rating.

Sincerely,

Marilyn Johnson
Office Manager

NORTHBOROUGH
FAMILY MEDICAL GR

(C)

Figure 20-4 *(continued)* (B) Second letter. (C) Third letter.

One service of the collection agency is to provide an intercept letter. For a nominal fee, this may be sent from the agency as the last resort before the account is turned over to collection. This communication alerts patients to the fact that if a response is not received, their account will go to collection. This often is the only action needed for the patient to pay the outstanding bill. Another service of a credit bureau or collection agency is to provide credit ratings of patients at the physician's request. Physicians who pay for this service are able to monitor patients' ability to pay their bills, as well as to trace a "skip," someone who leaves with an outstanding bill and no forwarding address.

When selecting a collection agency, be certain to hire one that is compatible with the medical office's philosophy. Ask for referrals from other physicians, ambulatory care centers, and hospitals. Ask the agency about its approach to collections and request sample letters and reminder notices.

USE OF SMALL CLAIMS COURT

In certain circumstances, the ambulatory care center may consider bringing a case to small claims court. Typically, small claims courts handle cases that involve only limited amounts of debt (these vary from state to state), they do not permit representation by an attorney, and they are generally efficient and streamlined in their proceedings. Nonetheless, preparing for small claims courts and taking time to appear will require a certain investment of staff. It is also important to note that, if the court finds in the medical office's favor, the medical office still must collect the money from the defendant.

SPECIAL COLLECTION SITUATIONS

In patient billing and collections, a number of special situations may arise.

Bankruptcy

If a patient has declared bankruptcy, statements may no longer be sent nor any attempt be made to collect delinquent accounts. Because a physician's fee is an unsecured debt, it is one of the last to be paid. Bankruptcy laws are federal and are subject to the Federal Wage Garnishment Law of attaching property to satisfy debt.

Estates

Collection of fees when a patient has died must be directed to the executor of the estate or the one responsible for overseeing the estate. Some general guidelines to follow include:

- Show courtesy by not sending a statement in the first week or so after a death.
- Address the statement to "Estate of (name of patient)" with the patient's last known address.
- If unsure of how to proceed, contact the office's attorney or the clerk of the probate court for advice.

Tracing "Skips"

As noted earlier in this chapter, a "skip" is a patient who has apparently moved with no forwarding address. If a statement is returned to your office marked "no forwarding address," first determine if there were any internal errors in addressing the envelope. If the address is determined to be correct, the medical assistant may try to call the patient with the number on the patient ledger; it is possible that the patient has retained the same number or there may be a new number given. If the medical assistant is unable to secure a telephone number, the office needs to decide whether to pursue the unpaid debt. This will depend on office policy and the amount that is owed. If it is decided to pursue an unpaid account, it could be turned over to a collection agency. If the medical assistant attempts to trace the skip by calling employers or relatives, it is very important not to violate any laws in doing so.

STATUTE OF LIMITATIONS

A statute of limitations is a statute that defines the period in which legal action may take place. When applying this concept to collections, the time period is usually defined by the class the account falls into. These include open book accounts, which may have periodic charges against them; written contracts; and single-entry accounts, which only have one charge against them. The time period in which legal action must take place against any of these accounts varies from state to state; if an unpaid account is more than three years old, it is wise to investigate the statute of limitations in your state before spending time and effort in collections.

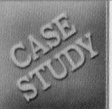

CASE STUDY 20-1

For patient accounts more than 60 days overdue, the offices of Doctors Lewis & King begin a series of collection proceedings to attempt to collect the monies. Initially, they place a telephone call to the patient to determine whether a billing problem might be present that can be clarified over the telephone. If they cannot reach the patient, or the patient does not respond to the call, then collections begin. Marilyn has assigned this function of the billing process to Ellen Armstrong because Ellen has a warm telephone manner and is good with patients.

CASE STUDY REVIEW

1. Why is Ellen's telephone manner of importance in the collection process?
2. In addition to telephone collections, what patient letters might Ellen send?
3. Ellen has come across an account that is delinquent and discovers that the patient has declared bankruptcy. What can Ellen do now?

SUMMARY

Billing and collection activities in the ambulatory care setting are intricately linked to daily financial practices and claims processing, and the medical assistant responsible for billing should also be well aware of these other functions. Billing need not entail a complex or elaborate system, but whether accomplished by manual or computer methodology, it needs to be precise, professional, and comprehensive, as all communications with patients should be. If collections become necessary, courteous and straightforward letters and telephone exchanges are the most effective. The goal of all billing and collections is to maintain the relationship with the patient while ensuring good cash flow and payment of accounts receivable in the ambulatory care setting.

REVIEW QUESTIONS

Multiple Choice

1. The Consumer Credit Protection Act:
   a. is designed to place limits on the amount of debt consumers are liable for
   b. is also known as the statute of limitations
   c. is also known as the Truth-in-Lending Act
   d. does not apply to medical facilities
2. Cycle billing is a system of billing:
   a. completed every fourth month
   b. done by computer
   c. completed by the 25th of the month
   d. in which accounts are divided alphabetically for billing purposes
3. One of the most common reasons patient bills go unpaid is:
   a. inability to pay because of financial hardship
   b. patients consider the cost of medical care too high
   c. patients think their insurance should cover all medical bills
   d. patients think physicians make too much money

4. Aging accounts:
   a. is a process of identifying overdue patient accounts
   b. describes patients that have a long-term relationship with the ambulatory care center
   c. describes elderly patients
   d. applies to accounts considered inactive
5. If an unpaid account goes to small claims court:
   a. the medical office must engage an attorney representative
   b. the medical office is still responsible for collecting even if the court finds in its favor
   c. there is no need to show up at court
   d. a very large sum of money must be at issue
6. A credit bureau:
   a. provides information about a patient's credit history
   b. collects outstanding debts
   c. produces database software
   d. provides information about a patient's medical history

7. The Truth in Lending Act requires disclosing any finance charges:
   a. when the agreement is unilateral
   b. when payment is to be received in more than 4 payments
   c. and requires the interest be expressed as an annual rate
   d. b and c above
8. It will be most difficult to collect past-due accounts from:
   a. those who just forgot their bill
   b. those who are unwilling to pay
   c. those who are having financial hardships
   d. those who have no insurance
9. A "skip" is defined as:
   a. the time period when legal action cannot be taken
   b. an estate involved in probate
   c. one who moves without a forwarding address and leaves an unpaid bill
   d. one who has paid a portion of a debt
10. Lack of payment is usually not considered serious until after:
    a. 120 days
    b. 45 days
    c. 60 days
    d. 90 days

Critical Thinking

1. Why is prompt and accurate billing important to the success of the ambulatory care setting and to the patient?
2. In establishing credit and collection policies, what issues should the ambulatory care center address?
3. Why is payment at time of service a good collection practice?
4. What information would you include in a complete statement?

5. What are the advantages and disadvantages of monthly billing? Cycle billing?
6. Describe a sample aging process for a patient with private insurance.
7. Write a series of collections letters, using the characters in this book.
8. With another student, role-play a telephone collections call. One student can be the medical assistant, one student, the patient.
9. Independently of one another, make notes on how the medical assistant handled the call in number 8. Then compare and discuss the observations.
10. Have a small group discussion on the ethics of collections. Each student can explain either a pro or a con position toward collections.

WEB ACTIVITIES

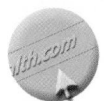

Research the World Wide Web for information on debt collections. Consider key words such as *credit law*, *collections*, *debt recovery*. What sources of information are found that might be helpful to an ambulatory care facility?

REFERENCES/BIBLIOGRAPHY

Andress, A. A. (1996). *Saunders manual of medical office management*. Philadelphia: W. B. Saunders.
Humphrey, D. D. (1996). *Contemporary medical office procedures* (2nd ed.). Albany, NY: Delmar.
Keir, L., Wise, B. A., & Krebs, C. (1998). *Medical assisting: Administrative and clinical competencies* (4th ed.). Albany, NY: Delmar.
Kinn, M. E., & Woods, M. A. (1999). *The medical assistant: Administrative and clinical* (8th ed.). Philadelphia: W. B. Saunders.
Murato, S. (1994, October 24). Practice management. *Medical Economics*. Montvale, NJ: Medical Economics Publication.

Chapter

21

ACCOUNTING PRACTICES

KEY TERMS

Accounting
Accounts Payable
Accounts Receivable (A/R) Ratio
Assets
Balance Sheet
Collection Ratio
Cost Accounting
Cost Analysis
Cost Ratio
Financial Accounting
Fixed Cost
Income Statement
Liability
Managerial Accounting
Owner's Equity
Utilization Review (UR)
Variable Cost

OUTLINE

Bookkeeping and Accounting Systems
Single-Entry
Pegboard
Double-Entry
Computerized Systems
Computer Service Bureaus
The Accounting Function
Cost Analysis
Fixed Costs
Variable Costs

Financial Records
Income Statement
Balance Sheet
Useful Financial Ratios
Accounts Receivable Ratio
Collection Ratio
Cost Ratio
Expenses of the Ambulatory Care Setting
Accounts Payable
Payroll

OBJECTIVES

The student should strive to meet the following performance objectives and demonstrate an understanding of the facts and principles presented in this chapter through written and oral communication.

1. Define the key terms as presented in the glossary.
2. Understand the purpose and range of the accounting function in the ambulatory care setting.
3. Describe the four different types of bookkeeping and accounting systems.
4. Compare and contrast financial, managerial, and cost accounting.
5. Explain the use and validity of the income statement and the balance sheet.
6. Recall three useful financial ratios and explain.
7. Identify proper steps in accounts payable management.
8. Discuss the impact of utilization review on reimbursement.

ADMINISTRATIVE

Practice Finances

- **Apply bookkeeping principles**
- **Document and maintain accounting and banking records**
- **Manage accounts receivable**
- **Manage accounts payable**
- **Process payroll**

GENERAL (TRANSDISCIPLINARY)

Legal Concepts

- **Document accurately**

Operational Functions

- **Apply computer techniques to support office operations**

When James Whitney, one of the physician-owners at Inner City Health Care, and Jane O'Hara, CMA, the office manager, decided to add a new medical assistant to the staff, they first reviewed the financial records for the previous year. While the volume of work in the center generated the need for an additional employee, Whitney and O'Hara had to be sure it was financially feasible. In addition to past records, they also had to make some projections for the upcoming year; with certain new managed care fees, they had to be sure that anticipated revenues would be sufficient to sustain the salary of a new employee.

INTRODUCTION

Medical financial management in the ambulatory care setting is most important in the daily functioning of the office business as it directly affects overall bookkeeping and accounting procedures. Accounting generates financial information for the ambulatory care setting and is defined as a system of monitoring the financial status of a facility and the specific results of its activities. It provides financial information for decision making.

Previous chapters have included the topic of proper daily financial practices (Chapter 17), the accurate coding and the specific processing of insurance forms (Chapter 18 and Chapter 19), and the efficient management of collecting on accounts (Chapter 20). All of this is essential to obtain maximum reimbursement and create profitability for the practice.

This chapter ties many of these elements together and creates a total picture of their interdependence. Each element is critical to the ambulatory care setting's accurate accounting practices.

BOOKKEEPING AND ACCOUNTING SYSTEMS

Medical offices utilize a variety of ways to monitor their financial accounts and the total financial operations of the business. Some small offices still use the single-entry bookkeeping and pegboard systems, while others prefer double-entry or computerized systems, or a combination.

Single-Entry

The single-entry system has been used in the physician's office for many years. This includes a daily journal or log, patients' statements, ledgers, checks, and disbursement (expenditure) records. Information is first recorded in the journal, which provides a chronological record of financial transactions. Information from the journal is then transferred to the ledger through the process of posting. All amounts entered in the journal must be posted to the accounts kept in the ledger to summarize the results. This system has been used extensively in ambulatory care settings because of its simplicity and inexpensive nature.

However, it is difficult to find errors, for there are no internal controls, which is a topic that will be further discussed in this chapter.

Pegboard

As discussed in Chapter 17, the pegboard system is often called "one write" or "write-it-once" system. The pegboard system is easier to use than the single-entry system and has greater internal controls. The pegboard system provides control over collections, payments, and charges. It utilizes No Carbon Required (NCR©) forms that are layered or shingled on pegs on the left of the board so that both income and disbursement entries need to be written only once. Many pegboard plans include a charge slip, which simplifies third-party payment processing for both the medical office and the patients. The charge slip is used to record the input needed during the patient's visit, while serving as the patient's receipt for services performed and fees charged. An advantage of the pegboard system is its accuracy; since data are entered at the time of service and not recopied, few errors can creep in.

Double-Entry

The double-entry system is based on the fact that each transaction has two aspects; that is, a dual effect on the accounting elements. This system is based on the accounting principle that assets equal liabilities and owner's equity. Assets are the properties owned by the business (supplies, equipment, accounts receivable, and so on). Liabilities include what is owed to creditors. Owner's equity is the amount by which the business assets exceed the business liabilities. Net worth, proprietorship, and capital are often used as synonyms for owner's equity.

The double-entry system requires that the two aspects involved in every transaction be recorded on each side of the equation and that the two sides always be in balance. Although this accounting system requires time and skill, it provides a comprehensive financial picture and has built-in accuracy controls. It is orderly, fairly simple, flexible, and accurate, making it impossible for certain types of errors to remain undetected for long. For example, if one aspect of a transaction is properly recorded but the other aspect is overlooked, the records are out of balance. This occurrence may be easily discovered and subsequently corrected.

Computerized Systems

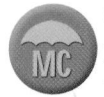 The majority of medical offices is relying on accounting software packages to prepare financial records, such as ledgers and reports, and to retrieve patient information. A computerized accounting system is most likely to be based on the principles of either the pegboard, write-it-once, or a double-entry bookkeeping system, or a combination of both.

Just as the pegboard system is customized to the individual ambulatory care setting, a computer system can also be customized to meet the needs of the practice. Most large multi-speciality clinics have a computer system designed particularly for their needs. Medical office software packages have the capabilities of including the most common procedure (CPT) and diagnostic (ICD-9-CM) codes within a database to be recalled when completing insurance claim forms or printing other computer-generated reports.

Computers also have the flexibility of assigning codes in other categories to indicate whether a bill has been paid with cash, a check, or by a third-party payer. Codes may also be assigned to place and type of service and the professional performing the service. This facilitates the tracking of payments and also allows for the analysis of specific sources that generate income for the practice. Adjustments to reflect discounts or reduced fees may also be entered into the computer. The computer is used in the preparation of billing statements, insurance forms, collection letters, and a number of financial ratios

and statements to assist in monitoring the practice's financial stability.

 Computers and Managed Care. Computerization of the medical facility has increased due to the emphasis placed on the importance of accurate documentation of medical records and the shift from fee-for-service contracts to managed care plans. As medical facilities realized they needed to monitor more information, an increasing number of offices opted for computerization.

Computer Service Bureaus

An option for ambulatory care settings that cannot afford the purchase of their own computers and software is to use a computer service bureau. In this case, the ambulatory care setting provides the data and the bureau provides basic billing and accounting services, furnishing financial statements, completed insurance forms, payroll materials, and checks.

Service bureaus handle accounts from the medical facilities in one of three ways:

1. Through the office's own computer terminal, on-line sharing occurs where the office is tied directly to the bureau's mainframe computer
2. Through on-line servicing, where the office has its own terminal which allows direct communication with the service bureau's computer
3. Through off-line batch processing, where the medical assistant or bookkeeper sends daily batches of data to the bureau to process

Many offices, however, prefer to have their own computerized system because dealing with a computer bureau sacrifices patient confidentiality and limits control over computer usage.

THE ACCOUNTING FUNCTION

Accounting is a system of monitoring the financial status of a facility and the financial results of its activities. Accounting may be divided into two major categories: financial and managerial. Financial accounting provides information primarily for entities external to the organization such as the government. In contrast, managerial accounting generates financial information that can enable more efficient internal management. Cost accounting helps to determine what it costs the ambulatory care setting to perform particular services and is an integral part of managerial accounting. A hospital cost report for Medicare is essentially part of financial accounting, since the report is generated for an external user—the Health Care Financing Administration (HCFA), which administers the Medicare program. However, it is also a part of cost accounting because a cost report on Medicare will show what it costs to care for patients on Medicare.

COST ANALYSIS

A very important aspect of the practice is the cost analysis. The purpose of the analysis is to determine the costs of each service. There are two factors to consider: fixed costs and variable costs.

Fixed Costs

Fixed costs are costs that do not vary in total as the number of patients vary. For example, the annual depreciation cost of the equipment is fixed because it will remain the same regardless of the number of patients who use it.

Variable Costs

Variable costs are those that vary in direct proportion to patient volume such as clinical supplies and laboratory procedures. Average costs to treat patients decline because of fixed costs not variable costs. The greater the volume, the more widely the fixed costs are spread and the less cost any one unit is responsible for.

Patient cost factors include administrative costs, such as the cost of billing and collections, personnel costs for office staff providing patient care, equipment costs, and costs for clinical supplies. The physician cost will include costs for interpreting tests, diagnosing illnesses, and the costs of professional liability insurance.

COMPUTERIZING THE AMBULATORY CARE SETTING

If the ambulatory care setting is to be more computerized, whether through a service bureau or a complete on-site system, it is important to remember:

- Computerization will require more time than estimated.

- The paper-pencil bookkeeping system will have to be maintained concurrently for a period of time.

- A poorly managed paper-pencil system will not be made better by computerization.

- Adequate on-site computer training for all staff is essential.

- Notify patients of the move to a computer system and the changes that will occur.

For more information on computers in the ambulatory care setting, see Chapter 11.

SPOTLIGHT ON AAMA ESSENTIALS THROUGH CAAHEP

- Maintaining the medical practice's financial profitability requires a medical assistant who is not only knowledgeable in this area, but who also maintains a high level of integrity and honesty.

- The medical assistant responsible for monitoring the accounts payable function of the office must be of high character, good moral standing, and above reproach in terms of handling money and other financial transactions.

- If required to perform any tasks related to employee salaries, the medical assistant needs to demonstrate a high degree of confidentiality and should never discuss topics related to specific employee salaries with anyone other than the employer-physician.

Calculating and reviewing costs provide the ambulatory care setting with data to set fees, market the practice, determine profit, and monitor the practice's performance.

FINANCIAL RECORDS

Indicators of the financial status of the medical facility include financial statements that reflect the daily operations of the business. These records comprise an accounting information system that is maintained for numerous reasons, one of which is to provide source data for use in the preparation of various reports. Two financial statements common to the ambulatory care setting are the income/expense statement and the balance sheet.

Income Statement

Figure 21-1 shows a sample income statement. The statement shows the cumulative profit and total expenses for the month. The statement is itemized to show operating expenses and employees' withholding taxes and retirement contributions. This statement enables the practice to monitor increases and decreases daily.

Balance Sheet

Sometimes called the statement of financial condition or statement of financial position, the balance sheet is an

INNER CITY HEALTH CARE
INCOME STATEMENT

	Month of ___, 20__	Year-to-Date	Budget for Year	Overhead Percentages
A. Revenue:				
1. Office #1	$	$	$	
2. Office #2	$	$	$	
B. Total Revenue:	$	$	$	100%
C. Expenses:				
1. Non–doctor (staff) salaries—gross	$	$	$	%
2. Staff fringes				
– Payroll taxes	$	$	$	
– Empl. benefits	$	$	$	
– Empl. seminars	$	$	$	
– Uniforms	$	$	$	
– Retirement plan	$	$	$	
	$	$	$	%
3. Occupancy costs:				
– Rent—Off. #1	$	$	$	
– Rent—Off. #2	$	$	$	
– Property taxes	$	$	$	
– Insurance	$	$	$	
– Utilities	$	$	$	
– Janitor/Grounds	$	$	$	
	$	$	$	%
4. Medical expenses:				
– Medications	$	$	$	
– Supplies	$	$	$	
– Lab fees	$	$	$	
	$	$	$	%
5. Office expenses:				
– Office supplies	$	$	$	
– Postage	$	$	$	
– Telephone	$	$	$	
	$	$	$	%
6. Malpractice ins.	$	$	$	%
7. Professional expenses:				
– Auto expenses (Doctors')	$	$	$	
– Dues/subscriptions	$	$	$	
– Books and videos	$	$	$	
– Dues/memberships	$	$	$	
– Entertainment	$	$	$	
– Professional development	$	$	$	
– Travel	$	$	$	
	$	$	$	%

(continues)

Figure 21-1 A sample income statement that shows profit and expenses for one month.

itemized statement of the assets, liabilities, and owner's equity of a medical facility as of a specified date. Its purpose is to provide information regarding the status of these basic accounting elements.

The balance sheet is made possible through the double-entry system of accounting since every transaction is recorded by two sets of entries made in a ledger or journal. Increases in assets are recorded as debits; decreases are recorded as credits. Increases in liabilities and owner's equity are recorded as credits; decreases are recorded as debits.

Debit and credit entries to one or more accounts make up the system. In any recording, the total dollar amount of the debit entries must equal the total dollar

	Month of ___ , 20__	Year-to-Date	Budget for Year	Overhead Percentages
8. Equipment costs:				
– Depreciation/amortization	$	$	$	
– Rent	$	$	$	
– Service/maintenance	$	$	$	
– Interest (if on equipment purchase loans)	$	$	$	
	$	$	$	%
9. Marketing expenses				
– Advertising	$	$	$	
– Other fees	$	$	$	
	$	$	$	%
10. Professional expenses:				
– Accounting	$	$	$	
– Legal	$	$	$	
– Consulting	$	$	$	
– Ret. Plan Admin.	$	$	$	
	$	$	$	%
11.				
12.				
13.				
14.				
D. Total Non–Doctor Expenses:	$	$	$	%
E. Operating New Income Before Doctors' Costs (B minus C)	$	$	$	%
F. Associate Physician's Costs:				
– Salaries—gross:	$	$	$	
– Benefits	$	$	$	
–	$	$	$	
–	$	$	$	
G. Total Non–Owner Doctors' Costs	$	$	$	%
H. New Income Available to Owner–Doctors (E minus G)	$	$	$	%
I. Owner–Doctors' Costs:				
1. Salaries—gross:				
–Dr. A	$	$	$	
–Dr. B	$	$	$	
2. Bonuses—gross:				
–Dr. A	$	$	$	
–Dr. B	$	$	$	
3. Retirement contributions:				
–Dr. A	$	$	$	
–Dr. B	$	$	$	
4. "Semi-personal" expenses:				
–Dr. A	$	$	$	
–Dr. B	$	$	$	
J. Total Owner–Doctors' Costs	$	$	$	
K. Net Income (H minus J)	$	$	$	

Figure 21-1   (*continued*)

amount of the credit entries. Each ledger or journal entry should have the:

1. Date of transaction
2. Journal or ledger account names involved
3. Dollar amount of the charges
4. Brief explanation of the transaction

USEFUL FINANCIAL RATIOS

There are a few financial ratios that can help evaluate how the practice is doing. Data from the current year and previous year's financial statements can be converted into ratios to highlight different financial characteristics.

Ratios should always be viewed in relationship to the total financial picture, however.

While two of these ratios were discussed in Chapter 20, some elaboration is in order in the context of this chapter.

Accounts Receivable Ratio

The **accounts receivable (A/R) ratio** formula measures the speed in which outstanding accounts are paid. The accounts receivable ratio provides a picture of the state of collections and probable losses. The longer an account is past due, the less likelihood of successfully making the collection.

$$\frac{\text{Total Accounts Receivable}}{\text{Monthly Receipts}} = \text{Turnaround Time}$$

> **Example:**
>
> $$\frac{\$120,000}{\$60,000} = \begin{array}{l}\text{2 Months Turnaround Time} \\ \text{for Payment on an Account}\end{array}$$

The goal of an efficient billing and collecting policy should be a turnaround time of two months or less.

Collection Ratio

The **collection ratio** shows the percentage of outstanding debt collected. The goal should be a 90 percent collection ratio. Total receipts divided by total charges give the unadjusted collection ratio, but adjustments may include federal and state insurance programs (Medicare and Medicaid, Workers' Compensation), managed care adjustments, and any other adjustments as directed by the physician.

Total Receipts	= $40,000
+ Managed Care Adjustments	$3,000
+ Medicare Adjustments	$2,000
TOTAL	$45,000
Total Charges	$52,000

$$\frac{\text{Total Receipts \$45,000}}{\text{Total Charges \$52,000}} = \begin{array}{l}\text{86.5\% Collection Ratio} \\ \text{after Adjustments}\end{array}$$

Cost Ratio

The **cost ratio** formula shows the cost of a procedure or service and can help in determining, for instance, the cost effectiveness of maintaining a laboratory in the ambulatory care setting. The ratio is:

$$\frac{\text{Total Expenses}}{\text{Total Number of Procedures for 1 Month}}$$

$$\frac{\text{Total Laboratory Expenses for September}}{\text{Total Number of Procedures Performed for September}}$$

$$\frac{\$48,000}{240} = \$200 \text{ per Procedure}$$

A conclusion might be reached that the lab is too costly because each procedure is not billed at $200.00.

EXPENSES OF THE AMBULATORY CARE SETTING

While the ambulatory care setting is trying to maximize its income, it is also responsible for overhead costs, such as payroll and other accounts payable. Good financial management ensures that these costs are always met in a timely fashion.

Accounts Payable

Accounts payable are an unwritten promise to pay a supplier for property or merchandise purchased on credit or for a service rendered. Accounts payable are the most common liability or financial obligation in a physician's office. These include expenses such as medical and office supplies, salaries, equipment, and services. Payments for these expenses are made by check to ensure complete, accurate records of all money received and disbursed. See Chapter 17 for information on writing checks.

The administrative medical assistant, the bookkeeper, or the office manager will monitor the accounts payable accounting functions. All bills received in the ambulatory care setting should be paid promptly. Some statements note that a discount of one or two percent is possible if paid within ten days of receipt of the bill. Such discounts should be noted and the bills paid within the time limit to warrant the discount.

The responsible person will check the accuracy of the statement, prepare the check, and mark on the statement date of payment, check number, and amount paid. The statements (noting payment) and checks are submitted for final approval and signature on the check by either the physician or office manager.

Payroll

The administrative medical assistant is likely to be involved in making certain the W-4 form, the Employee's Withholding Allowance Certificate, is completed by all employees. However, salary calculations, withholding taxes, and social security calculations are the responsibility of the office manager. See Chapter 45.

UTILIZATION REVIEW

In the present health care climate where there has been an increase in managed care plans with a corresponding decrease in the traditional indemnity fee-for-service contracts, more attention has been focused on how the billing and financial management process should proceed. Because of the influence of governmental mandates in the practice of medicine, and the growth of the utilization review industry, more accurate recordkeeping and documentation in all facets of the ambulatory care setting have become necessary. There are nearly 300 utilization review firms throughout the country. These companies aggressively sell their services to employers and to insurance carriers. Utilization review (UR) is actually a review of the service required before it may be performed. If the reviewer determines that the procedure or treatment is not needed, then it will not be approved or covered under the patient's insurance plan. Policies that once permitted medical decisions to be made solely by the physician are now made by other health professionals who are employed by UR firms. Some clinics may find it beneficial to have one medical assistant whose main responsibility is to present procedures to utilization review for acceptance or denial. Because of the increasing concern for quality of health care at low cost, more physicians also are realizing they need more documentation of both medical and financial information with more accessible means for retrieval.

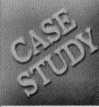

CASE STUDY 21-1

Because the owners of Inner City Health Care need to make adequate income to pay all overhead and share in a profit, they are instituting new measures to reduce their costs of operating. However, they have fixed costs that they cannot change. So they plan to look at their variable costs to determine where they can reduce expenses without any reduction in quality of service.

CASE STUDY REVIEW

1. What are some fixed costs that Inner City is likely to have?
2. What are some of the variable costs that should be considered when looking at profitability?
3. How may utilization review procedures affect the profitability of Inner City Health Care?

SUMMARY

Medical financial management is crucial to the profitability of the ambulatory care setting. It is necessary for each medical facility to decide on which accounting system best serves the individual practice. Careful monitoring of billing procedures and aging accounts, and accurately documenting both the medical and financial record will help in providing a sound financial analysis and a strong financial foundation for the ambulatory care setting.

REVIEW QUESTIONS

Multiple Choice

1. The "write-it-once" is a bookkeeping system also known as:
   a. single-entry
   b. pegboard
   c. double-entry
   d. disbursement

2. An example of a fixed cost is:
   a. salaries
   b. cost of supplies
   c. depreciation of equipment
   d. cost of treating patients

3. An itemized statement of financial position is the:
   a. income statement
   b. balance sheet

c. trial balance
d. collection ratio
4. The Employee's Withholding Allowance Certificate is the:
   a. W-2
   b. W-4
   c. FICA
   d. W-3
5. Utilization review:
   a. looks at the utility of all personnel
   b. examines how useful the ambulatory care center is to patients
   c. is a review of a procedure or treatment before it is performed to determine whether it is needed by the patient
   d. only affects hospitals
6. Assets include:
   a. equipment and supplies on hand
   b. building or property
   c. accounts receivable
   d. all the above
7. A computer service bureau:
   a. is the service you hire to care for the office computer system
   b. causes the office to sacrifice patient confidentiality
   c. can function through linkage of computers, on-line servicing or off-line batch processing.
   d. b and c above
8. In a medical facility where the total receipts including any adjustments are $83,500 and the total charges equal $97,750, the collection ratio:
   a. would be great at 94%
   b. would be quite good at 88%
   c. should be almost 85%
   d. shows a modest return at 75%
9. Money can be saved with accounts payable when:
   a. paid promptly
   b. discounts are realized
   c. realizing that buying in bulk is too expensive
   d. a and b above

Critical Thinking

1. Why is medical financial management important?
2. List one advantage and one disadvantage of the single-entry bookkeeping system.
3. Discuss the pros and cons of an on-site complete computer system and a computer service bureau.
4. How may fixed and variable costs differ?
5. Review the importance of financial records and identify and state the differences between the two primary records.
6. Identify three useful ratios in calculating how a practice is doing.
7. Give examples of the preceding three ratios.
8. How does utilization review affect financial reimbursement in the ambulatory care setting?

WEB ACTIVITIES

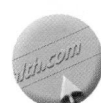

Using the World Wide Web, research companies producing and servicing medical software for use in the ambulatory care setting.

REFERENCES/BIBLIOGRAPHY

Andress, A. A. (1996). *Manual of medical office management.* Philadelphia: W. B. Saunders Company.

Kinn, M. E., & Woods, M. A. (1999). *The medical assistant: Administrative and clinical* (8th ed.). Philadelphia: W. B. Saunders Company.

Section

III

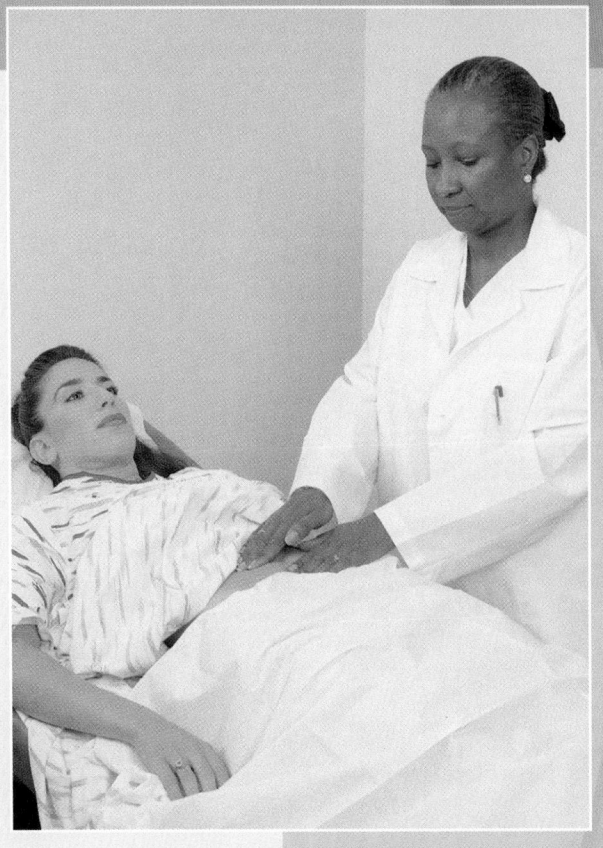

CLINICAL
PROCEDURES

331

INTEGRATED CLINICAL PROCEDURES

KEY TERMS

Acquired Immunodeficiency
  Syndrome (AIDS)
Airborne Transmission
Amniocentesis
Amoebic Dysentery
Antibodies
Antigen
Aspirate
Barrier
Biohazard
Bloodborne
Bloodborne Pathogen
Body Substance Isolation
Carrier
Cell-Mediated Immunity
Communicable
Contact Transmission
Contaminate
Contracting
Declination Form
Dermatitis
Disinfection
Documentation
Droplet Transmission
Endoscopy
Engineering Controls
Epidemiology
Epistaxis
Excoriated
Excretion
Fomite
Human Immunodeficiency Virus
Humoral Immunity
Immune System

(continues)

OUTLINE

KEY TERMS
(*continued*)

Immunity
Immunoglobulins
Immunosuppressed
Incinerate
Infection Control
Infectious Agent
Infectious Waste
Inflammatory Response
Invasive Procedures
Isolation
Isolation Categories
Jaundice
Lesion
Leukorrhea
Lochia
Lumbar Puncture
Malaria
Medical Asepsis
Menses
Microorganisms
Morbidity
Mortality
Normal Flora
Palliative
Parenteral
Pathogen
Phlebotomy
Regulated Waste
Resistance
Sanitization
Scabies
Secretion
Sharps
Sodium Hypochlorite
Spill Kit
Sputum
Standard
Standard Precautions
Surgical Asepsis
Thermolabile
Thoracentesis
Transmission
Transmission-Based Precautions
Trichomoniasis
Universal Precautions
Vaccine
Vacutainer®
Vector
Virulence
Virulent
Work Practice Controls

OBJECTIVES

The student should strive to meet the following performance objectives and demonstrate an understanding of the facts and principles presented in this chapter through written and oral communication.

1. Define the key terms as presented in the glossary.
2. Define and state the critical importance of infection control in the ambulatory care setting.
3. Outline the six links in the chain of infection.
4. Define the five classifications of infectious microorganisms.
5. Recall and elaborate on the four phases the immune system uses to defend against infectious disease.
6. State the four stages of infectious diseases.
7. Recall at least five infectious diseases, their agents of transmission, and symptoms.
8. Compare the routes of transmission of AIDS and hepatitis and discuss the risk of infection from needlestick.
9. Explain why Universal Precautions were introduced in 1985.
10. Describe the purpose of Standard Precautions and give six examples of ways health care providers should practice Standard Precautions.
11. Differentiate among the three types of Transmission-Based Precautions, defining what they are and how they are applied.
12. List eight types of body fluids and give an example of each.
13. Describe personal protective equipment.
14. Recognize five situations in which exposure to a patient's blood can occur and discuss why Standard Precautions are important.
15. Describe disposal of infectious waste.
16. Discuss components of the bloodborne standard. Analyze what the law covers.
17. List human fluids that may contain HIV and HBV.
18. Define medical asepsis.
19. Define surgical asepsis.
20. Compare and contrast medical asepsis and surgical asepsis.
21. State four methods of sterilization.
22. List supplies and equipment necessary to achieve surgical asepsis when using an autoclave.
23. Explain competent wrapping and operation of the autoclave.
24. State storage measures and expiration periods for autoclaved materials.

CLINICAL

Fundamental Principles

- Apply principles of aseptic technique and infection control
- Comply with quality assurance practices

GENERAL (TRANSDISCIPLINARY)

Legal Concepts

- Comply with established risk management and safety procedures
- Follow federal, state, and local legal guidelines
- Maintain awareness of federal and state health care legislation and regulations

Instruction

- Teach methods of health promotion and disease prevention

At Inner City Health Care, a multiphysician urgent care center, medical assistant Bruce Goldman, CMA, assumes responsibility for all infection control measures taken in the ambulatory care setting. In addition to his daily responsibilities related to medical and surgical asepsis, Bruce also makes it a point to stay current with infection control principles. Recently, he noticed that the Centers for Disease Control and Prevention (CDC) issued new guidelines, called Standard Precautions, that augment Universal Precautions. The CDC also issued another tier of precautions called Transmission-Based Precautions. When Bruce receives new information on any form of infection control, he makes it a point to become thoroughly familiar with the guidelines and to share his knowledge with other urgent care staff.

INTRODUCTION

Infectious diseases have plagued humans since the beginning of time. Recent scientific advances have changed our thoughts and behaviors regarding infectious disease. Advances such as antibiotic therapy and vaccination have significantly reduced risks of mortality from some previously fatal or debilitating infectious diseases. Infectious diseases that once were highly feared due to their likelihood of causing premature death are now preventable or treatable, causing us to forget the **virulence** and destructive potential of epidemics of infectious disease. The presence of AIDS as an incurable and fatal infectious disease has caused the world to realize the enduring impact of pathogens on the human race.

Although these medical advances have reduced the incidence of **mortality** and **morbidity** from infectious diseases, humans must never underesti-

mate the potential of resurgent infectious diseases. Tuberculosis has been the single leading cause of death in the history of mankind, yet was drastically reduced with the discovery of anti-tuberculosis drugs. Today, however, the tuberculosis organism may be found that has adapted to the drugs, thereby becoming resistant to our only line of defense. Medical assistants must pay close attention to the prevention of infectious diseases in the ambulatory care setting.

This chapter addresses the principles of the process of infection and control measures for use in ambulatory care settings. Since medical assistants deal directly with patients and other health care professionals, stringent adherence to the principles can greatly reduce **transmission**, or spread, of infectious disease. Continuous reliance on infection control measures ensures a clinical environment that is as safe as possible for employees, patients, and families. When infection control principles are not followed, infectious diseases may be transmitted to self, coworkers, or patients. The goals of infection control are to limit the presence of **infectious agents**, to create bar-

riers against transmission, and to decrease the risk to others of contracting infectious diseases. These goals can be achieved through medical asepsis and sterilization, by observation of all Standard Precautions and Transmission-Based Precautions set forth by the Centers for Disease Prevention and Control, and the Occupational Safety and Health Administration guidelines.

IMPACT OF INFECTIOUS DISEASES

Since the discovery of the germ theory by Louis Pasteur and Robert Koch in the nineteenth century, we have seen dramatic changes in global mortality and morbidity statistics from infectious diseases. Many scientists devoted their professional lives to the quest for the prevention and cure of infectious diseases, which were the main cause of death in earlier centuries. In developed countries, deaths from such diseases as tuberculosis, pneumonia, and smallpox have been significantly reduced due to pharmacologic agents such as antibiotics and **vaccines**. Antibiotic agents were widely introduced during World War II reducing deaths from traumatic wound infections. Edward Jenner is credited with the discovery of the first vaccine to protect against smallpox. Due to the vaccine, smallpox is considered to have been eradicated worldwide.

Epidemiology is the science that studies the history, cause, and patterns of infectious diseases. This field of medicine is credited to a Japanese bacteriologist in the late nineteenth century who correlated incidences of bubonic plague with rat infestation. Recent epidemiological studies have traced infectious diseases such as AIDS from the inception of the epidemic. The future of studies in infectious diseases will focus on increasing the pharmacological war against infectious diseases.

Reliance only on treatment of infectious disease does not address the crucial step in the spread of infectious diseases; that is, of prevention, or **infection control**. Emerging issues related to infectious diseases involve microorganisms that are resistant to present technology, **bloodborne pathogen** transmission, increased **immunosuppressed** populations, and global access to infection control and treatment. Developed countries become accustomed to anti-infectious medications, clean water, and laws that protect the public from infectious agents found in food and other consumables. These safety measures may not be present in other locations where political or economic factors limit access to infection control measures.

In the future, drug-resistant infectious diseases will place greater emphasis on prevention because there may never be a safe and universally effective drug for all infectious diseases.

Study of the history of infectious diseases allows us to realize the impact these diseases have on the lifestyles of people in various cultures. Infectious diseases such as AIDS and other sexually transmitted diseases have differing levels of social or cultural impact. Medical assistants should be aware of facts regarding the infectious process of specific diseases to reduce cultural isolation for the patient and to dispel myths regarding infectious diseases. Also see Chapter 6.

THE PROCESS OF INFECTION

Infectious diseases are caused by pathogenic microorganisms that are capable of causing disease. **Microorganisms** are microscopic living creatures capable of transmission and reproduction in specific circumstances. **Pathogens** are microorganisms that can cause infectious disease. Although all pathogens are capable of causing disease, not all microorganisms cause disease. Many microorganisms

are necessary for human, animal, and plant life survival. In the absence of microorganisms, life would not be possible. The term **normal flora** is used to recognize the beneficial role of microorganisms in certain parts of the body, in which microorganisms normally occupy space and use nutrients, thus retarding the potential of pathogenic growth in that specific body area. A fundamental concept in the study of infectious disease is that similar steps or phases occur in all infectious diseases; however, each specific microorganism causes unique characteristics and alterations in the process of infection. Medical assistants must apply the theoretical process of infectious disease growth and transmission in order to relate to specific pathogens. The goal is to reduce transmission and incidence of infectious diseases in patients, employees, and families.

CHAIN OF INFECTION

In order for infectious diseases to spread, several necessary steps must occur. These steps, or links, are known as the "chain of infection." Each link or step in the infectious process must occur for the spread of infection to take place. Infection control is based on the fact that the transmission of infectious diseases will be prevented when any of the levels in the chain are broken or interrupted (Figure 22-1). The steps are:

1. Infectious agent
2. Reservoir
3. Portal of exit
4. Means of transmission
5. Portal of entry
6. Susceptible host

Infectious Agents

Infectious agents are microorganisms that can be grouped into five classifications: viruses, bacteria, fungi, protozoa, and rickettsia. In order for an infection to occur, an infectious agent must be present. When infectious diseases are identified according to the specific disease-causing microorganism, the disease may be prevented with the use of anti-infective drugs or infection control practices. Each of the five classifications of infectious microorganisms will be explored.

Virus. Viruses are pathogens that require a living cell for reproduction and activity. These microorganisms are considered intracellular parasites, because they must live inside cells in order to multiply. They do so by altering particles of genetic material, such as DNA (deoxyribonucleic acid) or RNA (ribonucleic acid). Since viruses live

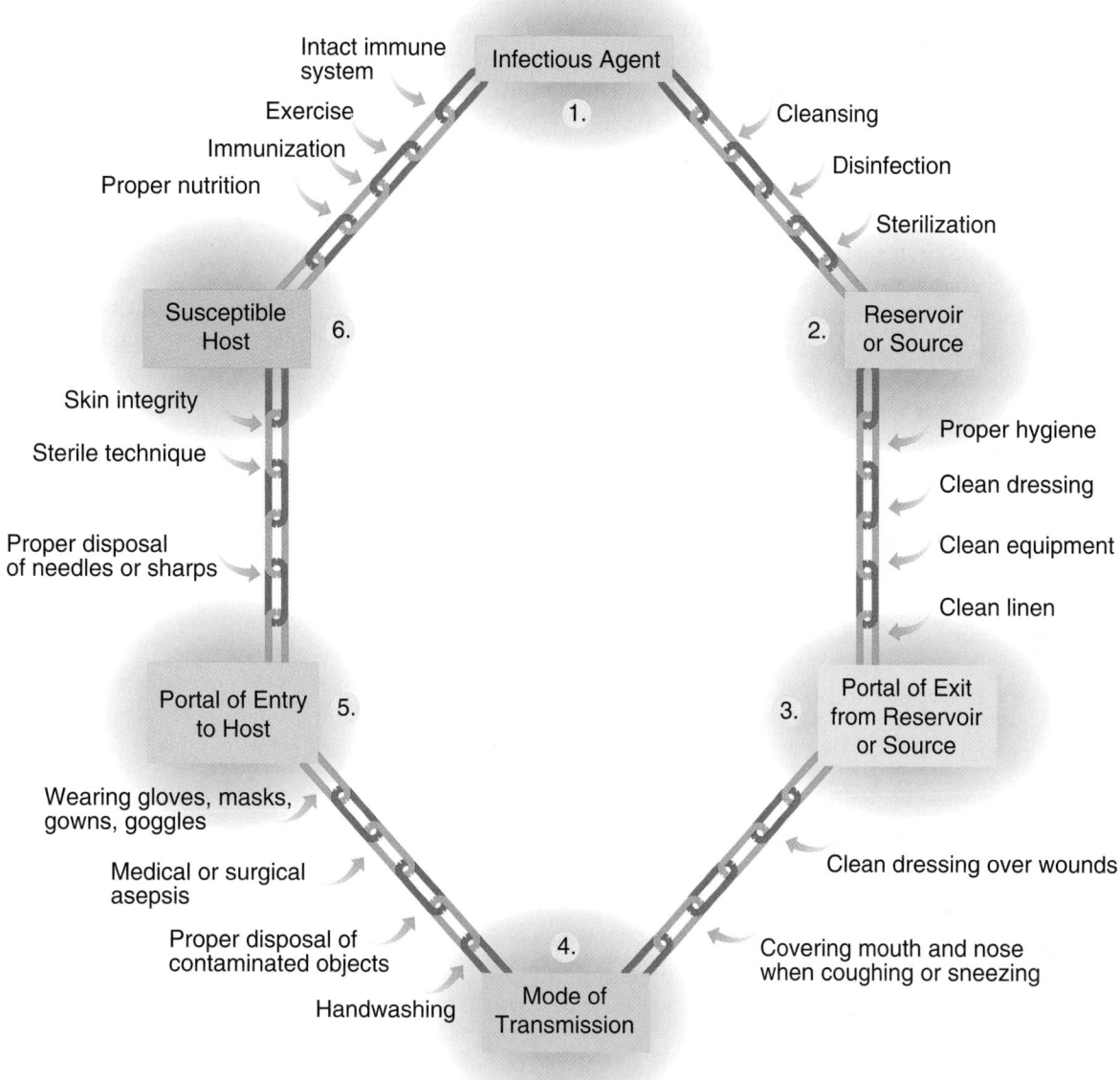

Figure 22-1 Health care worker's interventions used to break the chain of the infection transmission.

inside cells, they are protected against agents such as chemical disinfectants. Viruses are susceptible to heat. In order to survive, viruses have a notable characteristic of being able to change specific characteristics over time. For instance, viruses can adapt to their environment so they remain resistant to efforts to limit their growth. Viral infections have only a few pharmacological treatment agents, and usually these agents are **palliative** because they only relieve symptoms of the disease instead of curing the infection.

Bacteria. Bacteria are single-celled microorganisms that live in tissues rather than in body cells and are iden-

tified by characteristic shapes, or morphology. Bacteria may also be grouped according to ability to accept laboratory staining agents. Gram-negative bacteria stain visibly red under the microscope, whereas gram-positive bacteria stain purple. The bacteria that do not accept stain are considered spores, which are bacteria with a covering that protects them from many chemical disinfectants and higher levels of heat. The three classifications of bacteria are cocci (sphere or dot shaped); bacilli (rod shaped); and spirilla (spiral shaped). Bacteria are either pathogenic or nonpathogenic. Nonpathogenic bacteria normally reside on the skin of humans and in mucous membrane areas of the body. These are known as *normal flora.* The nonpathogenic bacteria use nutrients and occupy space, competing with the pathogenic bacteria. When nonpathogenic bacteria are reduced, the opportunity exists for pathogenic organisms to take over and cause infectious disease. A common cause of the reduction of nonpathogenic microorganisms is the use of anti-infectious drugs. Certain conditions favor bacterial growth and in fact are necessary for them to survive. They are darkness (promotes bacterial growth), oxygen (aerobic bacteria need oxygen to live, anaerobic bacteria live without oxygen), temperature (body temperature favors bacterial growth), and moisture (bacteria grow well in moist places). By depriving bacteria of their growth requirements they can be kept from causing an infection. This can be accomplished by providing light since certain bacteria will die in direct light or sunlight; providing or withholding oxygen according to the needs of the bacteria (aerobic or anaerobic); lowering temperatures to reduce bacterial growth; and keeping surfaces dry to inhibit bacterial growth. Examples of bacterial pathogens are listed in Table 22-1.

Fungi. Fungi are microorganisms that may be unicellular (single-cell) or multicellular (many cells). Mushrooms and molds are examples of fungi that are nonpathogenic.

Pathogenic fungi cause athletes' foot, ringworm, and candida infections. Other pathogenic fungi include histoplasmosis and toxoplasmosis, which are fungal infections spread through the air from infected fowl and bird waste.

Parasites. Organisms that live in or on another organism are classified as parasites. They may be single-celled or multicelled. Examples include protozoa (single-cell microscopic organisms that cause malaria, amoebic dysentery, and trichomoniasis); metazoa (multicellular organisms that cause pinworms, hookworms, and tapeworms); and ectoparasites (multicellular organisms that live superficially on another host, such as lice and scabies).

Rickettsiae. Rickettsiae are intracellular parasites, similar to the virus. However, they are larger than viruses and can be seen under conventional microscopes following staining procedures. These microorganisms are susceptible to antibiotic therapy. Examples of rickettsiae infections include typhus (transmitted by the body louse); Lyme disease (transmitted by ticks); and Rocky Mountain Spotted Fever (transmitted by ticks). Characteristic of rickettsia infections is a skin rash caused by the rickettsia invading the small blood vessels. This appears on the skin as a small hemorrhagic rash.

TABLE 22-1 INFECTIOUS BACTERIAL DISEASES

Disease	Infectious Agent	Mode of Transmission
Botulism (food poisoning)	Clostridium botulinum	Ingestion
Chlamydia (sexually transmitted disease)	Chlamydia trachomatis	Sexual contact
Clostridial myonecrosis (Gas gangrene)	Species of gram-positive clostridia	Wound entry
Gonorrhea (sexually transmitted disease)	Neisseria gonorrhoeae	Sexual contact
Legionnaires' disease (pneumonia)	Legionella pneumophila	Inhalation
Meningococcal meningitis	N. Meningitidis, S. Pneumoniae, or H. Influenzae	Direct contact, inhalation
Nosocomial (hospital-acquired) infection	Gram-negative bacteria	Normal flora transmitted during illness/procedures; opportunistic pathogens transmit during debilitated condition
Pulmonary tuberculosis	Mycobacterium tuberculosis	Inhalation
Samonellosis (food poisoning)	Salmonella	Ingestion
Shigellosis (bacillary dysentery) (diarrhea)	Shigellae	Fecal-oral
Staphylococcal infection (abscesses, food poisoning, urinary tract infections)	Staphylococci	Direct contact, ingestion, inhalation, bloodborne, vectors (animals)
Streptococcal infection (strep throat, otitis media, pneumonia)	Hemolytic streptococci (usually beta-hemolytic group A)	Inhalation
Syphilis (sexually transmitted disease)	Treponema pallidum	Sexual contact
Tetanus (lockjaw)	Clostridium tetani	Wound entry
Typhoid fever (enteric fever)	Salmonella typhi	Fecal-oral

Reservoir

The second level in the chain of infection is the reservoir or location of the infectious agent. Reservoirs are people, equipment, supplies, water, food, and animals or insects (known as vectors). Methods of infection control in the reservoir level include handwashing, environmental hygiene, disinfection, sterilization, and maintenance of employee health standards, such as annual tuberculosis skin testing.

Portal of Exit

Although the infectious agent is housed or living in the reservoir, it must leave the reservoir to infect another person. The portal of exit is the method by which an infectious agent leaves the reservoir. Microorganisms may leave the human body with normally occurring body fluids, such as excretions, secretions, skin cells, respiratory droplets, blood, or any body fluid. The portal of exit may be continuous, such as with respiratory droplets, or dependent on the body fluid exiting the body under unusual circumstances, such as when blood leaves the body during a surgical procedure or phlebotomy.

 Standard Precautions and Transmission-Based Precautions are infection control methods based on the knowledge that exiting infectious diseases can be spread to others. These precautions attempt to control the spread of infectious diseases as infectious agents exit the reservoir.

Means of Transmission

The means of transmission are specific ways in which microorganisms travel from one place (reservoir) to another (susceptible host). Transmission depends on the characteristics of the microorganisms. Types of routes of transmission include:

- Direct contact (touching an infected person)
- Airborne transmission (inhaling the microorganism into the susceptible host's respiratory system)
- Bloodborne transmission (infected blood enters susceptible host)
- Ingestion (eating or drinking contaminated items)
- Indirect contact (microorganism on a fomite, a nonliving object such as a table or piece of equipment that can absorb and transmit infection)
- Vector (a carrier of disease, usually an insect)

Infection control measures in the ambulatory care area specifically address the transmission stage of the process of infection.

 Methods that reduce the transmission of pathogens include adherence to Standard and Transmission-Based Precautions, handwashing, sanitization, disinfection, and sterilization. Methods of infection control are used in food handling, water and sewage processing, and child care.

Portal of Entry

Following transmission, the infectious agent must enter another person, or a susceptible host. The portal of entry allows the agent access to the next person. Common entrance sites to the human body include broken skin, mucous membranes, and systems of the body exposed to the external environment, such as the respiratory, gastrointestinal, and reproductive systems. Breathing in airborne microorganisms allows infectious diseases to be spread to the lungs. Eating or drinking contaminated water is the cause of gastrointestinal infectious diseases. Sexually transmitted diseases spread through vaginal, oral, and anal intercourse. Care of patients with infectious diseases includes careful consideration of infection control to limit further spread of the microorganism. Methods such as sterile wound care, transmission-based precautions, and aseptic technique limit the transmission of infectious microorganisms. The portals of exit and entry need not be the same.

Susceptible Host

Finally, infectious microorganisms must enter another person who is susceptible. This means that the person is able to contract the pathogenic organism. The susceptible host is therefore not resistant or immune to the organism. Causes of susceptibility include the presence of other diseases, immunosuppression (weakened immune system), surgical procedures, trauma, or the absence of immunity to the specific microorganism. Susceptibility of a person depends on several factors, including:

1. Number and specific type of pathogen
2. Duration of exposure to the pathogen
3. General physical condition
4. Psychological health status
5. Occupation or lifestyle environment
6. Presence of underlying diseases or conditions
7. Youth or advanced age (young and old at greater risk)

The goal of infection control at this level of the chain of infection is to identify patients at risk for susceptibility, treat their underlying conditions if possible, and isolate them from those reservoirs that could be hazardous to the susceptible person.

THE BODY'S DEFENSE MECHANISMS FOR FIGHTING INFECTION AND DISEASE

There are two primary defense mechanisms that protect the body from infection and disease. One is known as inflammation or the inflammatory response, a non-specific immune response; the other is an individual's immune system or specific response.

Inflammatory Response

Inflammation is the body's natural way of responding when invaded by a pathogen or trauma. The body goes through a distinct process in an attempt to destroy and get rid of the pathogenic microorganisms and their by-products, and if this is not possible, to restrict the amount of damage done. The response is identical whether the agent is a pathogen, trauma, foreign body, or extremes in temperature. The cardinal signs of inflammation are redness, heat, swelling, and pain. Inflammation is a response to infection (invasion by a pathogen) and the two should not be confused. Inflammation can occur without infection, but infection cannot exist without inflammation.

These are the steps in the inflammatory process:

- Local dilation of blood vessels increases blood flow to injured (infected) area causing redness or heat

- Plasma moves into the tissue causing swelling and pain due to pressure on nerve ending

- White blood cells move into injured tissue to fight infection and phagocytes destroy invading pathogens

Following destruction of the pathogen, tissue repair can begin. If the inflammatory response is not effective, the specific immune response is necessary.

Indications that an inflammatory process is inadequate are (1) the accumulation of purulent matter in the area (due to destroyed pathogens, white blood cells, and body cells), (2) lymph node enlargement (swollen glands), and (3) septicemia may result because pathogens have spread to the blood stream.

Immediate antibiotic therapy is indicated in these circumstances due to the inadequacy of the inflammatory response.

The Immune System and Immunity

In order to fight infectious diseases, our bodies are equipped with several effective physical and chemical barriers such as the skin, mucous membranes, body excretions and secretions, and a complex, highly specific immune system. The immune system's purpose is to protect against pathogens and abnormal cell growth. The system is composed of various cells that collectively recognize, subdue, attack, and eliminate pathogens. The two types of immune responses include cell-mediated immunity and humoral immunity. Cell-mediated immunity is usually involved in attacks against viruses, fungi, organ transplants, or cancer cells. This type of immunity does not produce antibodies. Humoral immunity produces antibodies that are capable of killing microorganisms and of recognizing the pathogen in the future. Generally, both types of immune responses occur in four phases:

1. *Recognition of the invader.* The immune system is equipped with cells that identify agents, pathogens, and abnormal cell growth as foreign substances. Macrophages and helper T cells recognize foreign invaders, whether they are pathogens, cancer cells, or transplanted tissues.

2. *Growth of defenses, which allows for multiplication of helper T cells and B cells.* Following foreign substance recognition, the immune system alerts T cells and B cells to multiply and move to the site of the foreign substance. In cell-mediated immunity, activation of helper T cells means that the T cells are specifically oriented to a unique antigen, a substance such as bacteria the body recognizes as foreign. Activated T cells divide, forming memory T cells and killer T cells. In humoral immunity, activated B cells are antigen-specific and divide into memory B cells and plasma cells.

3. *Attack against the infection.* Cell-mediated immunity uses killer T cells and macrophages to phagocytize, or engulf and destroy the pathogens. Humoral plasma cells have the ability to produce specific antibodies that lock on to specific antigens, which prevents the disease-producing characteristics of the pathogen from forming. These antibodies are called immunoglobulins and they render the pathogen unable to reproduce or continue growth.

4. *Slowdown of the immune response following death of the infectious agent.* Following the death of the foreign substance, the immune response is halted. T cells and B cells return to normal levels, and in the case of humoral immunity, the presence of antibody production causes the immune system to resist the specific infectious pathogen in future contacts with the pathogen.

Susceptibility to some infectious diseases is closely linked to the person's unique resistance, or immunity. Immunity means the ability of the body to resist specific pathogens and their toxins. Resistance occurs following an exposure to a pathogen, which is the antigen-antibody reaction. This natural body defense to fight infectious disease occurs gradually and over time as pathogens and other foreign substances such as antigens enter the human body. When the antigen enters the body, the immune system recognizes the antigen as foreign and attempts to contain and subdue the foreign invader. Specific chemical antibodies to the antigen are produced by B cells, which attempt to prevent the antigen from further growth. Following the completion of the stages of that infectious disease, the body retains the ability to produce antibodies in response to that specific microorganism or antigen. Therefore, immunity can last for some length of time, possibly to provide lifetime protection against specific infectious microorganisms. Several forms of immunity can occur in response to specific antigens:

- Acquired active immunity results from contracting an infectious agent and experiencing either an acute or subclinical infectious disease

- Artificial active immunity is achieved following administration of vaccines

- Congenital passive immunity occurs when antibodies pass to a fetus from the mother providing short-term immunity for the newborn

- Passive immunity may be achieved through administration of ready-made antibodies, such as gamma globulin used to treat or prevent infectious diseases

The Body's Natural Barriers. The body has several natural barriers that serve to help inhibit infection. The greatest barrier is intact skin. Other barriers include mucous membranes that line body orifices, the gastrointestinal tract with hydrochloric acid that inhibits infection, cilia in the respiratory tract that filter out potential infectious agents, and the lymph and blood systems that fight pathogens through phagocytosis.

Immunization. Immunizing individuals against specific infectious diseases provides immunity with active or passive vaccines. Although most of severe childhood communicable diseases can be prevented, the U.S. Department of Health and Human Services has estimated that only about three-fourths of U.S. preschoolers under two years old are fully vaccinated according to recommended schedules (U.S. Department of Health and Human Services, 1999). Several factors influence vaccination rates, such as access to health care, cost of vaccinations, and irregularity or confusion in maintaining young children on the recommended schedule. Since most of the vaccinations are administered in ambulatory health care settings, medical assistants may have the

SPOTLIGHT ON AAMA ESSENTIALS THROUGH CAAHEP

- It's important for the medical assistant to develop an inner sense for the need to practice good aseptic procedures, since this is one of the very few tasks that directly affect the health of the patient, the physician, and the entire office staff.

- A medical assistant needs to be aware of the importance of taking time to discuss proper medical asepsis and handwashing techniques, as well as the relationship of infection control to good hygiene, so that the patient understands the necessity of following these procedures.

- All patients coming into your office should have absolute assurance that they are being taken care of in an aseptic atmosphere, under aseptic conditions, free of pathogens and disease-producing microorganisms.

responsibility to administer, document, and monitor immunizations.

Vaccines produce active or passive immunity by stimulating the immune system to recognize antigens without having to contract the infectious disease to provide natural immunity as described previously.

There are various classifications of vaccines, depending on the method of immune stimulation:

1. *Live attenuated (changed) pathogens.* These pathogens stimulate the body's own antibody production. However, the patient does not contract the infectious disease (or only a mild or subclinical case) since the pathogen has been altered in some mechanical or chemical means by the manufacturer. Examples of live attenuated pathogens include OPV (oral poliovirus vaccine), to protect from poliomyelitis.
2. *Pathogenic toxins.* Some pathogens produce toxins (poisonous substances) that can stimulate antibody production. Examples of toxin vaccines include tetanus and diphtheria.
3. *Killed pathogens.* Inactivated pathogens stimulate antibody production; however, several vaccines may be required to provide sustained protection. Examples include pertussis and rabies.

STAGES OF INFECTIOUS DISEASES

Depending on the specific pathogen causing an infectious disease, several stages occur from the time of exposure until full recovery and the absence of infection. These stages are often predictable and offer guidelines for patient education and treatment opportunities.

Incubation Stage

The incubation stage is the interval of time between exposure to a pathogenic microorganism and the first appearance of signs and symptoms of the disease. Some infectious diseases have very short incubation stages, whereas other infections have lengthy stages, lasting for years. If an exposure to an infectious agent occurs, the patient will manifest the disease if the patient's immune system cannot contain the agent or if therapeutic medications are available to prevent disease progression. Not all infectious agents are treatable or preventable.

Prodromal Stage

Prodromal means vague or undifferentiated from symptoms of other illnesses. The prodromal stage is characterized by common, general complaints of illness, such as malaise and fever. It is the interval between the earliest symptoms and the appearance of fever or rash that suggest an impending disease process is occurring.

Acute Stage

Disease processes reach their peak during the acute stage. Symptoms are fully developed and can often be differentiated from other specific symptoms. Treatment modalities are useful to reduce patient discomfort, reduce possibilities of debilitation and adverse effects, and to promote healing and recovery.

The inflammatory process is the body's natural defensive reaction to the invasion by a foreign substance such as a pathogen, and it is in this acute state that the response is evident.

Declining Stage

Patient symptoms begin to subside or wane during the declining stage. The infectious disease remains, however, though the patient will demonstrate improving levels of health.

Convalescent Stage

Recovery and recuperation from the effects of a specific infectious disease are called the convalescent stage. The patient regains strength and stamina, and the overall goal of this stage is that the patient is returned to the original state of health.

DISEASE TRANSMISSION

When providing patients with health care, medical assistants run the risk of contracting, or acquiring, an infection from pathogens that are causing patients' illnesses. Such pathogens are viruses, bacteria, fungi, and others that can be found in patients' blood and body fluids. In medical offices, ambulatory care centers, and hospitals, many ill patients are seen every day. Pathogens can be easily transmitted to another person if care is not taken to prevent such an occurrence.

Consistent use and adherence to infection control measures significantly reduce the risk of disease transmission. The CDC recommends that health care providers consider each patient to be potentially infectious for AIDS, hepatitis B, and other bloodborne pathogens and to routinely and conscientiously apply the techniques of Standard Precautions as a means of infection control.

Infectious diseases are caused by unique infectious agents, are characterized by various symptoms, are transmitted by differing means, and have unique treatments and prognoses. Medical assistants must recognize the unique characteristics of specific infectious diseases to prevent their transmission and treat patients suffering from these infections. Table 22-2 classifies common infectious diseases by critical components. When patients have contracted an infectious disease or are exposed to the risk of transmission, patient education plays an important role in infection control. Although a family member may have an infectious disease, proper training and education may protect other family members and close contacts.

Medical assistants also are responsible for when specific infectious diseases are encountered in the health care setting. With the increasing risk of drug-resistant pathogens, all health care professionals must habitually use infection control measures as well as oversee prudent treatment of patients with existing infectious diseases. For instance, tuberculosis was only recently the major cause of death, and the discovery of effective antituberculosis drugs slowed death rates dramatically. However, we are experiencing resurgent strains of the mycobacterium, which in some instances are resistant to drugs.

ACQUIRED IMMUNODEFICIENCY SYNDROME AND HEPATITIS B

A great deal of attention is focused on the human immunodeficiency virus (HIV) that causes AIDS, because there is yet no cure for the disease. With the focus on AIDS, other potentially life-threatening and fatal illnesses do not come to mind so quickly. Hepatitis B and other viral hepatitis diseases are examples of other diseases that place health care providers at great risk for serious illness or death. Acute viral hepatitis also deserves close attention.

TABLE 22-2 COMMON INFECTIOUS DISEASES

Disease	Agent	Transmission	Symptoms	Diagnosis	Treatment	Comments	Patient Education
AIDS (Acquired Immunodeficiency Syndrome)	Human Immunodeficiency Virus (HIV)	• Bloodborne • Sexual contact • Intrauterine • Lactation	Opportunistic infections, lymphadenopathy, fatigue, malaise, fever	CD4 level less than 200 cells/mm³	Palliative care and treatment for opportunistic infections, antiviral drugs	WHO (World Health Organization) estimates 20–40 million people will be infected with HIV	1. Careful infection control to reduce contact with pathogens that cause opportunistic infections 2. Use of latex condoms in conjunction with effective spermicide 3. Support groups
Hepatitis B	Hepatitis B virus (HBV)	• Bloodborne • Sexual contact • Intrauterine	Fatigue, malaise, anorexia, headache, icterus, liver tenderness and enlargement, fever	Serum antibody tests; liver function studies elevated	Immunization of all those at risk of exposure, palliative therapy, monitor bilirubin levels, bedrest, frequent low-fat, high-carbohydrate diet	Mortality 1–10%	1. Follow-up required to monitor liver function studies 2. Close personal contacts of patient should receive HB vaccine or HBIG (HB immunoglobulin) 3. Teach infection control to patient to prevent spread to close contacts 4. Avoid alcohol, sedatives, or aspirin during acute phase
Tuberculosis (TB)	Mycobacterium tuberculosis bacillus	• Inhalation of contaminated airborne mucous droplets • Possibly ingestion	Productive cough, fatigue, fever, weight loss (elderly: behavior changes, anorexia, weight loss)	Sputum culture for M. tuberculosis, Mantoux skin test (PPD), chest X ray, pleural needle biopsy	Antituberculosis agents, airborne transmission-based precautions, until drug agents started, BCG vaccine for children at high risk (controversial)	Increase in incidence of TB, especially among persons with AIDS and the homeless; may be drug resistant; health care professionals should have annual skin testing	1. Encourage handwashing and proper sputum tissue disposal 2. Promote compliance with medications 3. Encourage close contacts to have skin tests 4. Well-balanced diet
Food poisoning and gastroenteritis	Bacteria or viruses (i.e. staphylococci, clostridium, botulinum, E. coli, shigella)	• Ingestion of contaminated food or water	Nausea, intestinal cramps, vomiting, diarrhea, dehydration, respiratory failure, death	Culture of emesis, feces, vomitus, or suspected food or water	Fluid balance restoration, medications, emergency treatment as required	Report outbreaks to local authorities	1. Teach proper food handling 2. Carefully washing hands prior to handling all food 3. Report to physician all signs of dehydration 4. Gastroenteritis usually communicable via feces for up to seven weeks following exposure
Influenza	Influenza viruses A, B, or C (various strains)	• Inhalation • Aerosolized • Mucous droplets	Acute upper/lower respiratory infection, severe cough, fever, malaise, sore throat, coryza	Tissue culture of nasal or pharyngeal secretions	Palliative therapy, active immunization (annual vaccine recommended for persons at risk [elderly, heart patients] for complications from infection)	Report cases to local health authority	1. Bed rest for two to three days after fever decline 2. Force fluids 3. Report signs of secondary infections
Chickenpox (Varicella)	Varicella-zoster virus	• Direct and indirect contact with respiratory droplets	Sudden onset fever, malaise, maculo-papular-vesicular skin rash	Vesicular fluid tissue culture during first three days after eruption; serology: increase antibodies two weeks after rash; lesion appearance characteristic of varicella	Acyclovir helpful to reduce severity of disease; zoster immune globulin (ZIG) for high-risk persons only within 96 hours of exposure; palliative therapy	Vaccine (varicella virus vaccine live) available in U.S. for children over 12 months of age	1. Communicable one to two days before rash until lesions crust 2. Avoid scratching lesions to prevent secondary infection and scarring

AIDS

Acquired immunodeficiency syndrome, or **AIDS**, is caused by a bloodborne virus, human immunodeficiency virus (HIV), and then ensuing infection directly affects the immune response. The HIV is responsible for T cell destruction; T cells are the white blood cells that provide immunity.

HIV is carried in semen, blood, and other body fluids, and the virus can penetrate mucous membranes. Once inside the body, the depletion of helper T cells leaves the patient vulnerable to a wide range of infections and malignancies. The infections that the patient contracts are devastating. There is no curative treatment for AIDS, but there are antiviral drugs such as AZT (azidothymidine), ZDV (zidovudine), Videx, and others that are used to halt cellular synthesis and incapacitate cell protein, which is important in the virus's reproduction.

Acute Viral Hepatitis Diseases

In any of the acute viral hepatitis diseases, the liver becomes inflamed and hepatic cells can be destroyed. Healthy persons can regenerate cells, but elderly patients cannot. There are several types of viral hepatitis, including hepatitis A (HAV); hepatitis B (HBV): hepatitis C (HCV); hepatitis D (HDV); and hepatitis E (HEV).

The hepatitis B virus (HBV) represents the greatest risk to health care providers. While a new type B vaccine that confers 96 percent immunity is available for high-risk groups, it is nonetheless critical to practice standard precautions to curtail the transmission of this very preventable disease.

Symptoms of Hepatitis B. Hepaptitis B (HBV) is considered the greatest **biohazard** for health care providers. The American Medical Association has said that loss of health care workers to HBV overshadows the risk of AIDS and is almost entirely preventable.

Hepatitis B (HBV) is easier to contract than HIV. Symptoms of HBV include loss of appetite, fatigue, nausea, headache, fever and **jaundice**, a yellow discoloration of the skin. The liver function is impaired and, in severe cases, may even be lost. It is important to note that in some individuals HBV may be asymptomatic and can still damage the liver and possibly lead to cancer of the liver. Usually, once patients become infected, they remain so for life, and are capable of transmitting the virus to others.

Transmission of HIV and HBV

HIV and HBV are transmitted essentially through the same means. Contracting either disease requires direct contact with the virus living in infected blood and body fluids. The viruses are transmitted primarily through the following means:

- Sexual contact with an infected person (heterosexual, homosexual, or bisexual). The virus enters the bloodstream through small tears in the mucous membrane of the vagina, rectum, penis, or mouth

- Sharing needles for intravenous (IV) drug use with an infected person

- Using unsterilized tattoo and body piercing tools after their use on an infected person

- Receiving blood or blood products from an infected person. (All blood collected for transfusions is routinely checked for HIV and HBV; therefore, risk from this is now rare.)

- Intrauterine infection of the fetus by a pregnant infected woman

- Human bite

Despite the similarities between HIV and HBV, the risk of contracting HBV is far greater than contracting HIV. See Figure 22-2 and Table 22-3.

Medical assistants and all other health care providers must understand the importance of protecting themselves from the viruses that cause AIDS and hepatitis B and other pathogenic microorganisms as well. Through strict adherence to Standard Precautions and routine infectious disease control measures such as those found in medical asepsis, the risk of contracting an infectious disease is minimized.

PRINCIPLES OF INFECTION CONTROL

By understanding the dependent nature of the chain of infection which holds that each link in the process must occur for infectious disease to occur, medical assistants may apply principles of infection control to eliminate or reduce the transmission of infectious microorganisms in the ambulatory care setting. Conscious and continual reliance on infection control is a professional standard and protects employees, patients, and families from contracting infectious diseases. There are two general types of infection control: medical asepsis and surgical asepsis. Each is indicated in specific circumstances and each is achieved by the various techniques that are described in this chapter and Chapter 31. Stringent application of infection control measures should be the foundation of clinical care in the ambulatory care setting.

THE CENTERS FOR DISEASE CONTROL AND PREVENTION, AND ITS ROLE IN INFECTION CONTROL

The Centers for Disease Control and Prevention (CDC) is responsible for studying pathogens and diseases in an

BLOODBORNE FACTS

WHAT IS HBV?

Hepatitis B virus (HBV) is a potentially life-threatening blood-borne pathogen. Centers for Disease Control estimates there are approximately 280,000 HBV infections each year in the U.S.

Approximately 8,700 health care workers each year contract hepatitis B, and about 200 will die as a result. In addition, some who contract HBV will become carriers, passing the disease on to others. Carriers also face a significantly higher risk for other liver ailments which can be fatal, including cirrhosis of the liver and primary liver cancer.

HBV infection is transmitted through exposure to blood and other infectious body fluids and tissues. Anyone with occupational exposure to blood is at risk of contracting the infection.

Employers must provide engineering controls; workers must use work practices and protective clothing and equipment to prevent exposure to potentially infectious materials. However, the best defense against hepatitis B is vaccination.

WHO NEEDS VACCINATION?

The new OSHA standard covering bloodborne pathogens requires employers to offer the three-injection vaccination series free to all employees who are exposed to blood or other potentially infectious materials as part of their job duties. This includes health care workers, emergency responders, morticians, first-aid personnel, law enforcement officers, correctional facilities staff, launderers, as well as others.

The vaccination must be offered within 10 days of initial assignment to a job where exposure to blood or other potentially infectious materials can be "reasonably anticipated." The requirements for vaccinations of those already on the job took effect July 6, 1992.

WHAT DOES VACCINATION INVOLVE?

The hepatitis B vaccination is a noninfectious, yeast-based vaccine given in three injections in the arm. It is prepared from recombinant yeast cultures, rather than human blood or plasma. Thus, there is no risk of contamination from other bloodborne pathogens nor is there any chance of developing HBV from the vaccine.

The second injection should be given one month after the first, and the third injection six months after the initial dose. More than 90 percent of those vaccinated will develop immunity to the hepatitis B virus. To ensure immunity, it is important for individuals to receive all three injections. At this point it is unclear how long the immunity lasts, so booster shots may be required at some point in the future.

The vaccine causes no harm to those who are already immune or to those who may be HBV carriers. Although employees may opt to have their blood tested for antibodies to determine need for the vaccine, employers may not make such screening a condition of receiving vaccination nor are employers required to provide prescreening.

Each employee should receive counseling from a health care professional when vaccination is offered. This discussion will help an employee determine whether inoculation is necessary.

WHAT IF I DECLINE VACCINATION?

Workers who decide to decline vaccination must complete a declination form. Employers must keep these forms on file so that they know the vaccination status of everyone who is exposed to blood. At any time after a worker initially declines to receive the vaccine, he or she may opt to take it.

WHAT IF I AM EXPOSED BUT HAVE NOT YET BEEN VACCINATED?

If a worker experiences an exposure incident, such as a needlestick or a blood splash in the eye, he or she must receive confidential medical evaluation from a licensed health care professional with appropriate follow-up. To the extent possible by law, the employer is to determine the source individual for HBV as well as human immunodeficiency virus (HIV) infectivity. The worker's blood will also be screened if he or she agrees.

The health care professional is to follow the guidelines of the U.S. Public Health Service in providing treatment. This would include hepatitis B vaccination. The health care professional must give a written opinion on whether or not vaccination is recommended and whether the employee received it. Only this information is reported to the employer. Employee medical records must remain confidential. HIV or HBV status must NOT be reported to the employer.

U.S. Department of Labor
Occupational Safety and Health Administration

Single copies of fact sheets are available from OSHA Publications, Room N3101, 200 Constitution Ave. N.W., Washington, D.C. 20210 and from OSHA regional offices.

Figure 22-2 *Bloodborne Facts,* published by the United States Department of Labor, Occupational Safety and Health Administration. This publication includes facts about hepatitis B virus, vaccination, declination, and steps to be taken by the employer should exposure to blood, body fluids, or OPIM occur.

TABLE 22-3   HEPATITIS VIRUSES A–E

	A	B	C	D	E
Etiologic Agent	Hepatitis A virus (HAV)	Hepatitis B virus (HBV)	Hepatitis C virus (HCV)	Hepatitis D virus (HDV)	Hepatitis E virus (HEV)
Transmission	Fecal-oral; contaminated water or food; person to person	Blood; sexual; perinatal; breast milk	Blood	Only persons with hepatitis B can get hepatitis D; blood and blood products; needlesticks; seldom sexual; rarely perinatal	Oral-fecal route; contaminated water; person-to-person uncommon
Risk Groups	Household/sexual contact with infected person; international travelers	Injection drug users; sexual/household contact with infected person; infants born to infected mothers; health care workers; multiple sex partners	Recipients of blood transfusions or organ transplants prior to 1992; people sharing needles; people exposed to blood and blood products	People sharing needles; health care workers	Travelers to countries where HEV is endemic
Incubation Period	15–50 days	45–160 days	14–180 days	15–60 days	15–60 days
Infectious Period	Usually less than 2 months	Before symptoms appear; lifetime if carrier	Before symptoms appear; lifetime if carrier	Not determined	Not determined
Diagnostic Tests	IgM anti-HAV	HBsAG	Anti-HCV; serum ALT increased 10x; HCVRNA	IgG anti-HDV	None available
Symptoms	Flu-like; jaundice; dark yellow urine; light-colored stools	Flu-like; may have jaundice; dark yellow urine; light-colored stools	Many have no symptoms; flu-like	Flu-like; may have jaundice; dark yellow urine; light-colored stools	Abdominal pain, anorexia; dark yellow urine; jaundice; fever
Prevention	Standard Precautions; enteric precautions; hepatitis A vaccine (entire series); immune globulin (for short term)	Standard Precautions; reduce risk behaviors; hepatitis B vaccine (entire series); immune globulin (for short term)	Standard Precautions; reduce risk behaviors; no vaccine	Standard Precautions; reduce risk behaviors; hepatitis B vaccine; if client already has hepatitis B, no prevention for hepatitis D	Standard Precautions; be sure water is safe when traveling; no vaccine
Treatment	Immune globulin within 2 weeks of exposure	Immune globulin (HBIg) Alpha interferon	Alpha interferon; ribavirin (Virazole)	Alpha interferon	None given
Prognosis	Rarely fatal; not a carrier	No cure; may become a carrier	85% or less have chronic infection; 70% develop chronic liver disease	Chronicity uncommon	No evidence of chronicity

(Courtesy Hepatitis Foundation International)

Data from: Centers for Disease Control and Prevention (CDC) (2000). Viral hepatitis. [On-line] Available: www.cdc.gov/ncidod/diseases/hepatitis; Lau, D. T., Kleiner, D. E., Park, Y., DiBisceglie, A. M., & Hoofnagle, J. H. (1999). Resolution of chronic delta hepatitis after 12 years of interferon alpha therapy. *Gastroenterology*, 117(5), 1229–33; National Institute of Diabetes and Digestive and Kidney Diseases (NIDDK) (1997). What I need to know about hepatitis A [On-line] Available: www.niddk.nih.gov/health/digest/pubs/hep/hepa/hepa.htm; NIDDK (1998). What I need to know about hepatitis B. [On-line] Available: www.niddk.nih.gov/health/digest/pubs/hep/hepb/hepb.htm; NIDDK (1999). What I meed to know about hepatitis C. [On-line] Available: www.niddk.nih.gov/health/digest/pubs/hep/hepc/hepc.htm; NIDDK (2000). Chronic hepatitis C: Current disease management. [On-line] Available: www.niddk.nih.gov/health/digest/pubs/chrnhepc/chrnhepc.htm; NIDDK (2000). The digestive diseases dictionary: E–K. [On-line] Available: www.niddk.nih.gov/health/digest/pubs/dddctnry/pages/e-k.htm.

effort to prevent their spread. A division of the United States Public Health Department, the CDC has issued a number of guidelines over the past twenty-five years that have enabled health care professionals to practice responsible infection control. As diseases evolve, and as new diseases are introduced into our society, the CDC revises and updates existing guidelines or issues new control measures to contain the spread of infection.

In 1970, the CDC developed a system of seven iso-lation categories for patients with known infectious diseases. This category system included strict isolation, respiratory isolation, protective isolation, enteric precautions, wound and skin precautions, discharge precautions, and blood precautions.

In 1985, the agency released a set of guidelines known as Universal Blood and Body Fluid Precautions, or simply Universal Precautions. These infection control practices were written in response to an increase in acquired immunodeficiency syndrome (AIDS) and hepatitis B, both bloodborne diseases, and to other infectious diseases as well.

Beginning in 1991, the CDC infection control guidelines were reviewed and subsequently revised. In 1996, a new set of guidelines was released. Standard Precautions reflect improved recommendations intended to protect all health care providers, patients, and their visitors from a wide range of communicable diseases. At the same time that the CDC issued the new Standard Precautions, they also released a second tier of precautions called Transmission-Based Precautions. These are intended to be used in addition to Standard Precautions when caring for patients with specific infectious diseases.

To understand the evolution and intent of these various CDC infection control guidelines, Universal Precautions, Standard Precautions, and Transmission-Based Precautions will be examined in more detail.

Universal Precautions

In an effort to curb the transmission of AIDS, hepatitis B, and other infectious diseases, in 1985 the CDC issued guidelines known as Universal Blood and Body Fluid Precautions or simply Universal Precautions. It is now known that consistent use and adherence to these guidelines greatly minimizes the risk of infectious disease transmission. At the recommendation of the CDC, health care providers were to consider every patient potentially infectious for AIDS, hepatitis B, and other bloodborne pathogens and to routinely and consistently use the techniques of Universal Precautions as a means of infection control.

While most of the basic tenets of Universal Precautions have now been incorporated into the new Standard

Precautions, it is nonetheless important to know and understand the primary preventive measures of these 1985 recommendations.

Following is a summary of the CDC's Universal Precautions and guidelines for control of AIDS, hepatitis B, and other infectious diseases:

1. Consider all (patients') blood and body fluids to be contaminated.
2. Always wash hands before and after (patient) contact.
3. Always wash hands if contaminated with blood or body fluids.
4. Wear gloves when handling or touching blood, body fluids, body tissue, mucous membranes, nonintact skin, or contaminated equipment and supplies.
5. Wear gloves when performing venipuncture and other blood access treatments or procedures.
6. Change gloves after each patient contact.
7. Wash hands after glove removal. Gloves do not replace handwash technique.
8. Wear gloves, gown, mask, goggles/face shield if splashing of blood or body fluids can occur or if exposure to droplets of blood or body fluids is a possibility. Examples of this are wound care and endoscopy.
9. Use extreme caution when handling needles, scalpels, and other sharp instruments (sharps) during procedures and when handling them after procedures are completed. Dispose of sharps in an approved puncture-proof container that should be located as close as practical to the work area.
10. Use a mouthpiece if performing cardiopulmonary resuscitation. The risk of transmission of human immunodeficiency virus (HIV) through saliva is very low.
11. Clean blood and body fluid spills with agency disinfectant or a 10 percent solution of sodium hypochlorite (household bleach).
12. Report needlesticks, splashes, and contamination by wounds or body fluids. Follow up with employee health services, physician, and other appropriate personnel.
13. Health care workers with open lesions (injury or wound) or dermatitis (skin rash) should avoid direct contact with patients and their supplies and equipment until healed.
14. Laboratory specimens and their containers are modes of disease transmission and gloves should be worn during handling.
15. Pregnant health care providers should be especially careful to adhere to the guidelines so as to protect themselves and the unborn child.

Standard Precautions

The CDC spent several years researching, improving, and developing recommendations to protect health care providers, patients, and their visitors from infectious diseases. This intensive period of research resulted in Standard Precautions, a set of infection control guidelines that should now be utilized by all health care professionals for all patients.

Standard Precautions combine many of the basic principles of universal precautions with techniques known as **Body Substance Isolation (BSI)**, a system that maintains that personal protective equipment should be worn for contact with all body fluids whether or not blood is visible. Although BSI was developed not by a federal or state agency but by a private hospital, its techniques nonetheless have been adopted by many health care facilities.

The rationale behind developing the new Standard Precautions was that while Universal Precautions and Body Substance Isolation provide a good degree of protection, the CDC recognized that both could be improved upon. Advantages of the new Standard Precautions are that they include all of the major recommendations of Universal Precautions and Body Substance Isolation, while incorporating new information; they simplify medical terminology to be as user-friendly as possible; they use new terms to avoid confusion with existing infection control and isolation systems; and they are intended to protect all patients, all health care providers, and all visitors.

According to the CDC, Standard Precautions are "designed to reduce the risk of transmission of microorganisms from both recognized and unrecognized sources of infection in hospitals" (CDC, 1997). They apply to:

1. Blood
2. All body fluids, secretions, and excretions regardless of whether or not they contain visible blood
3. Nonintact skin
4. Mucous membranes

To be effective, Standard Precautions must be practiced conscientiously at all times. Although Standard Precautions were intended primarily for use in acute care facilities such as hospitals, they can and should be applied in other types of facilities including the ambulatory care settings where many medical assistants are likely to be employed.

Figure 22-3 provides a comprehensive review of the Standard Precautions.

Transmission-Based Precautions

When the CDC was in the process of developing a new guideline for isolation precautions in hospitals, the agency arrived at what it terms two tiers of precautions. The first tier is called the Standard Precautions, discussed earlier in this chapter, designed for all patients regardless of their diagnosis or presumed infection status. The second tier of precautions is intended for patients diagnosed with or suspected of specific highly transmissible diseases. These are known as Transmission-Based Precautions.

Transmission-Based Precautions condense the seven existing categories of isolation precautions developed by the CDC in 1970 into three sets of precautions based on routes of infection. Released in 1996 to complement Standard Precautions, Transmission-Based Precautions reduce the risk of **airborne**, **droplet**, and **contact transmission** of pathogens and are always to be used *in addition to* Standard Precautions.

These airborne, contact, and droplet precautions also list specific syndromes that can appear in adult and pediatric patients who are highly suspicious for infection. They identify the appropriate Transmission-Based Precautions to be used until a diagnosis can be made. See Figures 22-4, 22-5, and 22-6 for specific information on these three Transmission-Based Precautions. Remember that these precautions are for specific categories of patients and are to be used in addition to Standard Precautions, which are used for all patients.

Blood and Body Fluids

In all infection control efforts, it is important to understand what is meant by blood and body fluids. Specifically, they are described as the blood, secretions, and excretions of a patient. Examples of blood and body fluids and some of the areas in which medical assistants may become exposed to them are:

Latex Sensitivity

Health care providers should be aware that some people, including professionals and patients, can be allergic to latex products. Some personal protective equipment (PPE) is made from latex; medical and surgical products also are often made from this product.

The allergic reaction can be a localized one such as dermatitis or a more severe systemic reaction such as anaphylaxis (see Chapter 9), a form of shock marked by vascular collapse, respiratory failure, hypotension, arrhythmia, and laryngeal edema. Vinyl gloves can be worn in place of latex for hypersensitive individuals. Any person with an allergy to latex should wear a bracelet or other form of identification indicating this fact since, in any emergency, medical personnel wear latex gloves.

STANDARD PRECAUTIONS
FOR INFECTION CONTROL

Wash Hands (Plain soap)
Wash after touching **blood, body fluids, secretions, excretions,** and **contaminated items.**
Wash immediately **after gloves are removed** and **between patient contacts.** Avoid transfer of microorganisms to other patients or environments.

Wear Gloves
Wear when touching **blood, body fluids, secretions, excretions,** and **contaminated items.** Put on **clean** gloves just **before touching mucous membranes** and **nonintact skin.** Change gloves between tasks and procedures on the same patient after contact with material that may contain high concentrations of microorganisms. Remove gloves promptly after use, before touching noncontaminated items and environmental surfaces, and before going to another patient, and wash hands immediately to avoid transfer of microorganisms to other patients or environments.

Wear Mask and Eye Protection or Face Shield
Protect mucous membranes of the eyes, nose and mouth during procedures and patient-care activities that are likely to generate **splashes** or **sprays** of **blood, body fluids, secretions,** or **excretions.**

Wear Gown
Protect skin and prevent soiling of clothing during procedures that are likely to generate **splashes** or **sprays** of **blood, body fluids, secretions,** or **excretions.** Remove a soiled gown as promptly as possible and wash hands to avoid transfer of microorganisms to other patients or environments.

Patient-Care Equipment
Handle used patient-care equipment soiled with **blood, body fluids, secretions,** or **excretions** in a manner that prevents skin and mucous membrane exposures, contamination of clothing, and transfer of microorganisms to other patients and environments. Ensure that reusable equipment is not used for the care of another patient until it has been appropriately cleaned and reprocessed and single use items are properly discarded.

Environmental Control
Follow hospital procedures for routine care, cleaning, and disinfection of environmental surfaces, beds, bedrails, bedside equipment and other frequently touched surfaces.

Linen
Handle, transport, and process used linen soiled with **blood, body fluids, secretions,** or **excretions** in a manner that prevents exposures and contamination of clothing, and avoids transfer of microorganisms to other patients and environments.

Occupational Health and Bloodborne Pathogens
Prevent injuries when using needles, scalpels, and other sharp instruments or devices; when handling sharp instruments after procedures; when cleaning used instruments; and when disposing of used needles.

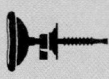

Never recap used needles using both hands or any other technique that involves directing the point of a needle towards any part of the body; rather, use either a one-handed "scoop" technique or a mechanical device designed for holding the needle sheath.

Do not remove used needles from disposable syringes by hand, and do not bend, break, or otherwise manipulate used needles by hand. Place used disposable syringes and needles, scalpels blades, and other sharp items in puncture-resistant sharps containers located as close as practical to the area in which the items were used, and place reusable syringes and needles in a puncture-resistant container for transport to the reprocessing area.

Use **resuscitation devices** as an alternative to mouth-to-mouth resuscitation.

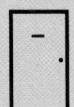

Patient Placement
Use a **private room** for a patient who contaminates the environment or who does not (or cannot be expected to) assist in maintaining appropriate hygiene or environmental control. Consult Infection Control if a private room is not available.

Figure 22-3 Standard Precautions for Infection Control issued by the CDC in 1997. (Courtesy Brevis Corp.)

AIRBORNE PRECAUTIONS
(in addition to Standard Precautions)
VISITORS: Report to nurse before entering.

Patient Placement
Use **private room** that has:
  Monitored negative air pressure,
  6 to 12 air changes per hour,
  Discharge of air outdoors or HEPA filtration if recirculated.
Keep room door closed and patient in room.

Respiratory Protection
Wear an **N95 respirator** when entering the room of a patient with known or suspected infectious pulmonary **tuberculosis**.
Susceptible persons should not enter the room of patients known or suspected to have **measles** (rubeola) or **varicella** (chickenpox) if other immune caregivers are available. If susceptible persons must enter, they should wear an **N95 respirator**. (Respirator or surgical mask not required if immune to measles and varicella.)

Patient Transport
Limit transport of patient from room to essential purposes only.
Use **surgical mask** on patient during transport.

Figure 22-4   Airborne Precautions, one category of Transmission-Based Precautions. (Courtesy of Brevis Corp.)

CONTACT PRECAUTIONS
(in addition to Standard Precautions)
VISITORS: Report to nurse before entering.

Patient Placement
Private room, if possible. Cohort if private room is not available.

Gloves
Wear gloves when entering patient room.
Change gloves after having contact with infective material that may contain high concentrations of microorganisms (**fecal** material and **wound drainage**).
Remove gloves before leaving patient room.

Wash
Wash hands with an **antimicrobial** agent immediately after glove removal. After glove removal and handwashing, ensure that hands do not touch potentially contaminated environmental surfaces or items in the patient's room to avoid transfer of microorganisms to other patients or environments.

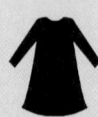

Gown
Wear gown when entering patient room if you anticipate that your clothing will have a substantial contact with the patient, environmental surfaces, or items in the patient's room, or if the patient is **incontinent,** or has **diarrhea,** an **ileostomy,** a **colostomy,** or **wound drainage** not contained by a dressing. **Remove** gown before leaving the patient's environment and ensure that clothing does not contact potentially contaminated environmental surfaces to avoid transfer of microorganisms to other patients or environments.

Patient Transport
Limit transport of patient to essential purposes only. During transport, ensure that precautions are maintained to minimize the risk of transmission of microorganisms to other patients and contamination of environmental surfaces and equipment.

Patient-Care Equipment
Dedicate the use of noncritical patient-care equipment to a single patient. If common equipment is used, clean and disinfect between patients.

Figure 22-5   Contact Precautions, one category of Transmission-Based Precautions. (Courtesy of Brevis Corp.)

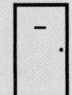

DROPLET PRECAUTIONS
(in addition to Standard Precautions)
VISITORS: Report to nurse before entering.

Patient Placement
Private room, if possible. Cohort or maintain spatial separation of **3 feet** from other patients or visitors if private room is not available.

Mask
Wear mask when working within **3 feet** of patient (or upon entering room).

Patient Transport
Limit transport of patient from room to essential purposes only.
Use **surgical mask** on patient during transport.

Figure 22-6 Droplet Precautions, one category of Transmission-Based Precautions. (Courtesy of Brevis Corp.)

Blood:

- Specimens drawn during venipuncture
- Open wounds of any kind
- **Epistaxis**, or nosebleeds
- Vaginal bleeding, including **menses** (menstruation), **lochia** (discharge following childbirth), and hemorrhage
- Feces and vomit or other body fluids with or without blood

Vaginal Secretions:

- Physiological **leukorrhea** (normal vaginal discharge)
- Vaginitis

Cerebral Spinal Fluid:

- Fluid **aspirated**, or withdrawn, during a **lumbar puncture**
- Leakage of fluid due to trauma to the brain and/or spinal cord

Synovial Fluid:

- Fluid aspirated during arthroscopic procedures

Pleural Fluid:

- Fluid aspirated during **thoracentesis**, a surgical puncture of the thoracic cavity
- Fluid leakage due to chest trauma

Pericardial Fluid:

- Fluid around the heart exposed during cardiac surgery or due to cardiac trauma

Peritoneal Fluid:

- Fluid exposed during abdominal surgery (least likely fluid that medical assistant will come into contact with), but exposure can occur during a paracentesis

Semen:

- Seminal fluid as a laboratory specimen for sperm count in examination for fertility level

Amniotic Fluid:

- Fluid aspirated during **amniocentesis**, a surgical puncture of the amniotic sac
- Vaginal leakage during pregnancy, labor, and delivery

Sputum:

- Material coughed up and expectorated from the respiratory tract

Saliva:

- Oral mucous gland fluid in mouth during oral/dental procedures
- Any other body fluid visibly contaminated with blood

Thus far, only blood and blood products, semen, vaginal secretions, and possibly breast milk have been directly linked to transmission of HIV, and the virus is not spread casually nor through close family contacts. There is not yet a vaccine to protect individuals from HIV.

HBV has been found in blood and blood products, vaginal secretions, semen, and saliva. Infection can spread through close family contacts, kissing, sexual contacts, intrauterinely, and during delivery. An infant may become a chronic **carrier**, one who has no symptoms but can transmit disease. If there has been an exposure to the virus, a prompt injection of immunoglobulin, an antibody, will help provide protection from the virus. Hepatitis B vaccine is available and the series of three injections usually immunizes an individual from an attack of hepatitis B for approximately 18 years.

Some states require health care providers and allied health students to be immunized prior to employment and prior to admission into a health program in an educational institution. Also, some states require infants to be routinely immunized with HBV vaccine.

Personal Protective Equipment

Universal, Standard, and Transmission-Based Precautions all make use of barriers or personal protective equipment (PPE). The barriers consist of gloves, mask, gown, and goggles/face shield. Gloves reduce the risk of contamination to hands but do not prevent needles or other sharp instruments from penetrating the skin. Masks and protective eyewear reduce the contamination risk to mucous membranes of the eyes, nose, and mouth. Gowns protect clothing from contamination. Barriers are used in various combinations depending upon the procedure or treatment being performed on patients. As a medical assistant, you may be exposed to infected blood and/or body fluids and must wear PPE (Figure 22-7).

Needlestick

One of the most common reasons for exposure to blood is caused by accidentally sticking oneself with a dirty (used) needle after performing invasive procedures such as injections and venipuncture. In the past, needlesticks were common due to the practice of needle recapping. Needles are no longer recapped, broken off, removed from syringes, or manipulated by hand in any way. They are disposed of in the approved puncture-proof container designated for sharps (Figure 22-8A). The risk to a health care provider of HIV infection caused by a needlestick is very slight; however, the risk for HBV infection caused by a needlestick can be significantly higher. OSHA has mandated the use of safer needle devices that can protect workers from needlesticks and sharp injuries; however, these are not yet being used widely enough to substantially reduce the number of yearly injuries. (See Chapter 36, Figure 36-15.) (Additional information regarding specific procedures to follow should an accidental needlestick occur as well as other safety procedures will be found later in this chapter and in Chapter 38, and are included in the OSHA and CLIA rules and regulations.)

Disposal of Infectious Waste

Infectious waste (contaminated items) is described as any item that has come in contact with patient blood or body fluids. These items must be handled with gloves and disposed of by placing them in the appropriate biohazard containers that are provided by an agency with which your employer has contracted (Figure 22-8B). Infectious waste is either incinerated (burned) or subjected to ster-

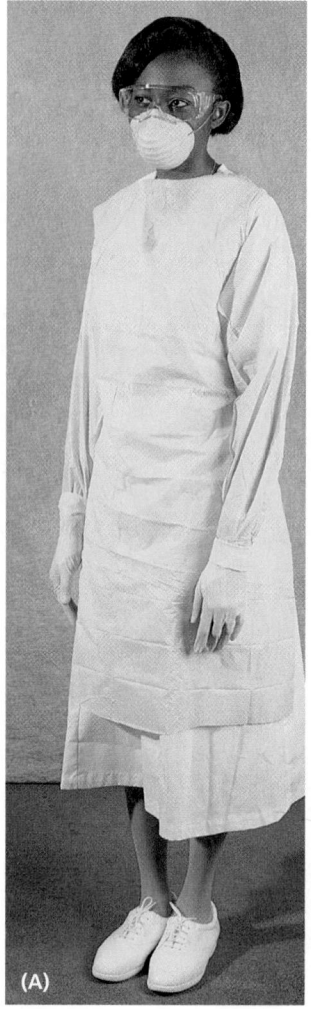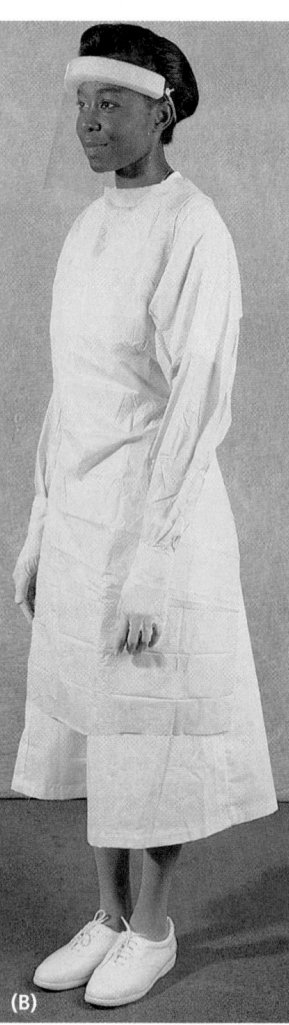

Figure 22-7   Medical assistant wearing personal protective equipment: (A) goggles, mask, gown, latex gloves; (B) full face shield, gown, latex gloves.

ilization by autoclave to render it harmless before it is disposed of in a sanitary landfill.

OCCUPATIONAL SAFETY AND HEALTH ADMINISTRATION (OSHA) REGULATIONS

 The Occupational Safety and Health Administration (OSHA) regulations are intended to ascertain that employers have a safe and healthful work environment for their employees. They represent requirements that employers must follow to ensure employee safety and health.

There are two **standards** that comprise the regulations, *The Occupational Exposure to Hazardous Chemicals in the Laboratory*, an amended version of the original standard *The Hazard Communication Standard*, and *The Bloodborne Pathogen Standard*. As with any standard, these

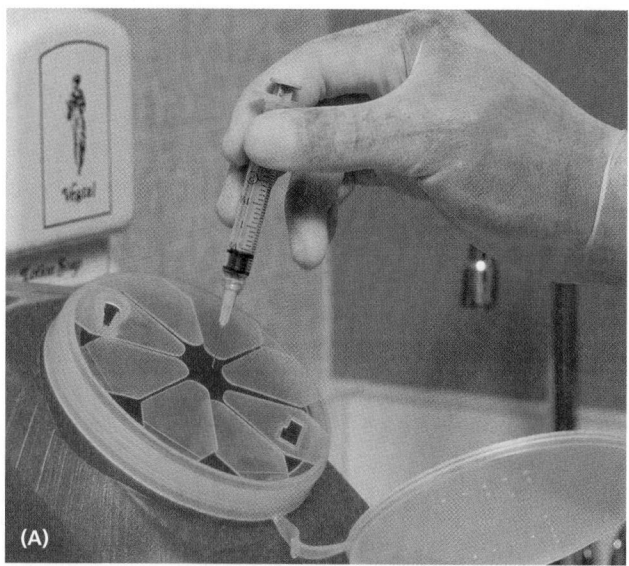

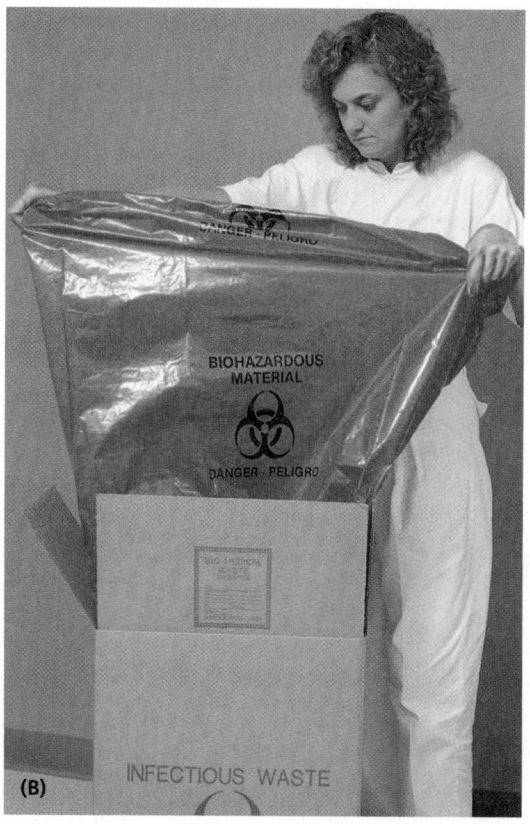

Figure 22-8 (A) Discard the entire disposable syringe with used needle intact in the biohazardous puncture-proof sharps container. (B) The medical assistant is placing a sturdy disposable plastic bag marked with the biohazardous waste symbol into a durable cardboard box for collection of infectious waste material. When full, these boxes are picked up by an agency for incineration or for autoclaving before disposal in a public landfill.

standards are rules established to measure quality, weight, extent, or value.

The Bloodborne Pathogen Standard

The Bloodborne Pathogen Standard became effective in March 1992. It came about principally in the hope of reducing the occupational-related cases of human immunodeficiency virus and hepatitis B infections among health care workers.

It covers all employees who can be "reasonably anticipated" to come into contact, as a result of performing their job duties, with blood and other potentially infectious materials (OPIM). It seeks to limit exposure to the pathogens. The law covers:

- Exposure determination
- Methods of control of exposure, especially Standard Precautions
- HBV vaccine
- Post-exposure follow-up
- Disposal of biohazardous waste
- Labeling
- Housekeeping and laundry functions
- Training for employee safety and documentation

Blood and Other Potentially Infectious Material (OPIM). Blood and OPIM are defined by the Centers for Disease Control and the Occupational Safety and Health Administration as the following human fluids:

- Blood and blood components
- Semen
- Vaginal secretions
- Cerebral spinal fluid
- Synovial fluid
- Pleural fluid
- Pericardial fluid
- Peritoneal fluid
- Body fluids visibly contaminated with blood
- Saliva in dental/oral procedures
- Unfixed human tissue (alive or dead); e.g., breast tissue from a frozen section biopsy
- Any tissue culture, cells, or fluid known to be HIV- or HBV-infected
- When the origin of a specimen is unknown, it must be handled as if it were infectious.

It is possible for medical assistants to come into contact with the majority of the fluids listed. Refer to "Blood and Body Fluids" earlier in this chapter.

Bloodborne Pathogens.

Disease-producing microorganisms are called pathogens; **bloodborne** refers to the manner in which the microorganisms can be transmitted—via blood or OPIM. Two pathogens of particular importance to health care providers are hepatitis B virus (HBV) and human immunodeficiency virus (HIV).

Hepatitis B causes diseases that directly affect the liver; the virus can be transmitted through blood from exposure to a contaminated needle. HIV is responsible for acquired immunodeficiency virus (AIDS), a fatal illness. HIV can be transmitted through blood from a contaminated needle and through direct contact with blood via broken skin. For a more in-depth discussion of both HBV and AIDS, refer to "Disease Transmission" earlier in this chapter.

Exposure Determination.

Exposure determination requires an employer to list all of the job classifications and employees in those job classifications that are exposed to blood and OPIM in the course of performing their jobs (Figure 22-9). Existing job descriptions can be used by the employer to identify the job categories that are considered high risk for exposure to blood and/or OPIM (Figure 22-10). It is important to note that exposure determination is made without regard to the use of PPE.

Plan to Control Exposure.

Every employer who has an employee(s) who is identified and determined to be at risk because of exposure potential must have a written exposure control plan (Figures 22-11 through 22-13). The plan must consist of methods of compliance for prevention of exposure, hepatitis B vaccination and post-exposure evaluation, communication of hazards to employee(s), documentation of the bloodborne standard, and a procedure for the determination of the events surrounding the exposure occurrence. The written plan must be employee accessible, updated regularly (at least annually), and modified when necessary and appropriate, especially to reflect changes in employee positions.

Methods of Compliance to Prevent Exposure.

There are seven major strategies mandated by OSHA for the prevention of exposure to bloodborne pathogens and OPIM.

1. *Standard Precautions*
   Adherence to the CDC's Standard Precautions is required; i.e., treating ALL bodily fluids and materials as if they are infectious. Handwashing is stressed and employers must provide handwashing facilities and must ascertain that employees use them frequently and especially following exposure to blood or OPIM.

2. *Engineering Controls and Work Practice Controls*
   Engineering controls and **work practice controls** consist of the physical equipment and mechanical

SAMPLE

Exposure Activity Form for Category 2 Employees.
Tasks Involving Occupation Exposure to Blood and Body Fluids

Employee at Risk and Job Title	Task Involving Risk and PPE	Risk Rating

Figure 22-9 Sample Exposure Activity Form for Category 2 Employees (no exposure to blood or body fluids), including tasks and risk rating. (Courtesy of POL Consultants)

SAMPLE

Exposure Classification Record of Employee

The following employee was classified according to work task exposure to certain body fluids as required by the current OSHA infection control standard on (Date) _____ as follows:

Employee Name: _____ SS# _____

_____ Category 1. "All procedures or other job related tasks that involve an inherent potential for mucous membrane or skin contact with blood, body fluids, or tissues, or a potential for spill or splashes of (blood or body fluids)."

_____ Category 2. Tasks in which "The normal work routine involves no exposure to blood, body fluids, or tissues, but exposure or potential exposure may be required as a condition of employment." For example, receptionists, accounting, or insurance staff or others who may, as a part of their duties, be asked to help in clean up, instrument recirculation, laboratory, or other similar procedures where exposure may result.

_____ Category 3. Tasks in which "The normal work routine involves no exposure to blood, body fluids, or tissues. Persons who perform these duties are not called upon as part of their employment to perform or assist in emergency medical care or first aid or to be potentially exposed in some other way."

Employer Signature _____

Because of a change of job assignment, the above employee was reclassified according to tasks exposure on (Date) _____ as follows:

_____ Category 1
_____ Category 2
_____ Category 3

Employer's Signature _____

Because of a change of assignment, the above employee was reclassified according to task exposure on (Date) _____ as follows:

_____ Category 1
_____ Category 2
_____ Category 3

Employer's Signature _____

NOTE: This record should be retained for length of employment plus thirty years.

OFFICE WORK PRACTICE EXPOSURE CONTROL PLAN

Effective Date: _____

Office of _____

As of the above date the office will follow the rules below to reduce exposure and contamination:

Observe Standard Precautions.

Wear gloves when drawing blood and performing procedures/tests.

Wash hands after removing gloves.

Change gloves frequently during the day and between patients.

Not answer phone or type while wearing gloves.

Not cap or break needles.

Dispose of all needles in sharps containers.

Not allow sharps containers to fill beyond ⅔ full.

Wear lab coats when performing tests.

Leave lab coats in laboratory/work area.

Dispose of all contaminated material in infectious waste container.

Disinfect the laboratory work surfaces frequently.

Disinfect the examining room surfaces, daily and as needed.

Sterilize nondisposable examination and testing equipment.

Monitor sterilization procedure.

Not eat or drink in work area.

Place gauze over tops of blood tubes when removing caps.

Clean up all specimen and chemical spills properly and immediately.

Label all chemicals according to OSHA regulations.

Label refrigerator that blood is stored in.

Centrifuges will have lids or specimens will be capped when spun.

Centrifuges will be disinfected regularly.

Hepatitis B vaccines will be offered to all employees.

Employees will take a safety training program.

Figure 22-10 Sample Exposure Classification Record of employee shows exposure categories into which employee's tasks fall. This record is kept for thirty years. (Courtesy of POL Consultants)

Figure 22-11 Office Work Practice Exposure Control Plan indicates a sample list of precautions to take to minimize employee risk exposure. (Courtesy of POL Consultants)

SAMPLE

Office Procedures Safety Form

PROCEDURE: _____

Type of hazard: _____

Person performing procedure: _____

Person assisting procedure: _____

Personal protective equipment used: _____
_____

Proper techniques for safety:
_____
_____
_____

What is done with used materials and soiled instruments?
_____
_____
_____

What chemical products are involved?
_____
_____
_____

What are the specific risks of procedure?
_____
_____
_____

Additional comments:
_____
_____
_____
_____

Prepared By: _____ Date: _____

Figure 22-12 Sample Office Procedures Safety Form lists procedures, type of hazard, employee performing procedure, employee assisting with procedure, and PPE. (Courtesy of POL Consultants)

SAMPLE

Safety/Work Practice Controls for Office Procedures

Each office has special safety procedures that are unique to that particular practice. These are also known as work practice controls. The fundamental work practice control is using Standard Precautions. Work practice controls reduce the likelihood of exposure to hazards. Many times the risks can be eliminated by changing the way a procedure is performed. Make copies of the PROCEDURES SAFETY FORM. Fill in the information for any procedure that involves exposure to potentially infectious body fluids. File these procedures in the office operation section of your manual. Do not limit this section to only body fluid exposures. General safety for other hazards such as chemicals and X-ray should be listed as well. Common examples are listed below. Check the ones you do and add to this list.

____ Patient exams	____ Arthroscopies
____ Aspirations	____ Vaginal exams
____ Inoculations	____ PAP smears/
____ Taking blood	IUDs
samples	____ OB care
____ Lab testing	____ Norplants
____ Lesion excisions	____ Vasectomies
____ Wound care	____ Biopsies
____ Dressing changes	____ Sigmoidoscopies
____ Colposcopies	____ _____
____ Surgical	____ _____
procedures	____ _____
____ X-rays	

Figure 22-13 Sample Safety/Work Practice Controls for Office Procedures lists procedures that involve exposure to blood, body fluids, and OPIM. (Courtesy of POL Consultants)

devices an employer provides in an attempt to safeguard and minimize employee exposure. A common example of an engineering control is sharps disposal containers (Figure 22-14). Others are mechanical pipettes, fume hoods, and splash guards. If and when occupational exposure continues after the engineering controls are in place, PPE must be used. Handwashing facilities or appropriate antiseptic hand cleanser (when handwashing facilities are unavailable) must be readily available. If antiseptic hand cleanser is used, hands must be washed with running water and soap as soon as possible. Employers must ascertain that employees wash their hands as soon as possible following the removal of gloves or other PPE, that employees wash hands and other skin surfaces with soap and water, flush eyes at the eyewash

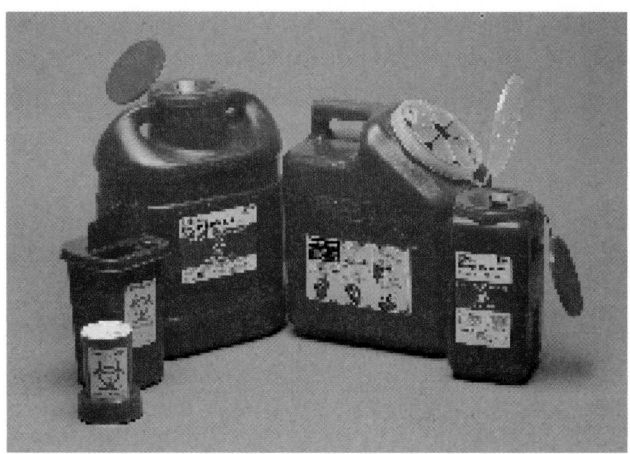

Figure 22-14   Various sizes of puncture-proof sharps containers. These and other biohazard waste containers are autoclaved when full and sent out to a biohazard agency for safe disposal.

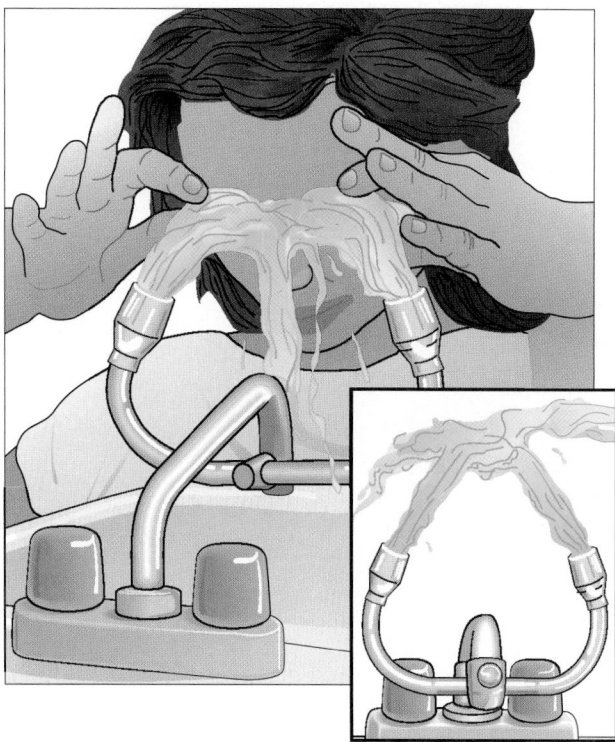

Figure 22-15   Emergency eyewash station: two streams of water wash both eyes simultaneously and continuously.

station, and flush mucous membranes with water as soon as possible following contact of these body parts with blood or OPIM (Figure 22-15).

Contaminated or used needles and other sharps must not be recapped, bent, nor removed unless required by a specific medical procedure. In such circumstances, a one-handed technique using a mechanical device must be used. (*In this instance, the needle has not been used on a patient.*) Contaminated sharps and needles must be placed immediately following use in a puncture-resistant container that is leak-proof and properly labeled with a biohazard label.

Eating, drinking, applying makeup, and so on are not allowed in areas when there is a possibility of exposure. Foods and drinks must be kept in a different refrigerator from one being used to store blood or OPIM.

Splashing, splattering, and spraying of blood or OPIM during procedures must be avoided if possible.

Mouth pipetting is not permissible.

Specimens must be put into containers that are labeled as biohazardous and the container must be leak-proof to prevent exposure during transport, handling, and collecting.

If equipment is contaminated with blood during its use, it must be decontaminated before it is serviced on-site or before it is sent out for service. It must also be labeled as biohazardous.

3. *Personal Protective Equipment* (PPE)
   When workplace exposure still exists after using engineering and work practice controls, employers must provide PPE at no cost to the employee. PPE is used to place a barrier between the employee and

blood and/or OPIM that can contaminate skin, mucous membranes, or non-intact skin. PPE consists of such items as latex gloves, masks, goggles, face shields, gowns, laboratory coats, and plastic mouthpieces used during cardiopulmonary resuscitation (Figure 22-16). PPE provides protection only if it prevents blood or OPIM from permeating through it onto clothes, eyes, skin, mouth or other mucous membranes.

The employer must be certain that PPE is available and accessible and provide an alternative type of glove if an employee is allergic to those originally provided. Cleaning and laundering and disposal of PPE is the responsibility of the employer and the employee does not incur any expense for such.

All PPE must be removed before the employee leaves the work site and placed in an appropriate container that is supplied by the employer.

Gloves must be worn when there is a possibility of hand contact with blood or OPIM, with mucous membranes and nonintact skin, and when performing such procedures as phlebotomy. Disposable gloves cannot be decontaminated. They must be discarded into a biohazard container used for **regulated waste**.

Masks, face shields, and goggles must be worn if there is a possibility of splashing or splattering of

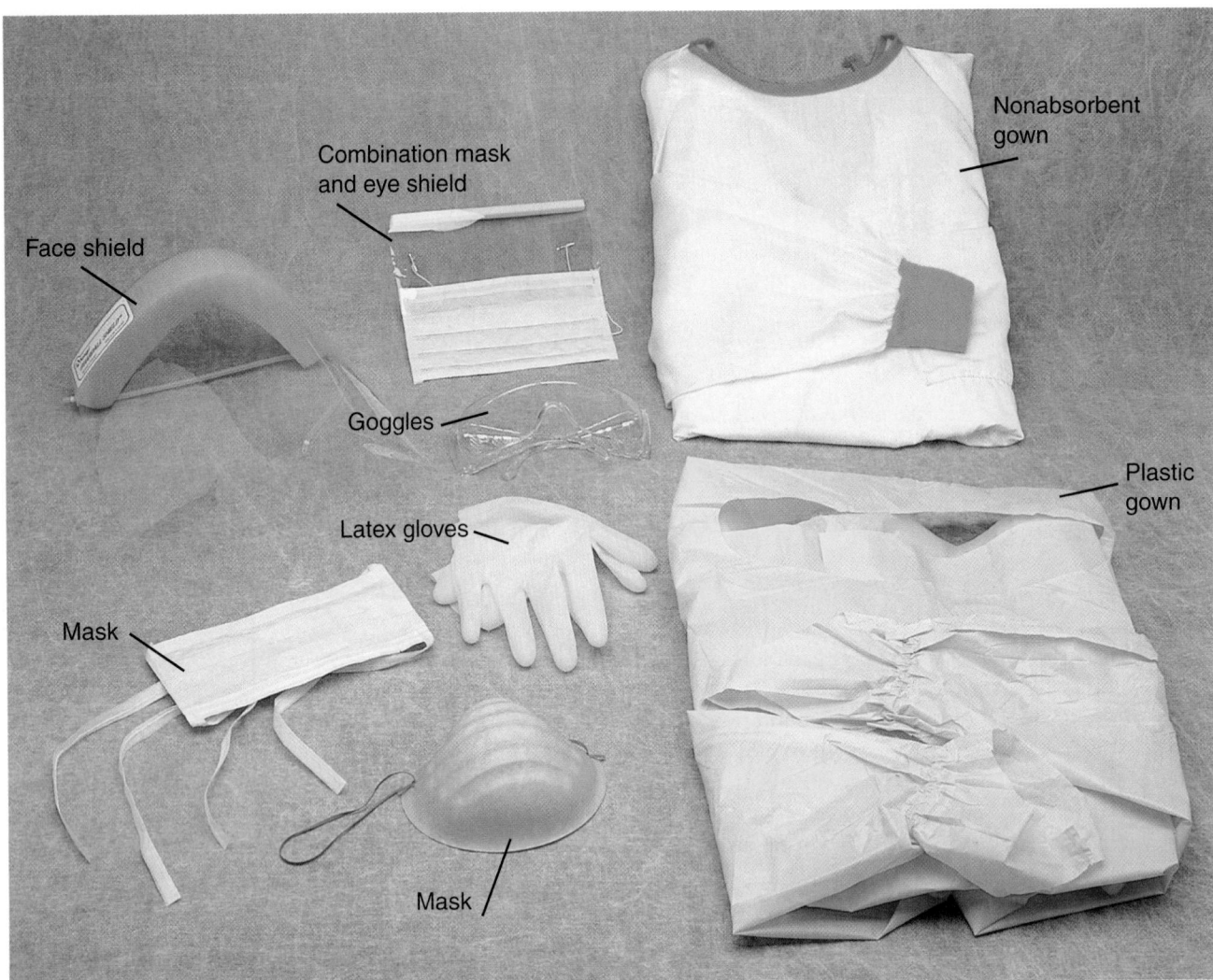

Figure 22-16   Personal protective equipment (PPE).

blood or OPIM. Gowns, laboratory coats, and other clothing must be worn to protect against exposure and must be left at the work site in an area set aside for their storage.

4. *Cleanliness of Work Areas*

The employer must maintain a work site that is clean and sanitary and have a written schedule for cleaning and decontaminating the work area after contact with blood and/or OPIM. Work surfaces that can become contaminated with blood or OPIM must be decontaminated after the work procedures are completed, after surfaces are contaminated, or at the end of the work shift. Some of the areas include counter tops, floors, examination tables, and wastepaper baskets.

When cleaning a work surface where there is the possibility of blood or OPIM present, latex gloves must be worn. A 10 percent solution of household bleach is used; alcohol is ineffective. Gloves should be worn when the spill is wiped with paper towels.

Both the towels and gloves are disposed of in a biohazard container and then the area is decontaminated (Figure 22-17).

Broken glass is placed in a sharps container after using cardboard or a dust pan and brush to remove it.

Laundry that is contaminated is handled with gloves and placed in a labeled container. If the laundry is damp or wet, gloves and other appropriate PPE must be worn and the damp/wet laundry must be placed in a plastic bag(s) to prevent blood or OPIM from leaking through it. PPE cannot be laundered at home (Figure 22-18).

Contaminated needles and other sharps must be disposed of into a puncture-resistant, leak-proof, and closable container immediately after use. The container must be labeled as biohazardous or orange-red in color and must be readily accessible to employees.

All other regulated waste must be placed into containers that are leak-proof and labeled as biohazardous or color coded orange-red.

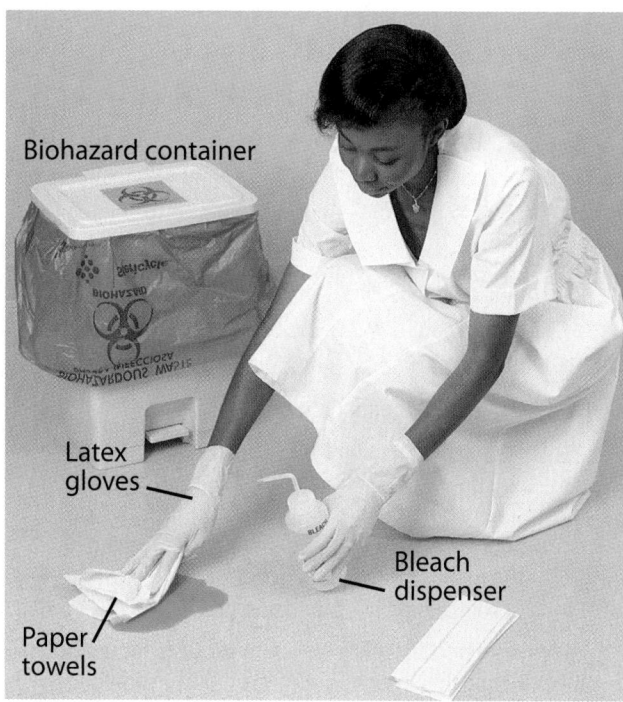

Figure 22-17   Medical assistant is wearing latex gloves to clean up a specimen spill. The biohazard waste bag is used to dispose of contaminated materials. The spill area is then cleaned with a 10 percent bleach solution.

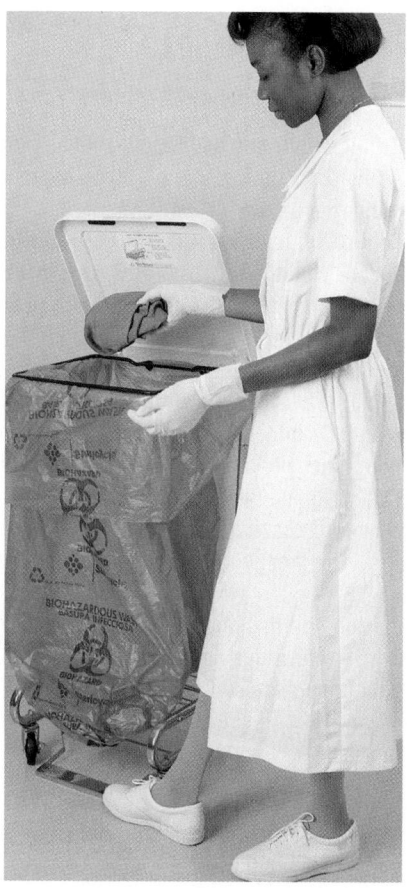

Figure 22-18   Medical assistant disposing of contaminated laundry in a covered laundry hamper containing a plastic biohazard bag.

5. *Hepatitis B Vaccine*

   Hepatitis B vaccine must be made available free of charge to every employee, full-time, part-time, or temporary within ten days of work assignment (Figure 22-19). This refers to employees who have the potential for occupational exposure, and who can "reasonably" be expected to have skin, eye, mucous membrane, or **parenteral** contact with blood or OPIM. The vaccine is given in three doses over a six-month time period and is used to protect the employee from infection with the hepatitis B virus. It is an intramuscular injection with an approximate 96 percent rate of effectiveness.

   An employee has the right to decline taking the vaccine, but must sign a **declination form**. There is the option to reconsider receiving the vaccine at a later time.

6. *Follow-Up After Exposure*

   An accidental exposure is broadly defined as one in which blood, blood-contaminated body fluids, or body fluids or tissues to which Standard Precautions apply are introduced onto a mucous surface, onto nonintact skin, or to the conjunctiva via a needle-stick, skin cut, or direct splash. If an incident exposes an employee to any of these, the employer must make available a confidential medical evaluation in which is documented:

- The circumstances surrounding the event
- The route or routes of exposure
- The identification of the person who was the source of the exposure

The following procedure describes the steps to take following an exposure incident:

- Immediately wash exposed area with soap and warm water.
- If mouth area is exposed, rinse with water or mouthwash.
- If eyes are exposed, flush with large amounts of warm water.
- Report incident to a supervisor immediately for **documentation** (Figure 22-20).

Additionally, OSHA requires the following information:

- The exposed employee must be tested for HBV and HIV only if consent is given. An employee may refuse or may have blood drawn and stored for ninety days at which time the choice can be made whether to have the blood tested.

SAMPLE

Hepatitis B Employee Vaccination Form

MEMO: To all employees with occupational exposure to blood or other infectious materials on an average of one or more times per month.

OSHA and the CDC have identified the potential exposure of health care workers to hepatitis B virus (HBV) in the course of performing their duties in this office. For the protection of our employees, we are offering prescreening testing and the HBV vaccination with follow-up evaluation to all employees who are exposed to blood or other potentially infectious materials on an average of one or more times per month. *In accordance with recommended OSHA guidelines, this vaccine and testing will be offered at no cost to the employee.* You have the ability to decide whether or not you want the testing and/or vaccine.

At the bottom of this memo, you may indicate your choice. Please return this memo with your signature and date to your immediate supervisor.

[ ]   I want to receive the prescreening (optional)
[ ]   I want to receive the vaccine and follow-up evaluation testing
[ ]   I *do not* want the vaccine and testing and have read the following statement:

I understand that due to my occupational exposure to blood or other potentially infectious materials I may be at risk of acquiring hepatitis B virus (HBV) infection. I have been given the opportunity to be vaccinated with hepatitis B vaccine at no charge to myself. However, I decline hepatitis B vaccination at this time. I understand that by declining this vaccine I continue to be at risk of acquiring hepatitis B, a serious disease. If in the future I continue to have occupational exposure to blood or other potentially infectious materials and I want to be vaccinated with hepatitis B vaccine, I can receive the vaccination series at no charge to me.

_____	_____
NAME	DATE
_____	_____
SIGNATURE	SS#

PRESCREENING DATE _____   RESULTS _____
DATE OF VACCINATIONS _____
DATE OF FOLLOW-UP EVALUATION _____
RESULTS _____
NOTES:

Figure 22-19   Sample Hepatitis B Employee Vaccination Form provides employee information regarding hepatitis B vaccine and space to sign indicating whether employee wants to receive the vaccine or whether employee declines vaccine. (Courtesy of POL Consultants)

SAMPLE

Post-Exposure Management Record

The following employee was the subject of an infectious exposure incident on (date) _____ and was examined and treated as follows:

Employee Name: _____ SS# _____
Type of Incident (describe) _____
_____

Route of Exposure: _____

Source Patient Information:

____   Source patient could not be identified.
____   Source patient was identified but refused to contribute blood.
____   Source patient was identified and blood was secured from such patient. Results of blood testing of source patient's blood are attached to this form.

Employee hereby grants permission for tests for antibodies of human immunodeficiency virus (HIV-1) and/or hepatitis B virus and acknowledges that the employee has been counseled concerning such tests.

Employee Signature _____ Date _____

The following test(s) were administered under supervision of a qualified physician:

____   Human Immunodeficiency Virus (HIV-1) Antibodies
____   Hepatitis B Virus Antibodies

Date(s) of Tests(s): _____ Results of Test(s)— See attached Physician's or Laboratory statement/ report.

Employee hereby acknowledges that the employee was counseled and a written copy(ies) of the results of the above test(s) were furnished to such employee on (date): _____

Employee Signature _____ Date _____

____   Additional follow-up was performed as indicated by attached reports.

NOTE: This record should be retained for length of employment PLUS thirty years.

Figure 22-20   Sample Post-Exposure Management Record can be used to document employee exposure to blood, body fluids, or OPIM, tests performed on the employee by a qualified physician, and their results. (Courtesy of POL Consultants)

- The source individual's blood, if permission is granted, is tested for HBV and HIV, and the employee shall know the results (unless protected by the law).
- The employee is offered prophylaxis, gamma globulin, and/or HB vaccine following the exposure according to the current recommendation of the United States Public Health Service.
- The employee is counseled regarding precautions to take to avoid possible transmission and is provided information on potential illnesses for which to be alert.
- An OSHA 200 form must be filed.

7. *Medical Records*

Medical records of an employee who has suffered an occupational exposure must be kept for the length of employment plus thirty years and confidentiality must be guaranteed.

The following information is to be included in the employee's record: name and social security number, HB vaccination status with dates, results of any examinations or tests, a copy of the health care provider's written opinion, and a copy of the information that was provided to the health care provider.

The records must be available to the employee, to OSHA, and anyone with the written consent of the employee, but *not* the employer.

Hazard Communication for Blood. The employer is required to label containers of regulated waste, refrigerators, freezers, and other containers that are utilized to keep or transport blood or OPIM with warning labels that are orange or orange-red in color and have the biohazard symbol affixed to them. Red bags may be used in place of labels. The labeling serves to warn employees of the hazard possibility of container contents (Figure 22-21).

Information and Training for Employees. Employers must ascertain that employees take part in training sessions during working hours at no cost to employees. The initial session must be provided when occupational exposure may occur and annually thereafter. If employee tasks and job description change, training must take place at that time.

Training consists of:

- An explanation of the bloodborne standard
- The symptoms of the bloodborne disease
- An explanation of the modes of transmission
- An explanation of the exposure control plan
- Appropriate engineering and work practices
- PPE to utilize to limit exposure

BIOHAZARD LABELS

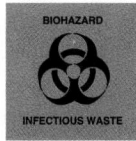

Containers that hold biohazardous materials must be properly labeled. Biohazardous materials include blood and body fluids as well as garments, gloves, masks, needles, gauze, wipes, aprons, and so on that may be contaminated with blood or other potential contaminated body fluids. Labels shall be used to identify the presence of an actual or potential biological hazard.

CONSIDERATIONS:

- Labels shall be fluorescent orange or orange-red, with lettering or symbols in a contrasting color.
- Labels should be affixed onto or as close as feasible to the container by adhesive, string, wire, or other method.
- Red bags or red containers may be substituted for labels.
- If blood or control serum is stored in a refrigerator, the refrigerator shall be marked with a biohazard label.
- If blood is stored in a refrigerator for transport or same-day shipment, it does not need to be labeled but should be put in containment bags.

Figure 22-21 Biohazard labels alert employees to biohazardous materials such as blood, body fluid, and OPIM.

- Information on the hepatitis B vaccine
- Procedures to follow should an exposure occur
- Information regarding post-exposure evaluation
- An explanation of the biohazard labels and color-coded containers

Documentation of training sessions must be available and kept for three years.

For an overview of the OSHA *Bloodborne Pathogen Standard*, see Figure 22-22.

OSHA REGULATIONS AND STUDENTS

With the passage of the OSHA law, all students with potential exposure to chemicals and bloodborne pathogens should follow all safety procedures as outlined by OSHA. Because students are not considered employees of a health care facility and are attending an educational institution, they do not fall under the OSHA guidelines. They should, however, take precautions to avoid contact with potentially infectious materials and toxic chemicals wherever learning is taking place.

Scope and Application

- The Standard applies to all occupational exposure to blood and other potentially infectious materials (OPIM), and includes part-time employees, designated first aiders, and mental health workers as well as exposed medical personnel.
- OPIM includes saliva in dental procedures, cerebrospinal fluid, unfixed tissue, semen, vaginal secretions, and body fluids visibly contaminated with blood.

Methods of Compliance

- General—standard precautions.
- Engineering and work practice controls.
- Personal protective equipment.
- Housekeeping.

Standard Precautions

- *All* human blood and OPIM are considered to be infectious.
- The *same* precautions must be taken with *all* blood and OPIM.

Engineering Controls

- Whenever feasible, engineering controls (devices that isolate or remove health hazards from the workplace) must be the primary method used to control exposure.
- Examples include needleless IVs, self-sheathing needles, sharps disposal containers, covered centrifuge buckets, aerosol-free tubes, and leak-proof containers.
- Engineering controls must be evaluated and documented on a regular basis.

Sharps Containers

- Readily accessible and as close as practical to work area.
- Puncture-resistant.
- Labeled or color-coded.
- Leak-proof.
- Closeable.
- *Routinely replaced* so there is no overflow.

Work Practice Controls

- Handwashing following glove removal.
- No recapping, breaking, or bending of needles.
- No eating, drinking, smoking, and so on in work area.
- No storage of food or drink where blood or OPIM are stored.
- Minimize splashing, splattering of blood, and OPIM.
- No mouth pipetting.
- Specimens must be transported in leak-proof, labeled containers. They must be placed in a secondary container if outside contamination of primary container occurs.

- Equipment must be decontaminated prior to servicing or shipping. Areas that cannot be decontaminated must be labeled.

Personal Protective Equipment (PPE)

- Includes eye protection, gloves, protective clothing, resuscitation equipment.
- Must be readily accessible and employers must require their use.
- Must be stored at work site.

Eye Protection

- Is required whenever there is potential for splashing, spraying, or splattering to the eyes or mucous membranes.
- If necessary, use eye protection in conjunction with a mask or use a chin-length face shield.
- Prescription glasses may be fitted with solid sideshields.
- Decontamination procedures must be developed.

Gloves

- Must be worn whenever hand contact with blood, OPIM, mucous membranes, nonintact skin, contaminated surfaces/items, or when performing vascular access procedures (phlebotomy).
- Type required—Vinyl or latex for general use.
    —Alternatives must be available if employee has allergic reactions (i.e., powderless).
    —Utility gloves for surface disinfection.
    —Puncture-resistant when handling sharps (i.e., Central Supply).

Protective Clothing

- Must be worn whenever splashing or splattering to skin or clothing may occur.
- Type required depends on exposure. Prevention of contamination of skin and clothes is the key.
- Examples—Low-level exposure lab coats.
    —Moderate-level exposure fluid-resistant gown.
    —High-level exposure fluid-proof apron, head and foot covering.
- *Note:* If PPE is considered protective clothing, then the *employer must* launder it.

Housekeeping

- There must be a written schedule for cleaning and disinfection.
- Contaminated equipment and surfaces must be cleaned as soon as feasible for obvious contamination or at end of work shift if no contamination has occurred.
- Protective coverings may be used over equipment.

(continues)

Figure 22-22   Overview of *The Bloodborne Pathogen Standard.* (Courtesy of the Occupational Safety and Health Administration, U.S. Department of Labor)

Regulated Waste Containers (non-sharp)

- Closeable.
- Leak-proof.
- Labeled or color-coded.
- Placed in secondary container if outside of container is contaminated.

Laundry

- Handled as little as possible.
- Bagged at location of use.
- Labeled or color-coded.
- Transported in bags that prevent soak-through or leakage.

Laundry Facility

- Two options:
  1. Standard precautions for all laundry (alternative color coding allowed if recognized).
  2. Precautions only for contaminated laundry (must be red bags or biohazard labels).
- Laundry personnel must use PPE and have a sharps container accessible.

Hepatitis B Vaccination

- Made available within ten days to all employees with occupational exposure.
- At no cost to employees.
- May be required for student to be admitted to college health program as well as for externship.
- Given in accordance with United States Public Health Service guidelines.
- Employee must first be evaluated by health care professional.
- Health care professional gives a written opinion.
- If the vaccine is refused, the employee signs a declination form.
- Vaccine must be available at a future date if initially refused.

Post-Exposure Follow-Up

- Document exposure incident.
- Identify source individual (if possible).
- Attempt to test source if consent obtained.
- Provide results to exposed employee.

Labels

- Biohazard symbol and word *Biohazard* must be visible.
- Fluorescent orange/orange-red with contrasting letters may also be used.
- Red bags/containers may be substituted for labels.

- Labels required on—Regulated waste.
  - —Refrigerators/freezers with blood of OPIM.
  - —Transport/storage containers.
  - —Contaminated equipment.

Information and Training

- Required for all employees with occupational exposure.
- Training required initially, annually, and if there are new procedures.
- Training material must be appropriate for literacy and education level of employee.
- Training must be interactive and allow for questions and answers.

Training Components

- Explanation of bloodborne standard.
- Epidemiology and symptoms of bloodborne disease.
- Modes of HIV/HBV transmission.
- Explanation of exposure control plan.
- Explanation of engineering, work practice controls.
- How to select the proper PPE.
- How to decontaminate equipment, surfaces, and so on.
- Information about hepatitis B vaccine.
- Post-exposure follow-up procedures.
- Label/color code system.

Medical Records

Records must be kept for each employee with occupational exposure and include:

- A copy of employee's vaccination status and date.
- A copy of post-exposure follow-up evaluation procedures.
- Health care professional's written opinions.
- Confidentiality must be maintained.
- Records must be maintained for thirty years plus the duration of employment.

Training Records

Records are kept for three years from date of training and include:

- Date of training.
- Summary of contents of training program.
- Name and qualifications of trainer.
- Name and job title of all persons attending.

Exposure Control Plan Components

- A written plan for each workplace with occupational exposure.

(continues)

Figure 22-22   *(continued)*

- Written policies/procedures for complying with the standard.
- A cohesive document or a guiding document referencing existing policies/procedures.

Exposure Control Plan

- A list of job classifications where occupational exposure control occurs (e.g., medical assistant, clinical laboratory scientist, dental hygienist).
- A list of tasks where exposure occurs (e.g., medical assistant who performs venipuncture).
- Methods/policies/procedures for compliance.
- Procedures for sharps disposal.
- Disinfection policies/procedures.
- Procedures for selection of PPE.
- Regulated waste disposal procedures.
- Laundry procedures.
- Hepatitis B vaccination procedures.
- Post-exposure follow-up procedures.
- Training procedures.
- Plan must be accessible to employees and be updated annually.

Employee Responsibilities

- Go through training and cooperate.
- Obey policies.
- Use universal precaution techniques.
- Use PPE.
- Use safe work practices.
- Use engineering controls.
- Report unsafe work conditions to employer.
- Maintain clean work areas.

Cooperation between employer and employees regarding *The Bloodborne Pathogen Standard* will facilitate understanding of the law, thereby benefiting all persons who are exposed to HIV, HBV, and OPIM by minimizing the risk of exposure to the pathogens.

Meeting the OSHA standard is not optional and failure to comply can result in a fine that may total $10,000 for each employee.

To obtain copies of *The Bloodborne Pathogen Standard*, contact OSHA at 800-321-6742 or www.osha.gov.

Figure 22-22 (*continued*)

Avoiding Exposure to Bloodborne Pathogens

Students can come into contact with blood and OPIM whenever in direct contact with patients or patients' specimens. The potential for exposure and contact increases whenever **invasive procedures** are being performed. Some examples of invasive procedures are:

- **Phlebotomy**, the process of withdrawing blood
- Administering an injection
- Performing or assisting with medical/surgical procedures such as suturing of wounds, removal of sutures, assisting with certain procedures such as Pap smears, arthroscopies, amniocentesis, thoracentesis, or lumbar puncture. Dressing changes, colposcopies, vaginal exams, obstetrical care, vasectomies, biopsies, and sigmoidoscopies are other examples in which students can contact blood and OPIM.

Students must be aware of and think about the procedures they are involved in and be certain that they use essential safety equipment (PPE) and procedures when necessary. Students should adhere to the same responsibilities that employees do.

PPE should be available in the student laboratory and used as necessary. Standard precautions must be strictly adhered to.

Gloves must be worn:
- During phlebotomy
- When giving injections
- When performing or assisting with invasive procedures
- When processing blood specimens

Eye protection with side projections must be worn:
- Whenever there is the potential for chemical exposure or the possibility of spray, splash, or splatter from blood or body fluids

Face shields or masks must be worn:
- When there is a chance of spray, splash, or splatter from blood or body fluids

Gowns or **aprons** must be worn:
- Where there exists any potential for exposure to contaminated materials

Lab coats must be worn and buttoned:
- When performing laboratory procedures

Students should always be on guard and make safety a priority by taking all precautions to avoid injuries. Some of the precautions are:

- No recapping of needles
- No bending or breaking needles
- Do not remove a needle from a syringe or a **Vacutainer®**
- Immediately dispose of needles and other sharps into a puncture-proof container
- No eating, drinking, smoking, or applying makeup in the area where there are patients or human specimens being handled and processed
- Never handle contaminated glass
- Clean spills with a device such as a shovel, cardboard, or paper towels, even if wearing gloves
- Know how to use a **spill kit**
- Know where the eyewash stations and showers are and know how to operate them

Students should decontaminate work areas with a 10 percent bleach solution and place contaminated waste into clearly marked biohazard containers. Some examples of contaminated waste items include disposable vaginal specula, patient swabs, gauze or dressing materials, and disposable suture removal kits, and any other equipment and supplies used during invasive procedures.

An exposure to blood or OPIM suffered by a student must be immediately reported to the instructor if the accident occurs at the college or to the supervisor of the clinical agency if the student is exposed during externship. OSHA procedures as outlined earlier in this chapter should be followed with the exception of the filing of the OSHA 200 form.

Many colleges require students studying the health professions to obtain the hepatitis B vaccine since it is approximately 96 percent effective against HBV. Because the vaccine is given in three doses over a period of six months, students should plan to have the injections in a timely fashion in order to be prepared for college laboratory courses and the externship period.

MEDICAL ASEPSIS

Medical asepsis is the destruction of pathogenic microorganisms after they leave the body. These techniques are used to decrease the risk of transmission to others. Objects should be medically aseptic if they are to be used in procedures that are on the external body or if they will enter a usually contaminated body part, such as the mouth. Medical asepsis also involves

environmental hygiene measures such as equipment cleaning and disinfection procedures. Careful attention to methods of medical asepsis greatly reduces the presence of pathogens that could cause disease in others. Specific procedures to achieve medical asepsis include adherence to standard and transmission-based precautions. Standard Precautions and Transmission-Based Precautions are considered methods of medical asepsis. These precautions should be followed stringently to provide barriers between potentially infectious blood and body fluids and those people who may come into contact with the fluids. Use of PPE, disinfection and waste control are crucial steps in practicing these precautions. Handwashing, sanitization, and disinfection of instruments or equipment are also essential.

Handwashing

Handwashing is perhaps the most important aspect of all infectious control procedures. Proper handwashing reduces pathogens that could be transmitted by direct or indirect contact to others. Since handwashing is frequently required, the use of a mild antibacterial lotion is acceptable to reduce the possibility of skin breaks due to dryness.

Procedure 22-1 outlines the steps of a medical asepsis handwash.

Sanitization

Sanitization of instruments and equipment, another procedure used in medical asepis, is needed to rid contaminated reusable instruments and equipment of tissue, debris, blood, secretions, excretions, or other contaminates. **Sanitization** is physically cleaning and scrubbing to remove contaminated debris. Mild instrument detergent is used with a scrub brush on an instrument, paying careful attention to interior surfaces, hinges, crevices, and serrations. Disposable gloves should be worn by the medical assistant to protect from blood and body fluids. Use of a special detergent designed for a medical setting ensures that instruments will be more easily and thoroughly rinsed to protect them from corrosion. A critical component to promoting effective sanitization is to complete the procedure as soon as possible following contamination, so tissue or body fluids do not have the opportunity to dry on the instruments. Dried debris are more difficult to remove and may require much scrubbing. Instruments may be left to soak in disinfectant solution or water with a solvent if sanitization cannot be performed immediately following use.

To avoid the risk of punctures or cuts from sharp instruments during sanitization, heavy-duty gloves should be worn. Some facilities use an ultrasonic cleaner for sanitizing instruments prior to sterilizing them. Goggles are worn to protect eyes from splashing of contaminated debris during the scrubbing procedure. A plastic apron provides protection from splashing of clothing. (See Chapter 31.) Hot water may be used for rinsing in order to remove all residue and aid in the drying process. Drying thoroughly will prevent damage from rust or water spots.

Larger items such as instrument trays or Mayo stands, stools, chairs, examination tables, and lamps should also have a decontaminating sanitization process with thorough washing, rinsing, and drying.

See Procedure 22-2 for instrument sanitization and Procedure 22-3 for removing contaminated gloves. Gloves contaminated with biohazard substances should be removed carefully in order to contain the contamination. Procedure 22-3 describes how to remove contaminated gloves while preventing further exposure to biohazard substances.

Also see Latex Sensitivity on page 348 for a description of allergic reactions to latex products such as disposable gloves.

Disinfection

Disinfection, a third procedure used in medical asepsis practices, consists of various chemicals that can be used to destroy many pathogenic microorganisms but not necessarily their spores. Chemicals are used on inanimate objects. Because of their caustic nature, chemicals can irritate the skin and mucous membranes. Chemicals can be used to disinfect items or equipment made from materials that could be damaged by heat or that are too large to fit into an autoclave such as glass mercury thermometers, percussion hammers, examination tables, and Mayo stands. These and other items are used during *external* physical examination or procedures.

Boiling water (temperature 212°F) is considered a form of disinfection because it will kill some forms of microorganisms. It is important to note that this method *cannot* be used as a technique to sterilize goods because the temperature is not high enough to kill the hepatitis virus or microbial spores. Articles such as nasal and aural specula can be disinfected by vigorous boiling for at least fifteen minutes. The only reasonable use for boiling as a means of disinfection in today's medical setting is for items that:

1. Will *not* be used in invasive procedures
2. Will not be inserted into body orifices nor be used in a sterile procedure

Prior to either chemical disinfection or disinfection by boiling, articles must first be thoroughly sanitized. Of special note are stainless steel gynecological and proctologic examination instruments. These instruments are not sanitized with other instruments due to the risk of transmission of sexually transmitted diseases (STDs). They are sterilized in the autoclave following sanitization to eliminate transmission of microorganisms.

Fiberoptic endoscopes are sanitized and chemically sterilized. See chemical sterilization in this chapter. (See also Chapter 31.)

Chemical disinfectant solutions must be carefully prepared and used according to the manufacturer's instructions in order to ensure effective disinfectant properties. Medical offices should use the disinfectant solution that best meets the needs of the ambulatory care setting as to quantity of instruments to be disinfected, preparation requirements, storage needs, and handling procedures. When choosing a chemical disinfectant solution, pay close attention to the manufacturer's report of the chemical disinfectant properties of the product. Some solutions are effective against a wide spectrum of microorganisms, whereas other solutions may be selective for certain common microorganisms. If instructions for use are closely followed, the chemical disinfectant properties will be considered to have been met. Environmental hygiene procedures ensure disinfection of large pieces of equipment, furniture, and other fomites. Protocols for agency disinfection should address the frequency, solutions, and fomites (substances that absorb and transmit infectious material) for disinfection.

Procedure 22-4 outlines steps involved in chemical disinfection of instruments.

Some specific examples of appropriate use of medical asepsis include:

- Wash hands before and after handling equipment and supplies and before and after working with each patient even if gloves were worn.

- Handle all specimens as if they were contaminated.

- Use disposable equipment whenever possible and dispose of it properly in a biohazard waste container. All equipment is contaminated after patient use.

- Use personal protective equipment (PPE) as outlined in Standard Precautions and wash hands after removal of any PPE.

- Keep contaminated equipment and supplies away from clothing to prevent transmission of pathogens to self and others.

- Place dressing materials, gauze, cotton balls, and any other absorbable material that is damp or wet in a waterproof bag prior to disposal in the biohazard waste container.

- Any break in the medical assistant's skin should be covered with a sterile dressing.

- Items that fall to the floor are contaminated. Either discard or sanitize and disinfect or sterilize before using.

● If uncertain whether equipment or supplies are clean or sterile, clean or sterilize them before use.

For surfaces such as countertops, the least expensive and most readily available chemical is a 1:10 solution of ordinary household bleach (sodium hypochlorite). However, besides the obvious disadvantage of bleaching clothing, bleach is not easily rinsed and it is only effective if the solution is mixed fresh daily. Nevertheless, its effectiveness is so highly respected that many medical laboratories depend almost entirely on bleach to chemically kill pathogens on countertops.

In summary, medical asepsis includes procedures for which all medical assistants must be qualified and responsible to incorporate into daily work practices. The responsibility for maintaining medical asepsis is the combined goal of the office staff and physician.

Refer to information presented earlier in this chapter for information on environmental hygiene and daily work practices.

SURGICAL ASEPSIS AND STERILIZATION

Surgical asepsis means all microbial life, pathogens and nonpathogens, are destroyed before an invasive procedure is performed. Therefore, all equipment used is sterile. The terms *surgical asepsis* and *sterile technique* often are used interchangeably. (See Chapter 31.)

The main purpose of surgical asepsis is to prevent organisms from entering the patient's body during an invasive procedure. An invasive procedure is either creating or treating an opening in the skin such as a surgical incision, laceration, or an injection; or exposing a sterile inner surface to possible invasions of microorganisms such as when a urinary catheter is inserted through the urethra and into the urinary bladder.

Because the microorganisms are on virtually every surface such as the skin, instruments, surgical instrument trays, clothing, and even in the air, it is necessary to destroy as many of them as possible prior to doing any surgical (sterile) procedure. Any item that will come into contact with the sterile field (the area in which the sterile procedure will be performed or where sterile supplies will be maintained during the procedure) must be sterilized using physical or chemical agents. Once the surfaces are sterilized, every precaution must be taken to prevent contamination of the sterile areas either from a nonsterile surface or from airborne contamination. To **contaminate** is to make impure; e.g., by the introduction of microorganisms or infectious material.

● Before items can be sterilized, they must first be thoroughly sanitized. The contaminated instruments are taken to a work area designated for that purpose. See Procedure 22-5 regarding sanitation of instruments. Care must be taken to prevent contamination of self. Heavy-duty gloves, goggles, and a plastic apron are worn for protection. Always check instruments for their working condition. Check ratchets, serrations, alignment, and ensure that they open and close readily. Separate improperly working instruments. Instruments are now ready to be wrapped for sterilization.

Living tissue surfaces such as skin cannot be sterilized but can be rendered as free of pathogens as possible before the use of a sterile covering. One example of this concept is preparing the patient's skin with a surgical scrub solution prior to applying sterile drapes around the intended surgical site (see Chapter 31). Another example is the use of surgical handwashing technique prior to applying sterile gloves. The differences between handwashing for medical asepsis as discussed in this chapter (Procedure 22-1) and handwashing for surgical asepsis are addressed in Chapter 31.

There are four methods of sterilization:

1. Gas sterilization
2. Dry heat
3. Chemical sterilization
4. Steam sterilization (autoclave)

Gas Sterilization

Gas sterilization is accomplished in a gas oven large enough for wheelchairs and beds and takes hours for the extremely toxic gases to permeate and dissipate. These features make the gas oven very useful in a large hospital setting, but much too costly for the office.

Dry Heat Sterilization

Dry heat sterilization requires higher temperatures than steam sterilization and requires longer exposure times as well (at least one hour at 320°F). This method can be used for instruments that easily corrode such as sharp cutting instruments. Powders, oils, ointments, rubber goods, and plastic tubing may be sterilized using the dry heat method. Procedures for wrapping are the same as when wrapping for steam sterilization, see Procedures 22-5 and 22-6.

Chemical Sterilization

Chemical sterilization, or cold sterilization (see Chapter 31), uses the same chemical agents used to chemically disinfect instruments or fomites. However, the exposure time for sterilization is achieved through prolonged immersion. The handling of instruments following chemical sterilization differs from handling procedures for instruments that are steam sterilized.

Chemical sterilization (also see Chapter 31) is a very effective method used in many medical offices when the object being sterilized is too large or too heat sensitive for autoclaving (see following information on autoclaving). Fiber-optic endoscopes are one of the most common items sterilized with the use of chemicals. These items are delicate and unable to withstand the high heat of an autoclave. The necessary equipment for chemical sterilization is a container or basin of adequate size for the intended item (and should be maintained for that purpose only) with a well-fitting lid and the chemical of choice. Two of the most popular brands available through medical supply sources are Wavecide and Cidex. Both have advantages and disadvantages. Offices must make individual choices based on convenience, expense, and other personnel preferences.

The effectiveness of any of these products depends greatly on the strength of the solution. If the strength is a 1:1 ratio of water to chemical, effectiveness will be lost if the solution is not mixed according to that dilution. Any attempt to cut cost by mixing a weaker solution will greatly compromise the effectiveness. Sometimes solutions are weakened unintentionally by placing wet items into them, thereby adding more water than is intended. For this reason, wet items must be carefully dried prior to chemical sterilization. To avoid evaporation, which also interferes with the strength of the solution, a well-fitting lid is essential. The lid also lessens the chance of dust and airborne microbes from falling into the solution.

Another factor influencing the effectiveness of the sterilizing chemicals is exposure time. The manufacturer will provide specific time charts for each purpose. Manufacturer's directions will also include a time frame for replacing the solution. The ability of the solution to kill pathogens will be directly related to its freshness or shelf life. Regardless of the chemical used for sterilization, ventilation is very important.

 When using commercial chemicals, make certain the lid is placed on the soak basin at all times except when placing or removing items. Care must be taken to avoid contact with skin, eyes, and mucous membranes. Wear protective gloves, goggles, and apron if splashing is anticipated. The effects on skin can range from slight irritation to serious caustic burns. See Procedure 31-1 in Chapter 31.

Before any chemically sterilized items are used for patient contact, the chemicals must be thoroughly rinsed off using sterile transfer forceps to remove the item from the container. In order to maintain sterility, sterile water must be used for the rinsing process. Then dry with a sterile towel, and place onto a sterile field with new sterile transfer forceps.

Steam Sterilization (Autoclave)

Steam sterilization is the most widely used method of sterilization in the medical office. An autoclave, basically a pressure cooker, is used to achieve sterilization. The autoclave uses steam under pressure to obtain higher temperatures than can be achieved with boiling (Figure 22-23). Water reaches a maximum temperature of 212°F through boiling. When under pressure, water is converted to steam and is then able to reach a temperature of 250–254°F. Exposing items to this extremely high heat and at least 15 pounds of pressure for a specific amount of time assures that all microorganisms and their spores are eradicated. The autoclave is actually an inner sterilizing chamber surrounded by a metal jacket. This creates a middle steam chamber between the inner sterilizing chamber and the jacket. Inside the jacket is a reservoir for water. When water is poured into the reservoir, the autoclave door closed and secured, and the autoclave turned on, several processes occur. The water in the reservoir heats until vapor is produced. The vapor enters the middle steam chamber inside the jacket. The air in the steam chamber is pushed out and replaced with steam. Since the air has been pushed out, the pressure increases. The increase of pressure causes the steam to then enter the inner sterilizing chamber (this is where the surgical instruments are placed) which pushes out the air. With the air being displaced with steam, the pressure increases in the inner chamber. The steam under pressure is able to reach a much higher temperature than boiling water. When the steam is able to reach all surfaces of the items placed in the autoclave and exposure is maintained for adequate amounts of time, sterility of those items is assured.

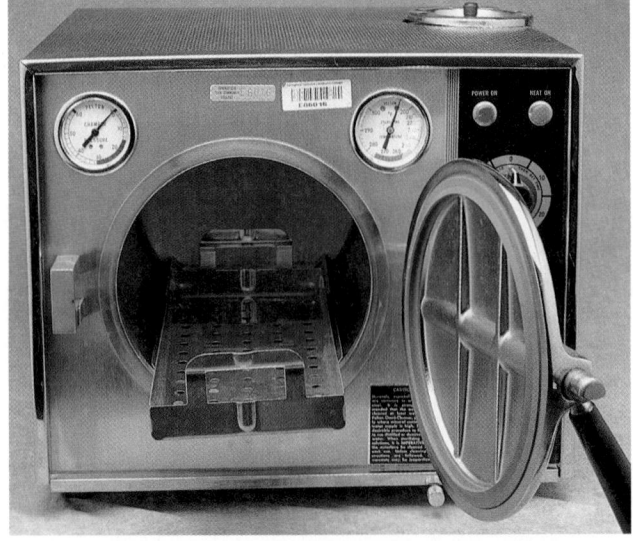

Figure 22-23 Commonly found in physician's offices, autoclaves are used for sterilization by steam pressure, usually at 250–254°F (121°C) for a specified length of time.

The recommended temperature for effective sterilization in an autoclave is 250–254°F. Unwrapped items should be sterilized for 20 minutes, loosely wrapped items for 30 minutes, and tightly packed items for at least 40 minutes. When uncertain about the proper amount of time necessary, the medical assistant should refer to the manufacturer's recommendations. The overall effectiveness of the autoclave in sterilizing contents is totally dependent on the medical assistant following proper operating procedure.

How to Load Packages. It is of extreme importance that instruments and materials be positioned properly in the autoclave in order for the steam to circulate through and between packs and penetrate them. Do not overload the autoclave. Place items as loosely as possible inside the chamber. Leave a one- to three-inch space between packs and the walls of the autoclave. Correct positioning and spacing allows sterilization to take place provided the medical assistant adheres to proper temperature, pressure, and time requirements.

Autoclave Maintenance and Cleaning. The autoclave, like any piece of equipment in the medical office, needs regular cleaning and maintenance. Frequency of cleaning the autoclave will depend somewhat on its usage. If the autoclave is used every day, the inner chamber should be washed with a mild detergent and cloth, rinsed, and dried on a daily basis. The outer jacket should be wiped clean of dust and soil. Follow the manufacturer's instructions and recommendations for cleansers. Omni cleanser is a well-known brand of autoclave cleanser.

At least once a week the autoclave should be drained of water and cleaned thoroughly. Cleaning the autoclave requires that it be drained, filled with cleaning solution, run through a 20-minute heated cycle, drained of solution, filled with distilled rinse water, run through another 20-minute heated cycle, drained of rinse solution, and filled with distilled water again. Then the inner shelves are removed and scrubbed and the inner chamber is wiped clean. Since this process is fairly time-consuming and will certainly put the autoclave out of use for a while, consideration should be given to scheduling the weekly cleaning at a time when personnel can devote the time and when the autoclave is not in demand for sterilization processes.

Distilled water is inexpensive, readily available, and always recommended to prevent mineral build-up. During the cleaning process, attention should be given to inspecting the rubber seal for cracks or wear. An extra replacement

---

General rules to ensure proper sterilization using an autoclave:

- Articles placed into the autoclave must have been sanitized and dried.
- The articles are wrapped and placed to allow adequate exposure of all surfaces (Figure 22-24). Instrument hinges should be opened and serrations exposed inside packages.
- To avoid trapped air pockets, containers should be placed on their sides with lids loosely in place.
- Any wrapping material used must be approved for autoclave use.
- Timing should not start until the gauges reach 15 pounds of pressure and 254°F.
- When the cycle is complete, the door must be opened slightly to allow steam to escape. The sterile wrapped articles will be hot and damp and should be left in the autoclave to cool and dry. Microorganisms can contaminate the sterile articles through the damp wrapping if the door is opened too wide or if articles are handled while damp.

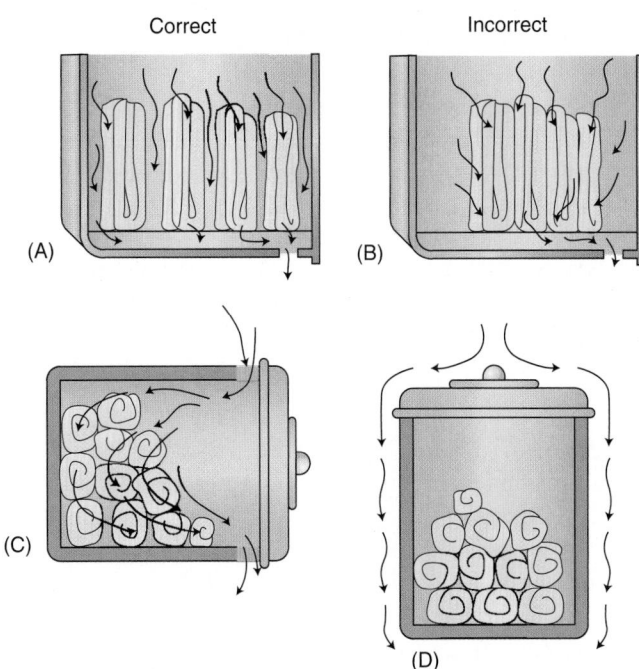

Figure 22-24 (A) Proper placement of instruments in the autoclave allows steam to circulate and penetrate from all sides. (B) Packages incorrectly loaded in autoclave. (C) When placed correctly, the jar should lay on its side with the cover loosely in place to allow steam to freely circulate through the jar and properly sterilize the dressings. (D) Incorrect method. (Courtesy of Steris Corporation, Mentor, OH)

rubber seal should always be kept on hand. The seals are available through medical supply sources. Refer to the manufacturer's instructions for regularly scheduled replacement of the rubber seal and other recommended maintenance procedures.

Quality Control and Assurance for Autoclave.

Quality control when using an autoclave consists of proper maintenance, proper operation, and observation of the temperature and pressure gauges. Equally important is the regular use of sterilization indicators and culture tests. Several types of sterilization indicators and culture methods are available:

- *Sterilization strips.* Contain a **thermolabile** dye that darkens when exposed to steam at the proper temperature and pressure for the proper amount of time. These indicators are placed in the center of the wrapped article (Figure 22-25).

- *Culture tests.* Available as a culture strip containing heat-resistant spores. The strip is placed in the center of a wrapped article and placed in a fully loaded autoclave. After processing is complete, the article is unwrapped and the strip is placed into a culture medium. If the autoclave is functioning properly and the medical assistant has followed proper operating procedure, no growth should occur. Also available through Becton-Dickinson Microbiology Systems is an ampule called the Kilit Ampule. These biological indicators are ampules that contain spores of the thermophile "Bacillus stearothermophilus." After being processed through the autoclave, the Kilit Ampule is sent to a cooperating laboratory for week-long observation for survival of the bacilli spores. A written report of the results is generated by the laboratory and sent to the office for its records.

Autoclave Wrapping Material and Packaging Supplies.

Wrapping or otherwise packaging surgical instruments and other surgical and medical articles prior to placing them in the autoclave will extend their shelf life up to six months. Before these articles are wrapped, they must first be sanitized, rinsed, and dried. Several materials are available for wrapping. Cost, convenience, visibility, time, space, and ease of use will help determine which to use. Many offices will utilize a combination of materials.

- Muslin is a cloth wrap available in several sizes and colors. Even with the cost of the initial purchasing, occasional replacements, autoclave tape, and laundering, muslin is still a very economical option. Besides these cost-effective advantages, many surgi-

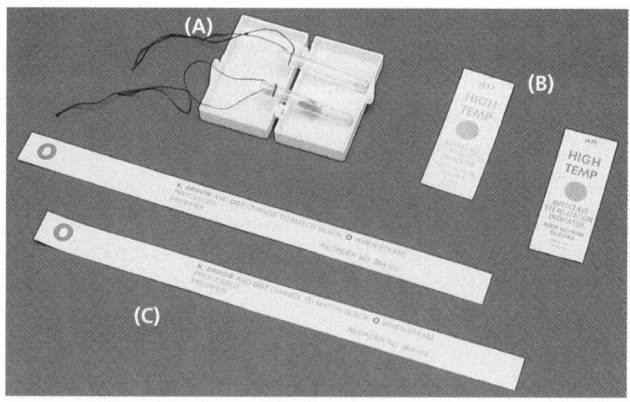

Figure 22-25 Types of sterilization indicators. (A) Commercially available pellets sealed in a glass container with string attached. Pellets melt when placed inside a package in the autoclave when proper temperature time and pressure have been attained. (B) Indicators are inserted into a holder and then placed into the center of a package to be sterilized. Indicator changes color when proper time, temperature, and pressure have been obtained. (C) Sterilization strips are placed in the center of packages to be sterilized. Strips change color when proper temperature, time, and pressure have been attained.

cal instruments may be wrapped together in muslin, making up a convenient surgery/procedure set. One of the main disadvantages of muslin is the inability to view the contents. Another disadvantage is the need for constant examination for holes, tears, and wearing out of the cloth. Patching is not a reasonable option since iron-on patches impede penetration of steam and sewn-on patches create their own set of perforations. A defective muslin cloth should be discarded. Wrapping space and training of personnel are necessary when using cloth.

- Paper sterilization wrapping squares are available in many different sizes and types. This disposable type of material requires that a new paper be used each time autoclave tape is needed, but eliminates the need for laundering. Similar to cloth wrapping, paper wraps also lend themselves to larger sets of articles being wrapped together for surgery or procedural packs. As with muslin cloth, wrapping space and some personnel training are necessary. Paper wraps are opaque, making viewing of the contents impossible.

- Sterilization pouches or bags may be either plastic or paper or a combination (Figure 22-26). They are fairly inexpensive and very easy to use. Since no wrapping is involved, additional work space is not required. Another advantage of bags is the visibility of the items inside. Some pouches are packaged on a continuous roll and are available in a variety of

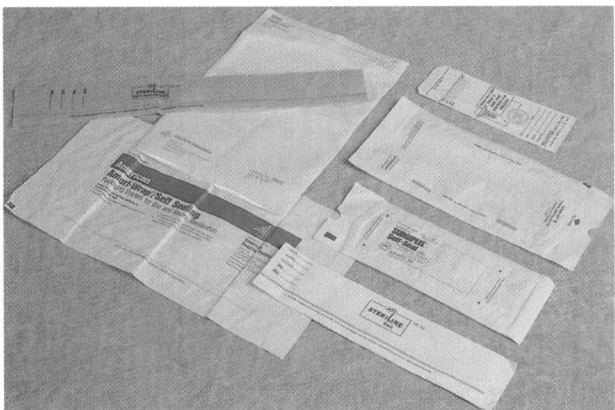

Figure 22-26 Various types and sizes of self-sealing bags for sterilization.

widths. This allows the medical assistant to cut the bag to fit the article. Since both ends need to be taped closed, it is very difficult to remove the article while maintaining its sterility. Probably the best bag-type option is individual bags with the top end open for instrument placement and the bottom end factory closed with a peel-apart seal. The article is inserted into the top opening, the bag is taped closed, and the package is sterilized (Figure 22-27). When needed, the sterile article is removed through the factory-sealed bottom end in a peel-apart sterile fashion. These bags need to be purchased in several individual sizes and are expensive

but have the advantages of ease of use and item visibility and are probably the preferred method for most medical offices today.

Autoclave Tape. Autoclave tape is chemically treated to become "striped" when exposed to heat. The striped pattern indicates exposure to high temperature but does not measure pounds of pressure or duration of exposure. Because of these limitations, autoclave tape does not assure that the wrapped package is sterile, only that it has been heated. Since it is placed on the outside of the package, it does not assure that steam has penetrated to the inner article but does help to determine if a package has been processed (Figure 22-28).

Labeling Packages for Autoclave. Surgical packages should be clearly labeled. Clear bags usually have a designated place for labeling, and muslin- or paper-wrapped packages may be labeled across the autoclave tape. Proper labeling should include the names of the articles in the pack, the date of sterilization, and the initials of the medical assistant responsible for the wrapping. The name of the instrument or article should be as specific as possible, especially when using the opaque cloth or paper wraps. If many instruments have been wrapped together for a specific surgery or for a specific physician, the label should clearly state which surgery or surgeon. For example, a "laceration repair set" could contain all the necessary instruments for repairing a laceration. "Dr. Peterson's vasectomy set" would contain all the instruments Dr.

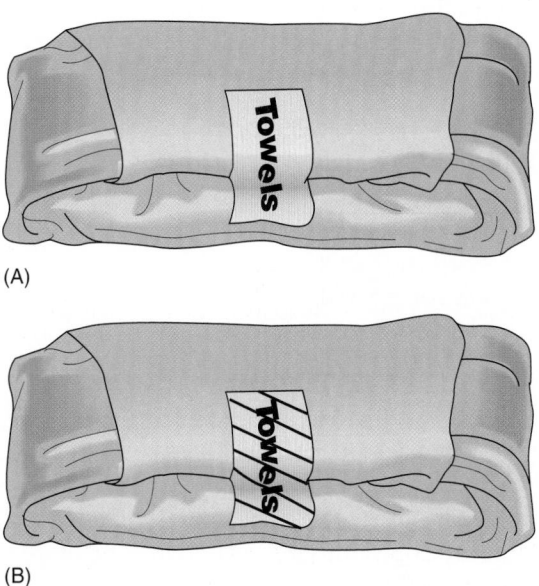

(A)

(B)

Figure 22-28 Package of towels (A) before and (B) after autoclaving. Note that the autoclave tape has a striped pattern indicating that the package was exposed to a high temperature. This does not assure sterility, however.

Figure 22-27 The medical assistant is placing a sanitized instrument into a sterilization bag for autoclaving by inserting the tips of the hemostat in first.

Peterson needs to perform a vasectomy, including, perhaps, personal preference instruments. The date of sterilization will help determine the expiration of sterility and determine a "pull date" for resterilizing. Initialing the package allows for accountability if necessary. Labels should always be written with a permanent marker. Ballpoint pen should never be used because the ink will smear when wet. Caution should be taken to avoid puncturing through the package during labeling.

Wrapping Techniques. Articles must be wrapped in a specific way in order to ensure they remain sterile when opened. Wrapped surgical instruments need to be double wrapped. Some methods advocate placing both layers of wrapping material together and double wrapping the pack in one process. A much more useful method is the "wrap-

ping twice" technique (see Procedure 22-5). The wrapping twice technique allows for additional options at the time of opening. Wrapping twice allows for a completely wrapped inner sterile package to be applied to the surgical tray. This wrapping twice technique eliminates struggling to control multiple instruments during the unwrapping process; and, if the inner package becomes contaminated during the unwrapping, the medical assistant has the additional option of unwrapping the inner package using the same technique without having to start over. All packs should be neatly and securely wrapped; firm enough to prevent the instruments from movement, but loose enough to permit adequate steam penetration.

See Procedure 22-5, Wrapping Instruments for Sterilization in Autoclave, and Procedure 22-6, Instrument Steam Sterilization (Autoclave).

Procedure 22-1   Medical Asepsis Handwash

STANDARD PRECAUTIONS:

PURPOSE:
To reduce pathogens on the hands and wrists, thereby decreasing direct and indirect transmission of infectious microorganisms. Average duration is two minutes before beginning to work with patients, 30 seconds following each patient contact.

EQUIPMENT/SUPPLIES:
Sink (preferably with foot-operated controls)
Soap (preferably liquid soap in foot-operated container; bar soap discouraged)
Water-based antibacterial lotion
Disposable paper towels
Nail stick or brush

PROCEDURE STEPS:
1. Remove all jewelry (plain wedding band is only acceptable jewelry). RATIONALE: Jewelry harbors microorganisms on the hands.
2. Prepare disposable paper towel (if using pull-down dispenser, prepare the amount of paper towel necessary for drying hands following wash; if using folded towels, have accessible). RATIONALE: Following the handwashing, you may not touch any contaminated surface, such as the

handle on a paper-towel dispenser or the water faucets.
3. Never allow your clothing to touch the sink; never touch the inside of the sink with your hands. RATIONALE: The sink is considered contaminated at all times (Note: sinks must be sanitized and disinfected at the end of each day).
4. Turn on the faucet with a dry paper towel (Figure 22-29A). Discard paper towel. Adjust water temperature to lukewarm. RATIONALE: Lukewarm water is best for handwashing because excessively hot water may overdry the skin.
5. Wet hands and apply soap using a circular motion and friction; rub into a lather (Figure 22-29B). RATIONALE: This initial handwash is to remove visible soil and some microorganisms. Interlace fingers to clean between them (Figure 22-29C).
6. Use an orange stick or brush at the first handwashing of each day (Figures 21-29D and E). RATIONALE: Nails harbor excessive numbers of microorganisms. Even with trimmed nails, this step must be performed on a daily basis.
7. Rinse hands with hands pointed down and lower than elbows (Figure 22-29F). RATIONALE: When hands are held lower than elbows, pathogens and contaminated water run off the hands and not up on the forearms.

(continues)

Procedure
22-1   *(continued)*

8. Repeat soap application and lather; interlace fingers well, wash with vigorous, circular motions all parts of hands including wrists; wash for at least one minute or longer depending on degree of contamination. RATIONALE: Appropriate length of handwashing is required to provide enough friction to remove soil and pathogens.

9. Rinse well, keeping hands pointed downward. RATIONALE: Rinsing removes microorganisms, contaminated water, and soap from the hands.

10. Repeat handwashing for the first handwashing of the day or if necessary for contaminated or visibly soiled hands. Lather wrists using a circular motion and friction. Rinse arms and hands. RATIONALE: When the hands are excessively contaminated or soiled, two handwashings may be necessary to remove microorganisms from the hands.

11. Dry hands and wrists with disposable paper towel; do not touch towel dispenser following handwashing; blot instead of rubbing with towel; if sink is not foot operated, use a clean disposable towel to turn off water faucet. RATIONALE: Touching the towel dispenser contaminates the hands. Blotting the hands dry reduces drying of the skin. Turning faucet off with paper towel prevents recontamination from dirty faucet.

12. Discard paper towel in waste container. Do not leave contaminated towels for repeated use. NOTE: Repeat handwashing procedure prior to and following each patient contact, procedure, or meal. RATIONALE: Handwashing must be performed on a regular and frequent basis to ensure the reduction of microorganisms transmitted by hands.

Water-based antibacterial lotion can be applied to prevent chapped, **excoriated** skin. If skin is excoriated, the medical assistant may not be able to work due to breaks in the skin.

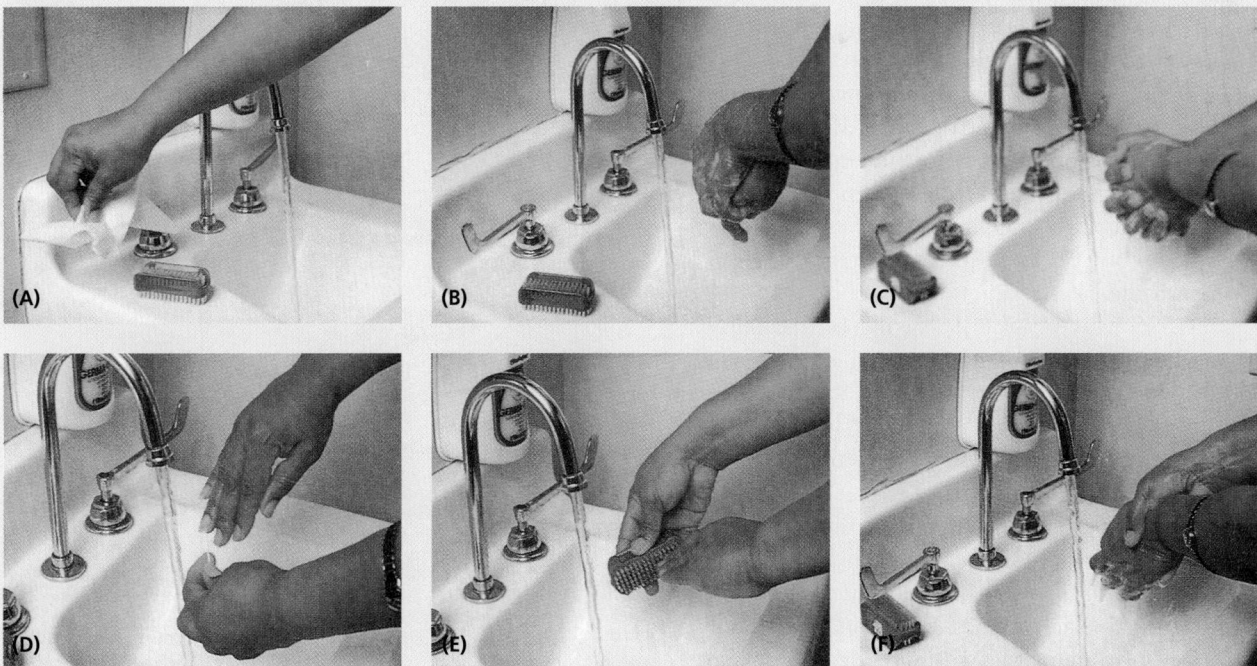

Figure 22-29   (A) Prepare towels for use. Turn on the faucet and adjust water to a lukewarm temperature. (B) Wet hands. Let water flow downward off hands and fingertips. (C) Use a circular motion to create friction and wash the palms and backs of hands. Interlace the fingers to clean between them. (D) Use an orange stick to clean under fingernails. (E) A hand brush may also be used to clean under fingernails. (F) Rinse hands thoroughly letting the water flow downward off your hands and fingertips.

Procedure

22-2 Sanitization of Instruments

STANDARD PRECAUTIONS:

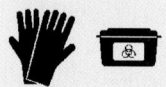

PURPOSE:

To properly clean contaminated instruments to remove tissue or debris.

EQUIPMENT/SUPPLIES:

Sink (or ultrasonic cleaner: follow manufacturer's instructions)
Sanitizing agent (low-sudsing detergent, approved chemical disinfectant, or blood solvent)
Brush
Disposable paper towels
Plastic apron
Disposable gloves, heavy-duty if cleaning sharps
Goggles
Biohazard waste container

PROCEDURE STEPS:

1. Wear disposable gloves, goggles, and apron. RATIONALE: Contaminated instruments pose a blood and body fluid precaution as indicated by OSHA standards. Disposable gloves must always be worn to sanitize instruments. Wear heavy-duty gloves if cleaning sharp instruments. Goggles are worn to protect eyes from splashing of contaminated debris during scrubbing procedure. A plastic apron provides protection from splashing of clothing.

2. As soon as possible following a procedure in which an instrument is contaminated, rinse the instrument in water and disinfectant solution; rinse again under running water. RATIONALE: Rinsing contaminated instruments as soon as possible following use removes debris and tissue that could quickly dry onto the instrument, making sanitization more difficult.

3. If contaminated instrument must be carried from one place to another for sanitization, place the instrument in a basin labeled "Biohazard." RATIONALE: Do not carry contaminated instruments in your hands. Biohazard basins must be sanitized and disinfected daily according to procedures for Standard Precautions.

4. Scrub each instrument well with detergent and water; scrub under running water, and be sure to scrub inside any edges and all surfaces (Figure 22-30). RATIONALE: Thorough scrubbing removes tissue and debris from all aspects of the contaminated instrument. If all tissue is not removed with scrubbing, the instrument may not be sterilized during sterilization procedures.

5. Rinse well with hot water. RATIONALE: Tissue and debris, as well as detergent, must be completely removed. Hot water will help remove all residue and aid in the drying process while rust and water spots will be eliminated.

6. After they are rinsed, place instruments on muslin or disposable paper towel until all instruments have been scrubbed and rinsed. RATIONALE: Often more than one instrument is sanitized; do not place sanitized instrument in the bottom of the sink or on a countertop without a disposable paper towel.

7. Dry instruments with muslin or disposable paper towels. RATIONALE: Wet instruments may rust or corrode. When preparing instruments for the sterilization procedures, they should be dry. Check instruments for working condition.

8. Remove gloves, wash hands.

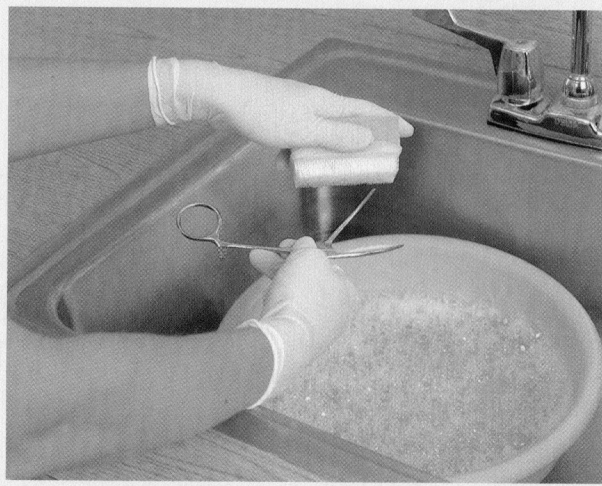

Figure 22-30 Medical assistant is using a scrub brush, plastic basin, and protein solvent detergent to sanitize surgical instruments. Note the medical assistant also is wearing gloves.

Procedure
22-3   Removing Contaminated Gloves

STANDARD PRECAUTIONS:

PURPOSE:
To carefully remove and dispose of contaminated gloves in order to contain exposure.

EQUIPMENT/SUPPLIES:
Biohazard waste container

PROCEDURE STEPS:
1. Grasp the palm of the used left glove with the right hand to begin removing the first glove.

Notice hands are held away from the body and pointed downward (Figure 22-31A and B). RATIONALE: Holding the hands away from the body will further prevent exposure to biological contaminants.
2. Turn the used left glove inside out and hold it in the right gloved hand (Figure 22-31C, D, and E). RATIONALE: Turning the glove inside out helps isolate the biological contaminants.
3. Holding the glove that has been removed with the hand that still has the glove on, the medical assistant inserts two fingers of the ungloved hand between her arm and the inside of the dirty glove (Figure 22-31F).

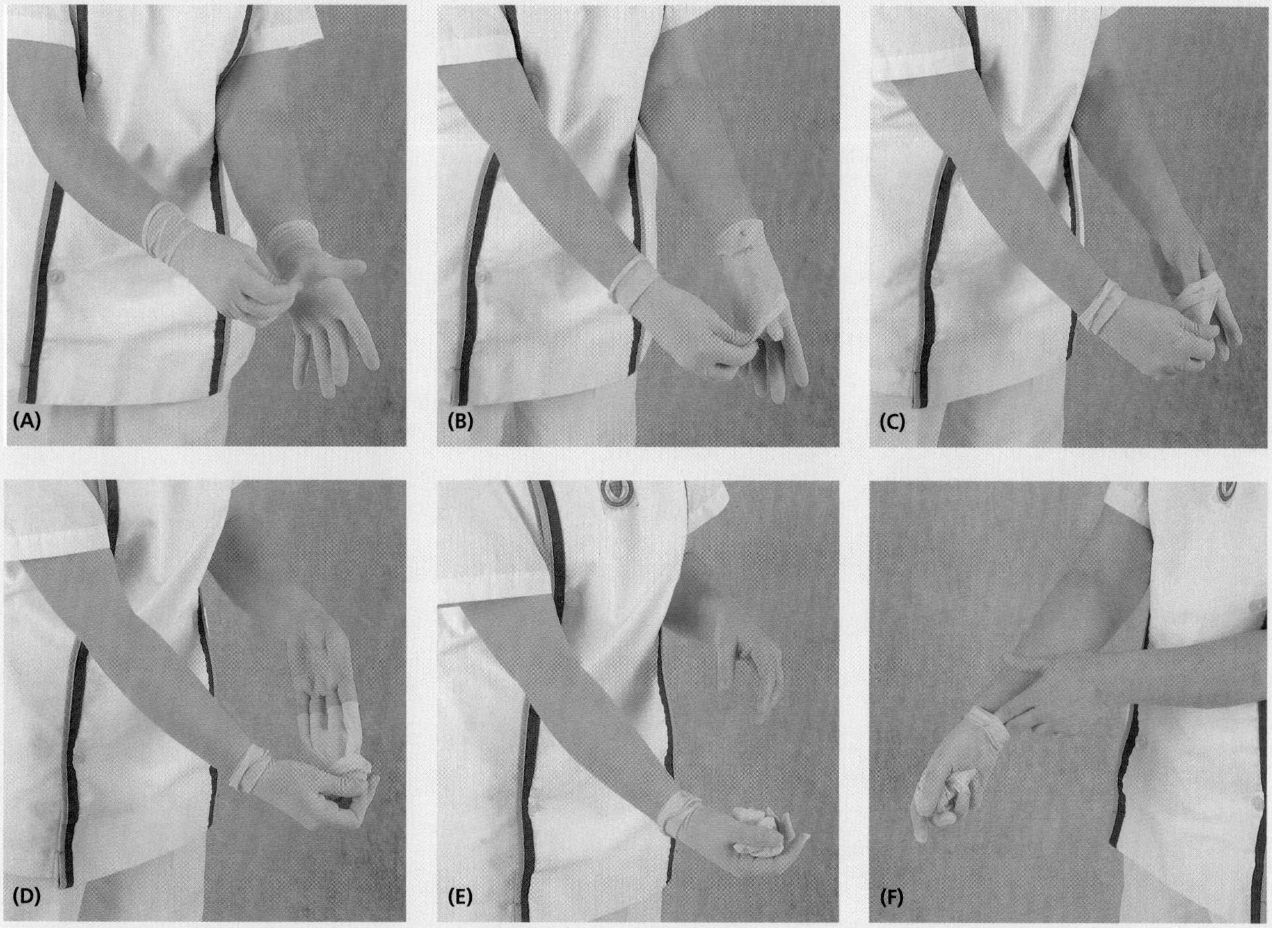

(A)

(B)

(C)

(D)

(E)

(F)

Figure 22-31   (A) Grasp the palm of the used left glove with the right hand. (B) Begin removing the first glove. (C and D) Turn the used left glove inside out. (E) Hold it in the right hand. (F) Hold the removed glove with the hand that is still gloved.

(continues)

Procedure
22-3 *(continued)*

4. Turn the right dirty glove inside out over the other. One glove is inside the other and the medical assistant can handle the gloves because the dirty, contaminated area is inside the gloves (Figure 22-31G and H). RATIONALE: Both gloves are inverted with the biological contaminates isolated.

5. Dispose of the inverted gloves into a biological waste receptacle (Figure 22-31I). RATIONALE: All biological waste should be placed into a red biohazard bag.

6. Wash hands thoroughly. RATIONALE: Immediate washing of hands is an additional precaution.

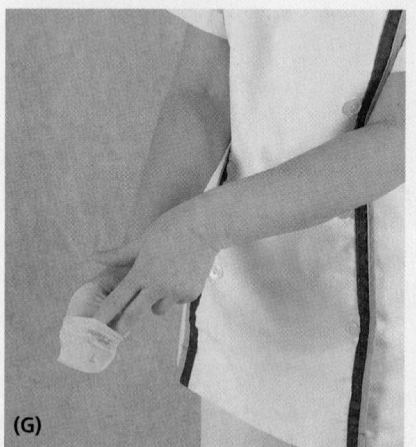 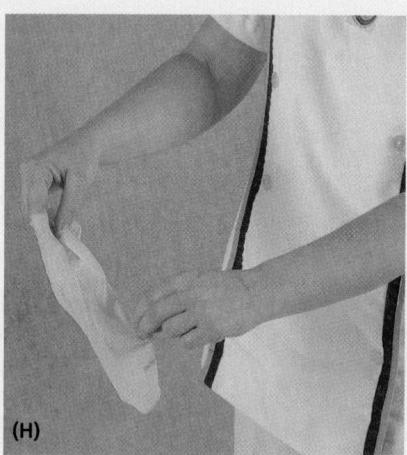 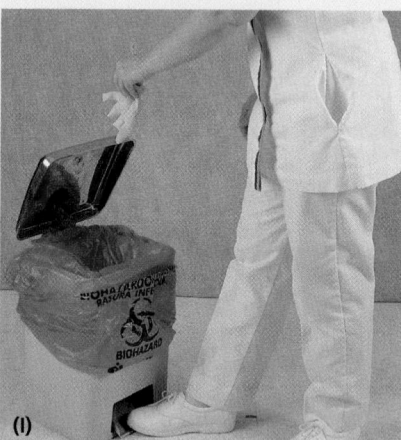

Figure 22-31 *(continued)* (G) Insert two fingers of the ungloved hand inside the dirty glove and turn it inside out over the other. (H) One glove is now inside the other. (I) Dispose of gloves in biohazard container.

Procedure
22-4 **Chemical Disinfection of Instruments**

STANDARD PRECAUTIONS:

PURPOSE:
Chemical disinfection is used to achieve medical asepsis for instruments that will be used during *external* physical examinations or procedures (i.e., thermometers, percussion hammers, nasal and aural specula).

EQUIPMENT/SUPPLIES:
Container with airtight lid (Figure 22-32A)
Disinfectant chemical solution (various brands and instructions for specific use)

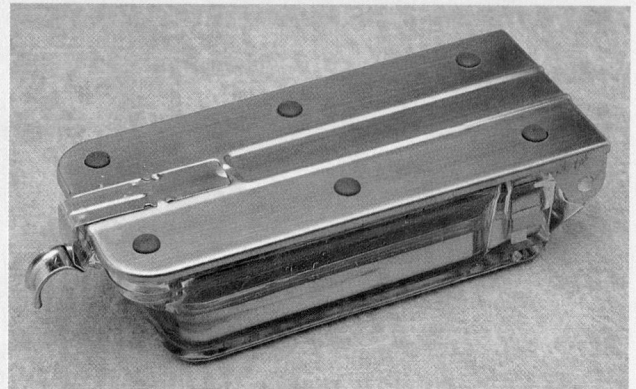

Figure 22-32 (A) Closed Bard-Parker® tray.

(continues)

Procedure

22-4   *(continued)*

Timer or clock
Water for rinsing following disinfection
Heavy-duty gloves
Biohazard waste container

PROCEDURE STEPS:

Chemical Disinfection:

1. Sanitize instruments that require medical aseptic chemical disinfection. RATIONALE: Recall that medical asepsis is not sterile and should not be used for instruments that will be used in invasive procedures requiring sterile technique.

2. Read the manufacturer's instructions on the original container of chemical disinfection solution. RATIONALE: Each brand of chemical disinfection solution has specific preparation instructions and germicidal properties; choose the solution that best fits the needs of the ambulatory care setting. Keep the solution in the original container to reduce chances of accidental poisoning.

3. Put on gloves. RATIONALE: Chemical disinfectant solutions are harsh on skin.

4. Prepare the solution as indicated by the manufacturer; place the date of opening or preparation on the container with your initials. RATIONALE: Following the manufacturer's instructions ensures proper germicidal properties. Note the expiration date of the prepared solution.

5. Pour the prepared solution into a container with an airtight lid; avoid splashing the solution (Figure 22-32B). RATIONALE: Disinfectant chemical solutions should not be left exposed to open air in order to prevent accidental inhalation or poisoning. Splashing solution may cause inhalation, skin, or mucous membrane contact and could cause injury.

6. Place sanitized instruments into solution; instruments must be completely covered; avoid splashing solution when putting instruments in tray. RATIONALE: If instruments are not covered with solution, disinfection cannot occur.

7. Close lid of container; label container with name of solution, exposure time, and initials. RATIONALE: Exposure time is the required time indicated by the manufacturer to achieve disinfection. Initialing work ensures accountability and responsibility.

8. Do not open or add additional instruments during disinfection period. RATIONALE: Adding instruments during a disinfection procedure limits the overall effectiveness of the disinfectant solution.

9. Following required exposure time, lift items from the container tray and rinse well under distilled water or tap water (according to the manufacturer's instructions). Do not use instruments without rinsing off chemical disinfectant solution; often solution is caustic and may corrode instruments over time.

10. Remove instruments and place on muslin or disposable paper towel.

11. Dry instruments with muslin or paper towel.

CAUTION: Use disinfection solution for only as many days as recommended by the manufacturer. Disinfectant properties will only last as long as reported by the manufacturer's instructions. (NOTE: Dispose of used solution as recommended by the manufacturer's instructions.)

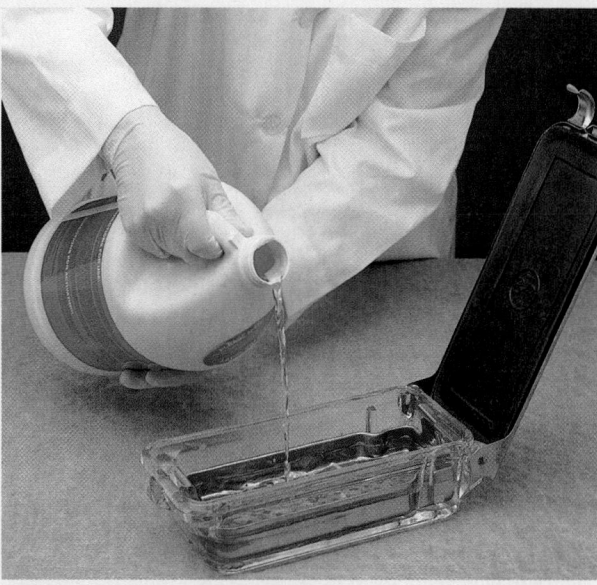

Figure 22-32 *(continued)* (B) With gloves on, carefully pour disinfectant solution into Bard-Parker® tray in preparation for soaking a sanitized instrument for disinfection.

Wrapping Instruments for Sterilization in Autoclave

Procedure **22-5**

PURPOSE:

To properly wrap sanitized instruments for sterilization in an autoclave.

EQUIPMENT/SUPPLIES:

Sanitized instruments
Wrapping material (muslin or disposable wrapping paper)
Sterilization indicator
2 × 2 gauze or cotton balls (if instrument has hinges)
Autoclave wrapping tape
Permanent marker or felt-tip pen (Figure 22-33A)

PROCEDURE STEPS:

1. Prepare a clean, dry, flat surface of adequate size to lay the wrapping material. RATIONALE: A clean area reduces risk of contamination. Adequate space is required for proper wrapping.
2. Select two wraps of adequate size in which to wrap instruments.
3. Place one square of wrapping material at an angle in front of you on the dry surface with one corner pointed directly toward you.
4. Place the sanitized instrument or articles to be placed in the autoclave just below the center of the wrap. Open instruments with hinges as wide as possible and place a 2 × 2 gauze or cotton ball in the opening (Figure 22-33B). RATIONALE: Instruments with hinged parts that are not spread open prior to autoclaving may not be properly sterilized.
5. Place one sterilization indicator with the instrument. RATIONALE: Sterilization indicators inside packages ascertain sterilization of each individual package. Indicators change colors when the required temperature has been reached, documenting the effectiveness of the sterilization. NOTE: quality control for autoclave operation can be evaluated with sterilization indicators.
6. Bring the corner of the wrap closest to you up and over the article toward the center. Bring the tip of the same corner back toward you until it reaches the folded edge, creating a fan-

fold effect. Smooth the edges of the fold. The article should remain completely covered (Figure 22-33C).

7. Fold one side edge toward the center line; fan-fold back to side, and crease (Figure 22-33D).
8. Repeat step 7 for the other side edge (Figure 22-33E).
9. Fold the package up from the bottom (Figure 22-33F).
10. Fold the top edge down and over the entire package (Figure 22-33G). RATIONALE: Final edge should wrap entire package for assurance of adequate coverage and protection once contents are sterilized. If wrap does not cover adequately, unwrap and start over with larger wrapping material.
11. To "wrap twice," place this package into the center of a second wrap (Figure 22-33H). Repeat steps 7 through 10. RATIONALE: Double wrapping allows more control of multiple instruments when setting up a surgical tray.
12. Tape with autoclave tape across the point left exposed. RATIONALE: Autoclave tape indicates whether or not the package has been through the autoclave; it is not a form of sterilization indicator or quality control.
13. Label the tape with the name of the instrument or type of pack (i.e., laceration repair pack), date of sterilization, and your initials (Figure 22-33I). RATIONALE: Proper instrument labeling is required to identify wrapped sterilized instruments. Instruments wrapped and sterilized in paper or cloth wrappers are considered sterile for four weeks from the date of sterilization. Initialing packages ensures accountability and responsibility.
14. Place wrapped instruments in autoclave. RATIONALE: If wrapped instruments are not to be immediately autoclaved, do NOT date the package. Leave the package on a clean, dry surface and date the package just prior to autoclaving.
15. Document the procedure.

(continues)

Procedure

22-5   *(continued)*

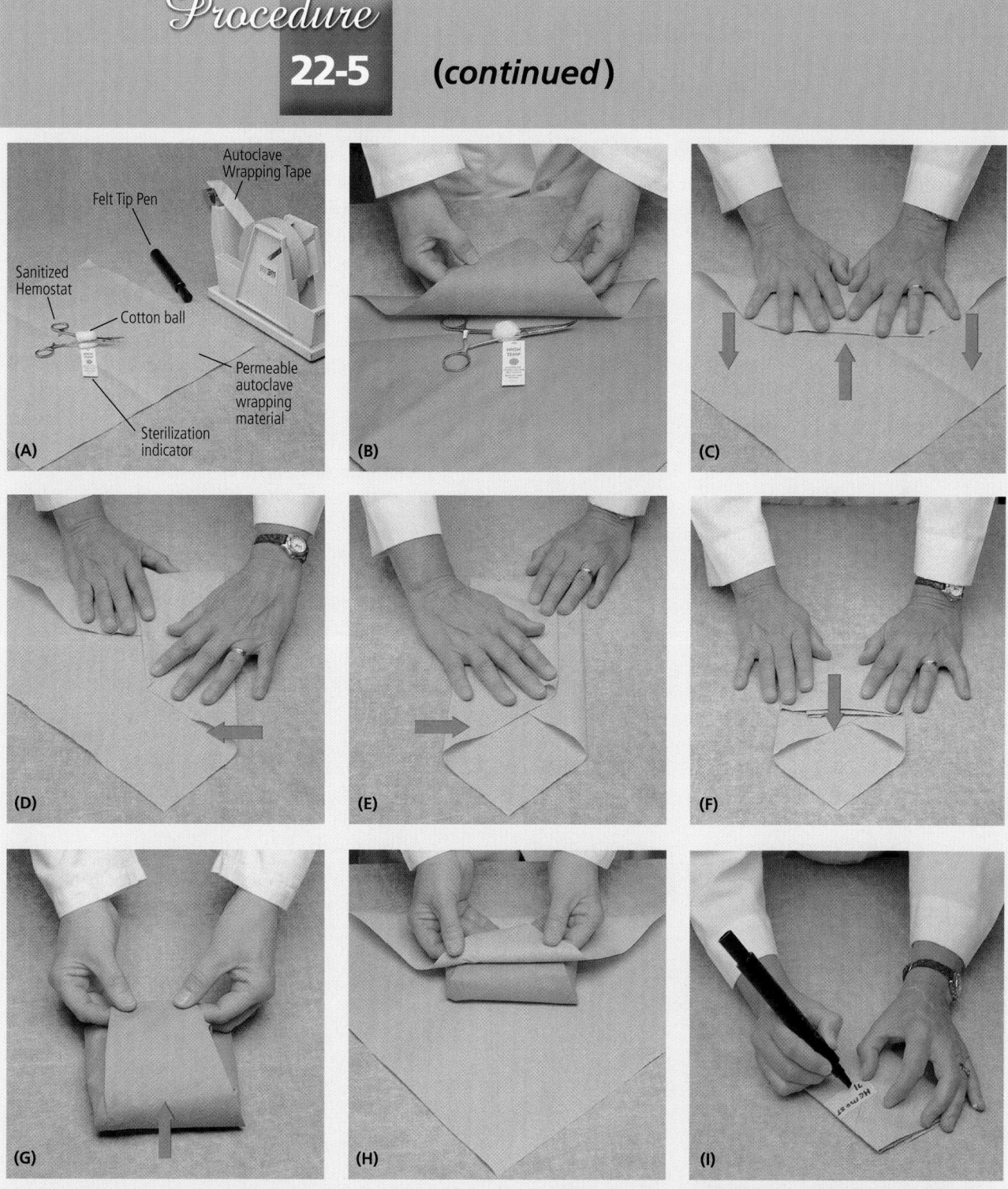

Figure 22-33 (A) Equipment needed to wrap surgical instruments or equipment for sterilization in an autoclave. (B) Place a cotton ball between the hinge joints of sharp instruments and a sterilization indicator in with the instruments to be wrapped. (C) The wrapping paper is folded toward center. A small corner is turned back on itself. (D) Fold one side toward center leaving a small corner turned back on itself. (E) Fold other side toward center leaving small corner turned back on itself. (F) The package is folded up from the bottom and secured. (G) Fold top down over package. (H) Wrap first package in another wrap. Double wrapping allows more control of multiple instruments when setting up a surgical tray. (I) Wrapped package is secured with heat-sensitive autoclave tape and labeled with the date, contents, and medical assistant's initials.

Procedure 22-6
Steam Sterilization of Instruments (Autoclave)

PURPOSE:
To rid instruments of all forms of microbial (microorganism) life for use in invasive procedures.

EQUIPMENT/SUPPLIES:
Steam sterilizer (autoclave)

Autoclave manufacturer procedure manual

Wrapped sanitized instrument package(s) with sterilization indicators placed inside package (or unwrapped item if removed with sterile transfer forceps)

PROCEDURE STEPS:
1. Load packages into autoclave tray; allow 3 inches between packages; avoid stacking directly on top of other packages (Figure 22-34). RATIONALE: Steam circulates in predictable patterns in an autoclave. When packages are loaded too closely or improperly, proper sterilization will not occur in individual packages.
   A. Load jars of dressings or cups on their sides, with tops ajar or loosely in place. RATIONALE: Steam is trapped within a jar when it is right side up; containers and goods will not be sterilized if loaded sitting up vertically.
   B. Load cloth or dressing packages vertically 3 inches apart.
   C. Load unwrapped items in similar fashion, not allowing item to touch any other item.
   D. Load unwrapped instruments flat with handles opened.
2. Close autoclave door and seal. RATIONALE: Pressure cannot be achieved without a proper seal.
3. Turn on autoclave and set temperature to achieve 250–254°F (121°C) and 15 pounds of pressure according to the manufacturer's guidelines. RATIONALE: Proper heat and pressure levels must be achieved in order to kill all microorganisms within the autoclave.
4. When the temperature dial indicates 250–254°F (121°C) and 15 pounds of pressure has been achieved inside the autoclave, begin necessary exposure time by setting timer. RATIONALE: Exposure time is required to kill all microorganisms. Careful note should be given to setting exposure time only after the proper temperature and pressure settings have been achieved.

Item	Required exposure time
wrapped instrument packages or trays	30 minutes
unwrapped items	15 minutes
unwrapped items covered with cloth	20 minutes

5. Do not attempt to open the door during the autoclave cycle. RATIONALE: Opening the door prematurely will allow the steam under pressure to cause injury.
6. Following completion of the autoclave cycle, exhaust steam pressure from the autoclave by following the manufacturer's instructions. RATIONALE: Read the manufacturer's instructions carefully.
7. Open the door approximately one inch after the pressure gauge indicates zero (0) pressure and the temperature gauge indicates a decrease to at least 212°F. RATIONALE: Do not open the door until these standards have been reached; injury may occur upon premature opening of the door.

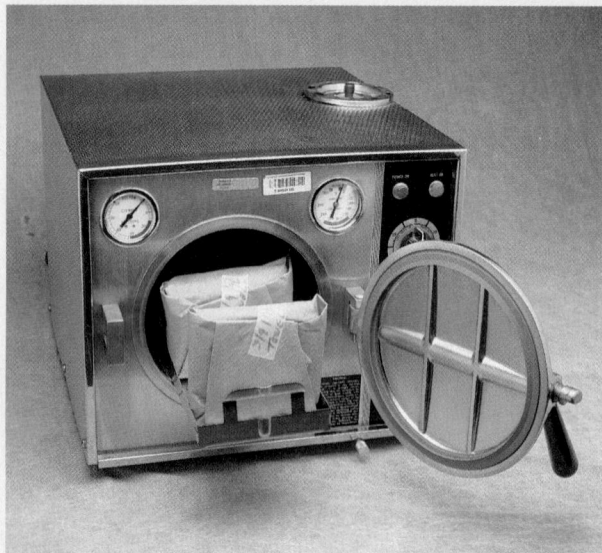

Figure 22-34 Carefully load packages into the autoclave so that the steam is able to penetrate all sides of the package allowing proper sterilization.

(continues)

Procedure
22-6   *(continued)*

8. Allow the contents to completely dry, approximately 10–15 minutes; do NOT touch contents until completely dry. RATIONALE: If packages are still wet or damp, microorganisms can enter a wrapped package, rendering it contaminated. Liquids travel along paper or cloth by capillary action and will be contaminated by microorganisms on countertops or from hands.

9. Remove wrapped contents with dry, clean hands and store in clean, dry area for sterilized packages only. RATIONALE: Sterilized wrapped packages can be held with clean hands, since only the interior contents require maintenance of sterility. If the outer wrapper is required to remain sterile, remove with sterile transfer forceps and place on a sterile field or in sterile storage areas.

10. Remove unwrapped contents with sterile transfer forceps; resanitize and resterilize the transfer forceps following use. RATIONALE: Sterile transfer forceps must have been sterilized immediately prior to or along with the unwrapped item.

11. Perform quality control on a regular basis, based on usage. RATIONALE: Quality control and maintenance of an autoclave is critical to assurance of proper operation. Accountability and responsibility to monitor quality control should be the responsibility of the medical assistant(s) most often responsible for sterilization.
    A. Monitor sterilization indicators with each use of sterilized instruments.
    B. Weekly perform quality control by documenting sterilization indicator outcome on a log; date and initialize quality control log entries.

12. Service the autoclave regularly according to the manufacturer's guidelines. When sterilization is not being achieved, take equipment out of service and contact a service agency for repair. RATIONALE: It is the responsibility of the medical assistant to take out of service any equipment that is not operating properly as a component of risk management.

13. Document the procedure.

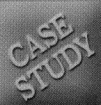
CASE STUDY 22-1

Your physician employer asks you to help develop an exposure control plan. Include the measures the employer must take to eliminate or lessen an employee's risk of exposure to blood or OPIM. How often will the plan be reviewed?

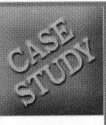
CASE STUDY 22-2

Considering the growth requirements for pathogens, describe how to discourage bacterial growth in the clinical area of the ambulatory care setting.

SUMMARY

Effective infection control measures are the first defense against the transmission of infectious diseases in the ambulatory care setting. Reliance on standard and transmission-based precautions, protective barriers, and basic principles of disinfection and sterilization promotes professional and responsible clinical care for patients. When the processes of infection control are applied to all clinical procedures, the chain of infection may be broken by many varied means. Remember that an infectious disease will not spread to another person if the chain is broken at any stage.

Infectious diseases and accidents occur through lack of education and carelessness. Medical assistants must understand the importance of the regulations and guidelines set forth by the federal government and follow through by helping employers implement them. In doing so, the health and safety of patients and health care workers can be protected, the spread of infectious diseases can be kept under control, and the risk of contracting an infectious disease such as AIDS or hepatitis B will be greatly minimized.

Every medical office and ambulatory care setting must, by law, have clearly written and readily available manuals containing information about Standard Precautions and OSHA for the safe handling, storage, and disposal of blood, body fluids, and chemicals.

Through consistent use of Standard Precautions and adherence to OSHA laws, health care providers can acquire the behaviors and techniques needed to safeguard themselves and their patients.

Because of frequent changes in the laws, it is necessary for medical assistants and all other health care providers to keep abreast of the government mandates.

REVIEW QUESTIONS

Multiple Choice

1. The bloodborne virus considered to pose the greatest threat to health care workers is:
   a. hepatitis B (HBV)
   b. human immunodeficiency virus (HIV)
   c. hepatitis A
   d. hepatitis C
2. Standard Precautions are issued by:
   a. HHS
   b. CDC
   c. HCFA
   d. OSHA
3. The Bloodborne Pathogen Standard is primarily concerned with:
   a. reducing the transmission of HIV and hepatitis B infections
   b. protecting the employer
   c. regulating the use of personal protective equipment
   d. taking blood samples from patients
4. In the chain of infection, the location of the infectious agent is known as the:
   a. reservoir
   b. portal of exit
   c. portal of entry
   d. means of transmission
5. The stage in infectious disease in which symptoms are vague and undifferentiated is called the:
   a. incubation stage
   b. prodromal stage
   c. acute stage
   d. onset of disease stage
6. An autoclave is an instrument used during:
   a. chemical sterilization
   b. steam sterilization
   c. dry heat sterilization
   d. gas sterilization

Critical Thinking

1. Analyze the importance of infection control and give five examples of how a medical assistant would practice responsible infection control in the ambulatory care setting.
2. Identify and describe the steps in the chain of infection.
3. Describe four types of infectious agents.
4. Explain sanitization and its function in the ambulatory care setting.
5. Describe three autoclave wrapping materials and packaging supplies.
6. Give eight examples of body fluids considered to be biohazardous substances. Explain how medical assistants could become exposed to blood and/or body fluids.
7. Describe needlestick and its relevance to HIV and HBV infection.
8. Discuss infectious waste and its disposal.
9. What is the purpose of OSHA's standard for bloodborne pathogens and who does it cover?
10. What is PPE? Name several types of PPE. Who is responsible for providing it?

WEB ACTIVITIES

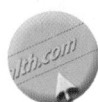

Go online to the Centers for Disease Control and Prevention and find the most current information about Standard Precautions. What is the procedure that must be followed in the event of a needlestick?

REFERENCES/BIBLIOGRAPHY

Bonewit, K. (2000). *Clinical procedures for medical assistants* (8th ed.). Philadelphia: W. B. Saunders Company.

Hegner, B., & Caldwell, E. (1999). *Nursing assistant: A nursing process approach* (8th ed.). Albany, NY: Delmar.

Ignatavicius, D. D., Workman, M., & Mishler, M. (1999). *Medical-surgical nursing: A nursing process approach* (3rd ed.). Philadelphia: W. B. Saunders Company.

Kinn, M. E., & Woods, M. A. (1999). *The medical assistant: Administrative and clinical* (8th ed.). Philadelphia: W. B. Saunders Company.

Lewis, M. A., & Tamparo, C. D. (1998). *Medical law, ethics, and bioethics in the medical office* (3rd ed.). Philadelphia: F A. Davis Company.

Marshall, J. (1995). *Fundamental skills for the clinical laboratory professional.* Albany, NY: Delmar.

Marshall, J. (1997) *Medical laboratory assistant.* New Jersey: Brady, Prentice Hall Division.

Occupational Safety and Health Administration Bloodborne Pathogen Regulation Section 1910.1030.

PDR generics (1st ed.). (1995). Montvale, NJ: Medical Economics Data Production Co.

Phipps, W. J., Sands, J., & Marek, J. F. (1999). *Medical-surgical nursing: Concepts and clinical practice* (6th ed.). St. Louis, MO: Mosby-Year Book, Inc.

Rice, J. (1999). *Principles of pharmacology for medical assisting.* (3rd ed.). Albany, NY: Delmar.

Smeltzer, S. C., & Bare, B. G. (2000). *Brunner and Suddarth's textbook of medical-surgical nursing* (9th ed). Philadelphia: J.B. Lippincott Company.

Taber's cyclopedic medical dictionary (18th ed.). (1999). Philadelphia: F.A. Davis Company.

Thompson, J. M., McFarland, G. K., Hirsch, J. E., & Tucker, S. M. (1998). *Mosby's clinical nursing* (4th ed.). St. Louis: C. V. Mosby.

U.S. Department of Health and Human Services, Centers for Disease Control and Prevention. (1997, November 7). *Draft guideline for isolation precautions in hospitals.* (Federal Register). Washington, DC: U.S. Government Printing Office.

Zakus, S. (1995). *Clinical procedures for medical assistants* (3rd ed.). St. Louis: Mosby-Year Book Inc.

TAKING A MEDICAL HISTORY, THE PATIENT'S CHART, AND METHODS OF DOCUMENTATION

KEY TERMS

Allergy

Chart

Chief Complaint

Clinical Diagnosis

Debridement

Objective

Problem-Oriented Medical Record (POMR)

SOAP

Source-Oriented Medical Record (SOMR)

Subjective

OUTLINE

OBJECTIVES

The student should strive to meet the following performance objectives and demonstrate an understanding of the facts and principles presented in this chapter through written and oral communication.

1. Define the key terms as presented in the glossary.
2. Understand the necessity and function of the medical history in patient treatment.
3. Define the parts of the medical history.
4. Identify and use effective methods of interacting with a patient.
5. Obtain a medical history from the patient.
6. Explain the different methods of charting/documentation.

(continues)

7. Define the meaning and function of SOAP.
8. Understand some issues of cultural sensitivity in taking a medical history.
9. Describe the contents of a medical record.
10. State five reasons why the medical record is important.
11. Document accurately.

ROLE DELINEATION COMPONENTS

CLINICAL

Patient Care

- Adhere to established triage procedures
- Recognize and respond to emergencies

GENERAL (TRANSDISCIPLINARY)

Professionalism

- Project a professional manner and image
- Adhere to ethical principles

Communication Skills

- Treat all patients with compassion and empathy
- Recognize and respect cultural diversity
- Adapt communications to individual's ability to understand
- Use professional telephone technique
- Use effective and correct verbal and written communications
- Recognize and respond to verbal and nonverbal communications
- Use medical terminology correctly
- Receive, organize, prioritize, and transmit information
- Serve as liaison   (*continues*)

SCENARIO

When clinical medical assistant Audrey Jones, CMA, of Doctors Lewis & King takes a patient history, she typically uses a form custom-designed for the office. Audrey uses the form as a guideline to be sure she gathers all pertinent information. However, she has learned that she must tailor her questions to the patient and sometimes will rearrange the order of the questions if necessary. While Audrey is adept at gathering specific and necessary patient information, she also is aware of patient concerns and sensitivities and adapts her approach to accomplish the task while making the patient feel at ease.

INTRODUCTION

In order to treat a patient effectively, the physician must know the patient's past medical history. If the patient is already established in the ambulatory care setting, the physician can work from the existing chart (record) with additional information obtained at the time of the office or clinic visit.

For a new patient, however, or for an established patient who has not been in for some time, an updated medical history form is of vital importance. Information contained in this history includes past medical problems, current medications and medication allergies, as well as other factors contributing to the patient's health.

Often the family practice clinic will have a broad questionnaire for patients to complete or the physician may tailor the medical history form to a particular specialty. The specialist physician will often mail the form to the patient prior to the appointment so that the patient can answer the questions in a quiet environment and have access to some of the information requested such as names and addresses of other physicians that they have seen.

The role of the medical assistant in taking the patient history is to be as thorough as possible while being as sensitive as possible. Respect for the patient's privacy must be balanced with the need for the kind of complete information that results in informed medical treatment and care.

The patient chart or medical record is a legal document that is a collection of confidential patient information. Should a patient's medical record be introduced in court, it becomes a legal record of care given. It is important that charting in the record be accurate, clear, concise, and complete.

ROLE DELINEATION
COMPONENTS (*continued*)

Legal Concepts

- Maintain confidentiality
- Prepare and maintain medical records
- Document accurately
- Use appropriate guidelines when releasing records or information

Instruction

- Explain office policies and procedures

THE FUNCTION OF THE MEDICAL HISTORY

The medical history is the basis for all treatment rendered by the physician, any on-call physician, and any specialist consulted to treat the patient. During the history-taking process, the physician often will discover information that helps guide treatment for the patient. The medical history in the **chart**, or record, makes it easier for the physician to recall previous treatment. Notes and laboratory results in the chart quickly show the progress of the treatment.

In addition, the charts give a base for statistical analysis: for the physician's own research, for insurance records, and for the health department, especially for infectious diseases. The health history and chart notes also become a legal record of the treatment rendered to the patient. This is especially important if the patient is making an injury claim against another party or if the patient makes a malpractice claim against the physician. If the records in the chart are precise and correct, the chart becomes a good defense; however, if the charting or documentation is sloppy or incomplete, the entire record could be set aside as an insufficient or incorrect record of treatment. The best procedure is to document everything concerning a patient including all treatment rendered, telephone calls, missed appointments, and discussions with other specialists regarding the patient's treatment. Also see Chapter 14 for information on medical records management.

THE CROSS-CULTURAL MODEL

It is important for the medical assistant to understand that every physician-patient interview is a cross-cultural one. Physicians and patients view the gathering of the patient history and the personal visit quite differently. Health and illness are inseparable from social and cultural beliefs. Who patients are—their background, their belief system, their family orientation, and their cultural heritage—influences their choices in health care. Physician and patient have different concerns and anticipations and the medical assistant conducting the interview needs to be aware of these varying perspectives. Consider the following perspectives.

- *Patient's chief concern:* The illness. The personal and social significance and the problems created by a perceived illness are important to the patient.

- *Physician's chief concern:* Disease. The physician is concerned with the malfunctioning and maladaptation of biological and psychological processes.

- *Patient's idea of treatment success:* Being able to successfully manage an illness and its problems is often more important to the patient than the curing of the disease.

- *Doctor's idea of treatment success:* Treatments, medications, and procedures that control disease problems and evaluating outcomes in these terms.

The medical assistant may find it helpful to ask certain questions of patients to help them move across cultures:

1. What do you think caused your problem?
2. When do you think it started?
3. What does it do to your body?
4. What do you expect from the course of this problem?
5. What do you fear from this problem?
6. What kind of treatment do you expect?

All these questions involve and respect the patient's perception. When conducting an interview with a patient, it is also wise to remember that the dominant form of care in the world is not the physician or medical staff but the family.

PATIENT INFORMATION FORMS

There are two sets of information forms in the medical office.

Administrative or Demographic Data Forms

The first set of forms includes the patient demographic data form and the financial information form. The demographic data form (Figure 23-1) registers the patient's full name, address, mailing address if different, home and work telephone numbers, date of birth, social security number and all insurance information, person to be contacted in case of emergency, and a release of information signature. Some medical offices include a second form, the financial information form (Figure 23-2), to be signed regarding the financial policy of the practice including billing, insurance billing, copayment billing, and any finance charges added to monthly billings.

PATIENT INFORMATION

TODAY'S DATE _____
　Patient's name (Last) _____ (First) _____ (M.I.) _____
　Address _____
　Phone (home) _____ (work) _____ (message)_____
　Please circle: Single/Married/Divorced/
　　　　　　　Widowed　　Male/Female
　Date of Birth ____ / ____ / ____
　Social Security # _____ / _____ / _____
　Occupation _____ Employer _____
　Spouse or Guardian Name _____

PRIMARY INSURANCE:
　Insurance Company Name_____
　Insurance Company Address _____
　Subscriber's Name_____
　Subscriber's Social Security # ____ / ____ / ____
　Group # _____

SECONDARY INSURANCE:
　Insurance Company Name_____
　Insurance Company Address _____
　Subscriber's Name_____
　Subscriber's Social Security # ____ / ____ / ____
　Group # _____

Person to notify in case of emergency
Name _____ **Phone (____)** _____

ASSIGNMENT AND RELEASE: I authorize my insurance benefits be paid directly to the physician. I understand that I am financially responsible for any balance due. I authorize the physician or insurance company to release any information required for this claim.

　Signed _____ **Date** _____

Figure 23-1 Patient information forms typically include demographic data, insurance information, emergency contact, and patient's signature for acceptance of financial responsibility.

FINANCIAL POLICY

In order to reduce confusion and misunderstanding between our patients and the clinic, we have adopted the following financial policy. If you have any questions about this policy, please discuss them with our Billing Manager. We are dedicated to providing the best possible care and service to you and we regard your complete understanding of your financial responsibilities as an essential element of your care and treatment.

Unless other arrangements have been made in advance by yourself or your health coverage carrier, full payment is due at time of service. For your convenience, we accept Visa, MasterCard, or we can arrange a payment schedule.

YOUR INSURANCE:

We accept assignment of benefit from Medicare. We also have direct billing agreements with many insurance companies. We will bill those plans for whom we have an agreement and will only require that you pay the copayment at the time of service.

If your medical plan determines a service is "not covered," you will be responsible for the entire charge. Payment is due upon receipt of statement from this office.

MINOR PATIENTS:

The adult accompanying the patient and the parent or guardian with custody will be billed for all services rendered to minor patients.

MISSED APPOINTMENTS:

In order to provide the best service and availability to our patients, we ask you to notify us 24 hours in advance if you know that you will be unable to keep the appointment. We reserve the right to charge for missed appointments.

I have read the financial policy and I understand it and agree to be bound by its terms.

_____　　　**Date** _____

Figure 23-2 A sample financial information form. Ambulatory care settings will have different financial policies depending on their practice and the insurance companies they work with.

Medical Forms

The second set of forms is the medical history form, which can be as short as one page (8½″ × 11″) or as long and detailed as six to eight pages. This form includes information on:

1. The current problem (chief complaint or CC) for which the patient is being seen
2. The patient's past medical history
3. The patient's family medical history
4. Social history including marital status or sexual orientation and occupation

The best form is neither too long nor too complicated. Patients may feel overwhelmed with a long form and will not finish it or will give up, stating they cannot remember all the information. The form that is simple and brief can provide the most information. Some patients find a history form too intimidating. It is easier for these patients to talk directly with the medical assistant or the physician about social history, feeling a one-to-one exchange is more personal and private.

A sample of a short history form is included in Figure 23-3. This form asks the reason for the visit (chief

Please take a moment to fill out this form. It will give us more detailed information about your medical history than would be obtainable in a normal office visit, and will also free up time to discuss the more current problems, and answer any questions about your health that you may have. This information is entirely confidential.

NAME_____

Why you are here today (chief complaint) _____
_____

Please circle any of the following symptoms that you have experienced recently:

Chest pain		Cough	
Chest pressure		Phlegm	
Chest heaviness		Coughing up blood	
Circulation problems		Shortness of breath	
Palpitations		Wheeze	
Rapid heartbeat		Change in exercise tolerance	
Irregular heartbeat			
Ankle swelling		Burning or pain on urination	
		Difficulty starting or stopping urination	
Change in appetite		Dribbling after urination	
Unexpected weight loss		Incontinence of urine	
Nausea		Blood in urine	
Vomiting		Cloudiness of urine	
Difficulty swallowing			
Belly pains		Skin rash	
Gas pains		New or changing moles	
Change in bowel habit:		Excess bruising or bleeding	
change in frequency		Mouth sores	
change in shape		Denture problems	
change in color		Sinus drainage or stuffiness	
change in consistency		Facial pain	
size of stool			
Blood, mucus or slime		Panic attacks	
Rectal pain or discomfort		Anxiety	
Hemorrhoids		Depression	
		Sadness	
Disturbance of sleep		Seizures	
Insomnia		Problems with concentration or memory	
Early wakefulness			
		Dizziness	
Fatigue		Fainting	
Fever/chills/sweat		Lightheadedness on standing	
Change in energy level		Vision problems	
Swollen glands		Hearing problems	
Sinusitis or chronic allergies		Numbness or tingling in arms or legs	
		Weakness in arms or legs	

PLEASE TURN PAGE OVER

Figure 23-3 Sample medical history form. (*continues*)

Have you ever had an allergic reaction to any medication?   YES   NO

If yes, what was/were the name/s of the medication/s? _____

What was/were the reaction/s? _____

_____

Past Medical History

Health Problem List	When first identified	Is the problem active?

List of surgeries	When performed?

Current Medications	Dose	Frequency	Date Started

Family History: Does any family member have the following conditions?

Condition	Who?	Age at onset? Age now?
Heart disease before age 60		
High cholesterol		
High blood pressure		
Diabetes		
Tuberculosis		
Cancer		
Other illness		
Depression		
Suicide		
Other psychiatric illness		

Social History:

Occupation: _____ Employer: _____

Marital status: **single**   **married**   **widowed**   **divorced**

Children: **male** ages now _____   **female** ages now _____

Do you smoke? _____ How many cigarettes per day? _____

Do you drink alcohol? _____ How many drinks per day? _____

Do you use recreation drugs or chemical substances? _____ Which ones? _____

        How often? _____

Do you have a sexual preference? _____ Male _____ Female _____

Do you have any sexual problems? _____ What kind(s)? _____

Figure 23-3 *(continued)*

complaint); symptoms the patient may be experiencing; past medical history including allergies to medications, past medical problems and surgeries, current medications; family history; and social history. Depending upon the ambulatory care setting, this form can be tailored to include vaccines and immunizations, usage of recreational drugs, exercise and diet regimens, accident information (especially if patient was hurt on the job), and any other information suited to the practice's specialty.

COMPUTERIZED HEALTH HISTORY

Some health care facilities use computerized health histories. These can be of two types: patient-generated and health care provider-generated. In patient-generated health histories, the patient responds on the computer to various questions, and then reviews information with the medical assistant for completeness. When using a health care provider-generated health history, the medical assistant completes the information on the screen after the patient interview. Frequently these programs are user-friendly and save time for both the patient and medical assistant. Some patients may not want to use a computer, however, and should be given the option of answering questions face to face.

THE FIRST OFFICE CONTACT

Telephone Contact

The first contact with a medical assistant in the ambulatory care setting is usually a telephone call. The patient or a relative of the patient calls to get information about the physician and the practice. When this occurs, primary administrative information is obtained including the patient's full name, telephone number, medical problem, insurance company, and sometimes the address as well. The administrative and medical history forms are given to the patient to complete upon coming into the office. If there is a long period of time between the telephone contact and the actual office visit, these forms may be mailed to the patient for completion. Also see Chapter 12 for information on telephone techniques.

Personal Visit

At times a physician will refer a patient to a specialist. When this happens, the patient may come to the specialist's office in person to bring records, X rays, or a referral and to make an appointment. If the patient is a member of a health maintenance organization, a referral from the primary care physician is usually mandatory. When the patient has a referral, the information forms are given to the patient to fill out in the office or to take home to complete in a quiet, undisturbed environment where the patient has access to records of past medical care.

Emergency Visit

When an acutely ill patient is referred by another physician to be seen immediately, or if an office or urgent care center accepts new patient emergency visits, the medical assistant usually knows about the visit in advance. In order to facilitate the history-taking process, the medical assistant may take the patient directly to an examination room where the atmosphere is quieter and private. This puts the patient at ease, which helps in preparing the forms. Depending upon the nature of the emergency, the medical assistant can help by asking the questions on the forms and writing down the patient's responses.

COMPLETING THE MEDICAL HISTORY FORMS

Interacting with the Patient

When the medical assistant is taking the medical history, the first responsibility is to put the patient at ease. A comfort level must be developed between medical assistant and patient. The medical assistant must guide the conversation, keeping it on track in order to obtain the most information for the physician. Allowing conversation to wander, talking about other people, or letting the patient tell anecdotes does not help to complete the history. Explaining a term or concept that the patient does not understand is helpful to the patient. The medical assistant must remain professional and not be embarrassed or made uncomfortable by the patient's answers, whether regarding illness, actions, or lifestyle. Refer to Table 23-1.

If the patient is already an established patient but has not seen the physician for several months or longer,

TABLE 23-1	GENERAL APPROACH TO THE HISTORY

1. Ensure an appropriate environment that is well-lighted, at a comfortable temperature, quiet, private, and free of distractions.
2. Sit facing the patient at eye level; the patient should be seated. Ensure that the patient is as comfortable as possible, since obtaining the health history can be a lengthy process. Figure 23-4 illustrates an appropriate setting.
3. Ask the patient if there are any questions about the interview before you begin.
4. Avoid the use of medical jargon. Use terms the patient can understand.
5. Reserve asking intimate and personal questions (social history) until rapport is established.
6. Remain flexible in obtaining the health history. It does not need to be obtained in the exact order it is presented in this chapter or on the form.
7. Remind the patient that all information will be treated confidentially.

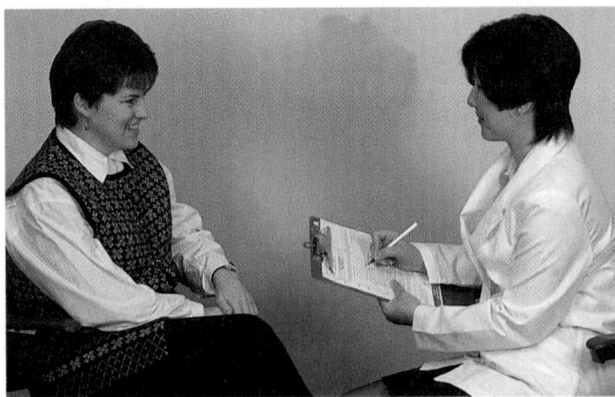

Figure 23-4 Showing concern for the patient's well-being can put the patient at ease while the medical assistant takes the medical history.

update the medical history by asking if any illnesses have occurred in the months elapsed, if any new allergies to any medications or other substances have occurred and the reaction to each. The chief complaint for the current visit should always be documented. The chief complaint is the problem that brings the patient to the physician this particular visit. Sometimes when patients know they are going to be seen, they save several problems to discuss. Depending on the appointment schedule for the day, the medical assistant may need to remind patients that an appointment for a specific problem was made and that the physician can see them for only that particular problem this visit. Another appointment can be made to discuss the remaining concerns on the list if necessary. The medical assistant should always note the chief complaint before the physician sees the patient to assure the main problem is addressed.

Displaying Cultural Awareness

As the medical assistant begins the encounter with the patient, awareness of cultural differences and other problems that may inhibit communication is important. Any number of situations may arise which the medical assistant must be prepared to address. The medical assistant has already overcome major obstacles if it is known that the patient does not speak English as a first language or needs an interpreter, if the patient is deaf and needs an interpreter, if the patient is from a culture in which the female patient does not disrobe for the physician, or if the patient has a mental disorder making communication difficult.

If there is a language difficulty, the medical assistant may be required to arrange for an interpreter. There are language interpreters in most areas; especially in large urban areas, an interpreter might be found for nearly any language. If the patient is receiving medical care through Medicaid, special arrangements can be made for an interpreter through the state agency administering the program. Often the patient will bring a family member to interpret; however, if the matter is intensely personal, the patient may not want to reveal personal matters with the family member present and may prefer an outside, objective interpreter.

The medical assistant should be accessible and should listen to the patient. Sometimes the patient will be uneasy talking to the physician but may be more comfortable telling the medical assistant about the problem. Med-

Patient Teaching Tip

In some cultures (e.g., Chinese, some Native Americans), it is disrespectful to speak of the dead. Thus, the patient may be reluctant to provide detailed information on the family health history of dead relatives. In these cases, you can ask the patient if there has been any history of specific diseases in the family and not focus on the specific individual if that person is deceased. The patient may be willing to share in which previous generation and which side of the family the condition existed. If these approaches are unsuccessful, explain to the patient the importance of this information, as it may provide clues to the patient's current health conditions.

Patient Teaching Tip

Some Asian cultures calculate age from conception, not from the actual birth date. For example, a newborn infant is considered to be one year old. The medical assistant needs to clarify the chronological age with the patient or caregiver. This is particularly important for pediatric patients because of the link between age and developmental milestones.

ical assistants can play a very important part in the medical practice by listening and communicating both with the patient and with the physician.

Handling a Difficult Patient

Some patients are frightened, hostile, or depressed. It is important to be open to nonverbal as well as verbal communication in answer to questions. Some patients react positively to a hand placed gently on the forearm; it calms and reassures them. Other patients have a negative response, pulling away from any such contact. The medical assistant needs to know when to touch the patient appropriately, always with permission either expressed or implied. (If the medical assistant tells the patient a blood pressure reading is next and reaches for the patient's arm and the patient extends an arm, permission to take the reading is implied. If, however, the patient pulls away and states no blood pressure is to be taken, permission is not given and the reading must not be done at that time.)

Trying to get information from a reluctant patient can be difficult and requires patience and understanding. If the patient is hesitant to discuss a problem with the medical assistant, it is better not to press for information. Pressing for information may make the patient become defensive or angry and can impair communication altogether.

A patient may come to the office upset and crying. This patient must be made to feel more in control, that no one is going to rush care being given. Sometimes just taking a few moments to sit with such patients until they feel more settled is enough to calm them and enable the history-taking interview to proceed.

Uncommunicative patients may require some special questioning techniques. The medical assistant may have to supply a sample of problems to get these patients to acknowledge the health concerns they have. Or they may shrug their shoulders at every question and be unresponsive. Some patients may simply say, "I don't know. I

just don't feel well." If a relative has accompanied the patient to the appointment, it may be appropriate initially to have the relative present with the patient. In this way the patient has a familiar face in the unfamiliar, often frightening, physician's office. It is always the patient's decision if anyone else is to be in the room.

Some patients may have particular needs which they often will state to the medical assistant. These may be as simple as not wanting to sit or wanting the door ajar. Meeting these needs is usually a minor matter and makes patients feel more comfortable.

Dealing with Sensitive Topics

Alcohol, drug use, and sexual practices are some of the most sensitive areas that are addressed in the health history. Some consideration in dealing with these sensitive topics include:

- Ask these questions in the later stages of the interview after rapport has been established.

- Use direct eye contact; this demonstrates the importance of the topic to the patient and your lack of embarrassment.

- Pose questions in a matter-of-fact tone.

- Adopt a nonjudgmental demeanor.

- Utilize the communication technique of "normalizing" when appropriate (e.g., "Some high school students drink alcohol/use drugs/engage in sexual relationships on a regular basis. Does this happen at your school? With you?").

- Observe an experienced medical assistant elicit sensitive information from patients; note the medical assistant's verbal and nonverbal behavior.

Patient Teaching Tip

Some patients may seem reluctant to answer your questions regarding birthplace or social security number. Noncitizens may fear deportation if they are identified in the health care system, especially if they are seriously ill. Remind these patients that you are there solely to assist them with their health care needs and encourage them to provide accurate information to assist you in appropriate diagnosis and treatment, since many diseases are specific to geographic locations.

If the medical assistant can enhance communication with the patient, communication between physician and patient will be more effective.

PARTS OF THE MEDICAL HISTORY

The components of the patient's medical history include:

- Personal data contained on the administrative form
- Chief complaint, which is noted at each visit by the medical assistant
- Present illness
- Past medical history
- Family history
- Social and occupational history
- Review of systems

Chief Complaint

The **chief complaint** (usually abbreviated CC) is the specific reason that brought the patient to see the physician. It should be noted in as few words as possible but be very specific. It can be a direct quote from the patient.

A good example of a chief complaint notation might be "nausea and vomiting × 3 days." This is a **subjective** complaint in that it is known by the patient but cannot be seen or measured by the physician. It is specific, however, in relating the patient's condition. The "×" is an abbreviation for the length of time since the symptom first occurred. Another example is "hurt ankle when tripped over curb yesterday." Again this is subjective but specific about cause, time of onset, and complaint. The ankle is visibly swollen and very painful to touch. The swelling is an **objective** sign, a manifestation that can be seen, heard, or measured by any observer.

On the other hand, a poor example of a chief complaint is "has not been feeling well." This notation tells the physician nothing about what symptoms or problems the patient has been experiencing. It gives no specific clue as to what the problem is from the patient's perspective. The medical assistant should try to pinpoint a complaint to a body system, to a time frame, to pain in a specific area. The patient usually will respond to questions that offer several options.

Nine characteristics of each chief complaint should be ascertained for a complete history. These characteristics are:

1. Location
2. Radiation
3. Quality
4. Quantity
5. Associated manifestations
6. Aggravating factors
7. Alleviating factors
8. Setting
9. Timing

Note that all chief complaints may not have all nine qualifiers; hoarseness, for example, may not be characterized by quantity.

Present Illness

The present illness is usually reflected in the chief complaint. Then the chief complaint is expanded upon to determine the onset of the illness, what the patient has done to treat the illness, and any current medications. In the preceding example of nausea and vomiting, the patient may indicate inability to eat or take fluids. This would alert the physician to possible dehydration. Often the present illness is based upon a prior health problem. For instance, a history of congestive heart failure gives a patient's symptoms of fluid retention, wheezing, and shortness of breath more importance since these are very common complications. Without this knowledge of the patient's past history, these symptoms could be confused with bronchitis, asthma, or pneumonia.

Past Medical History

The past medical history includes all health problems, major illnesses, and surgeries that the patient has had, all current medications including dosages and reasons for taking them, all allergies to any medications and the specific allergic reaction to each. These are very important to the present illness, for many health problems can overlap and affect the patient in several areas. A patient with a long history of diabetes mellitus may present with an ulcer on his foot. While the same ulcer in an otherwise healthy patient will heal with little intervention, the diabetic patient will require major treatment and attention including **debridement** (removal of dead or damaged tissue or foreign debris), antibiotics, and close monitoring.

Medications have side effects and contraindications that can affect patients. **Allergies** to medications can be serious and need to be noted in a readily visible part of the chart. Usually a red sticker is placed in a conspicuous area on the outside of the chart noting medication allergies. A notation is added inside the chart as well. The information needs to be updated at least annually. Also document herbal, vitamin, and mineral supplements the patient is taking.

Patients may be asked to complete a Release of Information form (Figure 23-5). This form is sent to their former physicians to obtain past medical records.

AUTHORIZATION TO RELEASE HEALTH CARE INFORMATION

Patient _____ Date of Birth _____
SSN _____ Previous Name _____

I request and authorize _____ to release the health care information of the patient named above to:

Name _____

Address _____

This request and authorization applies to:
(Please initial the appropriate box)

___ Health care information relating to the following treatment, condition, or dates of treatment:

_____

___ All health care information **EXCLUDING** specific information relating to sexually transmitted diseases (including HIV/AIDS), alcohol or drug use, or visits related to psychiatric disorders or mental health.

___ All health care information **INCLUDING** specific information relating to sexually transmitted diseases (including HIV/AIDS), alcohol or drug use, or visits related to psychiatric disorders or mental health.

___ Other: _____

I understand that my express consent is required to release any health care information relating to testing, diagnosis, and/or treatment of HIV (AIDS virus), sexually transmitted disease, psychiatric disorders/mental health, or drug and/or alcohol use. If I have been tested, diagnosed, or treated for HIV (AIDS virus), sexually transmitted disease, psychiatric disorders/mental health, or drug and/or alcohol use, you are specifically authorized to release all health care information relating to such diagnosis, testing, or treatment.

_____ / _____
Signature of patient or patient's   Relationship
authorized representative   to patient

_____
Date

Figure 23-5   Sample release of information form.

If the patient has several physicians, the examining physician will encourage the patient to choose one physician to manage primary medical care so that all medical care and records are concentrated in one office. Under most managed care insurance policies, patients have one primary care physician (women may also have an obstetrician/gynecologist) who coordinates the patient's health care.

Family History

The family history can provide clues to the patient's present condition. By asking open-ended questions about

Patient Teaching Tip

Patients who are adopted may have limited information about their biological parents. Encourage adopted patients to be frank with their family health history. If the family health history of the biological parents is unknown, this is documented. It is not uncommon for patients to seek out their birth parents in an attempt to learn more about their family health history.

The family health history of adoptive parents can be equally important. Certain environmental factors (smoking, drug and alcohol use, sanitation) can influence the health of the adopted child.

medical problems of siblings, parents, and grandparents, the physician will be alerted to hereditary and familial diseases and disorders such as coronary artery disease, hypertension, breast cancer, and so forth. Present ages of siblings, parents, and grandparents, or cause of their death and age at time of death are noted. For instance, a family history of diabetes together with the patient's symptoms of frequent urination and thirst may make a diagnosis of diabetes mellitus a possibility.

Social History

The social history of patients includes their marital status, sexual orientation, occupation, hobbies, and use of alcohol, tobacco, and recreational drugs or other chemical substances. This part of the history includes those lifestyles and behaviors that may put the patient at greater risk for injury or disease than would normally be found from factors in the family history and past medical history. If the patient's usage of alcohol exceeds an average amount and a hobby the patient pursues is auto racing, the physician will counsel the patient about the danger of the combination of these two behaviors.

Be aware that patients may refuse to answer questions pertaining to sexual history; attempt to return to these questions later. Ask the patient if a medical assistant of a different gender would make the patient more comfortable in discussing sexual practice.

For instance, the adolescent patient may refuse to answer questions of a sexual matter or provide false answers if the parent or caregiver is present. It may be best to ask the caregiver to leave the room at the completion of the health history so you can ask the patient if there is anything else to note in the sexual history.

Be alert for cues that demonstrate the patient's desire for knowledge of sexual education, such as questions or requests for written information. Answer the patient's questions, provide educational materials, and refer the patient to a specialist when indicated.

It may be necessary to inquire about the patient's home environment. You need to be attentive for clues that signal the necessity of performing an in-depth home environment assessment. Some clues include, but are not limited to, poor hygiene, frequent infections, smoke inhalation, burns, malnutrition, and falls (especially in the elderly).

Review of Systems

After the history is taken by the medical assistant, the review of systems (ROS) is performed by the physician during the physical examination. This is an orderly and systematic check of each part of the body and is recorded. The physician asks questions concerning each organ and system of the body during the examination of the patient. The ROS, in conjunction with the physical examination, helps elicit information that is essential to the diagnosis of disease. The physician usually begins with an overall assessment and proceeds to check each body system in an organized manner. The order in which this is done may vary from one physician to another, but all will check the cardiovascular, respiratory, gastrointestinal, genitourinary, and neurological systems as well as the extremities, the musculoskeletal system, and the skin.

Both positive and pertinent negative findings are documented in the ROS. When a response is positive, the physician asks the patient to describe it as completely as possible. Table 23-2 lists the symptoms and diseases that can be ascertained during the ROS. Many ambulatory care settings have preprinted ROS sheets. These are convenient, as positive findings can be circled and noted. Negative responses are not circled.

By the completion of this portion of the history, the physician usually has an idea about the patient's condition.

To complete the exam, the physician usually orders laboratory tests depending on the findings and the probable diagnosis. These results, together with the history,

---

TABLE 23-2   REVIEW OF SYSTEMS

General

Patient's perception of general state of health at the present time; difference from usual state; vitality and energy levels

Neurological

Headache, change in balance, incoordination, loss of movement, change in sensory perception/feeling in an extremity, change in speech, change in smell, fainting, loss of memory, tremors, involuntary movement, loss of consciousness, seizures, weakness, head injury

Psychological

Irritability, nervousness, tension, increased stress, difficulty concentrating, mood changes, suicidal thoughts, depression

Skin

Rashes, itching, changes in skin pigmentation, black and blue marks, change in color or size of mole, sores, lumps, change in skin texture, odors, excessive sweating, acne, loss of hair, excessive growth of hair or growth of hair in unusual locations, change in nails, amount of time spent in the sun

Eyes

Blurry vision, visual acuity, glasses, contacts, sensitivity to light, excessive tearing, night blindness, double vision, drainage, bloodshot, pain, blind spots, flashing lights, halos around objects, glaucoma, cataracts

Ears

Hearing deficits, hearing aid, pain, discharge, lightheadedness, ringing in the ears, earaches, infection

Nose and Sinuses

Frequent colds, discharge, itching, hay fever, postnasal drip, stuffiness, sinus pain, polyps, obstruction, nosebleed, change in sense of smell

Mouth

Toothache, tooth abscess, dentures, bleeding/swollen gums, difficulty chewing, sore tongue, change in taste, lesions, change in salivation, bad breath

Throat/Neck

Hoarseness, change in voice, frequent sore throats, difficulty swallowing, pain/stiffness, enlarged thyroid

Respiratory

Shortness of breath, shortness of breath on exertion, phlegm, cough, sneezing, wheezing, coughing up blood, frequent upper respiratory tract infections, pneumonia, emphysema, asthma, tuberculosis

Cardiovascular

Shortness of breath that wakes you up in the night, chest pain, heart murmur, palpitations, fainting, sleep on pillows to breathe better, swelling, cold hands/feet, leg cramps, myocardial infarction, hypertension, valvular disease, pain in calf with walking, varicose veins, inflammation of a vein, blood clot in leg, anemia

Breasts

Pain, tenderness, discharge, lumps, change in size, dimpling

Gastrointestinal

Change in appetite, nausea, vomiting, diarrhea, constipation, usual bowel habits, black, tarry stools, vomiting blood, change in stool color, excessive gas, belching, regurgitation or heartburn, difficulty swallowing, abdominal pain, jaundice, hemorrhoids, hepatitis, peptic ulcers, gallstones

Urinary

Change in urine color, voiding habits, painful urination, hesitancy, urgency, frequency, excessive urination at night, increased urine volume, dribbling, loss in force of stream, bedwetting, change in urine volume, incontinence, pain in lower abdomen, kidney stones, urinary tract infections

(continues)

TABLE 23-2 (continued)		
Musculoskeletal Joint stiffness, muscle pain, back pain, limitation of movement, redness, swelling, weakness, bony deformity, broken bones, dislocations, sprains, gout, arthritis, osteoporosis, herniated disc *Female Reproductive* Vaginal discharge, change in libido, infertility, sterility, pain during intercourse, menses (last menstrual period, age period started, regularity, duration, amount of bleeding, premenstrual symptoms, intermenstrual bleeding, painful periods), menopause (age of onset, duration, symptoms, bleeding),	obstetrical (number of pregnancies, number of miscarriages/abortions, number of children, type of delivery, complications), type of birth control, estrogen therapy *Male Reproductive* Change in libido, infertility, sterility, impotence, pain during intercourse, age at onset of puberty, testicular pain, penile discharge, erections, emissions, hernias, enlarged prostate, type of birth control *Nutrition* Present weight, usual weight, food intolerances, food likes, food dislikes, where meals are eaten	*Endocrine* Bulging eyes, fatigue, change in size of head, hands, or feet, weight change, heat/cold intolerances, excessive sweating, increased thirst, increased hunger, change in body hair distribution, swelling in the anterior neck, diabetes mellitus *Lymph Nodes* Enlarged, tenderness *Hematological* Easy bruising/bleeding, anemia, sickle cell anemia, blood type

examination, and patient symptoms, help to lead to a **clinical diagnosis**.

All of the components of the patient's medical history document integral parts of the patient's health. If any part is lacking, the current understanding of the patient's health is not complete. By using all the components, the physician can evaluate the patient's health completely and more easily.

See Procedure 23-1 for steps in taking a medical history.

THE PATIENT'S RECORD AND ITS IMPORTANCE

The patient's chart or record is a collection of confidential information that concerns the patient, care given to the patient, patient progress, and laboratory and other diagnostic test results that have been completed. This information is arranged in a file folder or a binder, or is held together by other suitable means. It is used for a variety of purposes, but primarily it is used to provide a foundation for planning patient care and making decisions about patient care. Other purposes for a medical record include using it as a basis for communication among care givers, for statistical analysis in research, and for reporting infectious diseases to the health department. It is also a legal document and belongs to the physician or the agency in which the physician is employed. See Chapter 7 regarding legal guidelines and medical records. Since it is a legal document, the medical record can be used to determine if patient care has been given according to the standards of care that the law recognizes; therefore, it must be complete, concise, accurate, and legible. Many important items of information must be written in the patient record and the medical assistant will be one of the professionals making chart entries.

Contents of Medical Records

Each patient has his or her own medical record. All patients' records hold standard information. In addition to the patient information forms previously mentioned, other important components of the record include:

- Informed consent forms
- Physical examination outcomes
- Laboratory and diagnostic test results
- The physician's diagnosis and plan of treatment
- Surgical reports
- Progress reports
- Follow-up care
- Telephone calls
- Discharge summary
- Other communications (from other physicians, laboratories, or agencies)
- Patient records from other physicians
- Medication history

METHODS OF CHARTING/ DOCUMENTATION

There are three primary ways to maintain chart notes. They are:

- Source-oriented medical records
- Problem-oriented medical records
- Computer-generated/modified records.

Source-Oriented Medical Records

The traditional or conventional method of charting, **source-oriented medical record (SOMR)**, consists of a chronological set of notes for each visit beginning with the patient's first visit (Figure 23-6). This form of charting makes it difficult to follow or track a specific patient problem. The caregiver must search through the record to locate information about a particular patient problem. Source-oriented notes may be typed by the medical transcriptionist from dictation after the physician has seen the patient.

The example of handwritten chart notes shows the complete history taken at the time of examination including the present illness (if any), the past medical history, allergies, family history, habits (social history), and review of systems. The physical examination follows with each area noted. Impressions and changes in medications and plan finish the examination notes.

Problem-Oriented Medical Records

A more efficient way of keeping chart notes is the **problem-oriented medical record (POMR)**. This method is used extensively today, especially by clinics or any medical practice where more than one physician may see the patient. This method calls for a list of problems to be made, dated, and numbers assigned to them. When a patient is seen, the problems are identified by number throughout the record. This system makes it easier for the physician to follow the patient's progress.

The problem-oriented medical record has four major components:

- *The database:* The patient's medical history, results from laboratory and other diagnostic tests, and results of physical examination are the core of the record.

- *The problem list:* Each problem is listed individually and assigned a number and dated.

- *The diagnostic and treatment plan:* This component addresses the laboratory and other diagnostic tests completed and the physician's plan for treating the patient.

- *Progress notes:* These notes are entered on every problem initially recorded. Documentation is done chronologically and includes patient's complaints, problems, condition, treatment, and responses to treatment and care given.

Physicians may dictate their notes to be typed by a medical transcriptionist and then filed in the chart (Figure 23-7). These notes may follow the form seen in the handwritten chart note or as in Figure 23-7.

Computer-Modified Records

The final example (Figure 23-8), shows a computer chart note that ties both methods together: the problems are

---

04/01/_ abdominal pain × 3 weeks
WT 192   BP 152/88   T 97.6   P78   R18
Pt complaining severe abdominal pain for 2 wks getting
progressively worse. Describes as burning. pressure.
Past Med. Hist.   chronic Peptic Ulcer Disease
                  quit smoking 3 yr ago – now back
                  to 2 ppd
Allergies–penicillin–hives 1950s
Family Hist   noncontributory
Habits   smokes 2 ppd
             beer–several daily
ROS
HEENT noncontributory–PERRLA OU correct to 20/20
        CR–clear, no rales, ronchi; murmurs
        GI–some guarding. No masses, tenderness lower
        abdomen. No nausea, vomiting, diarrhea
        GU–clear
PE alert; oriented to time & place
    HEENT–pupils   nat teeth
    fundi   thyroid   } ∅
    carotids
    chest–clear
    heart–no murmurs or enlargement
    abdomen–∅ masses
    rectal–soft brown stool in vault
    extremities–neg.
    neuro–reg.
    skin–clear
Impression–Chronic Peptic Ulcer Disease
            Hypertension, mild
Plan–Lab–CBC, Chem 7, UA, barium swallow
Rx–Omeprazole 20 mg qd
Return 3 days
M. Woo, MD

Figure 23-6   Sample of a handwritten chart note.

Leo McKay
Date of Birth 01/22/49
Office visit 04/01/__

This 52-year-old patient is seen after a several year absence because of abdominal pain which began approximately 2 weeks ago with progressively worsening abdominal pain. He has stopped eating to see if pain would improve, which it did not. Finally yesterday he stopped taking fluids as well. Until this episode, he was drinking several beers daily and smoking approximately 2 ppd.

Weight is 192. BP 152/88 P 78 R 18 T 97.6. He is a well-developed, moderately obese male in moderate distress. Abdomen is tense with some guarding at RUQ.

Abdominal pain - pt needs barium swallow, CBC, Chem 7 and UA. To restrict diet to clear liquids until seen in 2 days, omeprazole 20 mg qd.
        JW/tlm

Figure 23-7   Example of dictated and transcribed chart note.

Patient: Leo McKay
Date of Birth: 01/22/49
Visit Date: 04/01/___

Chief Complaint: Abdominal pain
History: Has been ill over the last 2 weeks with progressively worsening abdominal pain.
Review of Symptoms: Patient denies the following:
- Chest pain, Chest pressure, Chest heaviness, Circulation problems, Palpitations, Rapid heartbeat, Irregular heartbeat, Ankle swelling
- Cough, Phlegm, Coughing up blood, Shortness of breath, Wheeze, Change in exercise tolerance
- Burning or pain on urination, Difficulty starting or stopping urination, Dribbling after urination, Incontinence of urine, Blood in urine, Cloudiness of urine
- Change in appetite, Unexpected weight loss, Nausea, Vomiting, Difficulty Swallowing, Belly pains, Gas pains, Change in bowel habit: change in frequency, shape, color, consistency, size of stool; Blood, Mucus, or Slime, Rectal pain or discomfort, Hemorrhoids
- Skin rash, New or changing moles, Excess bruising or bleeding
- Mouth sores, Denture problems, Sinus drainage or stuffiness, Facial pain
- Panic attacks, Anxiety, Depression, Sadness, Seizures, Problems with concentration or memory, Disturbance of sleep, Insomnia, Early wakefulness
- Dizziness, Fainting, Lightheadedness on standing, Headaches, Vision problems, Hearing problems, Numbness or tingling in arms or legs, Weakness in arms or legs

Medications, including Herbal, Vitamin, and Mineral Supplements

Drug	Dose	Freq.	Started
none			

Medical Problem List

Problem	When Dx'd	Active?
Peptic Ulcer	1985	no

List of Surgeries

Surgical Procedure	When
none	

Family History: Parents deceased, father died of heart attack, mother of breast cancer.
Social History: Divorced, no children
Habits: Smokes 2 ppd, Several beers daily
Allergies: Penicillin _____

Physical Examination

GENERAL: Well developed and well nourished gentleman in no distress. No jaundice, cyanosis, clubbing, or edema.
VITALS: Weight = 192, Temp = 97.6, Pulse = 78, R = 18, BP = 152/88
HEENT: Normocephalic and without evidence of trauma, tympanic membranes and external auditory canals are normal. Pharynx and mouth are normal.
NECK: supple, no masses or thyromegaly.
NODES: No cervical nodes palpable. No axillary or inguinal adenopathy.
CARDIOVASCULAR SYSTEM: Heart sounds: no murmurs, rubs or gallops, carotids with good upstrokes, no bruits heard. Peripheral pulses including radials, brachials, and femorals intact. Posterior tibial, and dorsalis pedis pulses intact.
RESPIRATORY SYSTEM: resps 18/min, trachea central, expansion, fremitus, resonance, and breath sounds normal.
ABDOMEN: soft, no masses, organomegaly, or tenderness. No loin or costo-vertebral angle tenderness. Inguinal canals are intact without herniae. Bowel sounds active.
GENITOURINARY: Penis without lesions or discharge, scrotum, testicles, epididymis and cords all normal
RECTAL: no masses, tenderness, or hemorrhoids. Soft brown stool in vault. Prostate normal in size, and shape without nodules or tenderness.
MUSCULOSKELETAL SYSTEM: Joints with full ROM, no joint tenderness or swelling. Muscle bulk symmetric and normal.
SKIN: without masses, skin tags, rash, blisters or ulcerations. Nails are normal without splinter hemorrhages.
NEUROLOGICAL SYSTEM: Alert and oriented to place, person, and time. Communicates with good word recognition and appropriate word usage. Cranial nerves and spinal nerves grossly intact.

Assessment and Plan

Problem	Plan/Status
Abdominal pain	Reports about two weeks of epigastric and retrosternal chest pain radiating up and to the left. Episodes of pain occur usually during the day and last for 3-4 hours. No associated dyspnea, palpitations, sweats, dizziness. No nausea, vomiting or diarrhea. No blood in the stool. To get barium swallow, CBC, Chem 7 and UA. Begin omeprazole 20 m qd.

Follow-up appointment: 3 days
Mark Woo MD

Figure 23-8 Sample of computer-generated medical history and physical examination.

Leo McKay
Date of Birth 01/22/49
Visit Date: 04/04/__

S: Patient returns after undergoing barium swallow. He is not in as much discomfort as last visit. States he has been taking clear liquids only and is hungry.
O: Lab results are back. Chem 7 shows slightly elevated glucose at 133. CBC and UA normal. Barium swallow shows two small areas of ulceration.
A: Gastric ulcer.
P: Reduce omeprazole to 10 mg qd. Recheck glucose at return visit in 4 weeks.

MW/tlm

Figure 23-9 Sample of a dictated and transcribed SOAP follow-up visit note.

Leo McKay
Visit Date: 04/04/__

| Symptoms: | Feeling somewhat better. Abdominal pain is less on the Omeprazole. |
| Exam: | Weight = 185   BP = 150/84 Patient had barium swallow showing two areas of ulceration. Lab tests show normal findings for CBC and UA. Chem 7 shows slightly elevated glucose at 133. |

Assessment	Plan
Gastric ulcer	Omeprazole 10 mg qd. Recheck glucose at return visit.

Follow-up appointment: 4 weeks.

Mark Woo, MD

Figure 23-10 Sample of computer-generated follow-up visit note.

stated, but the record grows in chronological order. Note that the past health problems are shown at the top of each entry and all current medications are shown on each entry. Computer-modified records are advantageous if an agency has computer terminals in a network connected to a main computer. Records can be brought up on a terminal by a physician and reviewed, updated, and saved whenever the physician wants to do so. Records are available 24 hours a day and therefore can be accessed by the physician on a home computer.

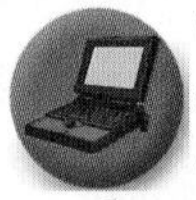

Protecting patient's confidentiality must always be a priority when medical records are computerized. See Chapter 11 regarding computers and confidentiality.

For more information on the SOMR and POMR charting methods, see Chapter 14.

SOAP Method of Charting

Charting under SOMR and POMR techniques for follow-up visits is accomplished most efficiently using a method with the acronym **SOAP**. In this method, the *subjective* complaint (patient's symptoms) is listed. This is the patient's description of the current problems. These problems are not discernible to an observer. The *objective* findings are those made by the physician during the physical examination, vital signs, and laboratory and other test results. These findings can be seen, felt, or measured, and the findings are observable. *Assessment* of the problem is next. The physician weighs the objective findings with the subjective information the patient has given and forms a diagnosis. The physician then formulates a *plan*. The plan includes further laboratory tests, X rays, medications, and instructions to the patient. Usually there is a follow-up appointment made for a few days or two to three weeks for a new problem, followed by a several

month follow-up for the problem once it has been brought under control.

Examples of the transcribed (Figure 23-9) and the computer-generated (Figure 23-10) follow-up visit notes are shown here.

Abbreviations Used in Charting

Abbreviations are used extensively in charting to document information. Some are used as a short-hand to save time and space, while other abbreviations are used to give an exact meaning to a finding. For instance, the abbreviation N&V indicates "nausea and vomiting" without having to write out the entire expression. See Table 23-3 for commonly used abbreviations.

Correcting an Error

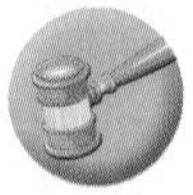

When an error has been made in the chart and it needs to be corrected, the proper procedure is to draw a line through the error, note "error" just above the line, and sign your initials and the date (Figure 23-11). Then enter the correct information. Do not erase, obliterate, or otherwise try to change the error because that will invalidate the legal and medical value of the patient's chart. As a medical assistant, you will be responsible for entering information in a patient's record and keeping it confidential. Remember that a patient's medical record is a legal document and it may be necessary to use it as evidence in a court of law.

TABLE 23-3	ABBREVIATIONS COMMONLY USED IN CHARTING
BP or B/P	blood pressure
c̄	with
CBC	complete blood count
CC	chief complaint
CPE	complete physical exam
D&C	dilation and curettage
dx	diagnosis
ECG, EKG	electrocardiogram
EEG	electroencephalogram
ER	emergency room
GI	gastrointestinal
GU	genitourinary
GYN	gynecology
HEENT	head, eyes, ears, nose, and throat
I&D	incision and drainage
L	left
MI	myocardial infarction
N&V	nausea and vomiting
NVD	nausea, vomiting, and diarrhea
OPD	outpatient department
OR	operating room
P	pulse
PERRLA	pupils equal, round, reactive to light and accommodation
PT	physical therapy
R	right
R	respiration
ROM	range of motion
ROS	review of systems
s̄	without
SOAP	subjective, objective, assessment, plan
SOB	short of breath
T	temperature
T&A	tonsillectomy and adenoidectomy
UCHD	usual childhood diseases
URI	upper respiratory infection
UTI	urinary tract infection
WNL	within normal limits
XR	X ray
>	greater than
<	less than
↑	increase
↓	decrease
Δ	change

Chart Organization

The chart notes are kept in chronological order for the primary physician. The laboratory tests, hospital notes, consultations by other physicians, and any correspondence should be kept in an orderly fashion. Figure 23-12 shows a chart with information easily found.

The chart order presents current medications on the left side of the chart with the laboratory reports and pathology reports underneath, each in chronological order. In the POMR system, often the list of medical problems is found above the current medications.

On the right side of the chart, the physician's notes are in chronological order with the most recent on top. The X rays and EKGs follow, including MRIs, mammograms, CT scans, exercise tolerance tests (ETTs), echocardiograms, and other similar tests. Following these are the hospital notes, including the history and physical, hospital consultations, and discharge summary. Consultations by other physicians are grouped next, again in chronological order.

The miscellaneous section may include anything from referrals for insurance companies to orders and updates from nursing homes or home health services. Finally, the correspondence section includes letters, insurance claim forms, and requests for prior medical records.

If a chart is kept in a specific order, information needed is easily gleaned by the medical assistant, the physician, or the front office administrative assistant.

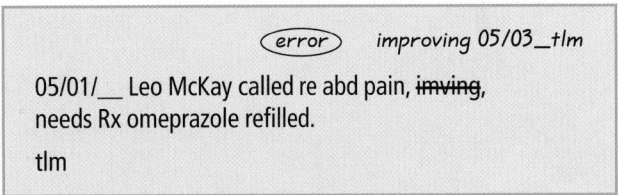

Figure 23-11 Correcting a charting error.

Current Medications	Primary Physician's Notes
Laboratory Results	EKGs - X RAYS
Pathology Reports	Hospital Notes
	Consultations
	Miscellaneous
	Correspondence

Figure 23-12 Sample chart organization.

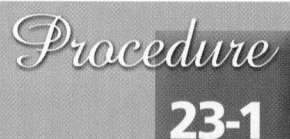

23-1   Taking a Medical History

PURPOSE:
To obtain a medical history from a patient new to the ambulatory care setting.

EQUIPMENT/SUPPLIES:
Patient history forms
Clipboard
Pens

PROCEDURE STEPS:
1. Introduce yourself to the new patient. Confirm identity of the patient and escort to the examination room or private area.
2. Make eye contact and use positive body language to put patient at ease.
3. Explain the purpose and importance of obtaining the patient information. Ask the questions on the form, trying to get as much information as possible without letting the patient wander from the subject.
4. Ask each question clearly. Be sure patient understands all questions. Ask about allergies.
5. Repeat patient answers when needed to confirm. Be specific when documenting answers. Do not just write "yes" for tobacco use. List "2 packs per day." Be specific.
6. Write legibly using dark ink (blue or black).
7. Recheck the medical history form to be sure all parts are complete. Note any additional information provided by patient. Make sure numbers, dates, spelling, and other information are accurate and legible.
8. Prepare the patient for the review of systems and physical examination if this is indicated.
9. Document the procedure.

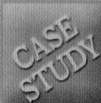

Maria Jover, a patient of Dr. Elizabeth King at Doctors Lewis & King, has finally convinced her teenage son to make an appointment for a physical. Adam Jover is 17, outgoing, fun loving, and apparently healthy. But Maria is concerned that he may be engaging in harmful social activities and hopes that by seeing Dr. Winston Lewis, Adam may discover ways to protect himself and his health. Adam agreed to the appointment but is adamant that his mother not accompany him. At the ambulatory care setting, it is decided that Adam might be more forthcoming with a male medical assistant, so Joe Guerrero is scheduled to take Adam's medical history before Dr. Winston does a review of systems.

CASE STUDY REVIEW

1. When Joe Guerrero first sits down with Adam to take the history, he notices that Adam is very ill at ease and nervous. What can Joe do to reassure Adam that his privacy will be protected?

2. When Joe attempts to take the social history, Adam seems evasive about answering Joe's questions and finally admits that he doesn't want his mother, Maria, to know about his social activities. What is Joe's response?

3. By the end of the interview, it becomes apparent that Adam may be engaging in some behaviors that put him at high risk for contracting the HIV virus. How can Joe provide Adam with guidance without alienating him?

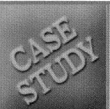

CASE STUDY 23-2

Harvey DiAntonio is a 46-year-old patient who lives at 45 W. Smith Avenue, Baltimore, Maryland, 21208. His date of birth is July 8, 1954. His phone number is 667-1870. He is a Baltimore City fire fighter and has been for 21 years. He has union medical insurance and Blue Cross/Blue Shield (BC/BS) is his carrier. His number is 211-67-87-56. He also carries major medical and his policy is Diagnostic #4. He has been referred by the fire department physician, Dr. Alan Byers. Mr. DiAntonio's complaint is severe "gripping" pain in the anterior mid-chest sometime radiating to the abdomen, neck, and both arms. Pain seems to occur with strenuous exercise, when walking uphill. Pain usually lasts 20 minutes with each episode. Pain does "ease up" when he ceases activity. Mr. DiAntonio states his episodes have occurred while he was shaving, climbing stairs at work, after a heavy meal, and during sexual intercourse. One episode last week was accompanied with dizziness, nausea, and fatigue. The episodes have been going on now once or twice a month for five months. Mr. DiAntonio's past history is essentially noncontributory. It is questionable whether this is due to good health or the fact that the patient has not had a physical examination for eight years. Surgeries include tonsillectomy and adenoidectomy, T & A, 1958, and appendectomy in 1964. Fractured rib, left side, in 1984 due to fire fighting incident. Usual childhood diseases. Hospitalized for observation, 1962, Sinai Hospital, for an unusually long episode of bronchitis. Social history shows that the patient is a pump operator on the job with much heavy exertion. Smokes 1½ to 2 packs of cigarettes per day and is a moderate drinker. He has a weight problem off and on and tends to eat too much while on duty. Lives in a one story home. Hobbies include carpentry and music. Some family problems and tension exist as both of his children are in adolescence. Patient describes himself as "fun-loving" with a "quick temper" and worries about meeting financial needs of the family. Is in a position to retire from active duty, but states he could not tolerate the boredom.

Family history shows both parents deceased—mother of heart attack, age 59, and father of unknown cause at age 49. Has two siblings, one brother with history of hypertension and one sister living and in good health. Has two children both living and well. Family history otherwise negative.

Physical examination revealed a well-nourished, well-developed male in no acute distress at this time. Patient does seem a bit anxious about this examination. T. 98.6 - P. 94 - R. 24 - BP 175/104. Ht. 69″, Wt. 198 pounds. HEAD, EYES, EARS, NOSE, THROAT—normal. NECK—supple. Trachea in midline. CHEST—normal in contour. Calcium deposit on left sixth rib probably due to history fracture. HEART—after careful examination with the patient recumbent and the scope placed lightly on the chest wall near the apex, a left atrial sound was heard (presystolic gallop). ABDOMEN—negative. EXTREMITIES—negative. GENITALIA—negative. SKIN—negative. NEUROLOGICAL—negative. Laboratory tests performed show a hemoglobin of 11.0 Gms. Awaiting results of serum cholesterol, calcium, phosphorus, and blood urea nitrogen. Chest X ray essentially negative. EKG report showed atrial sounds occurring presystolically with long P-R intervals. DIAGNOSIS: 1)Angina Pectoris. 2)Anemia 3)Hypertension. TREATMENT: Nitroglycerin tabs, sublingually as needed. To return to office in two weeks to follow medication effects. In consultation with patient, the patient was advised to control physical activity and quantity of food intake. Avoid extreme cold, 8 hours of sleep/night. Avoid emotional upsets. Attempt 4 meals/day. Low fat 1600 calorie diet. No smoking, moderate alcohol intake.

CASE STUDY REVIEW

1. Identify the following parts of the case study above and extract from the case study the portion that matches the appropriate medical history component.

   - Personal data
   - Chief complaint
   - Present illness
   - Past medical history
   - Family history
   - Social history
   - Review of systems

2. Using appropriate terminology and abbreviations, make a charting entry for Mr. DiAntonio by using the SOAP method of charting.

SUMMARY

The patient's medical chart or record is the mainstay of the medical practice. The history contained within it is the rationale for all decisions made by the physician for a patient. The more complete that information is, the better the physician can serve the patient. The more easily accessible the information in the chart is, the more efficiently the physician can treat the patient. The medical assistant must recognize the importance of documenting in the medical record information that concerns the patient, such as patient progress, care given, laboratory tests performed, prescription refills, and missed appointments. This collection of information must be accurate, concise, and complete and it must remain confidential.

REVIEW QUESTIONS

Multiple Choice

1. If the patient has difficulty with English, the medical assistant should:
   a. set up the appointment for the patient and obtain the services of an interpreter to be present as well
   b. not set the appointment until contact is made with the interpreter
   c. speak more loudly so the patient will understand
   d. suggest that the patient find a physician who speaks this language
2. If the patient's social history reflects exposure to sexually transmitted diseases including HIV, the medical assistant should:
   a. use standard precautions for this particular patient
   b. let the laboratory assistants know that there is a problem with this patient
   c. treat the patient the same as all other patients
   d. mark the chart somehow to alert to possible HIV patient
3. A helpful question to ask the returning patient is:
   a. Are you feeling bad today?
   b. Didn't you get better with the treatment prescribed last visit?
   c. Have you noticed any changes in your condition since your last visit?
   d. Do you realize you have gained six pounds since your visit last week?
4. When the patient complains of not feeling well, the medical assistant should:
   a. mark the chief complaint as "patient not feeling well"
   b. ask helpful questions to help the patient express specific problems or symptoms
   c. pin down the symptoms by guessing what the problem could be
   d. let the physician work with the patient

5. Source-oriented medical records:
   a. are chronological, and usually over a long period of time
   b. use lists such as lists of problems or lists of medications
   c. are the best for finding information quickly
   d. are best when many physicians see the patient

Critical Thinking

1. Name the sections of a medical history.
2. Define each section and state its importance.
3. What are the three main ways that new patients set up a first appointment?
4. How can a medical assistant help a patient provide a medical history?
5. What avenues of help are available to a medical assistant and physician for a patient with special needs?
6. What kinds of barriers should a medical assistant be prepared to encounter?
7. Name the methods of charting and compare them.
8. Where in a chart would you find a discharge summary? A follow-up visit for a consultation? A copy of the worker's compensation claim form?
9. What should be noted on the outside of the chart as well as in the chart notes?
10. What is the proper way to make a correction in a chart?

WEB ACTIVITIES

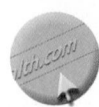

Using Case Study 23-2, go into the World Wide Web to research the treatment of Mr. Harvey DiAntonio's three diagnoses: coronary artery disease, hypertension, and anemia, using the National Institutes of Health as a resource.

REFERENCES/BIBLIOGRAPHY

Bonewit-West, K. (1995). *Clinical procedures for medical assistants* (4th ed.). Philadelphia: W. B. Saunders.

Frew, M. A., Lane, K., & Frew, D. (1995). *Comprehensive medical assisting: Competencies for administrative and clinical practice* (3rd ed.). Philadelphia: F. A. Davis.

Keir, L., Wise, B. A., & Krebs, C. (1998). *Medical assisting: Administrative and clinical competencies* (4th ed.). Albany, NY: Delmar.

Kinn, M. E., & Woods, M. A. (1999). *The medical assistant: Administrative and clinical* (8th ed.). Philadelphia: W. B. Saunders.

Prinkett-Ramutrowski, B., Barrie, A., Keller, C., Dazarow, L., & Abel, C. (1999). *Medical assisting: A patient-centered approach to administrative and clinical competencies*. New York: McGraw Hill.

Zakus, S. (1995). *Clinical procedures for medical assistants* (3rd ed.). St. Louis: Mosby LifeLine, Mosby-Year Book, Inc.

VITAL SIGNS AND MEASUREMENTS

KEY TERMS

Afebrile
Apical
Apnea
Arrhythmia
Baseline
Bradycardia
Bradypnea
Cheyne-Stokes
Diastole
Dyspnea
Emphysema
Eupnea
Febrile
Frenulum
Hyperpnea
Hypertension
Hyperventilation
Hypotension
Hypoventilation
Orthopnea
Pyrexia
Rales
Rhonchi
Stertorous
Stridor
Systole
Tachycardia
Tachypnea
Wheezes

OUTLINE

The Importance of Accuracy
Temperature
    Terms Used to Describe Body
        Temperature
    Types of Thermometers
    Recording Temperature
    Measuring Temperature
    Cleaning and Storage of
        Thermometers
Pulse
    Pulse Sites
    Measuring a Pulse
    Normal Pulse Rates
    Pulse Abnormalities
    Recording Pulse Rates

Respiration
    Respiration Rate
    Abnormalities
Blood Pressure
    Equipment for Measuring Blood
        Pressure
    Measuring Blood Pressure
    Recording Blood Pressure
        Measurement
    Normal Blood Pressure Readings
    Blood Pressure Abnormalities
Height and Weight
    Height
    Weight
    Significance of Weight
Measuring Chest Circumference

OBJECTIVES

The student should strive to meet the following performance objectives and demonstrate an understanding of the facts and principles presented in this chapter through written and oral communication.

1. Define the key terms as presented in the glossary.

2. Discuss normal and abnormal temperatures, including factors affecting temperature.

3. Identify and explain the procedures for using, caring for, and storing of the various types of thermometers.

4. Describe the locations and procedure for obtaining pulse rate.

5. Explain the procedure for obtaining respiration rates.

6. Identify and describe normal and abnormal pulse and respiratory rates and the factors affecting each.

7. Describe the appropriate equipment and procedure for obtaining a blood pressure measurement. *(continues)*

8. Identify normal and abnormal blood pressure, including factors affecting blood pressure.

9. Describe the procedures for obtaining height, weight, and chest measurements of adults.

10. Accurately record measurements on the patient chart.

ROLE DELINEATION COMPONENTS

CLINICAL

Fundamental Principles

- Apply principles of aseptic technique and infection control
- Comply with quality assurance practices

Patient Care

- Obtain patient history and vital signs
- Prepare and maintain examination and treatment areas
- Prepare patient for examinations, procedures, and treatments
- Assist with examinations, procedures, and treatments

GENERAL (TRANSDISCIPLINARY)

Legal Concepts

- Document accurately

SCENARIO

At Doctors Lewis & King, clinical medical assistant Joe Guerrero, CMA, assists both physicians in taking patients' vital signs. One of his favorite patients is Abigail Johnson, a friendly woman in her seventies who always has a kind disposition despite her financial and medical difficulties. Abigail is overweight and suffers from hypertension, so her blood pressure is monitored on a regular basis to be certain that it is under control. In reviewing Abigail's chart, Joe notices that her blood pressure has been quite stable for the last few visits. He also checks her weight and notices that Abigail is slowly losing weight. Abigail's chart, with its history of blood pressure and other measurements, informs Joe's perspective and is a helpful record when evaluating the progress Abigail has made since she became a patient three years ago.

INTRODUCTION

One of the most important and commonly performed tasks of a medical assistant is obtaining and recording patient vital signs. Vital signs, also sometimes referred to as cardinal signs, include temperature, pulse, respiration, and blood pressure, abbreviated TPR B/P. They are indicative of the general health and well-being of a patient, and with regular monitoring, may measure patient response to treatment. Vital signs, in total or in part, are an important component of each patient visit. Height and weight measurements, while not considered vital signs are often a routine part of a patient visit.

Patients will exhibit vital sign readings that are uniquely their own. As a result, baseline assessments of vital signs are usually obtained during the patient's initial visit. These baseline results are used as a reference point for future readings, differentiating between what is normal and abnormal for the patient.

 Two extremely important habits must be developed by the medical assistant before taking a patient's vital signs: aseptic technique in the form of hand washing and recognition and correction of factors that may influence results of vital signs. Proper hand washing before taking vital signs will assist in preventing cross contamination of patients. Refer to the discussion on standard precautions and medical asepsis in Chapter 22. Also, emotional factors of patients must be recognized and addressed. Explaining procedures and allowing the patient the opportunity to relax will ease apprehension that may affect readings.

THE IMPORTANCE OF ACCURACY

Vital signs may be altered by many factors. Medical assistants must recognize and correct factors that may produce inaccurate results. For example, patients may exhibit anxiety over potential test results or findings of the physician. They may be angry or may have rushed into the office. A patient may have had something to eat or drink prior to the visit or may have had a long wait in the reception area. Patient apprehension and mood must always be considered by the medical assistant, for these factors can affect vital signs. The medical assistant may be required to take vital signs more than once during an office visit to ascertain a baseline and obtain an impression of overall well-being of the patient.

Accuracy in taking vital signs is necessary because treatment plans are developed according to the measurement of the vital signs. Variations can indicate a new disease process or the patient's response to treatment. They may also indicate the patient's compliance with a treatment plan. Although taking vital signs is a task commonly performed by the medical assistant, it is never to be taken casually or lightly, and should never be rushed or incompletely performed. Concentration and attention to proper procedure will help assure accurate measurements and quality care of the patient. The following text will discuss procedures used to measure the vital signs of children and adults. Procedures used for infant examinations will be discussed in Chapter 27.

TEMPERATURE

Body temperature is maintained and regulated by two processes functioning in conjunction with one another: heat production and heat loss.

Body heat is produced by the actions of voluntary and involuntary muscles. As the muscles move, they use energy which, in response, produces heat. Cellular metabolic activities such as the process of breaking food-sugars down to simpler components (catabolism), are another source of heat.

The body loses heat by a combination of five processes:

1. *Convection.* The process by which heat is lost through the skin by being transferred from the skin by air currents flowing across it; such as a fan used on a hot day for cooling purposes.
2. *Conduction.* The transfer of heat from within the body to the surface of the skin and then to surrounding cooler objects touching the skin, such as clothing.
3. *Radiation.* Body heat lost from the surface of the skin to a cooler environment, much like a cool room becoming warm when occupied by many people.
4. *Evaporation.* A heat loss mechanism that uses heat absorption through vaporization of perspiration.

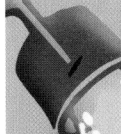

SPOTLIGHT ON AAMA ESSENTIALS THROUGH CAAHEP

- It is important to remember that some cultures may ingest certain foods or maintain specific lifestyles that could affect a patient's vital signs.

- Teaching the patient about methods of health promotion and disease prevention should be part of the process of measuring his or her vital signs.

- When you take vital signs, maintaining a positive attitude and attempting to get the patient to relax by explaining the procedure will help you to achieve a more accurate measurement.

5. *Elimination.* Heat that is lost through the normal functioning of the intestinal, urinary, and respiratory tracts.

The delicate balance between heat production and heat loss is maintained by the hypothalamus in the brain. The hypothalamus monitors blood temperature and will trigger either the heat loss or heat production mechanism with as little as 0.04°F change in blood temperature. Body temperature is measured in degrees and is influenced by several factors.

An increase of temperature may result from a bacterial infection, increased physical activity or food intake, exposure to heat, pregnancy, drugs that increase metabolism, stress and severe emotional reactions, and age. Age becomes a factor in that infants have an average body temperature that is one to two degrees higher than adults.

Decrease in temperature may result from viral infections, decreased muscular activity, fasting, a depressed emotional state, exposure to cold, drugs that decrease metabolic activities, and age. Age in this instance refers to the elderly, in that the elderly have decreased metabolic activity resulting in a decrease in body temperature.

Another factor that can increase or decrease body temperature is time of day. During sleep and early morning the temperature is at its lowest, while later in the day with muscular and metabolic activity the temperature increases.

Due to the many factors influencing body temperature and the uniqueness of individuals there is no "normal" temperature. The medical assistant must think of temperatures in terms of the "average," which for an adult is 98.6°F, or 37.0°C.

Terms Used to Describe Body Temperature

The following terms are used to describe body temperature:

- afebrile: absence of fever

- febrile: fever is present

- *fever:* body temperature elevated beyond normal range. Pyrexia is another term for fever.

- *onset:* time when fever begins

- *lysis:* body temperature gradually returns to normal following a period of fever

- *crisis:* body temperature drops suddenly to normal levels, the patient may perspire profusely (diaphoresis)

- *intermittent:* a fluctuating fever that returns to or below baseline, then rises again

- *remittent:* a fluctuating fever that does not return to the baseline temperature. It fluctuates, but remains elevated.

- *continuous:* a fever that remains above the baseline. It does not fluctuate, but remains fairly constant.

Figure 24-1 depicts types of fever.

Types of Thermometers

There are four types of thermometers available for use in the ambulatory care setting:

- mercury (or clinical)

- disposable

- digital

- tympanic

Mercury or Clinical Thermometers. These thermometers are made of glass with a bulb end containing mercury. As temperature increases, the mercury expands and rises in a column located within the thermometer. These have been used for many years. There are two types of mercury thermometers. One, commonly used in the United States, measures temperature in Fahrenheit (F) while the other measures in Celsius (C). There are charts

available that convert one scale to the other; however, the medical assistant can quickly and accurately calculate the conversion by using the following formulas:

To convert °F to °C = F temperature, subtract 32, then multiply by ⅝

To convert °C to °F = C temperature, multiply by ⅗, then add 32

Mercury thermometers are available in three styles: oral with a slender and elongated tip and blue color-coded end; rectal with a rounded tip and red color-coded end; and security for axillary measurement with a rounded tip with no color coding on the end. See Figure 24-2. Mercury thermometers are cleaned and disinfected with soap and cool water, rinsed, dried, and soaked in a disinfectant solution for at least thirty minutes. Oral and rectal thermometers are never placed in the same solution nor cleansed together as cross contamination with microorganisms from rectal to oral can occur.

 To prevent patient-to-patient cross contamination, a disposable plastic sheath is placed on all clinical thermometers when in use.

Disposable Thermometers. These are individually wrapped strips with heat-sensitive dots that change color to indicate temperature. They are used once and then discarded. There are strips for use on the forehead and others for oral use. Although strips are easy to use and prevent patient cross contamination, accuracy is questionable.

Digital Thermometers. These are widely used handheld battery-operated units that have easy-to-read digital display screens to indicate results (Figure 24-3). Digital thermometers are available in Fahrenheit or Celsius scales. Probes are attached and are color coded blue for oral, and red for rectal. The probes have disposable plastic covers. The plastic cover acts as a barrier to prevent contamination of the probe and is replaced for each patient to prevent cross contamination of the patient. An accurate result can be obtained in approximately ten seconds.

Tympanic Thermometers. The use of tympanic thermometers is becoming more popular as they are fast, provide no discomfort to the patient, can be used on infants as well as adults, and are usually accurate. They consist of a handheld unit with a probe tip that is inserted into the ear securely to make a seal. Disposable tips are used to prevent cross contamination. Accurate results are obtained in less than two seconds. With the tympanic method of measuring body temperature, the procedure is complete in a few seconds. It is comfortable for the

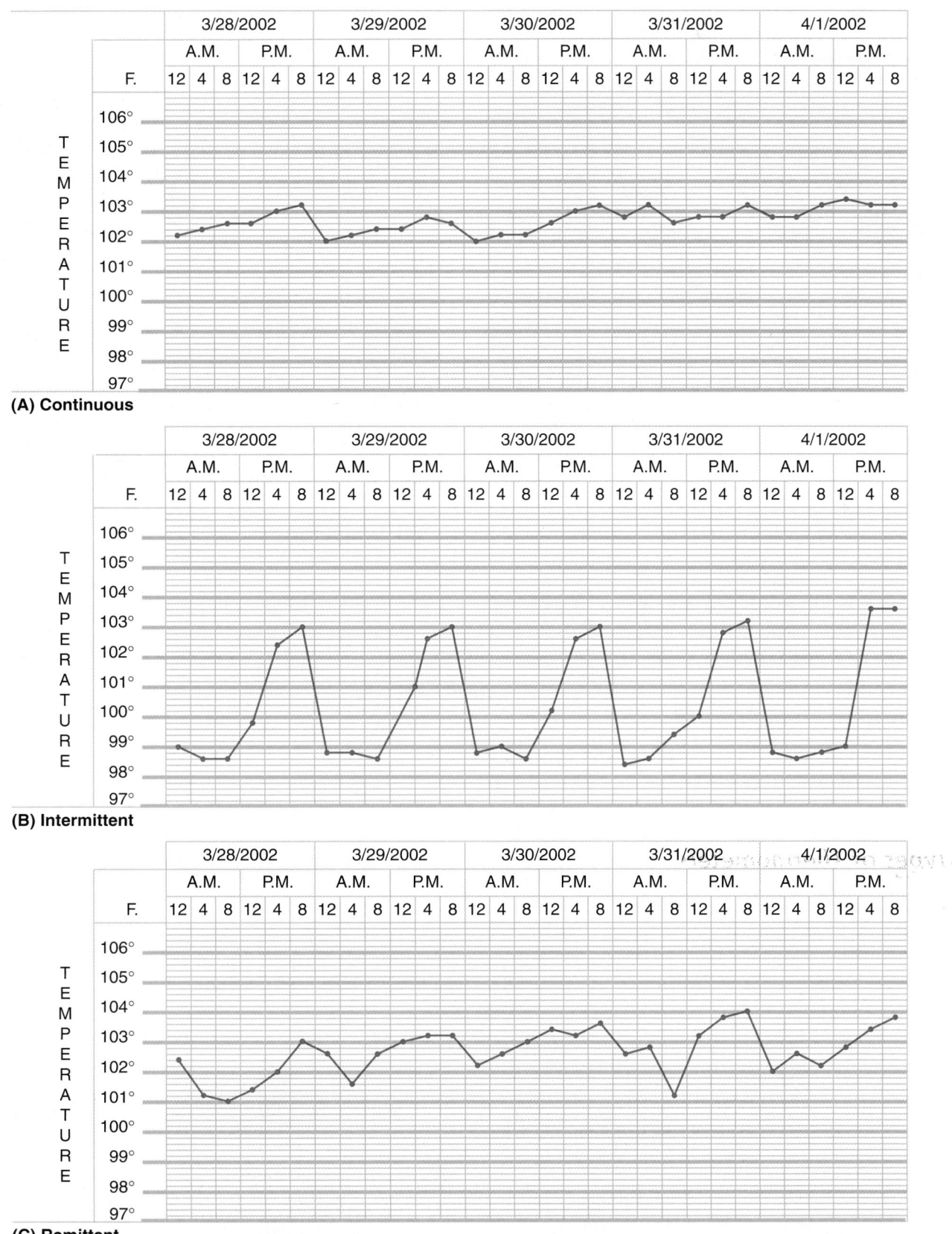

Figure 24-1 Types of Fevers. (A) Continuous—remains above baseline. Does not fluctuate. (B) Intermittent—a fluctuating fever. Returns to or below baseline, then rises again. (C) Remittent—a fluctuating fever, but does not return to baseline temperature. Remains elevated, but fluctuates.

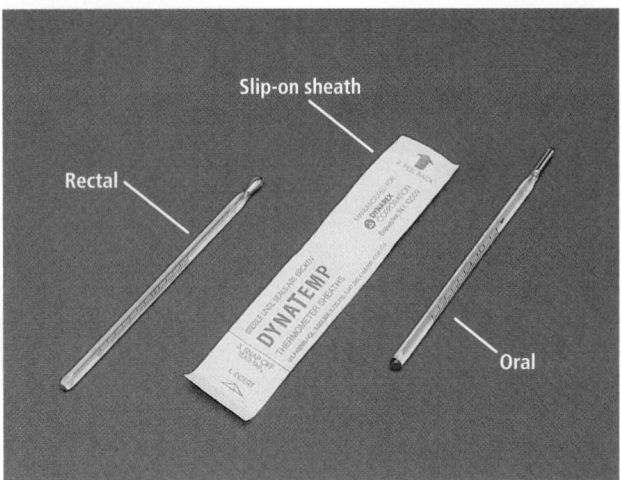

Figure 24-2   Mercury reusable thermometers with disposable plastic slip-on sheath.

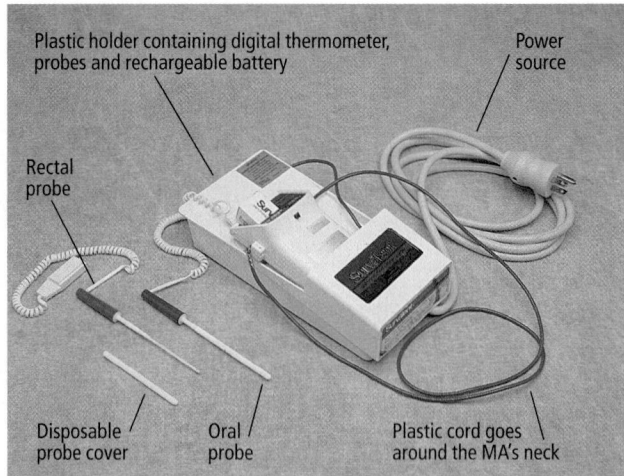

Figure 24-3   Digital thermometers have interchangeable oral and rectal probes attached to a battery-operated portable unit.

patient, nonthreatening to infants and children, and may be used when other methods are inappropriate. It is the thermometer of choice for pediatric patients over two years of age. However, physicians have found that inaccurate readings can result if patients have impacted cerumen in the ear of which they may be unaware. Also, if the patient has otitis media, a middle ear infection, the reading tends to be inaccurate.

Recording Temperature

Temperature may be taken on each visit to the physician's office in order to obtain a baseline for the patient. When recording the temperature, the scale used for the results must be designated (F) for Fahrenheit and (C) for Celsius. The route used must be labeled as well; methods other than oral must be labeled according to the route used as there is a difference in the measurement. Use (R) for rectal, and (A) for axillary.

Temperatures obtained by mercury and digital thermometers will be recorded as shown:

Oral   T 98.6°F
Rectal   T 99.6°(R) F
Axillary   T 97.6°(A) F

When a facility uses a tympanic thermometer exclusively, the route is known and therefore does not have to be labeled.

The medical assistant must read all manufacturer's instructions before using any digital or tympanic thermometer. Each may have a slight difference in operating procedure.

Procedures 24-1 through 24-7 detail steps involved in taking temperature by various routes.

Measuring Temperature

Oral Temperatures. To read a mercury thermometer, hold the thermometer at eye level and move it slightly until the mercury column can be seen. Note where the mercury is in relation to the numbers and lines on the thermometer. The longer lines on a Fahrenheit scale are calibrated by one full degree while the smaller lines are calibrated by two-tenths of a degree (Figure 24-4). On a Celsius thermometer, each long line represents a degree.

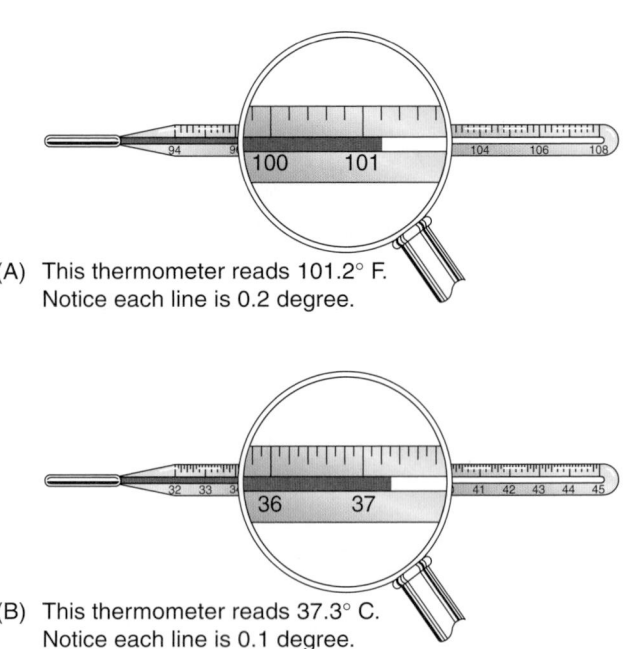

(A) This thermometer reads 101.2° F. Notice each line is 0.2 degree.

(B) This thermometer reads 37.3° C. Notice each line is 0.1 degree.

Figure 24-4   (A) Fahrenheit thermometer. (B) Celsius thermometer.

They are numbered consecutively, with nine lines between numbers, each line representing one-tenth of a degree. See Procedure 24-1 to take an oral temperature using a mercury thermometer.

To use an oral strip for taking a temperature, follow the same steps as with a mercury thermometer. Make certain that the package is not damaged then peel it back to reveal the strip. The strip is then inserted into the patient's mouth. After the appropriate time interval has elapsed, the thermometer is removed and the dots that have changed color are read using the scale located on the strip. While convenient to use, accuracy is not always assured with the strips and therefore they may not be appropriate for clinical use. See Procedure 24-2 to take an oral temperature using a disposable oral strip.

The procedure for obtaining an oral temperature with a digital thermometer (see Procedure 24-3) follows the same steps as when using a mercury thermometer. The digital thermometer is stored on a recharging base. When it is removed from the base, it is turned on and ready for use. A disposable cover is placed over the blue probe for oral temperatures. The probe is placed in the patient's mouth following the same procedures as used with a mercury thermometer. When the temperature has been obtained, the thermometer will beep at which time the temperature will be displayed on the screen. The probe cover is ejected into a biohazard container and the unit is returned to the base. The temperature is then recorded in the patient chart. Always read and follow the manufacturer's directions for use and care of a digital unit.

Aural Temperature.

Taking a temperature with a tympanic thermometer is a fast, safe method for obtaining a patient's temperature. This is becoming quite common in ambulatory care settings. Tympanic temperature can be obtained without discomfort for the patient whether elder, infant, or reluctant.

The tympanic thermometer measures the patient's temperature by measuring the infrared waves produced by the tympanic membrane and recording the temperature in less than two to three seconds on a digital screen. The tympanic membrane and the hypothalamus of the brain share the same blood supply, thus an accurate measurement of the body temperature can be obtained.

The greatest benefits of the tympanic thermometer are that it

- gives nearly instant results

- does not come into contact with mucous membranes, thereby minimizing cross contamination

- uses a site that is readily accessible

- is not affected by the patient smoking or drinking hot or cold liquids

- does not require that the patient be conscious

- is an easy instrument to use. The unit is battery operated and uses a disposable probe cover or ear speculum

Drawbacks to the tympanic thermometer have been demonstrated in pediatric patients with ear conditions such as otitis media. An inaccurate recording can result because the fluid buildup in the inner ear limits infrared wave transmission.

The tympanic thermometer is a handheld unit that is inserted into the outer third of the ear canal. See Procedure 24-4 to obtain an aural temperature using a tympanic thermometer.

Rectal Temperature.

The rectal method of obtaining a temperature is used on infants and young children and patients who are unable or incapable of cooperating with the oral method of temperature taking. Pediatric procedures are covered in Chapter 27. Patients experiencing breathing difficulties, such as an upper respiratory infection, asthma, or emphysema, or unable to follow instructions, as seen with senility, mental retardation, or Alzheimer's disease, will require a rectal temperature method. Rectal temperatures will have a reading that is approximately one degree higher than oral temperatures because the rectum is a closed body cavity. See Procedure 24-5 to measure a rectal temperature using a mercury thermometer.

See Procedure 24-6 for using a digital thermometer to measure the rectal temperature. The red probe is covered with a plastic cover and lubricated. Insert gently ½ inch for infants, 1 inch for a child, and 1½ inches for an adult. When the temperature registers, the thermometer will beep and provide a readout on the screen. The plastic cover is ejected into a biohazard container.

Axillary Temperature.

An axillary temperature may be used when the patient is an infant or for other reasons is unable to have an oral or rectal temperature taken. This method may be used for patients who display breathing difficulties or who are unable to follow directions as a result of mental incapacity. This is the least accurate method of obtaining a patient's temperature and should be used when other routes are unavailable or inappropriate. An axillary temperature is approximately one degree lower than an oral temperature because the axilla is an open body cavity.

Cleaning and Storage of Thermometers

Oral and rectal mercury thermometers must always be kept separated. Axillary security thermometers may be cleaned with the oral thermometers. The thermometer is rinsed immediately after use, then cleansed in a mild soap and cool water solution. Then the thermometer is dried and placed in a disinfectant solution, such as 70 percent isopropyl alcohol or solution of Zephiran Chloride for thirty minutes. Before storage or use, the thermometer must be rinsed and carefully dried. Storage will depend upon the policy of the facility. Containers used to store clean and uncleaned thermometers must be labeled to prevent possible improper use and cross contamination. Containers must be emptied and cleaned daily. New solution will be added according to the manufacturer's direction and at each cleaning.

Digital and tympanic thermometers are cleaned according to the manufacturer's directions. The covers protect the probes from contamination. Each type of thermometer will have a storage case or a wall-mounted base made specially for storing the unit. Disinfect these types of thermometers by wiping with a solution of 70 percent alcohol.

PULSE

The pulse rate consists of two phases of the heart action and can be felt when compressing an artery. As the heart contracts it increases pressure on the arterial walls. The increased pressure passes through the arteries in a wave-like movement resulting in a slight expansion in the arterial wall. When the heart relaxes, the pressure is decreased in the arteries, resulting in the wall returning to its previous position. One contraction and relaxation of the heart is equal to one heart cycle or heart beat. The pulse and heartbeat rate should be the same.

Pulse Sites

The pulse can be felt in those areas of the body where an artery is close to the surface and an underlying solid structure such as a bone. The common pulse sites include the radial, carotid, temporal, brachial, femoral, popliteal, and dorsalis pedis arteries (Figure 24-5). An apical pulse, located at the apex of the heart, may also be taken. Although the radial, brachial, and carotid arteries are the most frequently used sites for pulse rates, it is important to recognize pulse beats because circulation may be monitored by palpating the other sites. Pulse sites are also used when necessary as pressure points for controlling severe bleeding.

- The *radial* pulse is located at the thumb side of the wrist approximately one inch above the base of the thumb. This is the most commonly used site for obtaining a pulse rate.

- The *carotid* pulse, used during emergency situations and when performing CPR, is found between the larynx and sternocleidomastoid muscle in the front side of the neck on either side of the trachea.

- The *brachial* pulse is found in the inner aspect of the elbow called the antecubital space. This pulse site is the most commonly used site to obtain blood pressure measurements.

- The *temporal* pulse is located at the temple area of the head. It is rarely used to obtain a pulse rate but may be used to monitor circulation or control bleeding from the head and scalp.

- The *femoral* pulse is located in the groin area. It is a deep artery and must be compressed firmly to be felt.

- The *popliteal* pulse is located at the back of the knee. The patient must be in a supine position with the knee flexed for it to be felt as the artery is deep within the knee. This artery is the one used for leg blood pressure measurements and to monitor circulation.

- The *dorsalis pedis* pulse is felt on the top of the foot slightly to the side of midline next to the extensor ligament of the great toe, between the first and second metatarsal bones. It is commonly used to monitor lower limb circulation.

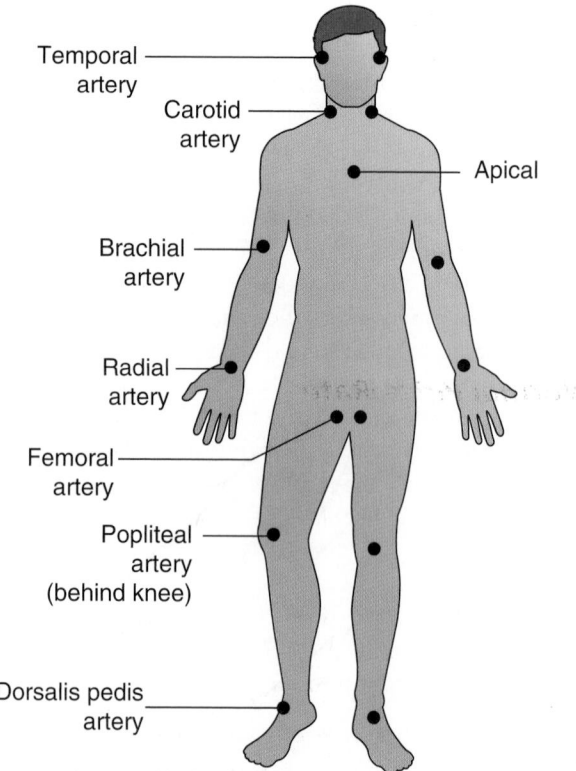

Figure 24-5   Pulse sites in the body.

Apical *pulse* is found at the apex of the heart, located at the fifth intercostal space left side, midclavicular line. That is, between the fifth and sixth ribs in the middle of the clavicle (usually below the nipple), left of the sternum. A stethoscope is required to obtain an apical pulse. Apical pulse is used on cardiac patients and to obtain infant pulse rates as they are difficult to obtain by the usual methods.

Measuring a Pulse

When measuring a pulse rate, other characteristics besides the rate must also be noted. These characteristics include rhythm, volume of pulse, and condition of the arterial wall.

The rate is the number of pulsations or beats felt for one minute. Pulse rates may vary according to age, activities, general health, gender, emotions, pain, and medications. The rate is lower when sleeping and higher when active or exercising. Rates for infants and children are higher than for adults. Well-conditioned athletes will have a lower than average resting rate as their cardiovascular system has been developed to function more efficiently.

Rhythm of the pulse refers to the time between pulsations and regularity of the beat. Normal rhythm occurs when the beats are felt at regular intervals. Abnormal rhythms, arrhythmias, are those rhythms in which the interval between pulsations is altered by either an increased or decreased time span. Arrhythmias must be noted and reported as they may indicate heart disease.

The volume of the pulse refers to the strength of the beat that is felt. The pulsations may feel full, strong, hard, soft, thready, or weak. A pulse may have a regular rate and yet have a variation in intensity or volume. Volume should be noted and reported.

Condition of the arterial wall can be felt as the pulse is taken. The normal artery feels soft and elastic. The abnormal artery may feel hard, knotty, wiry, or a combination of these. These should be noted and reported as they may indicate cardiac disease.

Normal Pulse Rates

Average pulse rates vary from birth to adulthood. At birth the pulse rate is much higher; as we age it generally decreases. Average rate by age group:

Birth	130–160 beats per minute
Infants	110–130 beats per minute
Children (between 1 and 7 years)	80–120 beats per minute
Children over 7 years	80–90 beats per minute
Adults	60–80 beats per minute

Pulse Abnormalities

Abnormalities may be in the rate, rhythm, and feel of the arterial wall.

Common pulse rate abnormalities include bradycardia, a pulse rate less than 60 beats per minute, and tachycardia, a pulse rate greater than 100 beats per minute. Common arrhythmias would include a pulsation felt before expected, which is called a premature ventricular contraction or PVC, and sinus arrhythmia. An occasional premature contraction can occur in response to stress, caffeine, nicotine, alcohol, or lack of sleep. Sinus arrhythmia is a variation of rhythm during respiration and may be found in children and young adults. The rate increases with inspiration and decreases with expiration. This usually does not require treatment.

When any pulse rate abnormalities or arrhythmias are felt, they must be noted, recorded, and the physician alerted. See Chapter 37 for information on electrocardiography.

Recording Pulse Rates

Pulse rates are normally recorded after the temperature, for example: T 98.6° P 72 regular. Any unusual findings should be recorded and reported to the physician.

Procedure 24-8 describes measuring a radial pulse; Procedure 24-9 describes measuring an apical pulse.

RESPIRATION

The function of respiration (breathing) is the exchange of gases: oxygen and carbon dioxide. External respiration occurs when oxygen is drawn into the lungs and carbon dioxide is expelled from the lungs. Internal respiration occurs when oxygen is used by the cells for cellular function. Carbon dioxide is a byproduct of cellular function and is expelled as a waste product. Respiration is an involuntary act controlled by the medulla oblongata of the brain. The medulla oblongata measures blood levels of carbon dioxide and triggers a respiration when the level of carbon dioxide increases. Although it is an involuntary act, respiration may be altered by holding the breath or when hyperventilation occurs. One inspiration (inhalation) drawing in of air, and one expiration (exhalation) expelling air, equals one respiration.

Characteristics of respiration such as rate, rhythm, and depth are noted when measuring respiration.

Respiratory rate is the number of respirations per minute. The normal respiratory rate, eupnea, varies with age, activities, illness, emotions, and drugs. The normal respiration rate to pulse rate is 1:4, one respiration to four pulse beats.

Respiratory rhythm refers to the pattern of breathing. This can vary with age, with adults having a regular pattern while infants have an irregular pattern. Rhythm may be altered by laughing and sighing.

Normal respiratory rates:

Infants	30–60 respirations per minute
Children (1–7 years)	18–30 respirations per minute
Adults	12–20 respirations per minute

Depth of respiration is the amount of air that is inspired and expired with each respiration. In the resting state, the amount should be consistent. Depth is noted by watching the degree of rise and fall of the chest wall when measuring respiration rate.

Respiration Rate

Procedure 24-10 describes steps involved in measuring respiration rate.

Abnormalities

Abnormalities of the respiration rate may be found in the rate, depth, rhythm, and sounds of respiration.

Rate abnormalities include apnea, tachypnea, bradypnea, and Cheyne-Stokes.

Apnea is the temporary complete absence of breathing. This may be a result of a reduction in stimuli to the respiratory center of the brain. Apnea will occur when the breath is voluntarily held and in Cheyne-Stokes respiration. It can be a serious symptom of other conditions of the cardiovascular and renal systems. It also can result from a head injury such as a concussion.

Tachypnea is a respiratory rate greater than 40 respirations per minute. It may be caused by hysteria or be transient in the newborn. Excessive loss of carbon dioxide may occur if tachypnea is prolonged; there is a potential for this to lead to more serious problems.

Bradypnea is a decrease in the number of respirations and is commonly seen during sleep or due to certain diseases.

Cheyne-Stokes is a regular pattern of irregular breathing rate. The cycle starts with a period of apnea lasting 10 to 60 seconds followed by increasing depth and rate of respiration, which is then followed by a decrease in rate with apnea starting the cycle once again. This cycle may be normal for children, but may indicate brain dysfunction.

Orthopnea is a respiratory condition of severe dyspnea (labored breathing). Breathing is difficult in any position *other* than sitting erect or standing. This may be seen in patients with heart failure, angina pectoris, asthma,

pulmonary edema, emphysema, pneumonia, and spasmodic coughing. Patients who experience orthopnea must be examined in a sitting position. Other positions will cause discomfort and not be possible.

Abnormalities in the depth of respiration may be divided into shallow abnormalities, such as hypoventilation, and deep abnormalities, such as hyperpnea and hyperventilation.

Hypoventilation occurs when respiration is decreased in rate and shallow in depth, and may result from a depression of nervous stimuli of the respiratory center in the brain.

Hyperpnea is respiration that is increased both in depth and rate. This is commonly seen with activities such as physical exercise. It can also be associated with pain, respiratory diseases, cardiac diseases, hysteria, and some drugs.

Hyperventilation is a type of breathing in which the amounts of oxygen drawn in during inspiration are greatly increased; this results in a decrease in the amount of blood carbon dioxide. Hyperventilation may be associated with asthma, pulmonary embolism or edema, and acute anxiety. The patient may be treated by reducing the amount of oxygen inhaled during an inspiration. The patient may be instructed to hold one nostril closed while breathing or may be instructed to breathe into a paper bag. Either procedure will reduce the amount of inspired oxygen and bring the oxygen and carbon dioxide blood levels back to within normal range.

Breath Sounds. The presence or absence of breath sounds can be indicative of respiratory problems. Sounds should be listened for and noted when taking the patient's respiratory rate.

Rales and rhonchi are rattling sounds heard during inspiration and expiration when the lung passageways contain secretions. The physician uses a stethoscope to listen for rales, which are associated with some lung diseases. Rhonchi are sounds similar to snoring, usually produced by a rattle in the throat.

Wheezes are high-pitched musical sounds heard on expiration. They can be the result of an obstruction in the bronchi and bronchioles of the lungs. Wheezes are commonly associated with asthma and emphysema, a chronic pulmonary disease characterized by dilated and damaged alveoli.

Stridor is a crowing sound heard on inspiration as a result of an obstruction of the upper airway. It is associated with laryngitis, a foreign body obstruction, and croup in children.

Stertorous respiration is described as a snoring sound with labored breathing. The sound is created by obstruction of air passages in the head.

BLOOD PRESSURE

Blood pressure measures cardiovascular function by measuring the force of blood exerted on peripheral arteries during the cardiac cycle or heartbeat. The measurement consists of two components. The first is the force exerted on the arterial walls during cardiac contraction and is called systole. The second is the force exerted during cardiac relaxation and is called diastole. They represent the highest (systole) and lowest (diastole) amount of pressure exerted during the cardiac cycle. Blood pressure is recorded as a fraction with the systolic measurement written, followed by a slash, and then the diastolic measurement.

Example: systole/diastole or 120/80

Blood pressure may be affected by many factors including blood volume, peripheral resistance, vessel elasticity, condition of the muscle of the heart, genetics, diet and weight, activity, and emotional state.

- Blood volume is the amount of blood in the arteries. Increased volume increases blood pressure, while a decrease in volume will decrease blood pressure as in the case of a hemorrhage.

- Peripheral resistance is the resistance to blood flow in the arteries. The resistance is in direct relationship to the lumen of the arteries. The smaller the lumen, the more pressure needed to push blood through, while the reverse is true: the larger the lumen, the less resistance and less pressure needed to push the blood through. The size of the lumen can become smaller from deposits of fatty cholesterol, resulting in an increase in blood pressure.

- Vessel elasticity refers to the ability of arteries to expand and contract to provide a steady flow of blood. As a person ages, elasticity of the vessels is reduced. It can cause an increase in arterial wall resistance resulting in an increase in blood pressure.

- The condition of the heart muscle is extremely important to blood flow and blood pressure. A strong heart muscle provides a forceful pump resulting in efficient blood flow and normal blood pressure. A weak heart muscle results in an inefficient pumping action of the heart leading to a decrease in blood pressure and blood flow. See Chapter 37, Electrocardiography.

Equipment for Measuring Blood Pressure

Blood pressure is measured by the auscultatory (listening) method using a sphygmomanometer and a stethoscope (Figure 24-6). There are two types of sphygmomanometers commonly used in the ambulatory care setting: mercury manometer and aneroid manometer (Figures 24-7 and 24-8).

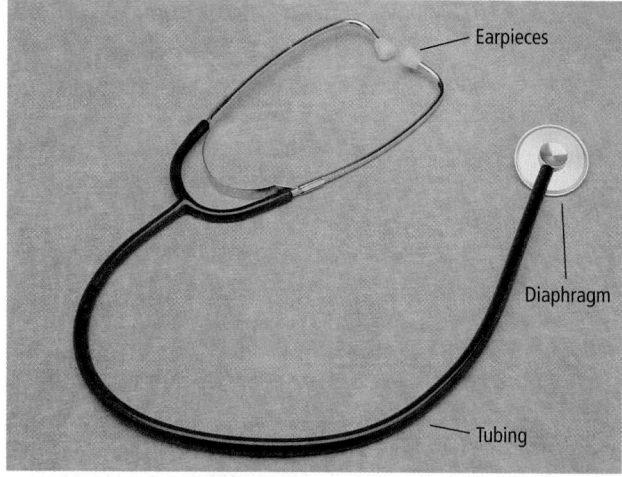

Figure 24-6 A single-head stethoscope. Used with a sphygmomanometer to measure blood pressure.

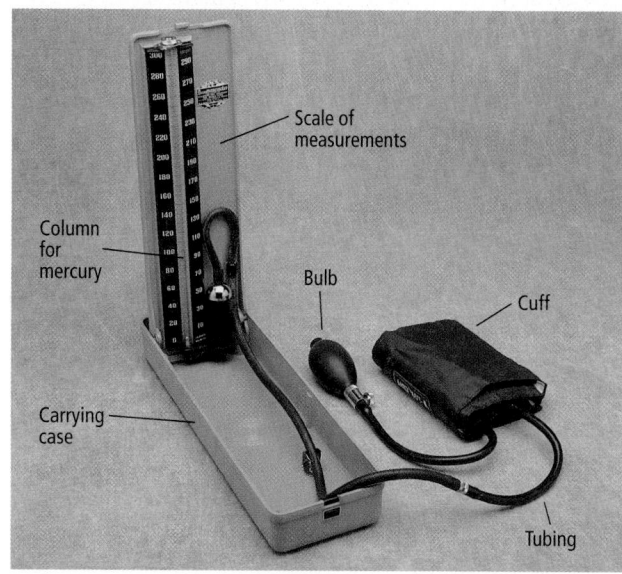

Figure 24-7 Mercury sphygmomanometer with cuff.

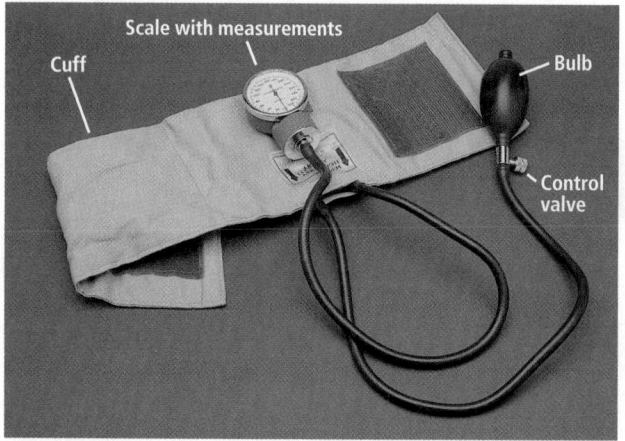

Figure 24-8 Aneroid sphygmomanometer.

The mercury manometer consists of a cuff containing a rubber bladder attached by rubber tubing to a glass column of mercury. The blood pressure is read at the meniscus of the mercury as it descends the column. Mercury manometers are the most accurate method of blood pressure measurement and are considered the standard as blood pressure is measured in millimeters of mercury. Although the most accurate, mercury manometers do have disadvantages: they are not as portable as aneroid manometers, and there is always the danger of a mercury spill should the glass column break. Mercury manometers need to be cleaned and checked regularly for accuracy by a professional technician. Care in handling and storage is important to prevent air bubbles and dirt from forming in the column or breaking the glass containing the mercury.

The aneroid manometer is a cuff containing a rubber bladder attached to a dial. The blood pressure is read at the level of the needle descending the dial. Aneroid manometers need to be calibrated regularly as they do not maintain calibration easily. Care in handling and storage will decrease the loss of calibration. While not as accurate as a mercury manometer, aneroid manometers are easily portable and there is no danger of a mercury spill.

Cuff sizes in both mercury and aneroid manometers range from the smallest cuff to the largest obese and thigh cuff (Figure 24-9). The appropriate cuff size is necessary in order to obtain an accurate blood pressure measurement. A cuff that is too small will give an artificially high blood pressure reading, while a cuff that is too large will give an artificially low reading. The selection of the cuff size depends upon the size of the arm, not the age of the patient. Due to the size of the arm, it may be necessary to use an adult-size cuff on a child or a pediatric-size cuff on an adult. Adult cuffs should have a width that covers one-third to one-half the circumference of the arm. The

length of the bladder should cover approximately 80 percent of the arm (about twice the size of the width). The cuff for a child should cover two-thirds of the upper arm.

Measuring Blood Pressure

The sounds heard during blood pressure measurement are named the Korotkoff sounds. The cause of the sounds is not known. They may be a result of distention of the vessels or the sound of the blood passing through the vessels. In either case, Korotkoff sounds have five distinct phases.

- *Phase I.* Begins with the first sound heard when deflating the cuff. It is a sharp tapping sound. Note this first sound as this will be the *systolic reading* of the blood pressure.

- *Phase II.* This sound is the result of more blood passing through the vessels as the cuff is deflated. The sound is that of a soft swishing sound.

- *Phase III.* More blood continues to pass through the vessels as the cuff is deflated. The sound is a rhythmic tapping sound. If blood pressure measurements are not carefully followed and Phases I and II are missed, Phase III may erroneously be reported as the systolic pressure.

- *Phase IV.* Blood is now passing through the vessels fairly easily as the cuff is deflated. The sounds heard will be a muffling and fading of the tapping sounds. This phase may be used to record the diastolic pressure in children and in those patients where a tapping sound is heard to zero.

- *Phase V.* Blood is flowing freely at this time, consequently all sounds disappear. The disappearance of sounds is noted and recorded as the *diastolic pressure*.

The procedure for taking blood pressure is a two-step method called the palpatory method. Step one of the method establishes the peak inflation level and is performed by placing the cuff on the patient's arm, palpating the radial pulse, and with a smooth pumping action inflating the cuff until the radial pulse can no longer be felt. The number where the radial pulse disappears is noted. The cuff is then deflated and the arm allowed to rest for a minute or two. The peak inflation level is then calculated by taking that number and adding 30 millimeters to it. This gives an indication as to the level to which to inflate the cuff when ausculating or listening to the sounds for the systolic and diastolic measurements. The purpose of this method is twofold: (1) patient comfort is assured as the cuff is not unnecessarily overinflated; (2) this procedure eliminates the possibility of missing an auscultatory gap. Auscultatory gap is heard in some patients. It is a time, usually between Phase I and II or III,

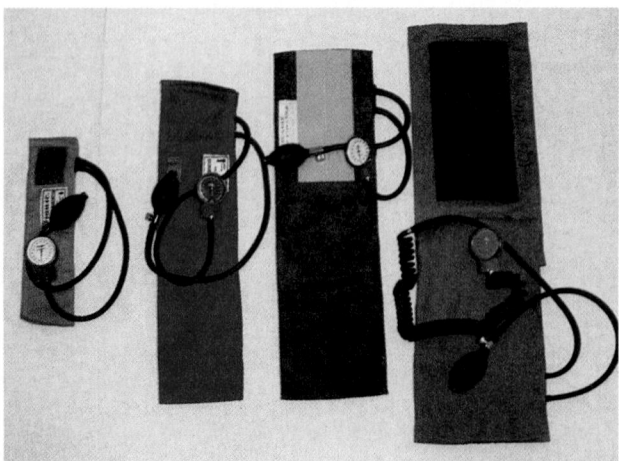

Figure 24-9 Blood pressure cuffs in sizes to fit the arm of a small child to an adult thigh. It is important to have the correct size to obtain an accurate reading.

when all sounds disappear. Within 20 to 30 millimeters, the sounds reappear. If the procedures are not followed carefully, the auscultatory gap is missed and the blood pressure measurement is incorrect in that systolic and diastolic readings may be in error according to the length of the gap. See Table 24-1.

Pulse pressure is the difference between the systolic and diastolic measurements. The normal range for pulse pressure is 30 to 50 mm. The difference should be no more than one-third of the systolic reading.

Recording Blood Pressure Measurement

The blood pressure is recorded on the patient chart in a fraction format. The position of the patient (sitting or lying down) may be noted. The arm used is also noted, particularly if the blood pressure has been taken in both arms.

Example: 120/80, rt. arm, supine

For children and those patients whose blood pressure can still be heard to zero, the beginning of Korotkoff Phase IV and zero are both recorded.

Example: 120/70/0

Procedure 24-11 outlines the procedure for measuring blood pressure.

Normal Blood Pressure Readings

Normal blood pressure is low at birth and gradually increases with age until adulthood, at which point it should remain fairly constant.

Newborn	50–52/25–30
Child 6 years	95/62
Child 10 years	100/65
Adolescent 16 years	118/75
Adult	Systolic below 140
	Diastolic below 89

Blood Pressure Abnormalities

There are only two possible blood pressure abnormalities: hypertension, blood pressure that is consistently above normal; and hypotension, blood pressure that is consistently below normal in which the patient is unable to function.

Hypertension. There are four types of hypertension: primary or essential, secondary, benign, and malignant.

TABLE 24-1 ERRORS IN BLOOD PRESSURE MEASUREMENT PROCEDURES

Errors in measuring blood pressure must be avoided. Common errors include:

1. Improper cuff size.
2. The arm is not at heart level. Do not hold the arm up or let the patient hold up the arm. Pressure is altered when this is done.
3. Cuff is not completely deflated before use or after palpatory method, resulting in a higher pressure measurement.
4. Deflation of the cuff is faster than 2 to 4 millimeters per second. Sounds are missed if this happens.
5. Reinflating the cuff during the procedure without allowing the arm to rest for 1 to 2 minutes.
6. Patient is not relaxed and comfortable. An anxious, apprehensive patient will have a reading that is higher than the actual blood pressure.
7. Improper cuff placement. Cuff is too loose, too tight, or not positioned correctly over the brachial artery.
8. Defective equipment in which there are air leaks in the bladder or valve, the mercury column is dirty, or air bubbles are present. Mercury and aneroid sphygmomanometers are not calibrated at zero.

All of these errors are easily corrected by following careful procedure and by having the manometers calibrated and/or cleaned according to a regular maintenance schedule.

- The most commonly seen form of hypertension is primary or essential. It is hypertension with no apparent cause or cure, but is treatable. Treatment is designed to control hypertension and is a lifelong process. It will not be cured, just controlled.

- Secondary hypertension is the result of some underlying problem such as renal disease, pregnancy, endocrine imbalances, obesity, arteriosclerosis, or atherosclerosis. Once the underlying problem has been removed, the blood pressure returns to normal. Secondary hypertension can be successfully treated.

- Hypertension that has a slow progression but may progress to the same endpoint as in malignant hypertension, is referred to as benign hypertension.

- Malignant hypertension progresses rapidly with severe damage to the cardiovascular system, possibly to the point of death.

Hypotension. Hypotension is blood pressure persistently below normal, usually below 90/60, although this may be normal for some healthy adults. Hypotension is defined as a blood pressure so low that the patient is unable to function normally. It is usually a result of various shock-like conditions such as hemorrhage, traumatic or emotional shock, central nervous system disorders, or chronic wasting diseases. With treatment for the underlying problems, the blood pressure usually will be in the range of normal readings.

Orthostatic hypotension occurs when a person rapidly changes position from supine to standing, when standing in one position for too long, or as a side effect of certain medications. In this instance, the blood pressure has momentarily dropped and the person will experience vertigo and may have blurred vision. These symptoms usually last only a few seconds, just long enough for the blood pressure to return to normal. Care should be taken when helping patients to an upright position from a supine position as orthostatic hypotension can lead to syncope and injury from falling.

HEIGHT AND WEIGHT

Although not considered a vital sign, height and weight are routinely measured if warranted by the age and the physical condition of the patient. Many physicians prefer that height and weight be measured as part of a yearly physical examination and otherwise may vary the frequency of patient height and weight measurements. Height and weight are normally measured simultaneously.

For children, height and weight are typically measured during each physician visit. The height of adults may be obtained on the initial visit only and weight taken on all visits. An adolescent or young adult may have height measured more frequently in order to plot body changes. Because elderly patients tend to lose the cushioning between vertebrae as part of aging, they may need to have their height measured more frequently to check the stage of any degeneration.

Elderly patients require special attention by the medical assistant when measuring height and weight. It is especially important to assist elderly patients both on and off the scale, for the scale platform is movable and elderly patients may lose their balance and fall if unassisted.

Height

To measure a patient's height, a scale with a measuring bar is necessary (Figure 24-10). A paper towel is placed on the scale as the patient's shoes should be removed for accurate measuring. The patient is asked to step on the scale and face away from the measuring bar. Assist patient onto the scale; the scale platform is movable and the patient could fall.

There are two reasons for having the patient's back to the scale. When the measuring bar is lifted, it could cause face or eye injuries if the patient were facing the

bar. Lifting the measuring bar prior to the patient stepping on the scale can also lead to eye and face injuries in that the patient could inadvertently walk into the bar. Another reason to have the patient's back to the scale is if the patient does not look straight ahead, the head is not level, which could result in a less than accurate measurement.

After the patient is on the platform, the measuring bar is placed firmly on the patient's head and the line between where the solid bar and sliding bar meet is read. The bars are measured in quarter inches (Figure 24-11). Children's heights may be recorded in inches, while adults will be recorded in feet and inches. Conversion from inches to feet is accomplished by taking the number of inches and dividing by twelve.

See Procedure 24-12 to measure height.

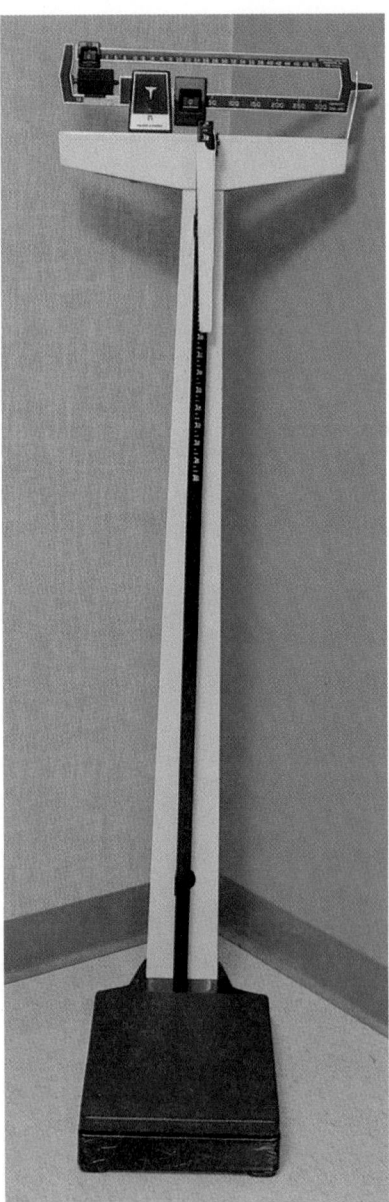

Figure 24-10 Traditional beam balance scale with measuring bar.

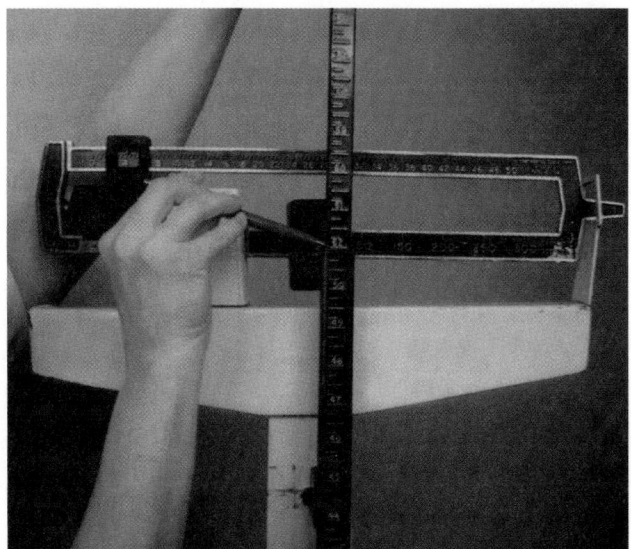

Figure 24-11   Read the height at the movable point of the ruler. The bars are measured in quarter inches.

Weight

Physician preference and patient health will dictate the frequency of measuring an adult's weight. Some physicians require the patient's weight measured on each visit while others do not if there are no health problems that require weight monitoring. Some health conditions that do require weight monitoring include obesity, eating disorders, hormone disorders such as diabetes and thyroid malfunction, hypertension, pregnancy, cancer, and some digestive disorders.

When measuring the weight of a patient, the medical assistant must maintain the patient's privacy. Most people are very conscious of their weight and may become embarrassed if the measurement is taken where others may see and hear. Privacy is important and often overlooked. The medical assistant must also be careful of comments regarding a patient's weight particularly with the obese patient and with those being treated for eating disorders. Encouragement for weight loss for the dieting patient is beneficial but must be done in privacy. Other comments are inappropriate.

Occasionally a patient will be instructed by the physician to monitor weight at home. It is important for the patient to understand the necessity of weighing at the same time each day as weight may vary significantly throughout the day. A normal routine is to measure weight before breakfast.

Before an accurate weight can be obtained, the scale must be calibrated. The point of the balance beam must be floating in the center when no weight is applied to the scale. Some scales are equipped with a screw at the end that can be turned slightly until the beam is in the correct floating position. Once it is centered, it is calibrated and ready for use.

The patient will wear normal indoor clothing, rather than disrobing, for weight measurement. Heavy coats or other outerwear should be removed. Heavy objects and purses should not be held during the procedure. A chair or counter should be provided to place these objects on while the procedure is being performed. Shoes should be removed.

See Procedure 24-13 for measuring adult weight.

Occasionally, as in the case of medication dosage, the medical assistant may be required to convert pound weight into kilogram weight.

> 1 kilogram = 2.2 pounds
> *To convert pounds to kilograms:*
> Take the number of pounds and divide by 2.2
> **Example:** 130 pounds divided by 2.2 = 59.09 kg
> *To convert from kilograms to pounds:*
> Take the number of kilograms and multiply by 2.2
> **Example:** 40 kilograms multiplied by 2.2 = 88 lb.

Significance of Weight

The careful monitoring of a patient's weight may provide an insight into metabolic, nutritional, and emotional problems.

MEASURING CHEST CIRCUMFERENCE

Occasionally, the medical assistant may be instructed to measure the chest of an adult. This procedure is done on patients with emphysema and as a requirement for insurance and truck driver licenses. Two measurements will be taken, one on the deepest inspiration and one on the deepest expiration. A comparison is then made to ascertain chest capacity. To perform the procedure, ask the patient to disrobe from the waist up. Place a tape measure around the chest at nipple level. Instruct the patient to inhale deeply while you measure, then ask the patient to exhale completely while you take the second measurement. Record the results as inspiration number and expiration number. The physician performs any necessary comparison.

Procedure 24-1
Measuring an Oral Temperature Using a Mercury Thermometer

STANDARD PRECAUTIONS:

PURPOSE:
To obtain an oral temperature.

EQUIPMENT/SUPPLIES:
Thermometer
Disposable thermometer sheaths
Gloves
Paper towels
Biohazard waste container

PROCEDURE STEPS:
1. Wash hands and follow standard precautions.
2. Assemble equipment.
3. Identify patient.
4. Position the patient in a comfortable position.
5. Determine if the patient has ingested hot or cold drinks or food or has been smoking within the previous half hour. RATIONALE: Ingesting hot or cold substances or smoking can result in an arbitrary increase or decrease in temperature results.
6. Explain the procedure. RATIONALE: To obtain patient cooperation and consent.
7. Shake the thermometer with a quick flip of the wrist until it reads below 96.0°F. RATIONALE:

To obtain an accurate result, the mercury must be below 96.0°F.
8. Cover thermometer with the sheath (Figure 24-12). RATIONALE: To prevent microorganism cross contamination.
9. Apply gloves.
10. Insert thermometer under the tongue to the side of the mouth. RATIONALE: Under the center of the tongue is the frenulum which impedes placement in this area.
11. Instruct patient to close mouth without placing teeth on thermometer (Figure 24-13). RATIONALE: To prevent air leakage and to avoid patient biting on thermometer.
12. Leave in place for 3 to 5 minutes.
13. Remove thermometer after appropriate time has elapsed.
14. Remove and discard sheath in biohazard waste container (Figure 24-14).
15. Holding the thermometer at eye level, read the thermometer (Figure 24-15).
16. Wash thermometer in cool water using friction, rinse, and dry. Place on clean paper towel.
17. Remove gloves and discard in biohazard waste container.
18. Wash hands.
19. Document on patient record.

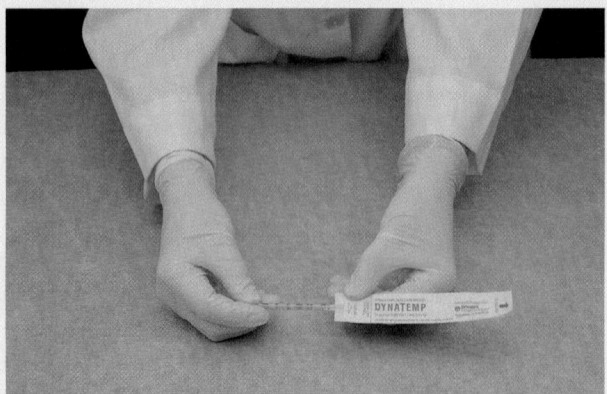

Figure 24-12 Cover the mercury thermometer with the disposable sheath.

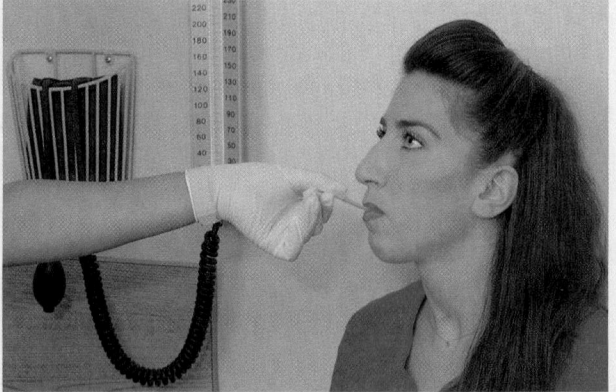

Figure 24-13 Place mercury oral thermometer sublingually (to the side of the mouth) in a heat pocket and ask patient to close mouth without placing teeth on thermometer.

(continues)

Procedure
24-1 **(continued)**

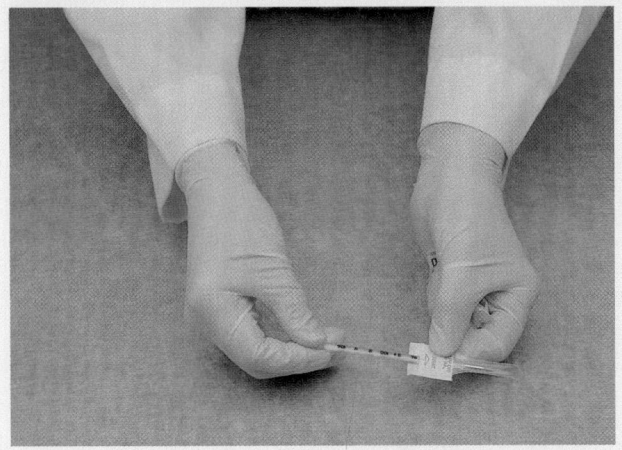

Figure 24-14 Remove the plastic sheath and discard in biohazard container before reading the thermometer.

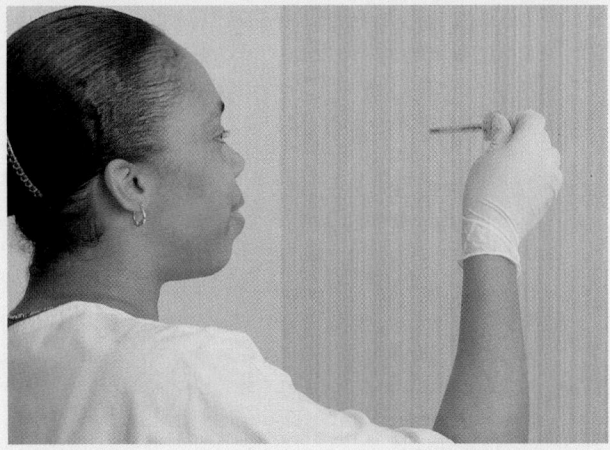

Figure 24-15 Rotate the stem slightly back and forth until you can see the silver mercury column in the middle. The point where the mercury stops is the reading to record.

Procedure
24-2 **Measuring an Oral Temperature Using a Disposable Oral Strip Thermometer**

STANDARD PRECAUTIONS:

PURPOSE:
To obtain an oral temperature.

EQUIPMENT/SUPPLIES:
Oral strip thermometer (Figure 24-16)
Gloves
Biohazard waste container

PROCEDURE STEPS:
1. Wash hands and follow standard precautions.
2. Assemble equipment.
3. Identify patient.
4. Position the patient in a comfortable position.
5. Determine if the patient has ingested hot or cold drinks or food or has been smoking within the

(continues)

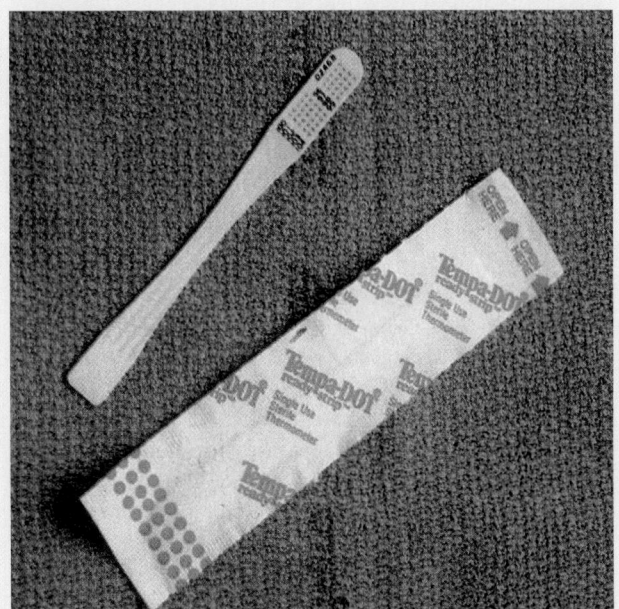

Figure 24-16 Disposable oral strip thermometer.

Procedure 24-2 *(continued)*

previous half hour. RATIONALE: Ingesting hot or cold substance or smoking can result in an arbitrary increase or decrease in temperature results.

6. Explain the procedure. RATIONALE: To obtain patient cooperation and consent.
7. Apply gloves.
8. Insert disposable oral strip thermometer under the tongue to the side of the mouth. RATIONALE: Under the center of the tongue is the frenulum, the fold of mucus membrane that attaches the tongue to the floor of the mouth, which impedes placement in this area.
9. Instruct patient to close mouth tightly. RATIONALE: To prevent air leakage.
10. Leave in place for 60 seconds.
11. Remove thermometer after appropriate time has elapsed.
12. Wait 10 seconds to read the dots.
13. Read temperature by locating the last dot that has changed color (Figure 24-17).
14. Discard strip in biohazard waste container.
15. Remove gloves and discard in biohazard waste container.
16. Wash hands.
17. Record temperature.
18. Document the procedure.

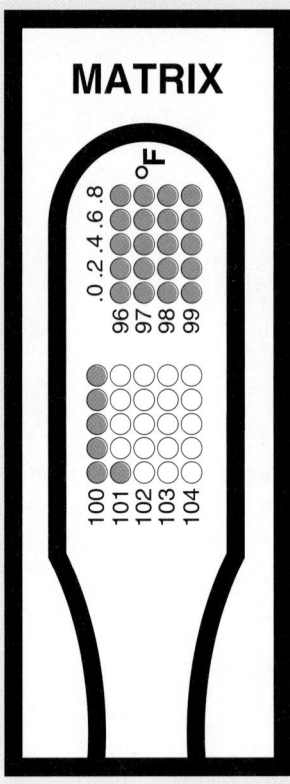

Figure 24-17   The reading on this disposable oral thermometer is 101°F.

Procedure 24-3 Measuring an Oral Temperature Using a Digital Thermometer

STANDARD PRECAUTIONS:

PURPOSE:
To obtain an oral temperature.

EQUIPMENT/SUPPLIES:
Digital thermometer
Probe covers
Biohazard waste container

PROCEDURE STEPS:
1. Wash hands and follow standard precautions.
2. Assemble equipment.
3. Identify patient.
4. Position the patient in a comfortable position.
5. Determine if the patient has ingested hot or cold drinks or food or has been smoking within the previous half hour. RATIONALE: Ingesting hot or cold substance or smoking can result in an arbitrary increase or decrease in temperature results.

(continues)

Procedure

24-3 *(continued)*

6. Explain the procedure. RATIONALE: To obtain patient cooperation and consent.
7. Select blue (oral) probe.
8. Cover with probe cover (Figure 24-18). RATIONALE: To prevent microorganism cross contamination.

9. Insert under the tongue to either side of the mouth (Figure 24-19). RATIONALE: Under the center of the tongue is the frenulum which impedes placement in this area.
10. Instruct patient to close mouth without placing teeth on thermometer. RATIONALE: To prevent air leakage.
11. Leave in place until the beep is heard.
12. Remove thermometer after appropriate time has elapsed.
13. Read the results on the digital display window.
14. Discard probe cover in biohazard waste container (Figure 24-20).
15. Replace digital thermometer in the base holder.
16. Wash hands.
17. Record temperature.
18. Document the procedure.

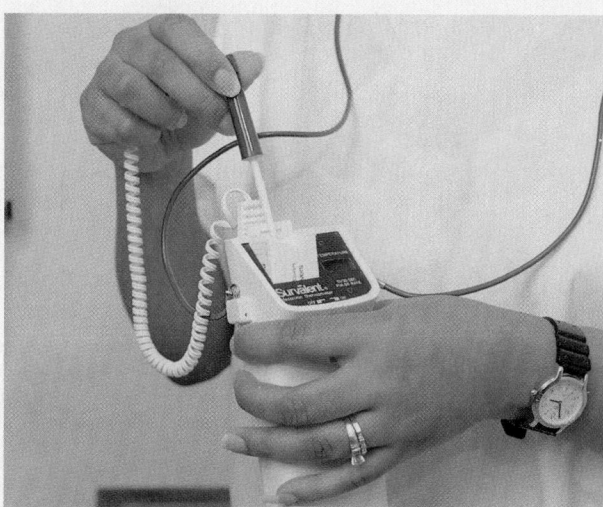

Figure 24-18 Slide the probe into the disposable cover, adjusting if necessary.

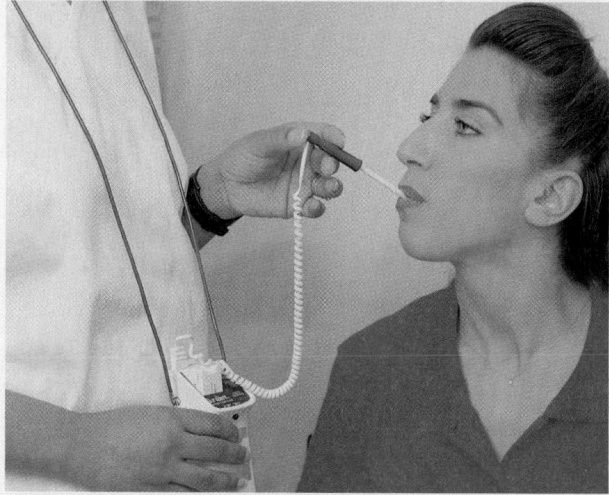

Figure 24-19 Insert the thermometer under tongue to either side of mouth.

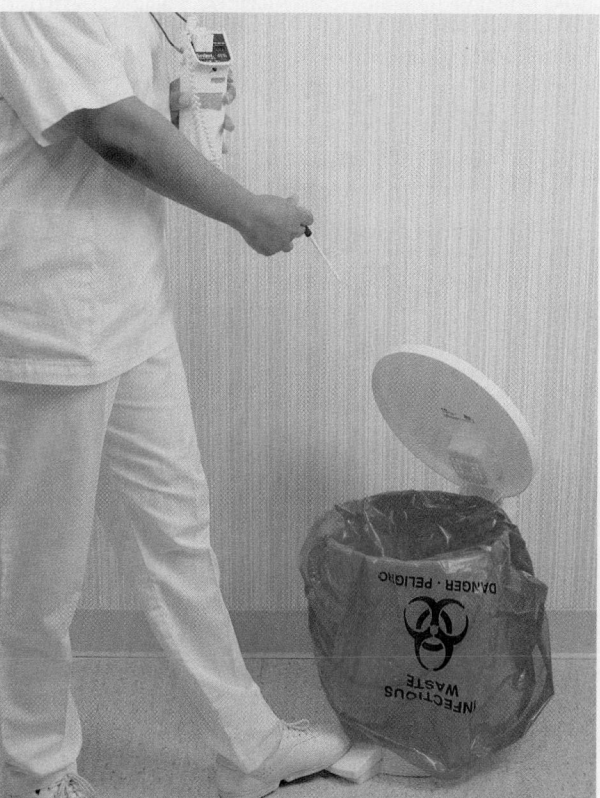

Figure 24-20 Discard probe cover in biohazard waste container.

Procedure 24-4 Measuring an Aural Temperature Using a Tympanic Thermometer

STANDARD PRECAUTIONS:

PURPOSE:
To obtain an aural temperature using a tympanic thermometer.

EQUIPMENT/SUPPLIES:
Tympanic thermometer (Figure 24-21)
Covers or ear speculum
Waste container

PROCEDURE STEPS:
1. Wash hands following standard precautions.
2. Assemble equipment.
3. Identify the patient.
4. Explain procedure. RATIONALE: This will help gain patient's cooperation and consent.
5. Place cover on thermometer (Figure 24-22).
6. Set thermometer to start.
7. Gently place probe into ear canal to seal the area and activate the system (Figure 24-23). RATIONALE: Air leaks will occur if the ear canal is not sealed.
8. Wait until the temperature is displayed on the screen.
9. Remove from the ear.
10. Discard cover into waste container by pressing the release button.
11. Wash hands.
12. Replace thermometer.
13. Record temperature in patient chart.

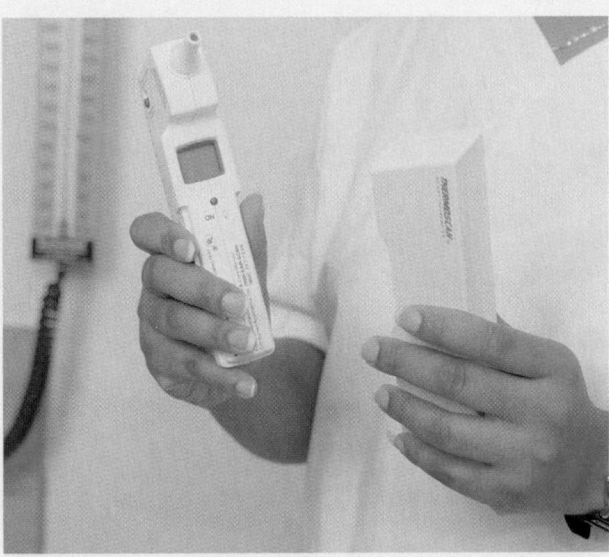

Figure 24-22   Attach the disposable speculum or cover to the tympanic thermometer to prevent spread of micro-organisms between patients.

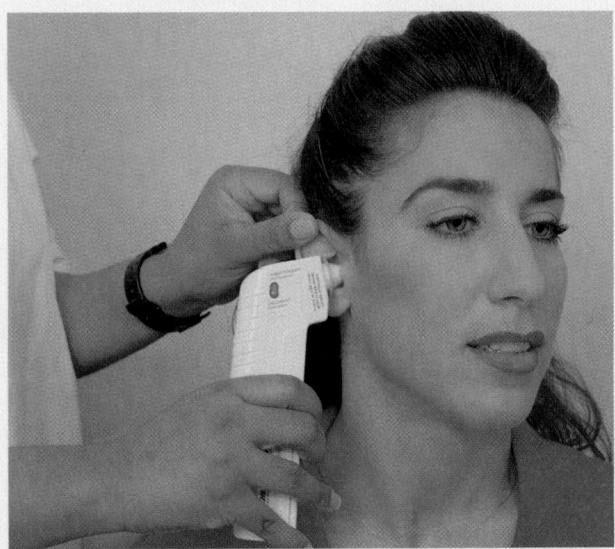

Figure 24-23   Pull up on the ear to straighten the auditory canal for an accurate reading.

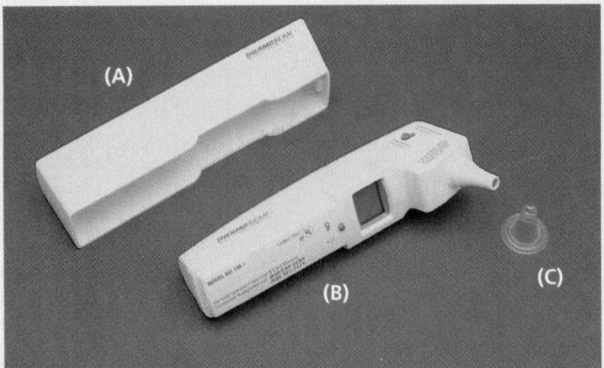

Figure 24-21   Tympanic thermometer: (A) holder, (B) tympanic thermometer, and (C) disposable speculum or cover.

Procedure 24-5 — Measuring a Rectal Temperature Using a Mercury Thermometer

STANDARD PRECAUTIONS:

PURPOSE:
To obtain a rectal temperature using a mercury thermometer.

EQUIPMENT/SUPPLIES:
Rectal thermometer (red tip)
Sheath
Lubricating jelly
Gloves
Clean paper towels
Biohazard waste container

PROCEDURE STEPS:

1. Wash hands, following standard precautions.
2. Assemble equipment.
3. Identify patient.
4. Explain procedure to patient. RATIONALE: Ensures understanding and gains patient cooperation and consent.
5. Remove clothing from the waist down, drape as necessary. RATIONALE: Maintains patient modesty, privacy, and warmth.
6. Position patient in Sims' position.
7. Place sheath on thermometer. RATIONALE: To prevent microorganism cross contamination.
8. Lubricate with lubricating jelly (Figure 24-24). RATIONALE: Easier insertion of thermometer and safety for patient.
9. Apply gloves.
10. Spread buttocks, gently insert thermometer into the rectum past the sphincter (1½ inches) for adult (Figure 24-25).
11. Hold buttocks together and keep the thermometer in place for 5 minutes. Do not let go of it. RATIONALE: Patient movement can cause thermometer to move in patient's rectum and cause injury.
12. Remove from rectum.
13. Place thermometer on gauze or tissue that was used to help lubricate thermometer.
14. Wipe lubricant from patient's anal area or offer tissue to patient. Place tissue in biohazard container.
15. Ensure patient's comfort and safety.
16. Remove sheath and place in biohazard container.
17. Read thermometer.
18. Wash, rinse, and dry thermometer.
19. Place thermometer on clean paper towel on shelf.
20. Remove gloves. Place in biohazard container.
21. Wash hands.
22. Immerse thermometer in container with alcohol marked "rectal" for thirty minutes.
23. Document on patient record, indicating a rectal temperature.

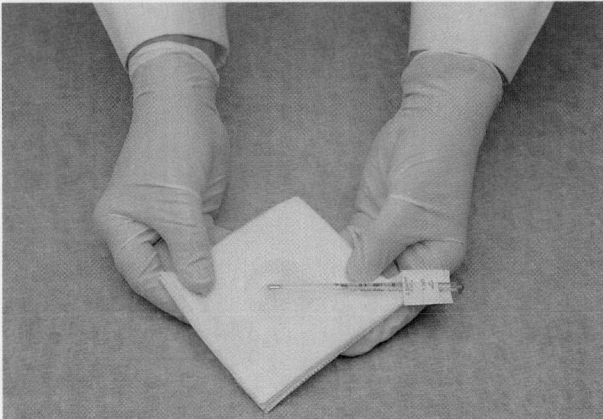

Figure 24-24 Lubricate thermometer by putting lubricant on tissue or gauze, then place first inch or two of the thermometer into the lubricant.

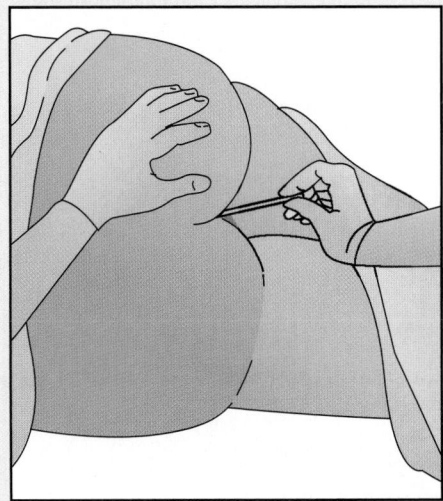

Figure 24-25 Gently insert thermometer into the rectum.

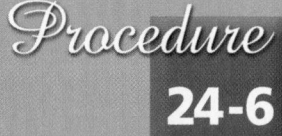

Measuring a Rectal Temperature Using a Digital Thermometer

STANDARD PRECAUTIONS:

PURPOSE:
To obtain a rectal temperature using a digital thermometer.

EQUIPMENT/SUPPLIES:
Digital thermometer with red probe
Probe cover
Lubricating jelly
Gloves
Biohazard waste container

PROCEDURE STEPS:
1. Wash hands and glove, following standard precautions.
2. Assemble equipment.
3. Identify patient.
4. Explain procedure to patient. RATIONALE: Ensures understanding and gains patient cooperation and consent.
5. Remove clothing from the waist down, drape as necessary. RATIONALE: Maintains patient modesty, privacy, and warmth.
6. Position patient in Sims' position.
7. Place probe cover on red probe (rectal). RATIONALE: To prevent microorganism cross contamination. Red probe indicates rectal thermometer.
8. Lubricate with lubricating jelly. RATIONALE: Easier insertion of thermometer and safety for patient.
9. Spread buttocks, gently insert thermometer into the rectum past the sphincter (1½ inches) for adult.
10. Hold buttocks together while holding the thermometer. Do not let go of thermometer. RATIONALE: Holding buttocks together prevents air leaks and inaccurate recording. Holding onto thermometer ensures patient safety.
11. Hold in place until the beep is heard.
12. Read results on digital display window.
13. Remove from rectum.
14. Discard probe cover into biohazard waste container by pushing the release button.
15. Replace thermometer on holder base.
16. Remove gloves, discard in biohazard waste container, and wash hands.
17. Offer tissue to patient to wipe anus. Assist patient in dressing and position as necessary.
18. Record on the patient chart labeled with (R) indicating a rectal temperature.

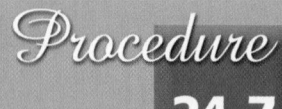

Measuring an Axillary Temperature

STANDARD PRECAUTIONS:

PURPOSE:
To obtain an axillary temperature using a mercury thermometer.

EQUIPMENT/SUPPLIES:
Mercury thermometer
Sheath
Towelettes
Paper towels

PROCEDURE STEPS:
1. Wash hands, following standard precautions.
2. Assemble equipment, place sheath on thermometer.
3. Identify patient.
4. Explain procedure. RATIONALE: This elicits patient cooperation and consent.

(continues)

Procedure 24-7 (continued)

5. Ask patient to remove clothing to provide access to axilla.
6. Gown as necessary to maintain patient modesty and warmth.
7. Wipe axillary area with dry towel or towelette to remove moisture. RATIONALE: Moisture in the axilla will cause inaccurate reading.
8. Place thermometer in axilla.
9. Ask patient to fold arm against chest or abdomen (Figure 24-26).
10. Leave in place for 10 minutes.
11. Carefully remove.
12. Remove sheath and discard.
13. Read thermometer.
14. Wash, rinse, and dry thermometer.
15. Place clean thermometer on clean paper towel or shelf.
16. Wash hands.
17. Immerse thermometer in container marked "oral" with alcohol for thirty minutes.
18. Document temperature in patient's record, indicating axillary temperature.

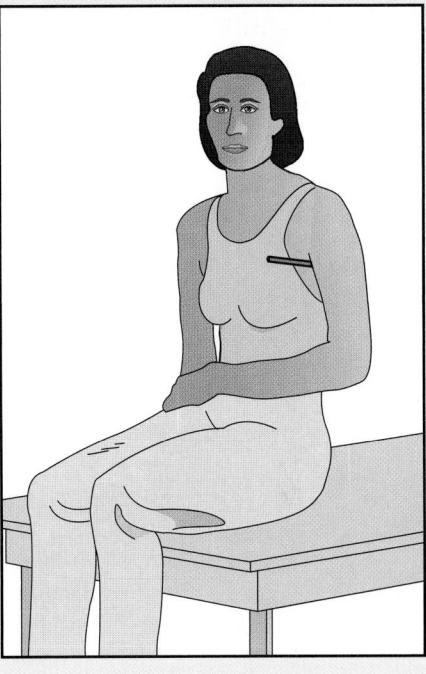

Figure 24-26 After placing thermometer in axilla, ask patient to fold arm against chest or abdomen.

Procedure 24-8 Measuring a Radial Pulse

STANDARD PRECAUTIONS:

PURPOSE:
To obtain a pulse rate.

EQUIPMENT/SUPPLIES:
Watch with a second hand

PROCEDURE STEPS:
1. Wash hands.
2. Identify patient.
3. Explain procedure. RATIONALE: Ensures patient cooperation and consent.

(continues)

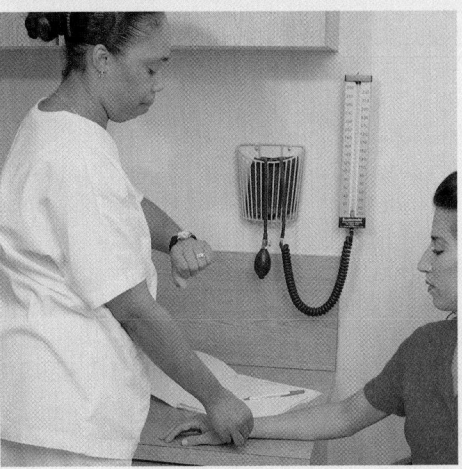

Figure 24-27 Position patient with wrist resting on table or lap.

Procedure

24-8 (*continued*)

4. Position patient with the wrist resting either on a table or on lap (Figure 24-27).
5. Locate the radial pulse with the pads of your first three fingers. Do not use thumb; it has its own pulse.
6. Gently compress the radial artery enough to feel the pulse.
7. Count the pulsations for one full minute.
8. Note any irregularities in rhythm, volume, and condition of artery.
9. Wash hands.
10. Record the pulse in the patient chart following the temperature, noting any irregularities.

Procedure

24-9 Taking an Apical Pulse

STANDARD PRECAUTIONS:

PURPOSE:
To obtain an apical pulse rate.

EQUIPMENT/SUPPLIES:
Stethoscope
Watch with second hand

PROCEDURE STEPS:
1. Wash hands.
2. Assemble equipment.
3. Identify patient.
4. Explain procedure. RATIONALE: Ensures patient cooperation and consent.
5. Assist patient in disrobing, removing clothing from the waist up.
6. Provide a gown or drape for patient modesty and warmth.
7. Position the patient in a supine position. RATIONALE: Easier access to apex of heart.
8. Locate the fifth intercostal space, midclavicular, left of sternum (Figure 24-28). RATIONALE: Location of apex of heart.
9. Place stethoscope on the site and listen for the lub-dup sound of the heart.
10. Count the pulse for one minute; each lub-dup equals one pulse.
11. Assist the patient to sit up and dress.

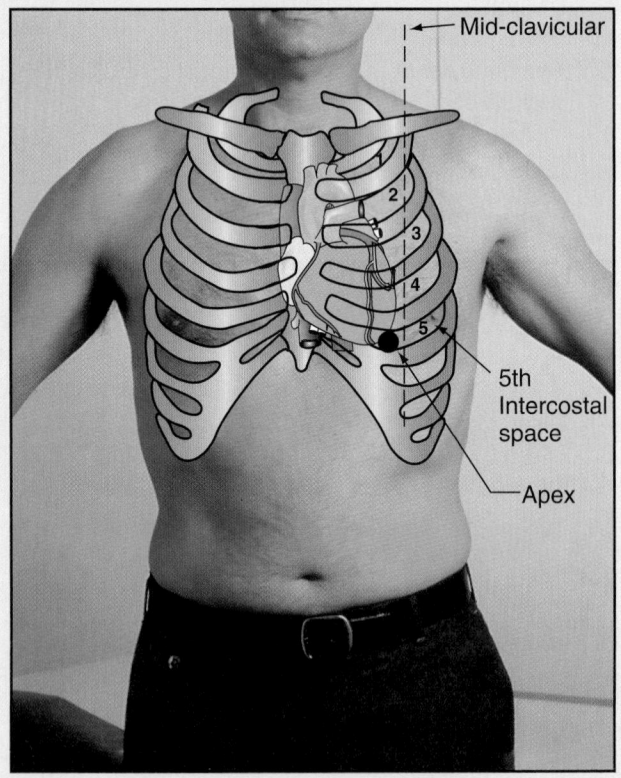

Figure 24-28   Locate the apical pulse by counting intercostal spaces. Locate the fifth intercostal space.

(*continues*)

Procedure 24-9 (*continued*)

12. Wash hands.
13. Record the pulse in the patient chart with the designation of (AP) to denote method of obtaining the pulse and note any arrythmias.

NOTE: Apical pulse and radial pulse are frequently taken simultaneously, with the radial pulse taken by another individual (Figure 24-29). Both pulse rates should be identical. A discrepancy may indicate a cardiac problem.

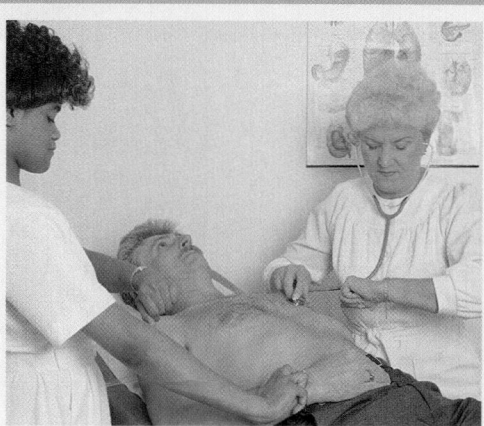

Figure 24-29 Sometimes apical and radial pulses are taken simultaneously.

Procedure 24-10 Measuring the Respiration Rate

STANDARD PRECAUTIONS:

NOTE: The respiration rate is normally taken immediately before or after the pulse rate. It should be taken without patient knowledge, as respiration can voluntarily be altered. While counting respiration, it is best to continue grasping the wrist as if still taking the pulse. This procedure will assist in preventing alteration of breathing by the patient.

PURPOSE:
To obtain an accurate respiratory rate.

EQUIPMENT/SUPPLIES:
Watch with second hand

PROCEDURE STEPS:
1. Wash hands.
2. Identify the patient.
3. Position patient in a comfortable position.
4. Watch the rise and fall of the chest wall for one minute, or, while holding the patient's arm, place it across the chest and feel for the rise and fall of chest wall. Alternatively, place a hand on the patient's shoulder and feel and watch for the rise and fall of the chest wall (Figure 24-30).
5. Note depth, rhythm, and breath sounds while counting.
6. Wash hands.
7. Record respiration rate in patient chart, noting any irregularities and sounds.

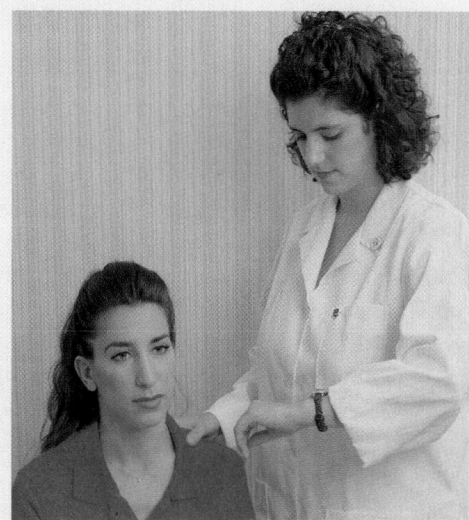

Figure 24-30 Place hand on patient's shoulder. Feel and watch for rise and fall of the chest wall.

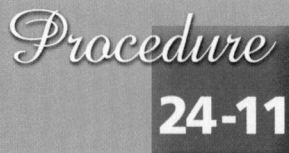

24-11   Measuring a Blood Pressure

PURPOSE:
To measure blood pressure.

EQUIPMENT/SUPPLIES:
Stethoscope
Sphygmomanometer
Alcohol wipes

PROCEDURE STEPS:
1. Wash hands.
2. Assemble equipment, making sure that cuff size is correct. RATIONALE: Inappropriate cuff size will result in inaccurate measurement.
3. Clean earpieces of stethoscope with alcohol wipe.
4. Identify patient.
5. Explain procedure. RATIONALE: May be the first instance where blood pressure is measured; to allay anxiety and ensure cooperation and consent.
6. Position patient comfortably; if sitting, feet flat on the floor, arm resting at heart level on the lap or a table. RATIONALE: Legs crossed may arbitrarily increase blood pressure; arm above heart level may result in inaccurate reading.
7. Bare the upper arm. If clothing is restricting, have patient remove it. RATIONALE: Tight clothing on the arm can produce inaccurate results.
8. Palpate brachial artery.
9. Securely center the bladder of the cuff over the brachial artery above the bend of the elbow. RATIONALE: Cuff should be high enough so stethoscope does not touch it. Extraneous sounds may be heard.
10. Palpate the radial pulse and smoothly inflate cuff until the pulse is no longer felt; note the number.
11. Quickly deflate the cuff and allow arm to rest for about 1 minute. Calculate peak inflation level. RATIONALE: This ensures that an auscultatory gap is not missed.
12. Make sure cuff is completely deflated.
13. Position stethoscope over the brachial artery and hold in position with the fingers only.

14. Inflate cuff smoothly and quickly to the peak inflation level (Figure 24-31).
15. Deflate the cuff at a rate of 2 to 4 millimeters of mercury per second.
16. Listen for Korotkoff Phase I; note when it appears.
17. Continue deflation, noting the Korotkoff Phases.
18. Note when all sounds disappear, Korotkoff Phase V.
19. Continue deflating the cuff at the same rate for at least another 10 millimeters after sounds have disappeared. RATIONALE: To hear an auscultatory gap should one be present.
20. The cuff may then be deflated quickly.
21. Remove the cuff.
22. Clean earpieces and diaphragm of stethoscope with alcohol wipes.
23. Wash hands.
24. Record the measurement in patient's chart.

NOTE: On a patient's initial visit and in hypertensive patients, the physician may want the blood pressure taken in both arms. There is normally a slight variation in pressure between the arms. If it is necessary to repeat the procedure, wait approximately five minutes before doing so.

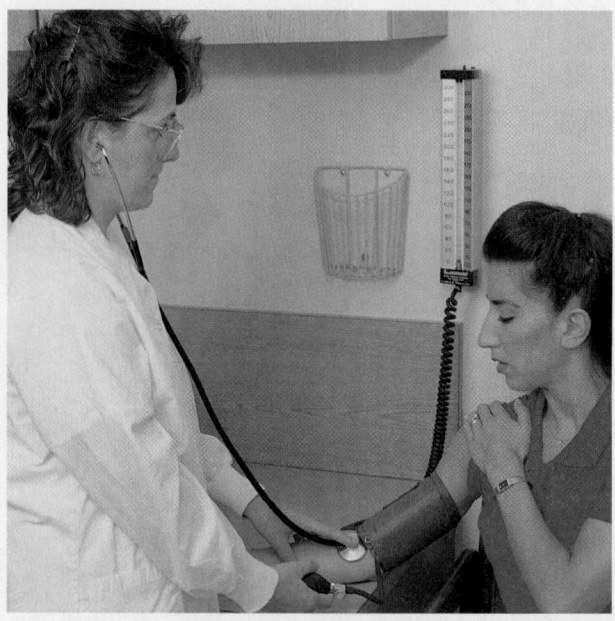

Figure 24-31   Inflate cuff smoothly and quickly.

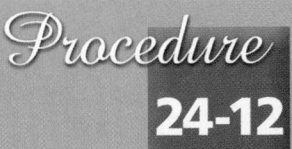

Procedure 24-12 Measuring Height

STANDARD PRECAUTIONS:

PURPOSE:
To obtain the height of a patient.

EQUIPMENT/SUPPLIES:
Scale with measuring bar
Paper towel

PROCEDURE STEPS:
1. Wash hands.
2. Identify patient.
3. Explain the procedure to patient to ensure understanding, cooperation, and consent.
4. Instruct patient to remove shoes and stand on paper towel on scale with back against scale, looking straight ahead. RATIONALE: Back against scale aids patient safety.
5. Assist patient onto scale. RATIONALE: Scale platform is movable and patient may become unsteady and lose balance and fall.
6. Lower measuring bar until firmly resting on top of head (Figure 24-32).
7. Assist patient to step off of the scale. Allow patient to sit and help with shoes if necessary.

8. Read line where measurement falls.
9. Lower measuring bar to its original position.
10. Wash hands.
11. Record height in patient chart.

Example: Ht. 5'6"

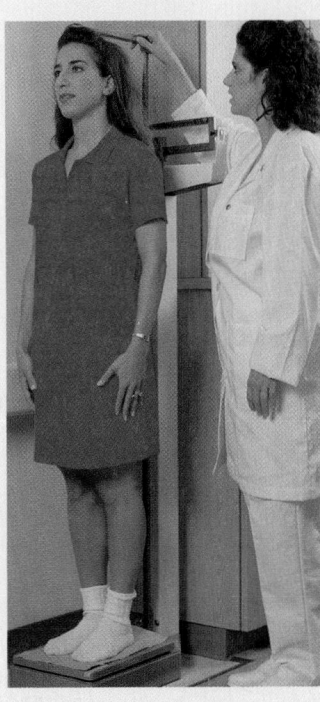

Figure 24-32
To measure height, have the patient stand with back against scale and keep head level.

Procedure 24-13 Measuring Adult Weight

STANDARD PRECAUTIONS:

PURPOSE:
To obtain the weight of the patient.

EQUIPMENT/SUPPLIES:
Balance beam scale
Paper towels

PROCEDURE STEPS:
1. Wash hands.
2. Identify patient.
3. Explain the procedure to patient to ensure understanding and cooperation.
4. Place a paper towel on scale. RATIONALE: Paper towel protects patient's feet.
5. Instruct the patient to place heavy objects on the area provided, including heavy objects that may be in their pockets.

(continues)

Procedure
24-13 *(continued)*

6. Instruct the patient to remove shoes, jackets, and heavy sweaters and step on the scale. Assist patient to the center of the scale. RATIONALE: The scale platform is movable and the patient may become unsteady, lose balance, and fall.
7. Move the lower weight bar (measured in 50-pound increments) to the estimated number (the patient may be asked for approximate weight).
8. Slowly slide the upper bar until the balance beam point is centered (Figure 24-33).
9. Read the weight by adding the upper bar measurement to the lower bar measurement.
10. Assist the patient to step off of the scale.
11. Provide a chair for the patient to sit to put on shoes. Return objects to the patient.
12. Return the weights to zero.
13. Wash hands.
14. Record measurement in the patient chart.

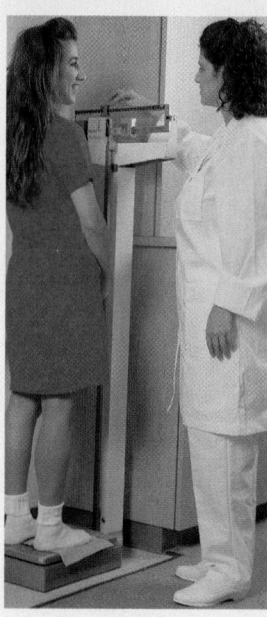

Figure 24-33 When weighing the patient, slide the upper bar until the balance beam point is centered.

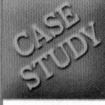

CASE STUDY 24-1

Herb Fowler, a regular patient of Dr. Lewis at Doctors Lewis & King, is an African-American man in his fifties. He has smoked for many years and only recently has thought about quitting smoking because of a chronic cough. Herb is also significantly overweight but has a hard time making the decision to give up smoking *and* change his diet. While his blood pressure has been stable for the last few years, clinical medical assistant Audrey Jones, CMA, is concerned when she takes Herb's vital signs during his most recent checkup. His weight is slightly up and his blood pressure has jumped from 140/90 to 156/100.

CASE STUDY REVIEW

1. Why is a blood pressure reading of 156/100 a cause for concern? Should Audrey take a second reading?
2. In addition to alerting the physician to the change in Herb's blood pressure and weight, Audrey feels she may be able to provide advice to the patient (with physician's permission). How can Audrey use her communication and medical assisting knowledge to counsel Herb Fowler on lifestyle changes?
3. To follow up, Audrey reviews her knowledge of hypertension and discusses the four types with the physician. What are the four kinds of hypertension and what are their characteristics?

SUMMARY

Throughout life, a patient will undergo various measurements to ascertain growth, development, and general health and well-being. The normal range for each of these measurements will vary according to the stage of life of the patient at the time of examination. The medical assistant must be aware of what to expect when measuring a patient in each life stage. Awareness of normal expectations for each stage of life will assist the medical assistant to perform the procedures in a more effective and efficient manner and aid in observing any abnormal signs and measurements.

Along with differences seen with age, the medical assistant will see differences in patients because each patient has unique medical problems.

The medical assistant has a great responsibility when performing patient measurements and must ensure patient safety and comfort while obtaining accurate results.

REVIEW QUESTIONS

Multiple Choice

1. The average adult oral temperature is:
   a. 96.2°F
   c. 98.6°F
   b. 97.8°F
   d. 99.5°F
2. The artery commonly used for taking a patient's pulse is:
   a. carotid
   c. radial
   b. brachial
   d. popliteal
3. A blood pressure cuff that is too small will:
   a. have no effect on the results
   b. give an arbitrarily low result
   c. give an arbitrarily high result
   d. have an effect on certain patients only
4. Rectal thermometers should be cleansed with:
   a. hot soapy water
   b. cool soapy water
   c. alcohol
   d. 10 percent bleach solution
5. The term used to indicate a pulse rate significantly above the average is:
   a. bradycardia
   c. arrhythmia
   b. tachycardia
   d. sinus rhythm

Critical Thinking

1. Discuss methods the medical assistant may use to obtain patient cooperation when taking vital signs.
2. Describe and demonstrate the appropriate charting procedure for normal vital sign results.
3. Discuss the responsibilities of the medical assistant in measuring vital signs.
4. Describe the care and use for each of the various types of thermometers.
5. Describe the procedure for converting temperatures from one scale to the other and calculate the following conversions:
   a. 98.6°F = _____ °C
   b. 39.1°C = _____ °F
6. Discuss the rationale for not using the thumb for taking the pulse rate of a patient.
7. Discuss the reasons for taking the respiratory rate of a patient without the patient's knowledge.

8. Discuss the importance of using the appropriate blood pressure cuff size when measuring a patient's blood pressure.
9. Discuss the normal vital signs differences expected between an infant and an adult.
10. Describe the following:
    a. hypertension
    c. apnea
    b. tachycardia
    d. remittent fever

WEB ACTIVITIES

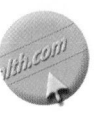

1. Access information on the Internet from the American Heart Association regarding essential hypertension and answer the following:
   a. What population of Americans is at greatest risk for essential hypertension?
   b. List four patient education tips for lowering blood pressure without the aid of medication.
   c. Check the list of normal blood pressure readings in this chapter and compare it to what the American Heart Association says are normal blood pressure measurements at various ages.
2. Access information on the Internet from the National Research Council and list its recommendations for weight of the following females:

Height	Age	Weight in Pounds
5' 2"	19–34 years	?
5' 4"	19–34 years	?
5' 6"	19–34 years	?

REFERENCES/BIBLIOGRAPHY

Keir, L., Wise, B. A., & Krebs, C. (1998). *Medical assisting: Administrative and clinical competencies* (4th ed.). Albany, NY: Delmar.

Kinn, M. E., & Woods, M. A. (1999). *The medical assistant: Administrative and clinical* (8th ed.). Philadelphia: W. B. Saunders.

Taber's cyclopedic medical dictionary. (18th ed.) (1999). Philadelphia: F. A. Davis.

Zakus, S. (1995). *Clinical procedures for medical assistants* (3rd ed.). St. Louis: Mosby-Year Book.

THE PHYSICAL EXAMINATION

KEY TERMS

Ataxia
Bruits
Catheterization
Cyanosis
Fenestrated Drape
Jaundice
Labyrinthitis
Pallor
Pyorrhea
Scleroderma
Symmetry
Tinnitus
Vertigo
Vitiligo

OUTLINE

Methods of Examination
   Observation or Inspection
   Palpation
   Percussion
   Auscultation
   Mensuration
   Manipulation
Positioning and Draping
   Examination Positions
Equipment and Supplies for the
   Physical Examination

Basic Components of a Routine
   Physical Examination
   Patient Appearance
   Gait
   Stature
   Posture
   Body Movements
   Speech
   Breath Odors
   Nutrition
   Skin and Appendages
   The Physical Examination
      Sequence

OBJECTIVES

The student should strive to meet the following performance objectives and demonstrate an understanding of the facts and principles presented in this chapter through written and oral communication.

1. Define the key terms as presented in the glossary.

2. Describe the six methods used in physical examinations.

3. Name and describe eight positions used for physical examinations.

4. Discuss the purpose of draping and demonstrate the appropriate draping procedure for each type of position.

5. Identify at least ten instruments and supplies used for examination of various parts of the body.

6. Identify eight basic components of a physical examination.

7. Describe the sequence followed during a routine physical examination.

8. Recall method of examination, instrument used, and position for examination of at least eight body parts.

At the multiphysician Inner City Health Care facility, five physicians are employed on a rotating basis, with two or three working at any one time. Clinical medical assistants Wanda Slawson, CMA, and Bruce Goldman, CMA, have developed a clear understanding of what each physician prefers in both room and patient preparation. Wanda and Bruce also coordinate with each other and with office managers Jane O'Hara and Walter Seals, both CMAs, to ensure patient comfort. Depending on the patient and the type of examination, Wanda will often assist with patient preparation when the patient is female and Walter will assist when the patient is a male.

INTRODUCTION

Physical examinations are performed to obtain a picture of the health and well-being of the patient. An initial examination will provide a baseline reference for future examinations. The examination follows a standard routine, usually starting at the head and following through the entire body, including all major organs and body systems. Although the sequence of events for the physical examination is relatively standard, variations will occur according to physician preference, type of practice, and patient's chief complaint. Diagnostic procedures such as laboratory and X rays may be ordered or performed in the facility or sent to an outside laboratory. At the conclusion of the physical examination, the physician will have an impression of the patient's general health, diagnosis if possible, and treatment plans. The physician uses information from three major sources to aid in making a diagnosis: the health history, the physical examination, and laboratory tests and diagnostic procedures.

The role of the medical assistant throughout the physical examination will greatly depend upon the physician. Some physicians will delegate many duties to the medical assistant, while others will require little assistance. Commonly performed medical assisting duties can be divided into two cate-

gories: patient preparation and room preparation. Patient preparation includes patient explanation and preparation, positioning, draping, vital signs, specimen collection such as urine and blood, and electrocardiogram (ECG). Room preparation includes assembling the appropriate instruments and equipment for the physician and assuring patient privacy and comfort.

Additional medical assisting duties include handing the physician instruments and equipment as required and taking notes dictated by the physician. Throughout and following the examination, the medical assistant will adhere to the principles of medical asepsis and standard precautions as required by OSHA. The effective medical assistant will establish an efficient but flexible routine providing for the needs of both the patient and physician.

METHODS OF EXAMINATION

There are six methods used by the physician to examine the body. They include observation or inspection, palpation, percussion, auscultation, mensuration, and manipulation. The physician will use all in total or in part depending upon the type of examination being performed.

Observation or Inspection

This is the process of observing the patient. The general health, posture, body movements, skin, mannerisms, and care in grooming are all noted. Closer observation will be focused on body **symmetry** (correspondence in shape and size of body parts located on opposite sides of the body) and contour. Deformities and skin rashes will be observed. Skin color is also noted (Figure 25-1).

Palpation

This is an examination of the body using touch and may be used to help verify observations. A body part or organ may be felt for size and condition. Abdominal masses may be felt through the abdominal wall. Skin texture, moisture, and temperature can be felt. The contour of limbs and rigidity and position of bones and joints may be felt. Palpation may be performed with the use of fingertips, one or both hands, or the palm of the hand (Figure 25-2).

Percussion

This is the process of eliciting sounds from the body by tapping with either a percussion hammer or fingers. The vibrations and sounds from underlying organs and cavities can be felt and heard. Using this method can determine the presence of air or solid material in the organ or cavity being checked. Healthy structures that are dense, such as the liver, produce a dull sound. Hollow structures such as the lungs should produce a more hollow sound. There are two methods used to perform percussion. The direct method is by tapping directly on the surface of the skin. The indirect method is performed by placing a finger or hand on the surface of the skin and tapping the hand (Figure 25-3).

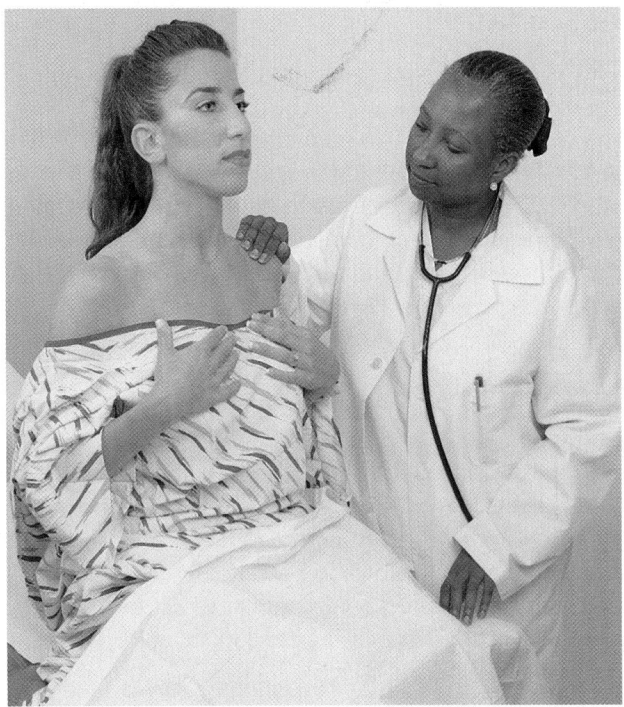

Figure 25-1 The physician observes the patient for signs of disease. This method of examination is known as observation or inspection.

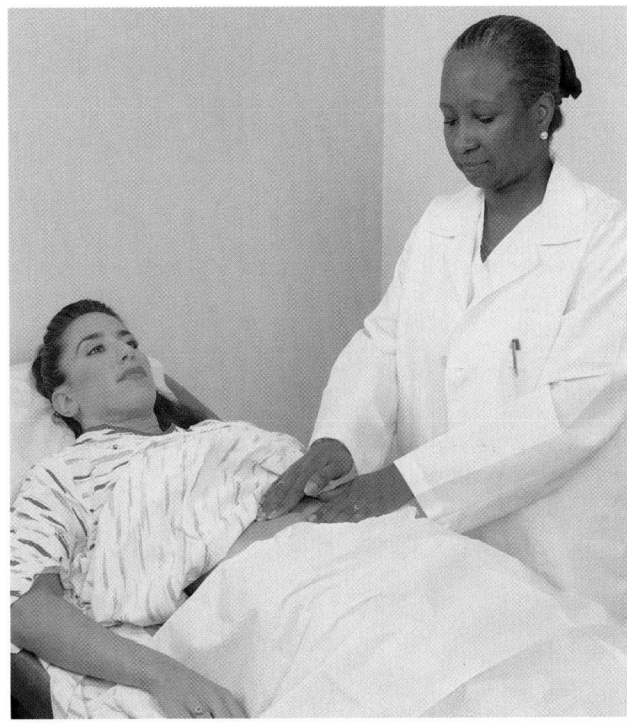

Figure 25-2 The physician palpates the abdomen during the physical examination to feel for abnormalities.

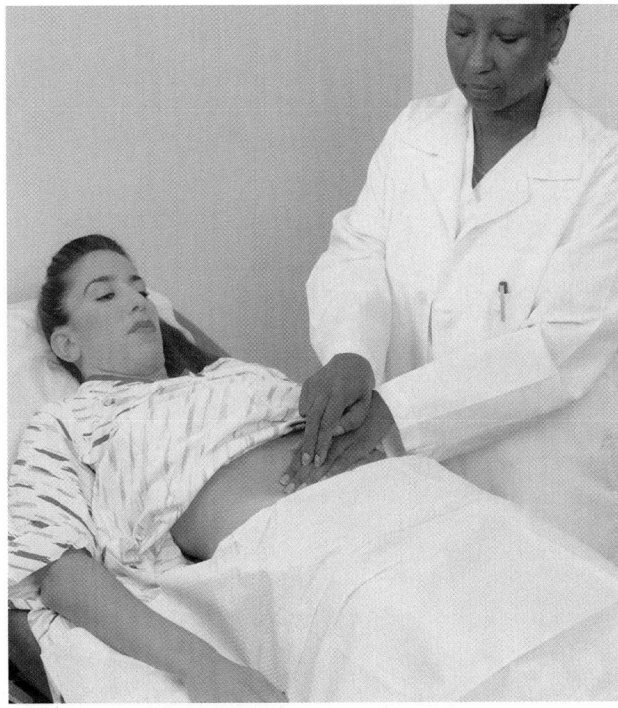

Figure 25-3 The physician uses percussion during the physical examination to tap the body to produce sounds that may indicate disease.

Auscultation

This is the process of listening directly to body sounds, normally with a stethoscope. The physician listens for lung and heart sounds such as murmurs, rales, or bruits, which generally are abnormal sounds heard on auscultation of an organ or vessel such as a vein or an artery. The abdomen will be examined for bowel sounds which include the clicks and gurgles of normal bowel activity, the sounds that occur with peristalsis (Figures 25-4 and 25-5).

Mensuration

This method of examination uses the process of measuring. The measurement of height and weight, the length of a limb, the amount of flexion and extension of an extremity are all forms of mensuration. Measurement of chest and infant head circumference are also forms of mensuration. In most instances, a tape measure is used to perform mensuration of an infant's head or circumference of a body part (Figure 25-6).

Manipulation

This method checks the amount of flexion and extension of a joint by applying forceful passive movement on the joint. Range of motion of some joints may be checked using this method. See Chapter 33 for information on range of motion.

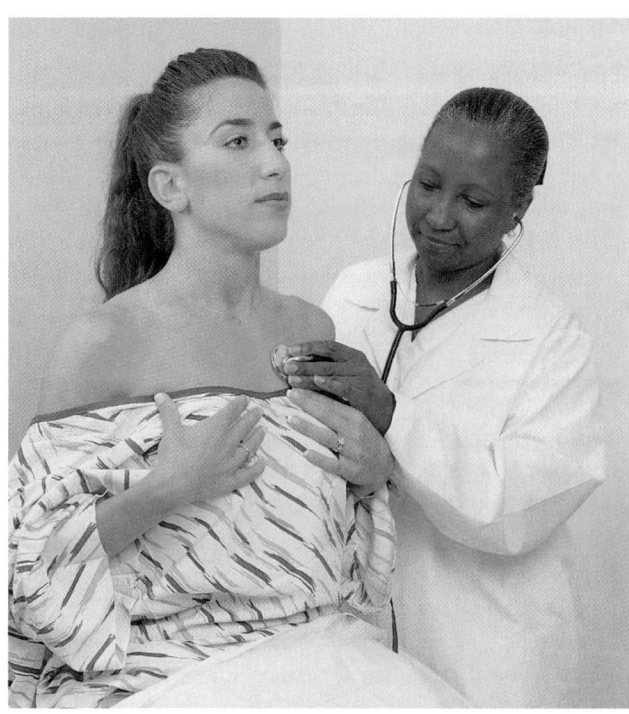

Figure 25-4   The physician uses a stethoscope to listen to sounds from the patient's body. This method of physical examination is known as auscultation.

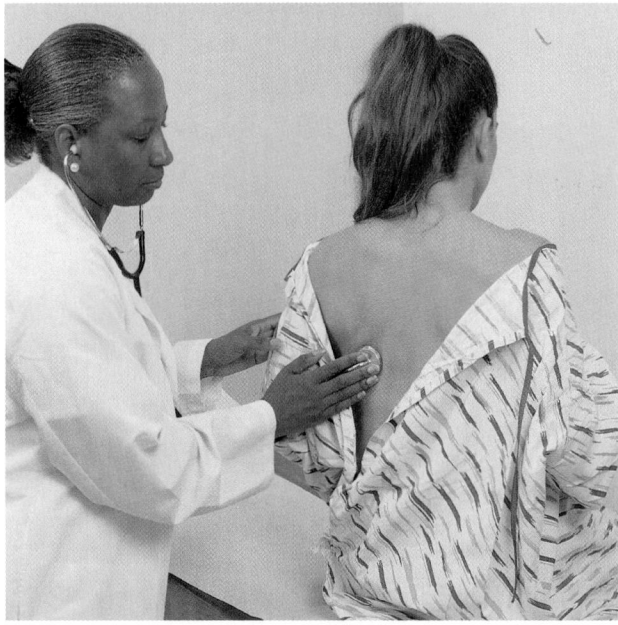

Figure 25-5   Auscultation is performed on the anterior and posterior portion of the body.

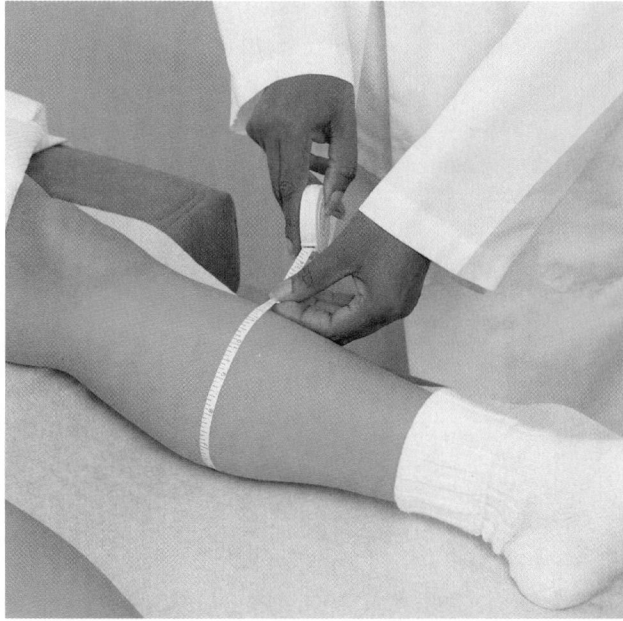

Figure 25-6   A tape measure may be used to measure the circumference of the calf of the patient's leg or other body part. This method of physical examination is known as mensuration.

POSITIONING AND DRAPING

Physical examinations may require the patient to be placed in various positions. Each position is designed to make examination of a particular area of the body easier and more efficient. The medical assistant may assist the patient in disrobing and will provide the appropriate drape and/or gown. The medical assistant also instructs the patient about the appropriate position required for the examination and may assist the patient into position by providing support and guidance. The patient experiencing pain should be allowed to assume the position with minimal help, as too much assistance by another may increase the pain. Always provide for patient safety.

Proper draping to protect modesty and prevent embarrassment is essential. If patients are capable of helping themselves, the medical assistant should leave the room while the patient disrobes and puts on a drape or a gown. If the patient is disoriented or extremely ill, the medical assistant must stay in the room; patient privacy can be provided by discreetly removing clothing and covering the patient as quickly as possible. When the patient is a child, the medical assistant should note the comfort level of the child while the child is getting disrobed. Children develop modesty at an early age and may be embarrassed by sitting on the examination table wearing only underwear. Respect a child's right to privacy by offering a gown or drape. The elderly will need assistance with disrobing and draping. Care must be taken to provide as much modesty and privacy as possible as you assist patients of all ages.

 Never turn your back on seriously ill or disoriented patients or young children. Ensure patient safety at all times.

Examination Positions

There are a number of positions that may be required of the patient during the physical examination. The posi-

tion used will depend on the type of examination. Eight common positions are outlined in Procedures 25-1 through 25-8. These include:

1. Supine (horizontal recumbent) (Procedure 25-1)
2. Dorsal recumbent (Procedure 25-2)
3. Lithotomy (Procedure 25-3)
4. Fowler's (Procedure 25-4)
5. Knee-Chest (Procedure 25-5)
6. Prone (Procedure 25-6)
7. Sims' (Procedure 25-7)
8. Trendelenburg (Procedure 25-8)

Supine (Horizontal Recumbent). This position is assumed when lying flat facing up (Figure 25-7). It is used for examination of the anterior surface of the body from head to toe. When the physician is performing a physical examination on a female, she should be provided with a gown and instructed to wear it with the opening in the front. A drape is then placed over the lap or from the waist down.

Dorsal Recumbent. The patient lies on her back (dorsal) face up, legs separated, knees flexed with feet flat on the table (Figure 25-8). This is the most comfortable position for patients with back and abdominal problems. Examinations performed in this position include rectal, vaginal, head, neck, and chest, as well as abdominal palpation. It can also be used for urinary catheterization. Preteen and early teen girls requiring a pelvic examination may be placed in this position and will require careful instructions and procedure explanations. The patient is covered with a drape that is diamond shaped. One edge of the diamond can be lifted to examine the genitalia without exposing the rest of the body.

Lithotomy. The patient is assisted to lie on her back similar to the dorsal recumbent position except the buttocks should be as close to the bottom edge of the table as

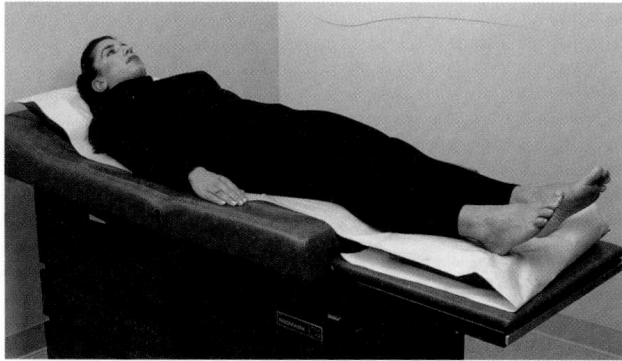

Figure 25-7 Supine or horizontal recumbent position.

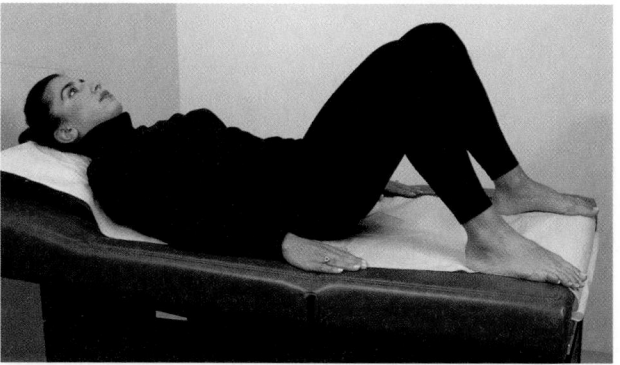

Figure 25-8 Dorsal recumbent position.

possible and feet placed in stirrups attached to the foot of the table (Figure 25-9). The lithotomy position is used for genital and pelvic examinations. It can also be used for urinary catheterization. At the conclusion of the examination, the patient should slide toward the head of the table before getting up from this position. Patients with special needs, such as the elderly and those physically challenged as with severe arthritis, may not be able to assume this position. If this is the case, assist patient into Sims' position (see Procedure 25-7) and the sigmoidoscopy, proctoscopy, or pelvic exam can be done in this position for these patients.

Fowler's. The patient sits in a position with the back of the examination table raised to either 45 degrees (Semi-Fowler's) (Figure 25-10) or 90 degrees (High-Fowler's) (Figure 25-11). Legs rest flat on the table. A pillow may be placed under the knees. This position is used for patients having cardiovascular or respiratory problems to facilitate their breathing, and for examination of the upper body and head.

Knee-Chest. This position puts the weight of the body on the knees and chest (Figure 25-12). The patient is instructed to kneel on the table and spread the knees shoulder width apart. The buttocks should be elevated, back straight with the chest resting on the table. The head is positioned to one side, with arms flexed on the side of the head and hands under the head. This is not a comfortable position and the patient may need assistance. If the position is too uncomfortable or difficult, have the patient rest on the elbows. This position is used primarily for proctologic examinations, sigmoidoscopy procedures, and in some instances vaginal examinations. Draping will require a large drape to cover the entire body. It may be necessary to use two smaller drapes, holding them together with towel clamps. A diamond- or triangle-shaped drape allows for one edge to be lifted to expose only the rectal area. Do not place the patient in knee-chest position until the physician is ready to begin the procedure.

Proctologic. This position requires the use of a specialized table known as a proctologic examination table (Figure 25-13). The patient is instructed to disrobe and to kneel on the knee board of the table. The patient then bends at the hips and rests the chest on the table. The head is supported by a head board. The table is then turned to elevate the buttocks. A triangular, diamond-shaped, or **fenestrated drape**

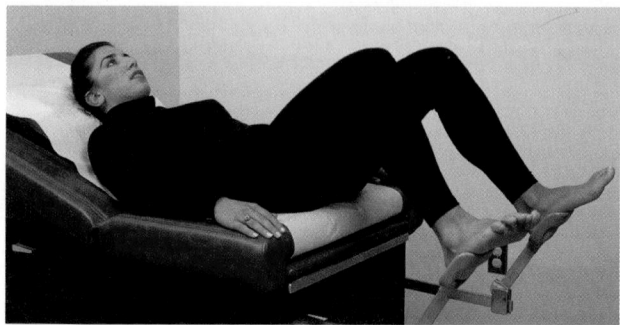

Figure 25-9   Lithotomy position.

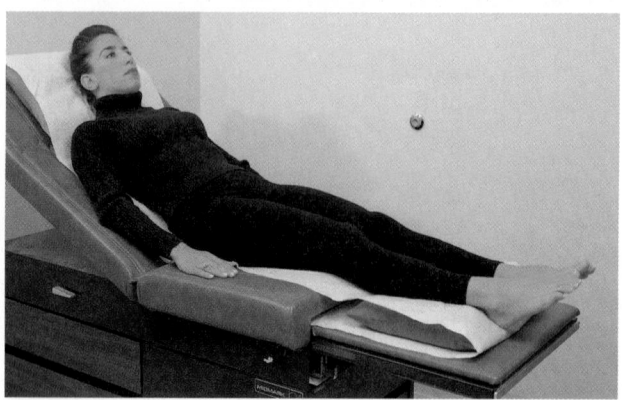

Figure 25-10   Semi-Fowler's position (45-degree angle).

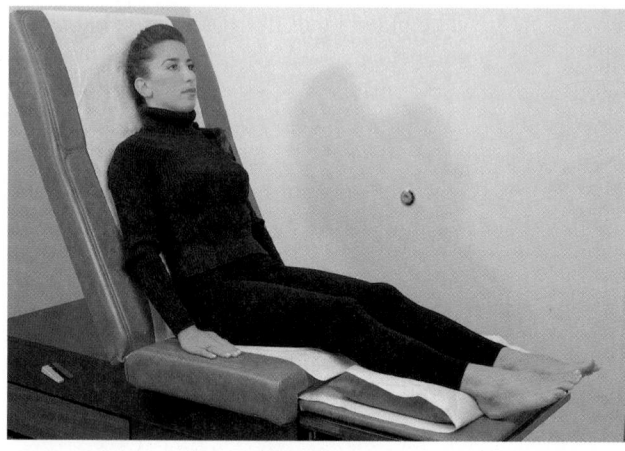

Figure 25-11   High Fowler's position (90-degree angle).

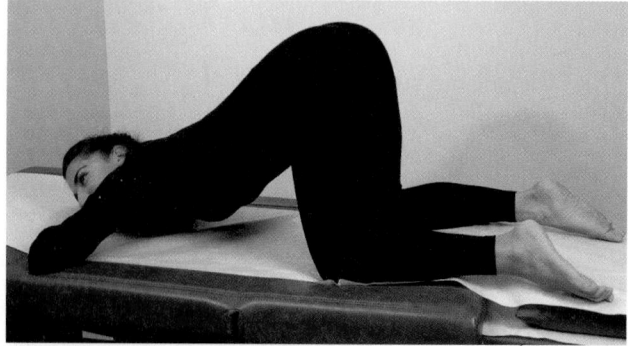

Figure 25-12   Knee-chest position.

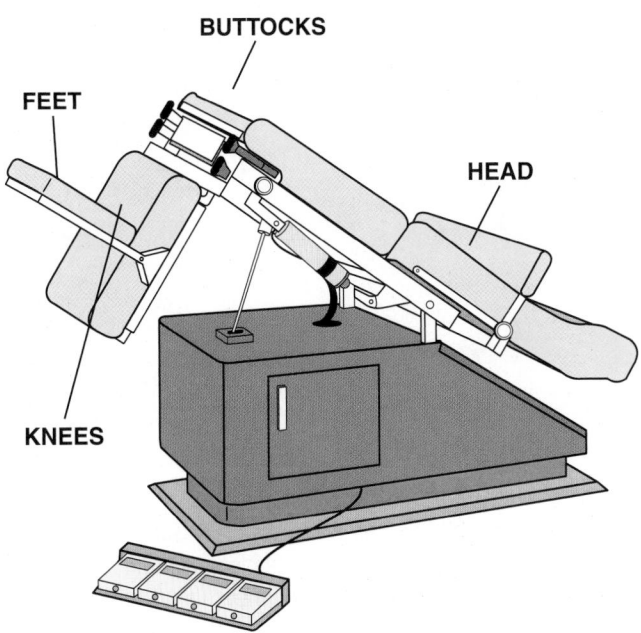

FEET

BUTTOCKS

HEAD

KNEES

Figure 25-13 Proctologic table.

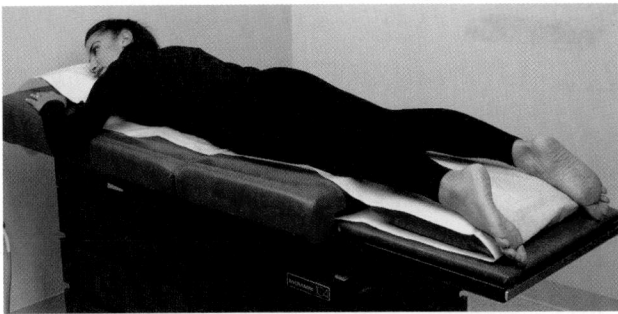

Figure 25-14 Prone position.

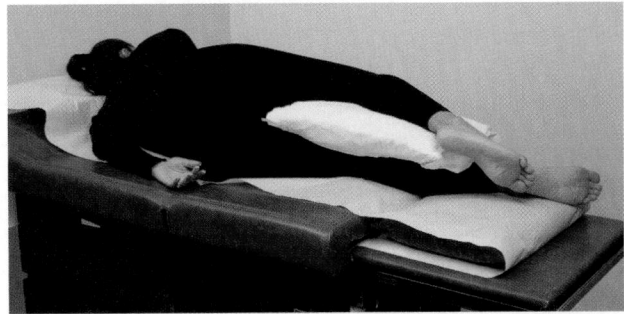

Figure 25-15 Sims' or lateral position.

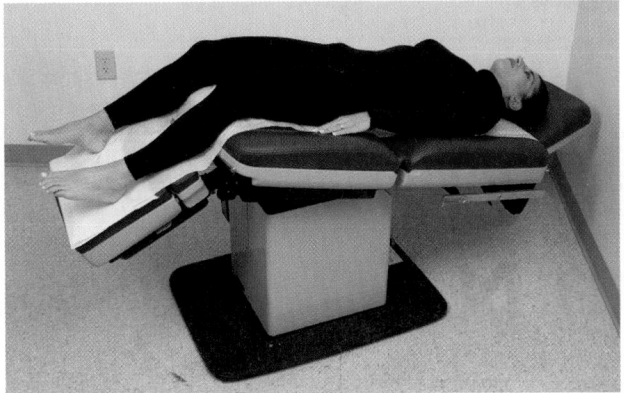

Figure 25-16 Trendelenburg position.

will cover the patient from the shoulders to the knees. This position is used for proctologic examinations.

Prone. The patient is instructed to lie face down on the table with head turned to side, arms may be placed above head or along side of body (Figure 25-14). The drape must cover from the mid-chest area to the legs. This position may be used for examining the posterior aspect of the body, including the back or spine.

Sims' (lateral). The patient is instructed to lie on the left side; the left arm and shoulder may be drawn back behind the body (Figure 25-15). The left knee is slightly flexed to support the body and the right knee is flexed sharply. A small pillow is provided for under the patient's head and a pillow may also be placed between the patient's legs if it does not interfere with the examination being performed. The drape should be large enough to cover the patient from the shoulders to the knees (triangle or diamond shape to expose rectum). This position may be used for vaginal or rectal examination, for rectal temperatures, sigmoidoscopy, or for enemas.

Trendelenburg. The patient lies flat on the back, face up, with the knees flexed and the legs hanging off the end of the table. Legs and feet are supported by a footboard (Figure 25-16). The table is positioned with the head 45 degrees lower than the body. The drape covers from the shoulders to the knees. This position is primarily used for surgical procedures of pelvis or abdomen. Variation of this position may be used for a patient in shock. (See Chapter 9 for information about emergency procedures.)

EQUIPMENT AND SUPPLIES FOR THE PHYSICAL EXAMINATION

Equipment and supplies used for physical examinations should be properly cleaned and ready for the physician's use. Refer to Chapters 22 and 31 for proper cleaning and care of instruments. The list of instruments and supplies in Table 25-1 includes those that may be used in the physical examination. However, this is a limited list. Actual equipment and supplies needed will vary with the physician and with the type of examination. Figure 25-17 shows some common instruments that may be used in the physical examination. For instruments used in specialty examinations, see Chapter 30.

TABLE 25-1 INSTRUMENTS AND SUPPLIES NEEDED FOR A PHYSICAL EXAMINATION	
Balance beam scales	Laryngeal mirror
Tape measure	Pharyngeal mirror
Thermometer	Examination lights
Stethoscope	Penlight
Sphygmomanometer	Gloves
Alcohol swabs	Emesis basin
Cotton balls	Percussion hammer
Gauze sponges	Patient gown
Otoscope	Drape
Tuning fork	Tissues
Ophthalmoscope	Specimen bottles/slides— request forms
Tonometer	
Nasal speculum	Biohazard and regular waste containers
Tongue depressors	

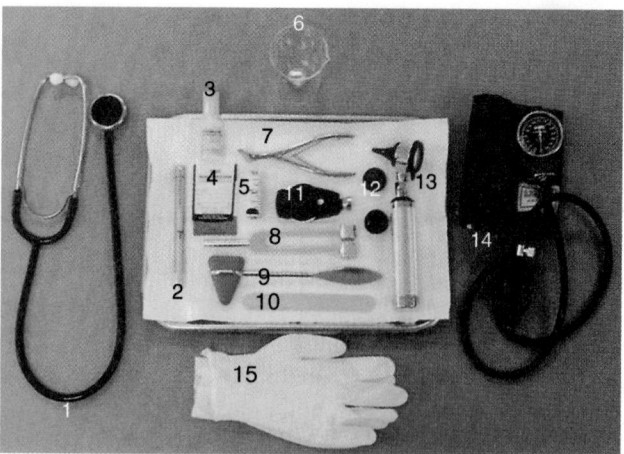

Figure 25-17   Instruments and supplies used in the physical examination: (1) Stethoscope. (2) Penlight. (3) Guaiac/occult blood test developer. (4) Guaiac/occult blood test. (5) Flexible tape measure. (6) Urine specimen container. (7) Metal nasal speculum. (8) Tuning fork. (9) Percussion hammer. (10) Tongue depresser. (11) Ophthalmoscope (head). (12) Okastic ear/ nose speculum. (13) Otoscope head attached to base handle. (14) Sphygmomanometer. (15) Latex gloves.

BASIC COMPONENTS OF A ROUTINE PHYSICAL EXAMINATION

The physical examination of the patient begins as soon as the patient enters the office. While the physical examination is performed by the physician, it is important for the medical assistant to be aware of the various examination components and the significance of each as an indicator of patient well-being.

Patient Appearance

General appearance and actions are noted as the patient is received by the medical assistant and during the patient history (see Chapter 23). Skin color is checked, general grooming, ease of conversation, and answers to questions are noted. The medical assistant should be alert to a patient with abnormal skin color, confusion or disorientation, or difficulty in movement. Such a patient may have a serious problem and should be placed in an examination room and the physician contacted immediately.

The following aspects of the patient's health are evaluated by the physician through the method of physical examination known as observation.

Gait

Gait pertains to the manner or style of walking. The patient may have a limp, walk with feet wide apart, appear to be dragging one leg, or have difficulty maintaining balance. The physician will observe the patient's gait by instructing the patient to walk on a designated straight line. Abnormal gait can include **ataxia**, uncoordinated

wide-based walk; steppage, in which the leg stepping forward is raised high enough to raise the toes off the ground; drag-to, in which the feet are dragged forward rather than lifted and moved; and spastic, in which the legs are held stiffly together and the feet are slightly dragged forward. Each of these gaits can indicate a disease process or health problem associated with neurological functioning.

Stature

The height of the patient is measured. The physician will look for height, trunk, and limb proportion.

Posture

Since normal posture is erect with the head held up, a patient in pain may exhibit postural differences. The spine might be in a fixed position, or there may be limited motion in an extremity. The physician will observe spine movement and alignment as the patient performs prescribed movements. Abnormalities can include kyphosis (humpback), which may be seen in the elderly, particularly women with osteoporosis; lordosis, abnormal curvature of the lumbar area, and scoliosis, curvature of the upper spine.

Body Movements

These may be either voluntary or involuntary. Voluntary body movements describe those movements intended to be made by the patient. Involuntary body movements are movements not controlled by the patient. Tremors are a form of involuntary movement that may be seen in the mouth, fingers, hands, arms, and legs of a patient. Tremors can indicate a neurological health problem. Involuntary body movements are usually easily observed.

Speech

The patient's speech may reveal abnormal conditions. Abnormalities include aphonia, loss of voice usually due to laryngitis, but which may have other causes; aphasia, the inability to express oneself through speech or writing, which may indicate brain injury or disease; and dysphasia, an inability to use appropriate speech patterns, such as using words in the wrong order. This may indicate a brain lesion.

Breath Odors

These may be detected when speaking with the patient or when obtaining vital signs. A sweet fruity odor may indicate acidosis. This may result from diabetes mellitus, starvation, or renal disease. A musty odor may indicate liver disease and an ammonia odor may indicate uremia.

Nutrition

There are various published charts containing guidelines for normal weight established by height and age. Overweight and underweight are defined as being above or below the published charts. Obesity and underweight have previously been mentioned in Chapter 24. Edema is a condition that causes weight gain and is an excessive accumulation of fluids in the body tissues. To test for edema, the physician will press a finger against the skin of the patient in an area over a bony prominence such as the ankle. If edema is present, pitting will be evident when the finger is removed. Fat tissue will not leave an indentation when pressed.

Skin and Appendages

Skin problems include abnormal skin color such as redness, pallor, cyanosis, jaundice, and vitiligo. Pallor is defined as lack of color or paleness; cyanosis is a slightly blue or gray discoloration of the skin, often seen in patients with severe anemia; jaundice is a yellowing of the skin, often due to obstructed bile ducts or liver disease; and vitiligo is characterized by white patches on the skin, observed against normal pigmentation. Other skin conditions are lesions, ulcers, and bruises. Texture may be smooth, rough, and scaly and have loss of elasticity. These findings may indicate health problems and/or excessive exposure to the sun. The nails can also indicate some forms of health problems. Infections, either local or sys-

SPOTLIGHT ON AAMA ESSENTIALS THROUGH CAAHEP

- Listening to how a patient says he or she feels is just as important as observing an irregularity during a physical examination.
- Always strive to maintain the patient's dignity and privacy by knocking before entering the examination room.
- Maintaining the patient's confidentiality will enable him or her to open up more readily and provide you with a better account of his or her chief complaint.

temic, may be observed in nails that are brittle, grooved, or lined. The appearance of the fingertips can be indicators of disorders as seen in a clubbing, which may indicate congenital heart disease; and spooning, which may be seen in severe iron deficiency anemias. Abnormal hair distribution as in facial hair on a female may indicate hormonal changes.

The Physical Examination Sequence

There is a sequence followed for a physical examination, although physician preference and the patient's chief complaint can produce a variation to this sequence.

The physical examination begins with the medical assistant taking and recording the patient's vital signs, height, weight, and visual acuity and auditory ability when appropriate. Additional laboratory procedures, such as urinalysis and blood analysis or electrocardiography, may be performed as directed by the physician prior to the physical examination. Prior to the examination, a patient will be instructed to empty the bladder saving a urine specimen for analysis. The patient is then told about the examination and what to expect during the examination. Any questions the patient might have should be answered by the medical assistant or referred to the physician. The patient should be instructed about disrobing (a private area should be provided for disrobing). The medical assistant should be explicit as to what clothing is to be removed and what can be left on. If a complete physical examination is required, all clothing should be removed. A gown and drape are provided for the patient. The medical assistant may leave the room while the patient disrobes unless the patient asks for help or is unable to manage alone. It is appropriate to knock before reentering the room.

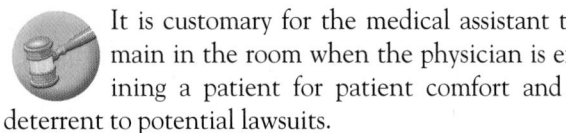

It is customary for the medical assistant to remain in the room when the physician is examining a patient for patient comfort and as a deterrent to potential lawsuits.

The medical assistant will place the instruments for the examination on the counter or Mayo stand, according to physician preference, but usually in order of use. When lamps are used for the examination, the medical assistant may turn them on and have them ready for the physician. Make sure that the light is not directed into the patient's eyes. Inform the physician that the patient is ready when the patient is comfortably positioned on the examination table. Normally the physical examination will start at the head and proceed downward. See Table 25-2 for a detailed review of the components of the physical examination.

TABLE 25-2 COMPONENTS OF THE PHYSICAL EXAMINATION

Body Part	Position	Instrument Used	Method of Exam	Physician's Findings	
				Normal	**Abnormal**
General appearance	Standing	—	Inspection	Patient is cooperative, good hygiene, good skin color, ease of gait.	Uncooperative, behavior inappropriate, unkempt appearance.
Skin	Supine	Flashlight	Inspection Palpation	Good color, warm to touch. No lesion such as warts, moles, abscesses, rashes.	Jaundice, cyanosis, pallor, redness, flakiness of skin, lesions, rashes.
Head and neck	Supine or Semi-Fowler's or sitting on edge of table	Light source	Inspection Palpation	Symmetry of head. Hair not dry or oily and distributed evenly. Scalp free of lesions and not dry.	Asymmetry of head. Alopecia, dry, flaky scalp. Swelling, lumps or pain in head or neck.
Eyes	Supine or Semi-Fowler's or sitting on edge of table	Flashlight Ophthalmoscope	Inspection Mensuration	Snellen test shows accurate visual acuity. Able to identify color plates. No tearing. Pupillary reaction to light equal. Retina pink and blood vessels healthy. Tonometer measurement of intraocular pressure within normal limits. No bulging of eyeballs.	Poor visual and color ability. Dull appearing eyes. Drainage. Unequal pupils. Clouded lens. Unequal papillary reaction. Intraocular pressure increased. Torturous, unhealthy retinal blood vessels. Bulging eyeballs.
Ears	Supine or Semi-Fowler's or sitting on edge of table	Otoscope Flashlight Tuning fork and/or audiometer	Inspection Percussion	Cerumen not impacted on tympanic membrane. Tympanic membrane gray and intact. No discharge or pain. Able to hear tuning fork or audiometer.	Impacted cerumen. Red, bulging tympanic membrane. Discharge (pus or blood). Inability to hear sound from tuning fork. Poor auditory ability when checked with audiometer.
Nose	Supine or Semi-Fowler's or sitting on edge of table	Nasal speculum Flashlight	Inspection	Mucous membranes moist and pink. Able to detect specific odors. Septum straight. Nostrils equal in size. No abnormal discharge. No lesions.	Dry, red swollen mucous membranes. Unable to detect odors. Deviated septum. Nostrils non-flaring. Discharge, polyps noted.
Mouth and throat	Supine or Semi-Fowler's or sitting on edge of table	Flashlight Tongue depressors Laryngeal and pharyngeal mirrors	Inspection	Gag reflex present. Mucous membranes moist and pink. Teeth intact, pink tongue. Tonsils nonswollen, pink.	No gag reflex. Tongue rough. Pallor of mucous membranes. Dental caries. Swollen tonsils.
Arms and hands	Supine or Semi-Fowler's or sitting on edge of table	Percussion hammer	Inspection Palpation	Good muscle tone. Normal range of motion. Nails pink, smooth. Ability to squeeze doctor's hands with equal strength.	Poor muscle tone. Poor range of motion. Nails cyanotic. Brittle, ridged nails.
Chest and lungs	Supine or Semi-Fowler's or sitting on edge of table	Stethoscope Tape measure	Inspection Palpation Auscultation Mensuration Percussion	Axillary lymph nodes not palpable. Lungs clear. No cough. Ribs nontender. Symmetrical chest wall. Respirations and heart rate normal. Normal chest sounds.	Enlarged axillary lymph nodes. Asymmetry of chest wall. Respiration and heart rate abnormal. Abnormal chest sounds.

(continues)

Head. The patient will be in a sitting position for this examination. The face will be checked for puffiness especially around the eyes. Facial skin will be checked for **scleroderma**, a tight and atrophied skin. The elderly patient may have fatty patches that appear raised and yellowish on the eyelids. The hair and scalp are checked. The head and neck are palpated for lumps and swelling.

Eyes. The appearance of the eyes is examined. The pupils of the eyes will then be checked for light accommodation. When a penlight or flashlight is placed in front of the pupil, the pupil will constrict. The other pupil should constrict equally. If they do not constrict and return to normal equally, it may indicate a problem in the brain. A tonometer may be used to measure the intraocular eye pressure of patients over the age of 35 years. Normal eye

TABLE 25-2 *(continued)*

Body Part	Position	Instrument Used	Method of Exam	Physician's Findings Normal	Physician's Findings Abnormal
Heart	Supine or Semi-Fowler's or sitting on edge of table	Stethoscope ECG	Auscultation Palpation Mensuration	Normal heart function per ECG. Regular rhythm, rate of heart sounds. No murmurs. Blood pressure normal range. Pulse points good quality.	Abnormal heart function per ECG. Irregularity of rhythm, rate. Murmurs. Blood pressure outside normal ranges. Poor pulse quality.
Breasts	Supine	—	Inspection Palpation	No lumps, tenderness, swelling, or thickening. No sores or lesions. No bleeding or discharge from nipples. No lymph node swelling in axilla. No dimpling or "orange peel" appearance.	Lumps, tenderness, swelling, thickening. Sores or lesions. Bleeding or discharge from nipple. Lymph node enlargement in axilla. "Orange peel" appearance to breast tissue. Dimpling of skin.
Abdomen	Supine	Stethoscope Measuring tape	Inspection Palpation Auscultation Mensuration Percussion	Liver, spleen not palpable. Symmetry to abdomen. No abnormal bowel sounds. No abnormal sounds from organs in abdomen. Abdomen soft. No abdominal or inguinal hernias.	Liver, spleen enlarged. Asymmetrical abdomen. Increased or decreased bowel sounds. Unusual sounds elicited from percussion of abdominal organs. Abdominal distention. Ascites. Presence of abdominal, umbilical, or inguinal hernia.
Female genitalia and rectum	Lithotomy or dorsal recumbent or Sims'	Vaginal speculum Light source	Inspection Palpation	External genitalia without lesions, sores, ulcerations. Vaginal mucosa pink and without discharge. Nontender ovaries. Cervix smooth, noneroded, noninflamed. Good muscle tone in perineal floor and rectum. Negative stool for occult blood. Non-palpable lymph nodes in groin.	Lesions, sores, ulcerations. Discharge from vagina, cervix. Painful ovaries. Cervix ulcerated, inflamed. Poor muscle tone in perineal and rectum floor. Prolapse of uterus or bladder into vagina. Hemorrhoids. Positive hemoccult. Enlarged inguinal lymph nodes.
Male genitalia	Supine Standing	—	Inspection Palpation	Penis pink, no discharge. No lesions, sores, ulcers. Testicles firm, nontender, and movable. Rectal musculature intact. Nonpalpable prostate. Nonpalpable lymph nodes in groin.	Discharge from penis. Ulcers, sores, other types of lesions. Testicles tender, swollen. Relaxed anal sphincter. Hemorrhoids. Positive hemoccult slide. Enlarged prostate. Enlarged lymph nodes in groin.
Legs and feet	Supine Prone	Tape measure	Inspection Mensuration Palpation	Normal muscle tone and range of motion. No edema. Pulses normal. No varicosities. Toenails smooth, no signs of fungus or other infection. Calves equal in size.	Muscle weakness. Poor range of motion. Edema. Diminished pulse. Varicose veins. Toenails ridged, infected. Unequal calf measurements.
Neurological exam	Supine	Percussion hammer Safety pin Cotton ball	Percussion Inspection	Normal reflexes oriented to time and place. Appropriate responses. Normal responses to sensation. Alert. Steady gait. No vertigo or syncope.	All reflexes disoriented. Inappropriate responses. Dulled response to pain and sensation. Lethargic. Unsteady gait. Poor coordination. Vertigo. Syncope.

pressure is 20 to 25 mm Hg. An increase above normal will be found in glaucoma. The physician will use an ophthalmoscope to view the retina of the eye. This is done by turning out the lights in the room allowing pupils to dilate. The patient is instructed to look straight ahead while the physician looks into the eye. Retinal changes indicate disease.

Ears. An otoscope is used by the physician to examine the ears. The external ear is checked for redness in the ear canal and buildup of cerumen. A healthy tympanic membrane has a pearly gray appearance. A red appearance to the tympanic membrane may indicate infection in the middle ear, known as otitis media. Vertigo may indicate that the patient has an inner ear infection or labyrinthitis. Tinnitus or ringing in the ears may indicate inner ear problems. Other symptoms of ear problems include pain, discharge, and deafness. The tuning fork is used in testing the sensations of hearing, including bone conduction and air conduction.

Nose. The nasal cavity will be visualized by the physician with the use of a nasal speculum. Discharge from the nose may indicate a postnasal drip in which the sinuses may be draining into the nose and throat. Other abnormalities may include obstruction due to a deviated septum. Polyps and ulcerations may be found in the nasal cavity. Epistaxis or nosebleed may be seen when the capillaries rupture on the surface of the nasal mucosa.

Mouth and Throat. The physician will use a tongue blade or depressor and a light source. The teeth and gums will be checked for dental hygiene such as caries and the gums will be checked for signs of pyorrhea (discharge of pus from the gums around the teeth). If the tonsils are present, they will be checked for signs of infection such as redness or white pockets of pus. The larynx and pharynx are examined in the same manner, using laryngeal and pharyngeal mirrors to look for abnormal redness and patches indicating a disease. The floor of the mouth is examined both visually and by palpation for indications of swollen glands and ulcerations.

Neck. The physician palpates the neck looking for swollen lymph nodes. The thyroid gland is palpated anteriorly and posteriorly for size, symmetry, and texture. The patient will be asked to swallow several times while the physician feels the thyroid gland. A small glass of water may be given to the patient to aid in swallowing. Range of motion will be checked by having the patient turn the head in each direction. Care must be taken with the elderly. The patient should be instructed to move the head slowly.

Chest. The symmetry of the chest is observed, both anteriorly and posteriorly. Chest measurement may have been performed prior to the examination. The chest of a patient with emphysema will appear barrellike in shape. While the patient is sitting, the physician will listen to the lungs with a stethoscope. The patient may be instructed to take several deep breaths during this process.

Carefully monitor the patient, particularly the elderly, as deep breathing may cause dizziness. The physician will be listening for abnormal lung sounds previously discussed. The physician may examine the lungs by percussion. Heart sounds will be auscultated both anteriorly and posteriorly. In cases of heart disease, the medical assistant may have been instructed to obtain an electrocardiogram.

Breast. The patient will be placed in a supine position and instructed to place the hand behind the head on the side on which the examination is taking place. The physician will examine the breast for masses by using a circular motion starting at the outer edge of the breast and working toward the center. The nipple will then be gently squeezed to see if there is any discharge. The patient is then instructed to change arm positions so that the other breast may be examined. With the patient in a sitting position, the physician will observe the breasts for symmetry. Female patients should be instructed on the procedure to follow for performing monthly breast self-examination. This may be an embarrassing procedure for the female. Maintain as much modesty as possible by carefully draping and giving emotional support. See Chapter 26 for more detailed information on breast examination.

Abdomen. The patient is placed in a dorsal recumbent or supine position with the arms at the sides for examination of the abdomen. The drape is lowered to just above the pubic hair. The female patient will wear a gown open in the front which can be pulled to the sides while still covering the breast. The physician will normally stand on the right side of the patient while performing this part of the examination. The abdomen will be examined by palpation, percussion, and auscultation. Following the quadrants of the abdomen, the physician will gently palpate the organs in each quadrant working from side to side. The physician will feel for organ size and location as well as the presence of masses, percuss the abdomen listening for sounds from abdominal organs, use the stethoscope to listen for presence of abdominal sounds, and will visually inspect the abdominal area for changes in skin color, scars, or other abnormalities. The contour of the abdomen may be flat or slightly convex. The presence of hernias will be checked both in the supine and standing positions. Patients with abdominal disorders may give a history of dyspepsia, dysphagia and/or excessive flatulence, nausea, and vomiting.

Genitalia. Also refer to Chapters 26 and 28 for more detailed information.

Female Genitalia. The patient is placed in the lithotomy position. The physician will examine both the external genitalia and reproductive organs. The rectum may be examined and a hemoccult test done at the conclusion of the pelvic examination. See Chapter 30 for information regarding the hemoccult slide test. After the examination, the patient is instructed to slide toward the head of the table and may be allowed to sit up slowly. Haste may cause orthostatic hypotension and dizziness.

Male Genitalia. Care must be taken to protect patient modesty and privacy. The physician will begin the examination by inspecting and retracting the foreskin of the penis if the patient is uncircumcised. The glans penis will be inspected for discharge and redness. The penis and scrotum will then be palpated for possible tenderness and masses. Due to the seriousness of testicular cancer, the patient will be instructed, usually by the physician, in the procedure to perform monthly testicular examinations. Refer to Chapter 28.

Rectal Examinations. The physician may examine the rectum as a part of the male genitalia exam. The patient is placed in either the Sims' or knee-chest position. The physician will perform a manual examination. The prostate gland is then examined by palpation. The physician inserts the gloved index finger into the rectum and palpates the prostate gland for any masses or swelling.

(See Chapter 28 for more information.) A lubricated rectal speculum may then be inserted for visual examination. Since this is uncomfortable for the patient, emotional support is important. The physician can visualize the rectum for any bleeding, fissures, polyps, or lesions.

Reflexes. The patient's reflexes are observed by the physician in both the supine and sitting positions. A percussion hammer is used. While sitting with the arm flexed, the elbow will be lightly tapped to elicit movement from the biceps. The patellar or knee-jerk reflex is tested by tapping the area just below the patella at the knee. The Achilles reflex or ankle-jerk is tested by tapping the Achilles tendon. The Babinski reflex is tested on the sole of a relaxed foot (the great toe will flex) with the patient in a supine position. Reflexes determine the integrity of the neurological system.

Procedure 25-9 outlines the steps in assisting with the physical examination.

Once the examination has been completed, the patient will be instructed to dress. The patient should be given privacy while dressing. Assist the patient as needed. Do not remain in the room to clean it while the patient is dressing. Remain in the room if the patient requires assistance. Further instructions regarding other testing procedures and treatment plans will be provided by the physician. Be specific with instructions to patients regarding what they should do after they are completely dressed.

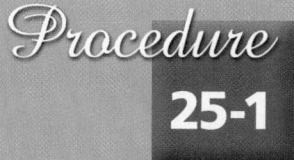 **Positioning Patient in the Supine Position**

25-1

STANDARD PRECAUTIONS:

PURPOSE:
To safely and properly assist patient into supine position for examination of anterior surface of the body from head to toe.

EQUIPMENT/SUPPLIES:
Drape
Gown

PROCEDURE STEPS:
1. Wash hands and follow standard precautions.
2. Assemble supplies.
3. Assist patient to sit on end of table.
4. Assist patient to lie back on table as you pull out the table extension. Support patient's feet and back while extending foot of table.
5. Cover patient with drape from shoulders to ankles.
6. Place small pillow under patient's head.
7. Upon completion of a procedure, assist patient to sitting position. RATIONALE: Allowing patient to remain seated helps to prevent dizziness caused by orthostatic hypotension.
8. Push table extension back into place while supporting patient's feet.
9. Once patient is stable (check color of skin, pulse), give further instructions as required.

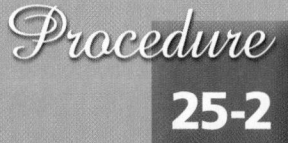

Positioning Patient in the Dorsal Recumbent Position

25-2

STANDARD PRECAUTIONS:

PURPOSE:
To safely and properly assist patient to dorsal recumbent position for catheterization or pelvic exam, head, neck, chest, abdominal, or lower limb examination.

EQUIPMENT/SUPPLIES:
Drape
Gown

PROCEDURE STEPS:
1. Wash hands and follow standard precautions.
2. Assist patient to sit on end of table.
3. Assist patient to lie back on table; extend the foot of the table while you support patient's feet and back.
4. Assist patient to bend knees and place feet flat on the surface of the table. Push in foot extension.
5. Cover patient with drape (diamond shape) from shoulders to ankles.
6. Place small pillow under patient's head.
7. Upon completion of procedure, assist patient to sitting position while you push table extension back into place and support patient's feet.
8. Have patient sit at end of table for a few minutes. RATIONALE: This helps prevent dizziness and possible fall from low blood pressure due to orthostatic hypotension.
9. Once patient is stable (check color of skin, pulse), give further instructions as required.

Positioning Patient in the Lithotomy Position

25-3

STANDARD PRECAUTIONS:

PURPOSE:
To safely and properly assist patient in lithotomy position for genital or pelvic examination or for urinary catheterization.

EQUIPMENT/SUPPLIES:
Drape
Gown

PROCEDURE STEPS:
1. Wash hands and follow standard precautions.
2. Have patient disrobe from waist down and put on gown.
3. Assist patient to sit on end of table. Cover patient's lap and legs with drape.
4. Assist patient to lie back on table as you support patient's feet and back while extending foot of table.
5. Position stirrups level with the table and approximately one foot from edge of table. Lock stirrups into position. RATIONALE: Facilitates patient examination and ensures patient safety.
6. Have patient slide down on table. Have patient move as close to edge of examination table as possible.
7. Assist patient to bend knees and assist her in placing feet in stirrups. Move drape to diamond shape to ensure privacy.
8. Place small pillow under patient's head.

(continues)

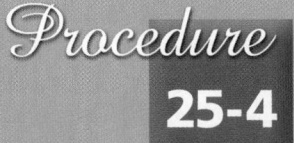

25-3 *(continued)*

9. Upon completion of procedure, extend foot extension of table.
10. Place feet on foot extension and assist patient to slide toward head of table.
11. Assist patient to sitting position while replacing foot extension.

12. Have patient sit at end of table for a few minutes. RATIONALE: This helps prevent dizziness and possible fall from low blood pressure due to orthostatic hypotension.
13. Once patient is stable (check color of skin, pulse), give further instructions as required.

Procedure 25-4 Positioning Patient in the Fowler's Position

STANDARD PRECAUTIONS:

PURPOSE:
To safely and properly assist patient into the Fowler's position for examination of upper body and head; often used for patients with cardiovascular or respiratory problems.

EQUIPMENT/SUPPLIES:
Drape
Gown

PROCEDURE STEPS:
1. Wash hands and follow standard precautions.
2. Provide gown and assist to disrobe if necessary.
3. Assist patient to sit on end of table. Cover lap and legs with drape.

4. Assist patient to slide back on table leaning against the back rest which has been raised slightly.
5. Support patient's feet while extending foot of table.
6. Position head of table at a 90° angle (45° for Semi-Fowler's).
7. Place pillow under patient's knees for comfort.
8. Cover patient with drape from shoulders to ankles.
9. Upon completion of procedure, replace foot extension.
10. Have patient sit at end of table for a few minutes. RATIONALE: This helps prevent dizziness and possible fall from low blood pressure due to orthostatic hypotension.
11. Once patient is stable (check color of skin, pulse), give further instructions as required.

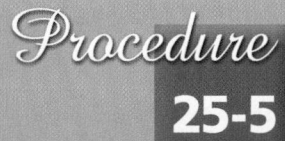

Procedure 25-5
Positioning Patient in the Knee-Chest Position

STANDARD PRECAUTIONS:

PURPOSE:
To safely and properly assist patient in knee-chest position for examination of the rectum, sigmoid colon, and in some instances the vagina.

EQUIPMENT/SUPPLIES:
Drape
Gown

PROCEDURE STEPS:
1. Wash hands and follow standard precautions.
2. Have patient completely undress. Provide gown.
3. Instruct patient to sit on end of table with drape over lap and legs.
4. Instruct patient to lie back on table while you support patient's feet and back and extend foot of table.
5. Assist patient to turn onto abdomen by turning toward you and being careful to stay in center of table to avoid a fall. Support patient by placing your left hand on patient's back and guide the patient toward you. Adjust drape.
6. Assist patient to rise to knees while bending at hips to place chest on table, keeping covered with drape.
7. Arms are bent to side of head with hands under head.
8. If this position is uncomfortable, have patient rest on elbows. Adjust drape from shoulders to ankles.
9. Upon completion of procedure, assist patient to lie flat on abdomen and then turn onto the back toward you and then return to sitting position.
10. Have patient sit at end of table for a few minutes. RATIONALE: This helps prevent dizziness and possible fall from low blood pressure due to orthostatic hypotension.
11. Once patient is stable (check color of skin, pulse), give further instructions as required.

NOTE: Since this is an embarrassing and uncomfortable position, it is best that the patient not be placed into this position until the physician is ready for the examination.

Procedure 25-6
Positioning Patient in the Prone Position

STANDARD PRECAUTIONS:

PURPOSE:
To safely and properly assist patient into the prone position for examination of posterior aspect of the body including the back, spine, or legs.

EQUIPMENT/SUPPLIES:
Drape
Gown

PROCEDURE STEPS:
1. Wash hands and follow standard precautions.
2. Have patient undress. Provide gown.
3. Assist patient to sit on end of table. Place drape over lap and legs.
4. Assist patient to lie back on table while you support patient's feet and back and extend foot of table.
5. Assist patient to turn toward you, then onto abdomen being careful to stay in center of table to avoid a fall. Place pillow under feet and head.
6. Adjust patient drape from shoulders to ankles.

(continues)

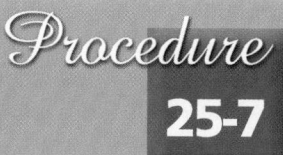

Procedure 25-6 *(continued)*

7. Upon completion of procedure, assist patient to turn toward you, then assist to sitting position.
8. Have patient sit at end of table for a few minutes. RATIONALE: This helps prevent dizziness

and possible fall from low blood pressure due to orthostatic hypotension.
9. Once patient is stable (check color of skin, pulse), give further instructions as required.

Procedure 25-7 Positioning Patient in the Sims' Position

STANDARD PRECAUTIONS:

PURPOSE:
To safely and properly assist patient into Sims' position for rectal examination, rectal temperature, proctoscopy, sigmoidoscopy, for an enema, and in some instances for vaginal examination.

EQUIPMENT/SUPPLIES:
Drape
Gown

PROCEDURE STEPS:
1. Wash hands and follow standard precautions.
2. Have patient undress. Provide gown.
3. Assist patient to sit on end of table. Place drape over lap and legs.
4. Assist patient to lie back on table while you support patient's feet and back and extend foot of table.

5. Assist patient to turn toward you onto the left side with left arm behind body, placing body weight on chest. Adjust drape.
6. Assist patient to slightly flex left knee and flex right knee to a 90° angle for support.
7. Right arm is bent in front of body with hand toward head at an angle to provide support.
8. Adjust drape from shoulders to ankles creating triangle or diamond shape.
9. Upon completion of procedure, instruct patient to turn toward you, then onto back, and then to sitting position.
10. Have patient sit at end of table for a few minutes. RATIONALE: This helps prevent dizziness and possible fall from low blood pressure due to orthostatic hypotension.
11. Once patient is stable (check color of skin, pulse), give further instructions as required.

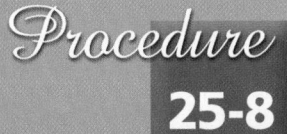

Positioning Patient in the Trendelenburg Position

STANDARD PRECAUTIONS:

PURPOSE:
To safely and properly assist patient into Trendelenburg position for certain abdominal and pelvic surgical procedures.

EQUIPMENT/SUPPLIES:
Drape
Gown

PROCEDURE STEPS:
1. Wash hands and follow standard precautions.
2. Assist patient to undress. Provide gown.
3. Assist patient to sit on end of table. Place drape over lap and legs.
4. Assist patient to lie back on table, with head at head board. Adjust drape.
5. Patient's feet are flexed over the end of the table.
6. Head of table may be lowered to a 45° angle.
7. Adjust drape from shoulders to ankles to ensure privacy.
8. Upon completion of procedure, assist patient to return to sitting position.
9. Allow patient to sit at end of table for a few minutes. RATIONALE: This helps prevent dizziness and possible fall from low blood pressure due to orthostatic hypotension.
10. Once patient is stable (check color of skin, pulse), give further instructions as required.

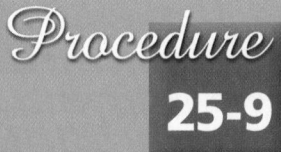

Assisting with a Complete Physical Examination

STANDARD PRECAUTIONS:

PURPOSE:
To assist physician in a complete physical examination.

EQUIPMENT/SUPPLIES:

Balance beam scales	Tape measure
Pharyngeal mirror	Thermometer
Lubricant	Stethoscope
Examination lights	Sphygmomanometer
Penlight	Alcohol wipes
Gloves	Cotton balls
Emesis basin	Gauze sponges
Percussion hammer	Safety pins
Patient gown	Otoscope
Drape	Tuning fork
Tissues	Ophthalmoscope
Specimen bottles/ slides—request forms	Tonometer Nasal speculum
Biohazard and regular waste container	Tongue depressors Laryngeal mirror

PROCEDURE STEPS:
1. Wash hands. Adhere to Standard Precautions.
2. Assemble equipment.
3. Place instruments in easily accessible sequence for physician use. RATIONALE: Efficient use of time and space.
4. Greet and identify patient.
5. Explain procedure to patient. RATIONALE: To obtain patient cooperation and allay apprehension.
6. Review medical history with patient. Refer to Chapter 23 for obtaining patient history. RATIONALE: To assure complete history has been obtained and is current.

(continues)

Procedure 25-9 (continued)

7. Take and record patient vital signs, visual acuity, and hearing test results.

8. Obtain a urine specimen. Refer to Chapter 42 for urine collection procedures.

9. Obtain all required blood samples. Refer to Chapters 40 and 41 for blood specimen collection procedures.

10. Perform electrocardiogram if directed by physician. Refer to Chapter 37 for ECG procedure.

11. Provide patient with appropriate gown and drape.

12. Assist patient to disrobe completely; explain where the opening for the gown is to be placed. RATIONALE: To assist patient in maintaining modesty, privacy, and warmth.

13. Assist patient in sitting at the end of the table; drape patient across lap and legs. RATIONALE: Always drape patient to maintain modesty.

14. Inform physician when patient is ready.

15. When the physician arrives, remain by the patient ready to assist patient and physician.

16. Position patient in a sitting or supine position for the head, throat, eye, ear, and neck examination.

17. Lights may be turned off to allow pupils to dilate for retinal examination.

18. Hand the physician instruments as required (some physicians will not require the medical assistant to hand the instruments).

19. The sitting position will be maintained for auscultation of the chest and heart.

20. Assist the patient into a supine position and drape for examination of the chest. Breast examination is discussed in Chapter 26.

21. Maintain a quiet atmosphere to enhance the ability of the physician in hearing heart and lung sounds. RATIONALE: Quiet is necessary to hear heart and chest sounds accurately.

22. Position patient in supine position and drape for abdominal examinations and examination of extremities.

23. Gynecological examination may then be performed. Refer to Chapter 26. Assist patient into lithotomy position for gynecological examination. Male genitalia examined.

24. If rectal examination is necessary, assist patient into Sims' position.

25. Place patient in prone position for examination of posterior aspect of body.

26. Upon completion of the examination, assist patient to sitting position and allow to sit at end of table for a few minutes. RATIONALE: Allows patients to recover from potential dizziness.

27. Assure patient stability (check color of skin, pulse) before allowing patient to stand up. RATIONALE: Prevents the possibility of a patient fainting from orthostatic hypotension.

28. Assist patient in dressing; provide privacy.

29. Chart any notes or patient instructions per physician orders.

30. Escort patient to physician's office for discussion of examination results.

31. Put on disposable gloves.

32. Dispose of gown and drape in biohazard waste container. RATIONALE: Prevent microorganism cross contamination; gown and drape may have body secretions on them.

33. Dispose of contaminated materials in biohazard container. RATIONALE: Prevent microorganism cross contamination of bloodborne pathogens and other potentially infectious materials (OPIM).

34. Remove table paper and dispose in biohazard waste container. RATIONALE: Prevent microorganism cross contamination.

35. Disinfect counters and examination table with a solution of 10 percent bleach. RATIONALE: Prevent microorganism cross contamination by blood and OPIM.

36. Clean, disinfect, or sterilize reusable instruments as appropriate (refer to Chapters 22 and 31). RATIONALE: Prevent microorganism cross contamination.

37. Remove gloves, discard in biohazard waste container. RATIONALE: Prevent microorganism cross contamination by blood and OPIM.

38. Wash hands.

39. Replace table paper and equipment in preparation for the next patient.

40. Document the procedure.

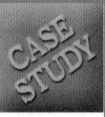

25-1 At Inner City Health Care, clinical medical assistant Wanda Slawson is helping Liz Corbin, a part-time administrative/clinical medical assistant, learn to prepare the examination room and patients for the physical examination. In addition to alerting Liz to physician preferences, Wanda wants to be sure that Liz has a solid understanding of the methods of examination, positions and draping, and the components of the physical exam.

CASE STUDY REVIEW

1. In reviewing with Liz the methods of examination used by physicians, what six primary methods would Wanda have Liz describe?
2. What patient positions would Liz need to know?
3. Wanda asks Liz to recall the various examination components and their significance. How should Liz respond?

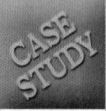

25-2 Mrs. Mason, a 72-year-old somewhat frail female with arthritis and hypertensive heart disease has an appointment today for a complete physical exam. It will include a basic physical exam and an exam of the pelvis because she has had bright red vaginal spotting.

CASE STUDY REVIEW

1. Discuss positions and draping for the physical exam including pelvic for this patient.
2. Discuss any special safety needs for Mrs. Mason.
3. What additional supplies and/or equipment should be available for the physician?

SUMMARY

A complete physical examination should be performed on the initial visit of the patient. Findings at this examination, both normal and abnormal, provide a baseline for future examinations.

The role of the medical assistant throughout the examination is twofold. The assistant assembles the necessary instruments and may hand them to the physician when requested. The medical assistant will also prepare specimens as required by the examination and physician. Responsibilities to the patient include explanations and careful positioning, protecting modesty by careful draping and, most important, providing comfort, emotional support, and safety ensurance. By performing these duties, the medical assistant can assure patient compliance and physician efficiency.

REVIEW QUESTIONS

Multiple Choice

1. The method of examination that is the process of listening directly to body sounds is called:
   a. percussion
   b. auditory
   c. auscultation
   d. the direct method

2. The supine position is also known as:
   a. horizontal recumbent
   b. dorsal recumbent
   c. knee-chest
   d. Sims'

3. During the physical examination, ataxia might be observed, which relates to:
   a. stature
   b. posture

c. body movement
d. speech
4. When the patient asks a question of the medical assistant, the medical assistant should:
   a. refer all questions to the physician
   b. try to answer all questions, even if uncertain
   c. answer questions to the extent of knowledge; refer others to the physician
   d. ask the patient to please hold all questions until the examination is complete
5. When the abdomen is being examined, the patient is typically in a:
   a. supine position
   b. prone position
   c. Fowler's position
   d. Sims' position

Critical Thinking

1. Discuss the responsibilities of the medical assistant during a physical examination.
2. Review the six methods used in the physical examination.
3. Give two reasons why positioning and draping are done.
4. Describe a type of examination that may be performed while the patient is placed in each of the following positions:
   a. lithotomy:
   b. Sims':
   c. knee-chest:
   d. supine:
5. List and describe the various components of a physical examination.
6. Explain the sequence for a physical examination.
7. List the instruments and/or supplies needed for examining the following body areas:
   a. head:
   b. reflexes:
   c. chest:
   d. abdomen:
8. Describe the cleaning process that the following instruments will need after their use in an examination:

a. nasal speculum
b. tuning fork
c. percussion hammer
d. reusable otoscope speculum
9. List and describe the three sources of information the physician uses to aid in making a diagnosis.
10. List two procedures or tests the medical assistant might perform as part of the patient's physical examination.

WEB ACTIVITIES

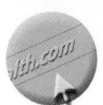

1. Using one of the "gateways" for general health and medical information and its links to other sites, gather information about the U.S. government's guidelines for average adult height and weight measurements. According to the government tables, what is considered an appropriate weight for your height?
2. Explore the Web for information about the following conditions and their possible causes:
   - changes in retinal blood vessels
   - enlarged liver
   - ascites
   - varicose veins
   - vertigo

REFERENCES/BIBLIOGRAPHY

Fremgen, B. F. (1998). *Essentials of medical assisting: Administrative and clinical competencies* (1st ed.). Upper Saddle River, NJ: Prentice Hall/Simon & Schuster.

Keir, L., Wise, B. A., & Krebs, C. (1993). *Medical assisting: Administrative and clinical competencies* (3rd ed.). Albany, NY: Delmar.

Kinn, M. E., & Woods, M. A. (1999). *The medical assistant: Administrative and clinical* (8th ed.). Philadelphia: W. B. Saunders.

Taber's cyclopedic medical dictionary (18th ed.). (1999). Philadelphia: F. A. Davis.

Thibodeau, G., & Patton, K. (1996). *The human body in health & disease* (2nd ed.). St. Louis: Mosby Year Book.

Zakus, S. (1995). *Clinical procedures for medical assistants* (2nd ed.). St. Louis: Mosby Year Book.

ASSISTING WITH SPECIALTY EXAMINATIONS AND PROCEDURES

OBSTETRICS AND GYNECOLOGY

KEY TERMS

Abortion
Amniocentesis
Bartholin Gland
Braxton-Hicks
Candidiasis
Carcinoma in situ
Cervical Punch Biopsy
Cesarean Section
Chlamydia
Colposcopy
Condylomata
Congenital Anomalies
Coupling Agent
Cryosurgery
Dilation
Dysmenorrhea
Dyspareunia
Dysplasia
Eclampsia
Ectopic
Effacement
Endometriosis
Fulgarated
Genitalia
Gestation
Gestational Diabetes
Gravidy
Human Chorionic Gonadotrophin
Hyperemesis Gravidarum
Hysterosalpingogram
Involution
Lamaze
Lochia   (*continues*)

OUTLINE

Obstetrics
Initial Prenatal Visit
Subsequent or Return Prenatal
 Visits
Complications of Pregnancy
Parturition
Postpartum Period

Gynecology
The Gynecological Examination
Gynecological Diseases and
 Conditions
Other Diagnostic Tests Used to
 Detect Female Reproductive
 System Diseases

OBJECTIVES

*The student should strive to meet the following performance objectives and demonstrate
an understanding of the facts and principles presented in this chapter through written and
oral communication.*

1. Explain the importance of prenatal care, and discuss what examinations
   will be performed as part of the initial visit.
2. Explain why the initial prenatal visit is important.
3. Describe what laboratory tests and procedures are performed during the
   initial prenatal visit.
4. List 12 conditions and/or diseases that can cause a pregnant woman and
   her fetus to be at greater risk for problems during the pregnancy.
5. List signs and symptoms and their possible corresponding conditions
   that the physician searches for during the prenatal history and physical
   examination.
6. Calculate an EDC (or EDB) using Nagele's Rule.
7. Explain the purpose of ultrasonography and amniocentesis.
8. List and describe six types of abortion.
9. Explain what occurs in each of the three stages of labor.
10. Describe what takes place during the postpartum examination.
11. List and describe the diseases and disorders that can affect the female.
12. Describe the laboratory tests and procedures that can help diagnose
    the diseases and disorders that can affect the female.   (*continues*)

Multigravida
Nagele's rule
Neonatal
Nullipara
Oxytoxin
Parity
Parturition
Patent
Pelvic Inflammatory Disease
Placenta Abruptio
Placenta Previa
Polycystic
Pre-eclampsia
Prenatal
Primigravida
Prostaglandin
Puerperium
Sickle Cell Anemia
Tay-Sachs
Thalassemia
Titer
Trichomoniasis
Trimester
Ultrasonography
Viable

OBJECTIVES (*continued*)

13. Describe seven sexually transmitted diseases.
14. Explain the medical assistant's responsibilities with a gynecological exam.
15. Describe breast self-examination and method of teaching patient breast self-examination.
16. Discuss menopause.
17. Explain hormone replacement therapy.
18. Describe several methods of contraception.
19. Explain reasons for impaired fertility.
20. Describe three therapies to assist in reproduction.

ROLE DELINEATION COMPONENTS

CLINICAL

Fundamental Principles

- Apply principles of aseptic technique and infection control
- Screen and follow up patient test results

Patient Care

- Obtain patient history and vital signs
- Prepare patient for examinations, procedures and treatments

Diagnostic Orders

- Collect and process specimens
- Perform diagnostic tests

(*continues*)

SCENARIO

At Inner City Health Care in the obstetrical department, Wanda Slawson and Bruce Goldman, both certified medical assistants, are preparing for the day's appointments. Both take responsibility for being certain all rooms have appropriate equipment and supplies needed for today's patients. There are three ultrasonograms in addition to the pelvic exams, Pap smear, and breast exams scheduled for the afternoon. Wanda is responsible for assisting the physician with each of them. She is careful to follow all safety precautions before, during, and after assisting with exams and procedures. She is careful to explain procedures to the patients and to direct any questions to the physician.

INTRODUCTION

Obstetrics is the medical specialty in which the physician treats the female from the prenatal period through labor, delivery, and during the six-week postpartum period. Gynecology is the specialty that treats the medical and surgical disorders and diseases of the female reproductive tract. Both specialties are usually combined, and the physician who practices them is known as an obstetrician/gynecologist, or simply, an OB/GYN physician. Knowledge of

ROLE DELINEATION COMPONENTS (*continued*)

**GENERAL
(TRANSDISCIPLINARY)**

Legal Concepts

- Document accurately

Instruction

- Instruct individuals according to their needs
- Teach methods of health promotion and disease prevention

the female anatomy, the laboratory tests and procedures for both specialties, the diseases and disorders that affect the female during her nonpregnant and pregnant states, and patient education are essential for the medical assistant who will care for these patients. The goal of the OB/GYN specialty is to promote the health and well-being of the woman and her baby.

OBSTETRICS

Obstetrics is the branch of medicine that provides care to the mother and fetus during pregnancy, labor, delivery, and the postpartum period known as the **puerperium**. Pregnancy is a period of approximately forty weeks from the day that conception takes place (Figure 26-1). The puerperium is the period of six weeks following delivery when the mother's body is returning to its prepregnant state. Visits to the physician for pre- and postnatal care are the initial **prenatal** visit, return visits, and the six-week postpartum checkup.

Initial Prenatal Visit

The initial prenatal visit is of utmost importance and usually occurs after a woman has missed a second menstrual period or after an at-home pregnancy test is positive. It is a time of health promotion for the expectant mother and her baby. It is also the time for diagnosis and treatment of maternal disorders that may have been present before the pregnancy or that may have developed during the course of the pregnancy. Growth and development of the fetus are followed and identification of problems that may

impede a normal labor are sought. There is ongoing assessment of the expectant mother and the fetus. Any abnormalities can indicate a problem or complication necessitating further testing and assessment. Early detection and management of conditions such as **gestational diabetes**, urinary tract infections, anemia, and **preeclampsia** can prevent serious complications.

The initial visit requires more time than subsequent visits because a thorough history and physical examination are done, including breast, abdominal, pelvic, and vaginal exams. Pelvic measurements are taken to help

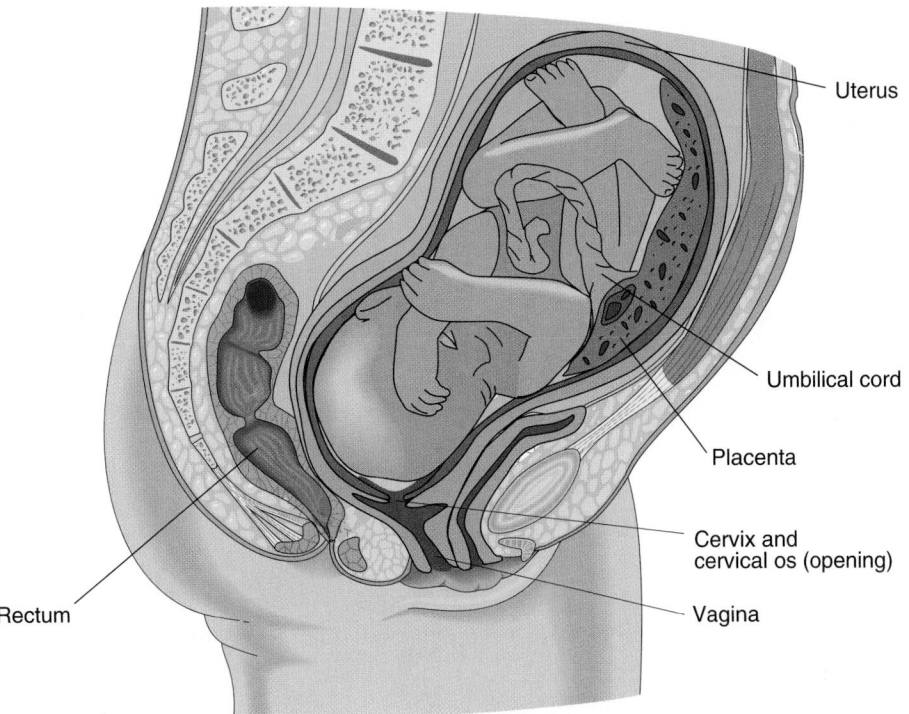

Uterus

Umbilical cord

Placenta

Cervix and cervical os (opening)

Vagina

Rectum

Figure 26-1   Normal uterine pregnancy.

ascertain if the pelvis is adequate for a fetus to be delivered vaginally.

The initial visit is followed by monthly visits and then weekly visits beginning about the twenty-eighth week. The routine visits consist of checking weight, blood pressure, testing blood and urine, education about nutrition, activity and rest, and preparing for childbirth.

Many groups of women do not receive prenatal care. Lack of financial resources, lack of transportation, and poor communication by health care providers are some of the reasons that some women do not participate in prenatal care. Modesty may deter some women from seeking prenatal care. Exposing the body to a male is viewed as a major violation of modesty in some cultures. This is why protecting the privacy of all patients is critical.

Certain cultures expect their women to observe practices believed to ensure a favorable pregnancy. Mexican women are advised not to watch an eclipse of the moon; the belief is that the baby will be born with congenital anomalies. Some Spanish women in the United States wear a braided cord around the midsection to ward off nausea and to ensure safe birth. Medals and beads, often worn by women, are believed to ward off evil spirits. Other cultures believe that inactivity during pregnancy will safeguard the mother and baby. There are also many dietary influences within different cultures. (See Chapter 34 for more information about culture and diet and food choices.) Respect for all cultures is of great importance and judgments should not be made that some women are ignorant or lazy.

All women should be fully involved in their care. Women with physical or emotional disabilities must have their particular needs addressed. When necessary, make adaptations whenever possible for women who are mentally challenged, blind, deaf, or physically incapacitated.

Laboratory Tests. The laboratory tests that are part of the initial prenatal visit are described in Table 26-1.

Patient Education. Patient education includes such topics as nutrition, dental care, rest, and exercise as well as discussion about over-the-counter (OTC) and prescription medications. Alcohol and tobacco and their dangers and potential harm to fetus and mother should also be discussed. Medications, alcohol, cigarettes, and mind-altering substances taken by the mother have deleterious effects on the fetus and should not be used.

Before the birth, the expectant couple is encouraged to choose a method of feeding the infant. During the initial prenatal visit, benefits of breast-feeding the newborn are discussed. Breast-feeding is encouraged because it offers many nutritional, psychological, and immunologic benefits. Because the immune system of newborns is not fully developed, the high level of immunoglobulins in breast milk gives them protection against some pathogenic diseases of the respiratory and gastrointestinal tracts. Close contact between mother and newborn is certain with breast-feeding, and bonding can readily take place. Breast-fed infants seem to have fewer allergic reactions. For the mother, one benefit of breast-feeding is that

TABLE 26-1   LABORATORY TESTS AT THE INITIAL PRENATAL VISIT

Laboratory Test	Disease or Condition
Complete blood count (CBC)	To detect anemia or infection
Urinalysis with microscopic examination (pH, specific gravity, color, glucose, albumin, proteins, WBC, RBC, casts, ocetone, human chorionic gonadotrophin [HCG])	To detect diabetes mellitus, renal disease, infection, hypertensive disease, pregnancy
Blood type, Rh factor	To detect Rh incompatibility
Rubella titer	To determine immunity to rubella
Renal function	Renal impairment evaluation in women with history of diabetes mellitus, hypertension, or kidney disease
Tuberculin skin test	Screens for tuberculosis
Venereal disease research lab (VDRL) and rapid plasma reagin (RPR)	To detect syphilis
Human Immunodeficiency Virus (HIV) with patient permission	Screens for HIV antibodies
Hepatitis B+C virus	Screens for hepatitis B and hepatitis C viruses
Glucose Tolerance Test (GTT)	Screens for gestational diabetes
Cardiac evaluation electrocardiogram (ECG), chest x ray, and/or echocardiogram	Evaluates cardiac function in women with history of heart disease or hypertension
Pap smear	To check for cervical dysplasia, herpes simplex virus 2
Vaginal and/or rectal smear or culture	To check for gonorrhea, chlamydia, human papilloma virus (HPV)

the uterus **involutes**, or returns more quickly to the nonpregnant state.

Formal childbirth education classes given in various languages teach the fundamentals of labor, delivery, and newborn care and feeding.

Prenatal History. The prenatal history will be comprehensive and include much of the same information that is obtained during the taking of a regular medical history. However, emphasis will be on identification of the high-risk patient. Particular attention is given to women who have a history of one or more of the following situations or conditions because they may place women at greater risk during pregnancy:

- Use of legal drugs (OTC, prescription, tobacco, caffeine, alcohol), illegal drugs (marijuana, cocaine), and herbal products

- Age under 16 and over 35 years

- Rh negative blood (particularly if father has Rh positive blood)

- A history of repeated premature labors and deliveries, abortions, or stillbirths

- Genetic diseases in the family

- Previous **Cesarean section**

- Diabetes

- Hypothyroidism or hyperthyroidism

- Sexually transmitted disease

- Hypertension

- Nutritional deficiencies

- Cardiac problems

- Kidney conditions

- Epilepsy

- Headaches

Any of these conditions or diseases place the woman and fetus at risk for serious complications.

During the initial prenatal visit, an obstetrical history is taken, which includes the **gravidy**, or total number of pregnancies, including the present pregnancy, regardless of duration. The history also includes the **parity**, the number of pregnancies carried to the point of viability regardless of whether the baby was born alive or dead. Multiple births, twins, and triplets count as one pregnancy (gravida) and one delivery (para). For example, a woman pregnant for the first time is referred to as Gravida 1, Para 0. After this woman delivers, regardless if the baby is born alive or dead, if it reached the age of **viability**, the

history of the woman is Gravida 1, Para 1. Viability is the ability to grow and develop after birth. The term **multigravida** refers to a woman who has been pregnant more than once. **Nullipara** describes a woman who has not carried a pregnancy to viability.

The present prenatal history includes information about the present pregnancy. The physician searches for problems indicative of high-risk factors. Identifying high-risk patients helps to limit maternal and newborn deaths and diseases. Some factors that indicate that a patient is at high risk are inadequate nutrition; use of drugs such as alcohol, tobacco, or cocaine; existing medical conditions such as high blood pressure or diabetes; sexually transmitted disease; and poverty. The physician watches for signs and symptoms that indicate a potentially serious condition. Examples are listed in Table 26-2.

TABLE 26-2	SIGNS AND SYMPTOMS OF POTENTIALLY SERIOUS CONDITIONS
Signs and Symptoms	**Possible Condition**
Rapid weight gain	Pre-eclampsia
Headaches	Pre-eclampsia
Hypertension	Pre-eclampsia
Vision changes	Pre-eclampsia
Severe nausea and vomiting	Hyperemesis gravidarum/dehydration
Bleeding, discharge, abdominal pain/cramping	Threatened abortion
Edema	Pre-eclampsia
One sided pelvic or abdominal pain	Ectopic pregnancy (Figure 26-2)
Chills, fever	Vaginal infection, sexually transmitted disease

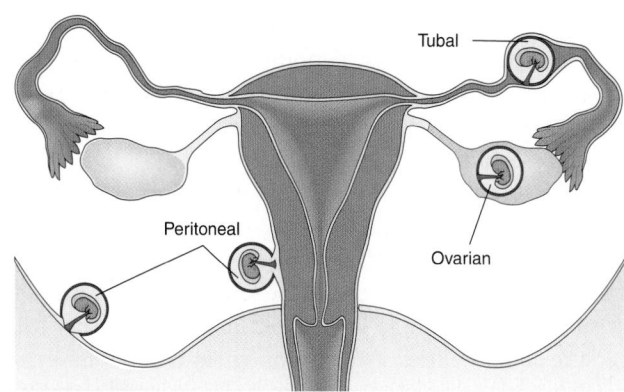

Figure 26-2 Sites of ectopic pregnancy.

Subsequent or Return Prenatal Visits

Each subsequent visit includes weight, blood pressure, urinalysis, complete blood count with hemoglobin and hematocrit, measurement of the height of the uterine fundus (a tape measure is used by placing it on the anterior symphysis pubis and the crest of the uterus), and fetal heart measurements. Generally, it is not possible to determine with accuracy the exact date of conception. Many formulas have been used for calculating the EDB (expected date of birth) or EDC (expected date of confinement). While none is foolproof, **Nagele's rule** is the usual method used because it is reasonably accurate. Nagele's rule is to add seven days to the first day of the last menstrual period (LMP), subtract three months, and add one year. An example is:

the first day of LMP = July 10, 2000
add 7 days = July 17
subtract 3 months = April 17
add one year = April 17, 2001

Another method to calculate EDB or EDC is to add seven days to LMP and count forward nine months. Most women give birth seven days before or after the EDB or EDC.

Vaginal exams are only done periodically up to two to three weeks prior to the EDB or EDC. Patients are encouraged to attend classes in the **Lamaze** method of childbirth as well as classes in the care of the newborn.

Tests and Procedures

Alpha Fetal Protein (AFP). Another test that may be done during a subsequent visit is a blood test known as alpha fetal protein blood test (AFP). It is done about the sixteenth week of pregnancy. It is a screening test only, done to rule out neural tube defects, abdominal wall defects, and chromosomal problems such as Down syndrome. If the test is positive, additional testing such as an **aminocentesis** or an ultrasound will be used to help make a diagnosis.

Chorionic Villi Sampling (CVS). Chorionic villi sampling (CVS) is a test performed on women who are over age thirty-five, have a history of chromosomal abnormalities, and are known carriers of a genetic disorder such as **thalassemia**, **sickle cell anemia**, or **Tay-Sachs**. The test is done at about 8 to 10 weeks **gestation** and has an advantage over amniocentesis because the latter cannot be done before the fourteenth week. For the CVS test, a sample of tissue that surrounds the fetus is taken by means of suction. The sample is analyzed in the laboratory for genetic abnormalities. An ultrasonogram is done simultaneously with an amniocentesis in order to avoid possible injury to the fetus or placenta.

Ultrasonography/Amniocentesis. Two tests can be done that can supply vital information: **ultrasonography**, or ultrasound, and amniocentesis. Ultrasound can be performed in the first, second, or third **trimester**. It uses high-frequency sound waves to produce an image of the fetus. A **coupling agent** is spread onto the mother's abdomen to enhance penetration of sound waves through the tissue, and the scanning mechanism is moved over the abdomen. An image of the fetus can be viewed on a screen similar to a television screen. Photos are taken during the exam. The technique usually takes about one half hour. There are no known side effects to the fetus or mother, and ultrasound uses no X rays. There is no pain involved, but slight discomfort can occur due to a full bladder. (A quart of fluid should be consumed one hour prior to the test and finished within 15 or 20 minutes.) A full bladder is essential to a good-quality ultrasound because it supports the uterus in position for good imaging. This procedure may be used to identify the number of fetuses, check the age of the fetus (number of weeks gestation), and detect some fetal abnormalities.

An amniocentesis is the surgical puncturing, with a long, thin needle, of the amniotic sac through the woman's abdomen. The purpose of this test is to obtain, by aspiration, a sample of amniotic fluid that contains fetal cells. The procedure can be done as early as fourteen weeks and helps to diagnose genetic mishaps, **congenital anomalies** (present at birth), and chromosomal defects. It also can be used to determine the lung capacity of the fetus.

Ultrasonography is performed while the physician is doing the amniocentesis to identify the position of the fetus and placenta, thereby avoiding injury to either. The procedure is not without risk and is not universally accepted. There can be bleeding, leaking of amniotic fluid, and infection.

Fetal heart rate is another test. Monitoring can be done in one of two ways: a nonstress test monitors the fetus's heart rate while it is moving spontaneously or a stress test monitors the fetal heart rate while the mother is stimulated with medication to have mild uterine contractions. Normally, the fetal heart rate will accelerate to a certain safe limit while it is being stressed.

Complications of Pregnancy

Abortion/Interruption of Pregnancy. The interruption of pregnancy before the fetus is viable is known as **abortion**. There are six types of abortion.

1. *Spontaneous:* Unknown etiology.
2. *Complete:* Expulsion of all products of conception, fetus, and placenta with no surgical intervention.
3. *Missed:* Fetus dies in the uterus and must be removed. Usually a dilation and curettage (D and C) is the surgical procedure performed.

4. *Incomplete:* Only parts of the fetus and placenta are expelled. Tissue remains in the uterus and a D and C usually must be performed.

5. *Threatened:* Bleeding from the uterus, but there are no contractions or dilation of cervix. Pregnancy continues.

6. *Induced:* Evacuation of the fetus and placenta from the uterus at the mother's request or because mother's health is in jeopardy.

Eclampsia. Eclampsia syndrome, also known as toxemia of pregnancy, can occur in pregnancy and result in convulsions unrelated to epilepsy or other brain conditions. It is a potentially life-threatening disorder characterized by hypertension, generalized edema, and proteinuria. It can put the woman and her fetus in grave danger. Preeclampsia is less severe. The symptoms are the same, except there are no convulsions. This is why weight is measured, blood pressure checked, and a urinalysis (including a check for protein) are routinely performed. Sudden significant weight gain, rise in blood pressure, and the presence of protein in the urine can indicate possible pre-eclampsia. The cause is unknown. The problem is seen more often in women who have received inadequate prenatal care, especially poor nutrition, in **primigravida** (pregnant for the first time) under age eighteen, in women with pre-existing cardiovascular and renal conditions, as well as in women who are diabetic.

Gestational Diabetes. Gestational diabetes first appears during the second or third trimester of the pregnancy and usually disappears after the woman has delivered her baby or when the pregnancy terminates for any other reason. This type of diabetes is usually a milder form of the disease. Prompt detection (through blood and urine glucose testing) and therapy are essential to avoid fetal and **neonatal** (newborn) illness and death.

Hyperemesis Gravidarum. Hyperemesis gravidarum, or excessive vomiting during pregnancy, can be very harmful and is more than morning sickness, which is a common complaint during the first trimester. The cause of the condition is not known, but it is thought to be related to the cells that become the placenta and to the production of pregnancy hormones. The symptoms include uncontrollable nausea and vomiting, inability to eat and exhaustion from inability to sleep. Severe dehydration can result and starvation may ensue. This complication is usually not fatal, but it is a severe problem that warrants immediate treatment. Treatment includes intravenous fluids to replace those lost through vomiting and mild sedation to aid rest and sleep.

Placenta Previa. Placenta previa occurs when the placenta implants low in the uterus and partially or com-

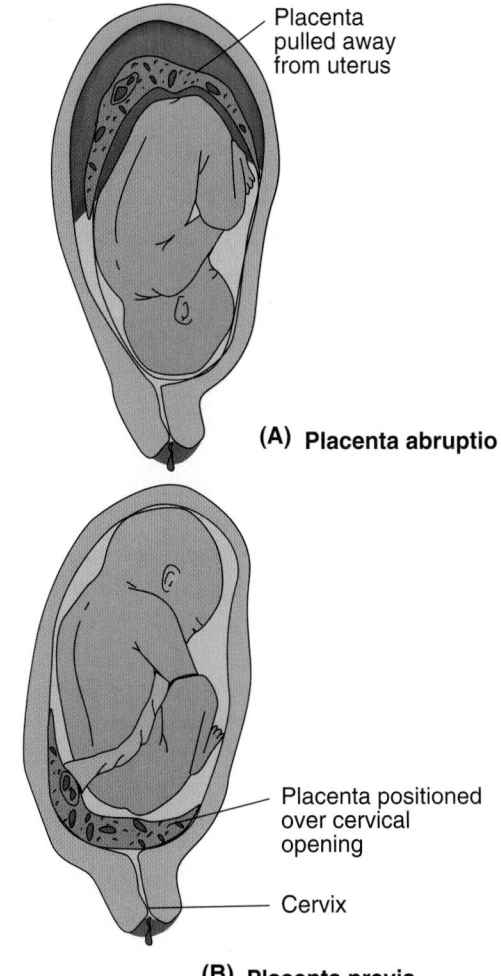

Figure 26-3 (A) Placenta abruptio. (B) Placenta previa.

pletely covers the cervical os. It is an emergency. The cause is unknown. When labor ensues and the cervix begins to dilate, the placenta is pulled away from the wall of the uterus and causes bleeding. On occasion, the bleeding, which comes on suddenly and is painless, will stop spontaneously. If it continues, significant maternal blood is lost, and the fetus may suffer anoxia and die when the placenta separates from the blood supply (Figure 26-3).

Ultrasonography will determine where the placenta is attached at which time the diagnosis can be made and treatment begun. Treatment depends on the gestational age of the fetus and the percent of placenta that covers the cervical os. Cesarean section may be necessary to remove the placenta, control bleeding, and deliver the fetus safely.

Placenta Abruptio. Placenta abruptio occurs when the placenta prematurely and abruptly separates from the uterine lining (see Figure 26-3A). It can result in fetal distress and death, and maternal shock. It usually occurs late in pregnancy but can occur during labor.

Factors that contribute to this complication are multiple pregnancies, chronic hypertension, trauma to the uterus, and sudden release of amniotic fluid. Delivery as soon as possible either vaginally or by Cesarean section is indicated. The prognosis of the newborn depends on the extent of hypoxia suffered during labor and delivery.

Impaired Fertility. The inability to conceive and bear a child after a period of unprotected sex is known as impaired fertility. Some reasons for this problem can be that many couples delay pregnancy until later in life when fertility is naturally lower. The increase in the incidence of **pelvic inflammatory disease** (PID), the increase in substance abuse, and environmental conditions such as pesticides and lead all can contribute to impaired fertility.

Diagnosis and treatment of impaired fertility requires a physical, emotional, and financial investment over a long period of time. To diagnose impaired fertility in the female, a complete history and physical exam are performed. Endocrine system and anatomic and physiologic abnormalities are sought. Laboratory tests on urine and blood are performed. Proof of ovulation can be determined by retrieving an ovum from the uterine tube, performing an endometrial biopsy, assessing mucus characteristics, and taking the basal body temperature. Levels of estrogen, progesterone, follicle-stimulating hormone, and lutenizing hormone are also measured. A **hysterosalpingogram**, an X ray of the uterus and tubes after the injection of dye, reveals defects in either the uterus or tubes.

Laparoscopy can be performed to visualize the internal pelvic structures. Tubal patency, **endometriosis**, pelvic adhesions, or **polycystic** ovaries can be seen. Endometrial biopsy is done to examine the tissue to determine whether the endometrium is capable of accepting a fertilized ovum for implantation. Ultrasonography, either abdominal or transvaginal, can assess pelvic organs for abnormalities.

Tests that can be performed on a male to diagnose impaired fertility are semen analysis, hormone analysis, and biopsy of a testicle. Once a diagnosis of impaired fertility has been made, a number of therapies are available to assist in reproduction. Some of them are:

- In vitro fertilization (IVF), indicated for fallopian tube blockage and endometriosis: Eggs are retrieved from ovaries, fertilized with sperm in the laboratory, then transferred to her uterus.

- Gamete intrafallopian transfer (GIFT): Eggs are retrieved from ovaries. An egg and sperm are aspirated into a special catheter then placed into the fallopian tube where fertilization can occur naturally.

- In vitro fertilization and gamete intrafallopian transfer (IVF + GIFT) with donor sperm: Eggs are retrieved from ovaries, fertilized with donor sperm in the laboratory, aspirated into a special catheter, then placed into the fallopian tube where fertilization can take place naturally.

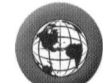 In some cultures, a woman is deemed the responsible party for impaired fertility, and the impairment is thought to be caused by her sins, evil spirits, or her own deficiencies. The virility of a male is questioned unless he is able to manifest his sexual potency by having a child.

Parturition

Parturition or labor is the process during which the uterus, through contractions, expels the fetus and placenta. There are three stages of labor:

Stage I Dilation: From onset of labor until complete **dilation** (expansion) and **effacement** (thinning and shortening) of cervix

Stage II Expulsion: From complete dilation and effacement through the birth of fetus (expulsion)

Stage III Placental: From birth of fetus through expulsion of the placenta

Labor is believed to be triggered by the release of **oxytoxin** and **prostaglandins** after the level of other hormones drop. When the oxytoxin is released, it causes the muscles of the uterus to contract. **Braxton-Hicks** contractions, often referred to as false labor, can usually be differentiated from real labor because of their irregularity and tendency to disappear when the woman moves about and changes positions.

Signs and symptoms to watch for during labor that indicate complications are heavy vaginal bleeding, sudden rise or drop in blood pressure, increased activity by the fetus, headache, extreme restlessness, and visual changes. Meconium in the vaginal discharge can indicate fetal distress.

Postpartum Period

The postpartum period is the time known as the puerperium during which the body returns to nonpregnant state. It is usually 4 to 6 weeks after delivery. The body undergoes changes during this time. The uterus involutes (returns to normal size) and healing of any injuries takes place.

A vaginal discharge, known as **lochia**, appears during the puerperium. It consists of tissue, blood, white blood cells, mucus, and bacteria. It can be described by its appearance. Lochia rubra is bright red and appears the first three days following delivery. Lochia serosa is pink or brown in color and is indicative of less blood. By about 10 days, the flow decreases, becomes whitish-yellow, and is known as lochia alba. Lochia usually disappears by the third week postpartum but may last for up to 6 weeks. Menstruation usually begins in a nursing mother 3 to 6 months after delivery, 2 months for non-nursing mothers. The mother is told to avoid heavy lifting, not to become fatigued, to eat a well-balanced diet, and to continue to take her prenatal tablets. An appointment in six weeks will evaluate the mother's general health, and the physician will discuss infant care, breast feeding, the importance of exercise and good nutrition, and birth control. The medical assistant can stress the importance of yearly Pap smears and of monthly breast self-examinations as these are important aspects of patient education.

Contraception. Voluntary prevention of pregnancy is known as contraception. The opportune time to discuss contraception with the mother is soon after delivery and before discharge from the hospital. She should know what method of contraception she and her partner will use before resuming sexual activity. To discuss contraception at the six-week postpartum checkup can be too late. Sexually transmitted disease (STD) protection should also be reviewed before discharge.

Written instructions about methods of contraception are important and help the patient understand options that are available.

Some nonprescription kinds of contraception are the various barrier methods: latex condoms, contraceptive foam, spermicide (nonoxynol-9) used with a condom to help prevent STDs, vaginal sponges that contain a spermicide, and abstinence.

Prescription methods of contraception include hormonal contraception in the form of oral birth control pills or Norplant®, a surgical implant of progestin in the upper arm, which provides up to five years of contraception. Other prescription methods include a diaphragm used with a spermicide, a cervical cap to fit over the cervix, and an intrauterine device (a small device made of copper or progesterone-medicated plastic).

Sterilization is a surgical procedure that renders the individual infertile. The woman's uterine tubes are **fulgarated** (destroyed by means of an electric current) or bands and clips are placed around the tubes to block them (ligation). Both fulgaration and ligation are considered to be permanent methods. Female sterilization can be performed immediately after birth or any time afterward during any phase of the menstrual cycle. Laparoscopic surgery is the usual approach.

The surgical procedure performed on a male to render him sterile is a vasectomy. It can be performed on an outpatient basis under local anesthesia. Small incisions are made into the scrotum above and to the side of each testicle. Each vas deferens is identified, ligated twice, and then severed. It is important for the patient to realize that sterility is not immediate because some sperm remain in the sperm ducts following vasectomy. One week to several months may elapse before the ducts are sperm free. Some form of contraception is necessary until two consecutive sperm counts are zero. (See Chapter 28.)

Another method of contraception recently approved by the Food and Drug Administration is a medication known as RU 486, which is used to cause or induce an abortion. It prevents a fertilized egg from implanting in the uterus.

GYNECOLOGY

Gynecology is the specialty that studies diseases of the female reproductive tract and the breasts. The gynecological examination is routinely performed in an office or clinic and usually includes abdominal, pelvic and breast examination, and a Pap smear. It can be done as part of the female's complete physical exam, or it can be a separate exam performed in the gynecologist's office or gynecology clinic. Early diagnosis and treatment of problems associated with the female reproductive organs helps the female to achieve optimum health of these organs and is the goal of the OB/GYN physician.

The Gynecological Examination

It is recommended that a gynecological exam and Pap smear be done annually on all women beginning when they become sexually active or by age 20. It is done to assess the female's health and to screen for cancer of the reproductive organs. It includes a breast examination by the physician and instructions for the patient about how to perform her own breast self-examination (BSE). It also includes a pelvic examination and Pap smear. Pap tests are done to detect cervical cancer. Women should be especially conscientious in scheduling annual Pap tests if they have a family history of uterine or cervical cancer. Early detection of cervical cancer and appropriate treatment can cure the disease. Others feel that in healthy women a Pap test done every 1 to 3 years is sufficient. The American Cancer Society recommends that females have a Pap test at least every 3 years, beginning when they become sexually active, or at age 20, if there have been two initial negative Pap test results 1 year apart. Encourage patients to have regular Pap tests. Women at high risk should have a Pap test every 6 months. If the patient is experiencing a vaginal discharge and there is a suspicion of a vaginal infection, smear(s) and cultures of discharge will be done to aid in diagnosis. See Chapter 43, Basic Microbiology, for more information.

Other gynecologic problems that may arise between annual gynecological examinations may require that an appointment, in addition to the annual gynecological checkup that is routinely done, be made and may include such symptoms and problems as severe **dysmenorrhea** (painful menses), lower abdominal pain, bleeding between menstrual periods, **dyspareunia** (painful intercourse), sexual dysfunction, infertility, and discomfort from menstrual symptoms. Women experiencing these problems will have a gynecological examination, and the physician will determine a diagnosis based upon the examination, patient's history, symptoms, signs, and laboratory data.

Breast Examination. The physician performs a breast examination on the patient as part of a gynecological examination. The physician looks for redness, dimpling, and puckering, and palpates each breast and axilla feeling for lumps or thickening. Part of the medical assistant's responsibility is to teach patients how to perform the BSE. Figure 26-4 provides illustrations for performing the BSE. The physician may also provide several pamphlets and/or a breast model with lumps and thickening for enhancing patient education and awareness about the importance of the examination (Figure 26-5A and B). (See Procedure 26-2.)

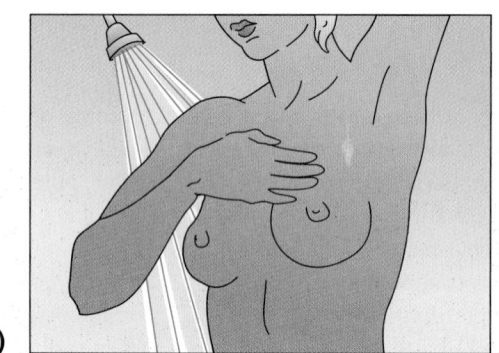

(A)

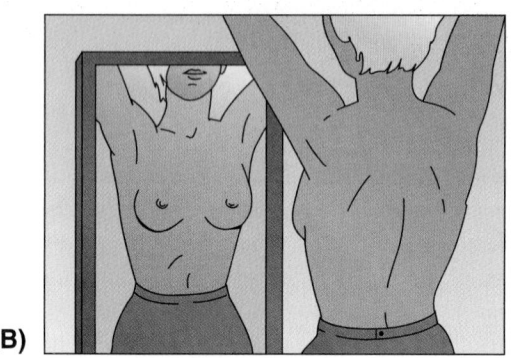

(B)

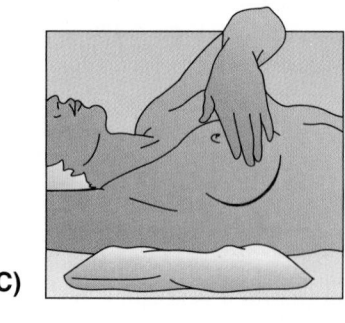

(C)

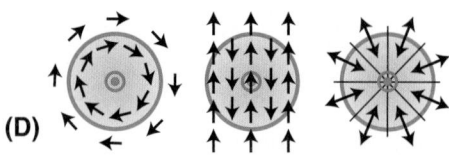

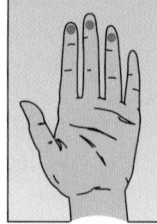

Finger pads

(D)

Figure 26-4 (A–D) Breast self-examination. (Courtesy of American Cancer Society)

Patient Teaching Tip

Breast Self-Examination
1. Breast self-examination (BSE) should be done in three different positions.
   a. In a warm shower (soaping each breast) checking for lumps, thickening, or changes that differ from previous self-exam. Refer to Figure 26-4A.
   b. In front of a mirror, checking for changes in appearance. Refer to Figure 26-4B.
   c. Lying flat in a supine position helps breast tissue spread allowing better palpation of outer tissue. Refer to Figure 26-4C. Use pads of fingers.
   d. Examine the breasts in a circular motion starting at 12 o'clock and moving around the breast clockwise. Use an up and down motion or an inward and outward motion from nipple outward or chest wall inward (Figure 26-4D).
2. Do the breast self-examination at the same time each month, 7 to 10 days after menses. Repeating the exam the same time each month provides familiarity with the contours of the body and allows for hormonal levels to return to premenstrual status. The breasts may be swollen, tender, and have thickening due to hormonal influence around the time of the menstrual cycle and for 7 to 10 days following menses.

Physician Breast Examination. The American Cancer Society recommends that:
a. Women ages 20 to 39 have a breast physical examination by a physician every 3 years and women age 40 and over have one yearly.
b. Women without symptoms of breast cancer ages 40 to 49 should have a mammogram every 1 to 2 years, and women age 50 and over, once a year (Figure 26-6 and 26-7). A tumor or mass can often be seen with a mammography up to 2 years before either the physician or patient notices or feels a tumor.

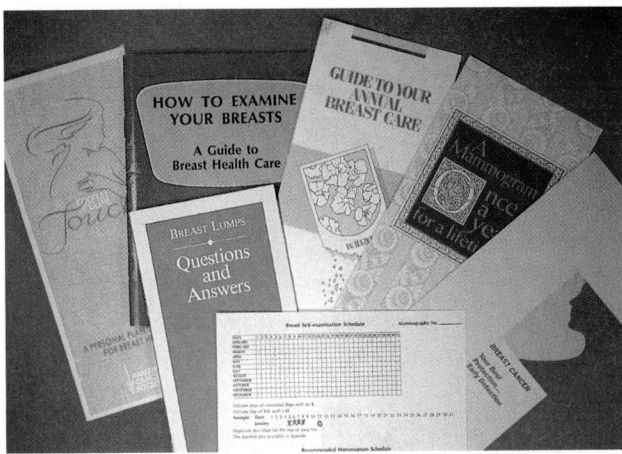

Figure 26-5A Informational pamphlets detailing the breast self-examination and its importance can be very helpful to patients.

Assisting with a Gynecologic Examination.

The gynecologic (GYN) exam consists of either four or five parts depending on whether the Pap test is done with the GYN exam. These parts include:

1. Inspection of external **genitalia** (labia minora, labia majora, urinary meatus, clitoris, **Bartholin glands,** and vagina) for swelling, lesions, or ulcerations.
2. Pelvic examination of cervix, uterus, tubes, and ovaries including a bimanual examination.
3. Rectal examination.
4. Breast examination.

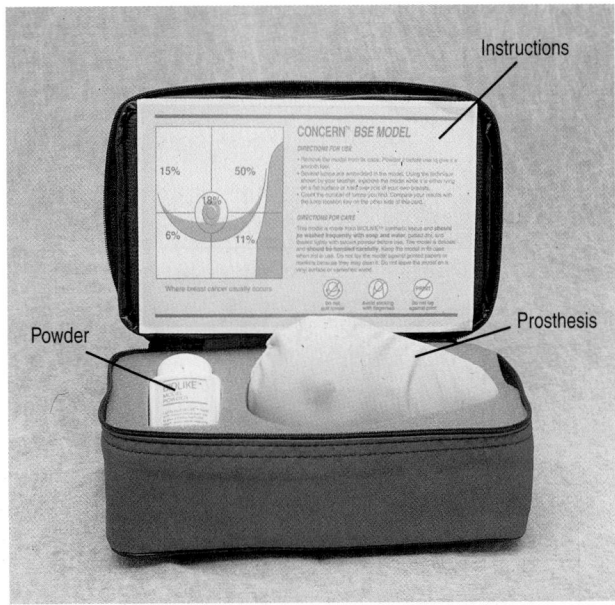

Figure 26-5B Breast self-examination model kit contains instructions for breast self-examination and powder to aid fingers in gliding over the breast prosthesis. The prosthesis contains lumps and thickened areas for identification and location.

5. The gynecologic pelvic examination can be performed with or without a Pap test. A Pap smear is taken during the gynecologic examination (Figure 26-8). The patient must refrain from sexual intercourse, using vaginal medication, and douching for 24 hours prior to the Pap test. These activities can interfere with obtaining a good sample of cervical

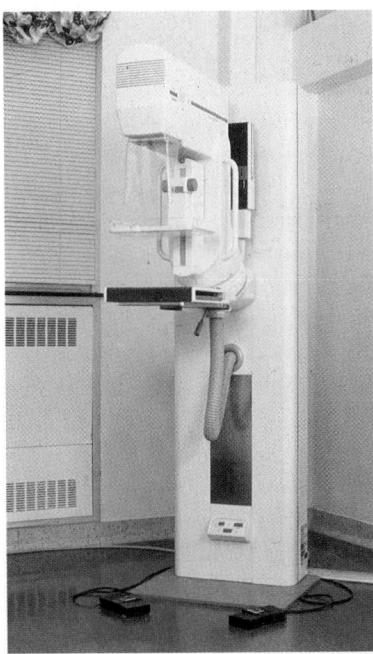

Figure 26-6 Breasts are compressed by the plates of mammographic x-ray unit.

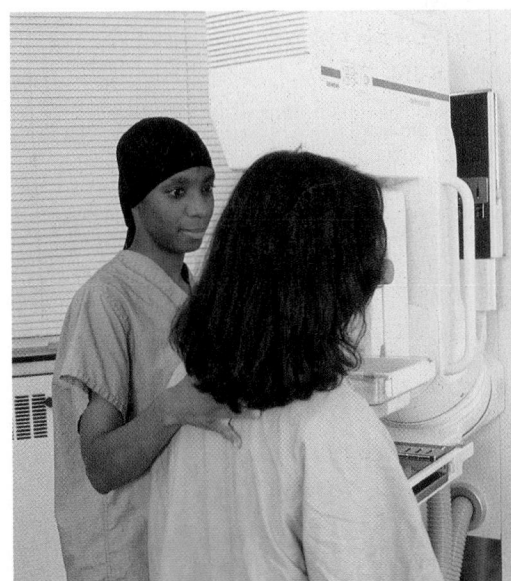

Figure 26-7 The technologist positions the patient for a mammography. The procedure requires the patient to move into various positions so different angles of the breast tissue may be x-rayed.

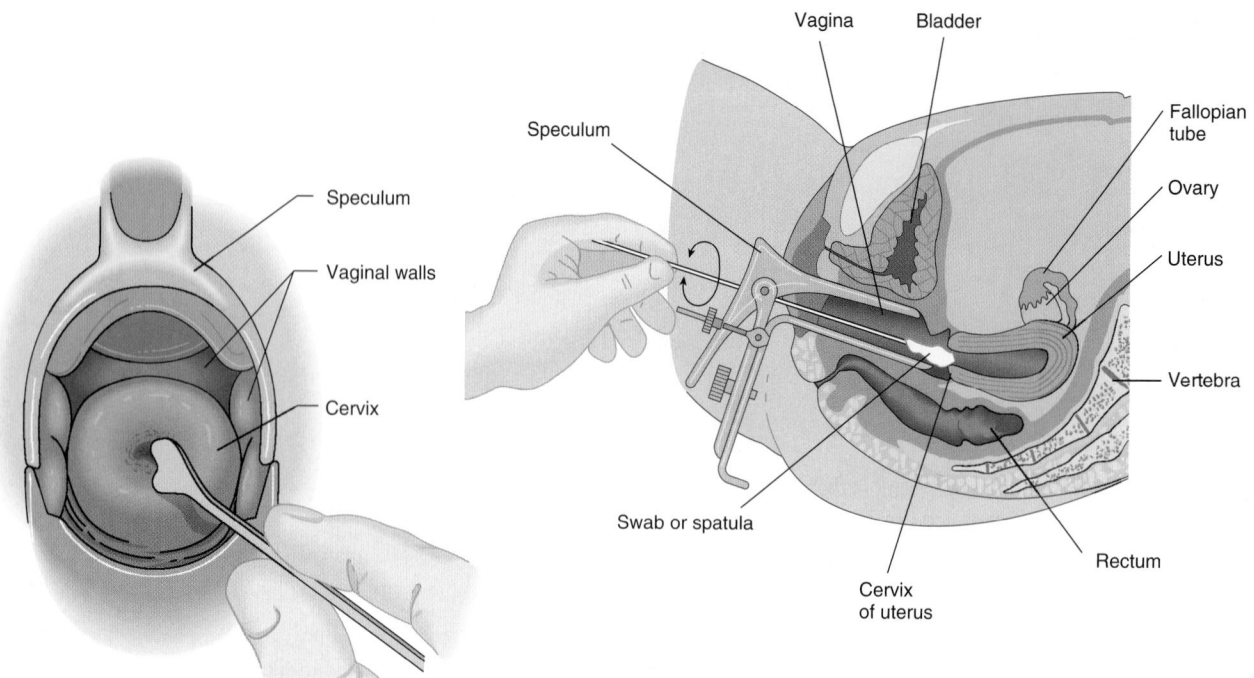

Figure 26-8   Use of speculum and obtaining a Pap smear.

cells. Also, a Pap smear cannot be done during menstruation because the red blood cells obscure the cervical cells.

The medical assistant should prepare the patient, equipment, and room prior to the examination.

Gynecologic Examination with Pap Equipment.

On a Mayo tray near the end of the exam table, place the instruments and supplies the physician needs to perform the gynecologic or pelvic examination with Pap test. Figure 26-9 shows the equipment commonly needed

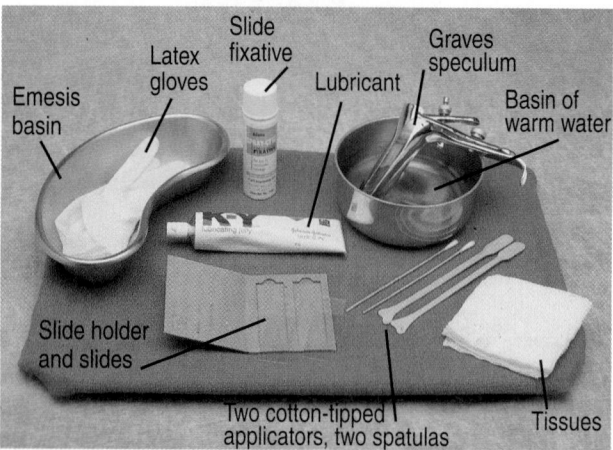

Figure 26-9   Setup for gynecologic examination including Pap smear.

for the examination. To aid in the inspection portion of the examination, a gooseneck lamp should be placed at the foot of the table behind the stool on which the physician will sit. (See Procedure 26-3.)

Pap Smear. The federal government regulates laboratories that perform testing on Pap smears. There are requirements placed on the individuals who test the specimens for malignant cells, and they include specialized training. Limits are placed on the number of slides that can be read in one day. Proficiency testing, mandated by the Clinical Laboratory Improvement Act of 1988 (CLIA '88) ensures accuracy and precision of test results and is a requirement for Pap smear examination. See Chapter 38 for more information about CLIA '88.

A computerized method, known as PAPNET, is used to retest Pap smears that have been analyzed by technologists. The method duplicates the process that the technologists perform. It is hoped that eventually the PAPNET will replace Pap smears done manually.

Another test, known as Virapap, can be used to screen for the human papiloma virus (HPV) in a Pap smear. There is higher incidence of cervical cancer in women who have HPV, and the test can help identify these women who are at greater risk for cervical cancer.

A system for cytologic reporting of a Pap smear is a descriptive report that tells the physician exactly what cellular changes have taken place. The classification includes the grades of cervical intraepithelial neoplasia (CIN).

CIN 1 = mild **dysplasia** (abnormal tissue development)

CIN 2 = moderate dysplasia

CIN 3 = severe dysplasia or **carcinoma in situ**

Pap Smear Results. The Pap smear will usually be sent to a reference laboratory where a pathologist will examine it and record the results on the cytology report form. The form will be returned to the physician.

Gynecological Diseases and Conditions

The female reproductive system is affected by many diseases and conditions caused by hormonal imbalance, cysts, infection, and tumors. Some of the more common disorders and diseases are covered here.

Infertility. Most women, with unprotected intercourse, will be able to conceive within a year. The inability to conceive can be caused by a problem with either the male or the female. Some common causes of infertility in a female are:

- Endometriosis
- Certain medications
- Blocked fallopian tubes
- Problems ovulating
- Chronic stress
- Scar tissue from surgery, infection, or ectopic pregnancy
- Tumors

A woman who is having difficulty conceiving and has a history of any of the above will have a physical examination by a physician who specializes in infertility. The specialist will decide what tests and/or procedures are necessary. Hormone levels may be measured to look for hypothyroidism and ovarian function determined through a surgical procedure, such as laparoscopy. A test for **patency** (openness) of the fallopian tubes can be performed by a hysterosalpingogram, a radiographic procedure done following injection of dye into the vagina, through the cervix, into the uterus, and out the fallopian tubes. The dye will pass through all of these organs if there is no blockage in any of them. (See Impaired Fertility, page 466.)

Menopause. The period of time that marks permanent cessation of menstrual activity is known as menopause. It usually occurs between the ages of 35 and 58. There may be a gradual decline in monthly menstrual flow, or a woman may suddenly cease to menstruate. Natural menopause occurs when the ovaries produce less and less estrogen. This causes the ovaries to cease ovulation and, therefore, menstruation stops. Surgical menopause is caused by the surgical removal of both ovaries (bilateral oophorectomy). Symptoms occur soon after ovulation ceases with both natural and surgical menopause. Symptoms may last for a few months to several years and include mild to severe symptoms. Hot flashes, chills, nervousness, fatigue, apathy, mental depression, crying episodes, insomnia, palpitations, and headache are some common symptoms experienced by some women. The long-term effects on lower estrogen levels are osteoporosis and atherosclerosis. Hormone replacement therapy (HRT) helps to prevent these diseases and reduce patient symptoms. There is some controversy regarding HRT benefits. Some studies show an increase in cancers of the female reproductive system in patients using HRT. Many authorities recommend HRT for most women unless they have a family history of breast cancer. Physicians believe that the benefits outweigh the risks for most women. When HRT is combined with a healthy lifestyle, well-being and health improve.

Endometriosis. This painful, common condition is characterized by endometrial tissue adhering to tissue and organs outside of the uterus. It is primarily found in the pelvis, adhering to an ovary, fallopian tube, or pelvic peritoneum. It also can be found outside of the pelvis, even in the abdomen adhering to tissue and organs, such as the bowel. The cause is unknown. The abnormal and engorged endometrial tissue responds to hormonal stimulation (estrogen) and builds up along with the normal endometrium of the menstrual cycle. It sloughs off at time of menstruation and is very painful. The blood has not had a way to leave the body and is discharged into the pelvic or abdominal cavities.

Endometriosis symptoms may respond to contraceptive medication because these pills suppress menstruation and no further treatment is necessary (see Figure 26-10). However, long-term hormonal treatment may help alleviate symptoms. Hysterectomy may be necessary if the woman does not respond to hormonal therapy.

Ovarian Cysts. Cysts that appear on the ovary are common. As part of the menstrual cycle, the ovarian follicles enlarge and become graafian follicles. Only one of these graafian follicles ruptures at the time of ovulation. The follicles that do not rupture, but remain, are filled with fluid. They may enlarge and become cysts (Figure 26-11).

Ultrasonography will aid in viewing the ovaries. Most ovarian cysts resolve without treatment. Laparoscopy can be done to either drain or remove the cyst. Contraceptive therapy many times is helpful in resolving the cyst without surgery.

Direct viewing of the ovaries and surgery may be necessary because cancer of the ovary must be ruled out.

Ovarian Cancer. Because the symptoms of ovarian cancer do not appear until the disease has had an opportunity to become established, it is difficult to make a diagnosis early in the disease process. Therefore, if a woman has any symptoms, the cancer has been present for some time. Symptoms may be pressure in the pelvis, lower abdominal discomfort, weight loss, and fluid in the abdomen. Diagnosis can be made by laparoscopic surgery and a biopsy. Hysterectomy and bilateral salpingo-oophorectomy are done followed by radiation therapy and/or chemotherapy. The cause is not known.

Pelvic Inflammatory Disease (PID). This disease involves some or all of the female reproductive tract and can be a mild to serious infection. The causative microorganism is usually a sexually transmitted pathogen. The microorganism enters through the vagina and ascends through the cervix into the body of the uterus. It can spread out through the fallopian tubes into the pelvic cavity. Culture and sensitivity of the vaginal discharge are performed, and appropriate antibiotics are prescribed. Early treatment helps to lessen damage caused by scar tissue that forms in the pelvis and organs. Delayed treatment can cause septic shock, which can be life-threatening. Infertility and ectopic pregnancy are long-range problems that can occur (see Tables 26-3, 26-4, and 26-5).

Other Diagnostic Tests and Treatments for Reproductive System Diseases

Colposcopy. Colposcopy is the examination of the vagina and cervix by means of a lighted instrument that has a three-dimensional magnifying lens called a col-

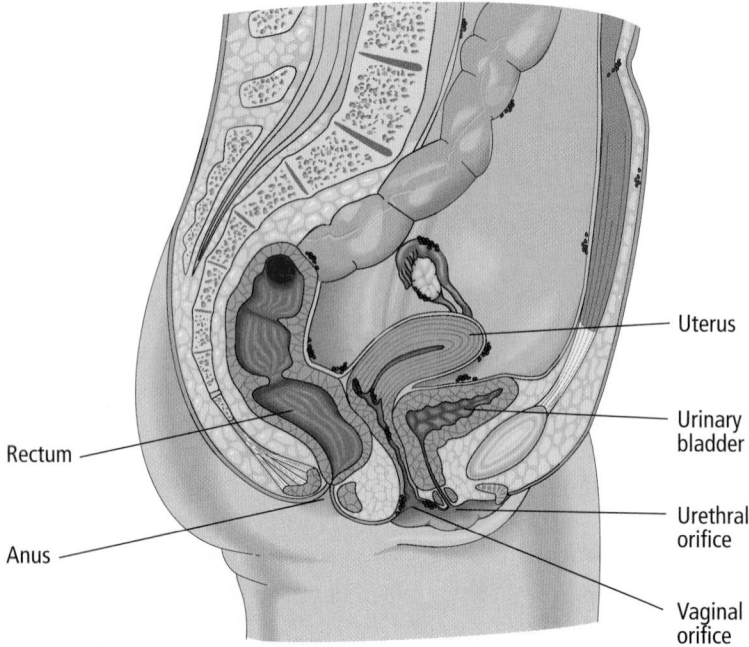

Figure 26-10   Endometriosis—common sites of endometrial implants.

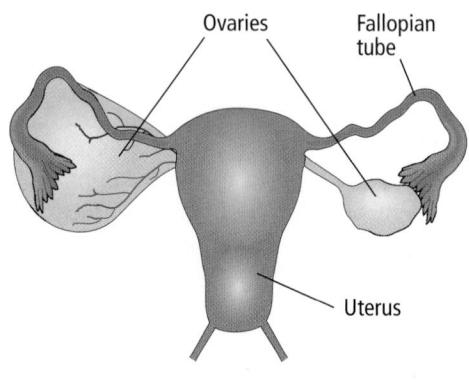

Figure 26-11   Ovarian cyst.

TABLE 26-3   FEMALE REPRODUCTIVE SYSTEM

Disease/ Disorder	Laboratory Diagnostic Tests			Radiography	Surgery	Medical Tests or Procedures
	Blood	Urine	Other			
Bartholin Gland Infection			Exudate culture and sensitivity		Incision and drainage	Pelvic exam
Breast Cancer	Breast cancer gene detection BRCAI			Mammography Ultrasonography	Biopsy of breast lesion	Monthly breast self-exam
Cervical Cancer			Pap smear		Cone biopsy Dilation & curettage (D&C)	Pelvic exam Colposcopy
Endometriosis		Urinalysis		Abdominal ultrasonography Chest x-ray	Laparoscopy Hysterectomy	Pelvic exam
Fibrocystic Breasts				Mammography Ultrasonography	Biopsy	Monthly breast self-exam
Pelvic Inflammatory Disease	Complete blood count and differential (CBC)	Urinalysis	Culture and sensitivity of vaginal discharge	Pelvic ultrasonography	Laparoscopy	Pelvic exam
Sexually Transmitted Diseases						
• Chlamydia	Serology	Urinalysis	Direct urethral and/or cervical smear using monoclonal antibodies			Pelvic exam
• Condylomata (genital warts)		Urinalysis		Excisional biopsy		Pelvic exam Pap smear
• Neisseria Gonorrhea	Complete blood count and differential (CBC)	Urinalysis	Direct smear of vaginal discharge, anal canal, and oropharynx Thayer-Martin culture	Pelvic ultrasonography		Pelvic exam
• HVB & HIV						
Vaginitis						
• Candidiasis	Blood glucose	Urinalysis	Wet mount: direct vaginal smear with potassium hydroxide (1 drop)			Pelvic exam
• Trichomoniasis		Urinalysis	Wet mount: direct vaginal smear with isotomic saline (1 drop)			Pelvic exam

TABLE 26-4   DESCRIPTION OF FEMALE REPRODUCTIVE SYSTEM DISORDERS AND CONDITIONS

- Bartholin Gland Infection. Infection of the gland(s) that open near the vaginal opening.
- Breast Cancer. Most common site of cancer in females. A genetic cause has been identified for some breast cancers. Some symptoms are lump, thickening, swelling, dimpling, pain, and nipple discharge.
- Cervical Cancer. A carcinoma of the cervix of the uterus caused by a progressive cervical dysplasia. Most common in women aged 30 to 40. A significant risk factor is seen in women who become sexually active early in their lives and who have multiple sex partners.
- Endometriosis. Presence of endometrium in sites other than inside the uterus. May be found on the ovaries, fallopian tubes, large bowel, lungs, and pleura. Causes pelvic pain, dysmenorrhea, and infertility.

(continues)

TABLE 26-4 *(continued)*

- Fibrocystic Breasts. Benign cysts in breast tissue that increase or decrease in size during menses. Thought to be a normal variation in breast tissue due to monthly hormonal influence prior to onset of menses.
- Pelvic Inflammatory Disease (PID). Pelvic reproductive organs become inflamed and infected by bacteria, viruses, or parasites. An ascending infection can ensue involving the vagina, cervix of uterus, body of uterus, fallopian tubes, and ovaries. Causes vaginal discharge, pain, fever. May cause infertility.
- Premenstrual Syndrome (PMS). Cluster of symptoms that occur monthly prior to the onset of menses thought to be caused by progesterone-estrogen imbalance. Symptoms include fluid retention, weight gain, irritability, and mood swings.
- Sexually Transmitted Diseases (STDs). Several diseases caused by bacteria, viruses, protozoa that are transmitted through sexual intercourse (vaginal, anal, oral).
  - Chlamydia. An invasion by an intracellular parasite causing urethritis, cervicitis, pelvic inflammatory disease, proctitis, infant pneumonia, and conjunctivitis.
  - Condylomata (Human Papilloma Virus). Genital warts caused by a virus. Grow around the external genitalia, rectum, cervix. Associated with abnormal Pap smears.
  - Neisseria Gonorrhea. An infection by a bacterium that can involve the cervix, urethra, fallopian tubes and ovaries, rectum, mouth.
- Vaginitis. Inflammation of the vagina may be caused by bacteria, fungus, protozoa, chemical irritants, irritation from foreign bodies, vitamin deficiency, uncleanliness, and intestinal worms.
  - Candidiasis. A yeast (fungal) infection of the vagina caused by prolonged antibiotic therapy, pregnancy, or diabetes which can change the normal vaginal flora leading to overgrowth of the fungus.
  - Trichomoniasis. An infection by a protozoan most commonly spread through sexual intercourse or may come from fecal contamination of the vagina.

TABLE 26-5   COMMON SEXUALLY TRANSMITTED DISEASES

Pathology	Symptoms	Test	Treatment
AIDS	Flu-like, lymphadenopathy, infections, malignancies, pneumonia	HIV	Medication—AZT, DDI—but disease is fatal
Chlamydia	Usually asymptomatic	Culture	Doxycyline
Condylomata	Warts on external and internal genitalia	Visual exam	Cryocautery or chemocautery preferred but electrocautery can be used. Keratolytic agents used such as Podofilox
Gonorrhea	Usually asymptomatic; yellowish-green discharge with dysuria in advanced stages	Gram stain or Thayer-Martin culture	Penicillin
Herpes Simplex II	Itching and soreness followed by genital vesicles, which heal in 10 to 14 days	Visual exam with blood test for confirmation	Acyclovir®
Syphilis	Stage I: papule develops into ulcer, which develops into chancre of vulva. Stage II: fever, general malaise, dermal and mucosal lesions. Stage III: degeneration of CNS, lesions of internal structures	VDRL, RPR, FTA, or TPI	Penicillin
Trichomonas	Milky white, frothy, malodorous discharge with genital burning and itching	Potassium wet hydroxide mount for microscopic exam	Oral Flagel®, partner(s) must also be treated

poscope. The examination is done to determine if areas in the vagina or the cervix contain precancerous cells or tissue. The procedure is performed following an abnormal Pap test. It can also be performed to evaluate a lesion noted during a pelvic examination and to follow up after treatment of cervical cancer. Because the instrument has

the ability to magnify tissue, the cervix can be more readily examined and a biopsy taken.

The patient is placed in lithotomy position and is prepared as she would be for a gynecologic examination. A nonlubricated speculum is inserted into the vagina. The vagina is swabbed with a long cotton-tipped applicator that has been moistened with saline. (This provides better visualization of the cervical tissue.) The cervix is then swabbed with acetic acid to dissolve mucus and provide a good contrast between normal and abnormal tissue. A staining medium can be used as another means of identifying abnormal cells. If the physician finds an area of abnormal tissue, a biopsy can be performed using cervical punch biopsy forceps. The specimen is examined by a pathologist to determine whether or not malignant cells are present.

Cervical Punch Biopsy. The **cervical punch biopsy** is usually done in conjunction with a colposcopy to obtain a sample of cervical tissue for pathological examination. The specimen is examined for malignant cells and the biopsy usually follows an abnormal Pap smear report.

The procedure is performed with the patient in lithotomy position and with a vaginal speculum in place. The physician may stain the cervix to aid in identifying abnormal tissue. If the colposcope is being used, it illuminates and magnifies the cervical tissue and the physician will take several tissue samples using the cervical punch biopsy forceps. If bleeding ensues, it can be controlled with a vaginal packing, or the area can be cauterized to stop the bleeding. The specimen is placed in a container with formalin, a completed requisition form is attached to the container, and it is sent to the pathology laboratory for examination. The patient may expect a small amount of bleeding and should notify the physician if bleeding ensues that is greater than a menstrual period. A discharge that has a strong, foul odor is to be expected and can last for up to one month following the procedure.

Cryosurgery. **Cryosurgery** is used to treat tissue by freezing temperatures. Chronic cervicitis and cervical erosion are two common problems treated in this manner. (Also refer to Chapter 31 for information on cryosurgery.) The freezing temperature causes cells to die and they are

---

Patient Teaching Tip

Post Cryosurgery of Cervix
1. Expect a clear, watery, heavy discharge for up to one week, tapering off for up to four weeks.
2. Use only sanitary pads, not tampons. Change often, cleansing perineal area with each pad change.
3. Report signs of infection: fever, foul discharge, pain, nausea, or vomiting.
4. Do not engage in sexual intercourse, douche, or use tampons for four weeks.
5. Expect a heavier than usual menstrual period the following month.

---

then cast off from the cervix and eventually replaced with healthy cells about a month following the procedure.

The procedure is performed with the patient in lithotomy position and the cervix is swabbed to remove mucous. The probe is placed against the affected area of the cervix and the machine is turned on. The liquid nitrogen flows over the area for about three minutes and freezes the tissue. The patient may have some pain similar to dysmenorrhea that may last for about one-half hour. There should be no strong, foul odor but there can be a discharge for up to one month. Patients should report any foul smelling discharges as this may indicate an infection. Healing usually takes 4–6 weeks.

Patient Teaching Tip

Post Cervical Biopsy
1. Rest for 24 hours following the procedure.
2. Do not lift heavy objects for two weeks.
3. Leave packing in place for 24 hours or as directed. Do not insert another tampon unless told to do so by the physician.
4. Report any bleeding greater than a normal menstrual period.

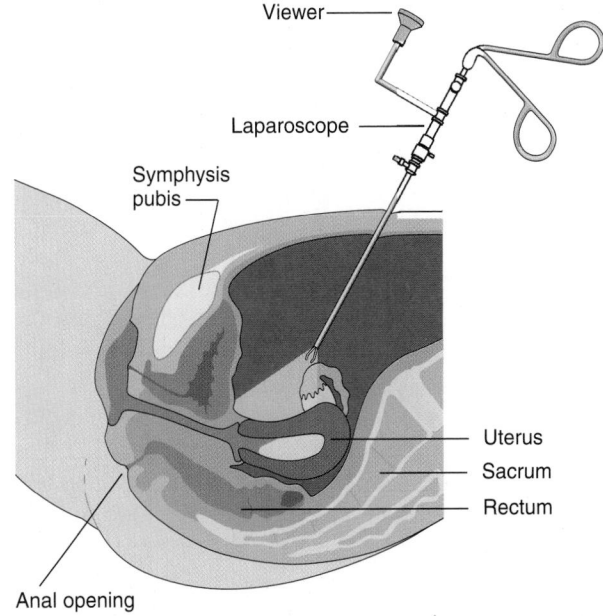

Figure 26-12 Laparoscopy.

Laparoscopy. Laparoscopy is a procedure in which a lighted instrument is used to view the inside of the pelvic cavity. It can be helpful in diagnosing endometriosis and ovarian cysts. A tubal ligation, severing of the fallopian tubes, can be done laparoscopically (Figure 26-12).

Dilation and Curettage (D and C). Dilation and curettage (D and C) is a surgical procedure that involves the dilating and scraping of the endometrial tissue. It is commonly performed to remove any remaining tissue following an incomplete abortion or to examine the tissue if the female has had abnormal uterine bleeding.

Procedure 26-1 — Assisting with Routine Prenatal Visits

STANDARD PRECAUTIONS:

PURPOSE:
To monitor the progress of the pregnancy.

EQUIPMENT/SUPPLIES:
Scale
Disposable gloves
Tape measure
Sphygmomanometer
Stethoscope
Doppler fetoscope and coupling agent
Urine specimen container
Biohazard waste container

PROCEDURE STEPS:
1. Wash hands.
2. Set up equipment.
3. Identify patient.
4. Obtain urine specimen. RATIONALE: A urine specimen for analysis is necessary. An empty bladder facilitates the exam and is more comfortable for the patient.
5. Measure blood pressure.
6. Weigh patient. RATIONALE: Assesses gain or loss of weight to help determine fetal development and maternal nutrition.
7. Have patient disrobe from waist down and put on a gown open in the front. RATIONALE: An open gown facilitates access to the abdomen for exam and measurement of the fundal height.

8. Test the urine specimen while waiting for the physician. RATIONALE: Urinalysis is done for detection of glucose and/or protein, which can indicate disease.
9. Assist patient onto exam table and drape her. RATIONALE: The patient may be off balance and unsteady on her feet due to the enlargement of the abdomen. Provide for her safety.
10. Assist the physician as the exam is performed.
    - Hand the physician the tape measure to measure height of fundus
    - Hand the physician the Doppler fetal pulse detector for measurement of fetal heart rate. The medical assistant may spread the coupling agent onto the patient's abdomen.
11. After the exam, assist patient to sit for a few moments. Assess her color, pulse. RATIONALE: Orthostatic hypotension can occur when a patient rises from a recumbent position. Give the patient time for the blood pressure to go back to normal so she will not experience dizziness from lowered blood pressure.
12. Provide any instruction or clarification of physician's orders.
13. Apply gloves. Discard disposable supplies per OSHA guidelines. Disinfect equipment used.
14. Remove gloves.
15. Wash hands.
16. Set up for the next patient.
17. Record all information in patient's record.

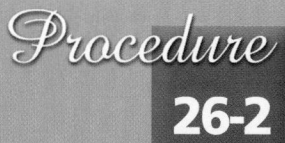

Instructing Patient in Breast Self-Examination

PURPOSE:
To properly instruct a woman in the procedure for performing a breast self-examination.

EQUIPMENT/SUPPLIES:
Breast model
Breast self-exam pamphlets
Pamphlet on breast self-examination

PROCEDURE STEPS:
Shower:
1. Examine breasts in a warm bath or shower. RATIONALE: Warm water softens the skin and hands glide easily over wet skin.
2. Using the flat pads of the three middle fingers moving in a circular motion, use the right hand to examine the left breast and left hand to examine the right breast. Beginning at the top outside edge using a circular, clockwise motion, examine part of each breast, ending at the nipple.
3. Check for lumps, thickening, and anything that is different from previous exams.

Mirror:
1. Inspect the breasts with arms at sides.
2. Raise arms high overhead.
3. Look for any change in contour of each breast.
4. Observe for swelling, hard lump, dimpling of skin (orange skin), or changes in nipple (retracting, swelling, or discharge).
5. Rest both hands on hips and pressing down flex chest muscles.

Lying Down:
1. Place a pillow or towel under right shoulder with the right hand behind the head to examine the right breast.
2. With left hand and fingers flat, press gently in small circular motions, starting at the top of the breast and moving toward the nipple.
3. Examine every part of the right breast tissue.
4. Repeat the procedure on the left breast using a pillow or a towel under the left shoulder and examine using the right hand.
5. Squeeze the nipple of each breast gently between thumb and index finger.
6. Report any abnormalities to the physician.

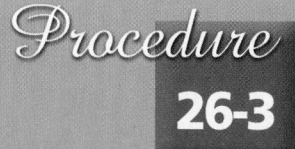

Assisting with Gynecologic or Pelvic Examination and a Papanicolaou (Pap) Test

STANDARD PRECAUTIONS:

PURPOSE:
To assist the physician in collecting cervical cells for laboratory analysis for early detection of malignant cells of the cervix and to assess the health of the reproductive organs to detect diseases leading to early diagnosis and treatment.

EQUIPMENT/SUPPLIES:
2 pair nonsterile gloves	Light source
2–3 frosted end glass slides	Drape sheet
Vaginal speculum (plastic or metal)	Marking pencil
	Lubricant
Basin of warm water	Slide holder
Long cotton-tipped applicator or cytology brush	Lab requisition
	Urine specimen container
Cervical scrapers	Tissues
Fixative	Biohazard waste container

(continues)

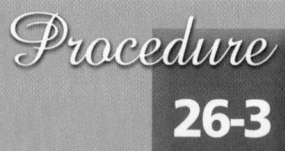

Procedure
26-3 *(continued)*

PROCEDURE STEPS:

1. Wash hands and assemble necessary supplies near patient.
2. Request that patient empty her bladder. (Instruct patient to save urine specimen and provide specimen container if ordered by physician.) RATIONALE: An empty bladder facilitates examination of the uterus and a urine specimen is frequently used for a urinalysis.
3. Provide patient with gown and request her to completely undress.
4. Explain procedure to patient.
5. Instruct patient to sit at end of table when ready. Drape patient for privacy. Label the frosted end of the slide with a marking pencil. Include patient's name on slide. Indicate site from where specimen is collected c = cervix, v = vagina, e = endocervical.
6. Assist patient into lithotomy position. Patient's knees should be relaxed and thighs rotated out as far as comfortable. Drape for privacy and warmth.
7. Encourage patient to breathe slowly and deeply through the mouth during exam. RATIONALE: Allows for relaxation of pelvic muscles and easier insertion of vaginal speculum.
8. Warm stainless steel vaginal speculum with warm water or place on a heating pad. Note: Do not lubricate speculum. Lubricant obscures exfoliated cervical cells when Pap test is being performed.
9. Hand speculum and spatula or cytology brush to physician.
10. Apply gloves.
11. Hold slides for physician to apply smear of exfoliated cells, one for vaginal (v), one for cervical (c), and one for endocervical (e) in that order.
12. Spray fixative over slide within 10 seconds at a distance of about 6 inches. Allow to dry for at least 10 minutes. RATIONALE: This maintains cell appearance and avoids contamination of cells. Avoid getting too close to slide with spray since this may destroy or damage cells. Slides must be fixed before they dry to protect the appearance of the cells.
13. Place lubricant on physician's gloved fingers without touching gloves, for bimanual and rectal exams. The physician will insert the index and middle fingers into the vagina. The other hand is placed on the lower abdomen. The size, shape, and position of the uterus and ovaries are palpated.
14. The physician will insert one gloved finger into the rectum to check the tone of the rectal and pelvic muscles. Hemorrhoids, rectal fissures, or other lesions may be palpated.
15. Assist patient to wipe genitalia and rectum.
16. Help patient to a sitting position, allowing her to rest awhile. Check her pulse and skin color. RATIONALE: Some patients, especially elderly, can experience orthostatic hypotension.
17. Discard disposable supplies per OSHA guidelines. If stainless steel speculum was used, soak in cool water. Sanitize and sterilize as soon as convenient.
18. Remove gloves and wash hands.
19. Assist patient down and off the table if necessary.
20. Instruct patient to dress. Inform patient of how and when test results will be reported to her.
21. Prepare laboratory requisition (cytology request) form. Include physician name and address, date, source of specimen, patient's name, address, date of last menstrual period (LMP), and hormone therapy. Place slides in slide container, attach requisition to container, and send to laboratory.
22. Wash hands.
23. Document procedure in the patient's chart.

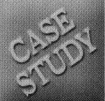

Maria Rodriguez has an appointment to see Dr. King today. It is her initial prenatal visit. She tells Liz Corbin, the medical assistant, as she is escorted from the reception area that she has been feeling, "pretty good."

26-1 CASE STUDY REVIEW

1. Explain the importance of the initial prenatal visit. Discuss.
2. Name five specific diseases and conditions for which Dr. King will be on the alert during Maria's pregnancy.
3. What laboratory and other procedural tests may be performed at the initial visit?
4. Discuss areas of patient education and health promotion that Liz will discuss with Maria at the initial visit.

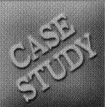

Emily Harris is scheduled to have a cervical punch biopsy.

CASE STUDY REVIEW

26-2

1. Explain the postbiopsy instructions she will need.

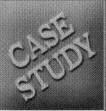

Annette Sanderson has made an appointment with Dr. King because she has had symptoms of vaginitis. When she arrives at the clinic, you take her chief complaint and history. She tells you that she has a milky-white, frothy, vaginal discharge and that she itches in the genital area.

26-3 CASE STUDY REVIEW

1. What tests/procedures will you prepare for Dr. King in consideration of Annette's symptoms?
2. What is the most likely causative microorganism for these symptoms?
3. Describe the treatment that Dr. King may prescribe.

SUMMARY

Obstetrics and gynecology are two specialties that are usually practiced by the same physician. The OB/GYN physician will care for the health and well-being of the female in her pregnant and nonpregnant states. Knowledge of the numerous tests and procedures that are performed to diagnose and treat problems in the female patient are essential. Health promotion and patient education are of extreme importance whether the patient is an obstetrical patient and scheduled for her initial prenatal visit or a gynecological patient scheduled for yearly pelvic, Pap, and breast examinations.

REVIEW QUESTIONS

Multiple Choice

1. Which of the following conditions or diseases that a obstetrical patient experiences is considered to place her in the high-risk category?
   a. urinary tract infection
   b. 19 years of age
   c. both partners Rh negative
   d. poor nutritional habits
   e. poor hygiene

2. Using Nagele's Rule, calculate the expected date of confinement (EDC) of a patient whose last menstrual period (LMP) was August 20, 2000.
   a. November 27, 2001
   b. December 13, 2001
   c. May 27, 2001
   d. April 20, 2001

3. The primary test performed at about the sixteenth week to check the fetus for neural tube defects is known as:
   a. alphafetal protein analysis (AFP)
   b. amniocentesis
   c. chorionic villi sampling (CVS)
   d. rubella titer
   e. Rh factor

4. The release of which of the following hormones is thought to cause labor to begin?
   a. progesterone
   b. estrogen
   c. oxytoxin
   d. thyroxine

5. Ultrasonography is done to check for which of the following?
   a. gestational diabetes
   b. pre-eclampsia
   c. degree of effacement
   d. number of weeks of gestation

6. Following a cervical punch biopsy, it is normal for the patient to experience which of the following?
   a. bleeding greater than a normal menstrual period
   b. no odor to vaginal discharge
   c. a strong, foul odor to vaginal discharge
   d. severe abdominal cramps

7. To make the diagnosis of trichomoniasis, the medical assistant will need to prepare for which of the following?
   a. Pap smear
   b. ultrasonography
   c. wet mount
   d. culture and sensitivity
   e. blood glucose

8. To diagnose pelvic inflammatory disease (PID), the physician may order which of the following?
   a. wet mount
   b. Pap smear
   c. urinalysis
   d. rubella titer
   e. ultrasonography

9. Which of the following is/are primarily associated with abnormal Pap smears?
   a. endometriosis
   b. Bartholin cyst
   c. condylomata
   d. ovarian cysts
   e. pelvic inflammatory disease

10. The primary purpose of colposcopy is to:
    a. treat advanced cancer of the vagina and cervix
    b. detect dysplastic cells of cervix following a positive Pap smear
    c. detect an ectopic pregnancy in the fallopian tube
    d. treat endometriosis of the pelvic cavity

Critical Thinking Questions

1. A pregnant woman who has had no prenatal care has not had a period for six months. She has called the OB/GYN clinic to schedule an appointment because she has had vaginal bleeding. She continues to feel fetal movement. a) What laboratory tests or procedures will the doctor order? b) What diagnosis is the physician most likely to make?

2. A 17-year-old female has missed her period and has called the clinic complaining of sharp right quadrant pain. What tests/procedures will help the physician make a diagnosis?

3. A 38-year-old woman has been diagnosed with human papilloma virus (HPV) infection. What is the significance of this infection?

4. A 27-year-old woman wants to schedule an appointment because she has had some bright red bleeding following intercourse.

5. Lower abdominal and back pain that increases just prior to and during menses may be caused by what condition?

WEB ACTIVITIES

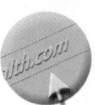

Obstetrics

Access a web site for expectant parents to locate information about the following:

1. Obtain fact sheets about each trimester.
2. Compile a list of tests, complications, and postpartum recovery.

Gynecology

Locate a web site specific to cancer of the female reproductive tract to complete the following:

1. What treatment options are available for cancer of the endometrium?
2. What tests are available to help diagnose the cancer?
3. Print a list of local support groups for women with endometrial cancer.

REFERENCES/BIBLIOGRAPHY

Bobak, I., Lowdermilk, D., Jensen, M., & Perry, S. (1999). *Maternity Nursing* (5th ed.). St. Louis, MO: Mosby-Year Book, Inc.

Damjanov, I. (1996). *Pathology for the health related profession* (1st ed.). Philadelphia: W. B. Saunders Company.

Ehrlich, A., & Schroeder, C. L. (1997). *Medical terminology for health professions* (4th ed.). Albany, NY: Delmar.

Frazier, M. S., Drzymkowski, J. A., & Doty, S. J. (1996). *Essentials of human diseases and conditions* (1st ed.). Philadelphia: W. B. Saunders Company.

Health Ink and Vitality. (August 2000). Your tour guide to health web sites, *Vitality, 14*(8), 12.

Health Ink and Vitality. (September 2000). Your tour guide to health web sites. *Vitality, 14*(9), 12.

Miller, B. F., & Keane-Brackman, C. (1992). *Encyclopedia and dictionary of medicine, nursing and allied health* (5th ed.). Philadelphia: W. B. Saunders Company.

Taber's cyclopedic medical dictionary. (18th ed.). (1999) Philadelphia: F. A. Davis Company.

Tamparo, C., & Lewis, M. (2000). *Diseases of the human body* (3rd ed.). Philadelphia: F. A. Davis Company.

Zakus, S. (1995). *Clinical procedures for medical assistants* (3rd. ed.). St. Louis: Mosby-Year Book, Inc.

Chapter 27

PEDIATRICS

KEY TERMS

Exudate
Myringotomy
Suppurative
Tympanostomy

OUTLINE

OBJECTIVES

The student should strive to meet the following performance objectives and demonstrate an understanding of the facts and principles presented in this chapter through written and oral communication.

1. Define the key terms as presented in the glossary.
2. Describe pediatric care including measuring height, weight, head, chest circumference, and vital signs.
3. Explain the process of collecting a urine specimen.
4. Describe common pediatric diseases and disorders.
5. Explain the importance of immunizations and scheduling of them.

At Inner City Health Care, clinical assistant Bruce Goldman is responsible for encouraging parents to keep track of their children's immunization records. Bruce teaches parents the importance of immunizations for long-term health protection and the importance of following recommended vaccination schedules for maximum benefit.

INTRODUCTION

New techniques and developments occur frequently in medicine and medical assistants must refine existing skills and learn new ones to be knowledgeable and proficient and to provide the most current, up-to-date quality care to patients. The medical assistant who works in a pediatrician's office or a pediatric ambulatory care setting that treats infants and children will need additional skills when providing pediatric care to patients.

Knowledge of the developmental stages and diseases of infants and children, the ability to gain the child's confidence and trust, and the caregivers' cooperation are all skills required to provide for the physiological, emotional, and psychological needs of the pediatric patient. This chapter covers the specialty examination and the appropriate clinical procedures in pediatrics.

WHAT IS PEDIATRICS?

Pediatrics is the branch of medicine that cares for newborns, infants, children, and adolescents. Pediatricians are physicians who diagnose and treat health problems and diseases specific to these age groups. This patient population has special needs, and medical assistants must be knowledgeable about the growth and development phases of life and diseases unique to pediatric patients. Children form judgments and have fears about health care providers. They need an atmosphere that is comfortable and one in which their physiological, emotional, and psychological needs are recognized and addressed.

Medical assistants must gain the confidence and trust of the child, allay fear, and help to promote positive relationships between the child and the physician and must themselves develop a positive relationship with the child. Children are likely to be cooperative when being examined or during a procedure if good rapport has been established. It is important to be honest with young patients and approach them at their level of understanding. Allow children to touch and hold a "safe" instrument, such as a stethoscope, and explain its purpose to them. By doing so anxiety and fear can be reduced (Figure 27-1).

The first physical examination of a newborn is performed immediately after delivery. The pediatrician

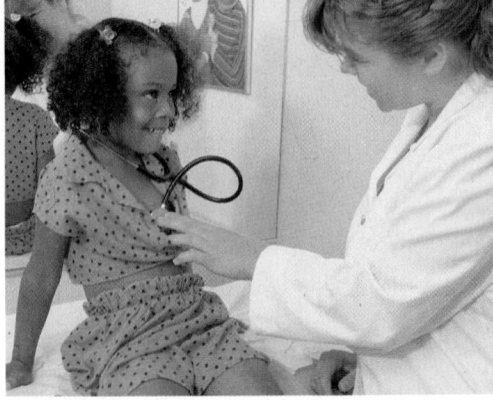

Figure 27-1   The medical assistant is making a game of a procedure to gain the child's cooperation.

will assess the infant's ability to exist outside of the mother's uterus. A scoring system is used to determine the infant's physical condition at one minute and five minutes after birth. It is known as the APGAR score. Muscle tone, skin color, respiration, heart rate, and response to stimuli are given a score 0, 1, 2, and so on, with the highest score 10. Infants with low APGAR scores need immediate attention, such as stimulation, oxygen, medication, and so on. Their condition is closely monitored.

Many patients seen in the pediatric setting are babies or children who are not ill. They are considered "well-baby" or "well-child" patients and are having routine checkups. Ill babies or children seen in the pediatrician's office or pediatric clinic are often called "sick-child" or "sick-baby" patients. Well-baby appointments are regularly scheduled appointments during which time the physician examines the child and evaluates the growth and development of the child. Most offices schedule well-baby appointments after birth according to the following time frame: 1, 2, 4, 6, 9, 12, 15, 18, 24 months, and yearly thereafter.

The goal of well-baby visits or checkups is prevention of health problems and diseases. Typically, immunizations are given during these appointments. The chart shown in Figure 27-2 includes immunization schedules

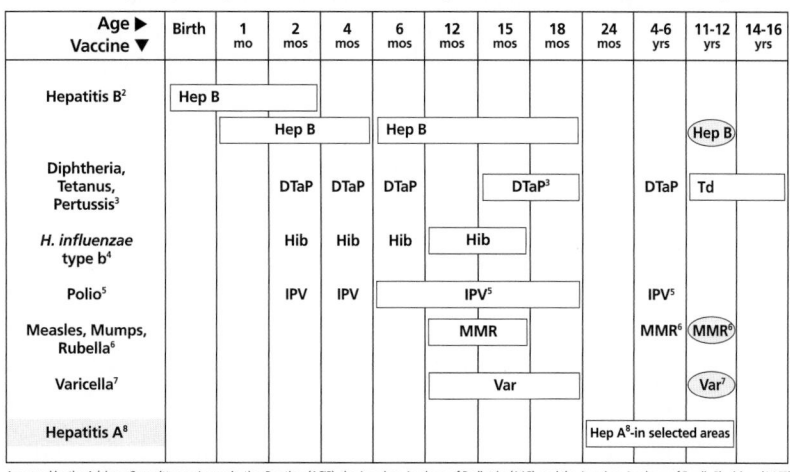

Recommended Childhood Immunization Schedule
United States, January – December 2000

Vaccines[1] are listed under routinely recommended ages. [Bars] indicate range of recommended ages for immunization. Any dose not given at the recommended age should be given as a "catch-up" immunization at any subsequent visit when indicated and feasible. (Ovals) indicate vaccines to be given if previously recommended doses were missed or given earlier than the recommended minimum age.

Age ▶ Vaccine ▼	Birth	1 mo	2 mos	4 mos	6 mos	12 mos	15 mos	18 mos	24 mos	4-6 yrs	11-12 yrs	14-16 yrs
Hepatitis B[2]	Hep B		Hep B		Hep B						(Hep B)	
Diphtheria, Tetanus, Pertussis[3]			DTaP	DTaP	DTaP		DTaP[3]			DTaP	Td	
H. influenzae type b[4]			Hib	Hib	Hib	Hib						
Polio[5]			IPV	IPV		IPV[5]				IPV[5]		
Measles, Mumps, Rubella[6]						MMR				MMR[6]	(MMR[6])	
Varicella[7]						Var					(Var[7])	
Hepatitis A[8]									Hep A[8]-in selected areas			

Approved by the Advisory Committee on Immunization Practices (ACIP), the American Academy of Pediatrics (AAP), and the American Academy of Family Physicians (AAFP).
IS 5081

(For **necessary footnotes** and important information, see reverse side.)

On October 22, 1999, the Advisory Committee on Immunization Practices (ACIP) recommended that Rotashield (RRV-TV), the only US-licensed rotavirus vaccine, no longer be used in the United States (MMWR Morb Mortal Wkly Rep. Nov 5, 1999;48(43):1007). Parents should be reassured that their children who received rotavirus vaccine before July are not at increased risk for intussusception now.

[1] This schedule indicates the recommended ages for routine administration of currently licensed childhood vaccines as of 11/1/99. Additional vaccines may be licensed and recommended during the year. Licensed combination vaccines may be used whenever any components of the combination are indicated and its other components are not contraindicated. Providers should consult the manufacturers' package inserts for detailed recommendations.

[2] <u>Infants born to HBsAg-negative mothers</u> should receive the 1st dose of hepatitis B (Hep B) vaccine by age 2 months. The 2nd dose should be at least 1 month after the 1st dose. The 3rd dose should be administered at least 4 months after the 1st dose and at least 2 months after the 2nd dose, but not before 6 months of age for infants.
<u>Infants born to HBsAg-positive mothers</u> should receive hepatitis B vaccine and 0.5 mL hepatitis B immune globulin (HBIG) within 12 hours of birth at separate sites. The 2nd dose is recommended at 1 to 2 months of age and the 3rd dose at 6 months of age.
<u>Infants born to mothers whose HBsAg status is unknown</u> should receive hepatitis B vaccine within 12 hours of birth. Maternal blood should be drawn at the time of delivery to determine the mother's HBsAg status; if the HBsAg test is positive, the infant should receive HBIG as soon as possible (no later than 1 week of age).
<u>All children and adolescents (through 18 years of age)</u> who have not been immunized against hepatitis B may begin the series during any visit. Special efforts should be made to immunize children who were born in or whose parents were born in areas of the world with moderate or high endemicity of hepatitis B virus infection.

[3] The 4th dose of DTaP (diphtheria and tetanus toxoids and acellular pertussis vaccine) may be administered as early as 12 months of age, provided 6 months have elapsed since the 3rd dose and the child is unlikely to return at age 15 to 18 months. Td (tetanus and diphtheria toxoids) is recommended at 11 to 12 years of age if at least 5 years have elapsed since the last dose of DTP, DTaP, or DT. Subsequent routine Td boosters are recommended every 10 years.

[4] Three *Haemophilus influenzae* type b (Hib) conjugate vaccines are licensed for infant use. If PRP-OMP (PedvaxHIB or ComVax [Merck]) is administered at 2 and 4 months of age, a dose at 6 months is not required. Because clinical studies in infants have demonstrated that using some combination products may induce a lower immune response to the Hib vaccine component, DTaP/Hib combination products should not be used for primary immunization in infants at 2, 4, or 6 months of age unless FDA-approved for these ages.

[5] To eliminate the risk of vaccine-associated paralytic polio (VAPP), an all-IPV schedule is now recommended for routine childhood polio vaccination in the United States. All children should receive four doses of IPV at 2 months, 4 months, 6 to 18 months, and 4 to 6 years. OPV (if available) may be used only for the following special circumstances:
1. Mass vaccination campaigns to control outbreaks of paralytic polio.
2. Unvaccinated children who will be traveling in <4 weeks to areas where polio is endemic or epidemic.
3. Children of parents who do not accept the recommended number of vaccine injections. These children may receive OPV only for the third or fourth dose or both; in this situation, health care professionals should administer OPV only after discussing the risk for VAPP with parents or caregivers.
4. During the transition to an all-IPV schedule, recommendations for the use of remaining OPV supplies in physicians' offices and clinics have been issued by the American Academy of Pediatrics (see *Pediatrics*, December 1999).

[6] The 2nd dose of measles, mumps, and rubella (MMR) vaccine is recommended routinely at 4 to 6 years of age but may be administered during any visit, provided at least 4 weeks have elapsed since receipt of the 1st dose and that both doses are administered beginning at or after 12 months of age. Those who have not previously received the second dose should complete the schedule by the 11- to 12-year-old visit.

[7] Varicella (Var) vaccine is recommended at any visit on or after the first birthday for susceptible children, ie, those who lack a reliable history of chickenpox (as judged by a health care professional) and who have not been immunized. Susceptible persons 13 years of age or older should receive 2 doses, given at least 4 weeks apart.

[8] Hepatitis A (Hep A) is shaded to indicate its recommended use in selected states and/or regions; consult your local public health authority. (Also see *MMWR Morb Mortal Wkly Rep.* Oct 01, 1999;48(RR-12); 1-37).

Immunization Protects Children
Regular checkups at your pediatrician's office or local health clinic are an important way to keep children healthy.
By making sure that your child gets immunized on time, you can provide the best available defense against many dangerous childhood diseases. Immunizations protect children against: hepatitis B, polio, measles, mumps, rubella (German measles), pertussis (whooping cough), diphtheria, tetanus (lockjaw), *Haemophilus influenzae* type b, and chickenpox. All of these immunizations need to be given before children are 2 years old in order for them to be protected during their most vulnerable period. Are your child's immunizations up-to-date?

The chart on the other side of this fact sheet includes immunization recommendations from the American Academy of Pediatrics. Remember to keep track of your child's immunizations—it's the only way you can be sure your child is up-to-date. Also, check with your pediatrician or health clinic at each visit to find out if your child needs any booster shots or if any new vaccines have been recommended since this schedule was prepared.
If you don't have a pediatrician, call your local health department. Public health clinics usually have supplies of vaccine and may give shots free.

American Academy of Pediatrics

The information contained in this publication should not be used as a substitute for the medical care and advice of your pediatrician. There may be variations in treatment that your pediatrician may recommend based on individual facts and circumstances.

Figure 27-2 Recommended vaccination schedule for infants and children. (Courtesy of American Academy of Pediatrics)

from the American Academy of Pediatrics. The Academy urges that all children be immunized because the vaccines provide the best defense against many dangerous childhood diseases. Immunizations protect children against hepatitis B, polio, measles, mumps, rubella, pertussis, diphtheria, tetanus, haemophilus influenza type b, and chicken pox. All of these need to be given before age two to protect children during the period of their lives when they are more susceptible to infectious diseases.

Preparation of Vaccines for Administration

Careful attention to both proper storage of vaccines and thorough patient preparation for immunization will promote effective vaccination results. Access to vaccination should be available to all patients, especially to families with young infants and children. Most of the recommended vaccines are administered in the child's first 15 months of life. Access involves cost of vaccines, appointment requirements, and time required to receive vaccines. Some offices permit walk-in vaccination administration with free or low co-pay fee only. Routine well-infant examinations should be scheduled according to the recommended vaccination schedule to promote and facilitate maintenance of the schedule.

Vaccine storage should follow specific manufacturer's guidelines. Some vaccine preparations require refrigeration or protection from light.

Vaccines stimulate the immune system to produce antibodies against pathogens. Some patients may have conditions or pre-existing conditions that would contraindicate vaccine administration. Safe vaccine administration requires assessment and recognition of conditions that would contraindicate vaccine administration at any specific time. Contraindications for each vaccine are presented in Table 27-1. When any vaccine is not given because of an existing contraindication, careful documentation and notification of the physician are required.

Recommended Vaccination Schedule

The recommended vaccination schedule for infants and children is based on the premise that repeated doses for several vaccines are required and vaccine manufacturers recommend administering only compatible vaccines at any one visit to avoid drug interactions. If no contraindications are present at the following ages, vaccines should be administered according to the schedule to ensure complete vaccination by the age of 15 to 18 months, with booster vaccines upon school entry and again every ten years throughout adult life. Should any vaccine be missed

TABLE 27-1   VACCINE ADMINISTRATION GUIDELINES

Vaccine	Disease	Route of Administration	Contraindications	Side Effects and Adverse Reactions	Comments
DTP	Diptheria, tetanus, pertussis	IM	Fever, inconsolable or high-pitched crying, neurological disorders or family history of neurological disorders, acute polio outbreak	Mild fever, drowsiness, anorexia, fretfulness. **Risk of severe neurological damage is 4.2% within 3 days of administration.**	Boosters required
MMR	Measles, mumps, rubella	SC (needle free of alcohol) (use only supplied diluent)	Immunosuppression, allergy to eggs, active untreated TB, febrile illness, pregnancy	Fever, few side effects	Vaccine promotes immunity in 95 to 99% of patients
Inactive Polio Virus (IPV)	Poliomyelitis	IM	Immunosuppression, acute illness, debilitated condition	Rare	Vaccine does not protect from pre-existing or incubating polio
Hib	Meningitis caused by H. influenza b	IM (use only supplied diluent)	Acute illness	Minimal side effects	Immunity not attained for several days to a week
HBV	Hepatitis B Vaccine	IM	Allergy to yeast, serious active infection, severe cardiovascular disease	Malaise, headache, nausea, vomiting, pain at site, upper respiratory infections, fever	Antibody response greater in children and young adults than in older adults (99% for children under 1 year)
Varicella	Chicken pox	IM	Avoid if allergic to eggs or neomycin		Need for booster unknown at this time

Patient Teaching Tip

Encourage patients to be aware of different vaccines and keep track of vaccination schedules by posting recommended schedules in visible locations in the ambulatory care setting.

Figure 27-2 illustrates the recommended vaccination schedule for infants and children, which is supported by the American Academy of Pediatrics, the Advisory Committee on Immunization Practices (ACIP), the Committee on Infectious Diseases (COID), the Commission of Public Health and Scientific Affairs (COPHSA), and the American Academy of Family Physicians (AAFP).

for any reason, vaccine schedules are available to ensure adequate vaccine administration.

Sick-baby or sick-child visits are those appointments that have been arranged for ill babies or children who will be examined by the pediatrician in order to determine a diagnosis and appropriate treatment for a particular problem.

Clinical responsibilities for medical assistants during either type of visit include the same or similar procedures as the adult examination. The instruments used for the pediatric physical exam are similar to those used for an adult physical exam. Vital signs are taken, visual acuity is measured, a urine specimen may be obtained, blood drawn and processed, height and weight measurements are taken, and head circumference is measured. To gain the child's confidence, begin the exam at the feet and work up to the head. These are some of the skills and procedures medical assistants will perform or with which they will assist during the pediatric office or clinic visit.

GROWTH PATTERNS

Growth patterns provide valuable information to the pediatrician regarding the infant's physical progress. They are also used to calculate pediatric doses of medication. Height and weight and head circumference are measured at each regularly scheduled appointment at the pediatric facility. The measurements are then plotted on a physical growth percentile chart that is part of the patient's permanent record (Figure 27-3).

Developmental Patterns

Infants develop very quickly in their first year of life. Motor skills progress rapidly and children also learn to speak. Children's vocabulary increases quickly, and they learn not only how to talk, but also how to walk. They are becoming toilet trained by about age three.

As preschoolers, children have been able to master many motor skills and are exhibiting signs of developing social skills.

School-age children have perfected their motor skills and their intelligence is growing quickly. Self-worth and a sense of achievement are developing. Social skills continue to improve.

By the time children become adolescents, they attempt to establish an identity as adults. Peer pressure is powerful and is important to adolescents. They may be torn between parental values versus peer values. This stage of development is the time when most adolescents mature emotionally and are becoming more capable of making beneficial choices and decisions. See Figure 27-4 for an illustration of growth and development of infants and toddlers.

Infant/Child Failure to Thrive. The failure of an infant or a child to grow and thrive may have many organic and inorganic causes. There may be social and emotional causes. Many of the causes for an infant or a child failing to grow and thrive may be treated if found in time. The emotionally deprived infant needing affection will not grow, as there will be a lack of growth hormone production. Once this child is given physical and emotional warmth, the growth hormone is produced and the child will grow. Other reasons for an infant failing to thrive may be because the infant has a chronic disease, a diet that is inadequate in calories and proteins, a disorder of the heart, brain, or kidneys, or has been improperly fed.

MEASURING THE INFANT OR CHILD

Careful measuring of the infant or child and monitoring of growth pattern are essential and should be done in a consistent and accurate manner.

Height and Weight Measurements

To record or plot height and weight measurements, first locate one growth value either length (highlighted yellow) or weight (highlighted red) in the vertical columns of the Physical Growth Percentile Chart in Figure 27-5. Find the child's age in months in the horizontal rows (highlighted green). Locate the area where the growth value lines intersect on the graph and plot the height and weight by marking with a dot. Connect dots from previous examination with a ruler to provide a neat and accurate graphic recording. The date, age, measurements, and

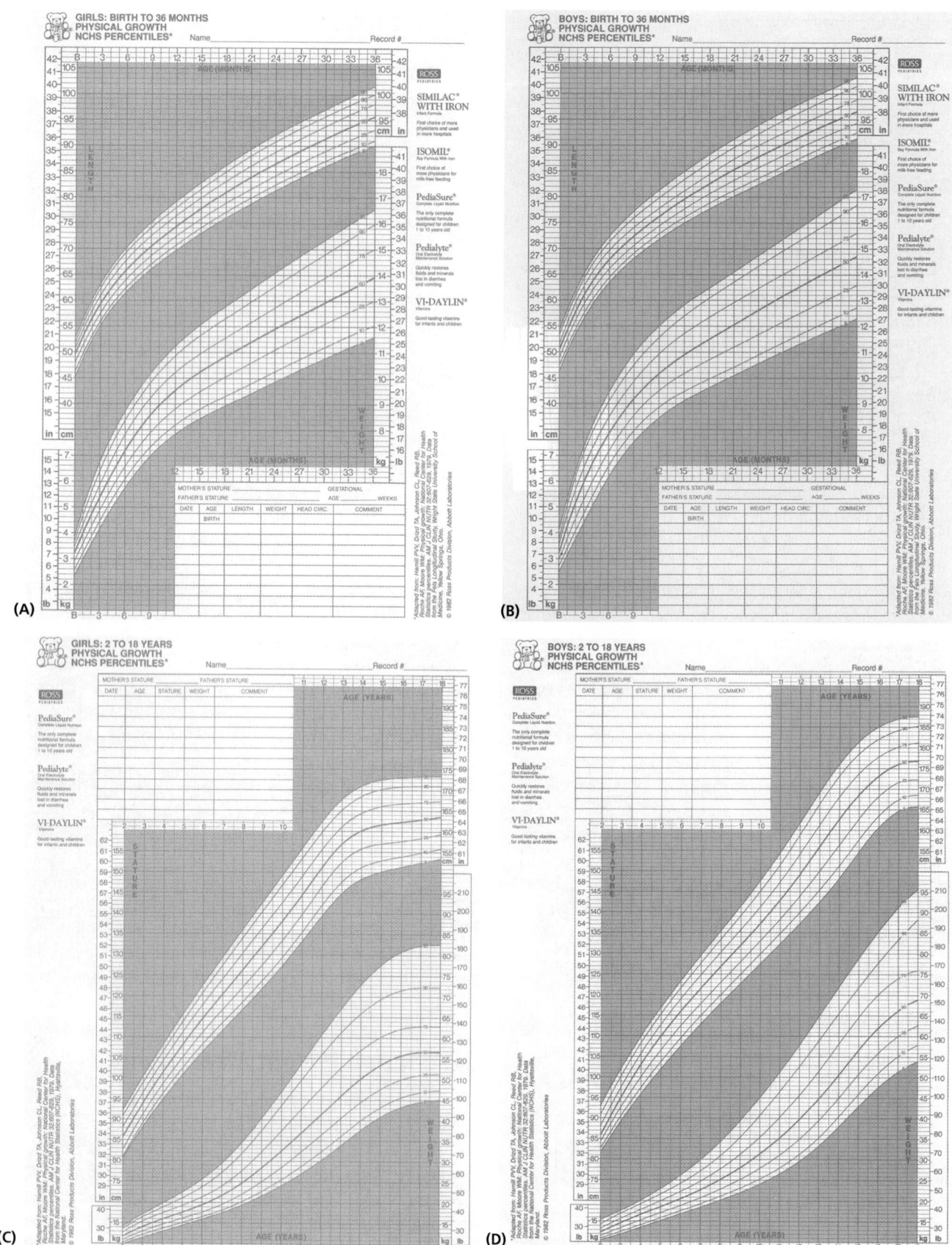

Figure 27-3   (A) Growth chart for girls' height and weight, age birth to 36 months. (B) Growth chart for boys' height and weight, age birth to 36 months. (C) Growth chart for girls' height and weight, age 2 to 18 years. (D) Growth chart for boys' height and weight, age 2 to 18 years. (Reprinted with permission of Ross Laboratories, Columbus, OH 43216, from NCHS Growth Charts)

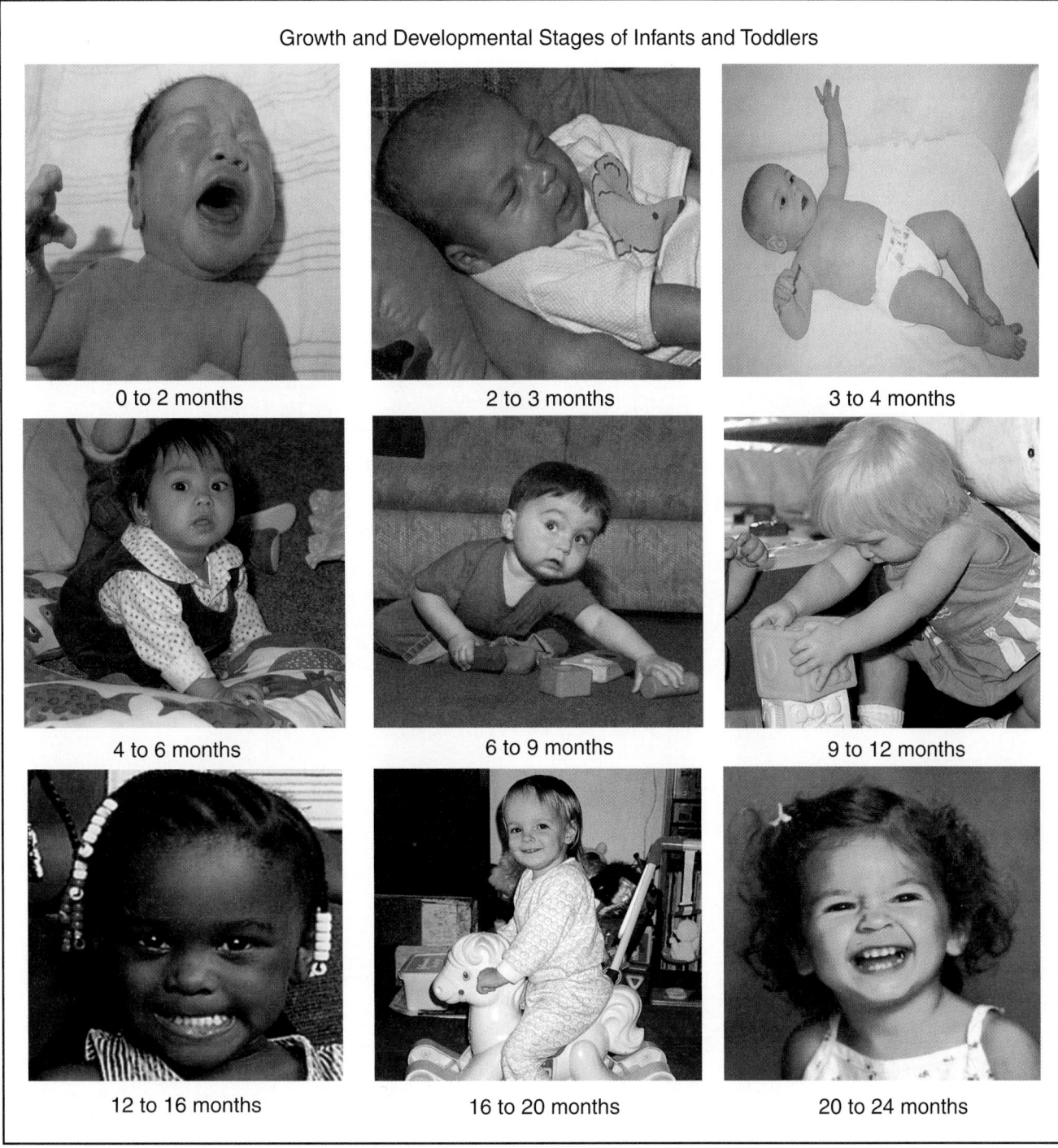

Growth and Developmental Stages of Infants and Toddlers

0 to 2 months

2 to 3 months

3 to 4 months

4 to 6 months

6 to 9 months

9 to 12 months

12 to 16 months

16 to 20 months

20 to 24 months

Figure 27-4 Growth and developmental stages of infants and toddlers.

comments should also be indicated at the bottom of the chart.

The curved lines printed across the growth charts show the normal range of growth of infants and children in the United States. The numbers on the right side of the chart, in the vertical boxes between age 34 and 35 months, show the percentiles of other children the same age. To determine into which percentile the infant falls in relation to other infants of the same age, follow the line (percentile) upward to the percentage values along the edge of the graph. The National Center for Health Statistics (NCHS) growth charts become a permanent record of the child's development. These give the physician a quick way to check the child's growth in relation to that of other children the same age. Growth charts aid in the diagnosis of growth abnormalities and nutritional disorders

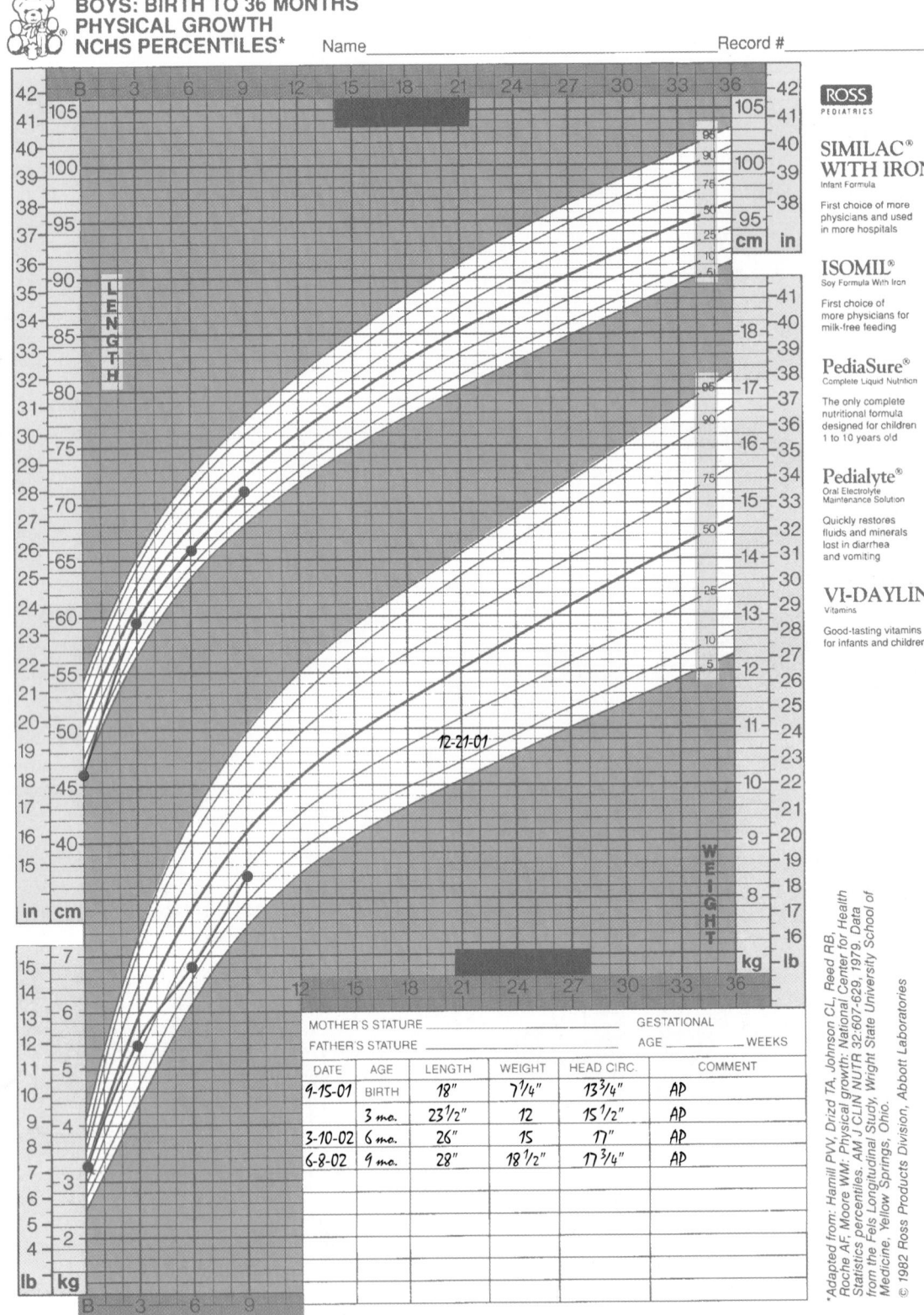

Figure 27-5 Sample growth chart with information plotted at birth, 3, 6, and 9 months. Sections in this figure have been highlighted to help you locate the values: length (yellow), weight (red), age (green), and percentiles (white). (Reprinted with permission of Ross Laboratories, Columbus, OH 43216, from NCHS Growth Charts)

and disease. Hereditary factors also influence growth patterns; therefore, having the family's history is important.

Height and Weight Measuring Devices

Various devices are available for measuring height and weight in children. Infants and small children are weighed on an infant platform scale, which provides a measurement in pounds and ounces and kilograms and grams (Figure 27-6). The scale has a platform with curved sides in which the child may sit or lie. Weigh the infant or child in as few clothes as possible, removing the diaper and shoes or slippers. A small sheet, cloth diaper, or paper towel should be placed on the scale before weighing the infant or child, to avoid the transfer of microorganisms from bare skin.

Infant length can be measured using an infant measuring board, which consists of a rigid headboard and movable footboard. Place the measuring board on a table and position the infant on his back on the board, with the head touching the headboard. Move the footboard up until it touches the bottom of the infant's feet.

An infant can also be measured on a pad by placing a pin into the pad or making a pencil mark at the top of the head and a second pin or mark at the heel of the extended leg. The length is the distance between the two pins. A tape measure can also be used. Note: 1 inch = 2.54 cm

A stature-measuring device may be used to measure height once the child is able to stand erect without support. The device consists of a movable headpiece attached to a rigid measuring bar and platform (Figure 27-7). A paper towel should be placed on the platform before use to avoid the potential transmission of microorganisms from bare feet.

Measuring Head Circumference

Head circumference measurement is routinely recorded on an infant's chart to alert the physician to any abnormal development. This procedure should be performed during routine visits until the child is 36 months old. Thereafter it should be measured on a yearly basis until the age of 6 years. Head circumference measurement requires a flexible paper or metal measuring tape. A cloth tape may stretch and give a false measurement. Head circumference is plotted similarly to height and weight but on separate Growth Percentile Charts for head measurements (Figure 27-8). Generally, head and chest circumference are equal at about 1 to 2 years of age. Rapid growth above the normal percentile may indicate hydrocephalus, a disorder in which excessive fluid accumulates around the brain causing an increase in intracranial pressure and possible brain damage. This could lead to mental and physical problems. Conversely, the growth of the head which falls below the normal percentile may indicate microencephaly caused by a premature closure of the fontanels. In this instance, there is not enough room for the development of the brain, and mental retardation can result. Head circumference for a newborn should be between 12.5 to 14.5 inches or 31.75 to 36.83 cm.

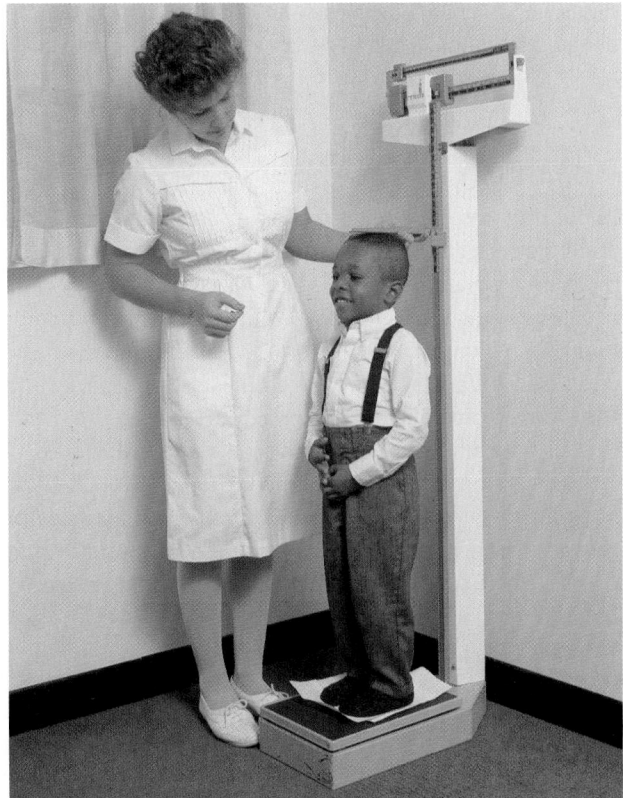

Figure 27-7 Young children who are able to stand erect without support can be measured on a scale that has a stature-measuring device attached.

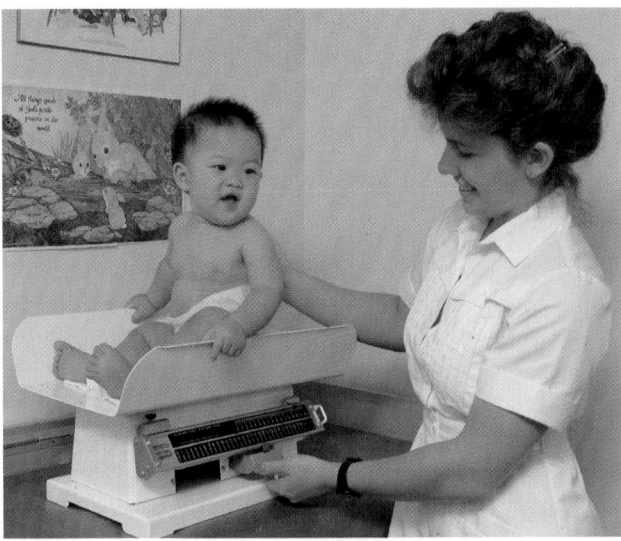

Figure 27-6 Infants who are able to sit and small children can be weighed on a platform scale.

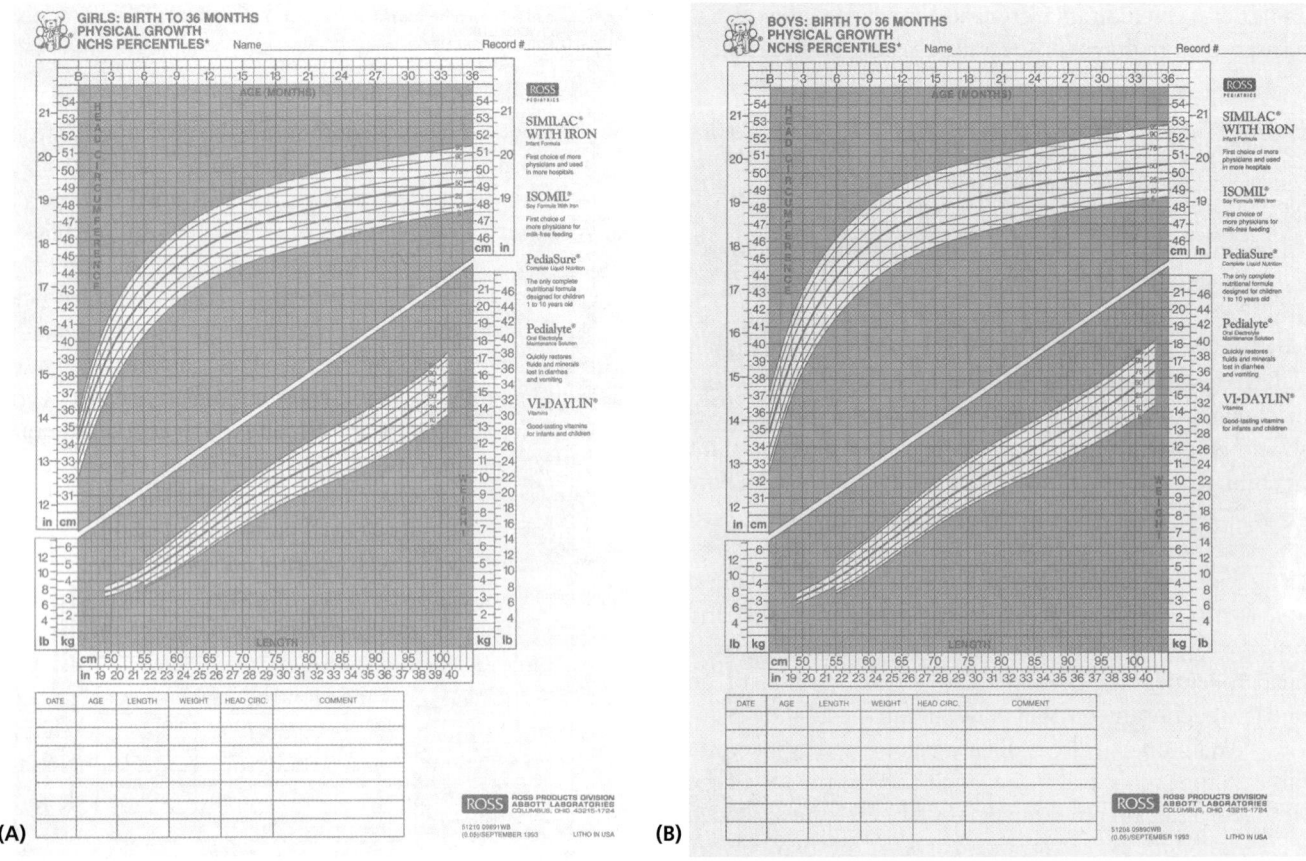

Figure 27-8   (A) Growth chart for girls' head circumference, birth to 36 months. (B) Growth chart for boys' head circumference, birth to 36 months. (Reprinted with permission of Ross Laboratories, Columbus, OH 43216, from NCHS Growth Charts)

Measuring Chest Circumference

Measuring the chest circumference of an infant is not normally performed during routine examinations. It may be performed and monitored when there is a suspicion of overdevelopment or underdevelopment of the heart and/or lungs, or calcification of rib cartilage. To measure the chest of an infant, snugly wrap the measuring tape around the chest at nipple level. It is preferable to read the measurement during the resting phase between respirations.

Occasionally it may be necessary for the medical assistant to convert measurement results into inches or centimeters. To accomplish the task accurately, note that 1 inch equals 2.54 cm. (See Procedure 27-1 for measuring infant chest and head circumference and weight and height.)

To convert inches to centimeters, multiply the number of inches by 2.54:

Inches × 2.54 = Centimeters

To convert centimeters to inches, divide the number of centimeters by 2.54:

Centimeters ÷ 2.54 = Inches

PEDIATRIC VITAL SIGNS

As with older children and adults, pediatric vital signs are commonly taken by the medical assistant. The vital signs are more fully covered in Chapter 24 for adult patients; however, specific procedures for taking an infant's temperature, pulse, respiration, and blood pressure are explained here. These procedures are done very differently for infants than for older children and adults.

Temperature

Body temperature may be measured in Fahrenheit (F) or Celsius (C) through oral, rectal, axillary, or tympanic routes. Many types of thermometers are used. Mercury (glass) thermometers have been replaced in ambulatory care areas and most offices by digital thermometers, electronic thermometers, and tympanic membrane sensors or aural, which provide accurate temperature readings in less time. Broken mercury thermometers release vapors into the air, which are toxic when inhaled and lead to mercury poisoning. Proper disposal of the mercury is regulated by the health department and varies from state to state. Electronic and digital thermometers can display temperature within 15 to 60 seconds, depending on the model used. A reading can be obtained by infrared tympanic membrane sensor in as little as 2 seconds.

Oral Temperature. The oral route is used for children over 5 years of age. Caution the child against biting down on the thermometer. If a mercury thermometer is used, wait about 3 minutes before removing the thermometer. Do not take an oral temperature if the child has a history of seizures.

Aural Temperature. The aural route uses the tympanic membrane thermometer. It is used on children over the age of two because it is considered less accurate for children under two years. Otitis media and impacted cerumen are two other reasons why this route may not be selected. A reading can be obtained in a matter of seconds.

Rectal Temperature. Rectal temperatures may be taken with caution in infants and toddlers when other methods or routes are not advised. Place the child prone or on the side, with the knees flexed. An infant can also lie prone on a parent's lap. Do not force the thermometer. When using a mercury thermometer, allow approximately 3 to 5 minutes to obtain an accurate reading. Rectal temperatures are not indicated for children who have had rectal surgery or for those who have diarrhea. (See Procedure 27-2.)

Axillary Temperature. Axillary temperatures are often preferable to rectal or oral temperatures for toddlers and preschoolers because they are safe and nonintrusive to take. Place the mercury thermometer or probe of the digital thermometer in the axillary space and have the child hold the arm close to the trunk. If a mercury thermometer is used, keep in place for 5 minutes before reading (Figure 27-9).

Pulse

The apical pulse is heard at the apex of the heart, located at the fifth intercostal space left side, midclavicular line.

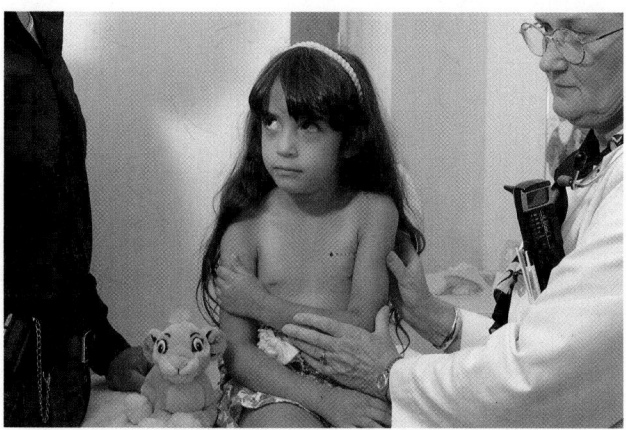

Figure 27-9 Taking an axillary temperature of a young child.

TABLE 27-2	NORMAL HEART RATE RANGES FOR CHILDREN	
Age	Heart Rate Range	Average Heart Rate
Infants to 2 years	100–160	110
2 to 6 years	70–120	100
6 to 10	70–110	90
10 to 16 years	60–100	85

That is, between the fifth and sixth ribs in the middle of the clavicle (usually below the nipple), left of the sternum. A stethoscope is required to obtain an apical pulse. The apical pulse is generally preferred over other pulse locations for infants and small children (under 5 years of age). Each "lub-dub" sound is counted as 1 heart beat. The pulse is counted for 1 full minute. (See Procedure 27-3.)

The normal pulse rate varies with age, decreasing as the child grows older (Table 27-2). The heart rate may also vary considerably among children of the same age and size. The heart rate increases in response to exercise, excitement, anxiety, and fever and decreases to a resting rate when the child is still.

Listen to the heart rate, noting whether the heart rhythm is regular or irregular. Children often have a normal cycle of irregular rhythm associated with respiration called sinus arrhythmia. In sinus arrhythmia, the child's heart rate is faster on inspiration and slower on expiration. Record whether the pulse is normal, bounding, or thready.

Respirations

In older children and adolescents, respiratory rate is counted in the same way as in an adult. In infants and young children (under 6 years of age), however, the respiratory rate is assessed by observing the rise and fall of the abdomen. Inspiration, when the chest or abdomen rises, and expiration, when the chest or abdomen falls, are counted as 1 respiration. Because these movements are often irregular, they should be counted for 1 full minute for accuracy. Normal respiratory rate varies with the child's age (Table 27-3). (See Procedure 27-4.)

TABLE 27-3	NORMAL RESPIRATORY RATE RANGES FOR CHILDREN
Age	Respiratory Rate per Minute
1 year	20–40
3 years	20–30
6 years	16–22
10 years	16–20
17 years	12–20

Blood Pressure

The blood pressure of an infant is not normally taken unless requested by the physician. In children 3 years of age and older, blood pressure should be measured annually as part of a routine vital sign assessment.

Blood pressure may be measured using mercury gravity, electronic, or aneroid equipment and a pediatric cuff. The size of the blood pressure cuff is determined by the size of the child's arm or leg. A general rule of thumb is that the width of the inflatable bladder should be 40 percent of the circumference of the extremity used. If the cuff is too small, pressure will be falsely high; if too large, falsely low. Sometimes it is difficult to hear the blood pressure in an infant or small child. Use a pediatric stethoscope over pulse sites if possible.

If the pulse still cannot be auscultated, the blood pressure can be measured by touch. Palpate for the pulse. Keeping your fingers on the pulse, pump up the cuff until the pulse is no longer felt. Slowly open the air valve, watching the column of mercury, and note the number where the pulse is again palpated. This is called the palpated systolic blood pressure.

COLLECTING A URINE SPECIMEN FROM AN INFANT

Occasionally the medical assistant may be required to obtain a urine specimen from an infant for laboratory testing. Special procedures and equipment are required for this procedure. The collection bag is clear plastic with adhesive tabs for application to the perineum of the infant (Figure 27-10). (See Procedure 27-5.)

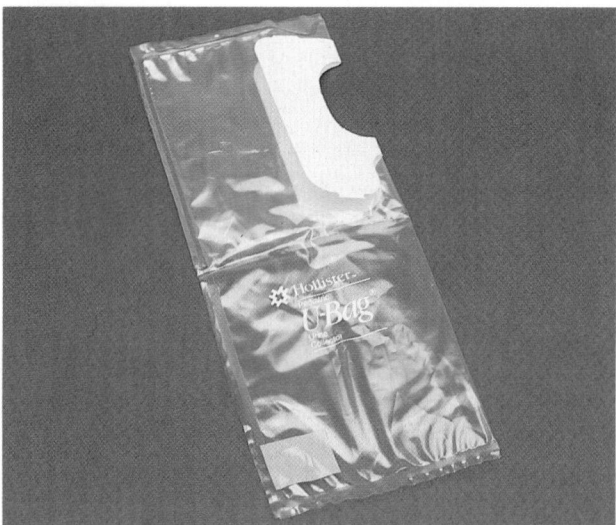

Figure 27-10   Pediatric urine collector. The collector is opened, and the paper backing is removed exposing the adhesive surface. The collector is firmly attached over the child's cleansed genitalia to prevent leakage.

SCREENING INFANTS FOR HEARING IMPAIRMENT

In some hospitals, infants are screened for hearing impairment immediately following delivery. An automated system for checking hearing ability is used by some clinics. It is a more complex screening requiring the use of sensors. As the infant moves in response to sounds produced by the system and recorded by sensors attached to the infant. This procedure is a more definitive screening process. The medical assistant must maintain a quiet environment while these screening procedures are being performed as extraneous sounds may invalidate the results.

SCREENING INFANT AND CHILD VISUAL ACUITY

Measuring the visual acuity of an infant is difficult and is not usually performed unless visual impairment is suspected. Newborns will respond to light by tightly shutting their eyes, keeping them closed until the light is removed. Older infants will follow an object up and down when it is placed directly in front of the eyes. It is estimated that a newborn has the vision equivalent to 20/150 which will reach the adult level of 20/20 by the age of 6 months. The medical assistant will be required to maintain a nonstimulating environment while the physician is screening the infant, as any interference may invalidate results.

The kindergarten chart is used to test visual acuity in young children. It contains pictures in descending size and the lines are labeled in the same manner as the Snellen Chart. The child is asked to identify the picture as the medical assistant points to it (Figure 27-11).

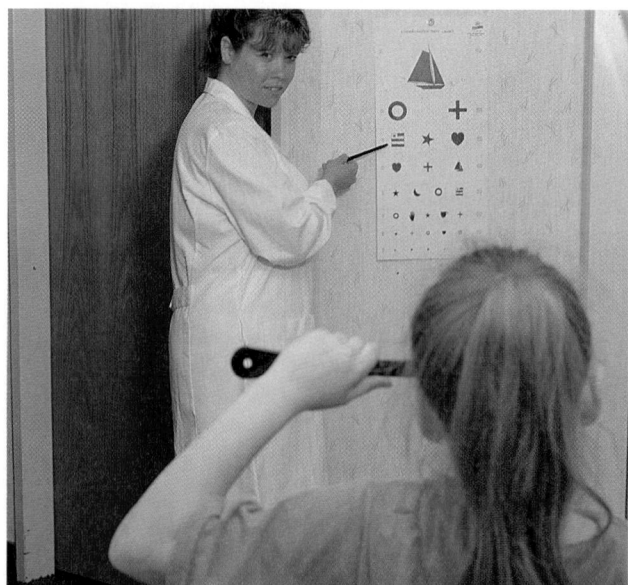

Figure 27-11   Measuring distance visual acuity of a child using a kindergarten vision screening chart.

The E chart is a series of "E"s pointing in different directions in descending size. The size and labeling are the same as the Snellen chart. This chart is used for older children. The child will be asked to point in the direction of the E as the medical assistant points to it (Figure 27-12).

Make a game out of measuring young children's visual acuity as their attention span is very limited.

COMMON DISORDERS AND DISEASES

Young children grow and physically change very quickly. Their immune systems develop normally when they are healthy infants and children. Immunizations, together with their own developing immune system give them protection from dangerous childhood diseases. Many life-threatening illnesses have been controlled because of scheduled immunization, the child's own developing immune system, and the use of antibiotics for infections.

Otitis Media

Otitis media is a commonly occurring disorder of infants and young children. It is characterized by inflammation of the middle ear. Fluid accumulates behind the tympanic membrane with a degree of temporary hearing loss. It is commonly known as a middle ear infection. Because of the infant and young child's eustachian tubes' connection to the nose and throat, bacteria that causes throat and res-

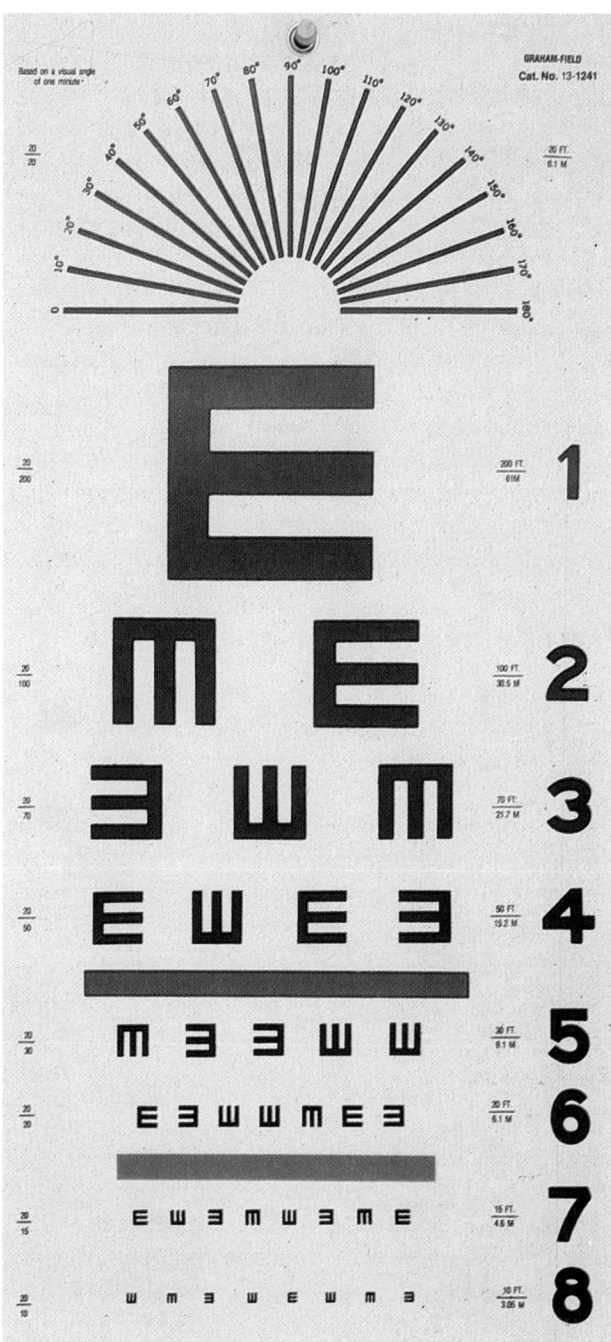

Figure 27-12 Snellen "E" or "Big E" chart for testing distance visual acuity of children.

piratory infections can easily access the inner ear via the eustachian tube. The fluid in the middle ear can become infected by the bacteria present in the nose and throat. The fluid turns to pus and is known as **suppurative** otitis media. Pain and loss of hearing are common symptoms. Many young children have eustachian tubes that are horizontal and narrow, which predisposes them to otitis media. As children develop physically, they can "outgrow" otitis media.

SPOTLIGHT ON AAMA ESSENTIALS THROUGH CAAHEP

- Gaining a child's confidence and trust during a pediatric examination will help to promote a positive relationship among the child, the physician, and the members of the medical staff.

- Protecting a child's space and modesty during an examination will help to encourage a more positive experience during the examination.

- Making a game out of a procedure and encouraging the child to take part in the examination will help to provide a more positive relationship between the child and the medical assistant.

The physician can diagnosis otitis media by visually examining the tympanic membrane with an otoscope. The membrane will be bulging and appear red and inflamed. If **exudate** or an oozing of pus is present, a culture and sensitivity can be done. The treatment for otitis media is antibiotics. To avoid antibiotic overuse and pathogen resistance, physicians will attempt to prescribe antibiotic therapy only when necessary. Decongestants are helpful in some children. For chronic otitis media, a **myringotomy**, incision into the tympanic membrane, may be necessary to avoid the rupture of the tympanic membrane and the scarring that results. Scarring can cause permanently impaired hearing ability.

Tympanostomy is a surgical procedure in which pediatric ear tubes are placed through the tympanic membrane to promote ongoing drainage. Chronic otitis media that is left untreated can result in permanent hearing loss.

The Common Cold

The common cold is aptly named because it is the most common and frequent disease that young children experience. Viruses are the usual microorganism that cause a cold, and they are spread by direct contact and droplets through the air when children cough and sneeze. Some symptoms are inflammation of the nasopharynx, coughing, nasal discharge, sneezing, and fever. Treatment consists of getting sufficient rest, forcing fluids, and eating a well-balanced diet.

Tonsillitis

The tonsils are located in the back of the nose and throat. They aid in protecting the respiratory tract from infection but frequently become inflamed and infected while doing their job. The cause most often is group A beta-hemolytic streptococcus. Fever, cough, sore throat, and red, swollen tonsils are common symptoms. Diagnosis can be made by doing a culture and sensitivity of tonsillar exudate. Antibiotics will rid the child of infection. Tonsillectomy is considered for older children who have chronic tonsillitis.

Pediculosis

Infestation with the head louse is known as pediculosis capitus and is common among school-age children. The parasites suck blood from humans and are highly contagious. Diagnosis can be made by visual examination of the hair and scalp and observing the eggs (known as nits) on the hair. Special medications applied to the hair is an effective treatment. Care should be taken to launder bed linens and clothing every day.

Asthma

Asthma has increased dramatically in the general population but especially in children. The cause of asthma is not known, but it can be brought on by environmental substances, such as pollen, chemicals, cigarette smoke, mold, and dog and cat hair. Its symptoms include wheezing, coughing, and shortness of breath. It is a serious chronic respiratory disease. Spasms of the bronchi trap air and mucus in the lungs. The child will complain of a tight chest and will have shallow respirations and a nonproductive cough. The asthma attack may become an emergency situation. The pediatrician may refer the child to an allergy specialist who will test the child for various allergies. Respiratory therapy is helpful for some children.

Child Abuse

Child abuse has risen significantly in recent years. By law, health care professionals, including medical assistants, as well as others must report suspected child abuse. The individual reporting the suspected abuse is protected against liability as a result of the reporting. If suspicion of abuse exists, the physician and health care professional should:

- Treat child's injuries
- Send child to hospital if necessary
- Inform parents of the diagnosis
- Inform parents that the incident will be reported to the public and social service agency
- Notify child protective agency
- Document all information
- Provide court testimony if requested

Some injuries commonly seen in child abuse include poor hygiene, bruises, welts, malnutrition, burns, fractures, head injuries, dislocated joints and neglected well-baby appointments.

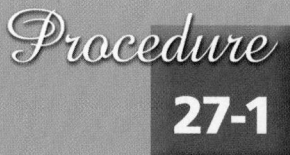

Measuring the Infant: Weight, Height, Head, and Chest Circumference

Procedure 27-1

STANDARD PRECAUTIONS:

PURPOSE:
To obtain an accurate measurement of an infant's weight, height, head, and chest circumference for medical records and to screen for growth abnormalities.

EQUIPMENT/SUPPLIES:

Infant scale	Patient's chart
Paper protector	Pen
Flexible measuring tape	Ruler
Growth chart	Biohazard waste container

PROCEDURE STEPS:

Measuring Infant Weight
1. Wash hands. Explain procedure to parent(s).
2. Undress infant (including the diaper).
3. Place all weights to left of scale to check balance.
4. Place a clean utility towel on scale, check balance scale for accuracy being sure to compensate for the weight of the towel. RATIONALE: The protection that the paper utility towel affords helps to reduce transmission of microorganisms and will provide warmth because the scale will be cool.

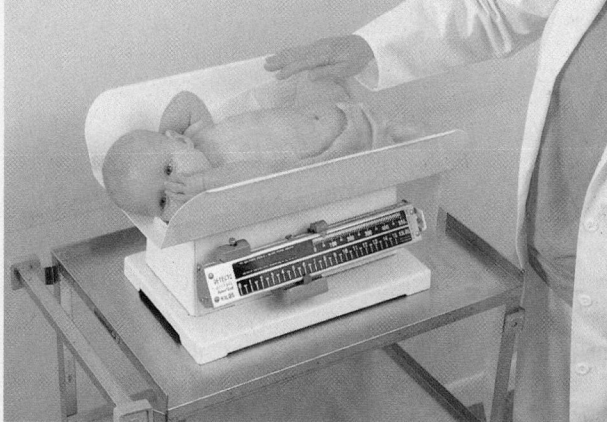

Figure 27-13 Infants who are unable to sit erect should be weighed on their back on a platform scale.

5. Gently place infant on her back on the scale. Place your hand slightly above the infant's body to ensure safety (Figure 27-13). RATIONALE: This will safeguard the infant from falling.
6. Place the bottom weight to its highest measurement that will not cause the balance to drop to the bottom edge.
7. Slowly move upper weight until the balance bar rests in the center of the indicator. A balanced scale will provide an accurate weight. Read the infant's weight while she is lying still.
8. Return both weights to their resting position to the extreme left.
9. Gently remove infant and apply diaper. (Parent can help with diapering and holding infant.)
10. Discard used protective paper towel per OSHA guidelines.
11. Sanitize scale.
12. Wash hands.
13. Document results according to office policy (pounds and ounces or kilograms) on growth chart, patient's chart, and parent's booklet if available. Connect dot from previous examination with a ruler to complete graph.

Measuring Infant Length/Height
1. Wash hands. Explain procedure to parent(s).
2. Remove infant's shoes.
3. Gently place infant on her back on the examination table. If the pediatric table has a headboard, ask parent to hold infant's head against (end) headboard of table at zero mark of ruler while you place infant's heels against footboard. Gently straighten infant's back and legs to line up along ruler. If there is no footboard (to place infant's feet against), use your right hand as a guide (Figure 27-14). If necessary, gently place your left hand over the child's legs at the knees to secure the child in place and straighten the legs so you can read the recumbent length from the head to the heel. RATIONALE: Sometimes it is difficult to straighten the legs.
4. Read length on the measuring device in inches or centimeters.
5. Wash hands.

(continues)

Procedure
27-1   *(continued)*

6. Document measurement on growth chart, patient's chart, and parent's booklet if available. Connect dot from previous examination with a ruler to complete graph.

Measure Head Circumference

1. Wash hands and explain procedure to parent(s).
2. Talk to infant to gain cooperation. Infant may be held by parent or lie on examination table for procedure. Older children of 2 or 3 years may stand or sit if they will remain still.
3. Place the measuring tape snugly around the head from the occipital protuberance to the supraorbital prominence. This is the largest part of the head (Figure 27-15).

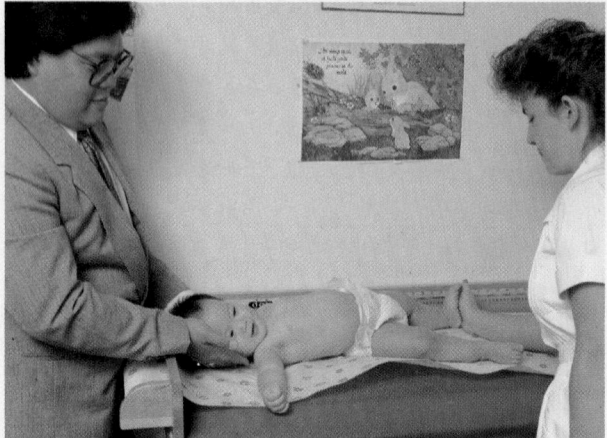

Figure 27-14   Measuring the recumbent length of an infant.

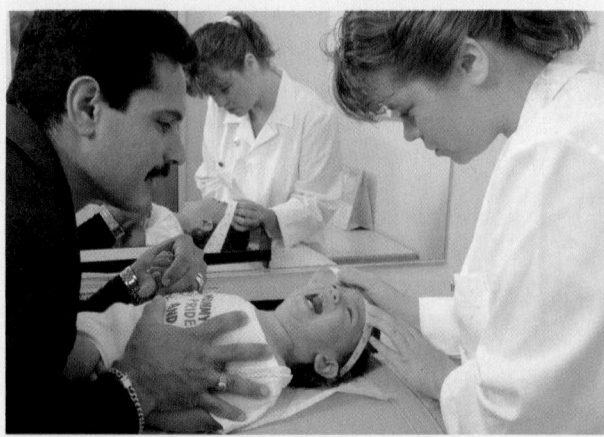

Figure 27-15   Measuring infant's head circumference.

4. Read the measurement which will be in either inches (to nearest ½ inch) or centimeters (to nearest 0.01 cm).
5. Wash hands.
6. Document results according to office policy on growth chart, patient's chart, and parent's booklet if available. Connect dot from previous examination with a ruler to complete graph.

Measure Infant's Chest Circumference

1. Wash hands and explain procedure to parent(s).
2. Use one thumb to hold tape measure with zero mark against the infant's chest at the midsternal area. With the other hand, bring the tape around/under the back to meet the zero mark of the tape in front. Take the measurement of the chest just above the nipples with the tape fitting around the child's chest under the axillary region. If you need assistance in holding the child still, ask the parent or another assistant. The measurement should be taken when the child is breathing normally and during the resting phase between respirations (Figure 27-16).
3. Read measurement to the nearest 0.01 cm or ¹⁄₁₆ inch.
4. Wash hands.
5. Document results in patient's chart.

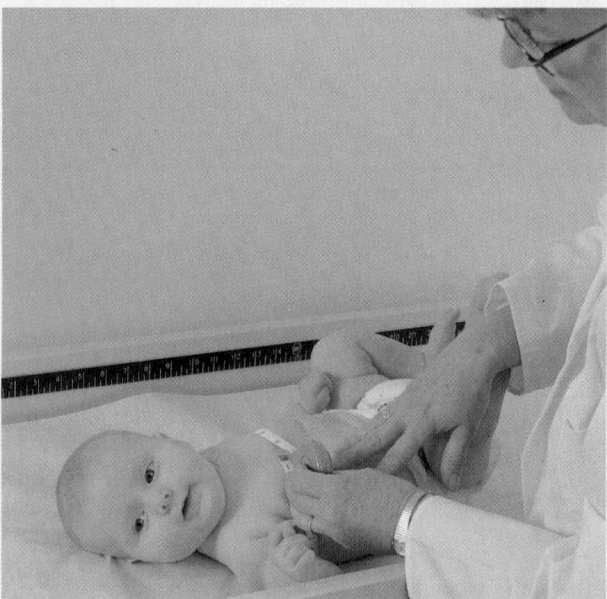

Figure 27-16   Measuring infant's chest circumference.

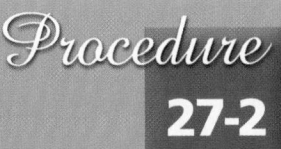

Taking an Infant's Rectal Temperature with a Mercury or Digital Thermometer

Procedure 27-2

STANDARD PRECAUTIONS:

PURPOSE:
To obtain a rectal temperature using a mercury or digital thermometer.

EQUIPMENT/SUPPLIES:
Mercury rectal thermometer (red tip) and sheath
 or
Digital thermometer (red probe) and probe cover
Lubricating jelly
4 × 4 gauze sponges
Gloves
Biohazard waste container

PROCEDURE STEPS:
1. Wash hands.
2. Assemble equipment.
3. Identify patient.
4. Explain procedure to parent(s). RATIONALE: Gain cooperation and assistance in disrobing infant and positioning properly.
5. Remove infant's diaper.
6. Position infant in a prone position having parent or another medical assistant safeguard infant.
7. Place sheath on thermometer. RATIONALE: Prevents microorganism cross contamination.
8. Lubricate with lubricating jelly. (Place lubricant on a 4 × 4 gauze sponge and place tip of thermometer in lubricant.) RATIONALE: Easier insertion of thermometer.
9. Apply gloves.
10. Spread buttocks, insert thermometer gently into the rectum past the sphincter; for an infant this is ½ inch (Figure 27-17).
11. Hold buttocks together while holding the thermometer. If necessary, restrain infant movement by placing your arm across infant's back. Parent can immobilize infant's legs. RATIONALE: Ensure infant's safety and comfort.
12. Hold in place for five minutes. Do not let go of the thermometer. RATIONALE: Movement by infant can cause thermometer to move and injure the infant.
13. Remove from rectum. Have parent attend to infant.

14. Remove sheath and place in biohazard container.
15. Read thermometer.
16. Wash, rinse, and dry thermometer. Place on clean paper towel.
17. Remove gloves, discard in biohazard waste container.
18. Wash hands.
19. Place thermometer in a disinfectant solution for rectal thermometers.
20. Assist parent in dressing infant if necessary.
21. Record on the patient chart labeled with (R) indicating a rectal temperature.

Using Digital Thermometer
1. Follow steps 1 through 11 for taking temperature with mercury thermometer.
2. Hold digital thermometer in place until the beep is heard.
3. Read results on digital display window.
4. Remove thermometer from rectum.
5. Discard probe cover into biohazard waste container by pressing the eject button on probe end.
6. Replace thermometer on holder base.
7. Remove gloves, discard in biohazard waste container, and wash hands.
8. Assist patient in dressing and position as necessary.
9. Record on the patient chart labeled with (R) indicating a rectal temperature.
10. Wash hands.

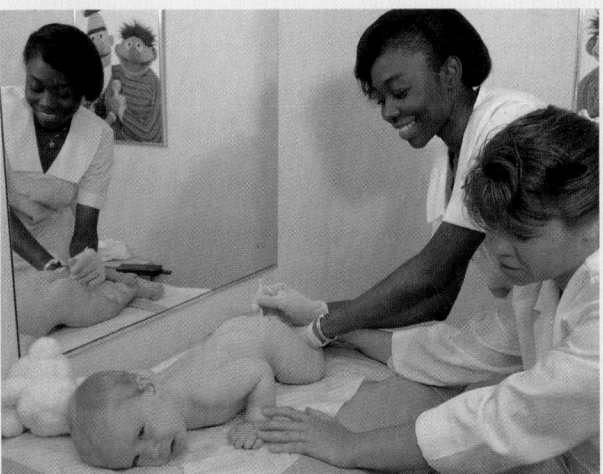

Figure 27-17 Taking the rectal temperature of an infant in the prone position.

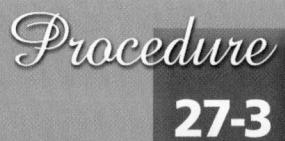

Procedure 27-3 — Taking an Apical Pulse on an Infant

STANDARD PRECAUTIONS:

PURPOSE:
To obtain an apical pulse rate.

EQUIPMENT/SUPPLIES:
Stethoscope
Watch with second hand
Alcohol wipes

PROCEDURE STEPS:
1. Wash hands.
2. Assemble equipment.
3. Identify patient.
4. Explain procedure to parent.
5. Assist in disrobing infant if necessary.
6. Provide a drape for infant's warmth if necessary.
7. Position the infant in a supine position or sitting in the parent's lap. RATIONALE: The supine position may offer easier access to apex of heart if the child is calm.
8. Locate the fifth intercostal space, midclavicular line, left of sternum. RATIONALE: Location of apex of heart.
9. Place warmed stethoscope on the site and listen for the lub-dup sound of the heart.
10. Count the pulse for one minute; each lub-dup equals one heartbeat or pulse.
11. Wash hands.
12. Record the pulse in the infant's chart with the designation of (AP) to denote method of obtaining the pulse.
13. Note any arrhythmias.
14. Assist patient as needed.
15. Clean earpieces and diaphragm of stethoscope with alcohol wipes. RATIONALE: Prevents cross contamination of microbes between patients.
16. Wash hands again.

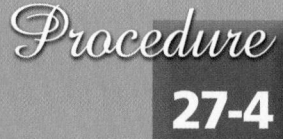

Procedure 27-4 — Measuring Infant's Respiration Rate

STANDARD PRECAUTIONS:

PURPOSE:
The respiration rate is normally taken immediately before or after the pulse rate to obtain an accurate respiratory rate.

EQUIPMENT/SUPPLIES:
Watch with second hand

PROCEDURE STEPS:
1. Wash hands.
2. Identify the patient.
3. Position infant in a supine position.
4. Place hand on the chest to feel the rise and fall of the chest wall for one minute.
5. Note depth, rhythm, and breath sounds while counting.
6. Wash hands.
7. Record respiration rate in patient chart, noting any irregularities and sounds.

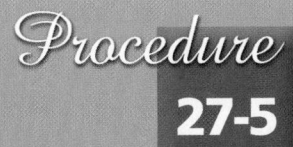

Obtaining a Urine Specimen from an Infant or Young Child

STANDARD PRECAUTIONS:

PURPOSE:
To obtain a specimen of urine from an infant or young child.

EQUIPMENT/SUPPLIES:
Urine collection bag
Laboratory request form
Gloves
Washcloth
Soap
Water
Towel
Biohazard waste container

PROCEDURE STEPS:
1. Wash and glove hands following standard precautions.
2. Assemble equipment.
3. Identify patient and explain procedure to parent(s).
4. Instruct parent to remove diaper.
5. Wash and dry perineal area. RATIONALE: Cleaning area reduces microorganism level and provides better quality urine specimen.
6. Apply collection bag, secure with adhesive tabs.
   a. Females: spread perineum, place bag over labia (Figure 27-18).
   b. Males: place bag over penis and scrotum.
7. Replace diaper carefully.
8. Frequently check bag for urine.
9. Once specimen has been collected, remove bag carefully.
10. Prepare specimen as required. Send to laboratory in a specimen container with a requisition or process the specimen in the office laboratory.
11. Remove gloves and discard in biohazard waste container.
12. Wash hands.
13. Record collection in patient's chart.

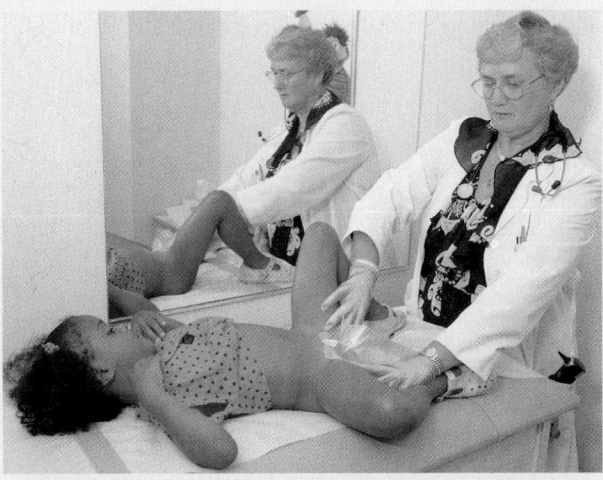

Figure 27-18 Applying the pediatric urine collector on a female. The opening of the bag should be directly over the urinary meatus. On a male, the scrotum and penis should project through the round opening of the bag.

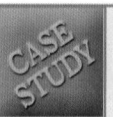

After examining Joey Little, Dr. King confirms the diagnosis of otitis media.

CASE STUDY REVIEW

27-1

1. Explain otitis media, the most common reason for its occurrence, and its treatment.
2. How can parents and caregivers be educated to help prevent otitis media?

SUMMARY

Caring for the health and well-being of infants and children through their various developmental stages and into adolescence is the responsibility of the pediatric practice.

Careful observation of the parent or caregiver and the child is helpful to the treatment and care given to the child. The medical assistant is responsible for reporting to the physician any suspicion of child abuse.

Opportunities abound for educating parents about topics that will keep their children healthy throughout life and include nutrition, sleep, immunization, and exercise. Pamphlets are available to share with parents and caregivers.

Children need respect and should be treated with empathy and love, and in doing so, a positive relationship can be developed with the child.

REVIEW QUESTIONS

Multiple Choice

1. At what age should the first polio vaccine be given?
   a. birth
   b. 1 month
   c. 2 months
   d. 3 months
   e. 6 months
2. One procedure done to treat otitis media is:
   a. suppuration
   b. tympanostomy
   c. ear irrigation
   d. otoscopy
   e. myringectomy
3. The pathogen usually responsible for causing tonsillitis is:
   a. staphylococcus aureus
   b. meningiococcus
   c. beta-hemolytic streptococcus group A
   d. beta-hemolytic streptococcus group B
4. Head circumference is measured on the child until what age?
   a. 1 year
   b. 2 years
   c. 4 years
   d. 6 years

5. An apical pulse is taken over which of the following sites?
   a. 3rd intercostal space on the left side
   b. 4th intercostal space on the left side
   c. 5th intercostal space on the left side
   d. 6th intercostal space on the left side

Critical Thinking Questions

1. You notice when you undress a two-year-old child to prepare for a physical examination that there are bruises on the buttocks and what appear to be burns on the feet. What course of action do you take?
2. Explain the importance of head circumference measurement.
3. Explain the importance of growth charts.
4. Describe the appropriate position in which to place an infant for a rectal temperature.
5. Describe the appearance of the pediatric urine collector bag. What is the best way to make certain it will adhere to the child's body?
6. Explain the type of chart used to test visual acuity in young children.
7. When is it appropriate to use the tympanic thermometer while taking a child's temperature?
8. When taking an infant's rectal temperature, what precautions should be taken?

9. Chest circumference measurements on an infant are performed for what purpose?
10. What do the curved lines printed across growth charts indicate?

WEB ACTIVITIES

Search for the American Pediatric Academy on the World Wide Web to answer the following:

1. What information is available about immunization for Hepatitis B?
2. What is the most recent recommendation that the American Academy of Pediatrics has made regarding varicella immunization?

REFERENCES/BIBLIOGRAPHY

Damjanov, I. (1996). *Pathology for the health related profession* (1st ed.). Philadelphia: W. B. Saunders Company.

Frazier, M. S., Drzymkowski, J. A., & Doty, S. J. (1996). *Essentials of human diseases and conditions* (1st ed.). Philadelphia: W. B. Saunders Company.

Fremgen, B. (1998). *Essentials of medical assisting: Administrative and clinical competencies*. Upper Saddle River, NJ: Brady-Prentice Hall.

Keir, L., Wise, B., & Krebs, C. (1998). *Medical assisting: Administrative and clinical competencies* (4th ed.). Philadelphia: W. B. Saunders Company.

Kinn, M. E., & Woods, M. A. (1999). *The medical assistant: Administrative and clinical* (8th ed.). Philadelphia: W. B. Saunders Company.

Tamparo, C., & Lewis, M. (2000). *Diseases of the human body* (3rd ed.). Philadelphia: F. A. Davis Company.

MALE REPRODUCTIVE SYSTEM

KEY TERMS

Cryptorchidism
Intravenous Pyelogram
Orchiectomy
Residual
Retention
Transilluminator
Transurethral Resection

OUTLINE

OBJECTIVES

The student should strive to meet the following performance objectives and demonstrate an understanding of the facts and principles presented in this chapter through written and oral communication.

1. Define key terms.
2. Describe common disorders and diseases of the male reproductive system.
3. Explain benign hyperplasia of the prostate.
4. Identify signs and symptoms of the various disorders and diseases of the male reproductive system.
5. Describe the common diagnostic tests and procedures used in the male reproductive system.
6. Explain testicular self-examination.

ROLE DELINEATION COMPONENTS

CLINICAL

Fundamental Principles

- Apply principles of aseptic technique and infection control
- Comply with quality assurance practices
- Screen and follow up patient test results

Diagnostic Orders

- Collect and process specimens
- Perform diagnostic tests

Patient Care

- Obtain patient history and vital signs
- Prepare and maintain examination and treatment areas
- Prepare patients for examinations, procedures, and treatments
- Assist with examinations, procedures, and treatments
- Coordinate patient care information with other health care providers

GENERAL (TRANSDISCIPLINARY)

Legal Concepts

- Document accurately

Instruction

- Instruct individuals according to their needs
- Teach methods of health promotion and disease prevention

SCENARIO

Joe Geurro, CMA, finds many situations daily to educate patients because he knows how important it is. He keeps abreast of the latest techniques and procedures about diseases and problems of the male reproductive system. He attends lectures, workshops and seminars when possible, and uses the World Wide Web for the latest information from the American Cancer Society about prostate cancer as a resource for people with prostate cancer. With Dr. Woo's permission, Joe shares that information with patients.

INTRODUCTION

The male reproductive system consists of a pair of testes in which sperm and hormones are produced, a system of tubes that transport the sperm to the outside of the body, and a penis that transports the sperm into the female reproductive tract. There are glands such as the prostate that secrete fluid and become part of the semen. The testes are suspended in the scrotum. Sperm are developed in tubules in the testes. Upon maturity, the sperm enter the epididymis, a convoluted tube resting on the surface of the testes. The epididymis leads to the vas deferens that passes into the abdominal cavity. The ejaculatory duct opens into the urethra. Semen is expressed through the urethral opening. Diagnostic tests, procedures, disorders, and conditions common to the male reproductive system are shown in Tables 28-1 and 28-2.

TESTICULAR EXAMINATION

Early detection of testicular cancer relies heavily on the patient's willingness to perform self-examination of these body parts on a regular basis. Patient teaching is valuable when used to educate the patient about self-examination for detection of abnormalities such as lumps or thickenings. Figure 28-1 illustrates a testicular self-examination and Procedure 28-1 outlines steps for instructions usually given by the medical assistant.

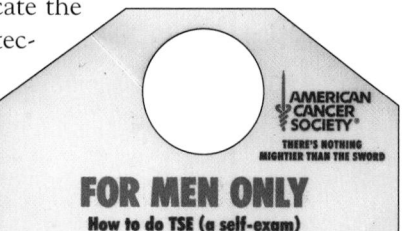

AMERICAN CANCER SOCIETY®
THERE'S NOTHING MIGHTIER THAN THE SWORD

FOR MEN ONLY
How to do TSE (a self-exam)

Cancer of the testicle can be cured if you find it early.

Use the shower check.

1. Check your testicles once a month.

2. Roll each testicle between your thumb and finger, like this:

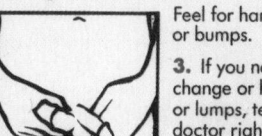

Feel for hard lumps or bumps.

3. If you notice a change or have aches or lumps, tell your doctor right away so something can be done about it.

Testicular cancer can be cured.

You should also know that prostate cancer is the most common cancer in men. Men over age 50 should have an annual health check-up that includes a prostate examination.

FOR MORE INFORMATION CALL THE AMERICAN CANCER SOCIETY TOLL FREE: 1-800-ACS-2345

Figure 28-1
Testicular self-examination.
(Courtesy of American Cancer Society)

Patient Teaching Tip

1. Testicular cancer is one of the leading causes of death in men under the age of 40.
2. Risk factors include an undescended testicle, **cryptorchidism**, and childhood mumps.
3. Prognosis is good when found in the early stages.

TABLE 28-1 MALE REPRODUCTIVE SYSTEM

Disease/Disorder	Laboratory Diagnostic Tests			Radiography	Surgery	Medical Tests or Procedures
	Blood	Urine	Other			
Benign Hyperplasia of Prostate	• PSA (rules out or detects prostate cancer)	• Urinalysis		• Intravenous pyelogram • Pelvic ultrasound	• Biopsy of prostate gland	• Rectal exam • Cystoscopy
Cancer of Prostate	• PSA (detects prostate cancer) • Acid phosphotase	• Urinalysis		• Intravenous pyelogram • Pelvic ultrasound	• Biopsy of prostate gland	• Rectal exam • Cystoscopy
Epididymitis	Complete blood count	• Urinalysis • Culture and sensitivity of urine	• Culture and sensitivity of urethral discharge	• Intravenous pyelogram • Pelvic ultrasound		• Rectal exam
Prostatitis	Complete blood count	• Urinalysis • Culture and sensitivity of urine				
Sexually Transmitted Diseases						
• Chlamydia		• Urinalysis	• Direct urethral smear using monoclonal antibodies			
• Genital Herpes (male or female)		• Urinalysis	• Culture of living tissue • Tzanck smear test			
• Gonorrhea	• Complete blood count	• Urinalysis • Culture and sensitivity of urine	• Direct smear of urethral discharge, anal canal, and oropharynx • Thayer-Martin culture	• Pelvic Ultrasound • Laparoscopy		• Cystoscopy
• Syphilis	• VDRL (Venereal disease research laboratory) • Treponema Pallidum Hemagglutination Test • Rapid plasma reagin	• Urinalysis • Culture and sensitivity of urine	• Culture of chancre			
• HVB and HIV See Chapter 4.						
Testicular Cancer					• Biopsy of testicle	

TABLE 28-2   DESCRIPTIONS OF MALE REPRODUCTIVE DISORDERS AND CONDITIONS

- Benign Hyperplasia of Prostate (BHP). Common in men over sixty years of age probably due to disturbance in sex hormones as the reproductive period of life declines. Because the gland surrounds the urethra, urinary flow is obstructed and can lead to urinary retention and urinary tract infection.
- Cancer of Prostate. Common malignancy. Most frequent cause of cancer in men after lung and colon cancers. Symptoms similar to BHP because the cancer causes the prostate to harden and obstruct the flow of urine.
- Epididymitis. Inflammation of the epididymis usually caused by gonorrhea. Epididymis becomes enlarged, hard, and painful.
- Prostatitis. Inflammation of the prostate gland that can result from an infection in an adjacent structure such as gonococcus of the urethra or *E-Coli* from the bladder. Seen in patients with frequent urinary tract infections (UTI) and sexually transmitted disease.

- Sexually Transmitted Disease (STD).
  - Chlamydial Infection. Common in males and females. A prevalent STD that often coexists with gonorrhea.
  - Genital Herpes. Painful, viral disease which is dormant and recurs periodically. There is no cure. Characterized by blisters similar to chicken pox. Common in men and women.
  - Gonorrhea. Caused by a bacterium and the infection can spread producing a stricture of the urethra or the vas deferens. Sterility can result if both vas deferens become involved.
  - Syphilis. Caused by a spirochete. Chancres develop. Can heal. If untreated, the disease progresses to stages two and three. Severe damage to the cardiovascular system, brain, vision, and hearing loss occur. General paralysis and death can result.
  - HVB & HIV see Chapter 4.
- Testicular Cancer. Primarily seen in males aged 15 to 35 and can be highly malignant.

DISORDERS OF THE MALE REPRODUCTIVE SYSTEM

Benign Prostatic Hypertrophy

Benign hypertrophy of the prostate gland or benign hypertrophic prostate gland also known as benign prostatic hyperplasia (BPH) is common in men age 50 or older. Symptoms include retention (the inability to completely empty the bladder), a diminished flow of urine, and difficulty starting to urinate. It is thought that the cause is aging and may be related to hormonal changes. The prostate enlarges and, because it surrounds the urethra, it causes constriction of the urethra and the associated symptoms. The physician can palpate the enlarged prostate gland when performing a rectal examination. This helps in making a diagnosis. Other tests may include a blood test known as prostate specific antigen (PSA), a urinalysis, and an intravenous pyelogram (an x-ray of the kidneys, ureters, and bladder using a contrast medium). If residual urine stays in the bladder, infections can develop, and kidneys may cease functioning because they can't drain urine properly into the bladder when it is full (Figure 28-2).

The PSA blood test is used to detect abnormally high levels of a protein substance that may indicate prostate cancer. The American Cancer Society recommends that men age 50 and over have an annual PSA blood test.

Ultrasound can be used to view the prostate, bladder, or kidneys. A biopsy of the prostate, done in conjunction with an ultrasound, can help diagnose either benign prostatic hypertrophy or cancer.

Treatment of BPH, in some cases, consists of medi-cation that can relax prostate muscles, hormones that block prostate growth, or bladder relaxants. Transurethral resection of the prostate (removal of prostate tissue using a device inserted through the urethra) is the most common surgical treatment. Instruments are inserted through the penis and a laser can be used to remove the excess tissue (Figure 28-3).

Prostatitis

Prostatitis, or inflammation of the prostate, occurs primarily in men over age 50. The prostate may enlarge and cause pain and discomfort, such as burning while urinating. There can be pain in the back, muscle aches, and urinary frequency. The cause may be bacterial, such as from gonorrhea, or may be caused by another pathogen that produced a urinary tract infection. Urinalysis, urine culture, and rectal exam (to palpate the prostate) help in making a diagnosis. Treatment is usually medication, such as penicillin and pain medication, and the patient will be told to force fluids by increasing fluid intake significantly.

Prostate Cancer

Prostate cancer is the third leading cause of cancer death in men, after lung and colon cancer. Metastasis to the spine or pelvis is not unusual. The symptoms, if present, are similar to urinary obstruction, difficulty urinating, frequency of urination, and inability to urinate. It is of value to check the blood level of PSA, but a biopsy is necessary to be certain. An ultrasonogram and CAT scan can help to determine if there has been any metastasis. Treatment consists of prostatectomy, hormonal therapy, radiation, and chemotherapy.

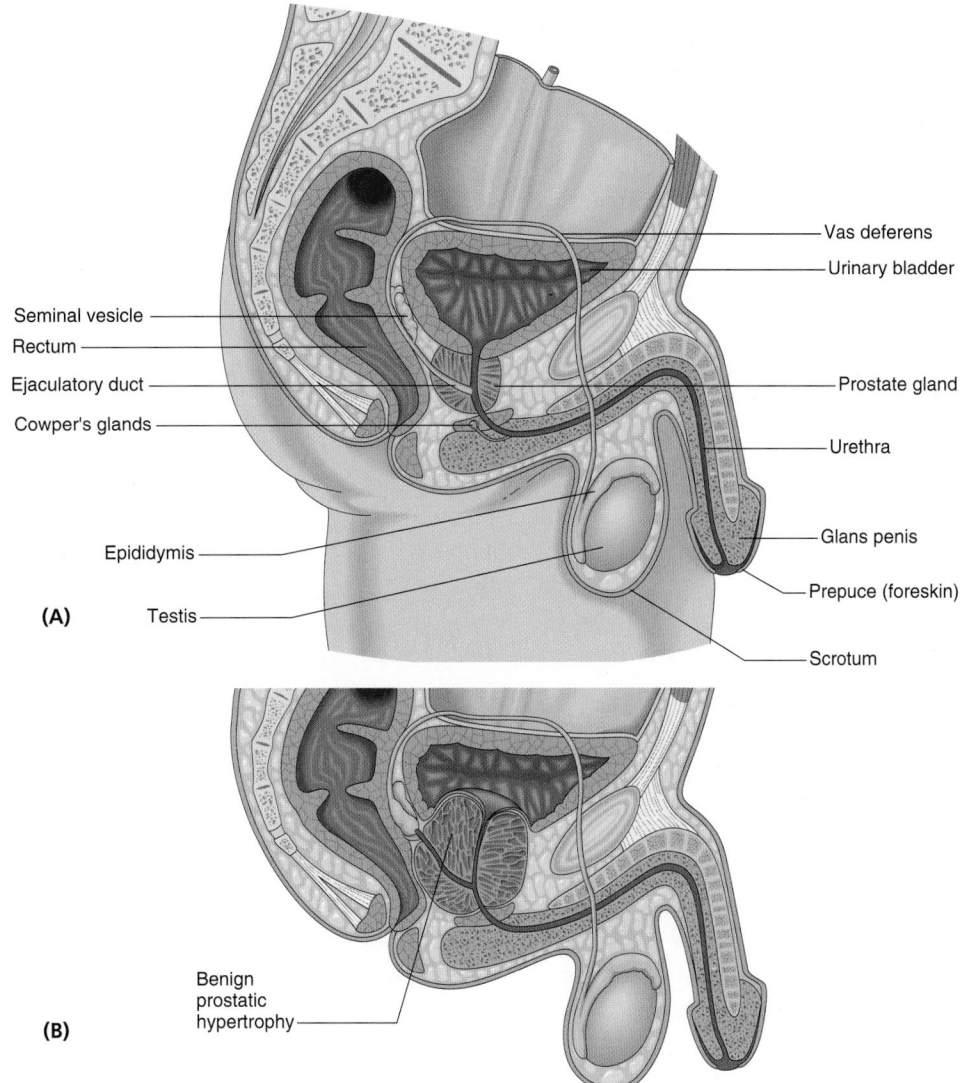

(A)

Seminal vesicle
Rectum
Ejaculatory duct
Cowper's glands
Epididymis
Testis

Vas deferens
Urinary bladder
Prostate gland
Urethra
Glans penis
Prepuce (foreskin)
Scrotum

(B)

Benign prostatic hypertrophy

Figure 28-2 Normal and enlarged prostate: (A) Normal; (B) Benign prostatic hypertrophy or hyperplasia.

Testicular Cancer

Testicular cancer is the most common kind of cancer in males between the age of 20 and 35 years, otherwise it is rarely seen. Usually a painless lump is found in a testicle. An undescended testicle, cryptorchidism, and a history of mumps are predisposing factors. Diagnosis can be made by performing a biopsy after palpation of the testicle finds a mass. Surgery to excise the testicle, orchiectomy, followed by radiation and chemotherapy is the usual course of action. Monthly testicular examinations are recommended by the American Cancer Society for all men and are considered the best preventive measure for testicular cancer. See Figure 28-1 and Procedure 28-1.

Sexually Transmitted Diseases

Sexually transmitted diseases (STDs) affect men and women, can damage health, and become life-threatening. Refer to Tables 28-1 and 28-2. Also see information in Chapter 26 regarding STDs.

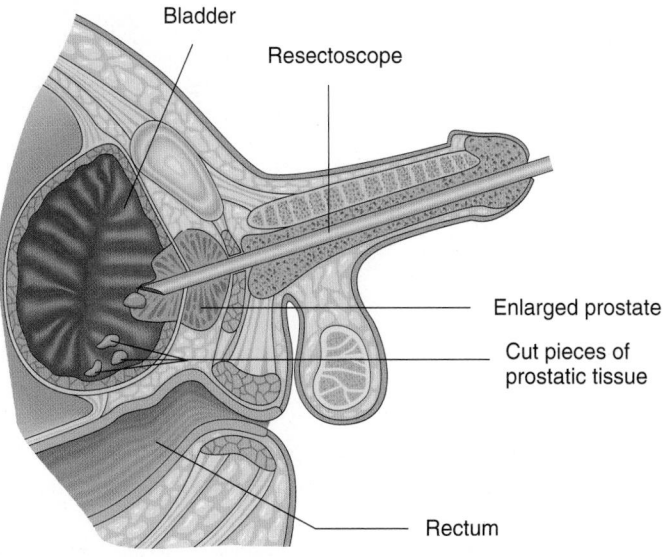

Bladder
Resectoscope
Enlarged prostate
Cut pieces of prostatic tissue
Rectum

Figure 28-3 Transurethral resection of prostate (TURP).

ASSISTING WITH THE MALE REPRODUCTIVE EXAMINATION

A female medical assistant may or may not be requested to assist the physician with the examination of the male reproductive system. The physician will examine the penis and the foreskin of the penis in an uncircumcised patient. The penis and testes are examined for swelling, masses, or discomfort. A transilluminator may be used by the physician to check the prostate gland. A lighted instrument used to inspect a cavity or organ, the transilluminator would be passed through the rectum to illuminate the prostate gland through the walls of the rectum. The physician will do a digital rectal examination to check the size of the prostate and will also check for an inguinal hernia.

DIAGNOSTIC TESTS AND PROCEDURES

Tests and procedures, in addition to those previously addressed, include vasectomy and a semen analysis.

Vasectomy

A vasectomy is performed to surgically sterilize the male. The vas deferens extends up into the abdomen where it connects to create the ejaculatory duct that opens into the urethra. By removing a portion of each vas deferens, sperm cannot travel to mix with semen, thereby causing the male to be sterile (Figure 28-4).

SPOTLIGHT ON AAMA ESSENTIALS THROUGH CAAHEP

- Being sensitive to the male patient's needs and emotions during an examination will help to provide a more positive relationship between the patient and the medical assistant.

- Helping the male patient establish a good rapport with the physician will promote a more positive experience during the examination process.

- Being aware of a patient's cultural diversity is extremely important and necessary to assist the patient in dealing with "old wives' tales" and rumors regarding disorders and illnesses affecting the male reproductive system.

Semen Analysis

Semen testing is frequently performed in the physician's office or clinic to determine sperm cell counts before referring patients to a specialist, such as a physician who treats infertility. It is also done as part of a complete fertility workup and to evaluate the effectiveness of a vasectomy. See Chapter 44 for extensive information about semen analysis.

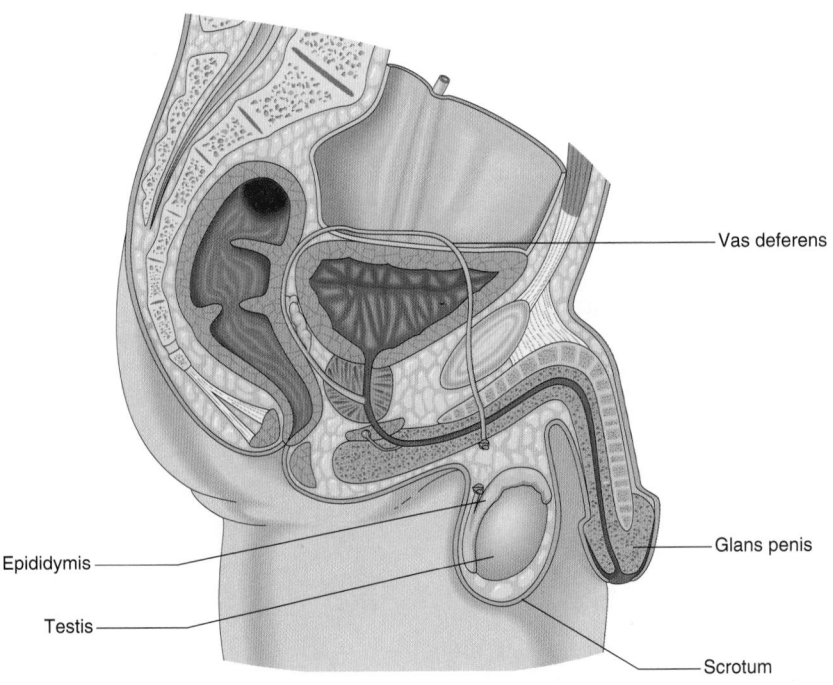

Figure 28-4 Vasectomy.

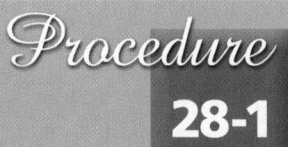

Procedure 28-1 — Instructing Patient in Testicular Self-Examination

PURPOSE:
To provide a patient with information concerning testicular screening for the presence of a painless mass in the scrotum.

EQUIPMENT/SUPPLIES:
Testicular self-examination card

PROCEDURE STEPS:
1. Instruct patient to examine his testicles in a warm shower. RATIONALE: The warmth causes the scrotal skin to relax.
2. Examine each testicle separately with both hands.
3. Place the index and middle fingers underneath the testicle and the thumbs on top. Roll the testicle gently between the fingers.
4. Locate the epididymis. Provide a chart to the patient that illustrates the testes and epididymis. RATIONALE: A lump can be similar in size to the epididymis and needs to be distinguished from the epididymis.
5. Look for swelling or changes in the scrotal area.
6. Encourage the patient to report anything unusual to the physician.

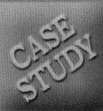

CASE STUDY 28-1

Adam Desmond has an appointment today in the clinic for a physical examination, and his chief complaint is that he has been having trouble sitting through ball games or movies without having to go to the bathroom to urinate several times.

CASE STUDY REVIEW

1. How can Dr. Woo make a diagnosis of benign prostatic hypertrophy?
2. What preliminary tests might Dr. Woo order for Mr. Desmond today?

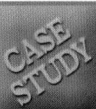

CASE STUDY 28-2

John Toomey called to say that he discovered "something hard in his right testicle, like a marble."

CASE STUDY REVIEW

1. What will Dr. King's examination consist of?

SUMMARY

A thorough knowledge of the diseases and disorders of the male reproductive system and the diagnostic tests and procedures that are performed for this specialty will enhance the quality of care given by the medical assistant.

REVIEW QUESTIONS

Multiple Choice

1. Cancer of the prostate may be detected early by which of the following?
   a. prostate-specific antigen
   b. transurethral resection
   c. semen analysis
   d. urine culture
2. The best preventive measure for testicular cancer is which of the following?
   a. yearly physical examination
   b. yearly intravenous pyelogram
   c. monthly self-examination
   d. monthly urinalysis with cultures
3. Benign prostate hypertrophy (BPH) is thought to be caused by:
   a. excessive consumption of alcohol
   b. aging and hormonal changes
   c. recurrent epididymitis
   d. chronic chlamydia infections
4. Which of the following is a symptom of prostatitis?
   a. painful urination
   b. low sperm count
   c. eruptions on the scrotum
   d. high testosterone level
5. The most definitive way to diagnose cancer of the prostate is by which of the following?
   a. ultrasonography
   b. intravenous pyelogram
   c. biopsy of the prostate
   d. semen analysis

Critical Thinking

1. Describe how a male should perform a self-testicular examination.
2. What is the purpose of severing the vas deferens?
3. List several symptoms of benign prostatic hypertrophy, and explain why the symptoms occur.

4. Describe the blood test that is helpful to diagnose prostate cancer.
5. Explain why benign prostatic hypertrophy is more common in men age 50 and over.
6. What age group is afflicted by testicular cancer, and how can the patient take action to detect it?
7. Describe two reasons why the physician orders a semen analysis.
8. List several sexually transmitted diseases that a male can contract.
9. How is a rectal examination on a patient useful to the physician in determining a diagnosis for a patient who has nocturia?
10. How is benign hypertrophy of prostate treated?

WEB ACTIVITIES

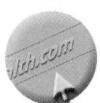

Search for information on the Internet regarding benign prostatic hypertrophy. Describe two surgical procedures that can be done for this condition.

REFERENCES/BIBLIOGRAPHY

Damjanov, I. (1996). *Pathology for the health related profession* (1st ed.). Philadelphia: W. B. Saunders Company.

Ehrlich, A. (1997). *Medical terminology for health professionals* (3rd ed.). Albany, NY: Delmar.

Frazier, M. S., Drzymkowski, J. A., & Doty, S. J. (1996). *Essentials of human diseases and conditions* (1st ed.). Philadelphia: W. B. Saunders Company.

Kinn, M. E., & Woods, M. A. (1999). *The medical assistant: Administrative and clinical* (8th ed.). Philadelphia: W. B. Saunders Company.

Neighbors, M., & Tannehill-Jones, R. (2000). *Human diseases*. Albany, NY: Delmar.

Taber's cyclopedic medical dictionary (18th ed.). (1999). Philadelphia: F. A. Davis Company.

Tamparo, C., & Lewis, M. (2000). *Diseases of the human body* (3rd ed.). Philadelphia: F. A. Davis Company.

GERONTOLOGY

KEY TERMS

Arteriosclerosis
Cognitive Functioning
Cystitis
Dementia
Empathy
Geriatrics
Gerontology
Hyperthermia
Hypothermia
Incontinence
Macular Degeneration
Pernicious Anemia
Presbycusis
Residual Urine
Senile
Transient Ischemic Attack

OUTLINE

OBJECTIVES

The student should strive to meet the following performance objectives and demonstrate an understanding of the facts and principles presented in this chapter through written and oral communication.

1. Define the key terms.
2. Identify expected physiological changes that occur as part of the aging process.
3. List five common functional changes that can occur.
4. Describe prevention techniques for complications arising from age-related disorders.
5. Explain two myths about aging.
6. Explain the importance of communication with the elderly.

Fundamental Principles

- Apply principles of aseptic technique and infection control
- Screen and follow up patient test results

Patient Care

- Obtain patient history and vital signs
- Prepare and maintain examination and treatment areas
- Assist with examinations, procedures, and treatments
- Coordinate patient care information with other health care providers

Diagnostic Orders

- Collect and process specimens
- Perform diagnostic tests

GENERAL (TRANSDISCIPLINARY)

Legal Concepts

- Maintain confidentiality
- Practice within the scope of education, training, and personal capabilities
- Document accurately
- Follow federal, state, and local legal guidelines
- Comply with established risk management and safety procedures

SCENARIO

Mrs. Johnson is an 82-year-old patient of Dr. King, and she is scheduled for an appointment in the cardiac clinic. She is being evaluated for congestive heart disease and has had hypertension for many years. It was difficult to control, but now it responds to medication. She has become a volunteer at the gift shop at St. Louis Hospital. She is an example of an elderly person with chronic illnesses who has changed some long-time behaviors that were harmful to her health.

INTRODUCTION

Gerontology is the scientific study of the problems associated with aging. Geriatrics is the branch of medicine that specializes in all aspects of aging: physiological, pathological, psychological, economic, and sociological. The importance of studying gerontology is becoming more recognized because the expected lifespan is increasing. Thousands of people are living to be 100 years old or older. The aging population is growing rapidly and according to the U.S. Census Bureau, by the year 2030, there will be 60 million people older than age 65. The 80 and above age group is currently the fastest growing group. As a medical assistant, you will be experiencing the impact on the health care system of this growing population of people.

Through knowledge of the physical and psychological changes that occur as an individual ages, as a medical assistant you will be better able to recognize the special needs of this group of people. You will draw upon and use effective communication skills and provide quality health care to the geriatric patients.

SOCIETAL BIAS

In our culture, there is a deeply ingrained bias about aging. Elderly people are systematically stereotyped, and there is much discrimination because of age. Myths and stereotypes are common and the medical assistant can be an advocate for the elderly and can be sensitive to these myths and stereotypes. Accurate information and useful concepts about aging must be communicated to the general public. Elderly oftentimes are viewed as sick, frail, powerless, sexless, and burdensome. As a society, we are obsessed with the negative aspects of aging rather than the positive. The most popular myth is, "to be old is to be sick." Recent studies indicate that older Americans are generally healthier than their counterparts of nearly a decade ago. Even in advanced old age, a majority of the older population has little functional disability. Years of research have debunked this myth. Because of better education about the practice of healthier lifestyles, to be old in America does not mean to be sick and frail. Thousands of people are living to be over 100 years old because of the recognition that healthy lifestyles are the most important factor in helping people to live long, healthy, productive lives. Such factors as good nutrition, regular exercise, stress reduction, yearly physical examinations, not smoking, and today's technology help suppress the aging process.

FACTS ABOUT AGING

- Aging is progressive and universal.

- There are no diseases specific to aging.

- As people age, not all functional changes are related to disease. Interest, personal, and financial resources, family structure, genetics, and attitude all play a part. The individual's lifestyle is also a factor. For example, smoking, misuse of chemicals such as alcohol or drugs, type of diet, and exercise all play a part in how people age.

- There is a wider range of what is considered "normal" function among older people than among younger people. There is a greater variability among older people in their physical abilities, sizes, and characteristics than among younger groups (Figure 29-1).

- All old age is not alike. People in their 60s, 70s, 80s, and 90s are all different.

PHYSIOLOGICAL CHANGES

Although aging is a normal process, not all individuals age in the same way or at the same rate, because no two people have exactly the same genetic inheritance, personal lifestyle, or experiences in life. All of these factors strongly influence the ways in which we grow older. Some believe that the body endures wear and tear and stress during life and that because of this, eventually the body loses its ability to function as well as it had. Others believe that as people grow older, the body produces smaller and smaller amounts of various hormones and other chemicals that keep the body functioning. The fewer of these kinds of substances that are produced, the more susceptible an individual becomes to disease.

Every body system undergoes changes as we age. The changes are physiological and psychological. As individuals move into their 60s and beyond, they will show physiological changes that are part of the aging process. As people age, their body systems function less effectively, causing them to have difficulty performing their ordinary, everyday tasks of living. Also, as people grow older, they become more susceptible to disorders and diseases. When taking the medical history of an older patient, it is evident that many have one or several chronic illnesses. Heart disease, diabetes, arthritis, hypertension, and vision and auditory impairments are common.

Although it is important to be knowledgeable about the physiological changes that occur as part of aging, it is important to realize that the majority of the elderly are free of serious, chronic health problems.

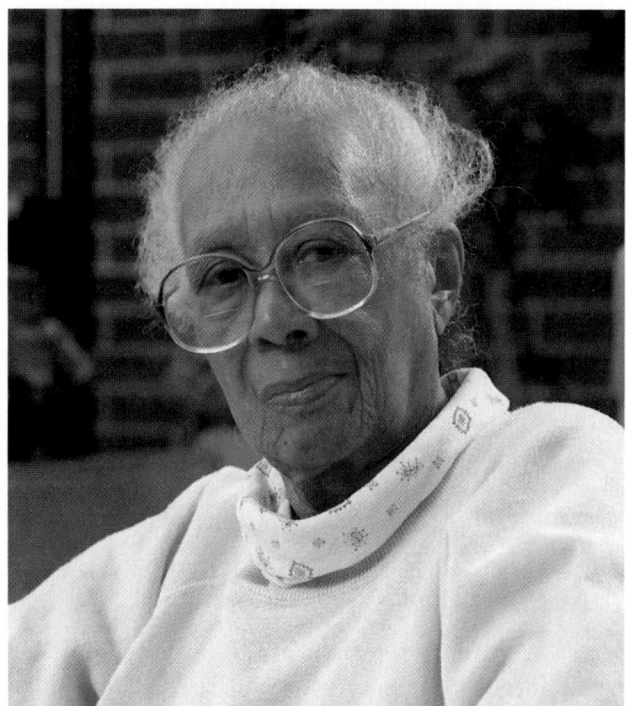

Figure 29-1 Note the many signs of aging.

Senses

Vision. Many changes occur in the eye's ability to function. Pupil size diminishes limiting the amount of light that can go through it to reach the retina. There is a diminished production of tears so the eye is dry, red, and irritated. The lens may become cloudy and the cornea thickens. There is increased sensitivity to glare. Several problems can occur as a result of these changes. There is less ability to see clearly at any distance and to discern various shades of colors. Older people will need eyeglasses to help correct their vision loss, but reading small print can remain very difficult. Glare can be minimized by incorporating a process known as polarization into corrective lenses.

Cataracts, **macular degeneration**, and glaucoma are common findings in the elderly. Cataracts can be surgically excised if they are large. Glaucoma can be treated medically or surgically, but if left untreated can lead to blindness. Macular degeneration can lead to vision impairment. The macular of the retina is an important area in the visualization of fine details. Degeneration of it is the leading cause of visual impairment over age 50, making it difficult to do fine work or such activities as threading a needle. Laser surgery may halt the progression of the degeneration.

Hearing. Loss of hearing in the aging process is not uncommon. It usually occurs over a period of years, and the older person may not be aware of the loss. Loss of hearing ability begins at about the third decade of life. Many times, individuals with hearing loss seem inattentive or confused and are thought to be mentally weak or senile. Presbyacusia or presbycusis is the progressive loss of hearing ability caused by the normal aging process.

Taste and Smell. Taste and smell diminish, making food less appealing because it no longer tastes as good as it once did (Figure 29-2). Taste buds decrease in size. Detecting odors becomes difficult and impaired and further lessens the desire for food. It is not unusual for older people to lose weight and even to become malnourished because of the loss of the ability to taste and smell. Lacking the sense of smell can be dangerous because of the inability to smell smoke or gas and other dangerous fumes.

Integumentary System

Aging individuals' skin becomes more fragile with less subcutaneous and connective tissue. Exposure to sunlight is the major cause of wrinkled skin, "liver spots," and leathery-looking skin.

Sweat glands become smaller and the body becomes nonsensitive to heat and cold. Hyperthermia, an unusually high fever, and hypothermia, an unusually low body temperature, are serious problems, and exposure to excessive hot or cold temperatures should be avoided. See Chapter 33, Rehabiliation and Treatment Modalities.

Hair loses color and becomes thinner. The skin dries and is less elastic. Fingernails and toenails thicken.

Nervous System

The brain shrinks in size as an individual ages because brain cells do not continue to divide throughout life as other cells do. Some loss of memory or delay in memory can be expected in many, but not all, aging people. Mental competence is the rule rather than the exception for older people. Sudden loss of memory accompanied by confusion and inability to do tasks once able to be performed could be an indication of an organic problem, such as transient ischemic attack, a temporary interference of the blood supply to the brain, or a brain lesion.

Problems with balance, temperature regulation, diminished pain sensation, and insomnia can occur as part of the physical changes of aging that affect the nervous system.

Chronic illnesses from which many elderly people suffer many times require several different medications to keep under control. Side effects of medication (over-the-counter and prescription) can cause decreased mental capacity as can malnutrition and substance abuse.

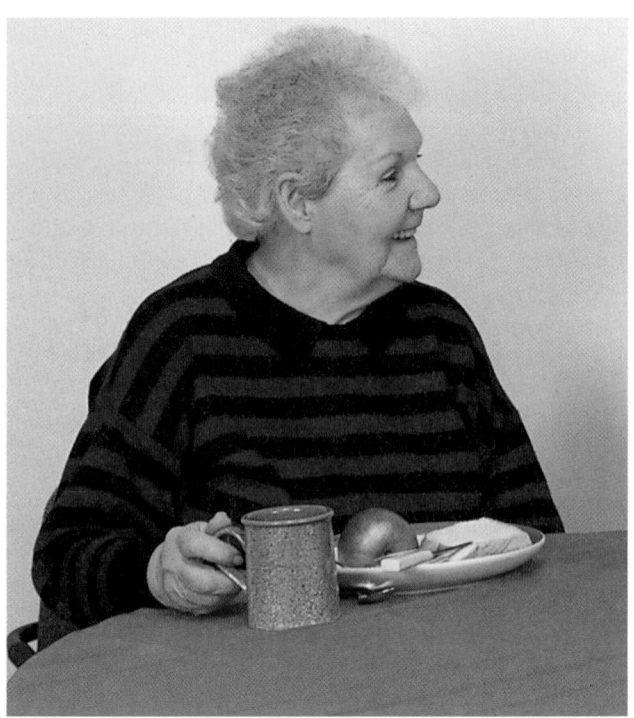

Figure 29-2 The elderly may tend to add more salt and sugar to their food to compensate for their diminished sense of taste.

Musculoskeletal System

The musculoskeletal system changes are evident because elderly people have less muscle strength. This results in loss of mobility and the activities of daily living (ADL) become more difficult. There is less flexibility and joints can stiffen. Loss of height and a stooped appearance can result. Arthritis and osteoporosis are not unusual, and the aging can suffer fractured bones more easily. Poor nutrition, malnourishment, and lack of exercise all contribute to these conditions and prolong healing time as well. See Chapter 33.

Respiratory System

Breathing capacity diminishes, and oxygen and carbon dioxide exchange is lessened. The rib and chest muscles become smaller and less efficient. Lungs lose their elasticity, and the older person may be dyspneic, short of breath (SOB), and more prone to pneumonia.

Cardiovascular System

Heart disease and blood vessel disorders are the major cause of death in the United States. Lifestyle has been implicated as the most significant cause of cardiovascular disease. Blood vessels lose their elasticity, become narrower, build up with plaque, and the arteries harden. This is known as **arteriosclerosis**. The myocardium loses some of its ability to pump effectively. This, together with narrowed and plaque-filled arteries, causes the heart to pump harder. Hypertension, or sustained high blood pressure, is a direct result of these factors. Hypertension can contribute to the accumulation of plaque in artery walls. Congestive heart failure is the inability of the heart to pump effectively to meet the body's demand for blood. Myocardial infarction, or heart attack, is another result of arteriosclerotic heart disease.

Gastrointestinal System

Stomach secretions and mobility slow as part of aging. Peristalsis slows and food moves through the gastrointestinal tract more slowly. **Pernicious anemia** is a disorder that can occur when cells of the stomach lining fail to secrete the intrinsic factor. Associated with the absence of hydrochloric acid, pernicious anemia affects the nervous system and red blood cell formation. Fewer calories are needed in the aging process because metabolism slows. Many overeat if they are lonely, gain weight, and may become obese. Eating is a social as well as physiological event, and if there is no one to eat with, many elderly will not prepare a meal or eat properly to have good nutrition. Loss of vigor and vitality occur. Malnourishment is not uncommon.

Poor eating habits, poor nutrition, overeating, or undereating can also lead to dental problems. Poor dental hygiene leads to gum disease and loss of teeth, many times making the chewing of food difficult and discouraging.

Urinary System

The kidneys decrease in size making urine production and output less. With cardiovascular arteriosclerosis, blood flow to the kidney is less. Filtering waste products from the blood is impaired. Medications are not excreted as quickly as they are in a young, healthy person. Levels of medication may rise to a dangerous level with poor filtration. The bladder walls become more inelastic, and the ability to empty the bladder completely becomes difficult. **Residual urine** remains in the bladder, and microorganisms can cause an infection. **Cystitis** is an inflammation of the bladder. Urinary **incontinence**, the uncontrollable loss of urine, can be the result of many factors, such as relaxed muscles in the female pelvic floor, cystitis, hypertrophy of prostate gland, and diabetes.

Reproductive System

Women experience menopause at about age 55. Estrogen produced by the ovaries ceases, and changes in the female genitalia are noticed. Hot flashes are not uncommon because of blood vessel dilation and contraction. Vaginal secretions diminish, the vagina becomes smaller, and infections are more likely. Estrogen replacement therapy helps to lessen symptoms and helps to protect women from heart disease and osteoporosis.

Men continue to produce sperm well after 50 years of age; however, testosterone levels diminish and may be the reason that many men over 50 suffer from benign hypertrophy of the prostate. Medication may help in some cases; otherwise surgery, a prostatectomy, may be performed.

Aging men and women maintain their sexual desires and many enjoy sexual intercourse more when there are no longer children in the home. There is more privacy and time to relax.

PREVENTION OF COMPLICATIONS

The elderly are at risk for complications as a result of changes in the structure and function of their body systems.

Accidents can happen because of impaired vision and the inability to see well or to hear a warning sound, such as a fire alarm.

Malnutrition and anemia can develop because of poor nutrition or poor absorption of food. This can be caused by lack of interest in food because of lack of sense of taste or smell.

Elderly people may have diminished sensitivity and lack the ability to feel pain as well as a younger person does. Heat and cold applications can injure an aging person if not watched carefully. Also, simple fractured bones may go unnoticed for some time. Loss of balance, disorientation, and confusion may be signs of impaired nervous system function.

Because many elderly suffer from osteoporosis, bones are more easily fractured. Falls are more common because of a loss of vision ability and balance.

Respiratory tract infections are not unusual. Pneumonia is a serious complication in this group of people. Encourage fluid intake and activity to keep the lungs healthy.

Urinary infections are more common. Adequate fluid intake (eight 8-ounce glasses of liquid per day) help keep infections at bay. Incontinence occurs when pelvic floor muscles are relaxed following childbirth.

Circulatory problems because of cardiovascular disease can cause poor circulation to the extremities, especially the legs. Fluid retention with noticeable edema are a common complication along with hypertension and congestive heart failure.

Vaginitis is more common because of vaginal dryness and irritation caused by lack of estrogen. The prostate gland enlarges making urination difficult for males.

PSYCHOLOGICAL CHANGES

There is a great deal of variation in the psychological functioning of the elderly. Among the factors that contribute are the person's health, psychosocial history, race, gender, and environmental aspects, such as education, support system, and social class.

The level of decline in an elderly person's intelligence is affected by social factors. People who maintain their intelligence tend to be in better health, have had more education, are in a high socioeconomic group, and are involved with others and in their community.

Dementia affects memory, personality, and cognitive functioning (awareness, reasoning, judgment, intuition). Alzheimer's is a common form of dementia. Some research has shown that there may be a genetic, as well as environmental, link to the cause of Alzheimer's disease. People who have had a stroke may suffer from dementia, impairing brain functioning.

Depression in the elderly can occur from loss of a spouse, chronic illness, or financial problems.

Personality seems to help determine how individuals adapt to changes that they experience as they grow older.

THE MEDICAL ASSISTANT AND THE GERIATRIC PATIENT

Many elderly suffer from dementia, mental illness, depression, stress, boredom, fear of the unknown, loss of independence, feelings of rejection and worthlessness, low self-esteem, loneliness, dependence, failed expectations, and disappointments. All of these factors coupled with the physiological changes that can occur offer a special challenge to the medical assistant caring for the health and needs of this group of patients. Allow patients time to ventilate and express their concerns, allow for private and confidential discussion, and empathize with their situation by being aware of their feelings, emotions, and behavior. Good communication is essential for quality care of the elderly. Do not talk to the elderly as if they are children. Speak slowly and clearly. Face the individual while talking. Write instructions in addition to verbalizing them.

Memory-Impaired Older Adults

Geriatric care poses challenges when attempting to communicate with impaired older adults. The inability to communicate on a meaningful level can be frustrating and challenging, especially for the older person who is struggling to communicate but can't find the right words. Following are some techniques that can be effective in improving verbal communication with older people experiencing memory impairment.

SPOTLIGHT ON AAMA ESSENTIALS THROUGH CAAHEP

- Being sensitive to a person's aging process also means being sensitive to their individual needs, such as loss of visual acuity, loss of hearing, and in some cases, loss of independence.

- By practicing good communication skills, the medical assistant can help to enhance the older person's self-esteem and self-worth.

- Holding a person's hand or just giving him or her a soft touch often helps to lessen the older patient's fears and thus helps facilitate the overall care and treatment by the physician.

1. Talk to the person in a nondistracting place. It can be very difficult for an older person to concentrate or to sort things out when there are environmental distractions, such as other conversations, equipment noises, or people walking by.
2. Begin conversations with orientating information. Identify yourself, and call the older person by his/her preferred name. Explain the purpose of your visit.
3. Use short words and short, simple sentences with no pronouns.
4. Speak slowly and say individual words clearly.
5. Never "talk down" or be condescending. This is demeaning. Speak in an adult manner as you would a co-worker or friend. Provide the dignity and respect you wish to receive yourself.
6. Lower the tone (pitch) of your voice. A raised pitch is a signal that one is upset. A lower pitch is also easier for people with hearing impairments.
7. Talk to the person in a warm and pleasant manner. Use nonverbal cues, such as facial expression, tone of voice, or touch, to show your feelings of affection and concern. Smiling, taking the older person's hand, or touching the person on the arm can vividly communicate that you are interested and really care.
8. When giving instructions, allow plenty of time for the information to be absorbed.
9. Give clear and simple instructions.
10. Ask the person to do one task at a time.
11. Listen actively. If you do not understand, apologize to the person by saying that you did not understand

exactly what was said. It is extremely important to phrase responses in a way that does not damage the self-esteem of the older person.

12. Avoid asking direct questions that require the person to remember a fact.

13. Focus on well behavior or things that we know the patient can still do.

14. Use humor when appropriate. If expressed naturally, humor brings much needed laughter, a dimension which is often lost in the health care setting.

15. Let the person know when you leave and if you are returning.

16. When discussing a case with another staff member, do so in private to protect patient confidentiality.

Visually Impaired Older Adults

Visually impaired people need to know you are present, but don't approach the individual until you make your presence known. Help by explaining his location, and identify others who may also be present (Figure 29-3).

Making Contact
Introduce yourself. Ask the visually impaired patient if he would like assistance. If he does, offer your arm by saying so and by touching your hand or forearm against his.

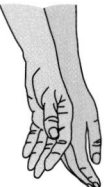

Pace
The pace should be comfortable for both of you. If the patient tightens his grip or pulls on your arm, slow down; your pace may be too fast or he may be anxious. You should alert the patient to obstacles such as curbs, stairs, doors, and thresholds. Be specific, but do not confuse him with too much information.

Grip
The patient grips your arm just above the elbow. The grip must be firm but not so tight that it becomes uncomfortable.

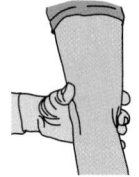

Stance
The patient stands next to you, slightly behind. His arm is bent and held close to his side. Relax your arm and let it hang naturally at your side.

Stairs
When approaching stairs, tell the patient. Let him know whether you are going to go up or down. Be sure you approach the stairs directly, not at an angle. Have the patient stand next to the handrail if there is one.

Pause at the top (or bottom) of the stairs and describe anything unusual about them. The patient will find the handrail and reach forward with his foot to locate the edge of the first step. Start down (or up) the stairs, keeping yourself one step ahead. Keep a steady pace.

When you reach a landing, stop immediately. (Do not take an extra step.) Doing so lets the patient know that there are no more steps, and he can then match his stride with yours.

The same procedure should be used when approaching curbs. Point out any changes in the terrain, even small ones.

Sitting
When guiding someone to a chair, walk up to it and place your hand on the back of the chair. Let the patient trail your arm down to its back. Tell him which way the chair is facing, and he can then seat himself.

If the chair lacks a back or is very large, bring the patient up to the chair so that his legs are against the front of it. He can then reach down to locate the arms and seat of it before he sits.

If the chair is at a table, describe the relationship of the chair, the table, and the patient. Place one of his hands on the chair and the other hand on the table.

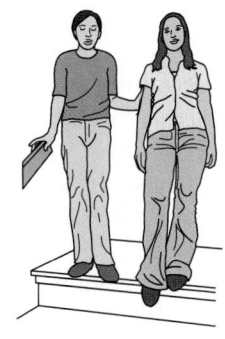
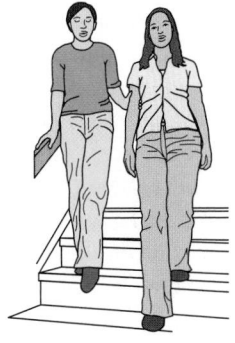
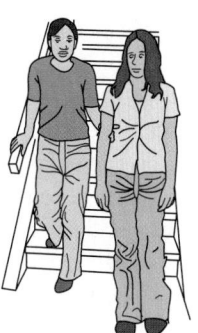

Figure 29-3 Sighted guide techniques.

(continues)

Doors

When approaching a closed door, tell the patient its position when open. For example, "The door opens away and to the left." Or say, "Take the door with your left hand." After you open the door and begin to walk through, the patient will have his hand ready to help hold it open as you walk through together. The patient will move his arm across the front of his body to find the door with the palm of his hand. He should close it behind you if it is not a self-closing door. Use the narrow passage technique in addition to this technique if the doorway is narrow.

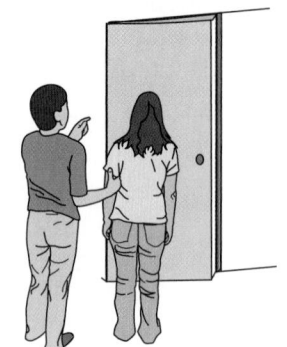

Narrow Passage Technique

When coming to a narrow passage, tell the patient. Move your guiding arm to the center of your back. Slow your pace. He will move behind you and extend his arm, placing you in a single-file position. Once you pass through the narrow passage, bring your arm forward and return to the normal stance.

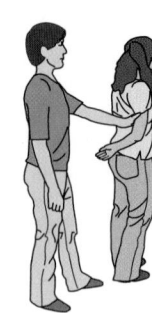

Figure 29-3 *(continued)*

Elder Abuse

What is elder abuse? Massachusetts law defines elder abuse as the committing or omitting of an act that results in serious physical or serious emotional injury to an elderly person. All states have elder abuse laws. Abuse includes physical abuse, emotional abuse, and neglect. The law protects elders abused or neglected by caretakers.

All persons age 60 and over living in the community are protected under the law. Who must report elder abuse? Physicians, medical interns, dentists, nurses, family counselors, police officers, psychologists, homemakers, licensed home health care aids, and many more are required to report abuse. Agencies are also liable. Any person required to report abuse who fails to do so is subject to a fine. Anyone who has reasonable cause to believe an elder has been abused may report and has a moral obligation to protect elders. In most states, the department responsible for elder affairs has established an elder abuse hotline to receive reports of abuse. Reports may also be made to the designated protective service agency in your community. Once reports are received by the elder protective services program, if appropriate, a caseworker will assess the situation to determine the nature and extent of the abuse. If abuse is confirmed, services will be provided to eliminate or alleviate abuse. Many social services are usually available. Mental health, legal, homemaker services, and alternative living arrangements may be provided. See Chapter 7.

Some signs and symptoms of mistreatment or abuse include:

Psychological Signs and Symptoms

- Increasing depression
- Anxiety
- Withdrawn/timid
- Hostile
- Unresponsive
- Confused
- New poverty
- Longing for death
- Vague health complaints
- Anxious to please

Physical Signs and Symptoms

- Lack of personal care
- Lack of supervision
- Bruises
- Welts
- Lack of food
- Beatings
- Neglect
- Unsatisfactory living conditions

There are many other signs and symptoms and not all of those listed by themselves indicate mistreatment, neglect, or abuse. If any seem to increase in number or severity, it may indicate a problem. By observing closely, you may be able to initiate corrective action or reduce or prevent the situation from deteriorating.

Usually the victim is frail (weak), physically and/or emotionally, and dependent upon the abuser for basic survival needs. The victim may be afraid to speak out for fear of retaliation.

Where should one call for information? Contact elder protective services programs in the Yellow Pages of your phone book, or call the Eldercare Locator toll free at (800) 677-1116.

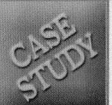

Adelaide Robinson, 83 years old, has an appointment Thursday morning for a recheck of her most recent complaint. She tells you that she is moving slower than she did just six months ago, and she has noticed less flexibility as well.

CASE STUDY REVIEW

1. What are the possible causes of Mrs. Robinson's complaints?
2. What effect will these problems have on Mrs. Robinson's daily routine?
3. What might Dr. King suggest Mrs. Robinson do to help alleviate symptoms?

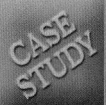

Sally Donovan, age 92, is in the gerontology clinic today. Her main concern, problem, and reason for appointment is that she "cannot taste or smell much anymore and food doesn't taste good." She wants suggestions from the physician about how to improve her taste and smell so she can enjoy food more freely.

CASE STUDY REVIEW

1. What are some reasons for the elderly to lose their sense of taste and smell?
2. Describe any dangers that can be associated with loss of taste and smell.

SUMMARY

Many aging people live well into their 80s, 90s, and even to 100 years of age. They remain physically and mentally stimulated. They learn a foreign language, learn to play a musical instrument, love to read, garden, and volunteer. Elderly are more aware today, than ever before, of the importance of a healthy lifestyle and of its significant contribution to their long and healthy lifespan.

Other elderly, due to genetic inheritance, wear and tear, stress, and loss of chemicals and hormones, seem to age quickly but have little control over these factors.

Many others practice poor health habits, some by choice and others by circumstance. These habits contribute to chronic diseases, disability, and a shorter and unhealthy lifespan.

Above all, dispel myths about the elderly. Be patient, kind, consistent, and thoughtful.

REVIEW QUESTIONS

Multiple Choice

1. The most chronic condition associated with the elderly is:
   a. arteriosclerotic heart disease
   b. cystitis
   c. presbycusis
   d. pernicious anemia
2. An eye disease common to the elderly that is characterized by fluid pressure buildup is:
   a. macular degeneration
   b. presbyopia
   c. cataract
   d. glaucoma

3. Why do joints in the elderly become worn?
   a. cartilage erodes in the joints
   b. osteoporosis makes bones brittle
   c. muscle fibers decrease
   d. vertebrae become thinner
4. Inability to cough deeply and raise mucous makes elders more susceptible to which of the following?
   a. emphysema
   b. asthma
   c. pneumonia
   d. bronchitis
5. Residual urine refers to:
   a. catheterized urine for urinalysis
   b. first-voided specimen
   c. amount of urine left in bladder after voiding
   d. total amount of urine in the bladder when full

Critical Thinking

1. How can an elder's food be made more appealing?
2. What are some strategies that seniors can do to keep mentally and physically stimulated?
3. What are some ways that the elderly can keep bones from becoming brittle?
4. Describe a vision problem that leaves the elderly having difficulty seeing color intensity.
5. What are four causes of urinary incontinence?
6. What is the most common myth about seniors?
7. What are your thoughts about this myth?
8. Give three ways to enhance communication with the elderly.
9. What is the best way to approach a visually impaired person?
10. Older Americans are generally healthier today than older Americans of 10 years ago. What are some of the reasons for this?

WEB ACTIVITIES

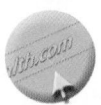

Search for a website that provides information publications about health issues surrounding the elderly.

1. Find the Patient's Bill of Rights. Summarize these rights.
2. Search for information about advanced directives. Find and describe two major types.

REFERENCES/BIBLIOGRAPHY

Cox, H. (2001). *Later life: The realities of aging* (5th ed.). Upper Saddle River, NJ: Prentice Hall.

Hegner, B., Caldwell, E., & Niedham, B. (1998). *Assisting in long-term care* (4th ed.). Albany, NY: Delmar.

Kinn, M. E., & Woods, M. A. (1999). *The medical assistant: Administrative and clinical* (8th ed.). Philadelphia: W. B. Saunders Company.

Markson, E., & Hollis-Sawyer, G. (2000). *Readings in social gerontology*. Los Angeles, CA: Roxbury Publishing Co.

Quadagno, J. (1999). *Aging and the life course*. New York: McGraw-Hill College.

Taber's cyclopedic medical dictionary (18th ed.). (1999). Philadelphia: F. A. Davis Company.

EXAMINATIONS AND PROCEDURES OF BODY SYSTEMS

KEY TERMS

Alimentary Canal
Allergen
Alveoli
Aphasia
Appendicular Skeleton
Aseptic
Auricle
Axial Skeleton
Biopsy
Bronchi
Calculi
Carbuncle
Catheterization
Closed Fracture
Colonoscopy
Comedone
Cystoscopy
Demyelination
Dislocation
Dysuria
Emaciation
Endoscopy
Equilibrium
Erosion
Erythema
External Respiration
Frequency
Furuncle
Gait
Guaiac
Hematemesis
Hematochezia
Hematuria
Hydronephrosis

(continues)

OUTLINE

Urinary System
  Signs and Symptoms of Urinary
    Conditions and Disorders
  Diagnostic Tests
  Urinary Catheterization
Digestive System
  Signs and Symptoms of Digestive
    Conditions and Disorders
  Diagnostic Tests
Sensory System
  The Eye
  The Ear

Respiratory System
  Spirometry
Musculoskeletal System
  Fractures, Casting, and Cast
    Removal
  Cast Care Guidelines
Neurological System
  Components of a Neurological
    Screening
Circulatory System
Blood and Lymph System
Integumentary System
  Allergy Skin Testing

OBJECTIVES

The student should strive to meet the following performance objectives and demonstrate an understanding of the facts and principles presented in this chapter through written and oral communication.

1. Define the key terms as presented in the glossary.
2. Describe how to perform a urinary catheterization.
3. State the proper protocol when collecting urine for a drug screening.
4. Describe patient preparation for occult blood testing.
5. Discuss patient instructions for three diagnostic digestive system tests: The upper GI series, a barium enema, and a cholecystogram.
6. Differentiate between an instillation and an irrigation.
7. Discuss the different types of visual acuity charts and how to use them appropriately.
8. Explain the medical assistant's role when assisting with audiometry.
9. Describe how to perform a nasal irrigation.
10. Describe the proper use of a metered dose nebulizer.

(continues)

Ingestion
Internal Respiration
Lesion
Malabsorption
Malaise
Melena
Nebulizer
Nitrogenous
Nocturia
Obturator
Occluder
Oliguria
Ophthalmoscope
Otoscope
Perforation
Peripheral Nerve
Peritonitis
Polycystic
Polyp
Proteinuria
Pyuria
Spirometry
Stratum Corneum
Uremia
Urgency
Wheal

OBJECTIVES (*continued*)

11. Briefly discuss the role of the medical assistant during spirometry.
12. Explain the medical assistant's role in cast application and cast removal and the guidelines for cast care.
13. List items required by a physician for a neurological exam and explain the medical assistant's role in the exam.
14. Identify patient education information for sputum collections.
15. Explain oxygen administration using a nasal cannula.

ROLE DELINEATION COMPONENTS

CLINICAL

Fundamental Principles

- Apply principles of aseptic technique and infection control
- Comply with quality assurance practices
- Screen and follow up patient test results

Diagnostic Orders

- Collect and process specimens
- Perform diagnostic tests

Patient Care

- Obtain patient history and vital signs

(*continues*)

SCENARIO

At Inner City Health Care, a number of specialty examinations are scheduled for Tuesday the 8th. Administrative medical assistant Jane O'Hara, who is office manager, is careful to schedule patients requiring specialty procedures so that times do not overlap; before she schedules, Jane makes certain examination rooms are available with an extra margin of time between patients. Clinical medical assistants Wanda Slawson and Bruce Goldman take responsibility to ensure that all supplies and equipment are assembled, that both physician and patient are comfortable with the physical environment, and that all safety precautions are followed before, during, and after the examination or procedure.

INTRODUCTION

New techniques and developments occur frequently in medicine and medical assistants must refine existing skills and learn new ones in order to be knowledgeable and proficient and to provide the most current, up-to-date quality care to patients. The medical assistant who works in a specialist's office or an ambulatory care setting that treats a variety of patient problems will need additional skills when providing specialty care to patients. Patients with complaints specific to a particular body system or body part need specialized care.

- Prepare and maintain examination and treatment areas
- Prepare patient for examinations, procedures, and treatments
- Assist with examinations, procedures, and treatments
- Coordinate patient care information with other health care providers

**GENERAL
(TRANSDISCIPLINARY)**

Legal Concepts

- Document accurately

Instruction

- Instruct individuals according to their needs
- Teach methods of health promotion and disease prevention

The medical assistant will assist the physician with a multitude of clinical procedures that are an integral part of each specialty examination.

This chapter covers specialty and body system examinations and the appropriate clinical procedures in urology; endoscopy; and the sensory, respiratory, musculoskeletal, neurological, circulatory, blood and lymph, and integumentary systems.

Each specialty description includes tables that contain information on diseases, disorders, and diagnostic tests and procedures used to confirm diagnoses. Other diseases and disorders and procedures related to each specialty are addressed in the body of the text.

URINARY SYSTEM

The urinary system includes the kidneys, ureters, and bladder. The main function of the kidneys is to form and excrete urine, which contains waste products harmful to body tissues. The kidneys also regulate water balance in the body and help maintain the acid base balance of body fluids.

Collecting and processing urine for laboratory analysis is covered in Chapter 41, Urinalysis. Several other clinical and diagnostic procedures of the urinary system will be covered in this section including urinary catheterization and performing a urine drug screen and a diagnostic X ray known as an intravenous pyelogram (IVP) used to diagnose disorders of the urinary tract.

Diagnostic tests, procedures, disorders, and conditions common to the urinary system are shown in Tables 30-1 and 30-2.

Signs and Symptoms of Urinary Conditions and Disorders

Signs and symptoms of urinary tract diseases include any abnormality in urine or in the ability to urinate. Some common signs and symptoms are: **dysuria**, **proteinuria**, **hematuria**, **pyuria**, **frequency**, **urgency**, **oliguria**, and **nocturia**. Patients may complain of flank or low back pain or experience fever, nausea, vomiting, general **malaise**, and fatigue.

Urinary tract infection (UTI) is the most common disorder of the system as it manifests itself with many of the above signs and symptoms. Urinary tract infection is a broad diagnosis covering any infection of the urinary tract including the urethra, bladder, and kidneys. UTIs may be caused by virus and fungus, but by far the most common infection is due to bacteria.

Bacteria may reach the urinary tract through the blood (hematogenous infection) or by entering the tract through the urethra (ascending infection). Hematogenous infection is less common and is usually the result of septicemia. In this case, the urinary tract is a site of secondary infection. Primary infection may begin in the respiratory or gastrointestinal tract and be carried to the urinary tract throughout the blood.

Diagnostic Tests

The most commonly performed test to diagnose urinary system disorders is a urinalysis. Many different disorders of the urinary system can be identified, making this test extremely valuable. A specimen of urine can be analyzed for many components such as pH, specific gravity, protein, glucose, leukocytes, and blood. The specimen can be further analyzed by examination under the microscope to look for bacteria, white and red blood cells, crystals, and cysts.

Urine culture and sensitivity can be performed and will indicate if a urinary tract infection is present so the appropriate antibiotic can be prescribed by the physician. To obtain a urine specimen for culture, there are two ways to collect the specimen, clean catch or by **catheterization**. See Procedures 30-1 and 30-3 and Chapter 42, Urinalysis.

Blood tests can be done to determine whether waste products are being adequately filtered out of the circulatory system. A test for kidney function confirms the status of glomeruli function.

Two **nitrogenous** waste products normally filtered from the blood are urea and creatinine. A blood urea nitrogen (BUN) test will check for levels of these two

TABLE 30-1 URINARY SYSTEM DISORDERS

Disease/ Disorder	Laboratory Diagnostic Tests			Radiography	Surgery	Medical Tests or Procedures
	Blood	Urine	Other			
Cancer of Urinary Bladder	• Complete blood count	• Urinalysis • Culture and sensitivity of urine		• Intravenous pyelogram • Pelvic ultrasound	• Biopsy of bladder	• Cystoscopy
Cystitis	• Complete blood count	• Nitrate • Urinalysis • Culture and sensitivity of urine		• Intravenous pyelogram		• Cystoscopy
Glomerulo-nephritis	• Blood urea nitrogen • Creatinine • Blood culture • Sedimentation rate • Electrolytes	• Urinalysis • Culture and sensitivity of urine		• Intravenous pyelogram • Ultrasound of kidneys		• Biopsy of kidney(s)
Polycystic Kidneys	• Blood urea nitrogen • Creatinine • Electrolytes	• Urinalysis		• Intravenous pyelogram • Ultrasound of kidneys • Computerized tomography (CT Scan)		
Pyelonephritis	• Blood urea nitrogen • Creatinine • Blood culture • Electrolytes	• Urinalysis		• Intravenous pyelogram • Ultrasound of kidneys		
Renal Calculi	• Complete blood count • Uric acid	• Urinalysis		• X ray of kidney, ureters, and bladder • Ultrasound of kidneys, ureters, and bladder • Intravenous pyelogram	• Lithotripsy	• Cystoscopy
Urinary Tract Infection (UTI)	• Complete blood count	• Urinalysis • Culture and sensitivity of urine				• Cystoscopy

TABLE 30-2 DESCRIPTION OF URINARY DISORDERS AND CONDITIONS

- Cancer of Urinary Bladder. Linked to cigarette smoking, industrial chemicals. Microscopic hematuria one of the first symptoms.
- Cystitis. Inflammation of the urinary bladder. More common in females due to the short length of the urethra. *E-Coli* may travel from the rectum to the bladder. Infectious organisms can invade the bladder during sexual intercourse. Frequency, burning, urgency are common symptoms.
- Glomerulonephritis. Seen in children and young adults post streptococcal infection; strep throat, scarlet fever. Causes degenerative inflammation of glomeruli. Chills, fever, weakness are common symptoms. Edema and albumin in urine are common.
- Polycystic Kidneys. A congenital anomaly. Kidneys contain multiple cysts and greatly dilated tubules do not open into renal pelvis. Hypertension, kidney failure, and death can result.
- Pyelonephritis. Caused by pyogenic bacteria such as *E. coli,* streptococci, or staphylococci. May originate in the bladder and ascend to the kidneys. Pyuria, chills, fever, sudden back pain are symptoms. Dysuria is common.
- Renal Calculi. May be present with or without symptoms. Cause intense pain when they lodge in the ureter(s). Formed by certain salts (perhaps calcium).

wastes. High levels of waste products can result in **uremia**, a toxic condition of the blood that, if not reversed, leads to death. (See Chapter 42, Urinalysis.)

An intravenous pyelogram (IVP), a kidneys-ureters-bladder (KUB), and cystogram are radiologic examinations of the urinary tract.

Intravenous Pyelogram (IVP).
An intravenous pyelogram (IVP) is used to examine the urinary tract (kidneys, ureters, and bladder) for blockage, narrowing, growths, and calculi. This urinary tract diagnostic X ray is also used to diagnose disorders such as lesions, **hydronephrosis**, and **polycystic** kidneys.

Patient Preparation for IVP. In studies of the urinary system, the IVP requires that the patient prepare with laxatives, enemas, and fasting (Table 30-3). The IVP consists of an intravenous injection of an iodine-based contrast medium that is used to define the structures of the urinary system. A retrograde pyelogram is a study of the urinary tract done by inserting a sterile catheter into the urinary meatus. Radiopaque contrast medium then flows upward into the kidneys. This diagnostic test is usually done in conjunction with cystoscopy. Patients should have iodine-sensitivity tests prior to the examination to determine the possibility of an allergic reaction. A voiding cystogram may be ordered in conjunction with an IVP. In this case, the contrast medium is injected into the bladder by catheter and no special patient preparation is needed. See Chapter 32, Radiology and Diagnostic Imaging.

Cystoscopy.
Cystoscopy is a procedure that uses a lighted scope (cytoscope) to view the urethra and bladder. Inflammation, **calculi**, and **polyps** can be seen using a cystoscope. A biopsy of the bladder can be done while performing a cystoscopy. See Figure 30-1.

Biopsy of the Kidney.
Biopsies of the kidney will help confirm a diagnosis. Using radiology, a fine-gauge

needle is inserted through the flank to remove a piece of kidney tissue for analysis and possible malignancy.

Urinary Drug Screening (Urine Toxicology Screening).
There may be circumstances when it is necessary to check a patient's urine specimen for traces of drugs. At times, employees and athletes are required to have their urine tested to qualify for employment or sports activities.

It is legally necessary to have a signed consent form from patients for all drug screening tests performed. It may also be necessary to identify the patient or donor before a test is performed by requesting a photo ID which can be copied and filed with the consent form.

Depending on the drug collection kit used, the urine sample volume can vary from 1 mL to 40 mL. Some kits may also supply a bluing agent that the medical assistant will need to place in the toilet and toilet tank prior to the urine collection. The collector should wait immediately outside the collection area to receive the sample directly from the donor. (See Procedure 30-1.)

TABLE 30-3	INTRAVENOUS PYELOGRAM	
Purpose	**Patient Education**	**Precautions**
To examine the urinary tract: kidneys, ureters, bladder, for blockage, narrowing, growths, calculi.	1. Light evening meal night before 2. Cathartic (laxative) 3. NPO after 9:00 P.M. 4. Cleansing enema(s) in A.M.	Contrast medium of iodine used for visualization (check with patient regarding seafood or iodine allergies) *Warn patients of possible warm flushed sensation when dye is injected and that they may experience a metallic taste.

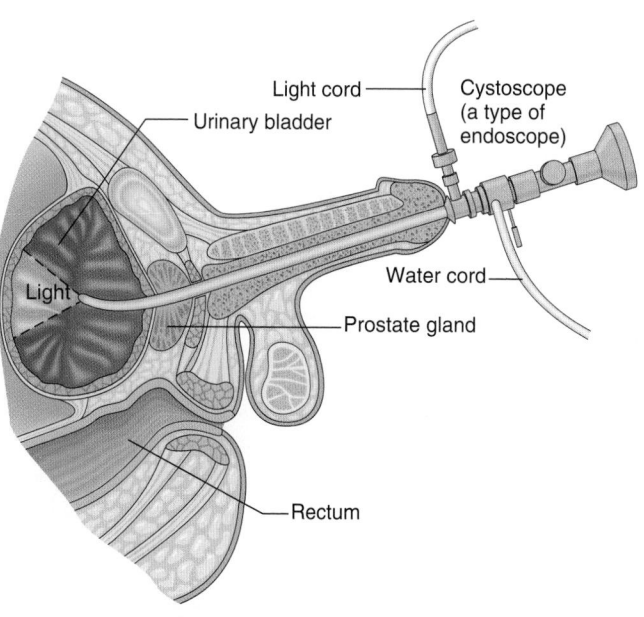

Figure 30-1 Cystoscopy.

Urinary Catheterization

The medical assistant may either perform or assist with the urinary bladder catheterization, which is the introduction of a sterile catheter (tube) through the urethra into the bladder for withdrawal of urine. See Figure 30-2 for male and female anatomy for catheterization. There are basically three reasons for catheterizing patients:

1. To obtain a sterile urine specimen for analysis
2. For relief of urinary retention
3. To instill medication into the bladder, after the bladder is emptied

In some cases, this procedure is done by a urologist; however, some physicians in obstetrics-gynecology and general and family practice may perform or have the medical assistant perform the catheterization. Catheterizing male patients is generally performed by physicians themselves. The physician may order a culture and sensitivity of the urine obtained from catheterization if the patient is experiencing dysuria, frequency, and urgency. This is done to determine if microorganisms are present and if so, what the causative microorganism is, in order to prescribe the appropriate antibiotics.

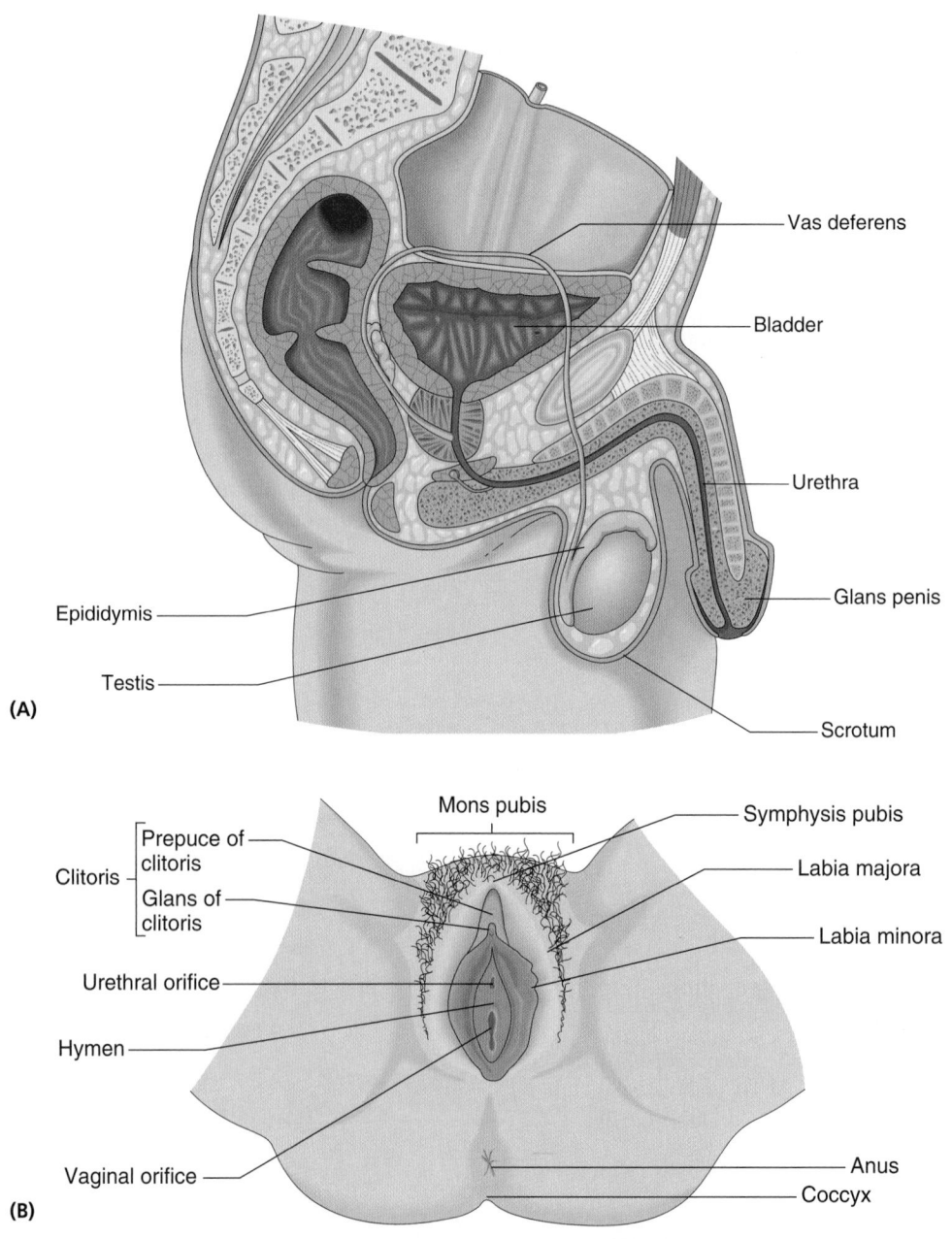

Figure 30-2   (A) Cross-sectional view of male anatomy showing urethra and bladder for catheterization. (B) External genitalia of the female.

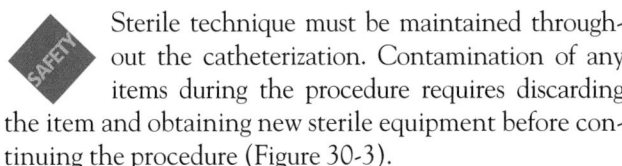

SPOTLIGHT ON AAMA ESSENTIALS THROUGH CAAHEP

● Maintaining a smile and offering a kind word can allay a patient's fears and do a lot to win a permanent customer and patient.

● Whenever the medical assistant is required to perform an examination or procedure, she or he should be friendly, outgoing, and explain the procedure to the patient.

● Concern for patients generally results in happier patients who return in the future for care.

Sterile technique must be maintained throughout the catheterization. Contamination of any items during the procedure requires discarding the item and obtaining new sterile equipment before continuing the procedure (Figure 30-3).

See Procedure 30-2 to perform a urinary catheterization on a female patient and Procedure 30-3 for male catheterization.

Catheterization Equipment. French catheters are used in performing catheterizations in which the catheter is removed following the procedure. The Foley catheter is used when the catheter will remain in the urinary bladder

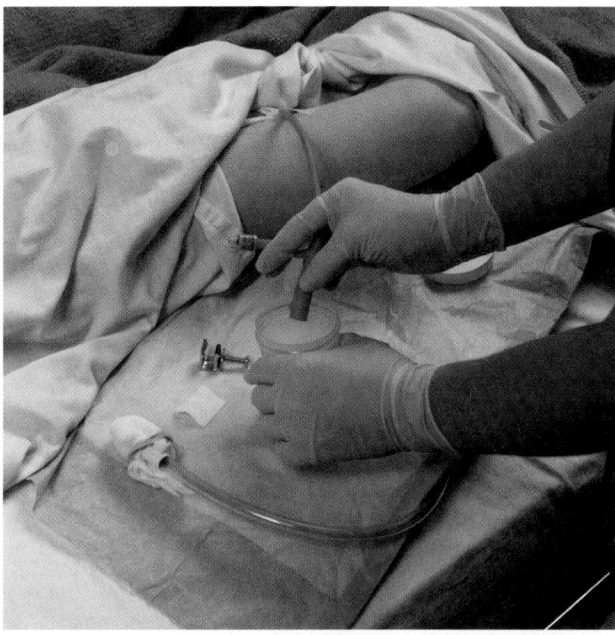

Figure 30-3 Urinary catheterization can be performed using a straight catheter, which is removed immediately after a urine specimen has been obtained, or it can be performed using a Foley catheter (an indwelling catheter). The indwelling catheter remains in the patient's bladder by means of a small inflated balloon at the bladder end of the catheter. A urine specimen can be obtained by disconnecting the tubing, being careful to make certain that asepsis is maintained.

(indwelling catheter). Sterile, disposable catheterization kits are available that contain all necessary items to perform the procedure. See Figure 30-4 for types of urinary catheterizations.

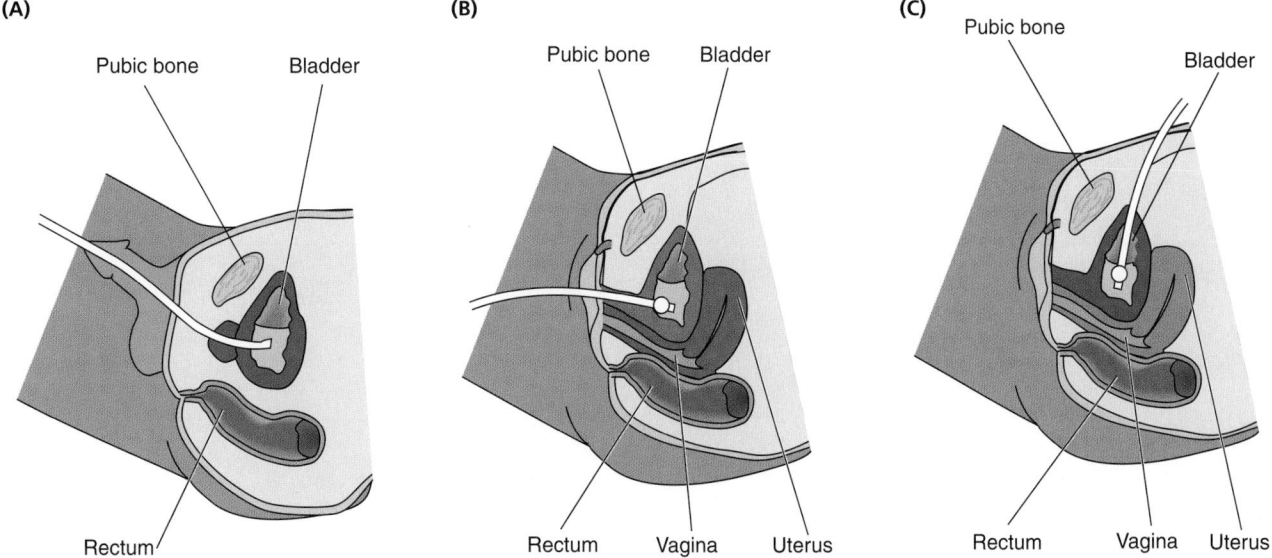

Figure 30-4 Types of urinary catheterizations: (A) In and out catheter. (B) Indwelling catheter. (C) Suprapubic catheter.

DIGESTIVE SYSTEM

The gastrointestinal system performs five functions which include:

1. **Ingestion** of food and breaking it into smaller particles
2. Passage of food through the digestive system (peristalsis)
3. Digestion through secretions of digestive enzymes
4. Absorption of nutrients into the bloodstream
5. Defecation of the solid waste products of digestion

When any of these functions is hindered, the digestive system malfunctions.

The digestive process begins in the mouth and concludes at the anus. As food passes through the **alimentary canal**, or digestive tract, it is mixed with gastric juices and enzymes allowing it to break down into smaller nutrients which allows absorption through the walls of the small intestine. Contents that have not been absorbed travel through the large intestine and are excreted through the anus. See Tables 30-4 and 30-5 for the common tests, procedures, disorders, and conditions of the digestive system. Figure 30-5 shows the major organs of the digestive system.

TABLE 30-4   DIGESTIVE SYSTEM DISORDERS

Disease/ Disorder	Laboratory Diagnostic Tests			Radiography	Surgery	Medical Tests or Procedures
	Blood	Urine	Other			
Anorexia Nervosa	• Complete blood count • Electrolytes • Blood glucose	• Urinalysis				• Electrocardiography
Appendicitis	• Complete blood count	• Urinalysis • Pregnancy test		• Abdominal ultrasound		• Rectal exam
Bulimia	• Complete blood count • Electrolytes	• Urinalysis				• Electrocardiography
Cholecystitis	• Complete blood count • Serum bilirubin	• Urinalysis		• Cholecystogram • Ultrasound of gall bladder		
Cholelithiasis	• Complete blood count • Serum bilirubin			• Cholecystogram • Ultrasound of gall bladder • I.V. cholangiogram		
Colon Cancer	• Complete blood count • Electrolytes			• Barium enema • Abdominal ultrasound	• Biopsy of colon	• Sigmoidoscopy • Colonoscopy
Crohn's Disease	• Complete blood count • Electrolytes			• Abdominal ultrasound • Barium enema	• Biopsy of colon	• Sigmoidoscopy • Colonoscopy • Stool culture
Diverticulitis	• Complete blood count • Erythrocyte sedimentation rate			• Barium enema		• Sigmoidoscopy • Colonoscopy
Duodenal Ulcer	• Complete blood count		• H. pylori	• Upper gastrointestinal series	• Biopsy duodenum	• Gastroscopy • Stool for occult blood
Gastric Ulcer	• Complete blood count		• H. pylori • Culture stomach secretions	• Upper gastrointestinal series	• Biopsy stomach lining	• Gastroscopy
Gastroenteritis	• Complete blood count • Electrolytes		• Stool culture	• Upper gastrointestinal series		• Gastroscopy • Colonoscopy

(continues)

TABLE 30-4 *(continued)*

Disease/ Disorder	Laboratory Diagnostic Tests			Radiography	Surgery	Medical Tests or Procedures
	Blood	Urine	Other			
Gastritis	• Complete blood count			• Upper gastrointestinal series		• Gastroscopy
Hemorrhoids	• Complete blood count				• Hemorrhoid-ectomy	• Physical exam • Proctoscopy
Hepatitis	• Protein • Bilirubin • Liver functions • Alkaline phosphotase • Gamma globulin	• Urinalysis			• Liver biopsy	• Liver scan
Hiatal Hernia				• Upper gastrointestinal series • Chest X ray	• Biopsy	• Esophagoscopy
Pinworms	• Complete blood count		• Stool sample for ova and parasites			• Perianal exam

TABLE 30-5   DESCRIPTION OF DIGESTIVE DISORDERS AND CONDITIONS

- Anorexia Nervosa. A disease of psychological origin. The individual does not eat and becomes emaciated and malnourished because of the need to avoid weight gain.
- Appendicitis. Acute inflammation of the appendix usually caused by infection or obstruction. Characterized by pain, nausea, vomiting, and fever.
- Bulimia. A syndrome in which an individual binges on food and then purges by inducing vomiting. The reason individuals engage in this behavior is to avoid weight gain, and it is of psychological origin.
- Cholecystitis. Inflammation of the gallbladder. Usual cause is gall stones, but other causes may be bacteria or chemical irritants.
- Colon Cancer. Common malignancy characterized by change in bowel habits, diarrhea or constipation and abdominal discomfort as tumor grows.
- Crohn's Disease. Chronic disease which exhibits inflammation of the ileum resulting in diarrhea, right lower quadrant pain and attacks of diarrhea and frequent blood in the stools.
- Diverticulitis. Inflammation of diverticula usually caused by impacted feces or bacteria in the sacs. Pain, cramp-like, usually in left side of abdomen. Obstruction can develop.
- Diverticulosis. Diverticula in colon without symptoms.
- Duodenal Ulcer. Lesion in the mucous membrane of the small intestine usually caused by hyperacidity.
- Gastric Ulcer. Caused by bacteria H. pylori.
- Gastroenteritis. Inflammation of the stomach and intestinal tract. Causes nausea, vomiting, diarrhea. May be caused by ingestion of pathogen.
- Gastritis. Inflammation of the stomach lining usually caused by an undefined irritant including alcohol, bacteria, or viruses. It can result in stomach discomfort, nausea and/or vomiting.
- Hepatitis. Inflammation of the liver caused by infection from a virus resulting in hepatomegaly, anorexia, and jaundice.
    Hepatitis A. Spread by fecal contamination of food or water.
    Hepatitis B. Spread by blood and body fluids contamination or sexual contact, contaminated needles, perinatal fluids, semen.
    Hepatitis C. Spread by blood (i.e., transfusion), contaminated needles, sexual contact.
    Hepatitis D. Intimate and sexual contact with intravenous drug users.
    Refer to Chapter 22 for more information about hepatitis.
- Hiatal Hernia. Congenital or traumatic protrusion of stomach through the diaphragm into the chest cavity (Figure 30-6).
- Pinworms. Intestinal parasites causing intestinal and rectal infection.

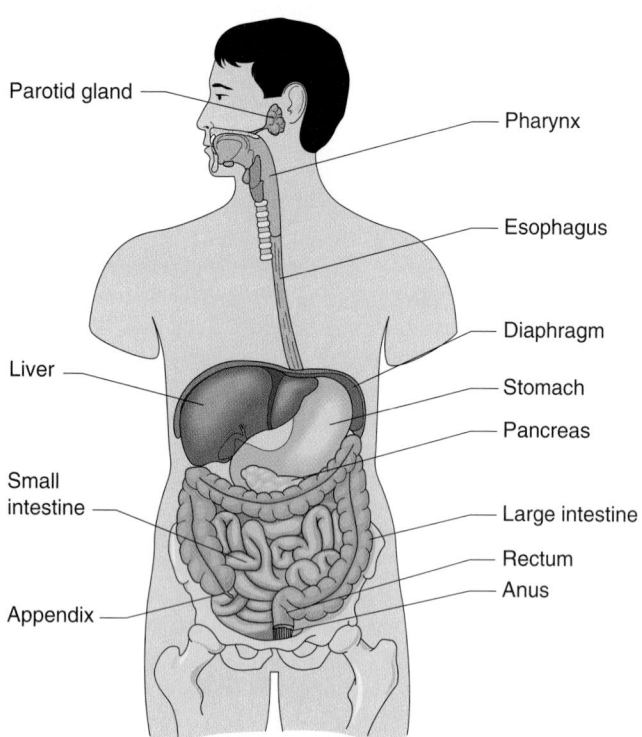

Figure 30-5 The digestive system.

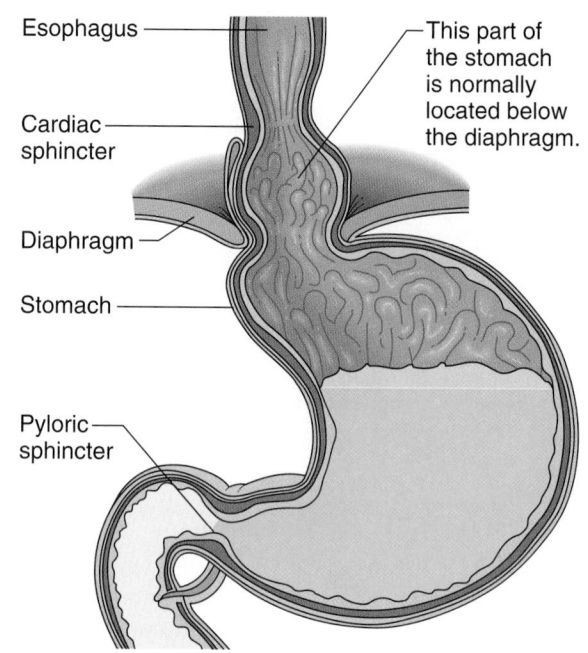

Figure 30-6 Hiatal hernia.

Signs and Symptoms of Digestive Conditions and Disorders

Common signs and symptoms of disorders and diseases of the digestive tract include nausea, vomiting, stomach cramping, diarrhea, heartburn, loss of appetite, weight loss, indigestion, fatigue, **hematemesis**, **melena**, and **hematochezia**.

There are many disorders and diseases of the digestive tract that can cause these signs and symptoms. Gastritis, a common ailment of the stomach, can be caused by caffeine, aspirin and other medication, spicy foods, and alcohol, and is characterized by epigastric pain, nausea, and vomiting of blood (hematemesis). Gastroenteritis, inflammation of the stomach and small intestine, another common ailment, is also known as food poisoning, intestinal flu, or traveler's diarrhea. It can be caused by infections from contaminated food or water, drug reactions, and allergic reactions to particular foods. Peptic ulcers found in the stomach are called gastric ulcers and can be caused by the action of pepsis, an enzyme. It is an **erosion** of the mucous lining of the stomach. Salicylates (such as aspirin), alcohol, smoking, oversecretion of hydrochloric acid, and stress seem to be implicated in this disease. Some gastric ulcers may be caused by the bacteria *H. pylori* and require antibiotic treatment. Ulcers found in the duodenum are called duodenal ulcers and are similar to gastric ulcers. A duodenal ulcer is an erosion of the mucous lining of the duodenum, a part of the small intes-

tine. If determined that the ulcer is caused by the bacteria, antibiotics will be prescribed. Both types of ulcers seem to run a chronic course and if they are not controlled, the ulcerated area can **perforate** and hemorrhage ensues. Contents of the stomach or intestine can spill out into the abdominal cavity and cause a serious complication called **peritonitis** (infectious organisms enter the membrane covering the internal organs). See Figures 30-7 and 30-8.

Diarrhea is characterized by frequent liquid bowel movements. Diarrhea and vomiting may have many causes such as allergic reactions, infections from food or water,

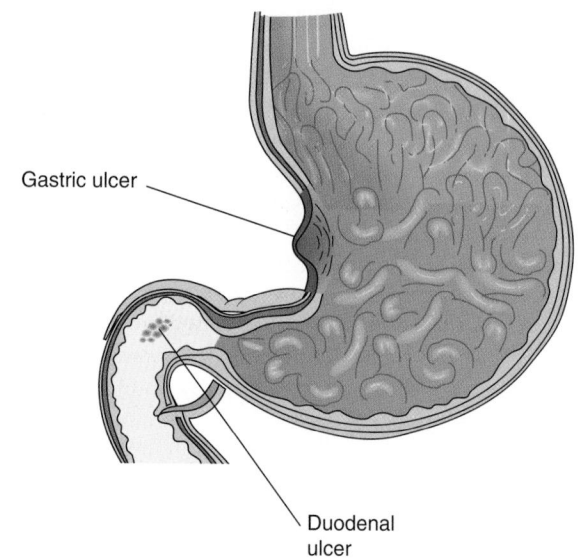

Figure 30-7 Peptic ulcers.

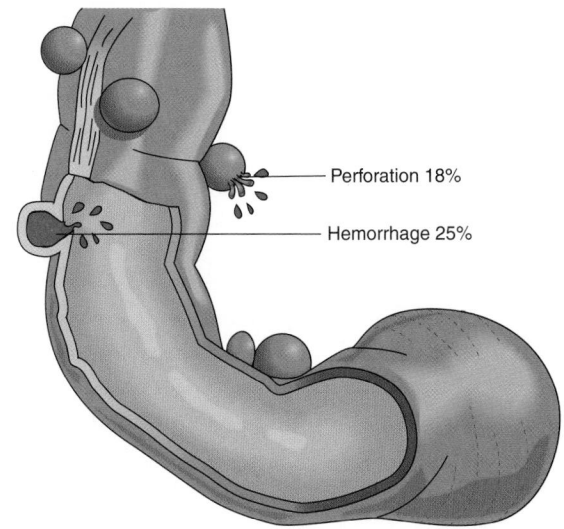

Figure 30-8 Diverticulosis.

— Perforation 18%

— Hemorrhage 25%

or from stress. Dehydration can become a problem if diarrhea continues for several days. Infants, children, and the elderly are especially vulnerable to dehydration from vomiting and diarrhea.

Diagnostic Tests

Diagnostic tests for the digestive system commonly include radiography and **endoscopy**. An upper GI series

(barium swallow) is done to visualize the esophagus, stomach, and upper portion of the small intestine. A lower GI series (barium enema) will visualize the large intestine. See Figures 30-9, 30-10, and Chapter 32, Radiology and Diagnostic Imaging.

Endoscopy allows the physician to look directly into the digestive organs with a lighted scope. Some examples of endoscopies used in the digestive tract are named by the organ being scoped:

stomach: gastroscopy

colon: colonoscopy

sigmoid colon: sigmoidoscopy

entire upper GI area: esophagogastro-duodenoscopy (EGD). (See Figure 30-11.)

Biopsies can be taken during an endoscopic procedure.

Sigmoidoscopy. Sigmoidoscopy is a diagnostic examination of the interior of the sigmoid colon. It is a useful aid in the diagnosis of cancer of the colon, ulcerations, polyps, tumors, bleeding, and other lower intestinal disorders. The sigmoidoscope is a metal or plastic (disposable) instrument with a light source and a magnifying lens, which permits the mucous membrane of the sigmoid colon to be seen.

The metal and plastic types of scopes may still be used in some offices (Figure 30-12), but the instrument

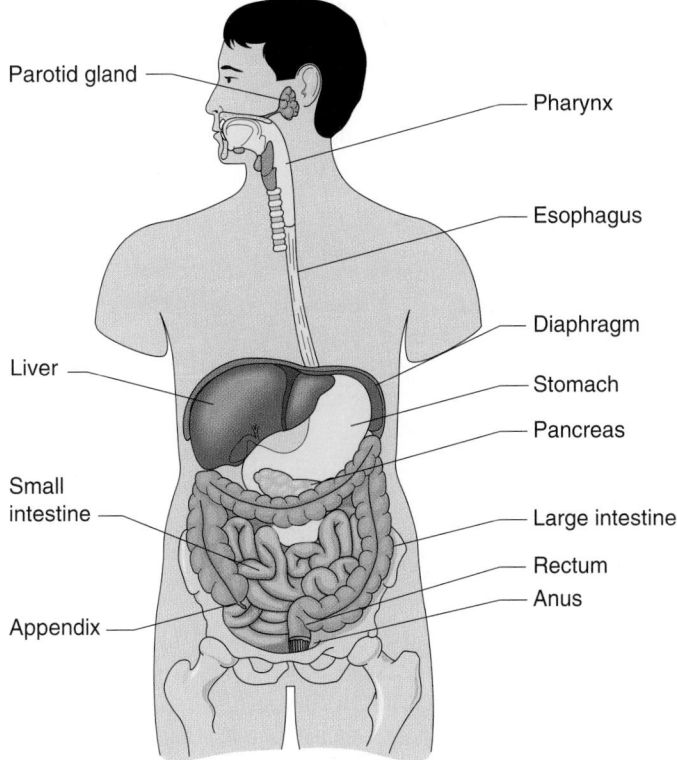

Figure 30-9 Lower GI; highlighted area is visualized.

Parotid gland
Pharynx
Esophagus
Diaphragm
Liver
Stomach
Pancreas
Small intestine
Large intestine
Rectum
Anus
Appendix

Figure 30-10 Upper GI; highlighted area is visualized.

Parotid gland
Pharynx
Esophagus
Diaphragm
Liver
Stomach
Pancreas
Small intestine
Large intestine
Rectum
Anus
Appendix

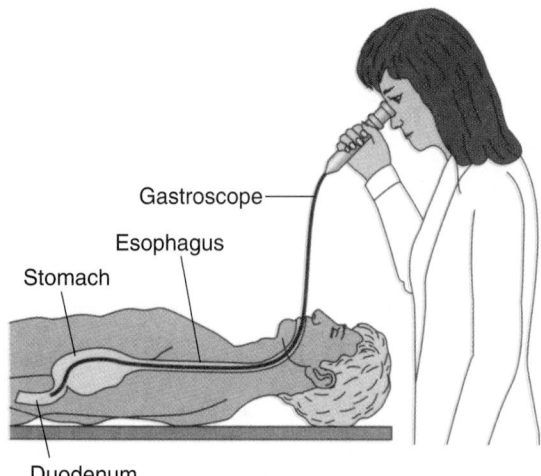

Figure 30-11 Esophagogastro-duodenoscopy procedure (EGD).

most commonly used by physicians is the flexible sigmoidoscope, which is shown assembled with items necessary for the procedure. Since it is flexible, it can be inserted much farther into the colon. This instrument makes it possible to view more of the mucous membranes of the intestines (Figure 30-13).

An **obturator** is inserted into the sigmoidoscope. The tip of the obturator and scope are lubricated and carefully inserted into the rectum. Then the obturator is removed so that the sigmoid colon can be seen. Patients find this an unpleasant procedure.

As with any examination of the abdominal cavity, you should advise the patient to empty the bladder and evacuate the bowel before the procedure begins. This will make the exam easier for both patient and examiner. During the procedure the patient should be instructed to

breathe through the mouth deeply and slowly to relax abdominal muscles. Patients may feel the urge to defecate during a colon examination because of the stretching of the intestinal wall from the instrument passing through and air being introduced with it. If patients use the breathing technique mentioned, this discomfort can be relieved. The procedure should last only a few minutes, especially if patients have followed preparation instructions.

Air is sometimes introduced into the colon (by the examiner's use of the inflation bulb attached to the scope with tubing) to distend the wall of the colon for easier placement of the lumen of the endoscope. Patients find this to be uncomfortable and sometimes painful. The physician may need to use suction to remove mucus, blood, or fecal material that is obstructing the view of the colon.

Assistance in handing necessary items to the physician and giving support to the patient are the medical assistant's roles during these exams.

It will also most often be the medical assistant who tells the patient how to prepare for the sigmoidoscopy and explains how the test is performed. For successful examination, proper preparation is essential. In addition to having patients restrict dairy products, raw fruits and

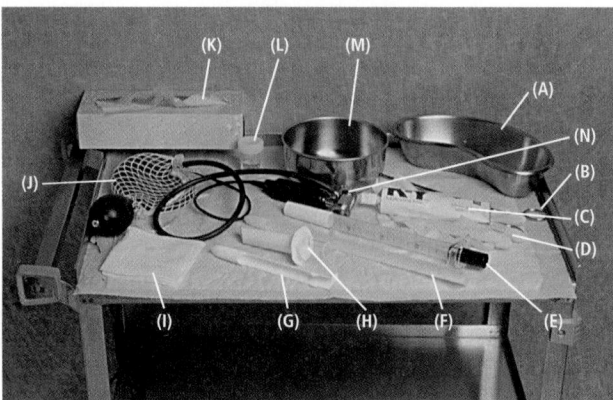

Figure 30-12 Setup for a proctosigmoidoscopy with a rigid sigmoidoscope and anoscope. (A) Kidney basin. (B) Sponge forceps. (C) Lubricant. (D) Gloves (latex). (E) Disposable sigmoidoscope. (F) Obturator for sigmoidoscope. (G) Obturator for anoscope. (H) Anoscope. (I) Gauze sponges. (J) Insufflator. (K) Tissues. (L) Biopsy container. (M) Basin of water. (N) Magnifying lens.

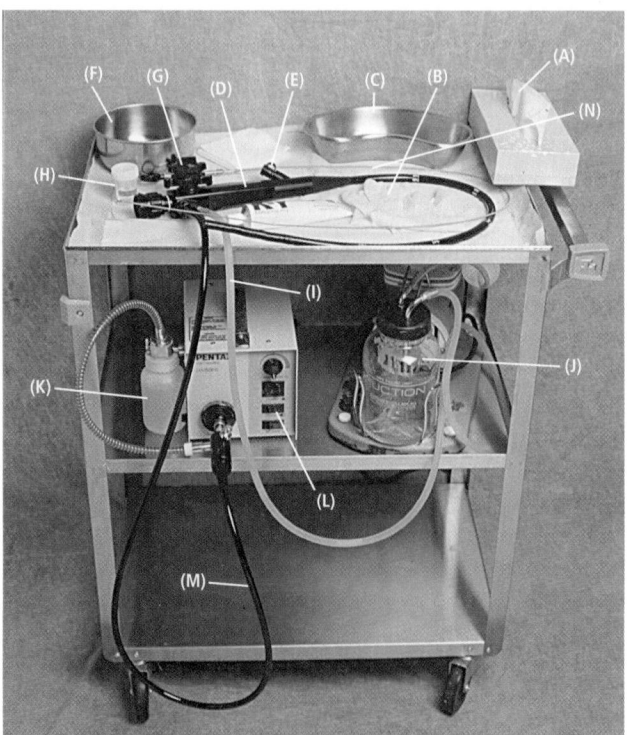

Figure 30-13 Setup for a proctosigmoidoscopy with a flexible sigmoidoscope. (A) Tissues. (B) Latex gloves. (C) Kidney basin. (D) Flexible sigmoidoscope insertion tube. (E) Eye lens. (F) Basin for water. (G) Control head. (H) Biology container with formalin. (I) Suction tubing. (J) Suction apparatus. (K) Water bottle. (L) Sigmoidoscope control panel. (M) Power cord.

vegetables, and grains and cereals from their diet, they should be encouraged to drink plenty of clear liquids and eat lightly the day before the scheduled appointment for the sigmoid colon exam. A plain commercial enema should be self-administered at home approximately 2 hours before the exam. Physicians may vary the instructions according to the patient's condition. If patients are not completely informed about preparations and the exam is attempted with unsatisfactory results, it will have to be repeated, which is both costly and inconvenient. Satisfactory results are obtained by giving patients both oral and written instructions.

There are occasions, during an appointment for which the patient was "worked in" to the schedules, when the physician feels that the patient's condition warrants the examination of the sigmoid colon. In this case, the physician will order an enema to be given to the patient in the office.

It is not a common procedure to administer an enema to a patient in the medical office or clinic, but is sometimes a necessity in the successful completion of a sigmoidoscopy or other rectal examination. Even though a patient may have received proper instructions and carried them out before the scheduled appointment, there is no guarantee that the patient achieved success. In the event that the patient comes in for the appointment and the colon is not sufficiently evacuated of feces for a sigmoidoscopy, the physician may order a cleansing enema so that the exam can be completed. It is generally best to proceed with the planned procedure, even with the delay of the enema. Usually this works out well for patient and staff, because rescheduling presents difficulties for everyone.

Often the patient did follow the list of instructions, but was not able to retain the enema solution long enough to get satisfactory results. You will more likely be able to encourage the patient to retain the contents of the enema longer. You may want to explain that the longer the contents are retained, the more successful the results will be. Otherwise, it may have to be repeated, or the exam rescheduled. Be certain that you use an examination room that is close to the rest room for the patient's convenience when you administer an enema. Your patience and understanding are needed, because many patients are embarrassed to have an enema administered to them. The procedure that follows will provide the information you need to carry out this procedure.

Some exams, such as diagnostic sigmoidoscopy and X rays, require the use of laxatives by the patient the day before or the morning of the exam. This may present a problem in the patient's personal or employment schedule if instructions are not made clear before the appointment is scheduled. Most patients are fearful of what the diagnostic examination will disclose. Helping them

Patient Teaching Tip

When patients come in for rectal or sigmoidoscopy examinations, here are a few informative topics that you may discuss with them with the physician's direction.

1. Remind them that laxatives and enemas should only be used by direction of the physician.
2. Constipation may be avoided/relieved by including fresh fruits and vegetables, cereals, and grains in the diet, drinking plenty of liquids (water), and getting regular exercise.
3. Instruct them that if they have any of the following symptoms persistently it could mean that a disease or an abnormal condition is present and consulting the physician is strongly advised: heartburn or indigestion, nausea and/or vomiting, constipation or diarrhea, excessive gas or bloating, stool that is tarry (black) or other than a normal brown color.
4. Inform patients who are age 40 and over that they should routinely test their stool for occult blood every 2 years for detection of cancer of the colon, or more often if advised by the physician (if family history indicates). All patients over age 50 should test annually.
5. Advise patients to include high-fiber foods in their diets, avoid fat (especially saturated fats) and cholesterol, and eat red meats very sparingly.
6. Urge patients to eat from a variety of foods (from the food pyramid) and to eat 4 to 6 small meals rather than 1 or 2 large meals daily to promote better utilization of nutrients and more energy.
7. Suggest to patients that it is better to select snacks and beverages wisely such as fruits, vegetables, and juices over coffee/tea/pop and high-calorie sweets or chips.

choose a convenient appointment time and explaining the reasons for the preparations they must undergo is usually appreciated.

Proper positioning of the patient during the sigmoidoscopy is important for both the physician's viewing of the rectum and sigmoid colon and the patient's comfort. Proctology tables are designed especially for this procedure (Figure 30-14). They provide support of the patient's chest and head with the arm resting against the head-

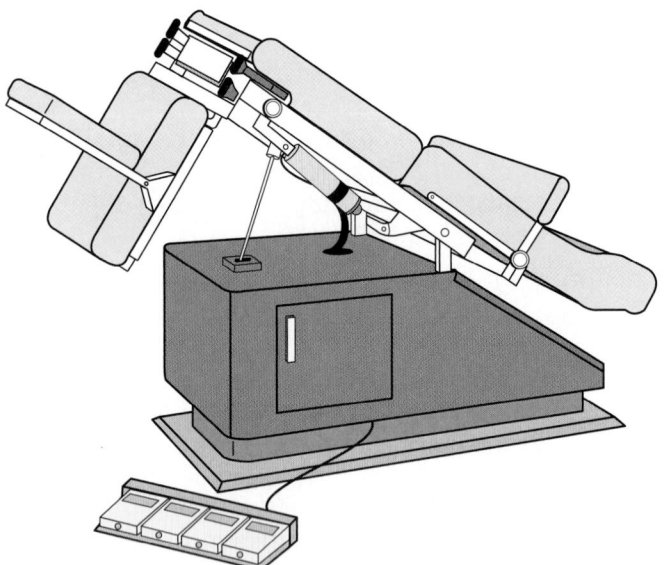

Figure 30-14 Proctologic table.

board as the table is tilted to the knee-chest position. Those who cannot tolerate this position are assisted into Sims' position for the exam. Many physicians find this acceptable and it is more comfortable for the patient. You should ask about the physician's preference in patient position since there are many variations.

The physician may wish to view the intestinal mucosa following a normal bowel movement. More often, the patient is instructed to eat a light diet containing plenty of clear liquids and avoiding dairy products for 24 hours before the exam, and to have a plain cleansing enema the morning of, or 2 hours before, the exam. Still other physicians may wish patients to use laxatives the day before and an enema the night before and also the morning of the exam. Patients have usually eaten little within the past few days because of their abdominal distress.

In the diagnosis of hemorrhoids, fissures, and ulcerations, the physician usually begins investigative procedures by examining the anus and the interior of the rectum with a proctoscope. During the sigmoidoscopy, the physician may want to take a biopsy of questionable tissue from the sigmoid colon to aid in confirming the diagnosis. It is a good rule to have all possible necessary items available. When the patient has been prepared and the physician is ready to begin the exam, the medical assistant hands the necessary instruments and supplies to the physician as needed. Remember to advise patients to report any problems, such as bleeding, discharge, swelling, or any other unusual discomfort following any procedure. A biopsy lab request form must be completed and accompany the tissue to the lab. Containers for biopsy specimens have a formaldehyde solution to preserve the tissue until the analysis is done.

Patient Teaching Tip

Following sigmoidoscopy, patients should drink plenty of clear fluids to help relieve the usual abdominal discomfort and flatulence. Patients may also find relief in lying in a prone position with a pillow across their midabdominal area to aid in the passage of gas.

See Procedure 30-4 to assist with a proctosigmoidoscopy.

While the proctosigmoidoscope examines the rectum and sigmoid colon with either a flexible or rigid (metal) scope, a procedure known as a **colonoscopy** can be scheduled in the outpatient department of the hospital or performed in the office or clinic. A flexible fiberoptic instrument is used and the entire length of the large intestine (colon) can be examined for lesions such as tumors, polyps, fissures, and so on. Biopsies which consist of small tissue pieces can be removed with a snare-type instrument inserted through the colonoscope. The tissue is microscopically examined by a pathologist to determine whether or not a malignancy is present in the colon. The patient receives a muscle relaxant/tranquilizer to facilitate the examination.

Fecal Occult Blood Test

Patients may be instructed to obtain three stool specimens at home to allow examination of a fecal sample for occult (hidden) blood. **Guaiac** slides, applicators, and envelopes will be given to the patient to take home (Figure 30-15). The patient will need to obtain a small stool sample from three separate bowel movements. Three separate samples are used to allow detection of blood from gastrointestinal lesions that exhibit intermittent bleeding. The medical assistant's role is to instruct the patient on how to properly collect the stool specimens on the test slides and care and store the slides until they are returned to the office. (See Procedure 30-5).

For patients who have daily bowel movements, this will not be a problem. For patients who have difficulty with daily elimination, it may take several days to collect the samples. Patients should not use laxatives unless directed by the physician.

Positive tests for occult blood require further testing such as sigmoidoscopy and colonoscopy to identify the source of bleeding. If a lesion is found either in the rectum or colon, a biopsy can be performed and sent to the laboratory for examination of cells for malignancy. (See Procedure 30-5.)

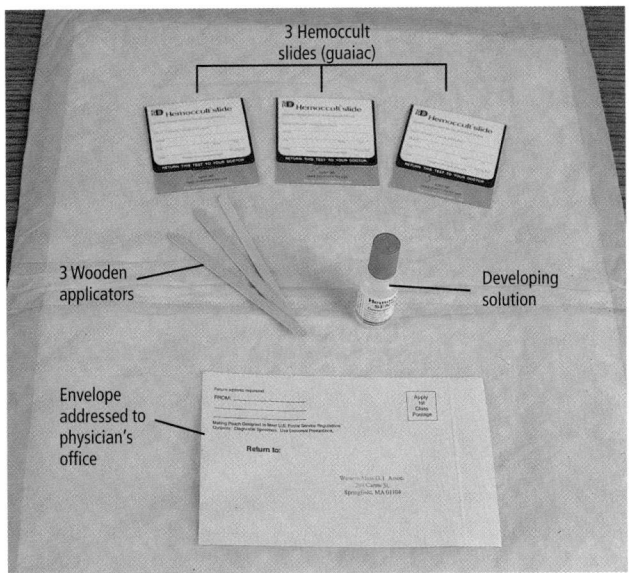

Figure 30-15 Supplies needed for the guaiac hemoccult test for fecal occult blood. The patient will take all supplies home except the developing solution.

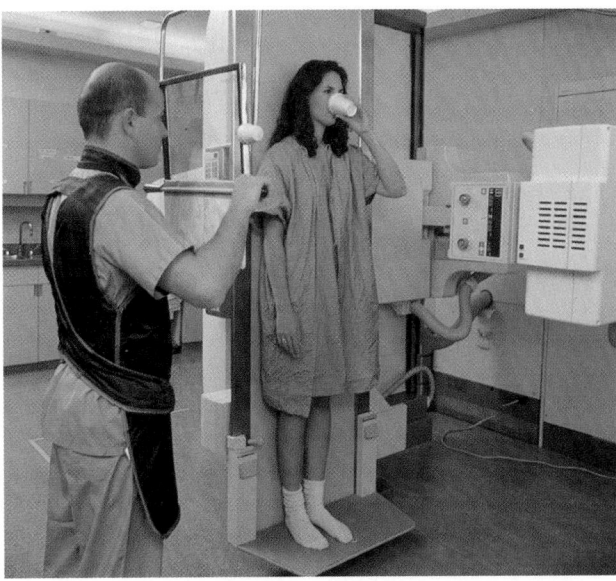

Figure 30-16 In a barium swallow test, barium sulfate is swallowed and X rays are taken of the esophagus, stomach, and small intestine. This is also known as an upper GI series.

Patient Teaching Tip

The following steps should be followed two days before the fecal occult blood test and continued until three slides have been prepared:

1. Avoid red meats, processed meats, and liver. These release hemoglobin which can produce a false positive result.
2. Avoid turnips, broccoli, cauliflower, and melons. These foods may contain a substance, peroxibase, that will cause a false positive result.
3. Avoid aspirin, iron supplements, and large doses of vitamin C for seven days prior to test. These substances may cause gastric bleeding that can mask bleeding from a lesion.
4. Consume a high-fiber diet. Fiber provides roughage to promote bowel movement and encourage bleeding from any lesion that may be present.
5. Do not begin test during menses, for three days after menses, or if bleeding from hemorrhoids.
6. Drink plenty of fluids to help avoid constipation.
7. Store slides at room temperature and protect from heat, sun, and fluorescent lights.

X-Ray Studies of the Digestive System. There are several diagnostic X-ray studies that can be performed to study digestive structures and functions for disease. They include the upper GI series (barium swallow) (Figure 30-16), lower GI series (barium enema), and the cholecystogram. Table 30-6 presents the purpose, patient preparation, and procedures for each of these studies.

SENSORY SYSTEM

The special senses of vision, hearing, equilibrium, smell, and taste permit the body to detect information about the environment. The eyes, ears, nose, and taste buds are all sense organs which contain specialized receptor organs. See Table 30-7 for diseases and disorders and diagnostic tests and procedures for eyes, ears, and nose.

The Eye

The eye is the primary organ for sight and is one of the few organs of the body externally exposed. Its accessory structures—the eyelids, eyelashes, lacrimal ducts, and extrinsic muscles—provide protection for the eye. The anterior portion of the eyeball protrudes outward and the remainder is protected by the orbit.

The intraocular structures consist of some parts of the eye visible externally and parts visible only through an ophthalmoscope. The intraocular structures include the following:

- Sclera: white area covering the outside of the eye except over the pupil and iris

TABLE 30-6   PATIENT PREPARATION AND PROCEDURE FOR X-RAY STUDIES OF THE DIGESTIVE SYSTEM

Test	Purpose	Patient Prep	Procedure	Time
Barium swallow (upper GI series)	To study the esophagus, stomach, duodenum, and small intestine for disease (ulcers, tumors, hiatal hernia, esophageal varices)	Day prior to X ray: 1. Light evening meal 2. NPO after midnight Day of test: 1. NPO Postprocedural: 1. Increase fluid intake 2. Take laxative as prescribed	1. The patient is asked to drink a flavored barium mixture while standing in front of the fluoroscope. 2. The radiologist observes the passage down the digestive tract 3. The patient is turned to various positions to allow good visualization of the intestine 4. X rays are taken	1 hr
Barium enema (lower GI series)	To study the colon for disease (polyps, tumors, lesions)	Clear liquid one day prior (allowed: carbonated beverages, clear gelatin, clear broth, coffee & tea with sugar). No milk or milk products 8 oz of water every hour until bedtime Prep kit: (usually supplied by physician's office) to include bottle of magnesium citrate, Dulcolax tab(s) Day prior to X ray: 1. Late afternoon drink bottle of magnesium citrate 2. Early evening take Dulcolax tab(s) as prescribed 3. Light eve. meal. NPO except water, after dinner Morning of procedure: 1. NPO 2. Cleaning enema Postprocedural instructions: 1. Increase fluid intake and dietary fiber 2. Report to physician if no bowel movement within 24 hours of test	1. The colon is filled with a barium sulfate mixture 2. The patient is turned in various positions to allow the barium to fill the colon. Air is injected to move the barium along the colon 3. When the colon is full, X rays are taken	1–2 hrs
Cholecystogram	To study the gallbladder for disease (stones, duct obstruction), inflammation	1. Evening before test fat-free dinner 2. Patient takes dye tablets with 8 oz water 3. Cathartic or cleansing enemas may be prescribed 4. NPO after dinner and tablets	1. A series of radiographs is taken 2. A fatty meal may be given to stimulate the gallbladder to empty 3. Other radiographs can then be taken to check gallbladder function	1 hr

- Cornea: clear tissue covering the pupil and iris
- Iris: round disk of smooth and radial muscles giving the eye its color.
- Pupil: round opening in the iris that changes size as the iris reacts to light and dark
- Anterior chamber: space between cornea and iris/pupil filled with clear fluid called aqueous humor
- Posterior chamber: space between the iris and lens that is filled with aqueous humor
- Lens: clear fibers enclosed in a membrane that refract and focus light to the retina
- Posterior cavity: the space in the posterior part of the eyeball filled with thick, gelatinous material called vitreous humor
- Posterior sclera: white opaque layer covering the posterior part of the eyeball
- Choroid layer: the layer between the sclera and retina containing blood vessels
- Retina: the inside layer of the posterior part of the eye that receives the light rays (visual stimuli)

The mechanism of vision occurs after impulses leave the retina and travel through the optic nerves to the

TABLE 30-7 SENSORY SYSTEM DISORDERS

Disease/ Disorder	Laboratory Diagnostic Tests			Radiography	Surgery	Medical Tests or Procedures
	Blood	Urine	Other			
Cataract						• Ophthalmologic exam
Chalazion					• Excision	
Color-Blindness						• Ishihara color plates
Conjunctivitis			• Culture and sensitivity of eye discharge			
Corneal Abrasion						• Fluorescein sodium
Diabetic Retinopathy					• Laser	• Fluorescein • Angiogram
Epistaxis	• Complete blood count					• Blood pressure
External Otitis	• Complete blood count		• Culture and sensitivity of exudate			
Glaucoma						• Ophthalmologic exam including intraocular pressure
Ménière's Disease						• Audiometry
Myopia						• Ophthalmologic exam
Hyperopia						• Astigmatoscopy
Presbyopia						• Snellen chart
Astigmatism						• Jaeger chart
Nasal Polyps					• Biopsy of polyp (lesion)	• Nasal exam
Otitis Media	• Complete blood count		• Culture and sensitivity of exudate		• Myringotomy • Tympanostomy	• Tympanography
Otosclerosis						• Audiometry • Rinne test
Retinal Detachment					• Laser or surgery to reattach	
Sinusitis	• Complete blood count		• Culture and sensitivity of exudate	• Sinus X rays		
Stye (Hordeolum)			• Culture and sensitivity if exudate present		• Incision and drainage	

brain. At the optic chiasm the nerve fibers cross and continue to the thalamus. These fibers synapse with other neurons that send the impulses to the right and left visual area of the occipital lobe of the brain. Since the tracts cross at the optic chasm, the stimuli coming from the right visual fields are translated in the visual area of the left occipital area, and the stimuli coming from the left visual fields are translated in the visual area of the right occipital lobe. See Table 30-8 for Common Eye Disorders. See Figure 30-17 and 30-18 for anatomy of the eye.

Signs and symptoms that are common to eye diseases and disorders are pain or burning in or around the eye, decreased visual acuity, any visual changes such as seeing sudden flashes of light, and eye redness.

Measuring Visual Acuity. A procedure commonly performed by the medical assistant is the measuring of a patient's visual acuity. This is only a screening process used when errors in refraction are suspected. The procedure must be performed in a well-lighted quiet area.

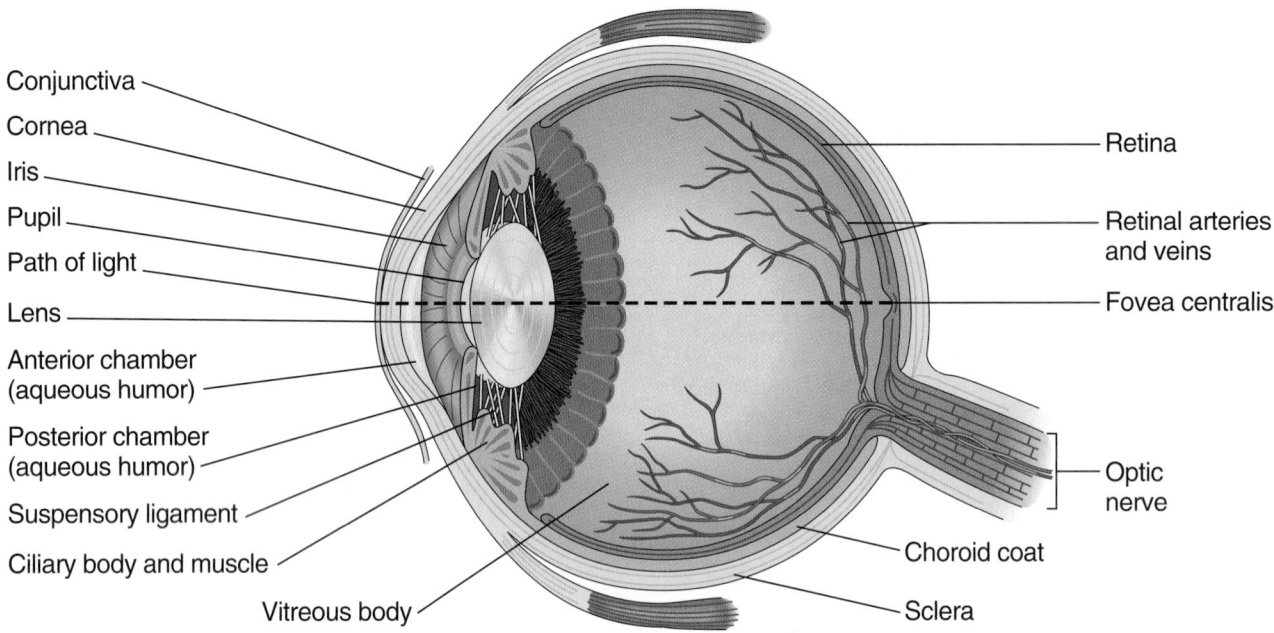

Conjunctiva
Cornea
Iris
Pupil
Path of light
Lens
Anterior chamber (aqueous humor)
Posterior chamber (aqueous humor)
Suspensory ligament
Ciliary body and muscle
Vitreous body

Retina
Retinal arteries and veins
Fovea centralis
Optic nerve
Choroid coat
Sclera

Figure 30-17   The eyeball—cross section view.

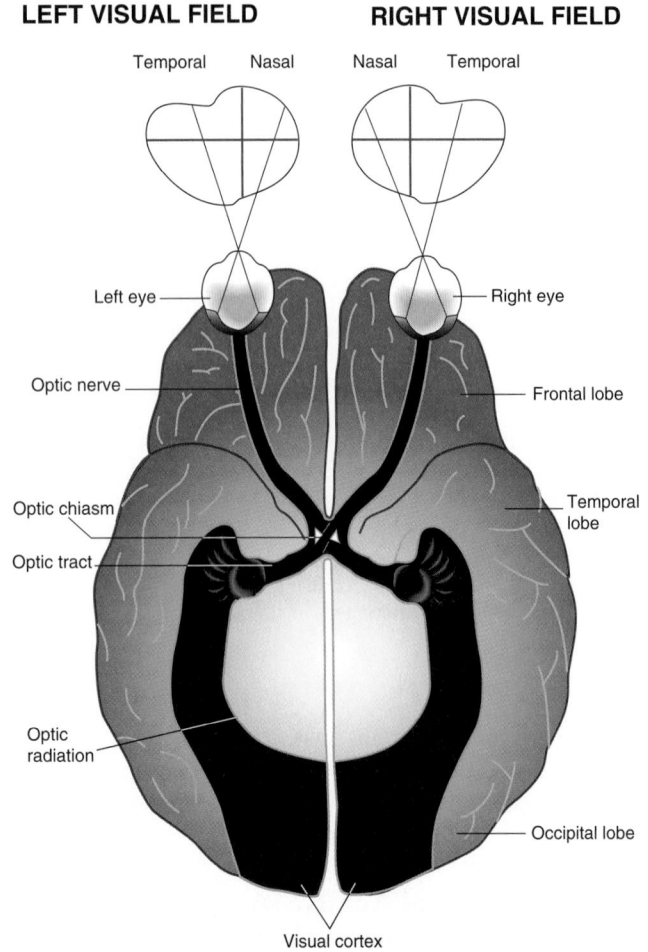

LEFT VISUAL FIELD   **RIGHT VISUAL FIELD**

Temporal   Nasal   Nasal   Temporal

Left eye   Right eye
Optic nerve   Frontal lobe
Optic chiasm   Temporal lobe
Optic tract
Optic radiation   Occipital lobe
Visual cortex

Figure 30-18   The visual pathways of the eye.

TABLE 30-8   DESCRIPTION OF EYE DISORDERS

Refraction and Other Disorders:

- Astigmatism. Irregular lens curvature or cornea shape causing improper focusing of objects.
- Cataract. Lens loses its transparent nature due to changes in its proteins. Usually brought on by aging.
- Color blindness. Inability to distinguish among colors. Caused by an absence of a cone photopigment, a genetic disorder.
- Conjunctivitis. Caused by a bacterial infection or irritant resulting in irritated and reddened conjunctiva. If caused by bacteria, conjunctivitis is highly contagious. See Figure 30-19.
- Corneal Abrasion. Caused by an injury to the cornea by a foreign body resulting in pain, tearing, redness, and possible infection.
- Glaucoma. Condition caused by increased intraocular pressure due to a buildup of aqueous humor. This results in mild visual disturbances with little or no pain but can lead to blindness if untreated.
- Nearsightedness (Myopia). Caused by an elongated eyeball and the image is focused in the front of the retina resulting in the inability to focus on objects at a distance.
- Farsightedness (Hyperopia). Caused when the eyeball is shortened and the image is focused behind the retina causing distance vision to be fuzzy.
- Presbyopia. Attributed to the aging process when the lens loses its elasticity, and the ability to accommodate. Vision is hampered when items are close.
- Stye (Hordeolum). Inflamed sebaceous gland of the eyelid caused by bacterial infection. Erythema, tenderness at site are common symptoms. See Figure 30-20.

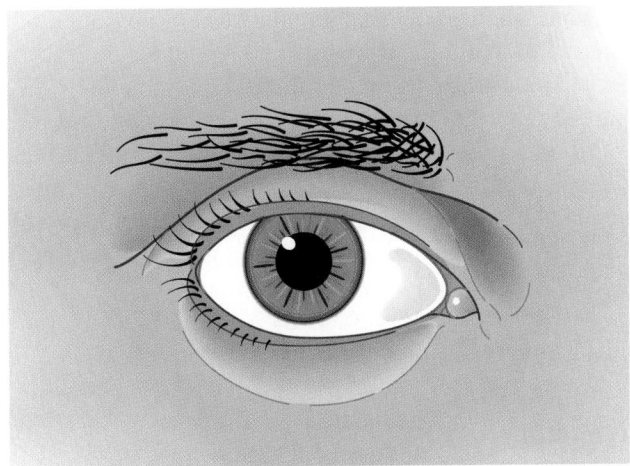

Figure 30-19 Conjunctivitis.

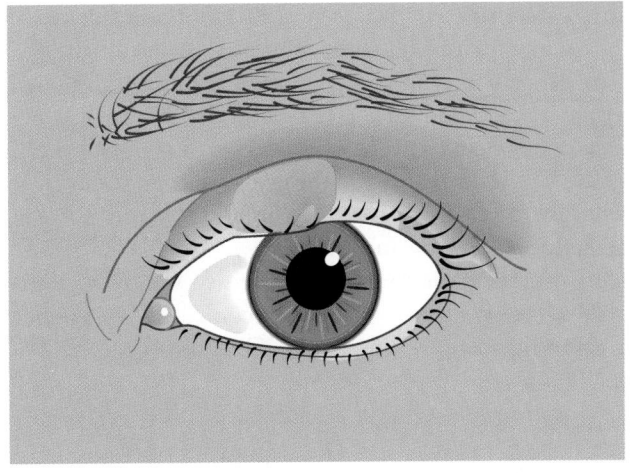

Figure 30-20 Stye (hordeolum).

While performing the procedure, the medical assistant must observe the patient for any action that may indicate difficulty with vision. These actions would include squinting, wiping of the eyes, or leaning toward the chart. In near-vision acuity, these actions would include holding the card nearer or farther than the stated position. The commonly used chart for distance visual acuity is the Snellen chart for the adult. Near-vision is commonly checked by using the Jaeger card.

The Jaeger chart used for checking clear vision is a small card that is held by the patient between 14 and 16 inches from the eye. The medical assistant measures the distance for accuracy. This is the distance from which a person with normal vision is able to read printed material such as a newspaper. The Jaeger test consists of a series of reading material, the letters of which gradually become smaller. Record the last line number that the patient can easily read. The patient is checked with and without corrective lenses and each eye is checked separately.

Errors in refraction is the term used to designate visual acuity abnormalities. The common visual abnormalities include: myopia (nearsightedness), the ability to see only near objects clearly; hyperopia (farsightedness), the ability to see only distant objects clearly; and astigmatism, uneven curvature of the cornea resulting in a scattering of light rays producing blurry vision. Presbyopia (associated with the aging process) is an increase in farsightedness and a loss of lens elasticity that is necessary to accommodate for near vision and is seen primarily in the older patient. (See Figure 30-21.)

The Snellen chart consists of the alphabet letters in various combinations starting at the top with a large E, and descending sized Es by line toward the bottom. Each line is labeled with the visual acuity measurement.

Recording Visual Acuity. Visual acuity, both near and far, is recorded in a fraction format. The numerator indicates

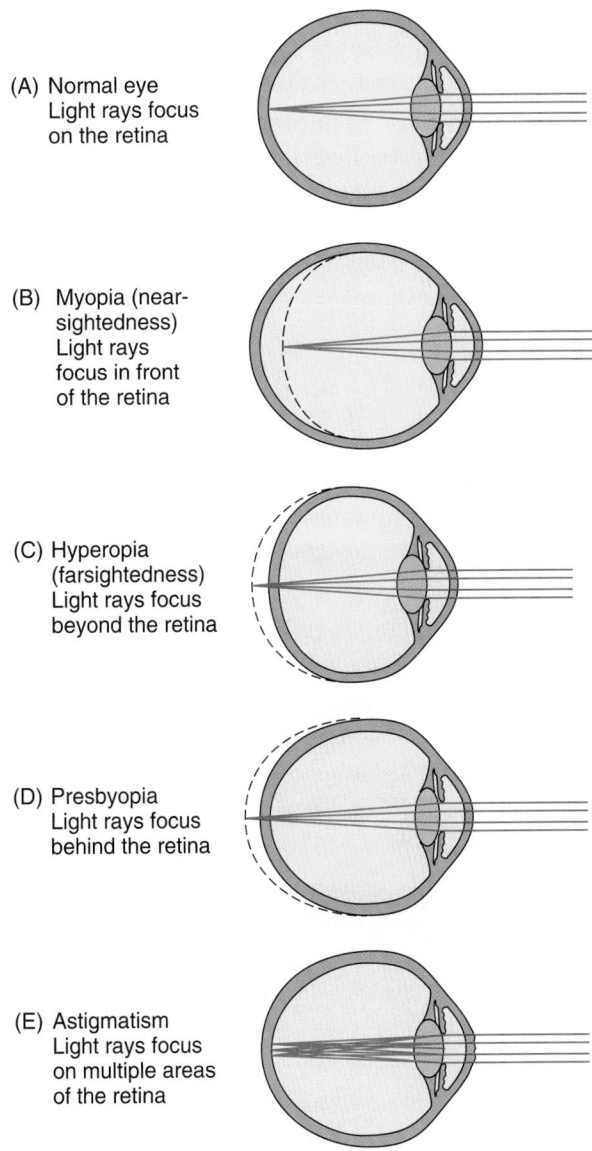

(A) Normal eye
Light rays focus
on the retina

(B) Myopia (near-sightedness)
Light rays
focus in front
of the retina

(C) Hyperopia
(farsightedness)
Light rays focus
beyond the retina

(D) Presbyopia
Light rays focus
behind the retina

(E) Astigmatism
Light rays focus
on multiple areas
of the retina

Figure 30-21 (A) Normal eye vision. (B) Myopia. (C) Hyperopia. (D) Presbyopia. (E) Astigmatism.

the 20-foot distance between the patient and the chart. The denominator indicates the visual acuity of the patient in relationship to the normal seeing eye. Normal vision is 20/20. This means that at 20 feet the eye is seeing what the normal eye would see at 20 feet. Should the vision be 20/30, this indicates that the eye is seeing at twenty feet what the normal eye would see at 30 feet away. A visual acuity of 20/15 indicates that the eye is seeing at twenty feet what the person with normal visual acuity would be able to see at 15 feet. Vision is recorded on the patient chart as right eye OD and left eye OS, both eyes OU.

Example: OD 20/20 OS 20/20 OU 20/20

Patients should be screened with and without their corrective lenses and results recorded as such in patients' records.

Color Vision. Checking color vision is not part of a routine examination. This procedure is usually performed on people who must distinguish color as part of their occupation, e.g., truck drivers, pilots, and salespeople. A commonly used color vision test is the Ishihara color graph. The Ishihara is a book containing pages comprised of varying sized and colored circles. Inside the circles are numbers or lines that can be traced. The patient is seated for the procedure with the book held 14 to 16 inches away and is instructed to identify the numbers as the page is turned or is instructed to trace the line from the indicated starting point to the end. Inability to see the number or follow the line may indicate color blindness. Should this occur the medical assistant must inform the physician as

to what number(s) could not be seen. The patient is referred to an ophthalmologist.

The medical assistant will be responsible for assisting the physician in ophthalmologic exams and performing the tests for visual acuity. Diagnostic procedures for the special senses involve the use of specialized instruments. The use of the ophthalmoscope (Figure 30-22) assists in identifying disease-related problems. The interior of the eye can be examined.

See Procedures 30-6, 30-7, 30-8, 30-9, 30-10, and 30-11 for specialty procedures for the eye.

The Ear

The structures of hearing and equilibrium are divided into the external ear, the middle ear, and the inner ear. The external ear includes the pinna (auricle) and the external auditory canal. The pinna is mostly cartilaginous tissue with a small amount of adipose tissue in the earlobe. The external auditory canal is about one inch in length and contains hair and wax (cerumen)-producing glands. The external ear and middle ear are separated by the tympanic membrane (eardrum).

The middle ear, also called the tympanic cavity, is a small space containing three bones, the malleus (hammer), incus (anvil), and stapes (stirrup). Next to the stapes is the oval window that leads to the inner ear. The eustachian tube connects the middle ear to the throat.

The inner ear is the most sophisticated part of the ear. It is responsible for both hearing and equilibrium (balance). The inner ear consists of a fluid-filled space housing the vestibule, the semicircular canals, the round

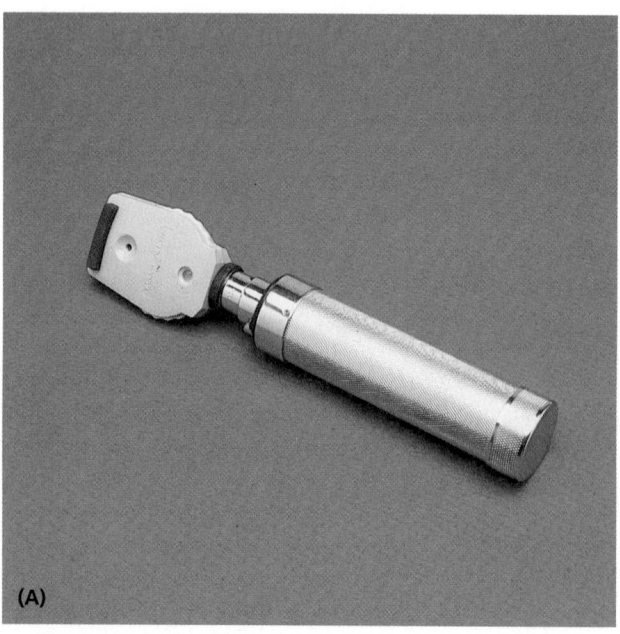
(A)

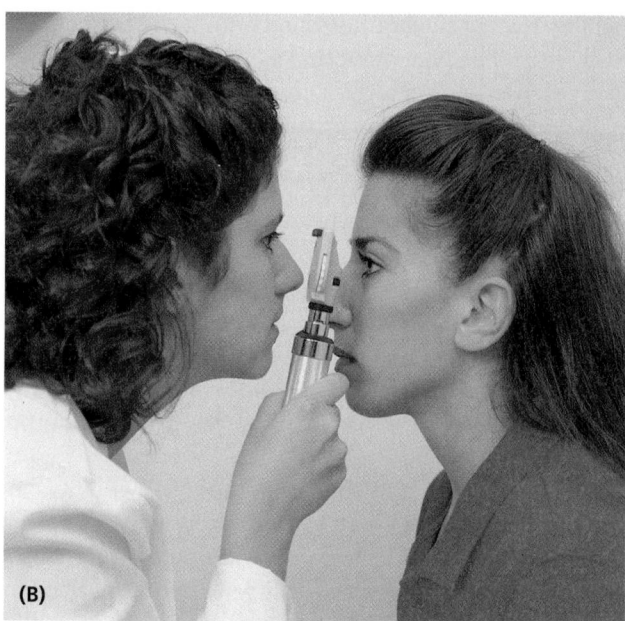
(B)

Figure 30-22   (A) The ophthalmoscope is used to identify eye disorders. (B) Here, the physician uses the ophthalmoscope to view the interior of the patient's eye.

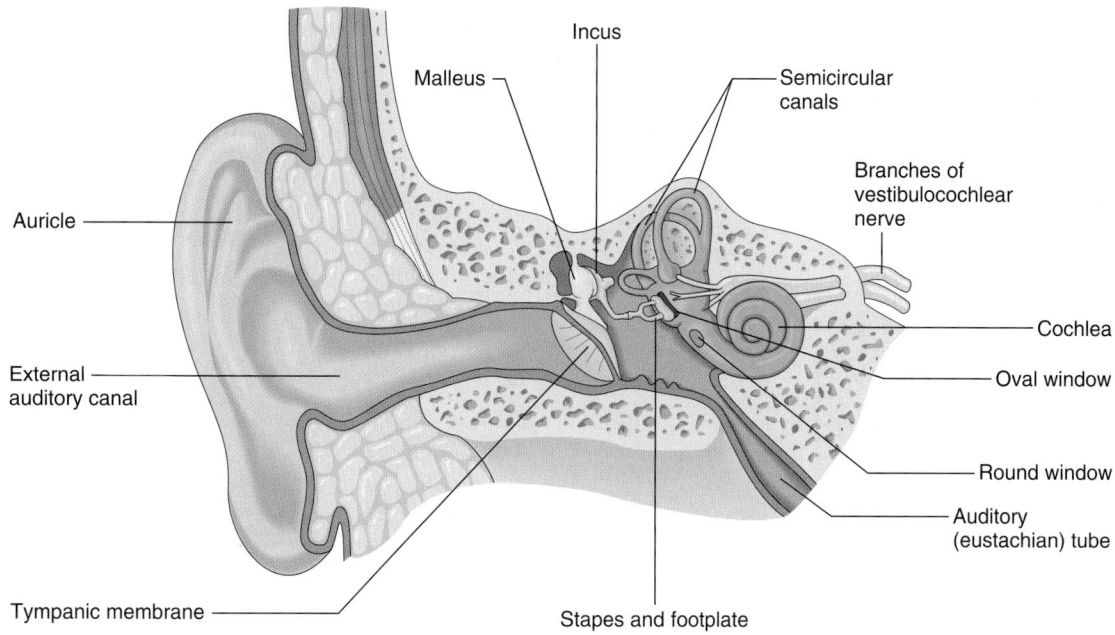

Figure 30-23 The ear.

window, and the cochlea. The structures in the vestibule are responsible for maintaining equilibrium during movement of the head. The semicircular canals assist the body to adjust to changes in direction. The movement of fluid in this area can cause symptoms of dizziness. The cochlea is the organ of hearing.

The outer ear (pinna) picks up sound waves that are sent through the external auditory canal to the tympanic membrane. The membrane vibrates in reaction to the sound striking it. These vibrations pass through the three tiny middle ear bones through the oval window and into the fluid in the cochlea. Receptor cells respond and transfer the sounds into electrical impulses that travel to the brain via the acoustic nerve. The receiving area of the brain for auditory impulses is in the temporal lobe. (See Figure 30-23.)

Diseases or conditions of the ear, if left untreated, can cause damage to nerves and tissues and can result in some degree of hearing impairment, from mild to deafness. Table 30-9 describes common diseases of the ear.

Measuring Auditory Ability. The simple methods of measuring hearing (gross hearing) are usually performed by the physician. The patient may be instructed to place a finger in one ear while the physician whispers one or two words in the other. The patient is then asked to repeat the words. A ticking watch may be placed by the patient's ear to ascertain hearing. A vibrating tuning fork may be placed on the mastoid process behind the ear and then on top of the head. The patient is asked if the sound vibrations could be heard or felt. This procedure will identify nerve or conduction deafness (Figure 30-24).

TABLE 30-9 EAR DISORDERS
• *External Otitis* (*swimmer's ear*). A buildup of fluid with inflammation of the surface of the eardrum. Symptoms are pain, fever, and decreased hearing acuity.
• *Otitis Media.* Acute infection of the middle ear usually caused by bacteria. Symptoms are pain, fever, discharge, and decreased hearing acuity.
• *Otosclerosis.* Conduction deafness caused by hardening of the stapes.
• *Ménière's Disease.* Characterized by deafness, vertigo, and tinnitus. Probable cause is edema of the labyrinth.
• *Impacted Cerumen.* Caused by accumulation of hardened cerumen that has built up against the tympanic membrane. Impaired hearing and tinnitus can result.

Conduction deafness occurs when the sound wave is not transmitted to the middle ear. This type of deafness may be a result of the presence of ear wax (cerumen) in the ear canal or a scarred tympanic membrane. Nerve deafness is a result of injury along the course of the nerves leading from the inner ear to the auditory centers of the brain.

A more complex procedure may be performed by the medical assistant using an audiometer. A quiet room with no distractions is required for the procedure to be accurate. The patient is seated facing away from the medical assistant and the audiometer, then ear phones are placed over the ears. The patient is instructed to raise a hand when a sound is heard. The audiometer has two dials, one for the various wave lengths and the other for wave intensity. Starting at the lowest pitch, the intensity is increased until the patient responds to the sound. The

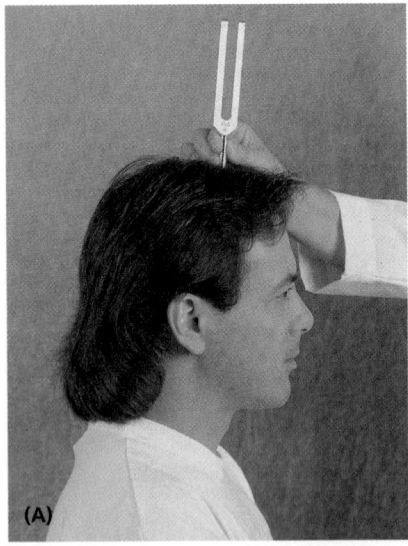
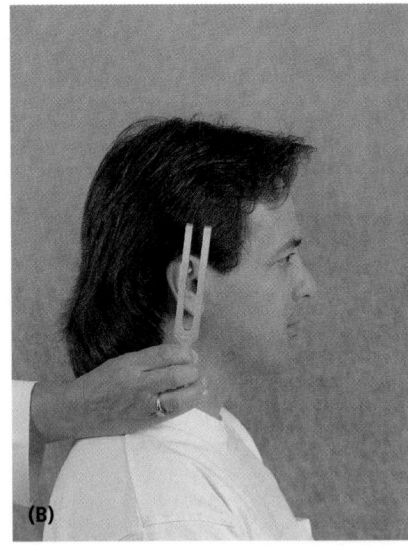
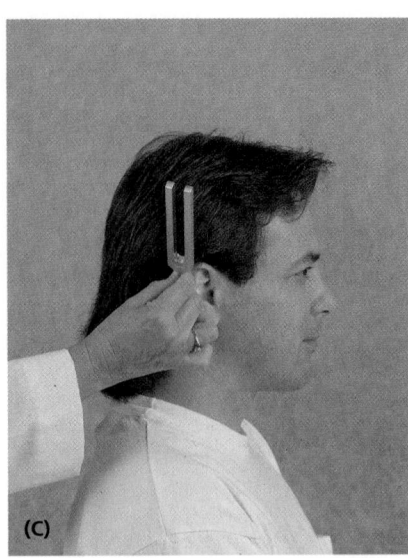

Figure 30-24 (A) The physician holds the tuning fork against the crown of the patient's head to determine which ear can hear the sound. (B) To check air conduction of sound, the physician holds the tuning fork one inch from the patient's auditory meatus. (C) The physician places the tuning fork on the bony prominence (mastoid bone) behind the patient's ear to check bone conduction of sound.

next pitch is then tested in the same manner. This process continues until the highest pitched sound is tested. The results are obtained by noting the number of intensity at which the sound was heard. When performing the procedure, the medical assistant must not develop a pattern that can be detected by the patient. The ears should be tested in an alternating fashion to ensure accuracy. (See Procedure 30-12.)

The medical assistant employed in an industrial medical facility may be required to monitor hearing of some employees. If this is the case, care must be taken to have the hearing test performed before the employee goes to work for the day. Hearing loss may result from the day's activities in some noisy facilities even when ear plugs are worn.

Tympanometry is a procedure used to ascertain the ability of the middle ear to transmit sound waves and is commonly performed on children to diagnose middle ear infections. A probe is inserted into the ear canal to measure the air pressure of the ear canal in relationship to the air pressure found in the middle ear. Tympanogram is the recording produced by this procedure. The waves and peaks are measured providing an indication of possible middle ear abnormalities.

During auditory testing, the medical assistant provides equipment to the physician and may perform irrigation or instillation to the external canal of the ear. Diagnostic procedures for the special senses involve the use of specialized instruments, including the **otoscope**, which assists in identifying disease-related ear problems (Figure 30-25).

Procedures 30-12, 30-13, and 30-14 describe steps in audiometry and ear irrigation and instillation.

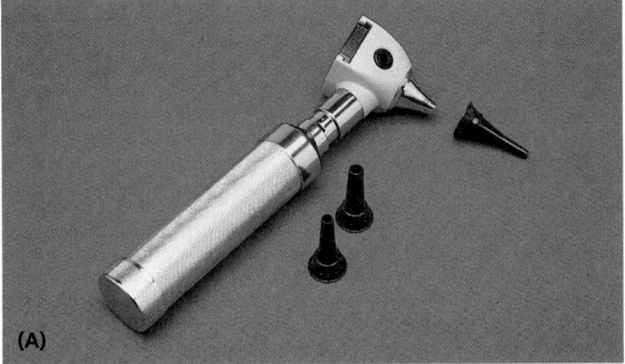

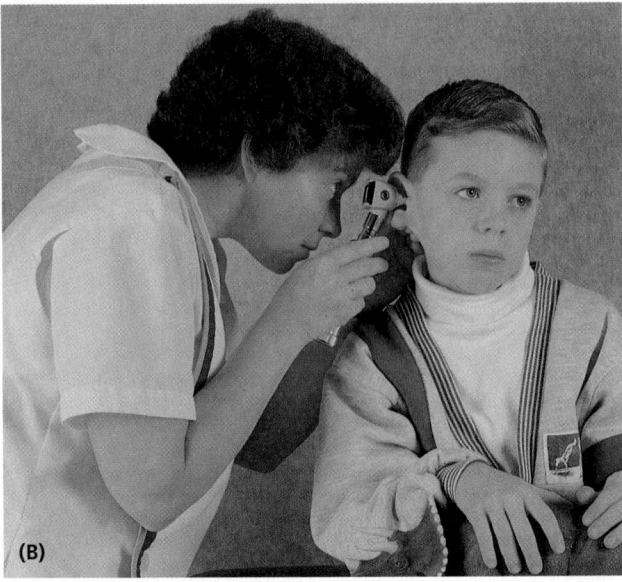

Figure 30-25 (A) An otoscope with three different sizes of reusable specula. (B) The otoscope is used to examine the patient's tympanic membrane.

RESPIRATORY SYSTEM

The respiratory process is all important to the life process. **External respiration** allows for the exchange of carbon dioxide and oxygen across the cell walls into the airspaces of the lungs. **Internal respiration** is the exchange of these gases at the cellular levels of the organs.

The respiratory process begins with air entering the nose or mouth, where it passes through the pharynx, down into the trachea, into the **bronchi**, and then enters the lungs. Gas exchange takes place when the blood filters through the **alveoli**. See Table 30-10 for respiratory diseases and disorders diagnostic procedures and Table 30-11 for a description of respiratory disorders.

Respiratory disorders are diagnosed with various X rays, bronchoscopy, blood studies, and pulmonary function studies. Cultures of sputum and the pharynx are widely used diagnostic tests. Irrigations of the nose, collection of sputum specimens, and assisting with pulmonary tests are the roles of the medical assistant. See Procedures 30-15, 30-16, 30-17, 30-18, 30-19, 30-20 and 30-21 for specialized respiratory examinations and procedures.

Spirometry

A commonly used tool in the medical office or clinic, **spirometry** assists the physician in the evaluation of signs and symptoms of pulmonary disease by measuring the air capacity of the lungs. Three components of lung functions are measured:

1. Forced virtual capacity (FVC), which represents the volume of air that can be exhaled from the lung after the lung is filled with air to meet its total capacity.
2. Forced expiration volume at 1 second (FEV), which is the volume of gas forcibly exhaled from the lungs the first second of expiration.
3. Mean expiration flow (FEF) rate, which is a measure on a volume-time curve.

Most spirometers are computerized and thus automatically calculate the lung functions.

See Procedure 30-21 to assist with spirometry.

TABLE 30-10   RESPIRATORY SYSTEM DISORDERS

| Disease/ Disorder | Laboratory Diagnostic Tests | | | Radiography | Surgery | Medical Tests or Procedures |
	Blood	Urine	Other			
Asthma	• Complete blood count • Arterial blood gases		• Sputum analysis	• Chest X ray		• Pulmonary function tests • Skin testing for allergies
Bronchitis	• Complete blood count		• Sputum culture and analysis	• Chest X ray		• Bronchoscopy
Emphysema	• Complete blood count • Arterial blood gases			• Chest X ray		• Pulmonary function tests
Influenza	• Complete blood count			• Chest X ray		
Laryngitis			• Throat culture			• Laryngoscopy
Lung Cancer	• Complete blood count		• Sputum cytology	• Chest X ray	• Biopsy of lung tissue	• Bronchoscopy
Pharyngitis	• Complete blood count		• Throat culture			
Pneumonia	• Complete blood count		• Blood culture • Sputum smear	• Chest X ray		
Pleurisy	• Complete blood count			• Chest X ray		
Tonsillitis	• Complete blood count • Streptococcal antibody test		• Throat culture			
Tuberculosis	• Complete blood count		• Sputum culture • Acid fast smear of sputum	• Chest X ray	• Biopsy of lung tissue	• Tuberculin skin test: Mantoux tine

---

TABLE 30-11 DESCRIPTION OF RESPIRATORY DISORDERS

- Asthma. Spasm of the smooth muscle of the bronchi brought on by an allergen and/or emotional upsets. Characterized by dyspnea and wheezing.
- Bronchitis. Inflammation of the bronchi, caused by viral or bacterial infection with a dry, painful cough, progressing to a productive cough of greenish-yellow sputum. Symptoms: cough, slight fever, chills, malaise, soreness under the sternum.
- Emphysema. Enlargement of the alveoli due to lost elasticity, usually brought on by a long-time irritant, such as cigarette smoking. Results in dyspnea, chronic cough, weight loss, and the appearance of a "barrel chest."
- Influenza. A viral infection of various strains of the upper respiratory tract (URI). Sudden onset of chills, fever, cough, sore throat, gastrointestinal disorders are common. Can range from mild to life-threatening.
- Laryngitis. Hoarseness, cough, aphonia caused by infections from nose or throat.
- Lung Cancer. Cancer that may appear in trachea, air sacs, and other lung tubes.
- Pharyngitis. Inflammation of the pharynx caused by a bacteria, virus, or an irritant. Difficulty in swallowing, pain, redness, and inflammation of the pharynx are some of the symptoms. Streptococcus is the most common bacterial infection, influenza virus and the common cold virus are the most common viruses involved. May be accompanied by fever, malaise, headache.
- Pneumonia. Inflammation of the lungs caused by bacteria, fungi, viruses, and chemical irritants. Usually has sudden onset and is characterized by chills, fever, chest pain, cough, purulent sputum. Symptoms include sore throat, fever, lymphadenopathy.
- Pleurisy. Inflammation of the pleura caused by bacteria or viruses. Symptoms include pain, fever, cough, chills and dyspnea.
- Tonsillitis. Inflammation of the tonsils usually caused by streptococcus. Tonsils become red and enlarged causing severe pharyngitis, fever.
- Tuberculosis. Inflammatory infiltrations, formation of tubercles, abscesses, fibrosis, and calcification. Can lead to infection of other body systems.

MUSCULOSKELETAL SYSTEM

The muscular system and the skeletal system interact to coordinate the supporting framework and movements of the body. The musculoskeletal system includes bones, joints, muscles, and surrounding tissue. The skeletal system provides support, protection for vital organs, and allows for the attachment of ligaments, tendons, and muscles. The muscular system gives the body form and shape and is responsible for the coordination of movement.

Bones of the skeletal system store minerals for later use by the body. They are classified according to their shape. Characteristics of bones are their marking, which provides for the attachment of muscles, joining of another bone, and which allows for the passage of nerves and blood vessels. The skeletal system is divided into two parts, the **appendicular skeleton** (126 bones) and the **axial skeleton** (80 bones).

One of the top four reasons a patient visits a physi-

cian is for back pain. During the visit, the physician will evaluate the patient for contributory factors for the pain by assessing the patient for any deformities, asymmetry, and/or signs of restricted motion. The physician will do a functional assessment by observing the patient's **gait** for indications of decreased mobility and postural changes associated with aging or injury. Flexion tests are done with a goniometer to detect the degree of resistance applied to a given force, thus defining restricted motion and the amount of discomfort associated with movement. Supine straight leg raising (SLR) tests are done to detect the amount of hamstring flexibility and can assess sciatic nerve damage.

There are over 600 muscles in the body. Muscles are comprised of bundles of muscle fibers, each with the ability to contract and relax. Any disease process that disrupts the balance between these two systems severely hampers a person's ability to move effectively and painlessly. See Tables 30-12, 30-13, and 30-14.

TABLE 30-12 MUSCULOSKELETAL SYSTEM DISORDERS

| Disease/ Disorder | Laboratory Diagnostic Tests | | | Radiography | Surgery | Medical Tests or Procedures |
	Blood	Urine	Other			
Carpal Tunnel Syndrome	• Erythrocyte sedimentation rate • Uric acid • Complete blood count				• Surgical repair	• Electromyography

(continues)

TABLE 30-12 *(continued)*

Disease/ Disorder	Laboratory Diagnostic Tests			Radiography	Surgery	Medical Tests or Procedures
	Blood	Urine	Other			
Dislocation				• X ray		
Gout	• Uric acid • Complete blood count • Erythrocyte sedimentation rate	• Urinalysis	• Synovial fluid analysis	• Skeletal X rays		
Herniated disk				• Computerized tomography • Magnetic resonance imaging		
Osteoarthritis	• Complete blood count • Sedimentation rate			• Skeletal X rays including vertebrae		
Osteoporosis	• Serum calcium • Alkaline phosphatase • Estrogen level • Total protein • Creatinine	• Calcium • Creatinine		• Bone scan		
Rheumatoid Arthritis	• Rheumatoid factor • Antinuclear antibody test • Lupus erythematosis test • Erythrocyte sedimentation rate • Complete blood count		• Synovial fluid analysis			
Rickets	• Serum phosphorus • Vitamin D • Creatinine	• Calcium • Phosphorus • Creatinine				

Spinal Curvatures
  Scoliosis
  Lordosis
  Kyphosis
				• X rays of spine		

TABLE 30-13 MUSCULAR/CONNECTIVE TISSUE DISORDERS

Disease/ Disorder	Laboratory Diagnostic Tests			Radiography	Surgery	Medical Tests or Procedures
	Blood	Urine	Other			
Back Pain		• Urinalysis		• X ray		• Computerized tomography (CT) • Magnetic resonance imaging (MRI)
Bursitis				• X ray affected joint for calcium deposits		
Fibromyalgia	• Rheumatoid arthritis antibody			• Skeletal X rays		• Electromyography
Strain, Sprain				• X ray affected body part to rule out fracture		
Tendonitis				• Arthrogram		

TABLE 30-14	DESCRIPTION OF SKELETAL AND MUSCULAR DISORDERS

Bone

- Carpal Tunnel Syndrome. Causes pain and weakness of hand and fingers. May cause paresthesia of hand and fingers. Caused by compression of the median nerve against the carpal bones. Usually results from repetitive tasks (such as typing or rolling hair).
- Cleft palate. Congenital disorder caused by nonunion of the maxillary bones. Surgical repair needed to close palate.
- Fractures. Break in a bone classified according to angle, usually caused by trauma or pathology.
- Herniated Disk. A rupture of the cushioning mass between two intervertebrae disks of the spine most often caused by injury. Causes back pain that may radiate into buttock(s) and down leg.
- Osteoporosis. Diminished bone mass caused by lack of calcium deposits in the bone, predisposing patients to fracture.
- Paget's Disease. Chronic disease marked by a high rate of bone destruction and irregular bone repair. The new bone fractures easily. Cause unknown, but may be hereditary.
- Rickets. Abnormal bone softening caused by inadequate utilization of vitamin D, inadequate intake or loss of calcium. One symptom is night fever.
- Spinal Curvatures. Spinal defects with exaggerated curves caused by diseases of the spine, faulty posture and/or congenital malformations.
    Scoliosis—right or left sideways curvature of the spine.
    Lordosis—inward curvature of the spine (swayback).
    Kyphosis—outward curvature of the spine (hunchback).

Joints

- Dislocation. A bone forcibly displaced from its joint usually caused by trauma.
- Gout. Form of arthritis caused by metabolic disturbances in purine metabolism resulting in uric acid crystal deposits in the joints. Causes periodic attacks of arthritis pain and joint inflammation.
- Osteoarthritis. Common, chronic inflammatory process of the joints, with overgrowth of bone and spur formation. Accompanies aging. Causes swollen joints and pain.
- Rheumatoid Arthritis. More serious and crippling form caused by inflammation of the synovial tissues of several joints, may be caused by antigen-antibody reaction. Systemic symptoms include fatigue, temperature elevation, sensory disturbances, pain, and joint deformities.

Muscle Disorders

- Back Pain. Localized discomfort in the lumbar area caused by stretching or straining of a muscle.
- Bursitis. Inflammation of the cavity found in connective tissue of a joint that is lined with synovial fluid usually caused by trauma.
- Fibromalagia. Discomfort of muscles, tendons, ligaments, and soft tissues brought on by trauma, strain, and emotional stress.
- Strain. Trauma to a muscle from violent contraction.
- Spasm. Sudden involuntary muscle contraction.
- Sprains. Caused by trauma to a joint with torn ligament if severe.
- Tendonitis. Inflammation of tendons and attachments caused by trauma such as strain.

Diagnostic procedures involving the skeletal system involve the extensive use of various forms of X rays and visual examination techniques. A bone biopsy may be ordered when additional diagnostic data are required. The muscular system employs the use of electrical stimulation to measure the neuromuscular activity and strength of muscles.

Therapeutic treatment of muscular system injuries caused by trauma is clinically handled by the use of hot and cold therapy and ultrasound therapy. These procedures are discussed in Chapter 33.

Fractures, Casting, and Cast Removal

A **closed fracture** or **dislocation** of the wrist, forearm, or upper arm is often treated in the ambulatory care setting. (See Table 30-15 for other types of fractures. Also refer to Chapter 9.)

Types of casting materials used are the plaster-of-Paris, synthetic or plastic cast, and the air cast. Plaster-of-Paris casts are formed by wetting bandage rolls impregnated with calcium sulfate and molding it to the injured body part. Synthetic casts (Figure 30-26) are formed by using tapes with either a polyester, cotton combination, fiberglass, or plastic resin imbedded in the tape. Air casts are a type of inflatable immobilizer and are used for sprains and postcast support. The type of casting material used is dependent upon physician preference and the body part to which a cast is being applied. Synthetic casts are lighter, stronger, and more water resistant.

- *Short arm cast.* Extends from the fingers to just below the elbow. (Fracture or dislocation of wrist and forearm.)

TABLE 30-15 TYPES OF FRACTURES
Fractures can be simple, or closed, so called because the bone is broken with no penetration of the skin; or they can be compound, or open, so called because the broken bone has protruded through the skin and there is an open wound in addition to the fracture.
Two of the most common fractures are both simple fractures: Colles fracture and Potts fracture.
Colles fracture is a fracture of the lower end of the radius. Potts fracture is a fracture of the lower part of the fibula and the malleolus of the tibia.
Fractures are described by their characteristics:
Greenstick. The bone is bent on one side and fractured on the other.
Oblique. The bone is fractured and runs obliquely to the axis of the bone.
Transverse. The bone is fractured at a right angle to the axis of the bone.
Comminuted. The bone is splintered into fragments.
Impacted. The bone is fractured into fragments and the fragments have been driven into the interior of another bone.

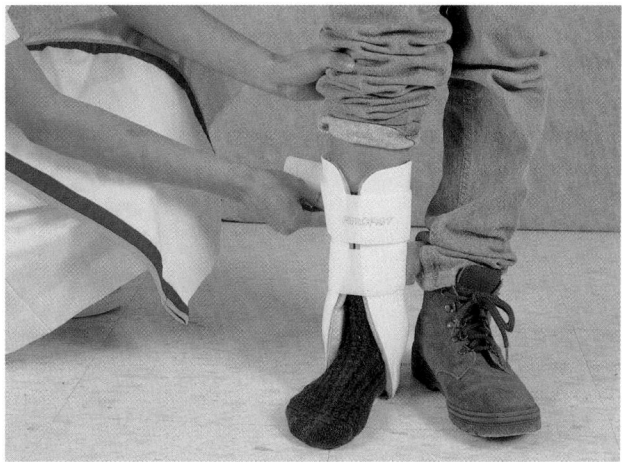

Figure 30-26 A synthetic cast being adjusted.

- *Long arm cast*. Extends from the fingers to the axilla, with a bend at the elbow. (Fracture of the upper arm.)

The medical assistant's role in cast application and removal is to offer assistance to the physician and to provide the required equipment and supplies. Patient teaching of cast care is also a primary function of the medical assistant. Procedures 30-22 and 30-23 outline steps in applying a plaster-of-Paris cast and assisting in cast removal.

Cast Care Guidelines

The medical assistant should instruct the patient on managing and caring for a cast.

- Allow the casting material to dry by exposing it to the air and keeping it uncovered, even during the night. Applying pressure to the cast prior to drying can result in tissue damage under the pressure area.

- Elevate the casted extremity to aid in reducing swelling and pain. This allows for a better fitting cast, and thus less discomfort.

- Observe the fingers or toes for changes in color, temperature changes, and decreased sensation and tingling. This could indicate the cast is too tight.

- Do not place objects into the cast to scratch irritated skin. A break in the skin will provide a breeding ground for bacteria. Do not use powder or creams.

- Do not get the cast wet. This could lead to a malformation of the cast, thus misalignment of the extremity. Cover with waterproof covering when bathing. If the cast gets wet, dry it with a hair dryer.

- Cleaning a cast can be accomplished by using a damp cloth.

- When decorating a cast, use only water-soluble paints or marking pens. This allows the cast to breathe, thus avoiding tissue damage.

- Do not cut or trim the cast. Use a type of masking tape if there is a sharp edge.

- Notify the physician if any of the following occurs:
  1. A bad odor coming from the cast. This may indicate an infection.
  2. Numbness, tingling, severe pain, difficulty moving, severe swelling, or cold fingers or toes. The cast may be too tight.
  3. A burning sensation over a bony area. The cast may be too tight.
  4. Bleeding or pink to red discoloration on the cast. There may be bleeding from a wound under the cast.

NEUROLOGICAL SYSTEM

The nervous system functions to coordinate the activities of body systems and allows for the body to adapt to its internal and external environment. Diagnosis and treatment of the brain, spinal cord, and **peripheral nerve** disorders are often difficult because of the interdependence of one part of the system on another.

The physician will screen the patient during a physical examination for neurological signs and symptoms. The medical assistant's role in a neurological screening is to observe and evaluate the patient's mental status and to assist or perform other tests as directed by the physician. Most of the exam is performed in conjunction with the

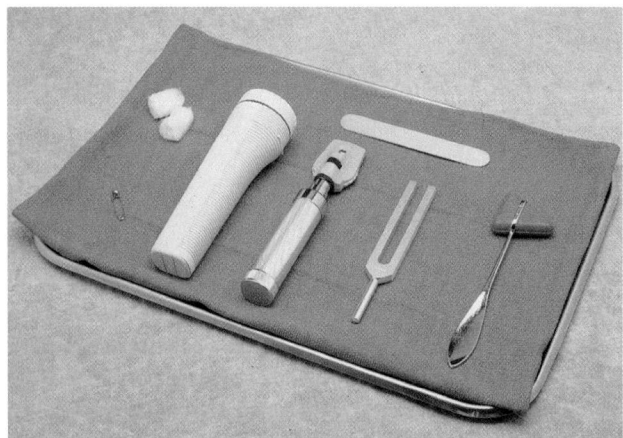

Figure 30-27 Equipment and supplies are used in the neurological screening to test reflexes, touch, smell, and coordination.

complete physical examination, but it can also be done when a patient is exhibiting specific signs and symptoms of a neurological problem such as lack of sensation, seizures, confusion, paralysis, or aphasia.

The equipment and supplies used in a neurological screening are those that test the patient's reflexes, touch, sense of smell, and degree of coordination to name a few (Figure 30-27). The physician pays particular attention to symmetrical strength and notes unequal weakness on either side of the body. A patient's gender and body build will be considered when examining muscle mass and tone. Table 30-16 describes neurological diagnostic procedures; Table 30-17 outlines neurological disorders.

Procedures performed to confirm a diagnosis of a neurological problem or disease are limited to the use of various X-ray and electrical impulse studies. The medical assistant will assist the physician during the procedures. Patient teaching by the medical assistant prior to a proce-

TABLE 30-16 NEUROLOGICAL SYSTEM DISORDERS

Disease/Disorder	Laboratory Diagnostic Tests			Radiography	Surgery	Medical Tests or Procedures
	Blood	**Urine**	**Other**			
Bell's Palsy	• Complete blood count					
Cerebral Vascular Accident				• Cerebral angiography • Computerized tomography • Magnetic resonance imaging		• Electroencephalography • Lumbar puncture
Epilepsy				• Computerized tomography • Magnetic resonance imaging		• Electroencephalography
Herpes Zoster	• Varicella-Zoster antibody					• Culture of cell scrapings from lesion
Multiple Sclerosis				• Computerized tomography • Magnetic resonance imaging		• Lumbar puncture
Rabies	• Complete blood count					
Reye's Syndrome	• Complete blood count • Serum ammonia		• Liver function studies		• Liver biopsy	• Lumbar puncture • Exam of cerebral spinal fluid
Sciatica				• Computerized tomography • Magnetic resonance imaging		
Tic Douloureux					• Biopsy of trigeminal nerve	

TABLE 30-17 DESCRIPTION OF NEUROLOGICAL DISORDERS

- **Bell's Palsy.** Paralysis of seventh cranial nerve caused by an acute inflammation. Usually characterized by unilateral facial paralysis and pain, but can be bilateral.
- **Cerebral Vascular Accident (CVA).** Loss of blood supply to the brain (anoxia). May be caused by a ruptured or clogged blood vessel in the brain and hypertension. Symptoms include sudden loss of consciousness and paralysis. Also referred to as a stroke.
- **Epilepsy.** Episodes of seizures caused by changes in electrical brain potentials which result in disturbed brain impulses or function.
- **Headache.** Diffuse pain in different parts of the head. May be acute or chronic with varying degree of pain and may be caused by a variety of reasons.
- **Herpes Zoster.** An acute infectious disease caused by varicella zoster virus. Painful vesicular eruptions.
- **Meningitis.** Inflammation of the membranes of the spinal cord or brain. Symptoms include a stiff neck, headache, anorexia, and irregular fever.
- **Multiple Sclerosis.** Chronic progressive disease characterized by demyelination of nerve fibers. The cause is unknown. First symptoms are visual disturbances and muscle weakness.
- **Parkinson's.** A slowly progressive disease, usually occurring in later life, caused by a degeneration of brain cells due to lack of dopamine in the brain. Muscle rigidity and akinesia are common symptoms.
- **Rabies.** Caused by a virus and transmitted to humans by scratches or bites from animals infected with the virus. The disease infects the brain and spinal cord and causes acute encephalitis.
- **Reye's Syndrome.** A neurologic illness usually seen in young children following a viral infection such as influenza, varicella, Epstein-Barr. There may be a connection between the viral infection and aspirin. Cause is unknown, but characteristic symptoms include vomiting, rash, lethargy and neurologic involvement, seizures and coma.
- **Sciatica.** Severe pain in the leg along the course of the sciatic nerve felt at the back of the thigh and running down the inside of the leg. Caused by compression of the nerve by a ruptured intervertebral disk or osteoarthritis. Characterized by sharp, shooting pain running down back of thigh. Leg movement aggravates the pain.
- **Tic Douloureux.** Degeneration of or pressure on the trigeminal nerve (fifth cranial) causing severe stabs of pain that radiate from the angle of the jaw along one of the branches. Pain may be felt in the eye, lip, nose, tongue. Pain may come and go for hours.

dure and active reinforcement during a procedure will promote patient cooperation. Procedure 30-24 outlines steps involved in removing cerebrospinal fluid from the lumbar area.

Components of a Neurological Screening

During the neurological screening examination, various functions are observed. Procedure 30-25 outlines the steps involved in a neurological screening examination.

- Mental status:
  Level of consciousness (alert)
  Memory (recall of past and present)
  Cognition (ability to calculate and remember current events)
  Mood (is it appropriate for the conversation)
  Ideational content (hallucinations)
- Cranial nerve function:

Cranial nerve I	Cranial nerve II
Aroma identification	Visual acuity
	Visual fields
	Optic disc

  Cranial nerves III, IV, and VI extraocular eye muscles

Cranial nerve V sensations of the face, scalp, teeth

Cranial nerve VII facial expressions, taste

Cranial nerve VIII ear—hearing and equilibrium

Cranial nerve IX and X gag reflex, saliva secretion, voice, slowing of heartbeat

Cranial nerve XI neck and shoulder muscle

Cranial nerve XII tongue

The physician continues with the neurological examination by checking the patient for the following:

- Cerebral function:
  Memory
  Muscle coordination
  Sensory interpretation
  Posture and gait
- Motor function:
  Muscle tone
  Strength
  Muscle mass
  Twitching
- Sensory function:
  Touch (pain, light touch, vibration, position sense)

- Deep tendon reflexes:

  Extremities:

  Upper—biceps, triceps

  Lower—quadriceps, achilles

  Additional Tests:

  Angiography provides visualization of the circulation of the blood throughout the brain.

  Computerized tomography (CT) helps to diagnose hemorrhage and tumors.

  Electroencephalography (EEG) records the electrical activity of the brain and helps to diagnose seizures and tumors.

  Magnetic resonance imaging (MRI) helps to diagnose tumors and hemorrhage. (See Chapter 32.)

CIRCULATORY SYSTEM

The circulatory system is comprised of the heart and a complex network of blood vessels. Their function is to pump and transport the blood to all parts of the body, thus supplying oxygen and removing waste products from body tissues. Table 30-18 reviews circulatory system disorders and diagnostic procedures; Table 30-19 provides a description of disorders of the circulatory system.

The variety of diagnostic procedures used to determine the patient's diagnosis are necessary because of the complexity of the cardiovascular system. The medical assistant assists with and performs some of the procedures used for clinical diagnosis. Electrocardiogram (ECG) procedure is found in Chapter 37.

TABLE 30-18   CIRCULATORY SYSTEM DISORDERS

Disease/ Disorder	Laboratory Diagnostic Tests			Radiography	Surgery	Medical Tests or Procedures
	Blood	Urine	Other			
Angina Pectoris				• Ultrasonography		• Electrocardiography • Stress test
Congestive Heart Failure				• Chest X ray		• Electrocardiography • Venous pressure
Coronary Artery Disease	• Electrolytes • Chemistry LDL, HDL, Cholesterol			• Angiography • Thallium stress test • Cardiac catheterization		
Essential Hypertension	• Electrolytes	• Urinalysis	• Kidney Function	• Chest X ray		• Electrocardiography
Mitral Valve Stenosis				• Echocardiography • Cardiac catheterization		• Electrocardiography
Myocardial Infarction	• Cardiac enzymes • Complete blood count			• Thallium stress test • Cardiac catheterization • Ultrasonography		• Electrocardiography
Pericarditis	• Complete blood count • Erythrocyte sedimentation rate • Cardiac enzymes • Bacterial antibodies	• Urinalysis	• Blood culture	• Chest X ray		• Electrocardiography
Rheumatic Fever	• Complete blood count • Streptococcal antibodies • Sedimentation rate • Cardiac enzymes • Kidney function • Liver function		• Throat culture	• Echocardiography		• Electrocardiography
Thrombo-phlebitis	• Bleeding and clotting time • Complete blood count	• Urinalysis		• Doppler ultrasonography • Angiography • Radioactive fibrinogen		
Varicose Veins				• Venography		

TABLE 30-19   DESCRIPTION OF CIRCULATORY SYSTEM DISORDERS

- **Angina Pectoris.** Chest pain caused by lack of oxygen to the myocardium. Usual cause is coronary arteriosclerosis.
- **Congestive Heart Failure.** A syndrome characterized by the heart's inability to pump blood adequately to the body tissues. Characterized by congestion in the lungs, or edema of lower extremities, dyspnea on exertion, cough and related edema.
- **Coronary Artery Disease.** Arteriosclerosis of the coronary arteries leading to impaired blood flow to the myocardium. Complete occlusion leads to myocardial infarction. May also be caused by thrombus in a coronary artery. Angina pectoris is the name of the chest pain that occurs due to lack of oxygen to the myocardium.
- **Essential Hypertension.** Consistently elevated blood pressure with no apparent cause.
- **Mitral Valve Stenosis.** Narrowing of mitral valve obstructing flow from atrium to ventricle. Usual cause is a rheumatic heart disease as a result of a streptococcal infection (throat or scarlet fever). Thrombi can form.
- **Myocardial infarction.** Death of myocardial tissue caused by anoxia to the myocardium. Symptoms include: dyspnea, chest pain, nausea, vomiting, diaphoresis.
- **Pericarditis.** Inflammation of the pericardium. Caused by tuberculosis, pyogenic organisms, uremia, myocardial infarction. Characterized by fever, dry cough, dyspnea, palpitations.
- **Rheumatic Fever.** A systemic disease affecting the heart, joints, and central nervous system following a Group A beta-hemolytic streptococcal infection. May occur without symptoms. Symptoms include fever, migratory joint pain, pericarditis, heart murmur.
- **Thrombophlebitis.** An inflammation of a vein with thrombus formation, may be caused by trauma. Symptoms: pain and swelling in affected vein.
- **Varicose Veins.** Enlarged, twisted and engorged veins, commonly occurring in the saphenous veins but may occur in any vein in the body. Caused by conditions that hamper venous return, such as pregnancy, standing for long periods of time and obesity. Symptoms: pain in feet and ankles, swelling, leg ulcers.

BLOOD AND LYMPH SYSTEM

The blood and lymph are excellent indicators of many underlying diseases. As blood circulates through body tissues and organs, it deposits nutrients and removes wastes. Failure to accomplish this leaves the body in a disease state. Blood cells include erythrocytes, leukocytes, and platelets and each has its own function. Studying the results of laboratory findings assists the physician in making a diagnosis.

Lymph is important because of its filtering properties. The body's immune system relies heavily on the fact that the lymph passes through the lymph glands and bacteria and other substances are filtered out. Table 30-20 describes diseases and disorders diagnostic procedures for

TABLE 30-20   BLOOD AND LYMPH SYSTEM DISORDERS

Disease/ Disorder	Laboratory Diagnostic Tests			Radiography	Surgery	Medical Tests or Procedures
	Blood	**Urine**	**Other**			
Anemias	• Serum iron • Complete blood count • Red blood cell count • Serum B_{12}		• Gastric analysis	• Ferrokinetic studies • Radioactive B_{12}		• Bone marrow
Hodgkin's Disease	• Complete blood count • Liver function			• Chest X ray • Lymphangiography	• Lymph node biopsy	• Bone marrow
Infectious Mononucleosis	• Complete blood count • Monoscreen • Heterophile antibody • Epstein-Barr virus • Liver Function					
Leukemia	• Complete blood count • Liver function • Platelet count • Bleeding time					• Bone marrow
Lymphedema			• Lymphangiography			

TABLE 30-21   DESCRIPTION OF BLOOD/LYMPH SYSTEM DISORDERS

- *Anemias.* All anemias are manifested by a reduction in circulating red blood cells and the amount of hemoglobin, which is the volume of packed red blood cells per 100 ml of blood. Symptoms include pallor of the skin, nailbeds, and mucous membranes; weakness; vertigo; headache; drowsiness; and general malaise.

    Iron Deficiency. Lack of reserve iron in the body and in red blood cells that lack hemoglobin resulting from inadequate dietary intake of iron, iron malabsorption, blood loss, or pregnancy.

    Pernicious anemia. Lack of intrinsic factor in the stomach secretions (hydrochloric acid). Vitamin B_{12} cannot be absorbed. Red cells cannot develop properly.

    Sickle cell anemia. A hereditary chronic anemia characterized by abnormal red blood cells causing lysis of the cells and the formation of clumps in the blood vessels, impairing circulation.

- *Hodgkin's Disease.* An idiopathic malignancy of the lymphatic system causing enlargement of lymphatic tissue, spleen, and liver. Symptoms include fever and night sweats.

- *Leukemia.* Overproduction of abnormal and immature white blood cells. Cause is unknown. Symptoms include anemia, fatigue, fever, and joint pain.

- *Lymphedema.* Abnormal accumulation of lymph in the extremities caused by obstruction of the lymphatics. Symptoms include edema in arms or legs.

blood and lymphatic system; Table 30-21 describes blood and lymph system disorders.

Common laboratory and diagnostic procedures requested by the physician include some of the following:

- *Complete Blood Count* (CBC). A routine test that includes a hemoglobin, hematocrit, and red and white blood cell count.

- *Differential.* Distinguishes among the various types of white blood cells.

- *Erythrocyte Sedimentation Rate* (SED Rate or ESR). Done to time the speed of red blood cells settling to the bottom of a test tube.

- *Platelet Count.* The number of platelets in a blood specimen.

- *Liver Function Studies.* Measure coagulation factors, prothrombin, and fibrinogen necessary for blood coagulation.

- *Schilling Test.* Radioactive vitamins B_{12} and intrinsic factor measured in 24-hour urine specimen.

Procedures to collect blood specimens and laboratory procedures are covered in Chapter 40, Venipuncture, and Chapter 41, Hematology.

INTEGUMENTARY SYSTEM

The integumentary system consists of the skin and its associated structures, such as hair, nails, nerve endings, and the sebaceous and sudoriferous glands. This system provides protection for the body against invasion of microorganisms and trauma and helps regulate body temperature. Nerve endings sense pressure, touch, and pain. Structurally, the skin consists of two layers (Figure 30-28),

which function differently from one another to perform specific activities.

- Epidermis is the outer layer of the skin that is comprised of squamous epithelium and produces keratin and the pigment melanin.

- Dermis is the inner layer of the skin made up of connective tissue and contains blood vessels, nerve endings, and glands. Provides strength and elasticity.

- Subcutaneous connective tissue (hypodermis) is the layer on which the skin and muscles lie and consists of elastic and fibrous connective tissue and adipose tissue. Guards against heat loss and provides insulation.

Skin disorders frequently produce a lesion unique to a specific skin disease, thus allowing for the diagnosis to be based on the appearance of the lesion, the patient's history, allergies, emotional well-being and inherited diseases. If the lesion appears suspicious, the physician may perform a biopsy for tissue analysis. This procedure aids in the diagnosis and treatment of specific skin disorders. Table 30-22 describes integumentary system diseases and diagnostic procedures; Table 30-23 describes skin disorders of the integumentary system.

Diagnostic procedures involving the skin range from the simple to the complex. Simple observations such as skin color, texture, size and shape of a lesion, and patient history can lead to a quick diagnosis. Confirmatory procedures such as clinical studies of urine and blood, culture of a purulent lesion, X rays, and biopsies of the affected tissues can further delineate the disease.

The clinical procedures most commonly performed by the medical assistant concerning the skin are obtaining wound cultures, the application of a sterile dressing to the wound site, and allergy skin testing.

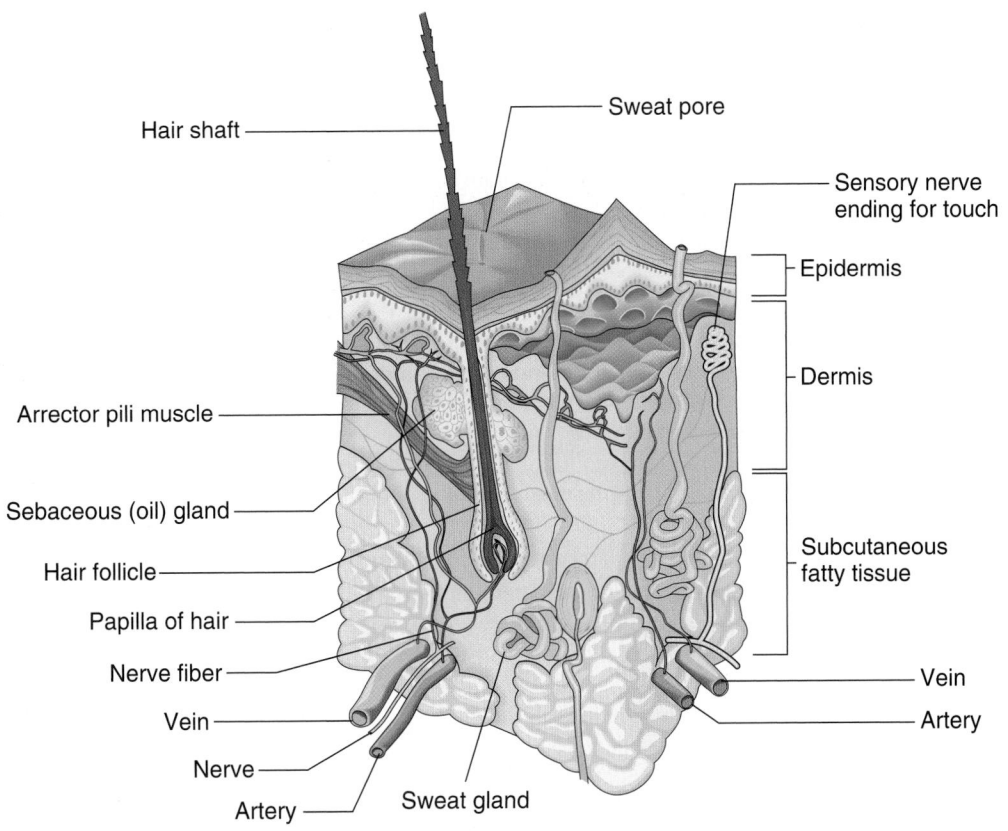

Hair shaft
Sweat pore
Sensory nerve ending for touch
Epidermis
Dermis
Arrector pili muscle
Sebaceous (oil) gland
Hair follicle
Papilla of hair
Nerve fiber
Subcutaneous fatty tissue
Vein
Vein
Artery
Nerve
Artery
Sweat gland

Figure 30-28 Cross section of skin.

TABLE 30-22	**INTEGUMENTARY SYSTEM DISORDERS**					
	Laboratory Diagnostic Tests					
Disease/ Disorder	**Blood**	**Urine**	**Other**	**Radiography**	**Surgery**	**Medical Tests or Procedures**
Abscess (Furuncle Carbuncle)	• Complete blood count • Blood glucose		• Culture and sensitivity of wound exudate		• Incision and drainage	
Acne			• Culture of skin lesions			
Corn, Callus, Wart (Verucca) Mole (nevus)					• Excisional Biopsy • Electrocautery	
Dermatitis	• Serum IgE				• Biopsy of lesion	
Dermato-phytosis			• Culture			• Wood's rays
Impetigo	• Complete blood count		• Gram stain of discharge from lesion			
Melanoma				• Chest X ray	• Biopsy of lesion	
Psoriasis					• Skin biopsy	
Scleroderma	• Sedimentation rate • Rheumatoid arthritis factor • Antinuclear antibodies	• Urinalysis • Kidney function		• Gastrointestinal • Chest		
Skin Cancer					• Biopsy of lesion	

TABLE 30-23   DESCRIPTION OF SKIN DISORDERS

- **Abscess.** Furuncle "Boil". Acute circumscribed infection of the subcutaneous tissues and surrounding tissues caused by staphylo-cocci.
  Carbuncle. A circumscribed inflammation and infection of the skin and deeper tissues accompanied by fever, leukocytosis, and sometimes prostration. Caused by staphylococcus and common in patients with diabetes.
- **Acne.** Chronic inflammatory disease caused by blocked sebaceous glands, characterized by comedones, papules, and pustules.
- **Corn and Callus.** Thickening and hyperplasia of the stratum corneum caused by pressure or friction to the affected area.
- **Dermatitis.** Caused by a specific irritant characterized by erythema or redness as in inflammation.
- **Dermatophytosis.** A highly contagious infectious fungus infection of the skin. Common on hands and feet. When feet are infected, it is known as athlete's foot or tinea pedis.
- **Herpes Zoster.** An acute infectious disease caused by varicella-zoster virus. Characterized by inflammation of the ganglia of the spinal or cranial nerves. Painful, vesicular eruptions occur along the course of the nerves.
- **Impetigo.** Contagious small pustules caused by a staphylococci or streptococci or a combination of both and spread by direct contact.
- **Melanoma.** A malignant pigmented mole. Virulent and invasive. Can be caused by ultraviolet light exposure.
- **Nevus.** A mole. Usually congenital.
- **Psoriasis.** Chronic, genetically determined dermatitis, characterized by flat reddened areas with silvery scales.
- **Scleroderma.** Progressive thickening of the skin involving collagen tissue. Systemic involvement occurs. Cause is unknown.
- **Skin Cancer.** Malignant lesions on the skin surface caused by exposure to ultraviolet rays.
- **Verruca.** A wart. Caused by a virus.

Allergy Skin Testing

When performing allergy skin tests, the likelihood of severe allergic reaction is a distinct possibility. Emergency treatment must be available immediately and consists of the following: 1) notify physician immediately; 2) have patient lie down; 3) apply constriction band above the site of allergen application to suppress absorption of allergen; 4) have epinephrine injection ready to be administered; 5) check patient's vital signs. See Chapter 9, Emergency Procedures and First Aid.

Scratch Test. The back and arms are used for this type of allergy testing. The skin surface is numbered in rows approximately 2 inches apart so that they can be identified. A small scratch is made on the surface of the skin and the allergen is placed on the scratch. As many as 50 allergens can be used at one time. A reaction to the allergen usually occurs within a half-hour. If the patient is allergic to a substance, a wheal or hive will develop at the scratch site. The site is compared to a scratch test with no allergens introduced into it, but rather an allergy-free fluid. The physician will read the results, which are graded on a scale from 2 to 4. A number 2 reaction indicates a wheal larger than the control scratch reaction (which is minimal). A number 3 is given to a larger reaction and a 4 is given to a reaction in which there are extensions of the wheal beyond the usual circumscribed area of the wheal. The allergen extract should be wiped away from the scratch area that is exhibiting a number 4 reaction.

Patch Test. The suspected allergen is placed on the skin and is covered with a square of cellophane and held in place by tape. As many as 25 tests can be done at one time and results are read in 24 to 96 hours.

Intradermal Test. A small dose (0.1cc) of an allergen is injected intradermally. Ten to fifteen tests can be done simultaneously on each arm, and the patient can suffer a severe reaction more quickly. This test is always done on the patient's forearm.

Radioallergosorbent Test (RAST). This laboratory test is obtained by venipuncture and uses radioisotopes to measure minute, specific antibodies present in the circulating blood. Scratch, patch, and intradermal testing provide immediate information about allergies and is less expensive.

Following any type of allergy skin test, the patient is told to remain in the office for 20 to 30 minutes in order to watch for an allergic reaction. If a reaction occurs, emergency medications and supplies must be readily available.

Common procedures with which the medical assistant can assist the physician are the cutaneous punch biopsy and wart and mole removal. The prime responsibilities of the medical assistant are to follow the principles of surgical aseptic technique, infection control, and standard precautions; provide the physician with the required supplies as needed; safely handle and transport the biopsy specimen; and document in patient record that biopsy was sent to the laboratory.

Procedure 30-1 — Performing a Urine Drug Screening

STANDARD PRECAUTIONS:

PURPOSE:
To accurately obtain a urine specimen from a patient for traces of drugs.

EQUIPMENT/SUPPLIES:
Urine Drug Kit (provide at least 2 choices)
Gloves
Biohazard waste container

PROCEDURE STEPS:

1. Ask patient to show a photo ID and have patient sign a consent form, keeping copies for the patient file. RATIONALE: Only the person scheduled to take the test will be able to do so.
2. Wash hands and explain procedure to the patient.
3. Supply at least two (2) collection kits from which the patient can choose one of them.
4. Have patient remove unnecessary outer garments, empty pockets, and wash and dry hands. RATIONALE: Patient cannot substitute another specimen.
5. Instruct patient to collect at least 40 mL of urine in the collection container.
6. Put on gloves. Record temperature of specimen, volume, and any contamination. RATIONALE: If fresh, specimen should be at least 98.6°F.
7. Label specimen and have patient initial specimen lid.
8. Seal specimen kit bag and have patient initial. RATIONALE: Kit bags are tamper-proof.
9. Secure sample in a locked container until pickup.
10. Collector and donor will need to sign off on the test collection procedure to document all procedure steps were followed.
11. Remove gloves and dispose of in biohazard waste container.
12. Wash hands.
13. Document procedure in patient's chart.

Procedure 30-2 — Performing a Urinary Catheterization on a Female Patient

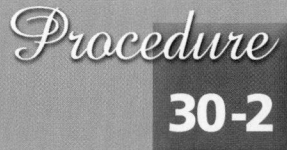

STANDARD PRECAUTIONS:

PURPOSE:
To obtain a sterile urine specimen for analysis or to relieve urine retention.

EQUIPMENT/SUPPLIES:
Catheter kit (commercially available)
Sterile gloves
Antiseptic solution (Betadine®)
Waxed paper bag
Lubricant
Sterile cotton balls
Sterile urine container with label
Sterile 2 × 2 gauze sponges
Forceps
Sterile absorbent plastic pad
Sterile catheter (size and type as ordered by physician)
Biohazard waste container
Laboratory requisition form

PROCEDURE STEPS:

1. Identify the patient and explain the procedure.
2. Instruct patient to breathe slowly and deeply during procedure. RATIONALE: This helps the

(continues)

Procedure

30-2   (*continued*)

patient relax the abdominal and pelvic muscles and facilitates easier insertion of the catheter.

3. Wash hands and assemble supplies.
4. Place catheter kit on Mayo stand near the patient.
5. Provide adequate lighting.
6. Have patient disrobe below the waist; provide a drape.
7. Position patient into a dorsal recumbent position on an exam table. RATIONALE: This allows for access to the urinary meatus.
8. Drape patient with sheet exposing only external genitalia.
9. Open outer wrapping of sterile kit.
10. Place sterile absorbent plastic pad under patient's buttocks. Place catheter tray between patient's legs.
11. Ask patient to keep knees apart. RATIONALE: This position provides good visualization of the urinary meatus.
12. Wash hands and put on sterile gloves.
13. Pour Betadine® over three cotton balls in appropriate compartment of the kit.
14. Open urine specimen container.
15. Apply sterile lubricant to a gauze sponge and place tip of catheter in lubricant and other end of catheter into the sterile basin.
16. Remind patient to breathe slowly. Spread labia with nondominant hand. Dominant hand remains sterile. With dominant hand and sterile forceps, wipe genitalia with each of the three antiseptic soaked cotton balls, with a front to back motion. First, wipe the right labia using front to back motion. Discard cotton ball into waxed paper bag that is placed away from sterile area. Second, wipe the left labia repeating procedure and last, wipe down the center discarding cotton ball after each wipe. Discard forceps. Continue to hold labia apart until catheter is inserted. RATIONALE: Holding labia open will keep urinary meatus from becoming contaminated from labia while inserting catheter.

17. Using sterile gloved hand, pick up catheter and hold it about 3 to 4 inches from lubricated end.
18. Gently insert lubricated tip of catheter into urinary meatus approximately 6 inches or until urine begins to flow. Move nondominant hand to hold catheter in place.
19. Interrupt urine flow by clamping off. RATIONALE: Stop flow of urine while specimen container is positioned.
20. Position end of catheter into urine specimen container.
21. Collect specimen by releasing clamp and collecting approximately 60 ml of urine.
22. Allow remaining urine to flow into basin until flow ceases. Pinch catheter closed.
23. Remove catheter gently and slowly.
24. Dry area with remaining cotton balls.
25. Tighten lid on the urine specimen container.
26. Remove procedure items.
27. Position patient for comfort.
28. Assist patient in sitting up or relaxing in a horizontal recumbent position.
29. Allow patient to remain lying down. Help patient to sit on edge of table. Check patient's color and pulse.
30. Discard disposable items per OSHA guidelines.
31. If collecting specimen for analysis, label specimen container and attach to completed laboratory requisition form.
32. Assist patient from exam table.
33. Clean room and table. Remove gloves and discard in biohazard waste container.
34. Wash hands.
35. Document procedure in patient's chart including the amount of urine collected. Document that specimen was sent to outside laboratory (if appropriate).

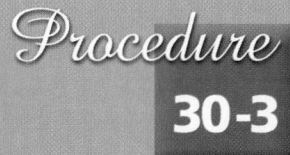 **Performing a Urinary Catheterization on a Male Patient**

30-3

STANDARD PRECAUTIONS:

PURPOSE:
To obtain a sterile urine specimen for analysis or to relieve urine retention.

EQUIPMENT/SUPPLIES:
Catheter kit (commercially available)
Sterile gloves
Antiseptic solution (Betadine®)
Waxed paper bag
Lubricant
Sterile cotton balls
Sterile urine container with label
Sterile 2 × 2 gauze sponges
Forceps
Sterile absorbent plastic pad
Sterile catheter (size and type as ordered by physician)
Biohazard waste container
Laboratory requisition form

PROCEDURE STEPS:
1. Identify the patient and explain the procedure.
2. Instruct patient to breathe slowly and deeply during procedure. RATIONALE: This helps the patient relax the abdominal and pelvic muscles and facilitates easier insertion of the catheter.
3. Wash hands and assemble supplies.
4. Place catheter kit on Mayo stand near the patient.
5. Provide adequate lighting.
6. Have patient disrobe below the waist; provide a drape.
7. Position patient into a dorsal recumbent position on an exam table. RATIONALE: This allows for access to the urinary meatus.
8. Drape patient with sheet exposing only external genitalia.
9. Open outer wrapping of sterile kit.
10. Place sterile underpad under patient's penis. Figure 30-29A. RATIONALE: Provides sterile field.
11. Wash hands. Put on sterile gloves.
12. Open fenestrated drape and, being careful not to contaminate drape or gloves, position drape opening over penis. Figure 30-29B.
13. Place sterile pad on table top or onto Mayo stand and empty contents of kit onto it.
14. Apply sterile lubricant to a sterile gauze sponge and place tip of catheter in lubricant and the end of catheter into sterile kit.
15. With nondominant hand, hold the penis below the glans. In uncircumcised males, the glans must be pulled pack to expose the meatus. This is done entirely with the nondominant hand. RATIONALE: The dominant hand remains sterile so as not to contaminate remaining sterile equipment.

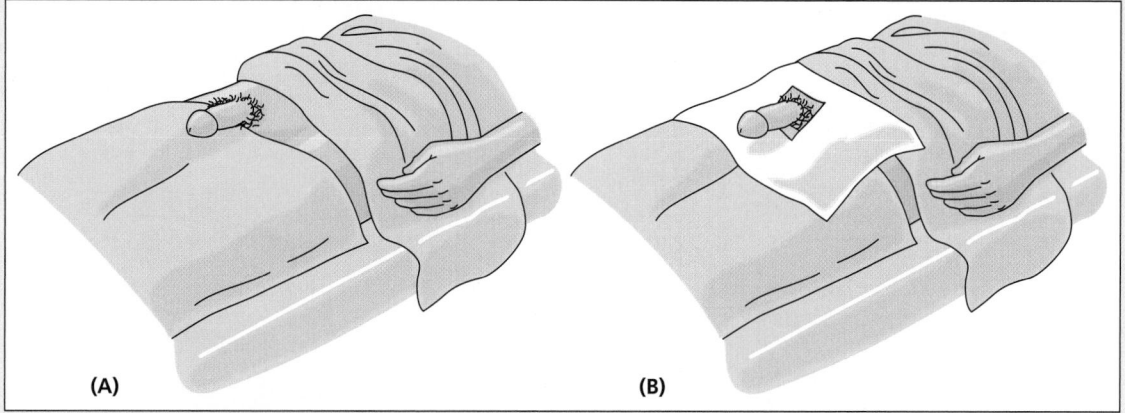

(A) (B)

Figure 30-29 (A) Place sterile underpad under patient's penis. (B) Open fenestrated drape. Being careful not to contaminate drape or gloves, position drape opening over penis.

(continues)

Procedure

30-3   *(continued)*

16. With the dominant hand, take the sterile forceps and a cotton ball that has been dipped in Betadine®, clean around the meatus in a circular motion from center toward outside. Use all three cotton balls and Betadine®. Figure 30-30.
RATIONALE: Assures that as many microorganisms as possible will be removed from the meatus and surrounding areas before insertion of sterile catheter.

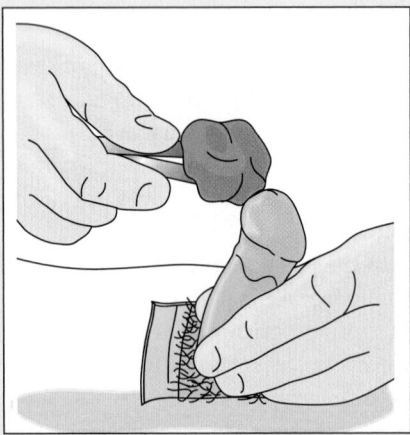

Figure 30-30 With the dominant hand, take the sterile forceps and a cotton ball dipped in Betadine® and clean around the meatus in a circular motion from center toward outside. Use all three cotton balls and Betadine®.

17. With the dominant hand, take catheter out of lubricant and while holding the penis upright and straight with the nondominant hand, insert the catheter approximately 6″ until the urine flows into the sterile kit. Figure 30-31A.
RATIONALE: Holding the penis upright and straight facilitates insertion of the catheter.
CAUTION: Do not force catheter. If problems arise attempting insertion, do not continue with procedure.
18. Obtain a specimen if ordered. Figure 30-31B.
19. After urine flow ceases, remove catheter gently and slowly.
20. Dry penis with remaining cotton ball(s).
21. Position patient for comfort.
22. Discard disposable items per OSHA guidelines.
23. If collecting specimen for analysis, label specimen container and attach to completed laboratory requisition form.
24. Assist patient from exam table.
25. Clean room and table. Remove gloves and discard in biohazard waste container.
26. Wash hands.
27. Document procedure in patient's chart including the amount of urine collected. Document that specimen was sent to outside laboratory (if appropriate).

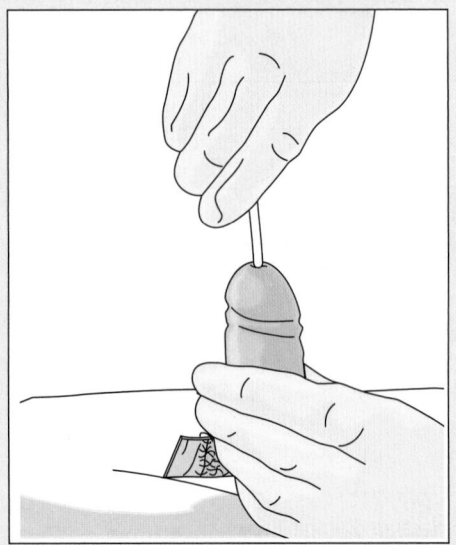

(A)

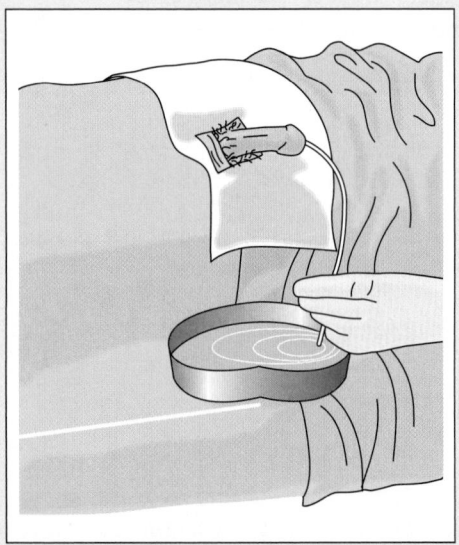

(B)

Figure 30-31 (A) With the dominant hand, take catheter out of lubricant and while holding the penis upright and straight with the nondominant hand, insert the catheter approximately 6″ until the urine flows into the sterile kit. (B) Obtain a specimen if ordered.

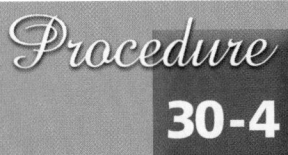

30-4 Assisting with Proctosigmoidoscopy

STANDARD PRECAUTIONS:

PURPOSE:
To assist the physician in assessing the status of the sigmoid colon and rectum for signs of disease such as tumors, polyps, ulcerations, hemorrhoids, or rectal bleeding.

EQUIPMENT/SUPPLIES:
Sigmoidoscope with obturator, either a flexible fiber-optic sigmoidoscope or a rigid sigmoidoscope
Sterile biopsy forceps
Patient gown
Sterile specimen container w/preservative
Laboratory requisition form
Tissues
Biohazard waste container
Patient drape
Small pillow
Anoscope
Rectal speculum
Insufflator
Suction machine and tip
Probe with bulb tip
Gloves
Finger cots
Long cotton applicators
Lubricating jelly
Basin of water
4 × 4 gauze sponges

PROCEDURE STEPS:
1. Wash hands and prepare equipment and supplies.
2. Check the lights on the illuminated instruments for loose bulbs by turning the bulb clockwise. Turn the switch to the on position to verify the light is working. Turn off light.
3. Label specimen container with patient's name, address, date, and source.
4. Check to see that obturators are correctly positioned.
5. Have a basin ready to receive used instruments.
6. Prepare a basin of water to rinse out suction tubing.

7. Test suction machine.
8. Prepare patient. Be sure patient has been properly prepared; i.e., necessary laxative taken, enema administered, and adequate results obtained from enema.
9. Identify patient.
10. Verify consent form has been signed.
11. Explain procedure to the patient. RATIONALE: Reassuring the patient promotes relaxation and reduces apprehension.
12. Ask patient to empty bladder and save specimen (if required). RATIONALE: Facilitates examination and is more comfortable for patient.
13. Ask patient to disrobe and put on gown.
14. Assist patient into the knee-chest position or Sims' lateral position which assures accessibility to the rectum and sigmoid colon. Some physicians have special proctologic tables that tilt the patient into knee-chest position. RATIONALE: Abdominal contents tip forward and away from pelvic area, making it easier to insert the sigmoidoscope.
15. Drape the patient and place small towel directly over the anus and under the perineal area or use a fenestrated drape over the anus.
16. Apply gloves and assist the doctor during examination.
17. Place lubricant on physician's gloves for digital examination.
18. Warm metal scope by placing in warm water for a few minutes.
19. Lubricate scope tip.
20. Plug in scope when physician is ready to use. RATIONALE: Plugging in too soon allows the light source to get too hot and may harm the patient.
21. Remind the patient to take slow deep breaths to promote relaxation of muscles to facilitate insertion of the sigmoidoscope.
22. Attach inflation bulb.
23. Attach light source.
24. Observe patient throughout procedure. Provide support and reassurance.
25. Take instruments from physician as needed.

(continues)

Procedure 30-4 (continued)

26. Pass long cotton-tipped applicators to the physician and assist with suction equipment.
27. Place suction tubing in basin of water.
28. Place instruments in basin.
29. Assist with collection of biopsy by handing biopsy forceps to the physician. Do not touch inside of specimen container. RATIONALE: Container is sterile and will become contaminated if inside is touched. Inaccurate results may occur.
    a. Receive and care for specimen. Label properly.
30. Clean patient's anus with tissue.
31. Remove gloves. Wash hands.
32. Assist patient to supine position after examination. Do not let patient rise too rapidly because of the possibility of dizziness. Check patient's blood pressure. RATIONALE: Vagal nerve stimulation may cause shocklike symptoms, or orthostatic hypotension can occur from lying flat for extended period.
33. Assist patient to dress if needed.
34. Apply gloves.
35. Transport specimen with completed lab requisition form.
36. Clean room and equipment following OSHA guidelines. Flexible sigmoidoscope should be sanitized and subjected to cold sterilization according to manufacturer's directions. Metal (rigid) sigmoidoscope must be sanitized and sterilized in the autoclave.
37. Remove gloves and wash hands.
38. Document procedure in patient's chart.

Procedure 30-5   Fecal Occult Blood Test

STANDARD PRECAUTIONS:

PURPOSE:
To test feces for occult blood.

EQUIPMENT/SUPPLIES:
3 guaiac slide test kits containing three slides, applicators, and envelope

PROCEDURE STEPS:
1. Check expiration dates on occult slides. RATIONALE: Outdated slides can give an inaccurate reading.
2. Identify the patient.
3. Fill out all information on the front flap of all three slides (Figure 30-32).
4. Explain the stool collection process; the patient will need to:

a. Keep slides at room temperature away from sunlight. RATIONALE: Sunlight destroys effectiveness of guaiac paper and could result in an inaccurate result.
b. Open the front flap of the first slide.

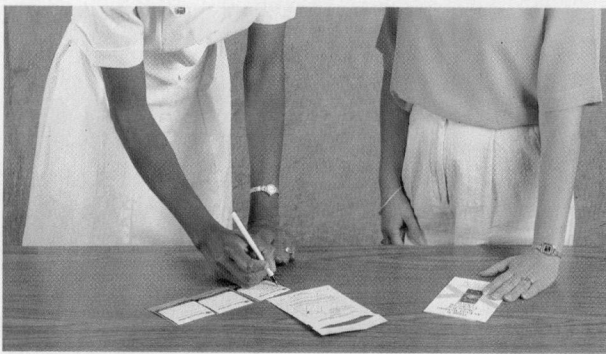

Figure 30-32   Medical assistant writes patient name, date, and specimen numbers on each hemoccult slide.

(continues)

Procedure 30-5 *(continued)*

c. Use one end of the wooden applicator to apply a thin smear of the stool sample from the toilet to Box "A." Note: *Do not collect during menstrual cycle or if hemorrhoids are present.*

d. Repeat the procedure using the other end of the applicator, taking a specimen from a different section of the same stool and applying a thin smear to Box "B." RATIONALE: Occult blood may be distributed differently throughout the bowel movement.

e. Dispose of the applicator in a waste container.

f. Close the cover after air drying overnight.

g. Date the front flap.

h. Repeat the process with the next two bowel movements, on subsequent days.

5. Provide the patient with an envelope to return the slides to the physician's office (Figure 30-33).

6. Record that the test kit and instructions were given to patient.

Developing the fecal occult slide

When the patient returns the fecal occult samples to the office, the medical assistant will be responsible for developing the slides. Although most slides may be stored for up to 14 days before developing, the medical assistant should develop them as soon as possible because the patient may have already stored them for several days. Test results are important to ensure prompt treatment should a problem be discovered.

EQUIPMENT/SUPPLIES:
Prepared fecal slides from patient
Occult blood developer
Reference card that accompanies kit
Gloves
Biohazard waste container

PROCEDURE STEPS:
1. Check the expiration date on the developer.
2. Apply gloves.
3. Open the window flap on the back of the slide.
4. Apply two drops of the developer to each Box "A" and "B," directly over each smear (Figure 30-34). RATIONALE: Paper contains the chemical guaiac, which will help identify occult blood.
5. Interpret the results within 30 to 60 seconds. Record the results.
6. A positive reaction will have a blue halo appear around the perimeter of the specimen.

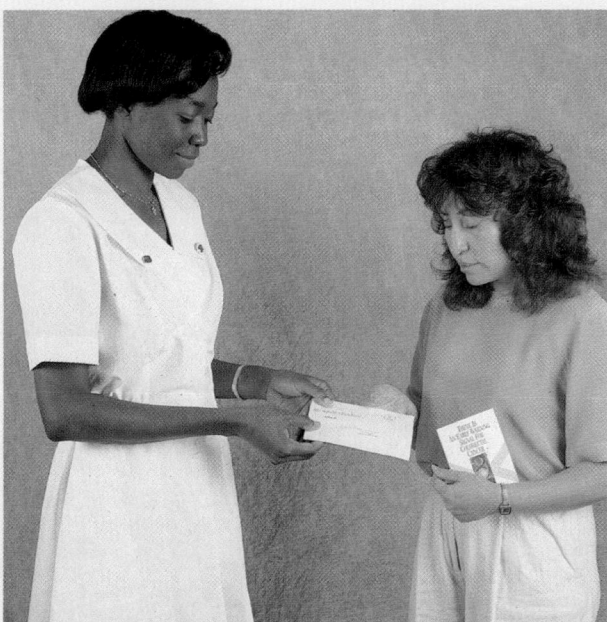

Figure 30-33 Medical assistant has put the three hemoccult slides and wooden applicators into a preaddressed envelope which the patient will use to return slides to the office. Patient also has been given instructions for collecting the three samples, which can be obtained at home.

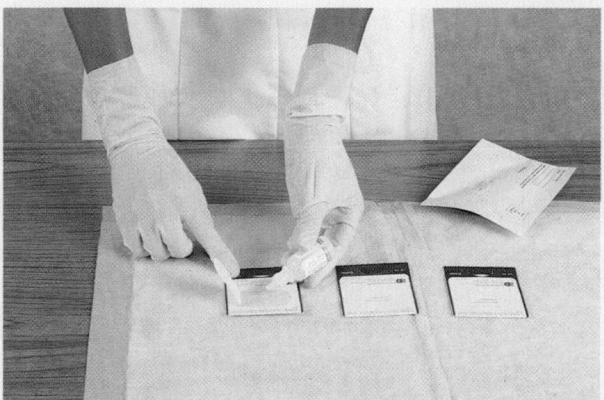

Figure 30-34 The medical assistant has removed three hemoccult slides from envelope received from a patient and places developing solution on the slide.

(continues)

Procedure 30-5 (continued)

7. Perform the quality control procedure by processing the positive and negative monitor strip on each slide to confirm the test system is functional. RATIONALE: Failure of the positive strip to turn blue or negative strip to remain neutral indicates faulty supplies. Recheck expiration dates on slide and developer. Repeat test if necessary.

8. Dispose of all supplies according to OSHA guidelines.
9. Remove gloves and dispose in biohazard waste container.
10. Wash hands.
11. Document results in patient's chart.

Procedure 30-6 Performing Visual Acuity Testing Using a Snellen Chart

STANDARD PRECAUTIONS:

PURPOSE:
To perform a visual screening test to determine a patient's distance visual acuity.

EQUIPMENT/SUPPLIES:
Snellen eye chart placed at eye level (appropriate for age and reading ability of patient)
Pointer
Occluder
Alcohol wipes

PROCEDURE STEPS:
1. Wash hands and assemble equipment.
2. Prepare a well-lighted room, free from distractions and with a distance mark 20 feet from the eye chart.
3. Explain the procedure to the patient. Patients should be tested with their glasses or contact lenses, unless otherwise indicated by the physician.
4. Instruct the patient to stand behind the mark and cover the left eye with the occluder (Figure 30-35). Instruct the patient to keep the left eye open under the occluder and not to apply pressure to the eyeball. RATIONALE: Closing of the eye not being tested may cause the person to squint when reading the chart.
5. Stand next to the chart and point to row 3 instructing the patient to read each letter with the right eye, verbally identifying each letter read (Figure 30-36). If unable to read line 3, go

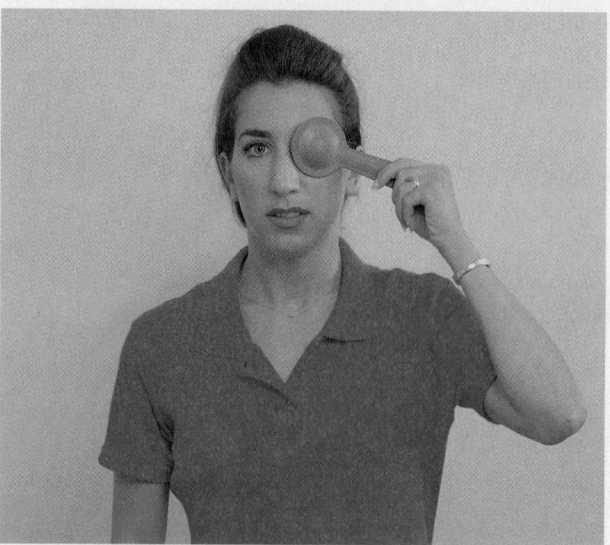

Figure 30-35 The patient covers the left eye with the occluder, keeping the eye open under the occluder.

(continues)

Procedure 30-6 *(continued)*

to line 2 or 1. RATIONALE: Pointing to each row helps the patient to focus on one row of letters at a time. Beginning at row 3 saves time.

6. Record the results at the smallest line the patient can read with two or fewer errors. Vision is recorded as right eye, left eye, both eyes.

   Examples: OD 20/25; OS 20/20; OU 20/20

   RATIONALE: Visual acuity is recorded as a fraction. The number above the line on the chart is the distance the patient is standing from the chart. The number below the line on the chart is the distance from which a person with normal vision can read that row of letters.

7. Record the patient's reaction during the test. RATIONALE: Leaning forward, squinting or straining, or eye tears may indicate eye problems.

8. When finished with the examination of the right eye, use the same procedure to test the left eye.

9. Wipe occluder with alcohol. Wash hands. Record the results.

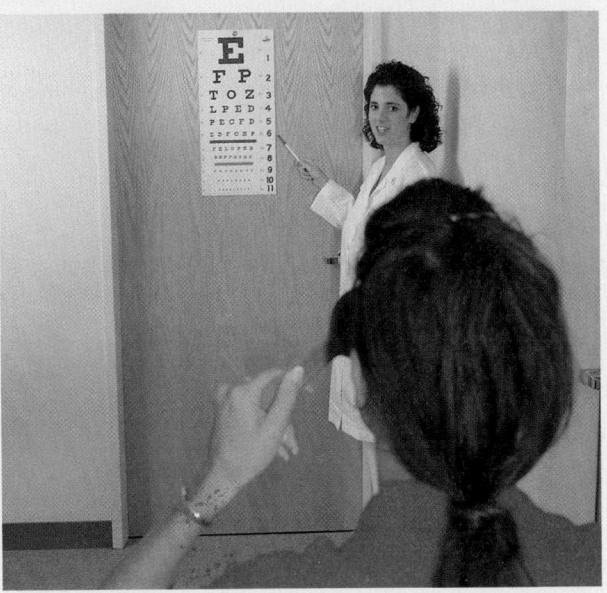

Figure 30-36 The patient uses the right eye to read the letters on the chart. The patient is instructed to start with row 3. Here she is reading row 6.

Procedure 30-7 **Measuring Near Visual Acuity**

STANDARD PRECAUTIONS:

PURPOSE:
To measure the near vision of the patient.

EQUIPMENT/SUPPLIES:
Appropriate near visual acuity chart
3 × 5 cards or occluder

PROCEDURE STEPS:
1. Wash hands.
2. Identify patient.
3. Explain procedure to patient; provide occluder. RATIONALE: To obtain patient cooperation.

4. Position patient in a comfortable position.
5. Position the near visual acuity card 14 inches from the patient by measuring with a tape measure. RATIONALE: To obtain accurate results.
6. Have patient lightly (no pressure) cover the left eye with the occluder. RATIONALE: Pressure will cause blurring of the other eye.
7. Have patient read the paragraphs printed on the card.
8. Once patient has reached a line where more than two mistakes are made, note the visual acuity for that eye (allow the patient to repeat the line to verify acuity).

(continues)

Procedure **30-7** *(continued)*

9. Repeat the process to measure the left eye.
10. Repeat the process to measure both eyes.
11. Record the result in the patient chart. Results are charted 14/14 for normal near visual acuity.
12. Discard the 3 × 5 card or disinfect the occluder. RATIONALE: To prevent microorganism cross-contamination.
13. Wash hands.
14. Record results.

Procedure **30-8** Performing Color Vision Test Using the Ishihara Plates

STANDARD PRECAUTIONS:

PURPOSE:
To assess a patient's ability to distinguish between the colors red and green.

Patient Education:
1. Explain that the purpose of the test is to determine if the patient has a color vision deficiency.
2. Show patient plate number twelve as an example of the test process.

EQUIPMENT/SUPPLIES:
Ishihara plates (1–12) (Figure 30-37)

PROCEDURE STEPS:
1. Wash hands and assemble the equipment in a room lighted by daylight. RATIONALE: Direct sunlight or electric light may produce errors in the results because of an alteration in the appearance of shades of color.

2. Hold each plate 75 cm or 30 inches from the patient and tilted so that the plane of the plate is at a right angle to the line of the patient's vision (Figure 30-38).
3. Record the number given by the patient on each plate.

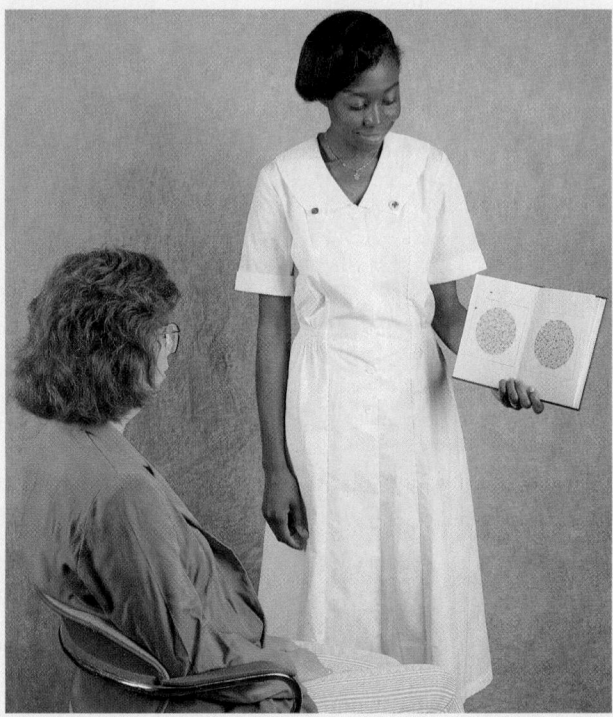

Figure 30-38 The medical assistant holds the plate 30 inches, or 75 cm, from the patient and tilts the card so that the plane of the plate is at a right angle with the line of the patient's vision.

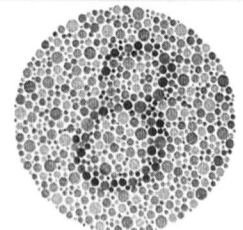 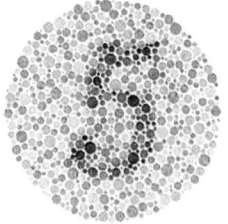

Figure 30-37 Ishihara plates are used to assess the patient's ability to distinguish between the colors red and green.

(continues)

Procedure 30-8 (continued)

4. Assess the patient's readings and record. RATIONALE: If ten or more plates are read correctly, the color vision is regarded as normal.
   Source for Error: Test plates should be kept covered when not in use. Undue exposure to sunlight causes a fading of the color plates, thus leading to inaccurate test interpretation.

Procedure 30-9 Performing Eye Instillation

STANDARD PRECAUTIONS:

PURPOSE:
To treat eye infections, soothe irritation, anesthetize, and dilate pupils. Ophthalmic medication is supplied in liquid or ointment form. Use separate medication for each eye, if both are affected.

EQUIPMENT/SUPPLIES:
Sterile eye dropper
Sterile ophthalmic medication as ordered by the physician, either drops or ointment
Sterile cotton balls
Sterile gloves

PROCEDURE STEPS:
1. Wash hands.
2. Assemble supplies using sterile technique.
3. Check medication carefully as ordered by the physician, including expiration date. Read label three times.
4. Identify patient.
5. Explain procedure to the patient and inform the patient that instillation may temporarily blur vision.
6. Position the patient in a sitting or lying position.
7. Instruct the patient to stare at a fixed spot during instillation of the drops.
8. Prepare medication using either drops or ointment.
9. Have the patient look up to the ceiling and expose the lower conjunctival sac of the affected eye by using fingers over a tissue to pull down (Figure 30-39).
10. Place the number of drops ordered in the center of the lower conjunctival sac or a thin line of ointment in the lower surface of the eyelid being careful not to touch the eyelid, eyeball, or eyelashes with the tip of the medication applicator. Carefully replace dropper in bottle to avoid contamination.
11. Have the patient close the eye and roll the eyeball. RATIONALE: Movement distributes the medication evenly.
12. Blot excess medication from eyelids with cotton ball from inner to outer canthus.
13. Dispose of supplies.
14. Wash hands.
15. Record procedure in patient's chart.

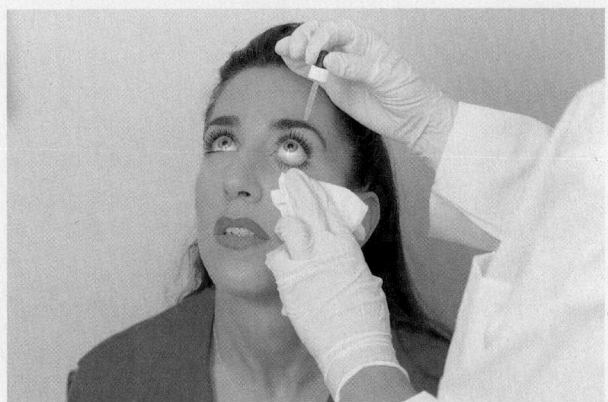

Figure 30-39 When instilling medication into the patient's eye, the patient should look up to the ceiling and the medical assistant should pull down on the lower lid. Contact with the eyeball should be avoided.

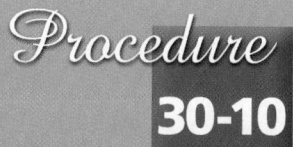

Performing Eye Patch Dressing Application

30-10

STANDARD PRECAUTIONS:

PURPOSE:
To apply a sterile eye patch.

EQUIPMENT/SUPPLIES:
Tape
Sterile eye patch
Sterile gloves

PROCEDURE STEPS:
1. Wash hands and assemble supplies.
2. Identify patient.
3. Explain the procedure.
4. Position the patient in a sitting or supine position.
5. Instruct the patient to close both eyes during the application of the patch. Prepare sterile area by opening the sterile package and using the inside of the package as a sterile field. Apply sterile gloves.
6. Place the patch over the affected eye using sterile gloves.
7. Secure the patch with 3 to 4 strips of transparent tape diagonally from mid-forehead to below the ear.
8. Remove gloves.
9. Wash hands.
10. Document the procedure and provide verbal and written care instructions to the patient.

Performing Eye Irrigation

30-11

STANDARD PRECAUTIONS:

PURPOSE:
To irrigate the patient's affected eye.
  a. To cleanse of a foreign object
  b. To cleanse discharge
  c. To remove chemicals
  d. To apply antiseptic
  e. To apply heat

EQUIPMENT/SUPPLIES:
Sterile irrigation solution as ordered by the physician
Sterile bulb syringe (rubber)
Kidney-shaped basin to catch irrigation solution
Sterile cotton balls
Sterile gloves
Biohazard waste container
Towel
Pillow

PROCEDURE STEPS:
1. Wash hands and assemble supplies. Note: If both eyes need to be irrigated, use separate equipment for each eye. RATIONALE: Avoid cross-contamination.
2. Identify patient.
3. Explain the procedure to the patient.
4. Position the patient in a supine position.
5. Check expiration date on solution bottle.
6. Check label three times. Warm solution to body temperature (98.6°F).
7. Tilt head toward affected eye. Place towel on patient shoulder. RATIONALE: Avoid cross-contamination of unaffected eye by allowing the solution to flow from the affected eye into the kidney basin.
8. Place the basin beside the affected eye. RATIONALE: Allows for the solution to drain into a catch receptacle.
9. Put on sterile gloves.

(continues)

Procedure 30-11 *(continued)*

10. Moisten 2 to 3 cotton balls with irrigation solution and clean the eyelids and eyelashes of the affected eye from inner to outer canthus. Discard after each wipe.
11. Expose the lower conjunctiva by separating the eyelid with your index finger and thumb.
12. Have the patient stare at a fixed spot.
13. Irrigate the affected eye with sterile solution by resting the sterile bulb syringe on the bridge of the patient's nose being careful not to touch the eye or conjunctival sac with the syringe tip. Allow the stream to flow from the inside canthus to the outer corner of the eye (Figure 30-40). RATIONALE: This avoids a flow of solution into the unaffected eye causing cross contamination.
14. After irrigation, dry the eyelid and eyelashes with sterile cotton balls.
15. Discard supplies in biohazard container if discharge or exudate is present.
16. Remove gloves.
17. Wash hands and document procedure.

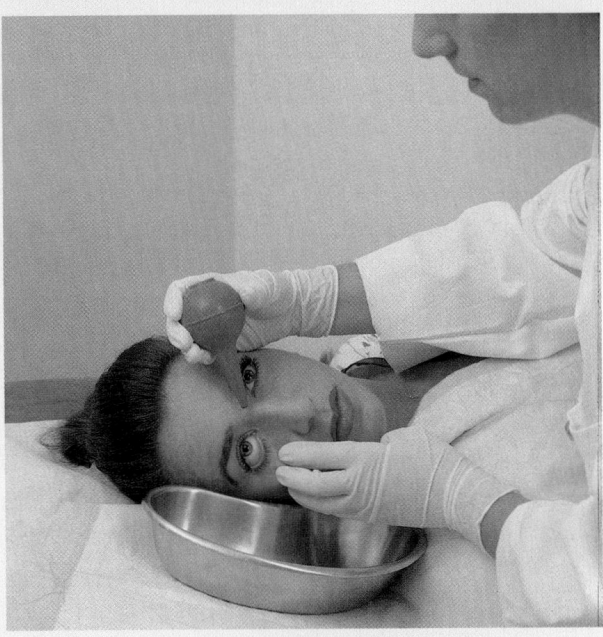

Figure 30-40 The medical assistant irrigates the patient's eye. Note that the solution will go from inner to outer canthus. The patient is turned toward the affected eye.

Procedure 30-12 **Assisting with Audiometry**

STANDARD PRECAUTIONS:

PURPOSE:
To assist in testing patient for hearing loss.
Patient Education:
1. Explain the use and purpose of the audiometer and that the test measures frequency of sound waves and ability of patient to hear various frequencies of sound waves (one frequency at a time).
2. When the patient hears a new frequency, he is to signal the tester.

EQUIPMENT/SUPPLIES:
Audiometer with head phones
Quiet room

PROCEDURE STEPS:
1. Wash hands and assemble equipment and supplies.
2. Prepare room. Test must be held in a room without outside noises. RATIONALE: Outside interference may cause inaccurate test results, especially in the lower frequencies which are more difficult to hear.
3. Explain procedure to patient.

(continues)

Procedure 30-12 *(continued)*

4. Position patient in a comfortable sitting position.
5. Have patient put on head phones. The procedure is done on each ear separately.
6. If the medical assistant has been thoroughly trained to do the procedure, the physician will allow the medical assistant to perform the audiometry. The audiometer is started at low frequency. The patient indicates when the sound is heard and the medical assistant plots it on the graph (the audiogram) (Figure 30-41).
7. The frequencies gradually increase until completed.
8. The other ear is checked in the same manner.
9. The results are given to the physician for interpretation.
10. Equipment is cleaned following manufacturer's instructions.
11. Wash hands.
12. Document procedure on patient's chart.

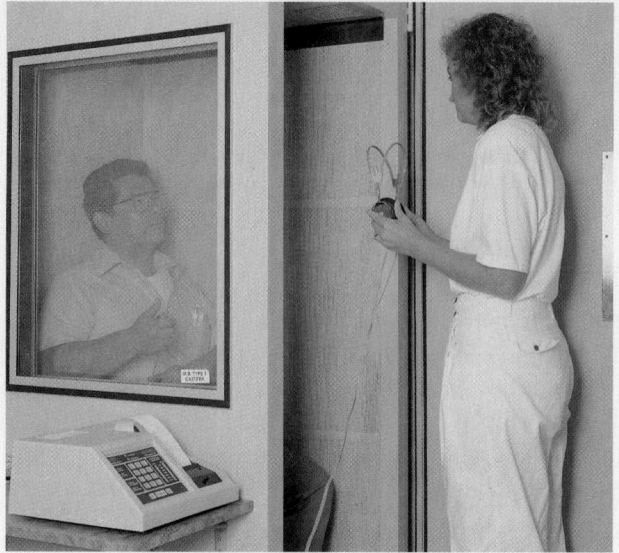

Figure 30-41 The patient presses the handheld control button each time he hears a sound. The medical assistant plots sounds heard on the audiogram.

Procedure 30-13 **Performing Ear Irrigation**

STANDARD PRECAUTIONS:

PURPOSE:
To remove impacted cerumen, discharge, or foreign materials from the ear canal as directed by the physician.

EQUIPMENT/SUPPLIES:
Irrigation solution as ordered by the physician warmed to body temperature (98.6°F).
Ear syringe or bulb
Ear basin or emesis basin
Basin for warmed solution
Towel
Cotton balls
Otoscope

PROCEDURE STEPS:
1. Wash hands and assemble equipment.
2. Identify patient.
3. Explain the procedure and inform the patient that during the procedure a minimal amount of discomfort and dizziness may be experienced caused by solution coming into contact with the tympanic membrane.
4. Place the patient in a sitting position with head tilted toward affected ear and use an otoscope to visualize the affected ear.
5. Cleanse the outer ear with a wet cotton ball moistened with irrigation solution.
6. Gently pull the auricle upward and back in order to straighten the ear canal.

(continues)

Procedure

30-13   *(continued)*

7. Tilt the patient's head slightly forward and to the affected side (Figure 30-42). RATIONALE: This position allows the solution to flow into the basin by gravity.

8. Place towel on the patient's shoulder of the affected side.

9. Place the ear basin under the affected ear and have the patient hold the basin in place.

10. Check label of solution three times for correctness and also check the expiration date of the solution.

11. Pour the solution into a basin and fill the syringe with the warmed irrigation solution as prescribed by the physician. Use about 30 to 50 cc of solution at a time. (Repeat Step 5.)

12. Straighten the external auditory canal by pulling back and upward on the auricle for adults.

13. Expel air from syringe and gently insert the syringe tip into the affected ear, being careful not to insert too deeply. Do not occlude external auditory canal. Direct the flow of the solution upward toward roof of canal. RATIONALE: This will avoid injury to the tympanic membrane and prevent occlusion of external auditory canal, allowing solution to drain out.

14. Repeat the irrigation allowing the solution to drain from the ear, noting the return. Allow for free flow of return each time.

15. Dry the outer ear and visualize the inner ear with the otoscope to verify the procedure has removed or dislodged the foreign body.

16. Notify the physician the procedure has been completed.

17. When the procedure is completed, remove the ear basin and towel.

18. Have patient lie on affected side on exam table for ear to continue draining.

19. Provide dry cotton balls to the patient to catch any further drainage if directed by the physician.

20. Dispose of supplies.

21. Wash hands.

22. Document the procedure noting return and amount. Provide postcare instructions:
    a. Report any pain or dizziness to the physician.
    b. Do not insert any foreign object (i.e., cotton applicator) into the ear canal.

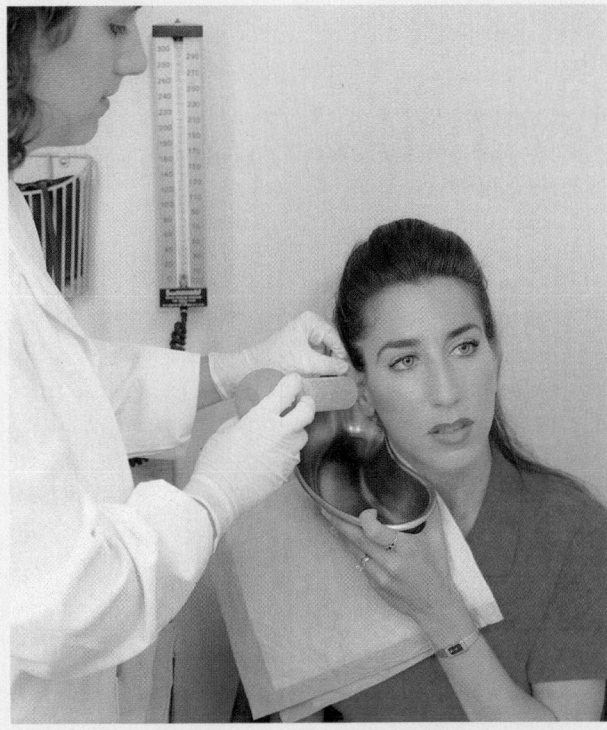

Figure 30-42   When irrigating the patient's ear, the affected ear is tipped to facilitate the flow of solution. The tip of the syringe does not occlude the opening to the external auditory canal.

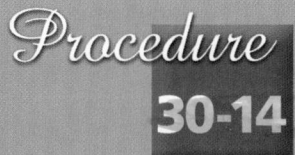

30-14   Performing Ear Instillation

STANDARD PRECAUTIONS:

PURPOSE:
To soften impacted cerumen, fight infection with antibiotics, or relieve pain.

EQUIPMENT/SUPPLIES:
Otic medication as prescribed by the physician
Sterile ear dropper
Cotton balls
Gloves

PROCEDURE STEPS:
1. Wash hands and assemble supplies.
2. Identify patient.
3. Explain procedure to the patient.
4. Position patient to either lie on unaffected side or sitting position with head tilted toward unaffected ear. RATIONALE: Facilitates flow of medication.
5. Check otic medication three times against the physician's order and check expiration date of the medication. RATIONALE: Only otic medication can be used in the ear. Checking the medication three times minimizes medication error.
6. Draw up the prescribed amount of medication.
7. Gently pull the top of the ear upward and back (adult) or pull earlobe downward and backward (child) (Figure 30-43).

8. Instill prescribed dose of medication (number of drops) by squeezing rubber bulb on dropper into the affected ear.
9. Have the patient maintain the position for about 5 minutes to retain medication.
10. When instructed by the physician, insert moistened cotton ball into external ear canal for 15 minutes. RATIONALE: Moistened cotton ball will not absorb medication and will help retain medication in ear.
11. Dispose of supplies.
12. Wash hands.
13. Document procedure.

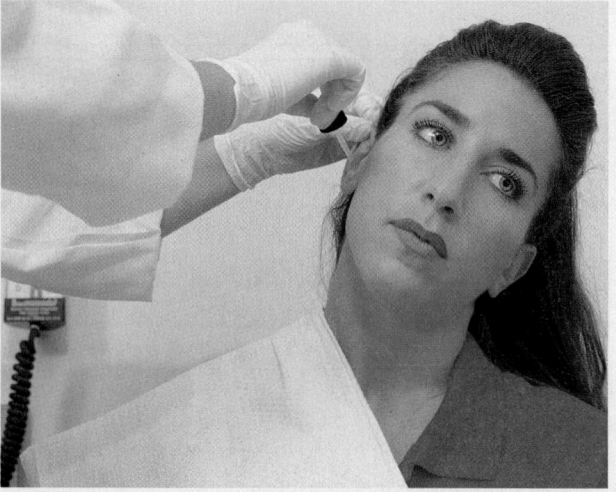

Figure 30-43   When instilling drops into patient's ear, have the patient tilt head so the affected ear is uppermost.

30-15   Assisting with Nasal Examination

STANDARD PRECAUTIONS:

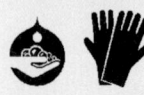

PURPOSE:
To assist the physician with the nasal exam when looking for polyps, engorged superficial blood vessels, and to assist in the possible removal of a foreign body.

(continues)

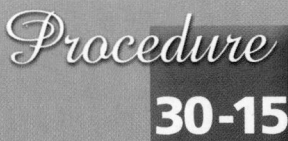

Procedure 30-15 (continued)

Patient Education:
When a foreign object is involved, instruct the patient not to blow the nose or to attempt to remove the object because this could cause tissue damage or push the object deeper into the nasal passage.

EQUIPMENT/SUPPLIES:
Nasal speculum
Light source
Gloves
Bayonet forceps
Kidney basin

PROCEDURE STEPS:
1. Wash hands and assemble supplies.
2. Identify patient.
3. Explain the procedure to the patient.
4. Place the patient in a sitting position.
5. Reassure the patient.
6. Hand the physician equipment and supplies as needed.
7. Clean equipment and dispose of supplies per OSHA guidelines.
8. Wash hands.
9. Document procedure noting foreign object if applicable.

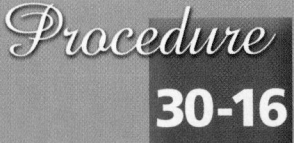

Procedure 30-16 Performing Nasal Irrigation

STANDARD PRECAUTIONS:

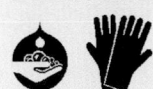

PURPOSE:
To remove a foreign body, relieve inflammation, or increase drainage.
Patient Education:
Instruct the patient not to blow the nose for 5 minutes after the procedure. RATIONALE: Blowing the nose could force the solution into the sinuses or ears.

EQUIPMENT/SUPPLIES:
Bulb-tip syringe
Emesis basin
Basins for irrigation solution
Towels
Nonsterile gloves

PROCEDURE STEPS:
1. Wash hands and assemble supplies.
2. Identify patient.
3. Explain the procedure to the patient.
4. Warm irrigation solution to 98.6°F.
5. Position the patient with head slightly tilted in a sitting position. RATIONALE: Promotes nasal drainage.
6. Place towel across patient's chest and shoulders to absorb solution that may splash.
7. Have the patient hold the emesis basin under the nose.
8. Pour warmed irrigation solution into a basin and withdraw the irrigating solution into the bulb syringe.
9. Insert the tip of the syringe into the affected nostril and gently squeeze the bulb. Do not occlude nostril.
10. Repeat until the required amount of solution has been used.
11. When complete, assist the patient. Give the patient a towel to wipe the face.
12. Dispose of supplies per OSHA guidelines.
13. Wash hands.
14. Document the procedure.

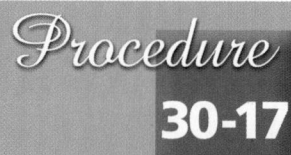

30-17   Performing Nasal Instillation

STANDARD PRECAUTIONS:

PURPOSE:
To provide medication to the nose as ordered by the physician.
Patient Education:
1. Instruct the patient to keep the head tilted back during the procedure to allow the medication to cover the nasal tissues.
2. Do not blow nose immediately following treatment. Medication will be forced out of nose.

EQUIPMENT/SUPPLIES:
Medication as ordered by physician
Medicine dropper
Cotton balls or 2 × 2 gauze sponges

PROCEDURE STEPS:
1. Wash hands and assemble equipment.
2. Identify patient.
3. Explain procedure to the patient.
4. Position the patient with the head lower than the shoulders.
5. Draw medication into dropper after checking medication three times and checking expiration date.
6. Place the dropper over the center of the outside of the affected nostril. Care should be taken not to touch the inside of the nostril. RATIONALE: Touching the inside of the nostril will lead to contamination of the dropper.
7. Repeat the procedure for the other nostril if required.
8. Instruct the patient to remain in position for 5 minutes.
9. Provide cotton balls or gauze sponges to the patient when the patient returns to a sitting position. RATIONALE: Medication may still drain from the nostrils.
10. Dispose of the supplies per OSHA guidelines.
11. Wash hands.
12. Document the procedure.

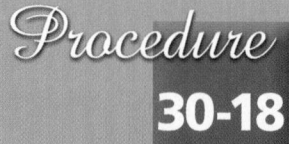

30-18   Obtaining a Sputum Specimen

STANDARD PRECAUTIONS:

PURPOSE:
To collect a quality sputum specimen for laboratory analysis to assist in diagnosing disease.
Patient Education:
1. If specimen must be collected at home, the container must be closed, labeled with date, time, and patient's name.
2. Encourage the patient to drink plenty of fluids. RATIONALE: Increased fluid intake keeps mucus moist.

EQUIPMENT/SUPPLIES:
Tissues
Small plastic bag to deliver specimen to laboratory
Sterile sputum container & label
Laboratory requisition
Nonsterile gloves
Goggles
Gown
Biohazard waste container

PROCEDURE STEPS:
1. Wash hands, assemble supplies, and label container.

(continues)

Procedure 30-18 *(continued)*

2. Explain procedure to the patient. If specimen is to be collected for AFB (acid-fast bacillus), three specimens are needed on three different days.
3. Identify patient.
4. Put on gloves, goggles, and gown.
5. Instruct patient to cough deeply and to expectorate directly into the sterile container (Figure 30-44). RATIONALE: The cough must be deep since this will bring up secretions from the lungs and bronchial tubes. Tell the patient to take several deep breaths in order to cough up sputum (not saliva).
6. Secure the top of the container.
7. Fill out laboratory requisition and secure it to the specimen container. Place in plastic bag and deliver to laboratory within 30 minutes after collection.
8. Dispose of supplies per OSHA guidelines.
9. Wash hands.
10. Document the procedure.

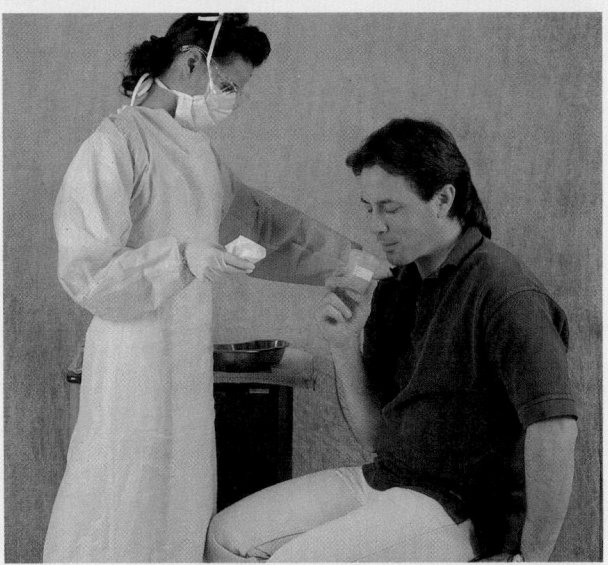

Figure 30-44 The patient should cough deeply and expectorate directly into the sterile container. Note medical assistant is wearing personal protective equipment.

Procedure 30-19 Administer Oxygen by Nasal Cannula for Minor Respiratory Distress

STANDARD PRECAUTIONS:

PURPOSE:

To provide a low dose of concentrated oxygen to a patient during periods of respiratory distress (e.g., chronic obstructive pulmonary disease).

Patient Education:

1. Demonstrate the position of the nasal prongs of the cannula into the nose. They face upward and the tab rests above the upper lip.
2. Describe how to clear the oxygen cylinder valve by turning it counterclockwise.
3. Oxygen supports combustion and a fire can start with oxygen in use. Friction, static electricity, or a lighted cigarette or cigar can cause ignition.

EQUIPMENT/SUPPLIES:

Portable oxygen tank with stand
Disposable nasal cannula with connecting tube
Flowmeter
Pressure regulator

PROCEDURE STEPS:

1. Wash hands and explain procedure to the patient.
2. Identify patient.
3. Open the cylinder one full turn, counterclockwise.
4. Check the pressure gauge. RATIONALE: This will determine the amount of pressure in the cylinder.
5. Attach the nasal cannula to the tubing and then to the flowmeter.

(continues)

Procedure **30-19** (*continued*)

6. Adjust the flow rate according to the physician's order.
7. Check for oxygen flow through the cannula.
8. Place the tips of cannula into the nares no more than 1 inch.
9. Adjust the tubing around the patient's ears (Figure 30-45) and secure it under the chin.
10. Answer patient's questions.
11. Wash hands.
12. Document the procedure.
    Note: Oxygen is usually humidified to prevent drying of respiratory mucosa.

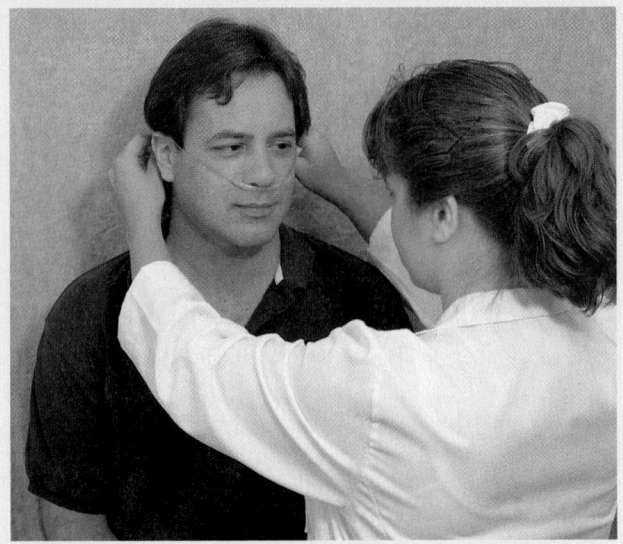

Figure 30-45 Position the nasal cannula, adjusting the tubing around the patient's ears and securing the cannula under the chin.

Procedure **30-20** Instructing Patient in Use of Metered Dose Nebulizer

STANDARD PRECAUTIONS:

PURPOSE:
To instruct a patient in the correct use of a handheld nebulizer, a device that delivers a fine mist of medication with or without the use of oxygen to the respiratory tract including the lungs.
Patient Education:
1. Remind the patient to inhale slowly.
2. Close the mouth and lips around the mouthpiece.
3. Clean the inhaler by rinsing the mouthpiece in warm water.
4. Adhere to prescribed dose.

EQUIPMENT/SUPPLIES:
Handheld nebulizer containing medication ordered by the physician

PROCEDURE STEPS:
1. Wash hands and assemble equipment.
2. Identify patient.
3. Demonstrate the use of the equipment to the patient and then have the patient return the demonstration.
4. Instruct the patient to exhale fully.
5. Holding the nebulizer upside down, close the mouth, lips, and teeth around the mouthpiece.
6. Tilting the head back, instruct the patient to take a deep breath and at the same time push the bottle against the mouthpiece.

(*continues*)

Procedure **30-20** *(continued)*

7. Instruct the patient to continue to inhale until the lungs are full.
8. Remove the mouthpiece and slowly exhale.
9. Repeat steps 4 through 7 if the physician has ordered more than one dose.
10. Wash hands.
11. Document patient was given instructions and has demonstrated to you the use of the nebulizer.

Procedure **30-21** **Spirometry Testing**

STANDARD PRECAUTIONS:

PURPOSE:
To prepare a patient for a spirometry to obtain optimum test results.

Patient Education:
1. Reinforce the importance of good posture during the process.
2. When blowing into the mouthpiece, the lips must seal tightly around it.
3. Explain the parameters needed for successful completion of the test.

Parameters:
- Patient must inhale deeply and quickly and exhale quickly and forcibly until no air can be expelled.
- Patient must refrain from the use of bronchodilators for 24 hours prior to test.
- Explain to the patient that maximum effort is required for accurate test results.

EQUIPMENT/SUPPLIES:
Spirometer
Disposable mouthpiece

PROCEDURE STEPS:
1. Wash hands and assemble equipment.
2. Identify the patient.
3. Explain the procedure and equipment to the patient. Allow the patient to breathe into the machine to become acquainted with the equipment.
4. Place the patient in a comfortable position (sitting/standing). Loosen tie or collar.
5. Instruct the patient not to bend at the waist when blowing into the mouthpiece.
6. Reinforce the inhalation process (deep breaths to fill the lungs to maximum capacity).
7. Instruct the patient to continue to blow into the mouthpiece until instructed to stop.
8. Be supportive and encouraging throughout the test.
9. Wash hands.
10. Attend to patient's needs.
11. Place the test results on the patient's chart after being reviewed by the physician.

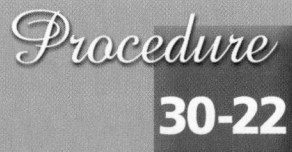

Procedure 30-22

Assisting with Plaster-of-Paris Cast Application

STANDARD PRECAUTIONS:

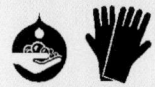

PURPOSE:
To assist physician in cast application.
Patient Education:
1. Instruct patient how to cover cast when bathing. Showersafe® is a type of waterproof material that can be used to cover a cast while showering.
2. Provide patient with dietary information for bone healing. Protein and high-calcium foods help the bone to heal.

EQUIPMENT/SUPPLIES:
Cast material:
Plaster bandage roll or synthetic tape
Container of 75°F water, which is lined with plastic or cloth to catch loose plaster
Water
Stockinette (3-inch width for arms, 4 inch for leg casts)
Webril (Sheet wadding)
Bandage
Scissors
Rubber gloves
Sponge rubber for padding

PROCEDURE STEPS:
1. Provide the patient with an explanation of the procedure.
2. Answer any questions about the injury or cast application within the scope of the medical assistant's training.
3. Wash hands and assemble the equipment and supplies.
4. Position the patient in a sitting position or as required by the physician.
5. Put on gloves.

6. Clean and dry the area to be casted, as directed by the physician. Chart any areas of bruising, redness, or open areas. RATIONALE: Appropriate documentation of skin condition is needed to assist in evaluation of the extremity at a later time.
7. Pad bony prominence with sponge rubber. RATIONALE: To protect from pressure.
8. Provide the correct width of stockinette for the area on which cast is being applied. RATIONALE: A stockinette that is too large will form creases, thus allowing for injury to tissues.
9. Provide physician with correct width of webril. RATIONALE: Webril provides protection to the patient's skin preventing pressure sores. Folds in the padding could lead to irritation of the skin.
10. Place the bandage in the container of warm water for 5 seconds. Remove from water and gently squeeze to remove excess water. Do not wring.
11. Assist with the application of the cast material as requested by the physician.
12. Reassure patient as needed.
13. After cast application, review cast care instructions and provide written instructions for cast care and isometric exercises (if prescribed by the physician). Reinforce any precautions given by the physician. RATIONALE: Reviewing possible complications with the patient enhances the immediate reporting of circulatory impairment and infection.
14. Discard water down the sink drain being cautious to keep plaster from going down the drain. Discard plaster in trash receptacle.
15. Clean work area.
16. Remove gloves and wash hands.
17. Schedule patient for next appointment to have cast checked.
18. Document the procedure.

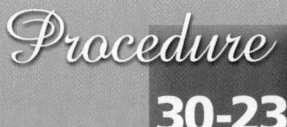

Procedure 30-23 Assisting with Cast Removal

STANDARD PRECAUTIONS:

PURPOSE:
To assist the physician with the removal of a cast.

EQUIPMENT/SUPPLIES:
Cast cutter
Cast spreader
Bandage scissors
Bag for disposing of cast materials

PROCEDURE STEPS:
1. Wash hands.
2. Explain the cast removal process to the patient. The cutter vibrates and does not spin. Some pressure and warmth may be experienced.

RATIONALE: Explaining the procedure reduces apprehension and fears about being cut with the blade.
3. Reassure the patient that skin color and muscle tone will improve with therapy.
4. Hand the physician the equipment as requested.
5. After the procedure provide written instructions for postcare.
6. Clean equipment.
7. Wash hands.
8. Document cast removal and appearance of body part from which cast was removed.

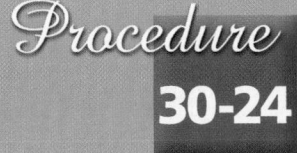

Procedure 30-24 Assisting the Physician During a Lumbar Puncture

STANDARD PRECAUTIONS:

PURPOSE:
To assemble supplies and position the patient for removal of cerebrospinal fluid from the lumbar area which will be sent to the laboratory for analysis.
Patient Education:
1. Review post-spinal tap instructions.
   a. The patient should remain in a prone position for 2 to 3 hours to allow tissues to close over the puncture site and minimize cerebrospinal fluid leakage.
   b. Reinforce the need to increase fluid intake since this helps to replace fluid loss.
   c. Report any severe headaches or alterations in neurological status (paralysis, numbness, tingling, and so on).

EQUIPMENT/SUPPLIES:
Drape
Xylocaine 1%–2%
Syringe and needle for anesthetic
Sterile gloves
Disposable sterile lumbar puncture tray (to include):
   Skin antiseptic with applicator
   Band-Aid
   Spinal puncture needle
   3 test tubes with corks or tops
   Drape
   Manometer
   Laboratory requisition
Examination light

PROCEDURE STEPS:
1. Reinforce physician's explanation of the procedure and answer questions.
2. Verify the patient has signed a consent form.

(continues)

Procedure **30-24** (continued)

3. Patient should be instructed to empty the bladder and bowel.
4. Wash hands and set up sterile field for the physician.
5. Cleanse the puncture site with antiseptic soap and water. Rinse.
6. Position the patient in a lateral recumbent position with the back at the edge of the exam table and a small pillow under the head. RATIONALE: Patient's alignment of the spine is best achieved in a horizontal position.
7. Drape patient for warmth and privacy.
8. Have the patient draw the knees up to the abdomen and grasp onto knees (Figure 30-46A) and flex chin on chest. RATIONALE: Position allows for easier needle insertion into the subarachnoid space of the spinal cord because this position widens the spaces between the lumbar vertebrae. Procedure is performed at the fourth intervertebral space of the lumbar region (Figure 30-46B).
9. The physician will swab the puncture site with antiseptic such as Betadine®.
10. The physician drapes area with fenestrated drape.
11. Assist physician to aspirate anesthetic.
12. Help the patient maintain this position until the needle has reached the subarachnoid space. RATIONALE: Movement by the patient could produce trauma to the spinal cord area.
13. Remind patient to breathe evenly, not to hold his breath or talk, since this may interfere with the pressure reading.
14. At the physician's direction, have the patient straighten his legs. RATIONALE: Muscle tension can give false pressure reading.

15. After the procedure has been completed, the physician will apply a Band-Aid to the puncture site. The patient is placed in a prone position for 2 to 3 hours, or as directed by the physician. RATIONALE: This helps prevent cerebrospinal fluid from leaking through the puncture site.
16. Apply gloves. Cap specimens tightly.
17. Label samples with date, patient's name, and number CSF #1, #2, #3.
18. Send the labeled specimen to the laboratory with the appropriate laboratory requisition. Store in incubator.
19. Clean area using standard precautions.
20. Remove gloves.
21. Wash hands.
22. Document procedure in patient's chart.

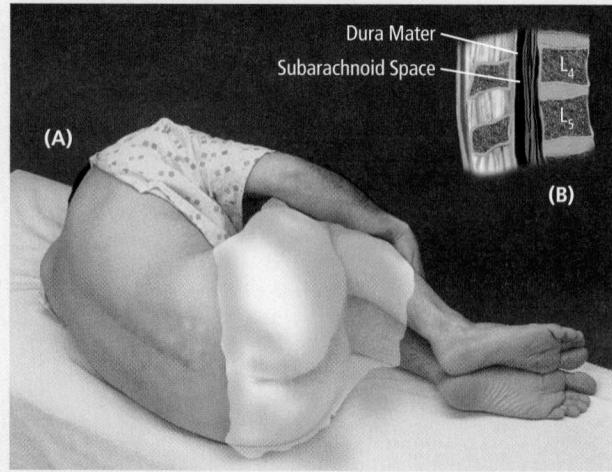

Figure 30-46   (A) Have the patient draw up the knees to the abdomen and grasp onto knees. Chin should flex on chest. (B) The site for the lumbar puncture.

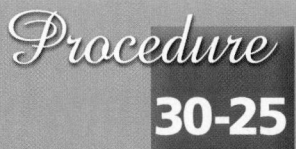 **Procedure 30-25**

Assisting the Physician with a Neurological Screening Examination

STANDARD PRECAUTIONS:

PURPOSE:
To determine a patient's neurological status.
Patient Education:
Inform the patient the purpose of the exam is to assess her response to pain and touch reflexes and other neurological functions.
a. The physician will use several supplies to test the functioning of each cranial nerve and to test the reflexes and the coordination of the patient.

EQUIPMENT/SUPPLIES:
Percussion hammer
Safety pin
Material for odor identification
Cotton ball
Tuning fork

Flashlight
Tongue blade
Ophthalmoscope

PROCEDURE STEPS:
1. Wash hands.
2. The mental status examination can be done by the medical assistant when taking the patient's medical history by observing the following:
   a. When taking patient's history, pay special attention to level of awareness, memory, cognition, and mood. When the patient answers questions during the history taking, note if behavior is appropriate for the circumstances.
3. The physician will evaluate the cranial nerve functions by using the results of the visual acuity tests as well as other tests.
4. Assist the patient as needed during and after the exam.
5. Document procedure in patient's chart.

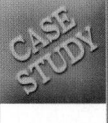 **CASE STUDY 30-1**

Corey Bayer is a fifteen-year-old patient at City Health Care. He sustained an injury to his right wrist today during soccer practice. Dr. Rice has examined him and ordered an X ray of the right forearm. The results show that Corey has sustained a Colles' fracture of the right wrist. Dr. Rice asks you to prepare the equipment to apply a cast.

CASE STUDY REVIEW

1. Describe assisting in cast application. What are the medical assistant's responsibilities?
2. Following Corey's cast application, describe the cast care instructions that will be given to Corey and his mother.

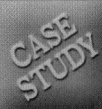 **CASE STUDY 30-2**

Dr. Rice has scheduled Anita Blanchette for a spirometry test and wants you to telephone her the day before the test to prepare her for it so that optimal results are obtained.

CASE STUDY REVIEW

1. What information can you give to Anita prior to her spirometry to obtain the best test results?

SUMMARY

Medical assistants are a vital link in the team of health care providers. A thorough knowledge and understanding of the various body system examinations and clinical procedures routinely performed as part of patient care will enhance the quality of care given.

Some of the specialty procedures will be performed on a routine basis in the ambulatory care setting; others will only be performed occasionally and perhaps only in the larger settings that offer special-

ized as well as primary care. Sometimes, in order to feel comfortable assisting with the less common procedures, medical assistants may need to broaden their base of knowledge by conducting independent research. Medical assistants who are willing to constantly expand their clinical understanding will not only fine-tune their professional skills but will derive greater satisfaction from their job performance.

REVIEW QUESTIONS

Multiple Choice

1. What are the elevated skin lesions affecting the epidermis caused by the papilloma viruses called?
   a. scleroderma
   b. moles
   c. calluses
   d. warts
2. What is the disorder that is characterized by discomfort of the muscles, tendons, ligaments, and soft tissues brought on by trauma, strain, and emotional stress?
   a. carpal tunnel syndrome
   b. bursitis
   c. gout
   d. fibromalagia
3. What type of fracture has its bone fragments driven into each other?
   a. greenstick
   b. impacted
   c. oblique
   d. comminuted
4. What disease is caused by a degeneration of brain cells caused by lack of dopamine, bringing about muscle rigidity and akinesia?
   a. multiple sclerosis
   b. Bell's palsy
   c. Parkinson's
   d. tic douloureux
5. An acute circumscribed infection of the subcutaneous tissues caused by staphylococcus is a:
   a. comedone
   b. carbuncle
   c. furuncle
   d. psoriasis

Critical Thinking

1. Describe how to perform a urinary catheterization.
2. Why are the rules of evidence always followed during a drug screen?
3. Phyllis Lomeli, a new patient of Dr. Reynolds, has been experiencing gastrointestinal problems. Dr. Reynolds has ordered fecal occult blood tests for the patient. What diet instructions does the medical assistant give to the patient? What directions and supplies does the medical assistant give to the patient? When the guaiac slides are returned, how does the medical assistant develop and interpret them?
4. List the patient preparation instructions for the following tests:
   a. barium enema
   b. upper GI
   c. cholecystogram
   d. intravenous pyelogram
5. List the steps the medical assistant must follow when performing the visual acuity test on an adult, a 9-year-old child, and a 4-year-old toddler.
6. What is the use and purpose of the audiometer? How is the test administered?
7. Explain the rationale when doing an eye irrigation that the flow of the irrigating solution is from the inside canthus to the outer canthus of the eye.
8. Differentiate among bronchitis, emphysema, and asthma.
9. Discuss how to obtain a sputum specimen.
10. What is the medical assistant's role when assisting in spirometry?
11. List the various types of casting material used in a physician's office. What are the cast care guidelines that the medical assistant gives to the patient?

12. List the components of a neurological screening.
13. When a mental status exam is given, what five areas are being reviewed?
14. Explain the medical assistant's role when assisting with a lumbar puncture.

WEB ACTIVITIES

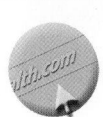

Use the Internet to search for information from a medical site to find answers to the following:

1. What is the most current treatment for kidney stones?
2. What are the long-term harmful effects of cigarette smoking?
3. What recommendations does the surgeon general of the United States have for quitting smoking cigarettes?

REFERENCES/BIBLIOGRAPHY

Bonewit-West, K. (2000). *Clinical procedures for medical assistants* (5th ed.). Philadelphia: W. B. Saunders Co.

Campeau, F. & Fleitz, J. (1999). *Limited radiography* (2nd ed.). Albany, NY: Delmar.

Damjanov, I. (1996). *Pathology for the health-related professions.* Philadelphia: W. B. Saunders Co.

Ehrlich, A. (1997). *Medical terminology for health professionals* (3rd ed.). Albany, NY: Delmar.

Frazier, M. S., Drzymkowski, J. A., & Doty, S. J. (1996). *Essentials of human diseases and conditions.* Philadelphia: W. B. Saunders Co.

Keir, L., Wise, B. A., & Krebs, C. (1998). *Medical assisting: Administrative and clinical competencies* (8th ed.). Albany, NY: Delmar.

Kinn, M. & Woods, M. (1999). *The medical assistant: Administrative and clinical* (8th ed.). Philadelphia: W. B. Saunders Co.

Neighbors, M., & Tannehill-Jones, R. (2000). *Human diseases.* Albany, NY: Delmar.

Taber's cyclopedic medical dictionary (1999) (18th ed.). Philadelphia: F. A. Davis Company.

Tamparo, C., & Lewis, M. (2000). *Diseases of the human body* (3rd ed.). Philadelphia: F. A. Davis Company.

Tortora, G., & Grabowski, S. (1996). *Principles of anatomy and physiology.* New York: Harper Collins.

Travaline, J., & Criner, G. J. (1994, August). Pulmonary function testing using a spirometer. *Hospital Medicine,* 57.

White, G. (1998). *Basic clinical lab competencies for respiratory care* (3rd ed.). Albany, NY: Delmar.

Wojciechowski, W. (2000). *Respiratory care sciences: An integrated approach* (3rd ed.). Albany, NY: Delmar.

Zakus, S. (1995). *Clinical procedures for medical assistants* (3rd ed.). St. Louis: Mosby-Year Book, Inc.

ADVANCED TECHNIQUES AND PROCEDURES

Chapter

ASSISTING WITH MINOR SURGERY

KEY TERMS

Allergy
Anesthesia
Antibacterial
Approximate
Bandage
Betadine®
Cautery
Contamination
Dressing
Epinephrine
Exudate
Fenestrated
Friable
Hibeclens®
Hydrogen Peroxide
Infection
Inflammation
Informed Consent
Isopropyl Alcohol
Ligature
Liquid Nitrogen
Mayo Stand/Instrument Tray
Ratchets
Silver Nitrate
Sitz Bath
Sodium Hydroxide
Strictures
Surgery Cards
Surgical Asepsis
Suture
Swaged
Volatile

OUTLINE

Surgical Asepsis
 Handwashing for Surgical Asepsis
Sterile Principles
Common Surgical Procedures
 Performed in Physicians'
 Offices and Clinics
Alternative Surgical Methods
 Electrosurgery
 Cautery
 Cryosurgery
 Laser Surgery
Suture Materials and Supplies
 Suture/Ligature
 Suture Needles
Instruments
 Structural Features
 Categories and Uses
 Care of Instruments
 Chemical "Cold" Sterilization

Supplies and Equipment
 Sponges and Wicks
 Solutions/Creams/Ointments
 Dressings and Bandages
 Anesthetics
Patient Care and Preparation
 Patient Preparation and Education
 Informed Consent
 Medical Assisting Considerations
 Postoperative Instructions
 Wounds, Wound Care, and the
  Healing Process
Basic Surgery Set-Up
 Basic Rules and Concepts for
  Setup of Surgical Trays
Minor Surgery Process
Preparation for Minor Surgery
 Using Dry Sterile Transfer Forceps

OBJECTIVES

The student should strive to meet the following performance objectives and demonstrate an understanding of the facts and principles presented in this chapter through written and oral communication.

1. Define the key terms as presented in the glossary.
2. Define surgical asepsis and differentiate between surgical asepsis and medical asepsis.
3. List eight basic rules to follow to protect sterile areas.
4. Explain the sizing standards of suture material and the criteria used to select the most appropriate type and size.
5. Given a variety of surgical instruments, be able to identify each and describe its intended use. *(continues)*

OBJECTIVES (*continued*)

6. Demonstrate the ability to select the most appropriate type of dressings for a given situation.
7. State advantages and disadvantages of Betadine®, Hibeclens®, isopropyl alcohol, and hydrogen peroxide when each is used as a skin antiseptic.
8. Define anesthesia, and explain the advantages and disadvantages of epinephrine as an additive to injectable anesthetics.
9. List five preoperative issues to be addressed in patient preparation and education.
10. List five postoperative concerns to be addressed with the patient and the caregiver.
11. Demonstrate applying sterile gloves.
12. Demonstrate setting up a surgical tray, including laying the field, applying supplies and instruments, pouring a sterile solution, using transfer forceps, and covering the sterile tray.
13. Explain what is meant by alternative surgical methods.

ROLE DELINEATION COMPONENTS

CLINICAL

Fundamental Principles

- Apply principles of aseptic technique and infection control
- Comply with quality assurance practices

Patient Care

- Obtain patient history and vital signs
- Prepare and maintain examination and treatment areas
- Prepare patient for examinations, procedures and treatments
- Assist with examinations, procedures and treatments
- Maintain medication and immunization records

(continues)

SCENARIO

It might be instructive to compare two different ambulatory care settings. At the multiphysician Inner City Health Care, minor surgery is performed on a routine basis. Certain days are dedicated to certain procedures. Because of the high volume of patients and different physician preferences, Inner City maintains two special rooms for minor surgery and has a large selection of instruments. At the smaller two-physician Lewis and King, however, minor surgical procedures are less frequent and are conducted in the patient examination rooms.

INTRODUCTION

Minor office surgery differs greatly from major surgery, not only in complexity but in the supplies, equipment, instruments, and personnel needed. Some minor office surgery is performed by the physician alone; some require the assistance of the medical assistant. Most ambulatory care settings do not need a large variety of surgical instruments, but will often need more than one of the more frequently used instruments. As a personal preference, special instruments may be purchased and maintained for a specific physician to use during a particular surgical procedure. These particular instruments are generally not used by any other physician.

The equipment and supplies used in minor office surgery are usually portable and easily maintained. It is the larger practices that perform many minor office surgeries that can afford the space and expense of maintaining a special room just for that purpose. Often patient examination rooms serve as small surgical suites with portable **Mayo stands/instrument trays**, supplies, and equipment brought into the room for the procedure.

Whether assisting with minor surgery is a routine or an infrequent event for the medical assistant, it is nonetheless important to be knowledgeable about the use and care of instruments and room as well as patient preparation for minor surgery. Medical assistants should also understand the preference of each physician on staff in order to make the minor surgical procedure comfortable and effective for both patient and physician.

SURGICAL ASEPSIS

Regardless of the number and complexity of minor surgical procedures performed in the office or ambulatory care center, surgical asepsis must be strictly maintained. Surgical asepsis uses practices known as sterile techniques. The primary purpose of surgical asepsis is to prevent microorganisms from entering the patient's body during an invasive procedure. Some examples of invasive procedures include creating an opening in the skin such as a surgical incision, closing a wound such as a laceration, giving an injection, or inserting a sterile catheter into a sterile body cavity such as the urinary bladder.

Because microorganisms are on virtually every surface such as skin, instruments, surgical instrument trays, clothing, and even in the air, it is necessary to destroy as many as possible before any surgical procedure. Surgical asepsis or sterile technique prevents microorganism entry into the body during an invasive procedure and, therefore, protects the patient from infection. Once the items and areas are sterilized, every precaution must be taken to prevent contamination of the sterile items or areas either from a nonsterile surface or from airborne contamination.

Living tissue surfaces such as skin cannot be sterilized but can be made as free of pathogens as possible before the use of a sterile covering. One example of this concept is the use of the surgical handwashing technique prior to applying sterile gloves (see Procedure 31-1). Another example of asepsis is preparing the patient's skin with a surgical scrub solution prior to applying sterile drapes around the intended surgical site.

Refer to Chapter 22 for more complete information on the concepts of asepsis and aseptic techniques including handwashing for medical asepsis and methods of sterilization for surgical asepsis.

The differences between handwashing for medical asepsis as discussed in Chapter 22 (see Procedure 22-1) and handwashing for surgical asepsis are addressed in the following section.

Handwashing for Surgical Asepsis

Handwashing for medical asepsis is defined as removing pathogenic microorganisms from the hands after contamination. Medical handwashing is used many times throughout the day to cleanse the skin after removing contaminated gloves, assisting with patient care, and touching unclean surfaces. Handwashing for surgical asepsis is defined as removal of as many microorganisms as possible prior to performing surgery or a sterile procedure. Handwashing for surgical asepsis consists of meticulously washing hands prior to applying sterile gloves. Both medical and surgical aseptic handwashing techniques are designed to prevent exposing patients, health care workers, and the public to potentially harmful microorganisms.

Proper protocol when assisting with minor surgery requires the use of surgical handwashing at the beginning of each workday as well as prior to sterile techniques, with the complementary use of medical handwashing before leaving the office and when returning and between patients and procedures. Any opening in the medical assistant's skin should be covered with a sterile adhesive dressing and gloves are worn during any direct patient contact. See Chapter 22 for information on standard precautions.

For a summary of how surgical handwashing differs from medical handwashing see Table 31-1.

STERILE PRINCIPLES

Sterile principles are a set of guidelines designed to designate what items and areas are considered sterile and what actions cause contamination. Some areas are logical and clear, some are subtle and less clear. It has already been noted that some surfaces, such as skin, cannot be sterilized. In addition, large items such as instrument stands and their trays cannot fit into an autoclave for sterilization. To create sterile areas and surfaces where sterility is not possible, sterile gloves can be worn over the hands and sterile drapes can be applied to trays once both have been washed with soap and water, rinsed, and dried.

TABLE 31-1 DIFFERENCE BETWEEN MEDICAL AND SURGICAL HANDWASHING	
Medical Handwashing	**Surgical Handwashing**
• 2 minute duration	• 5–6 minute duration
• Wash hands and wrists	• Wash hands, wrists, and forearms to the elbows
• Hands should be held down during rinsing	• Hands should be held up during rinsing
• Scrub nails with brush; clean under nails with cuticle stick	• Scrub nails with brush and clean under each nail with cuticle stick
• Apply lotion*	• Do not apply lotion*
• Glove for protection	• Glove for sterility and personal protection

*The use of lotions is encourage to help prevent chafing of the skin, especially with frequent hand washings. Nevertheless, recent studies have determined that lotions containing petroleum or mineral oil can break down latex and should be avoided if latex gloves are going to be worn within one hour after applying the lotion. If lotions are applied immediately prior to gloving, the use of water-based lotions is recommended. Of special interest to persons with latex sensitivities (see Chapter 22) is the fact that using lotions and creams actually increases the amount of latex protein that is transferred from the gloves into the skin, thereby increasing the symptoms of latex sensitivity.

Guidelines to protect sterile items and areas include:

- A sterile object may not touch a nonsterile object.

- Sterile objects must not be wet. Moisture will draw microorganisms into the sterile object.

- An acceptable border between a sterile area and a nonsterile area is one inch. The portion of a drape that hangs over the edge is considered nonsterile, no matter what its size. Sterile articles should be placed in the center of the sterile field and away from the edge as much as possible.

- Do not turn your back on a sterile field. If you cannot see the field, you cannot be aware of what touched it.

- Anything below the waist is considered contaminated. In support of this principle, all surgery trays should be positioned above the waist. All articles are to be held above the waist.

- All sterile objects (such as gloved hands) must be held in front and away from the body and above waist level.

- Do not cough, sneeze, or talk over a sterile field. Airborne particles may fall onto the sterile area and contaminate it.

- Do not reach over the sterile area. Clothing may touch and thereby contaminate the area. Spend as little time as possible reaching into the sterile area.

- Do not pass contaminated dressings or instruments over the sterile field.

- Arrange for the physician to place contaminated instruments into a separate container or area.

- Always be aware of actions in order to determine whether the sterile field has been contaminated. When in doubt, err on the side of safety.

- When opening sterile packages, the outer wrapper is contaminated. It should be opened without touching the inner contents, and the contents are then dropped onto the sterile field. Double wrapping can be used. (Refer to Chapter 22, Procedure 22-4.)

- Sterile solutions in bottles should be poured into sterile basins or cups on the sterile field without touching the rim of the bottle and without splashing solution onto the sterile field. If the sterile field is not polylined and becomes wet, it is considered contaminated, because when a field is wet it acts as a wick and draws microorganisms into the article. Using polylined drapes as sterile fields protects against contamination.

COMMON SURGICAL PROCEDURES PERFORMED IN PHYSICIANS' OFFICES AND CLINICS

All minor surgery has commonalities as well as specifics. The following specific minor surgery includes lists of needed instruments, supplies, and equipment as well as basic patient preparation and postoperative instructions for some of the more frequently performed minor surgery. The following procedures are suggested protocol only, as each physician will have preferences and techniques unique to them and their practices.

This section includes a general procedure for assisting with minor surgery and is followed by specific minor surgical procedures, including:

- Assisting with Minor Surgery (Procedure 31-2)

- Suturing of Laceration or Incision (Procedure 31-3)

- Dressing Change (Procedure 31-4)

- Suture Removal (Procedure 31-5)

- Application of Sterile Adhesive Skin Closure Strips (Procedure 31-6)

- Sebaceous Cyst Excision (Procedure 31-7)

- Incision and Drainage of Localized Infections (Procedure 31-8)

- Aspiration of Joint Fluid (Procedure 31-9)

- Hemorrhoid Thrombectomy (Procedure 31-10)

ALTERNATIVE SURGICAL METHODS

Alternative surgical methods refer to those methods not requiring the use of a surgical knife or scalpel, but which use other methods of cutting or destroying, such as electric current, heat, freezing, chemicals, or laser beam. Which method is used is determined by the physician's preference.

Electrosurgery

Electrosurgery uses an electric current in a concentrated area to either cut or destroy tissue whenever pathological examination is not required. The equipment for electrosurgery consists of a power source, usually a small boxed unit, and a detachable handheld applicator with removable tips. The tips are available in various sizes and are removable for cleaning and sterilizing.

Electrosurgery is very useful in removing benign skin tags and warts. The main advantage of electrosurgery is that the bleeding is controlled through the cauterization of the blood vessels as the electric current is applied. The terms *electrocoagulation, electrofulguration, electrodessication, electroscission,* and *electrosection* all refer to various uses of electric current to either coagulate blood vessels, destroy tissue either with a spark or by drying, or cut tissue.

Cautery

The word **cautery** comes from the term *caustic* and means the application of a caustic chemical or destructive heat. The burning of tissue, either chemically or electrically, is known as cauterization. Sometimes during surgical procedures unnecessary bleeding can be controlled by use of an electrocautery machine (Figure 31-1). Tissues that do not need to be pathologically examined, such as benign skin tags, can be destroyed using cauterization. Some common chemicals used to destroy tissue and stop bleeding are **silver nitrate**, **liquid nitrogen**, and **sodium hydroxide**.

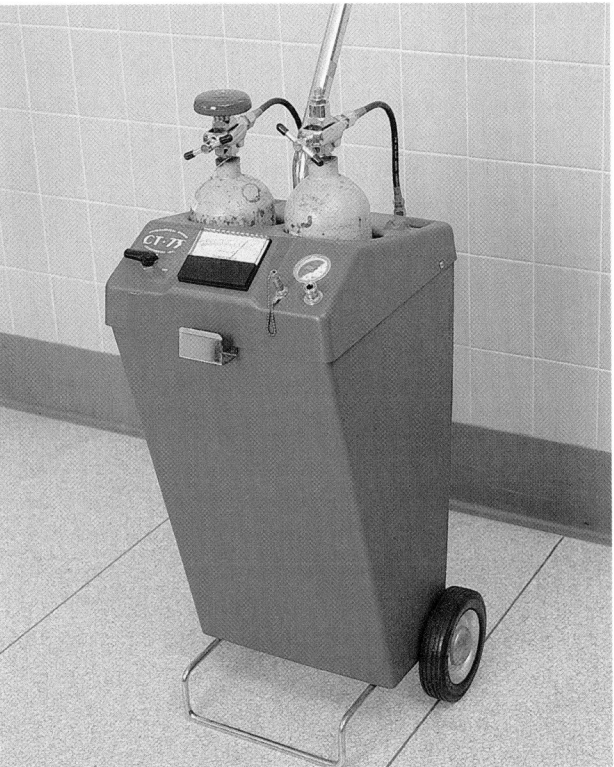

Figure 31-1 Electrocautery machines are used to burn tissue with electric current. This is done to destroy tissue, such as warts or polyps, or to cauterize small blood vessels to decrease blood loss during surgery.

Chemical Tissue Destruction. Silver nitrate is available in a solid form, impregnated on the end of a wooden applicator stick. Silver nitrate is especially useful inside the nose to cauterize **friable**, easily broken, blood vessels in the treatment of epistaxis (nosebleed).

Liquid nitrogen, often incorrectly referred to as dry ice is extremely **volatile**, easily evaporated, and must be kept in a covered insulated canister. Liquid nitrogen is obtained when nitrogen gas is compressed under very cold temperatures into a liquid. It is most often used to destructively "freeze" warts.

Liquid chemical caustic agents such as sodium hydroxide are used to permanently destroy the growth plates of toenails whenever total and permanent removal of the toenail is necessary.

Electrical Tissue Destruction. Electrical burning of tissue is performed with the use of an electrical instrument called an electrocautery. A wand on the end of a handheld apparatus is electrically heated and applied to tissues. The adjustable current is controlled by a foot pedal. Disposable battery-operated cautery units designed for one-time use are also available.

Cryosurgery

Cryosurgery refers to the destruction of tissue by freezing. Some types of tissues react differently to heat than cold in the rate of healing and level of scarring. The cryogenic substance most often used to destructively freeze tissue is liquid nitrogen. Liquid nitrogen may be applied to cervical erosions to facilitate the healing growth of normal tissue.

The cryogenic properties of solid carbon dioxide make it useful for freezing warts and nevi as well. Histofreezer is the trade name of an aerosol spray canister containing imethyl ether as the freezing agent. Hollow disposable cotton-tipped applicators attach to the Histofreezer canister. The applicator tip is placed on the lesion and the imethyl ether passes through the hollow core of the applicator and freezes the target tissue. More extensive tank units are available for more complex procedures. The tank units have a pistol-type adaptor with stainless steel tips of various sizes.

Laser Surgery

Laser is an acronym for Light Amplification by Stimulated Emission of Radiation. The laser instrument converts light into a very intense beam. By focusing the laser beam onto the target, the application can be extremely precise without damaging surrounding tissue. Over the past two decades, laser surgery has become less expensive, more readily available, and consequently much more widespread as a treatment of choice for surgery in dermatology, ophthalmology, and plastic surgery. Most specialty surgery is now using laser in various ways. With the advent of many physicians utilizing laser technology in the ambulatory care setting, the medical assistant must be familiar with the dangers involved with laser surgery and safety precautions must be implemented. Attending a laser education and safety workshop is recommended for all personnel intending to work with lasers.

 The following precautions are designed to heighten awareness and serve as a safety guide:

- When the laser beam is focused on the target tissue, the cells explode and vaporize. Care should be taken not to inhale the vapors.

- Whenever high levels of electricity are used, care should be taken to avoid burns and to assure that the equipment is always in good working order.

- Safety glasses should be worn by the physician, medical assistant, and, if possible, the patient.

- The patient should not have the skin prepared with flammable products such as alcohol-based antiseptics.

- Sterile water should be readily available to extinguish any fire if the beam accidently ignites cloth or paper in the area.

SUTURE MATERIALS AND SUPPLIES

Suture/Ligature

The word **suture** can be used as a verb to describe the motion of sewing or as a noun to describe the material—the thread—used to sew. Suturing, or sewing, a wound is a common procedure in physicians' offices. The purpose is to **approximate**, or bring together the edges of a wound. Suturing hastens healing and lessens scarring. Whether the wound is an accidental laceration or a surgical incision, the suturing process is basically the same. When thread is used for tying (e.g., ends of blood vessels during surgery) rather than sewing, it is termed **ligature**. The terms *suture* and *ligature* both refer to thread, but they are named according to their uses.

Most suture material, or thread, used in minor surgical procedures comes already fused, or **swaged**, to a needle and packaged in various lengths (see Figure 31-2). Eighteen inches is a preferred length because it is short enough to be manageable yet long enough to complete most suturing procedures. Combinations of sizes and types of suture materials and sizes and shapes of needles are endless, but most physicians will use a select few. Selection of the many different suture materials and needles is based on size, strength, and purpose. Suture ranges in size on a scale from the smallest gauge below 0 (aught) to the

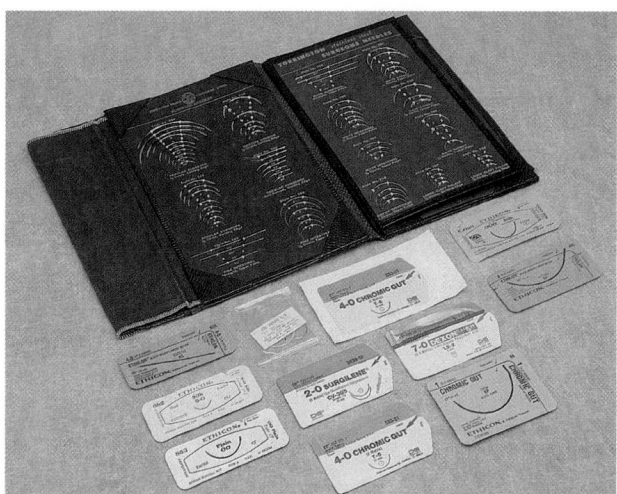

Figure 31-2 Top case displays a variety of curved and straight surgical needles. Bottom packages display a variety of prepackaged suture materials with needles of various sizes and shapes.

largest gauge above 0. The scale from 6-0 to 4 includes all sizes from the smallest to the largest:

6-0, 5-0, 4-0, 3-0, 2-0, 0, 1, 2, 3, 4

Sometimes 2-0 is labeled 00, 3-0 labeled 000, 4-0 labeled 0000, and so on.

If the tissue being sutured is delicate, as on the face or neck, the smaller suture material is used; the finer the stitch, the less scarring. Some sutures are made from materials that dissolve when they come in contact with the tissue enzymes. These are referred to as absorbable sutures. Surgical gut (also called cat gut) is made from sheep intestinal tissue. Left "natural" or uncoated, it is called plain gut suture and will dissolve or be absorbed in about one to two weeks. If more time is needed to heal, surgical gut may be coated with chromion salts. It is then called chromion gut and allows for a longer period of healing to take place before dissolving. Absorbable gut suture is used for underlying tissues where removal is not reasonable and areas where suture removal is inconvenient. Individual body chemistries will influence the exact absorption rate of both plain and treated gut suture. (Gut is rarely used now and has been replaced by an artificial absorbable suture called vicryl.) Suture is also made of nonabsorbable materials such as stainless steel, silk, cotton, nylon, and Dacron. Each type of suture material comes in a variety of options such as different colors for ease of visualization, braiding for additional elasticity and strength, and coatings for lubrications and to lessen irritability to tissues.

Suture Needles

The needles swaged to the suture material are also varied (Figure 31-2). In minor office surgery the needles are usu-

ally curved. They are categorized according to size, shape, radius of curve, and type of point. Needles may be termed cutting needles, round taper point needles, or blunt point needles.

INSTRUMENTS

Structural Features

Rarely does the phrase "form determines function" have as much meaning as when discussing surgical instruments. One can almost always correctly imagine function simply by close examination of the instrument's design. Handles designed to be squeezed between the thumb and finger are called "thumb" handles. "Ring" handles are designed for the insertion of the thumb and finger into rings. **Ratchets** are locking mechanisms located between the rings of the handles and are used for locking the instrument closed. Ratchets are designed to close in varying degrees of tightness. Serrations are the crevices etched into the surfaces of the jaws of hemostats, some forceps, and needle holders. The serrations provide a more secure grip during use with slippery tissues without actually puncturing the tissue. For the purposes of puncturing tissue, forceps with teeth are an option. Teeth may be numerous or few but are always sharp and should approximate tightly when the instrument is closed. To help delicate tips match up properly, some thumb instruments may have a guide pin built into the handle. Box-lock is the name given to a special type of hinge found on most ring-handled instruments, especially grasping instruments such as hemostats, forceps, and needle holders. Since the box-lock provides strength and aids in the prevention of warping, most instruments with ratchets also need the box-lock hinge. Other features include prongs, hooks, and loops (Figure 31-3).

Categories and Uses

Several companies publish and distribute large pictoral catalogs of well over 30,000 medical-surgical instruments. A glance through these references shows the many choices available. For ease of discussion, learning, and cataloging, most surgical instruments are placed according to their uses into three basic categories.

Cutting	Scissors and scalpels
Grasping/Clamping	Hemostats, forceps, clamps, and needle holders
Dilating/Probing	Specula, scopes, probes, retractors, and dilators

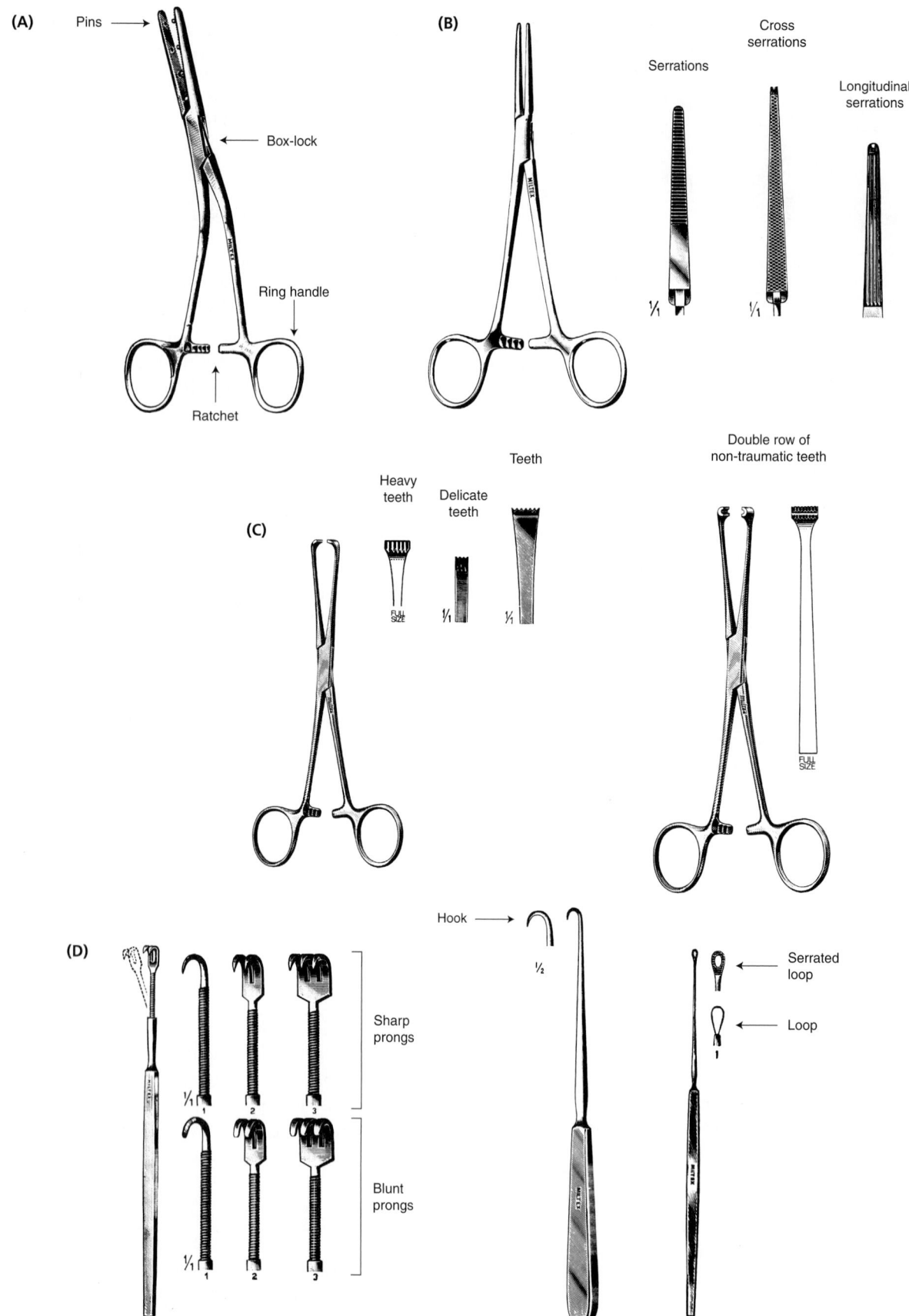

Figure 31-3 Structural features of instruments include (A) ratchets, box-locks, pins, and ring handle; (B) serrations; (C) teeth; (D) prongs, hooks, and loops. (Courtesy of Miltex Instrument Company, Inc.)

Instruments designed for specific purposes within medical specialties often do not readily fit into any one group and are called specialty instruments. This group includes long-handled gynecological instruments as well as other instruments designed to meet specific needs within specialty practices.

Scissors and Scalpels. Most of the cutting instruments are scissors. Scissors have ring handles, two blades, and vary in size, shape, and function. Because scissors have two blades, the word *scissors* is always plural. Bandage scissors have one rounded tip to allow insertion under a bandage without causing injury to the patient. The two most common styles are the Lister bandage scissors and the finer finger bandage scissors (Figure 31-4).

Operating scissors are used to cut tissues and generally have very sharp blades. The blades may be curved or straight, and the tips may be sharp, blunt, or a combination of each. They are described as sharp/sharp (s/s), blunt/blunt (b/b), or sharp/blunt (s/b) (Figure 31-5A). A special type of scissors, the Mayo dissecting scissors, may be straight or curved, but are never described as sharp or blunt since the tips are specifically designed to be neither but have a beveled edge with slightly rounded points (Figure 31-5B). Very useful, delicately bladed scissors are iris scissors, originally named for usefulness in eye surgery but now widely used in many procedures. Iris scissors may be either curved or straight (Figure 31-6A). Suture scissors, also called stitch or stitch removal scissors, have a distinctively

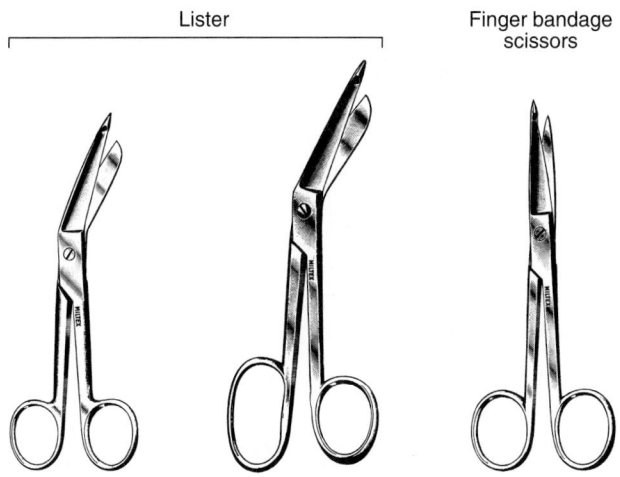

Figure 31-4   Bandage scissors: (A) Lister bandage scissors, small. (B) Lister bandage scissors, large, with one large finger ring. (C) Knowles finger bandage scissors, straight. (Courtesy of Miltex Instrument Company, Inc.)

notched blade to facilitate the insertion of one tip under a suture (Figure 31-6B).

Another common instrument in the cutting category is the scalpel. The scalpel is actually a blade secured to a handle which, when combined, becomes a surgical knife or scalpel. Disposable one-piece units are also available. The most common blade sizes are #10, #11, and #15, with #11 often referred to as a "stab blade" due to its sharp point (Figure 31-7A). Handles vary in size but the most popular are the sturdy #3 and #3L (long) and the more delicate #7 (Figure 31-7B).

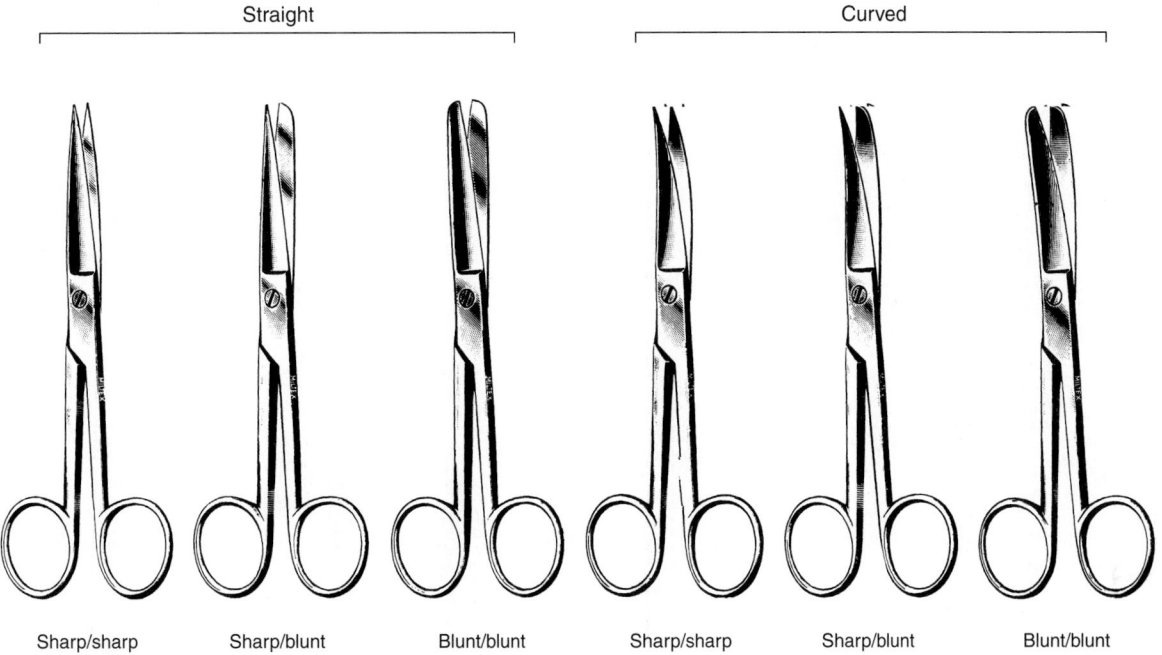

Figure 31-5A   **Standard operating scissors.** (Courtesy of Miltex Instrument Company, Inc.)

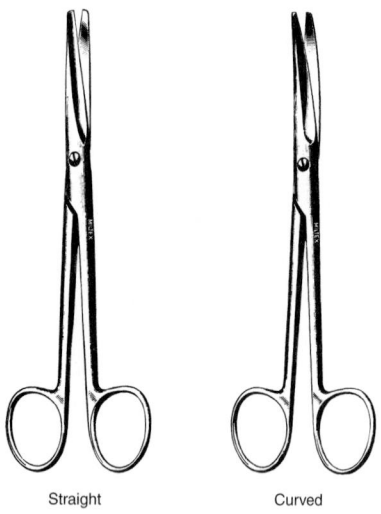

Figure 31-5B Mayo dissecting scissors. (Courtesy of Miltex Instrument Company, Inc.)

Straight   Curved

Hemostats, Forceps, Clamps, and Needle Holders. Grasping and clamping instruments are the largest of the instrument categories. These instruments are used for many different tasks. Included in this category are the towel clamps or clips, needle holders, and forceps. Forceps designed to hold tissue often have teeth and serrations in order to grasp firmly. Many forceps also have locking mechanisms called ratchets. Forceps may have ring handles or use a squeeze concept like a tweezer. Forceps number in the hundreds, but most offices need only a select few. Like the word *scissors*, the word *forceps* is always plural. Hemostatic forceps, or hemostats, are used to grasp and clamp blood vessels. Their name means literally to "stop blood." Since blood vessels are slippery, hemostatic forceps have serrations for grasping and ratchets for locking tightly. Mosquito hemostatic forceps have fine tips, with serrations along the entire length of the tips. The Kelly hemostats

Small   Large

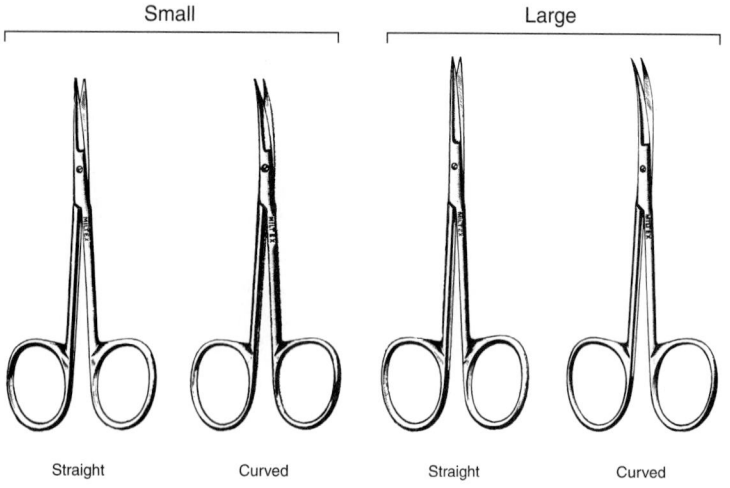

Straight   Curved   Straight   Curved

Figure 31-6A Iris scissors. (Courtesy of Miltex Instrument Company, Inc.)

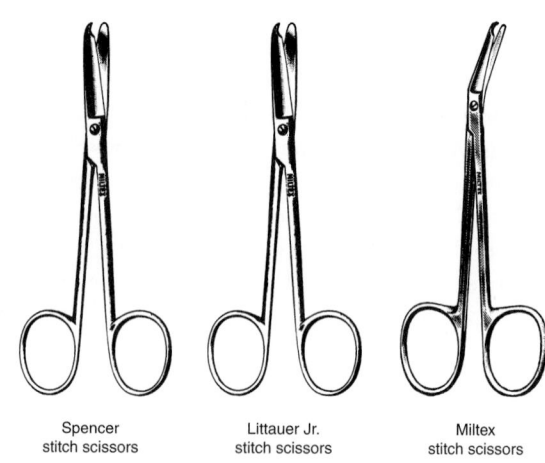

Spencer   Littauer Jr.   Miltex
stitch scissors   stitch scissors   stitch scissors

Figure 31-6B Suture or stitch scissors. (Courtesy of Miltex Instrument Company, Inc.)

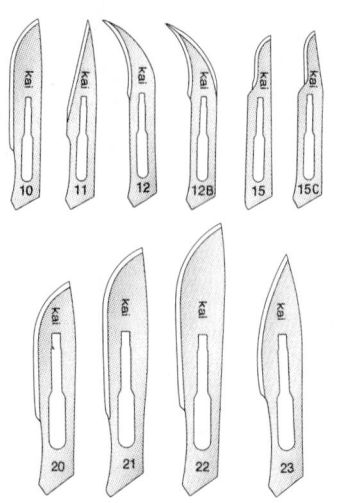

10   11   12   12B   15   15C

20   21   22   23

Figure 31-7A Surgical blades: #10, #11, #12, #12B, #15, #15C, #20, #21, #22, and #23. (Courtesy of Miltex Instrument Company, Inc.)

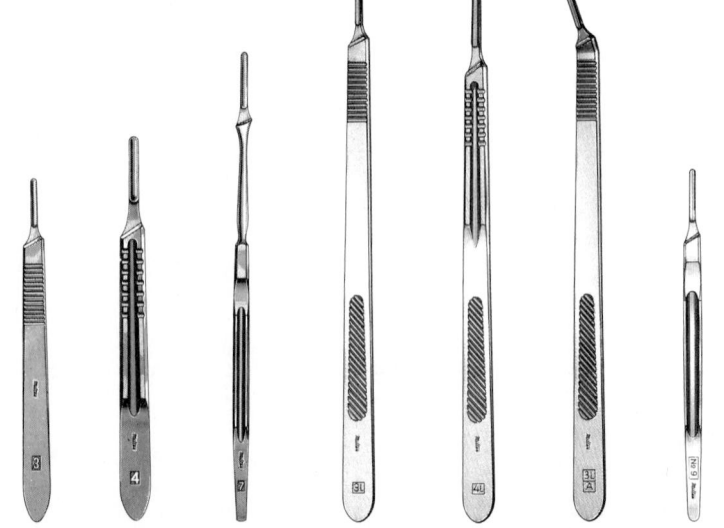

Figure 31-7B Scalpel handles: #3, #4, #7, #3L, #3LA (angled), and #9. (Courtesy of Miltex Instrument Company, Inc.)

have serrations only along partial length of the tips. Both the Kelly and Crile hemostatic forceps are sturdier, and the Rochester Ochsner hemostatic forceps have teeth. All types may be straight or curved (Figure 31-8).

Allis tissue forceps are of a similar design to hemostatic forceps but have unique angular jaws with teeth. Another type of grasping instrument are thumb forceps, sometimes referred to as "pick-ups." Thumb forceps do not have ring handles or ratchets but are more like the common tweezers. Thumb forceps with teeth are called tissue forceps because of their ability to grasp tissue. Dressing forceps do not have teeth and are very useful for dressing wounds and applying sterile skin closure strips. Dressing forceps are also used to insert sterile gauze packing strips into wounds to facilitate drainage. The Adson, a special type of thumb forceps, is easily differentiated by the shape. Adsons may have teeth or be plain.

The Lucae bayonet-type forceps, used in nose and ear procedures, have a thumb handle and are curved to allow the simultaneous use of other instruments and scopes and to facilitate viewing. In contrast, the Hartman ear forceps, Duckbill ear alligator-type forceps, and the Hartman nasal dressing forceps have ring handles but also are bent for ease in ear and nose procedures. See Figure 31-9 for examples of each.

Splinter forceps do not have teeth and are used for pulling splinters. Many splinter forceps such as the plain splinter forceps and the Walter are of the thumb-handled style, but the Physician's splinter forceps have ring handles and the Virtus have a spring-type handle (Figure 31-10).

Sponge forceps such as the Foerster may have rings on the tips and, as the name implies, are used to hold surgical gauze sponges. The sponge forceps may have long handles making them very useful for gynecological procedures and are then called uterine sponge forceps. Many medical offices will use the uterine sponge forceps as transfer forceps (Figure 31-11). See Basic Surgery Setup also in this chapter.

Towel clamps are used to attach surgical field drapes to each other and in some situations, such as when bisecting the vas deferens in a vasectomy, to clamp onto dissected tissue. In the case of a vasectomy, the Backhaus towel clamp is used to hold the dissected section of the vas deferens (Figure 31-12).

Needle holders are ratcheted instruments similar to hemostats but with a wider and more stout jaw. Often called needle drivers, they are designed to hold the needle firmly without crushing it. Most needle holders have a vertical ditch in the center of the jaw to disperse tension and help prevent slipping of the needle. Needle holders such as the Crile-Wood may have a special groove in which to place the needle during suturing. Some needle holders come equipped with a cutting edge which eliminates the need for a separate scissors to cut the suture material (Figure 31-13).

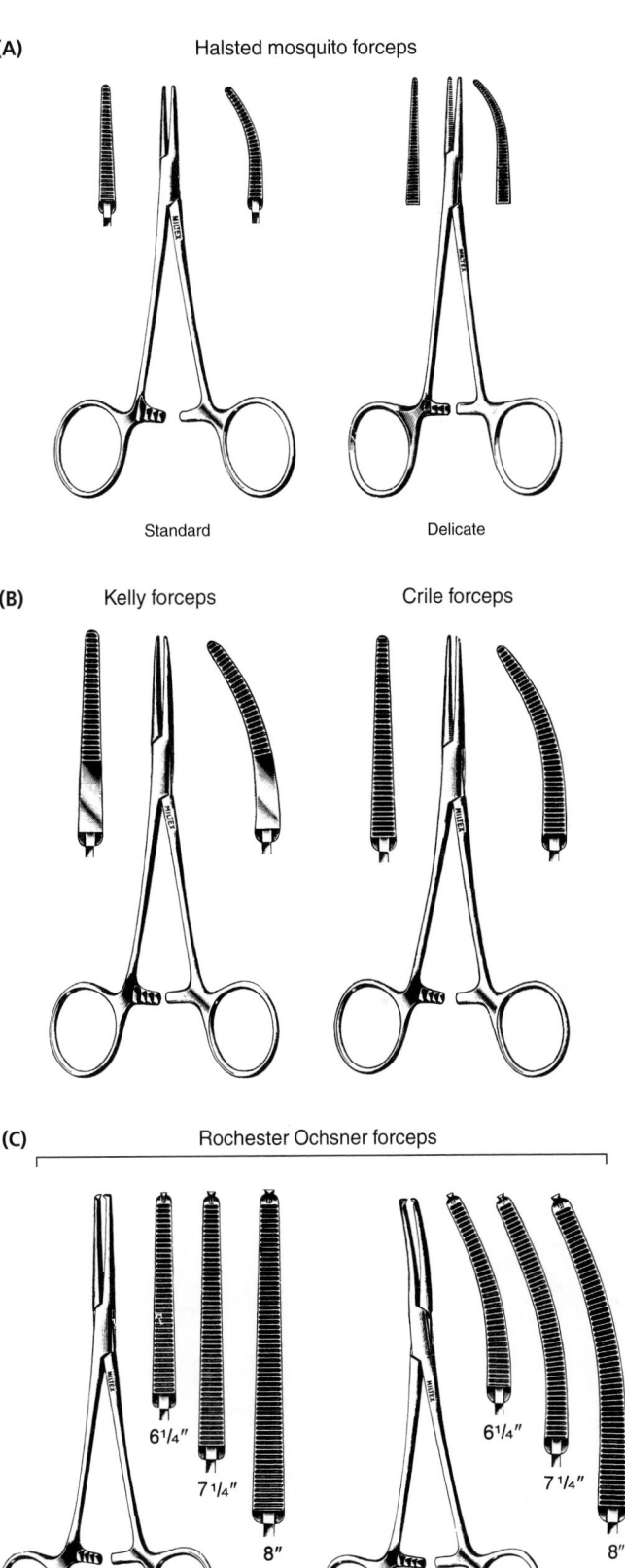

(A) Halsted mosquito forceps
Standard   Delicate

(B) Kelly forceps   Crile forceps

(C) Rochester Ochsner forceps
6¼″   7¼″   8″
6¼″   7¼″   8″
Straight   Curved

Figure 31-8 Hemostatic forceps include (A) Halsted mosquito forceps; (B) Kelly and Crile forceps; (C) Rochester Ochsner forceps. (Courtesy of Miltex Instrument Company, Inc.)

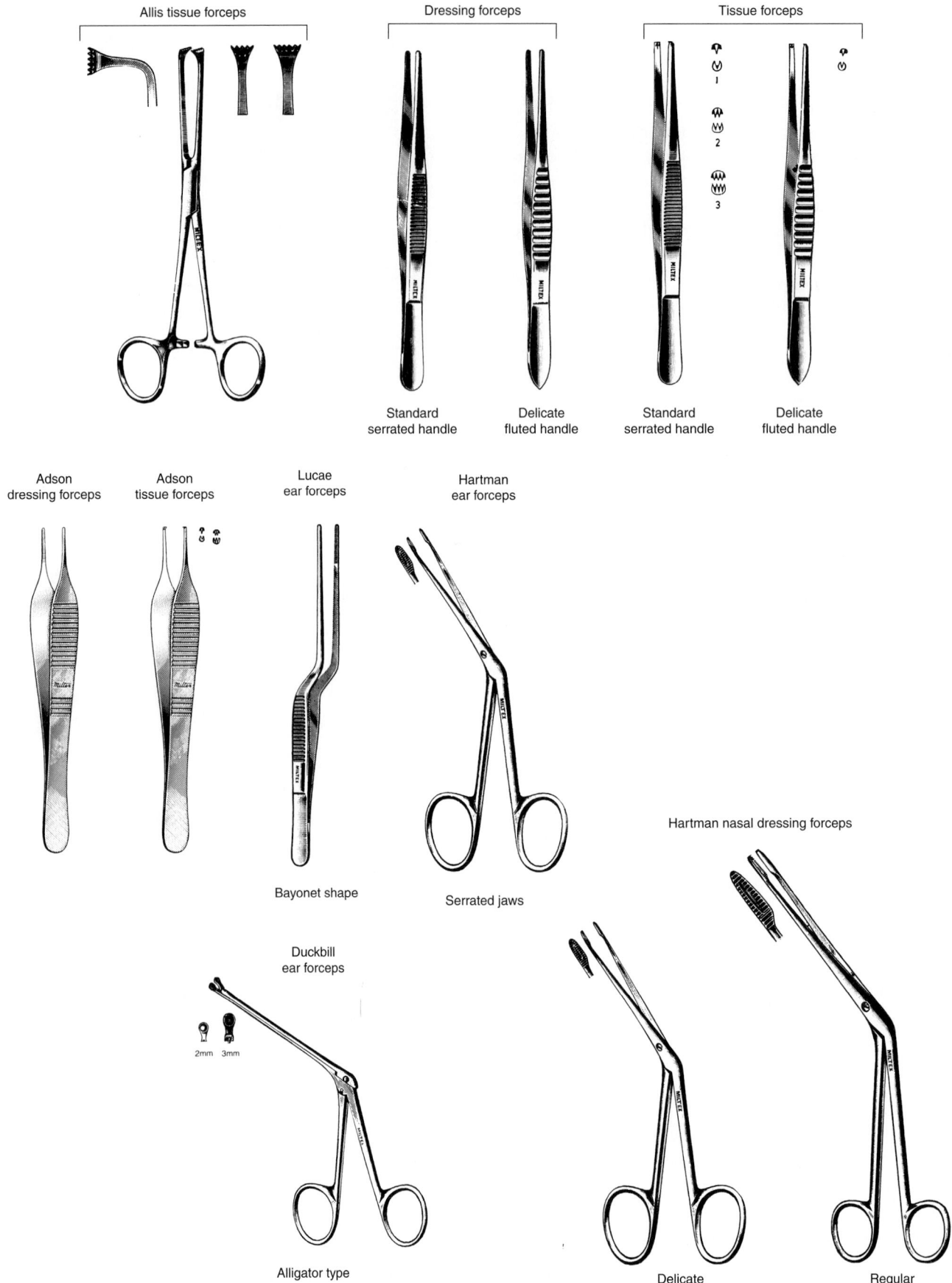

Figure 31-9 Tissue and dressing forceps. (Courtesy of Miltex Instrument Company, Inc.)

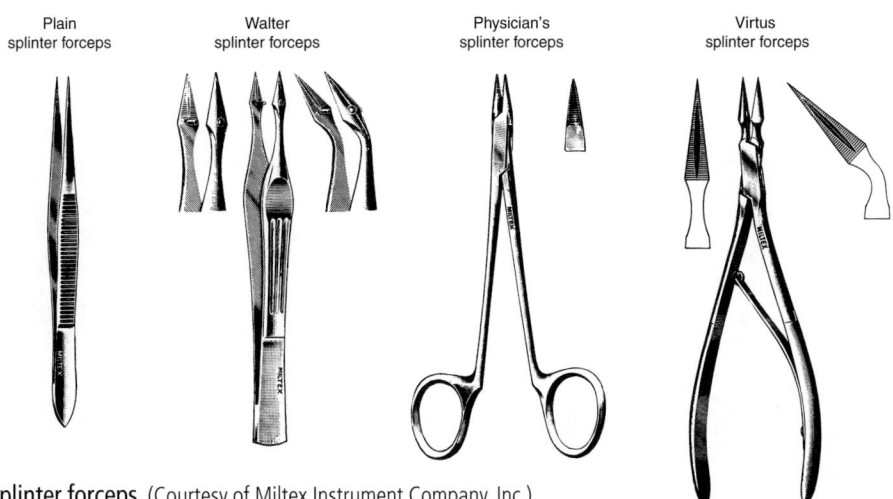

Plain splinter forceps   Walter splinter forceps   Physician's splinter forceps   Virtus splinter forceps

Figure 31-10   Splinter forceps. (Courtesy of Miltex Instrument Company, Inc.)

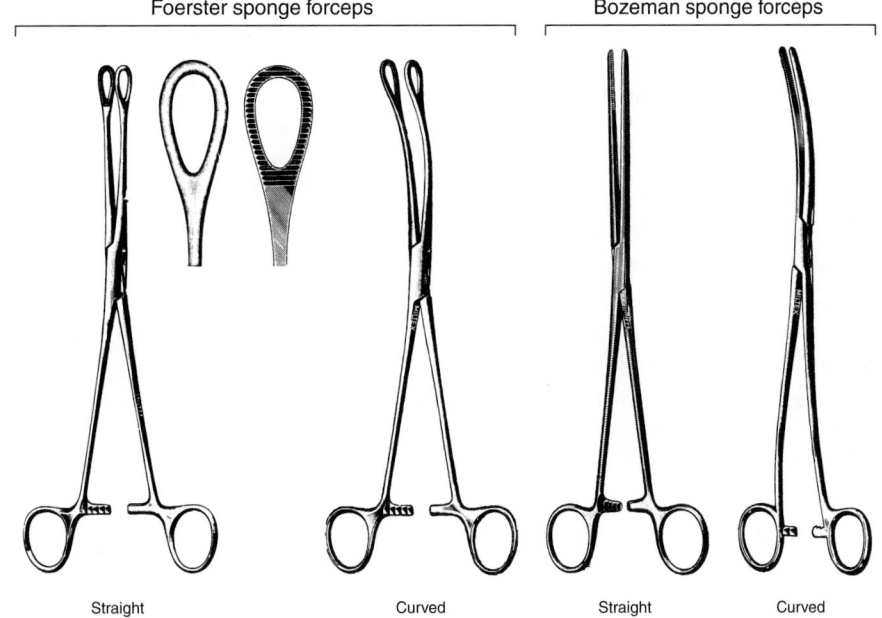

Foerster sponge forceps   Bozeman sponge forceps

Straight   Curved   Straight   Curved

Figure 31-11   Sponge forceps. (Courtesy of Miltex Instrument Company, Inc.)

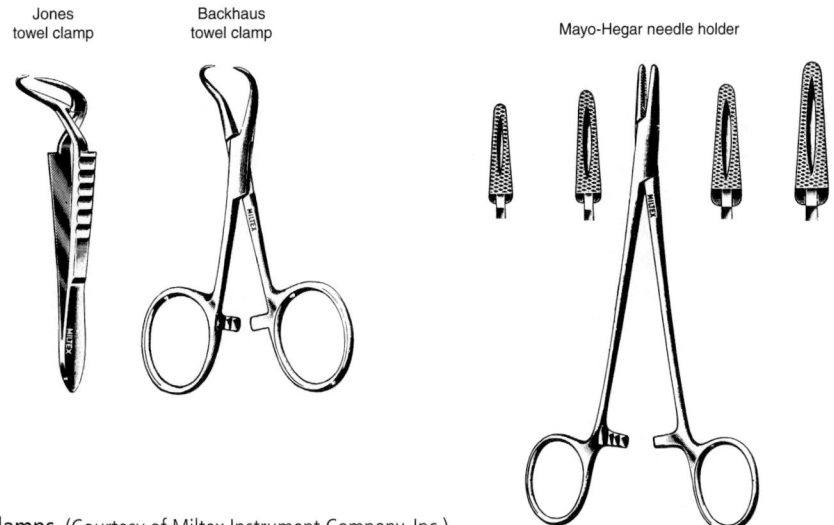

Jones towel clamp   Backhaus towel clamp   Mayo-Hegar needle holder

Figure 31-12   Towel clamps. (Courtesy of Miltex Instrument Company, Inc.)

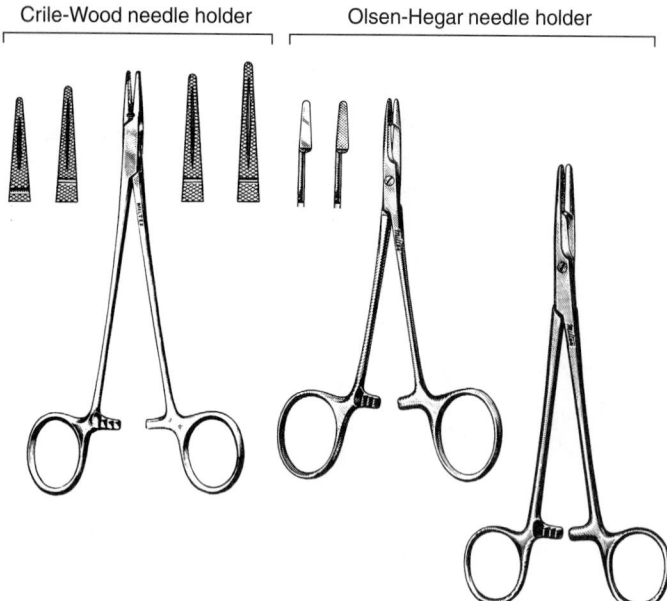

Figure 31-13 Needle holders. (Courtesy of Miltex Instrument Company, Inc.)

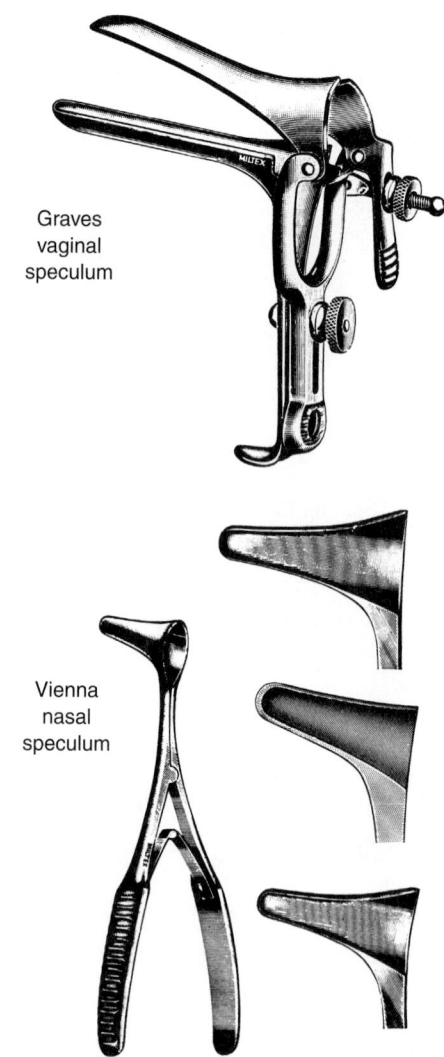

Figure 31-14 Specula are used to explore body canals. (Courtesy of Miltex Instrument Company, Inc.)

Specula, Scopes, Probes, Retractors, and Dilators.

The category of dilators and probes includes specula which are designed for enlarging and exploring body orifices (Figure 31-14). The vaginal speculum is available in various lengths and widths and may be made of metal or disposable plastic. The most common instrument for enlarging the nostril is the Vienna nasal speculum. This instrument is used with the Lucae bayonet forceps to perform procedures within the nose.

Scopes are defined as lighted instruments used for viewing. The otoscope, used to visualize the ear canal and eardrum, has a small light aimed into an ear speculum. Ear specula may be disposable or reuseable. If reused, they are sanitized, chemically disinfected, rinsed, and dried before reuse. Proctoscopes, anoscopes, (Figure 31-15) and rigid sigmoidoscopes are used for viewing the rectum, anus, and the sigmoid portion on the large intestine and have guides called obturators to ease insertion. The light source for the proctoscopes and anoscopes is usually a separate lamp. Although the light sources cannot be sterilized, they can be meticulously disinfected. The speculum portion that is inserted into the rectum may be disposable plastic or made of metal. Both the metal speculum and its obturator may be sanitized and sterilized in the autoclave.

There is another group of long flexible scopes that are much more complex and use fiber-optic light sources. Fiber-optic scopes are considered to be medical equipment rather than surgical instruments. Although considered to be medical equipment, these flexible scopes are inserted into body cavities and must be sanitized and sterilized.

Probes are slender instruments used to probe into a hidden area, body cavity, or wound. Sounds are long, slender probing instruments used to determine the size and shape of the area being probed or to detect the presence of an unseen foreign body. Sounds may be calibrated in centimeters or inches (Figure 31-16).

Retractors used in minor surgery are often called skin hooks and are used to hook onto and retract the edges of a wound to facilitate better viewing. Skin hooks are fine-tipped and delicate. As with all of the finer surgical instruments, special care should be taken to avoid damaging the delicate tips (Figure 31-17).

Dilators are double-ended metal rods with smooth rounded tips, ranging in calibrated sizes from small to large. Dilators are inserted into narrowed or constricted ducts and tubes for the purpose of gradually dilating or enlarging the opening. Hegar uterine dilators are used to dilate the cervix to gain access to the inside of the uterus.

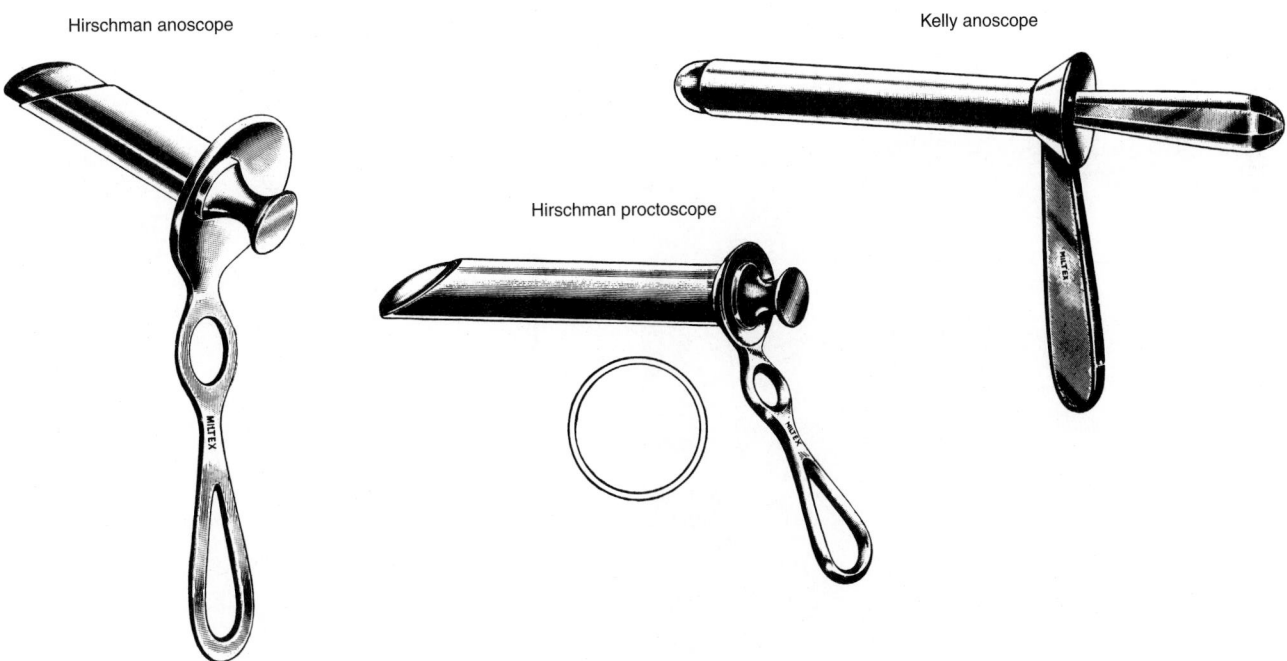

Hirschman anoscope

Kelly anoscope

Hirschman proctoscope

Figure 31-15 Scopes are used for viewing body orifices. (Courtesy of Miltex Instrument Company, Inc.)

Larry probe, groved director	Pratt rectal probe	Walther urethral sound	Sims uterine sound (maleable)	Volkman retractors	Miltex skin hooks

½

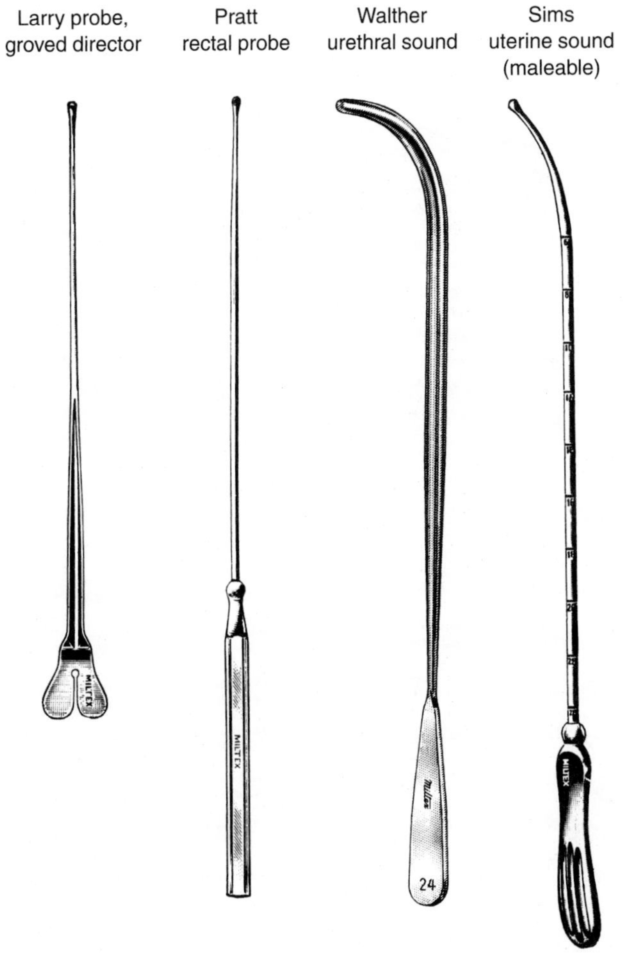

Figure 31-16 Various types of probes and sounds. (Courtesy of Miltex Instrument Company, Inc.)

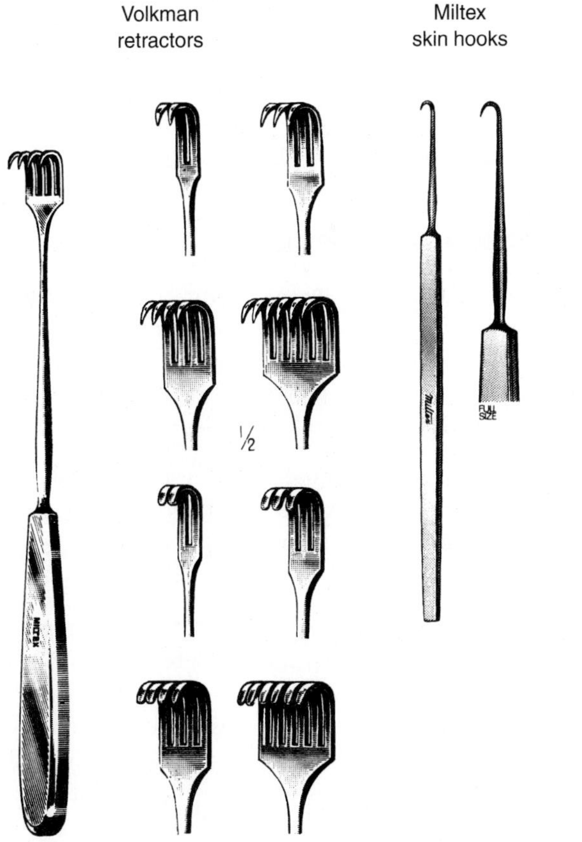

Figure 31-17 Various types of retractors. (Courtesy of Miltex Instrument Company, Inc.)

(continues)

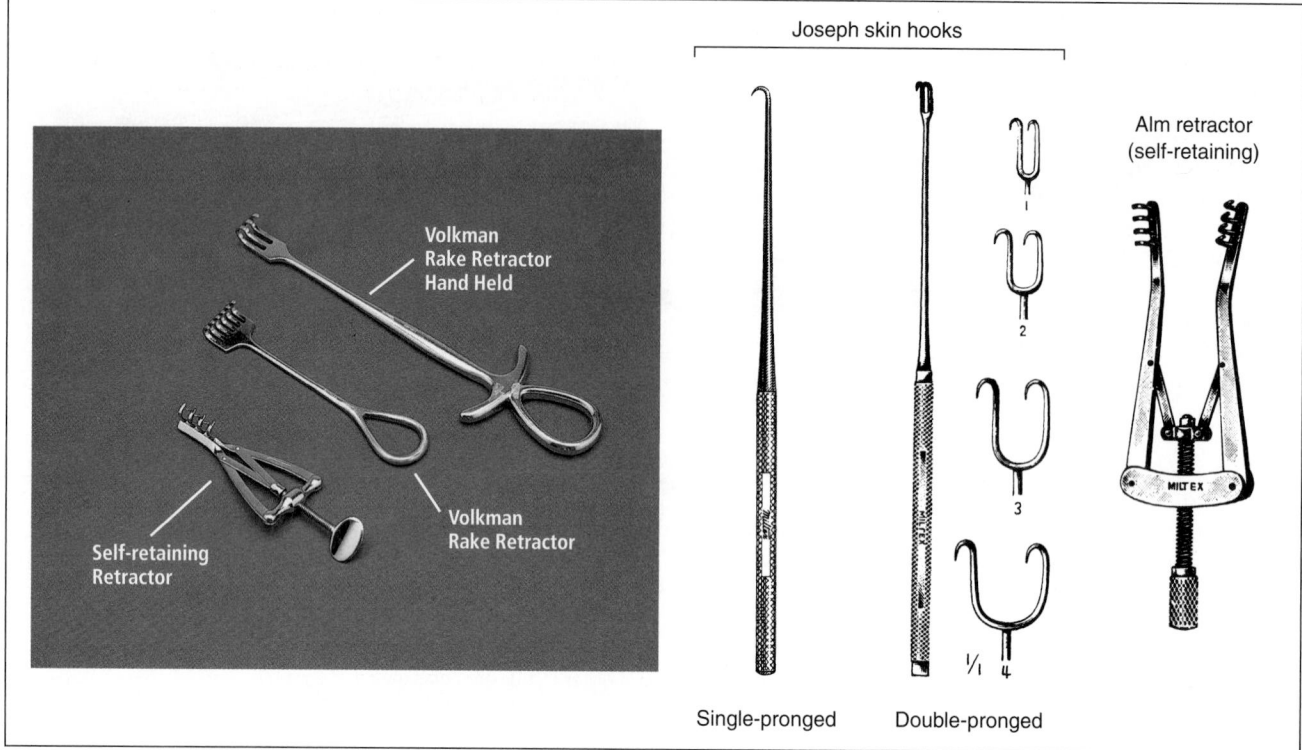

Figure 31-17 Various types of retractors. (*continued*)

Esophageal dilators are used to relieve **strictures**, or narrowing, of the esophagus. Urethral dilators are used to relieve strictures of the urethra (Figure 31-18).

Care of Instruments

Medical/surgical instruments require special care to prevent excessive wear and tear and unnecessary damage. Careful and frequent inspections will determine when instruments need to be replaced or repaired.

Some basic rules and rationales include:

● Immediately after use, soiled instruments should be soaked. This prevents blood and other body fluids from drying onto the working surfaces of the instruments.

● Soak solutions should be about room temperature and contain a neutral pH detergent with a protein/blood solvent. The proteins in the body fluids will not coagulate on the instruments in cool water and the neutral pH detergent will help prevent spotting and corrosion of the metals. Solvents will help break up the blood and proteins in the body fluids.

● Soak basins should be plastic to prevent damaging of points and edges. If a metal soak basin is used, placing a towel on the bottom as padding will help prevent damage to the instruments.

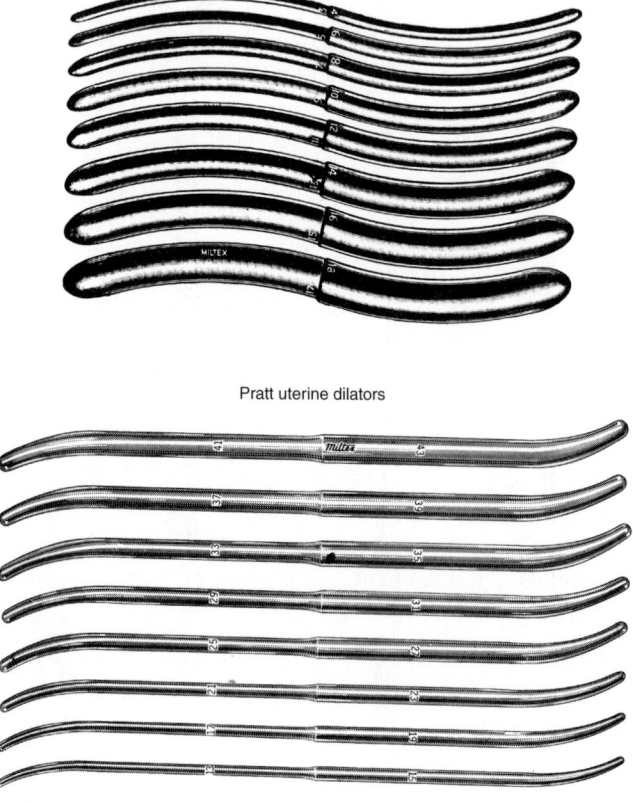

Figure 31-18 Two types of dilators. (Courtesy of Miltex Instrument Company, Inc.)

- Heavy-duty rubber gloves should be worn when cleaning instruments to lessen the likelihood of being stuck or cut with the sharp points and edges.

- Delicate instruments should be separated from heavier instruments to prevent the delicate instruments from being bent or otherwise damaged.

- Sharp instruments should be carefully separated from the other instruments and washed with extreme caution. The danger of being cut or punctured is greater when cleaning sharp instruments than at most other times and the sharp instruments are usually the most contaminated.

- A soft bristle brush should be used to scrub hinges, ratchets, and serrations. The brush should be firm enough to clean crevices thoroughly yet soft enough to prevent scratching instruments.

- Immediately after sanitization, instruments should be thoroughly rinsed and dried to prevent spotting and water damage.

- Carefully inspect all surfaces, edges, and points. Check for nicks, dulling, and warping. Test blades for sharpness. Be sure the instrument is not bent or pitted. Handles should also be checked for nicks that may snag and tear surgical gloves, thus disrupting the protective barrier and causing contamination.

- Damaged or malfunctioning instruments should be repaired or replaced.

Ultrasonic Cleaning. Surgical instruments can be cleaned (sanitized) by using an ultrasonic cleaner. Instruments are placed into a tank of water and detergent. Sound waves vibrate to loosen debris and contaminants. Place instruments with ratchets or hinges into the cleaner in an open position. The articles, when finished, are rinsed well, dried, and wrapped for sterilization. The process of sanitizing contaminated instruments by ultrasound is safe for all instruments including delicate instruments. Follow manufacturer's directions for use and care of the ultrasonic cleaner.

Sanitization by use of an ultrasonic cleaner eliminates cleaning instruments by hand, thereby reducing the risk of contamination to the medical assistant.

- Instruments should be processed in the cleaner for the full recommended cycle time—usually 5 to 10 minutes.

- Place instruments in open position into the ultrasonic cleaner. Make sure that "sharps" (scissors, knives, osteotomes) blades do not touch other instruments.

- All instruments have to be fully submerged.

- Do not place dissimilar metals (stainless, copper, chrome plated) in the same cleaning cycle.

- Change solution frequently—at least as often as the manufacturer recommends.

- Rinse instruments with water after ultrasonic cleaning to remove ultrasonic cleaning solution.

Chemical "Cold" Sterilization

This type of sterilization is sometimes referred to as "cold" sterilization which indicates that heat-sensitive items such as fiber-optic endoscopes and delicate cutting instruments can be immersed in a chemical solution. The chemicals used are reliable and capable of destroying bacteria and their spores and, used in strict accordance with the manufacturer's instructions regarding length of immersion time, sterility can be assured.

See Procedure 31-11. Also, see Chapter 22 for disinfection and sanitization procedures.

SUPPLIES AND EQUIPMENT

The supplies necessary for minor office surgery are often disposable and should be replenished as needed. Most medical/surgical supply companies have catalogs available for ordering and many companies have sales representatives who make regular stops or are available by telephone to assist in the ordering process. Sales representatives are familiar with the products their company markets and are extremely useful as a resource. Samples of new products are often available for trial, and optional choices are always offered. Medical/surgical supply companies frequently offer special prices for larger quantity purchases. If a medical/surgical supply item is being used frequently and storage space is available, buying in larger quantities might be more cost-effective. If a product currently being used is not meeting expectations, requesting optional trial products is usually the first step toward finding a better product. Following are some of the more commonly used supplies associated with minor surgery.

Sponges and Wicks

Surgical sponges are prepackaged squares of folded gauze used in surgery. Within the physician's office, sponges are more often referred to by their size. A gauze square measuring four inches by four inches is called a 4 × 4 (Figure 31-19). The other most useful sizes are 3 × 3 and 2 × 2. The 4 × 4s are either packaged in individual peel-apart packages of two or may be purchased in nonsterile bulk packages of one hundred. The individual packages are

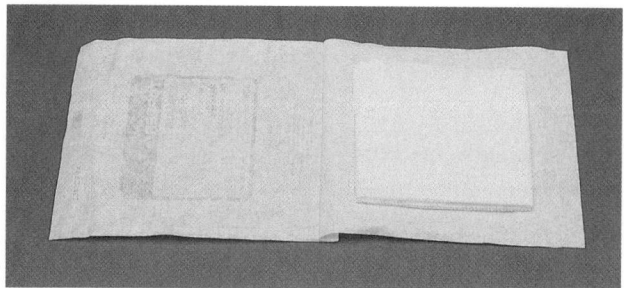

Figure 31-19 Peel-apart sterile open package of 4 × 4 gauze. These are also referred to as 4 × 4s or, in surgery, as surgical sponges.

convenient, sterile, and very useful for most purposes, but cost more per sponge than the non-sterile bulk packages. For larger surgical needs, the medical assistant may package bulk sponges in a canister and sterilize several sponges for later use (see Chapter 22). Most sponges are simply folded gauze, but some have cotton or rayon pads embedded in them to increase absorption ability and to create a softer texture. The medical assistant using the sponge will probably have a preference among the different types and uses. Gauze sponges are used in wound cleansing, in skin preparation, as absorbable sponges during surgery, as dressings and coverings, and for padding. The ambulatory care setting may prefer to have different sizes and types in stock to meet different needs.

Sterile surgical wicks or wound packing strips are used when an infected wound needs to remain open for drainage. The wicking material is made of narrow strips of gauze packaged in long lengths in opaque glass bottles. The most recognizable trade name is Iodoform®. The bottles are sterile and packaged for multiple-use purposes. Extreme care should be taken to prevent contamination during removal of individual lengths. The bottle is opened using sterile technique, sterile dressing forceps are inserted into the bottle, the strip is cut to the desired length using sterile scissors, and the lid is applied without compromising the sterility of the remaining wicking material in the bottle.

Solutions/Creams/Ointments

Many different soaps and solutions are available and effective as skin cleansers, preoperative scrubs, paints, soaks, and antiseptics. Betadine® (povidone-iodine) is a well-known antiseptic and is available as a surgical soap called a "scrub" and as a nonsoap solution for preoperative skin preparation/paint. Hibeclens® is another very effective antiseptic that does not have the staining tendencies of iodine. Medical/surgical supply companies will have

names and samples of other products. Consideration should be made to cost, effectiveness, ease of use, shelf life, and personal preferences. Isopropyl alcohol, a 70 percent alcohol solution, is of limited medical/surgical use although due to its rapid volatility rate and its ability to dissolve oils, it is still preferred for skin preparation prior to injections and venipuncture. Isopropyl alcohol is available in bottles for use with cotton/rayon balls or in convenient individually packaged pledgets. Isopropyl alcohol can be irritating and is not effective as a preoperative skin preparation. Hydrogen peroxide is a noncaustic mildly effective skin antiseptic. It bubbles on contact with mucous membranes and other moist skin surfaces, dissolving blood and proteins, and seems to have a mechanical cleansing action. Hydrogen peroxide is ineffective as a skin prep prior to surgery but is useful for cleaning after surgery.

Antibacterial creams and ointments are sometimes applied topically on wounds to aid healing. Antibacterial creams are usually white, water-based, and nongreasy. Antibacterial ointments are usually clear and oil based. If a wound requires thorough cleaning between dressing changes, an antibacterial cream is preferred due to the ease of removal.

Some examples of sterile solutions are sterile saline, sterile distilled water, and Betadine® solution.

Dressings and Bandages

Dressings are defined as the sterile material applied directly onto the surface of a wound or surgical site. Bandages are defined as the supportive material applied over the top of dressings and are nonsterile. A dressing, being sterile, should be handled with care to avoid contamination of the wound. Often a nonstick pad or topical medication will be applied to the wound to prevent the dressing from adhering to the wound.

Dressings are usually made of gauze and need to completely cover the wound. Dressings must be adequately absorbent.

Bandages are used to keep dressings in place, to provide padding and protection, and to immobilize. Bandaging may consist of rolled gauze wrapped around the wound area with an additional sturdier wrap applied overall. An elastic bandage may provide additional support, and a triangular bandage or sling even more. A unique type of bandage is the tubular gauze bandage. Tubular gauze bandages are used to cover appendages such as fingers, arms, toes, and legs and come in various sizes according to the size of the body part being covered. Refer to Chapter 9 for further information about bandages. See Figure 31-20 for examples and illustrations of various bandage-wrapping techniques.

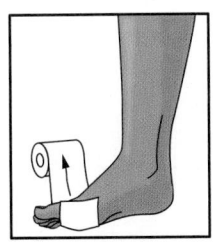

Foot and ankle Use 3-inch width. Hold foot at right angle to leg. Start bandage on ridge of foot just back of the toes.

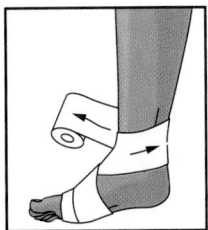

Pass bandage around foot from inside to outside. After two or three complete turns around foot, ascending toward the ankle on each turn, make a figure eight turn by bringing bandage up

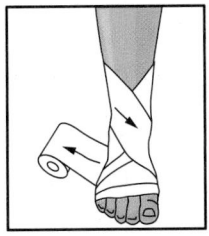

over the arch–to the inside of the ankle–around the ankle–down over the arch–and under the foot.

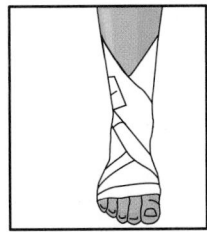

Repeat the figure eight wrapping two to three times. Fasten end by pressing the last 4 to 6 inches of unstretched bandage to the preceding layer.

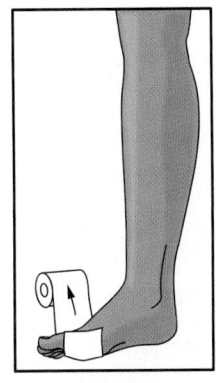

Lower leg: Use 3-4 inch width depending on the size of the leg. A leg wrap requires two rolls of bandage. Hold foot at right angle to leg. Start bandage on ridge of foot just back of the toes.

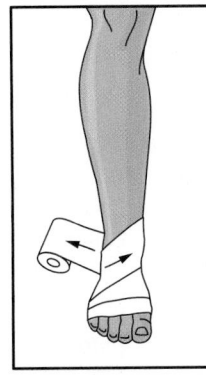

Pass bandage around foot from inside to outside. After two complete turns around foot, make a figure eight turn by bringing bandage up over the arch–to the inside of the ankle– around the ankle–

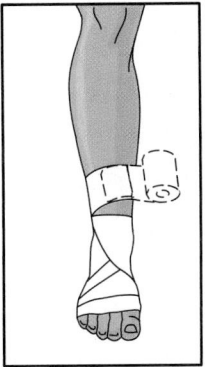

down over the arch–and under the foot. Start circular bandaging, making the first turn around the ankle. To begin the second roll of bandage, simply overlap the unstretched ends by 4 to 6 inches, press firmly, and continue wrapping.

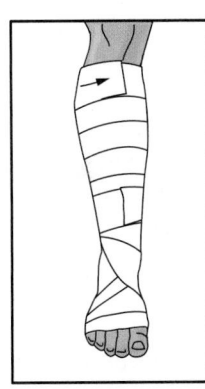

Wrap bandage in spiral turns to just below the kneecap. Fasten end by pressing the last 4 to 6 inches of unstretched bandage to the preceding layer.

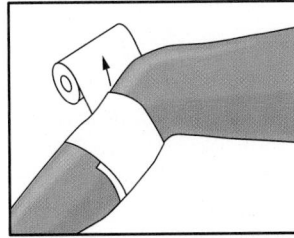

Knee: Use 4 inch width. Bend knee slightly. Start with one complete circular turn around the leg just below the knee.

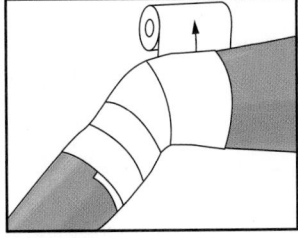

Start circular bandaging, applying only comfortable tension. Cover kneecap completely.

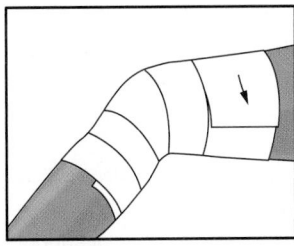

Continue wrapping to thigh just above the knee. Fasten end by pressing the last 4 to 6 inches of unstretched bandage to the preceding layer.

Figure 31-20 Bandage-wrapping techniques illustrating the circular, spiral, and figure-eight turns. The Peg Self-Adhering elastic bandage is used in these illustrations. (Courtesy Becton-Dickinson Division, Becton, Dickinson, and Co., Rutherford, NJ) *(continues)*

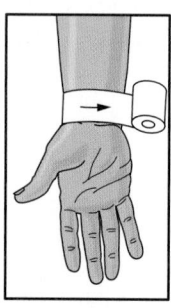

Wrist Use 2- or 3-inch width. Anchor bandage loosely at the wrist with one complete circular turn.

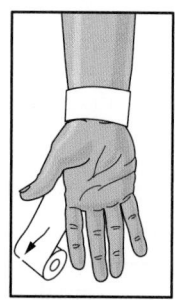

Carry the bandage across the back of the hand, through the web space between the thumb and index finger

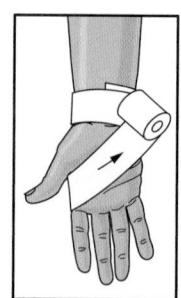

and across palm to the wrist, Make a circular turn around

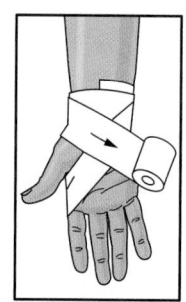

the wrist and once more carry the bandage through the web space and back to the wrist.

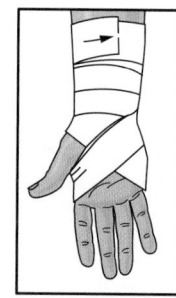

Start circular bandaging, ascending to the wrist. Fasten the end by pressing the last 4 to 6 inches of unstretched bandage to the preceding layer.

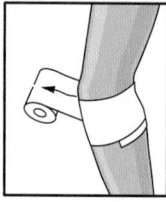

Elbow Use 3- or 4-inch width, depending on the size of the arm. Two rolls of bandage are required to complete the wrap. Start with a complete circular turn just below the elbow.

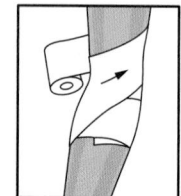

Wrap bandage in loose figure eights

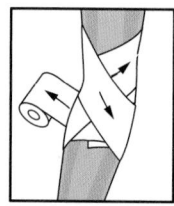

to form a protective bridge across the front of the elbow joint.

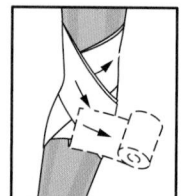

Fasten end by pressing 4 to 6 inches of unstretched bandage to preceding layer. Start second bandage with a circular turn below the elbow

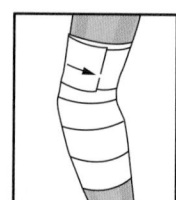

over the first wrap. Continue spiral bandaging over the elbow, ascending to the lower portion of the upper arm. Fasten end with circular turn.

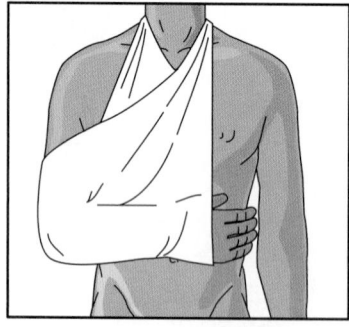

Shoulder A shoulder wrap is used to provide additional support for an arm in a sling. Use 4- or 6-inch width. One or two rolls of bandage may be used. Start under the free arm.

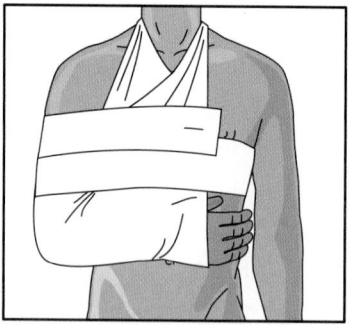

Carry the bandage across the back, over the arm in the sling, across the chest and back under the free arm in complete circular, overlapping turns. Fasten the end by pressing 4 to 6 inches of unstretched bandage to underlying bandage.

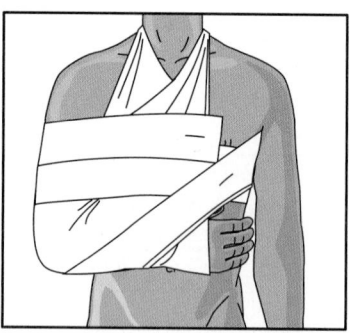

Additional support can be obtained with a second bandage. Start at the back just behind the flexed elbow in the sling. Carry the bandage under the elbow, up over the forearm, around the chest and back, and repeat. Fasten end.

Figure 31-20 *(continued)*

Anesthetics

The word **anesthesia** means the loss of feeling or sensation. An anesthetic is any mechanism that causes this loss of feeling. The application of extreme cold can be an anesthetic because it causes numbness to nerve endings and thus the loss of feeling. Anesthetics may be inhaled, topically applied or sprayed, or injected either directly into a vein (intravenously), the spinal column (intrathecally), or locally (subcutaneously) into the tissues at the site of the surgical procedure.

Injectable Anesthetics. Most anesthetics used in minor surgery are administered locally through injection into the subcutaneous tissues. The nerves exposed to the anesthetic become temporarily unable to conduct sensations and feelings to the brain, thereby causing a lack of pain sensation in the area during minor surgery. All synthetic local anesthetics have names that end in "caine." Some of the most common are Xylocaine (lidocaine), Novacaine (procaine), Marcaine, and Carbocaine. Local anesthetics are available in single-dose vials or ampules of 10 mL, but most medical offices prefer the cost-effectiveness of multiple-dose vials containing 30 to 50 mL. Local anesthetics are also available in varying strengths such as 0.5 percent, 1 percent, and 2 percent.

Injectable anesthetics may contain an additive called **epinephrine**. Epinephrine causes vasoconstriction and is used when reduced blood flow to the area is desired. The medical assistant is often delegated the responsibility of filling the syringe with the prescribed amount and strength of the ordered anesthesia or may assist the physician in drawing up the medication.

Drawing Techniques. If the physician plans to inject the anesthesia prior to applying sterile gloves, either the medical assistant or the physician may draw up the medication. The filled syringe is then placed on the side, rather than directly on the sterile field. This allows the physician to anesthetize the patient prior to beginning the sterile procedure. After the anesthesia has taken effect, the physician will perform a surgical handwash, apply sterile gloves, and begin the surgery.

When the physician applies sterile gloves prior to injecting the anesthesia, the sterile syringe may be placed directly on the sterile field either empty or filled. One person wearing sterile gloves may handle the syringe and draw up the medication while another person not wearing sterile gloves holds the vial. This method requires either that the syringe and needle be applied directly to the sterile tray or handed directly to a "sterile" person. Refer to Chapter 36 for the specific techniques for drawing up medications.

Topical Spray Anesthetics. Not all anesthesia is injectable. Topical (applied to the surface) anesthetics are available in liquid and spray. The most common topical anesthetic used in the medical office is ethyl chloride spray. Ethyl chloride freezes the skin to allow for simple piercing or lancing. The anesthetic action usually only lasts for a few seconds; therefore, the procedure must be performed quickly. One example for the use of ethyl chloride spray is to briefly numb an area prior to an injection. A lesion that is infected is extremely painful to inject with a local anesthetic; however, by using ethyl chloride spray before the injection, the patient is able to remain still. Ethyl chloride spray may also be used prior to installing intravenous lines.

See Table 31-2 for a summary of supplies and equipment.

TABLE 31-2	SUPPLIES AND EQUIPMENT COMMONLY USED IN MINOR SURGERY
Item	**Use/Description**
Sponges	Used in wound cleansing, skin preparation, as absorbable sponges during surgery, as dressings and coverings, and for padding. Also called 4 × 4s. Typically made of folded gauze, though some have cotton or rayon pads embedded in them to increase absorption.
Wicks	Used when an infected wound needs to remain open for drainage. Wicking material is made of narrow strips of gauze packaged in long lengths in opaque glass bottles, which should be opened using sterile technique.
Solutions	Used as skin cleansers, preoperative scrubs, paints, soaks, and antiseptics. Most common are Betadine, an antiseptic often used in soap form as a scrub; Hibeclens, an effective antiseptic without iodine's staining properties; isopropyl alcohol, a 70 percent alcohol solution favored for skin preparation prior to injections and venipuncture but not effective as a preoperative skin preparation; hydrogen peroxide, a mildly effective noncaustic skin antiseptic.
Creams and ointments	Antibacterial. May be used topically on wounds to promote healing.
Dressings	Sterile material applied directly onto surface of a wound or surgical site. Usually made of gauze. Must be adequately absorbent and completely cover the wound.
Bandages	Nonsterile supportive materials applied over dressings to keep the dressing in place. May be rolled gauze, elastic bandage, or tubular gauze bandage.
Anesthetics	A mechanism used to cause the loss of feeling. May be inhaled, topically applied, sprayed, or injected directly into a vein, the spinal column, or locally into the tissues at the site of the surgical procedure.

PATIENT CARE AND PREPARATION

Patient Preparation and Education

If the patient is having a planned surgical procedure performed, an opportunity for patient preparation and education is available. Patients may need to modify their diet, adjust medication, acquire special supplies, adjust their personal home and work situations, obtain prior approval from their insurance, and prepare for the postoperative period. If the patient is having an urgent procedure performed, such as a laceration repaired, there is less time for preparation. In either case, the medical assistant will need to follow an established protocol covering wound care, patient education, patient health consideration, and consent. In the case of an accidental wound, the medical assistant needs to determine the cause of the wound and the date of the last tetanus injection. See Chapter 22 for specific information about immunization schedules. The medical assistant must also check to determine whether or not the patient has allergies or sensitivities of any kind, in particular to medication.

Diet modifications include abstaining from eating and/or drinking for several hours prior to the surgical procedure as well as restricting the types and amounts of certain foods or liquids consumed prior to and directly after the procedure. When patients are aware of special dietary needs after surgery, they can shop early and be prepared. An example of a medication treatment includes prescribing an antibiotic to be taken as a precaution against acquiring an infection following surgery or adjusting anticoagulant medications to prevent excessive bleeding during surgery. Each clinic, physician, procedure, and patient will have individual requirements and preferences. The patient might be required to obtain special supplies for the convalescent period. For instance, immediately after a vasectomy a scrotal support is usually recommended. Crutches or special foot coverings might be necessary following foot or leg surgery. Specific wound dressing and bandages might need to be purchased prior to the surgery in anticipation of the postoperative need. Having another person accompany the patient to the clinic for the surgery is required for the safe return home. Knowing the planned period of time for recovery allows the patient to make the necessary arrangements for work, child care, and other personal situations.

Informed Consent

Prior to a surgical procedure, the patient's written consent must be obtained. In many medical and all surgical procedures, a written, **informed consent** form must be signed. An informed consent is a document that may be created specifically for a particular procedure or that may be an established document available for duplication. An informed consent document informs the patient of the medical or surgical procedure to be performed; describes to the patient, in lay terms, the actual procedure; cites alternative treatments; and lists the possible undesirable outcome and risks involved in the procedure. See Chapter 7 for additional information on informed consent.

The cost of the procedure is also important information. Any questions the patient has about the surgery should be answered completely by the physician and an assessment should be made that the patient understands the answers. Even in the best of circumstances, results cannot be guaranteed. Most of the difficult situations between physicians' practices and patients come from misunderstandings about unexpected outcomes. If patients are informed completely, even unplanned results are better tolerated.

Medical Assisting Considerations

The general health and condition of the patient prior to surgery is very important when planning the recovery. A frail, weak man living alone may need home health care following even a simple surgical procedure. Some people may not be able to follow standard preoperative or postoperative instructions. The recovery may depend on the availability of supplies beyond what the patient can financially afford. If difficult circumstances can be identified prior to the surgery, arrangements can be made with home health care services, community assistance services, or friends and family. This can help avoid complications. Prior medical history should also be established and questions should be asked regarding **allergies** and sensitivities to medications and medical substances.

Postoperative Instructions

Postoperative instructions should be written and clearly understood by the patient. If the patient has a caregiver at home, the postoperative instructions should be clearly understood by the caregiver as well. The telephone number of the clinic and an after-hours number should be written on the postoperative instructions and brought to the attention of the patient and caregiver. It is good practice to plan to call patients within the first postoperative day to check on their condition.

Wounds, Wound Care, and the Healing Process

There are many different types of wounds based on the type of injury incurred. Wounds may be classified as open or closed, accidental or intentional (surgical).

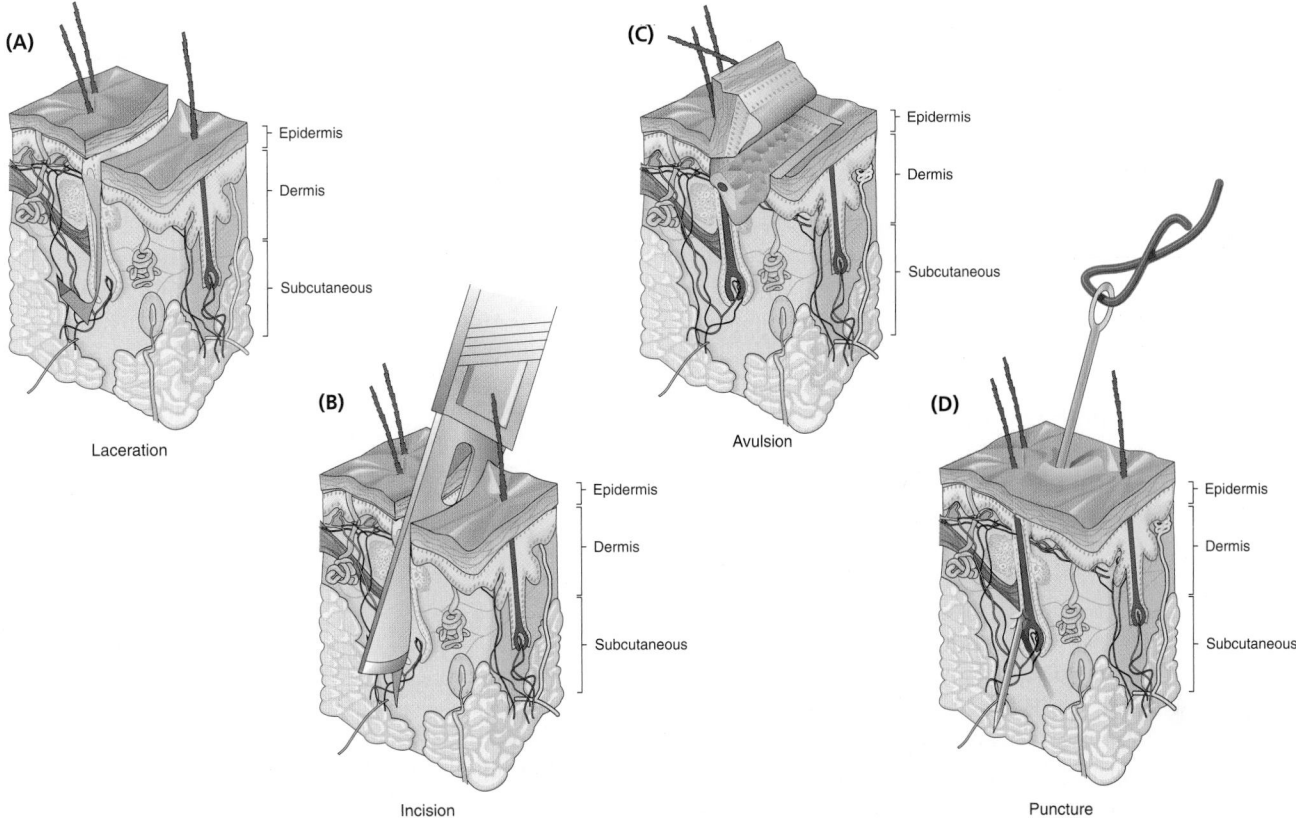

Figure 31-21   Open wounds. (A) Lacerations are accidental tearing of the body tissue usually made by sharp objects. The torn flesh may be smooth or jagged and is usually difficult to clean and suture properly. There is typically extensive bleeding. Paper cuts are examples of lacerations. (B) Incisions are intentional cuts typically made with a scalpel for surgical procedures. (C) Avulsions are accidental tearing away of a part or structures of the skin. (D) Punctures are holes or wounds made by a pointed object and can be either accidental or intentional. Puncture wounds have little bleeding because the point of entry is small. These wounds are typically not much larger than the instrument entering the skin. A puncture wound may also be the result of a bite or a gunshot wound.

Lacerations, incisions, avulsions, and punctures are all examples of open wounds (Figure 31-21). They are a result of tearing or cutting of the skin.

Ecchymosis (bruise), contusion, and hematoma are all examples of closed wounds. They are due to a blunt trauma that damages underlying tissues but leaves the skin intact (Figure 31-22).

Wounds are classified as superficial if the injury does not extend deeper than the subcutaneous tissues. Deep wounds extend beyond the subcutaneous layer. The size

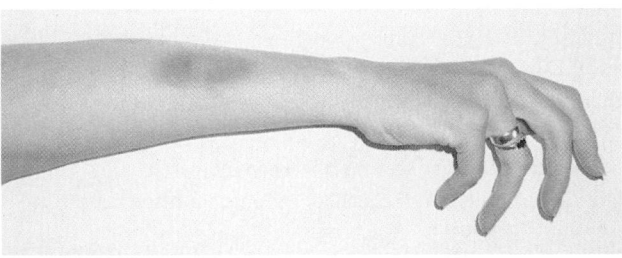

Figure 31-22   Closed wounds include contusions, ecchymoses, and hematomas. This photograph shows an ecchymosis.

and location as well as the depth of the wound are all important descriptors both for the medical record and for proper insurance reimbursement. A typical description of a patient wound that is an intermediate laceration might be, "patient sustained a deep 3.5 cm laceration to the anterior surface of the right knee caused by a fall onto a rock." A puncture wound might be described as, "patient presents with a 2 cm deep puncture wound on the plantar surface of the left foot obtained from stepping on a rusty nail." Both statements describe not only the size, depth, location, and type of wound, but also the causative factor.

Inflammation is the body's natural reaction to trauma. Inflammation is also a normal process of wound healing. Occasionally inflamed tissue will become infected if the trauma is caused by a pathogen. While a certain degree of inflammation is expected, prevention of infection is a primary goal (see Chapter 22).

See Chapter 9 for further description of wounds and emergency care of wounds.

The best treatment for infection is prevention. Instructing the patient about proper wound care is

Patient Teaching Tip

The basic signs of inflammation are redness, heat, swelling, pain, and loss of function. Any one or more of these may be present in varying intensities during an inflammatory process. Most wounds will have a mild inflammation described as slightly red or pink, mild warmth, slightly tender to the touch, and mildly swollen. The symptoms are caused by increased blood supply to the traumatized area and the infiltration of white blood cells in reaction to the trauma. Patients should be taught to watch for an increase in the intensity of redness, pain, swelling, and heat or any drainage, fever, or lymph gland swelling which indicates an infection from invading pathogens. The patient should be given instructions as to what actions to take if these symptoms of infection are noticed. The instructions should include a name and telephone numbers to call during the day or night. The medical assistant should reassure the patient not to hesitate to contact the center or physician if infection is suspected.

extremely important. Encourage the patient to keep the wound clean and dry. In certain circumstances, the physician may prescribe a warm soak solution or the application of a topical antibacterial medication. Protecting the wound from further trauma and contamination will also aid in the healing process. Opinions will differ on whether a wound is best left open to air or covered with a dressing. Most health care providers will agree that covering a wound is preferred whenever contamination is likely. (See Procedure 31-4.)

BASIC SURGERY SETUP

Preparing for surgery includes assembling supplies and equipment, setting up the surgery tray, getting the patient and room ready, and preparing to assist during surgery. The specific instruments, supplies, and equipment needed for each surgery should be listed on individual **surgery cards**. These cards may be 3 × 5 or 5 × 7 cards stored in a card file or full sheets of procedures compiled in a manual or notebook. Each physician will have individual sets for each surgical procedure performed. Information on the surgery card should include physician glove size, standing preoperative and postoperative instructions, and any additional information specific to the physician's needs or to the surgical procedure.

Basic Rules and Concepts for Setup of Surgical Trays

In addition to basic sterile principles, the guidelines in Table 31-3 will help ensure the sterile field remains sterile.

MINOR SURGERY PROCESS

For ease in understanding the individual tasks involved in minor office surgery, Table 31-4 provides generic steps for setting up the surgical tray, preparing the room, preparing the patient, assisting with the surgery, and the cleanup process. Table 31-4 is intended as a quick checklist only and does not include all the specific details necessary for each surgery. Refer to the individual surgical procedures that follow for more details.

PREPARATION FOR MINOR SURGERY

The following section includes the following procedures used in preparation for minor surgery:

- Applying Sterile Gloves (Procedure 31-1)
- Preparation of Patient Skin for Minor Surgery (Procedure 31-12)
- Setting Up and Covering a Sterile Field (Procedure 31-13)

TABLE 31-3   GUIDELINES FOR STERILE TRAY SETUPS
• Set up the sterile surgery tray just prior to the surgery to allow less chance of accidental contamination.
• Immediately after the tray is set up, cover it with a sterile drape.
• Once the tray is prepared and covered, move it directly into the surgery area rather than leaving it in a common area.
• Inform the patient and others in the surgery room that the tray is sterile and should not be touched. Patients are often curious about instruments and may attempt to look under the covers if not cautioned against it.
• If the medical assistant is interrupted while preparing the tray and it becomes necessary to leave the tray unattended, cover the tray and move it out of traffic paths to prevent it from being bumped.

TABLE 31-4 PREPARATIONS FOR MINOR SURGERY

Tray Setup

1. Wash hands.
2. Reference surgery card.
3. Gather equipment and supplies.
4. Sanitize and disinfect Mayo instrument tray.
5. Set up sterile field.
6. Place sterile instruments and supplies on the sterile field.
7. Apply sterile gloves.
8. Arrange instruments and supplies in an organized and logical manner.
9. Medication may be drawn up with assistance (optional).
10. Recheck tray for accuracy and completeness.
11. Remove gloves.
12. Cover and transport tray.
13. Add sterile solution (skin antiseptic) to tray if required.

Room Preparation

In preparing a room for a surgical procedure, all equipment should be clean and in good working order. Be certain to have spare parts such as light bulbs and filters readily available. Turn on equipment prior to the procedure to make sure all is working properly.

1. Check room equipment (light, stool, machinery, examination table, waste receptacle).
2. Check room supplies (tissue, extra gloves, and so on).
3. Arrange accessory supplies on the side counter in a logical order (pathology specimen bottle containing preservative, lab requisition, sterile glove package, dressings/bandages, postoperative medications).

Patient Preparation

1. Wash hands.
2. Greet patient and ensure identity.
3. Escort the patient to the procedure room and offer restroom facilities.
4. Discuss the patient's compliance to preoperative instructions.
5. Explain the procedure again and address any questions.
6. Review postoperative instructions.
7. Check for signed informed consent form.
8. Have the patient remove appropriate clothing and position the patient on the examination table. Offer a drape, gown, pillow, and blanket for comfort.
9. Prepare the skin for the surgical procedure (Procedure 31-12).

Assisting with Minor Surgery

1. Remove the sterile cover from the surgical tray while the physician applies sterile gloves.
2. Assist the physician with stool and lamp adjustment as needed.
3. If the medical assistant did not perform the skin preparation, assist the physician as needed during skin preparation and draping. The equipment and supplies for skin preparation are separate from the surgery tray and equipment (see Procedure 31-12).
4. Adjust the instrument tray and equipment around the physician.
5. Assist with drawing up local anesthetic or other medication as needed.
6. Apply clean gloves for protection or sterile gloves to assist.
7. Surgery begins.
8. The medical assistant either assists with sterile procedure or supports the patient as needed.
9. After surgery, assist with or perform dressing of wound.
10. Clean patient if necessary.
11. Dispose of biohazardous waste materials.
12. Remove contaminated gloves, wash hands.
13. Assist the patient postoperatively.

Assisting the Patient Postoperatively

1. Check patient vital signs.
2. Remain with patient to ensure patient safety. Allow to rest if necessary.
3. Assist patient off examination table and assist with clothing as necessary.
4. Review written postoperative instructions with patient and caregiver. Dressing should be kept clean and dry. Patient should report any signs of infection.
5. Clarify any medication orders with patient and caregiver.
6. If not previously arranged, schedule follow-up appointment.
7. Document postoperative instructions in patient record.

Room and Equipment Cleanup

1. Apply barrier gloves.
2. Dispose of drapes, table cover, pillowcase, and so on. Use biohazardous waste receptacle whenever appropriate.
3. Transfer contaminated surgical tray to cleanup area.
4. Using forceps, isolate sharps from surgical tray and dispose of them into designated sharps container.
5. Place instruments into a soak solution.
6. Sanitize Mayo instrument tray and all surfaces (examination table, stool, counter, lamp, machinery, and equipment).
7. Dispose of contaminated barrier gloves and apply protective gloves.
8. Disinfect all surfaces (examination table, stool, counter, lamp, machinery, and equipment).
9. Allow to dry.
10. Sanitize, dry, rewrap, and sterilize instruments.

Note: During most surgical procedures, if tissue is excised, it is placed in a biopsy specimen jar containing formalin (a preservative) and sent to the pathology laboratory with an appropriately completed requisition (Figure 31-23).

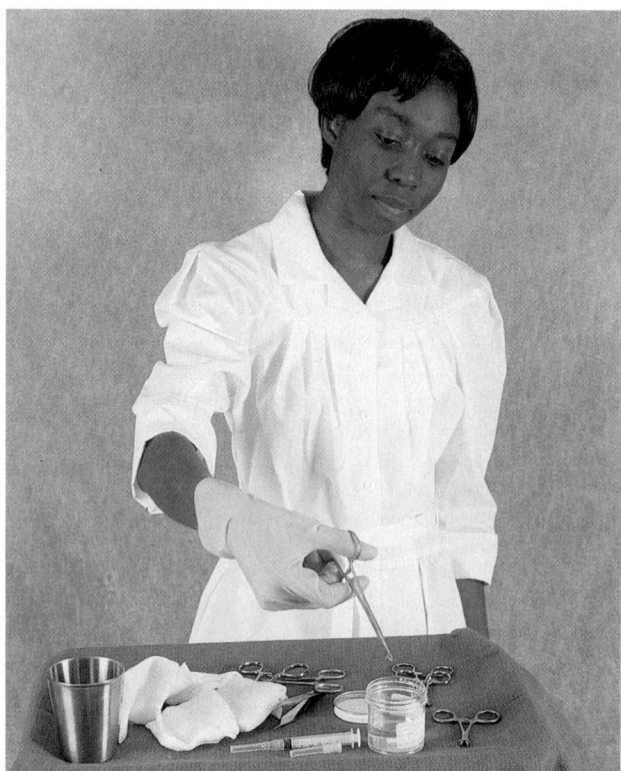

Figure 31-23 Medical assistant placing tissue for biopsy into specimen jar with formalin. The specimen will be sent to the pathology lab for examination.

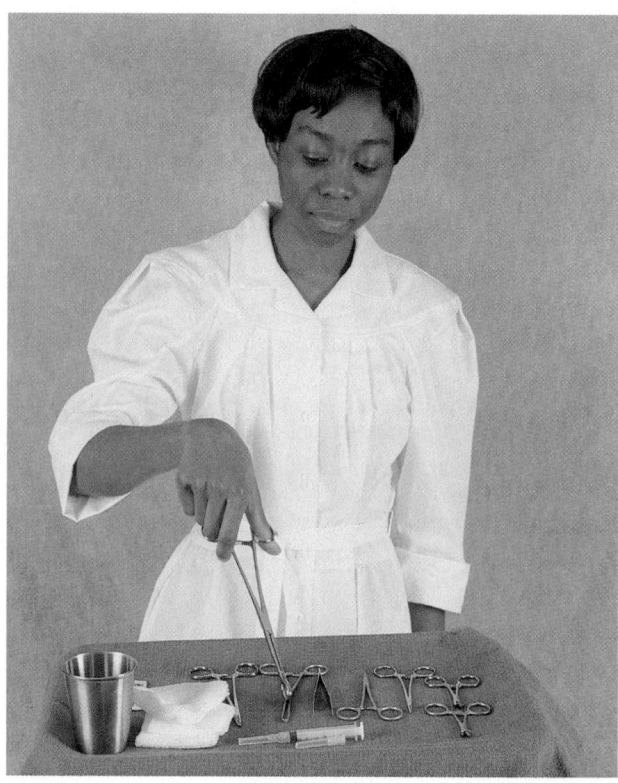

Figure 31-24 If sterile gloves have been removed, use dry sterile transfer forceps to apply or rearrange sterile items on the tray.

● Opening Sterile Packages of Instruments and Supplies and Applying Them to a Sterile Field (Procedure 31-14)

● Pouring a Sterile Solution into a Cup on a Sterile Field (Procedure 31-15)

Setting up surgical trays for specific surgeries will be addressed in a later section of this chapter.

A sterile tray is set up in the surgical area for immediate use. Therefore, a solution will be poured just prior to the tray being used because it will not have to be moved.

Using Dry Sterile Transfer Forceps

Occasionally after a sterile tray has been set up and sterile gloves removed, an additional item needs to be applied to the tray. The use of dry sterile transfer forceps allows sterile items to be applied or sterile items on the tray to be rearranged without the application of another pair of sterile gloves (Figure 31-24). The practice of using wet sterile transfer forceps is no longer recommended. Instead, when the use of sterile transfer forceps is needed, dry sterile transfer forceps are unwrapped, used only once, and then reprocessed for sterilization and subsequent use.

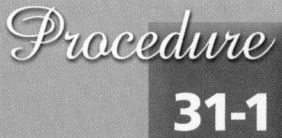

31-1   Applying Sterile Gloves

STANDARD PRECAUTIONS:

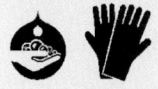

PURPOSE:
Since hands cannot be sterilized, everyone performing sterile procedures must wear sterile gloves. This procedure provides direction on how to apply sterile gloves without compromising sterility.

EQUIPMENT/SUPPLIES:
Packaged pair of sterile gloves

PROCEDURE STEPS:

1. Remove rings and watch. Wash hands using surgical asepsis. RATIONALE: Rings and watches can snag and tear gloves and therefore interfere with barrier protection.
2. Inspect glove package for tears or stains. RATIONALE: Tears and stains indicate that the gloves are no longer considered sterile and must be disposed of or used for a nonsterile purpose.
3. Place the glove package on a clean, dry, flat surface above waist level. RATIONALE: Using a contaminated surface could compromise the sterility of the sterile package.
4. Peel open the package taking care not to touch the sterile inner surface of the package. Do not allow the gloves to slide beyond the sterile inner border. RATIONALE: Care must be taken to maintain the sterility of the gloves.
5. The gloves should be opened with the cuffs toward you, the palms up, and the thumbs pointing outward. If the gloves are not positioned properly, turn the package around, being careful not to reach over the sterile area or touch the inner surface or the gloves. RATIONALE: Sterile gloves are packaged in this position for ease in application.
6. With the index finger and thumb of the nondominant hand, grasp the *inner* cuffed edge of the opposite glove. The glove should be picked straight up off the package surface without dragging or dangling the fingers over any nonsterile area (Figure 31-25A). RATIONALE: Picking up the glove by grasping the inner cuff prevents the outer glove from becoming contaminated. Strict adherence must be made to the sterile principles listed in the beginning of this chapter.
7. With the palm up on the dominant hand, carefully slide the hand into the glove. Do not allow the outside of the glove to come in contact with anything. Always hold the hands above the waist and away from the body (Figure 31-25B, C, D).

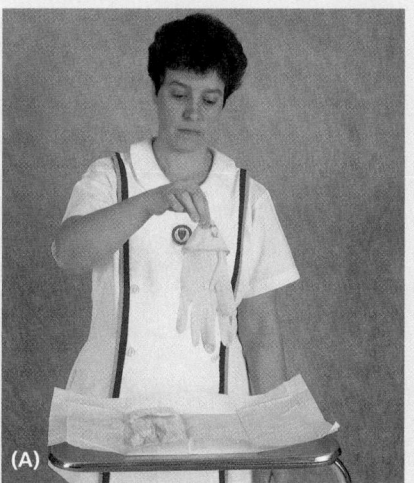
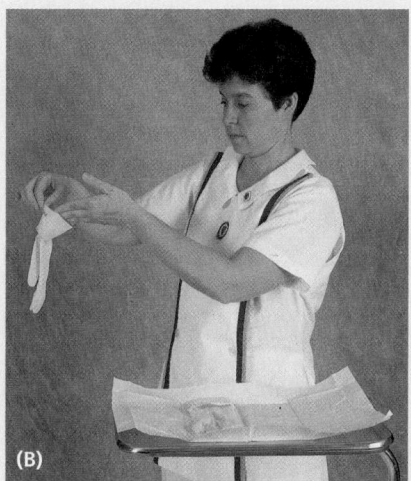
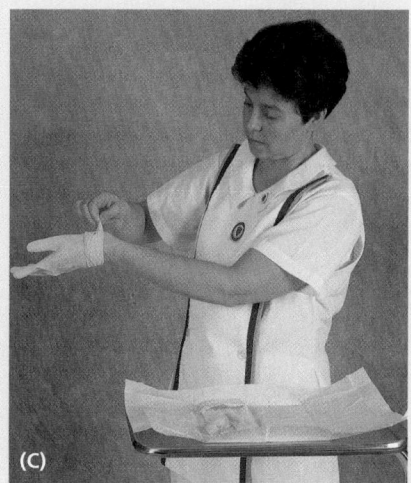

Figure 31-25 To apply sterile gloves: (A) With the nondominant hand, grasp the *inner* cuffed edge of the opposite glove. (B) With palm up on the dominant hand, slide the hand into the glove. (C, D) Hold the hand above the waist and away from the body.

(continues)

Procedure

31-1 *(continued)*

RATIONALE: Keeping the palm up allows the glove to remain sterile in the palm area if it rolls slightly on the back of the hand.

8. With the gloved hand, pick up the glove for the remaining hand by slipping four fingers under the *outside* of the cuff. Lift the second glove up, keeping it held above the waist and away from the body. Do not allow the glove to drag across the package or touch nonsterile surfaces (Figure 31-25E). RATIONALE: The outside of the second glove is sterile

and may only be touched by another sterile surface.

9. With the palm up, slip the second hand into the glove. Do not allow the outside of the gloves to touch nonsterile skin (Figure 31-25F).

10. Adjust the gloves on the hands as needed, but avoid touching the wrist area. Keep gloved hands above the waist and away from the body. Do not touch nonsterile surfaces with the gloved hands (Figure 31-25G, H, I).

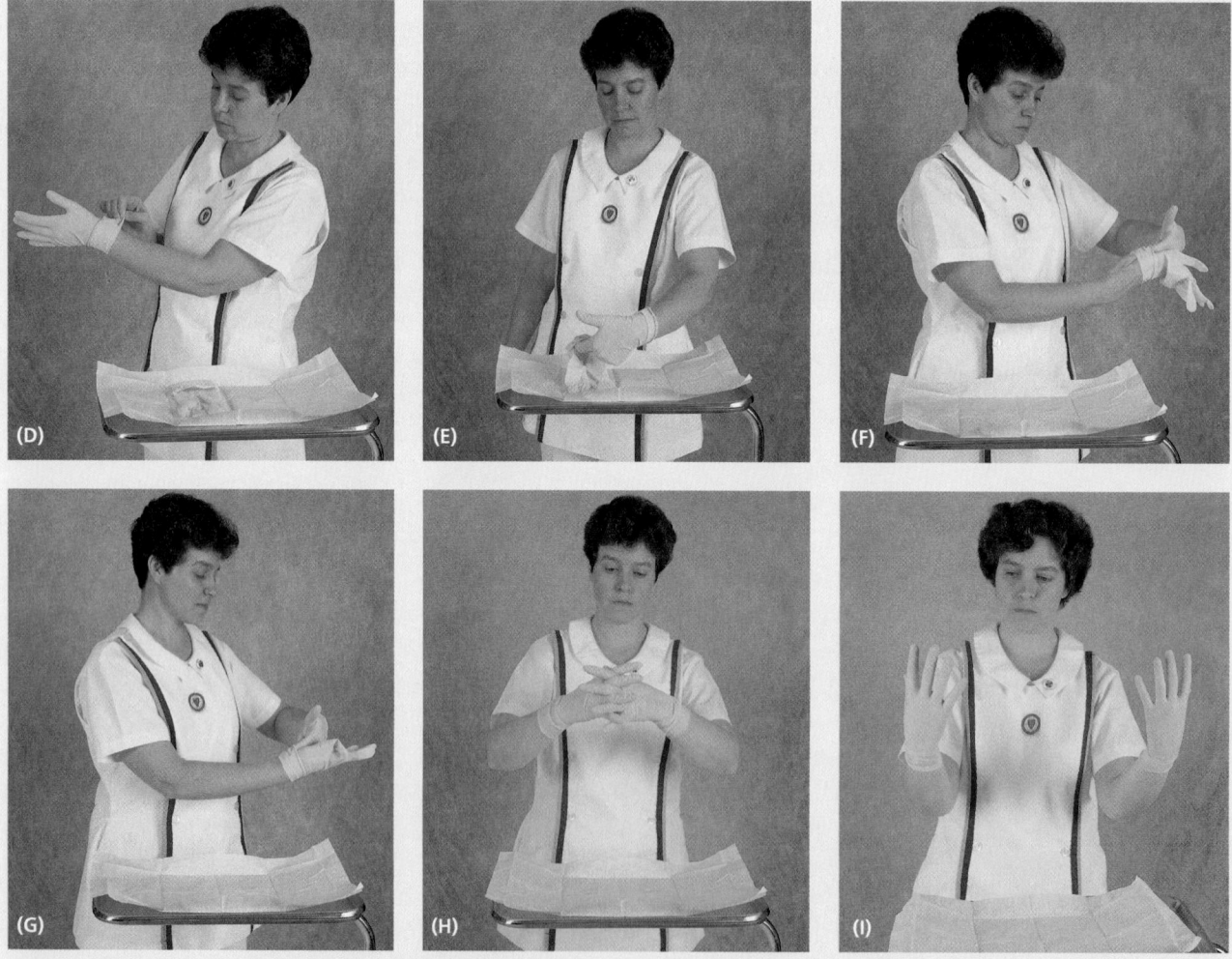

Figure 31-25 *(continued)* (E) With the gloved hand, pick up the glove for the remaining hand by slipping four fingers under the *outside* of the cuff. (F) With palm up, slip the second hand into the glove. (G, H, I) Adjust gloves. Avoid touching wrist area. Keep gloved hands above the waist and away from the body.

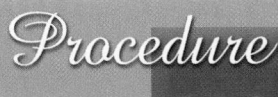

31-2　Assisting with Minor Surgery

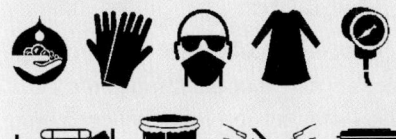

PURPOSE:

To maintain sterility during minor surgical procedures that require surgical excision of a neoplasm.

EQUIPMENT/SUPPLIES:

Mayo stand on which to create a sterile field that includes:

Needles and syringe	Tissue forceps
Bowl	Needle holder
Betadine solution	Skin retractor
Gauze sponges	Transfer forceps
Scalpel and blades	Side table:
Dissecting scissors	Sterile gloves
Operating scissors	Labeled biopsy containers
Forceps that hold	with formalin
the drapes or 4	Appropriate laboratory
sterile towels and	requisition
4 clamps	Anesthesia
Hemostats (2 curved	Alcohol wipes
and 2 straight)	Dressing tape, bandages
Thumb forceps	Biohazard container
Suture material	

PROCEDURE STEPS:

1. Check room for readiness and equipment for cleanliness.
2. Wash hands.
3. Set up side table of nonsterile items. RATIONALE: Nonsterile items cannot be placed onto a sterile field because they will contaminate it.
4. Perform surgical asepsis handwash.
5. Set up sterile field on a Mayo stand or on a clean dry flat surface.
   A. Use a commercially prepared sterile setup that is appropriate for the surgical procedure. Open the setup creating a sterile field from the inside of the sterile wrap. Add other articles such as instruments and supplies by using sterile transfer forceps or peel-apart packages that can be opened in a sterile fashion. (Refer to Procedure 31-14 on opening sterile packages.)

or

B. Remove a sterile fanfolded towel from a canister of sterile towels using sterile transfer forceps. Hold one edge of the sterile towel and allow it to become unfolded by gently shaking it. Grasp the other edge and gently place the towel on the Mayo stand from the farther side to the side nearest you. Add sterile articles as described in A. RATIONALE: This maneuver prevents leaning over the sterile towel and contaminating it as you lay it down.

6. Apply sterile gloves. Arrange instruments according to use.
7. Cover the sterile field with a sterile towel if not being used immediately. Gently place towel from the side nearest you to side farthest from you.
8. Identify patient, explain the procedure, and prepare the patient. Refer to patient preparation in Table 31-3.
9. Prepare patient's skin. Refer to Procedure 31-12.
10. Remove the sterile cover from the sterile setup as the physician applies sterile gloves.
    C. Lift the towel by grasping the tips of the corners farthest away from you and lifting toward you. Do not allow arms to pass over sterile field. RATIONALE: Avoids crossing over sterile field.
11. Assist the physician as necessary, being certain to follow the principles of surgical asepsis.
    - The physician will inject the local anesthetic, apply Betadine or other antiseptic to the surgical site, apply sterile drapes, and begin the surgery.
    - The medical assistant will hold the vial of anesthesia while the physician withdraws the appropriate dose.
    - Adjust the instrument tray and equipment around the physician.
    - Assure a good light source.
    - Comfort and support patient emotionally.
    - Assist with the surgery as directed by the physician (sterile gloves must be worn).
    - Hand instruments to the physician and receive used intruments from the physician and place in a basin or container out of patient's sight.

(continues)

Procedure
31-2   *(continued)*

- If necessary, hold biopsy container to receive specimen being excised.
- Do not contaminate the inside of the container.
- Hold the cover facing down. Tightly place cover on the container.
- Assist with or apply sterile dressing to the operative site.

12. Assist patient as necessary. Refer to Assisting the Patient Postoperatively in Table 31-4.
13. The specimen container must be handled with disposable gloves as recommended by standard precautions. The container must be tightly covered, labeled with the patient's name, date, type, and source of specimen and sent to the laboratory accompanied by the appropriate laboratory requisition.
14. Wearing appropriate personal protective equipment (PPE), clean surgical or examination room.
    - Dispose of used sponges in biohazard container and knife blades and other disposable sharps in puncture-proof sharps container.
    - Rinse used surgical intruments; soak, sanitize, and sterilize for reuse.
    - Remove gloves and other PPE and dispose of per OSHA guidelines.
15. Wash hands.
16. Document in the patient's record that the specimen was sent to the laboratory.

Procedure
31-3   Suturing of Laceration or Incision Repair

STANDARD PRECAUTIONS:

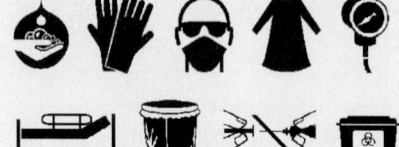

PURPOSE:
Suturing is recommended if a laceration or incision is gaping, bleeding uncontrolledly, or is located on the face, neck, or a bend of a body part or extends deep into underlying tissue. Suturing facilitates healing by approximating the edges. Suturing decreases scarring, helps decrease the likelihood of infection, and promotes healing. The wound and the surrounding area must be meticulously cleaned of any dirt and debris. Many physicians have standard orders for wound cleaning prior to suture repair of either a laceration or incision-type wound.

EQUIPMENT/SUPPLIES:
Surgical tray:
  Syringe and needle for anesthetic

Hemostats (curved)
Adson or tissue forceps
Iris scissors (curved)
Suture material and needle
Needle holder
Gauze sponges
Side table:
  Anesthetic as ordered by the physician
  Dressings, bandages, and tape
  Splint/brace/sling (optional)
  Sterile gloves

PROCEDURE STEPS:
1. Wash hands.
2. Identify the patient and explain the procedure. Check for signed consent forms.
3. Reassure and comfort the patient as needed.
4. Assess cause of wound and its severity.
   - Determine any known allergies and last tetanus booster.
   - Identify any health concerns to avoid possible complications.

(continues)

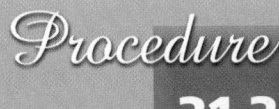

31-3 (continued)

- Soak wound in an antiseptic solution as ordered by physician.
- Clean and dry wound.
- Position patient comfortably, lying down.
5. Assist the physician as needed.
6. Support the patient as needed.

Give postoperative care:
7. Apply sterile gloves.
8. Clean area around the wound.
9. Dress/bandage/splint wound following physician's preference.
10. Remove gloves.

11. Wash hands.
12. Check patient's vital signs.
13. Explain wound care to the patient (and caregiver) and provide written instructions including symptoms of infection.
14. Assist the patient with any concerns or questions.
15. Arrange for follow-up appointment and medication as ordered.
16. Dispose of supplies per OSHA guidelines. Clean room, sanitize instruments, sterilize for reuse.
17. Wash hands.
18. Document the procedure.

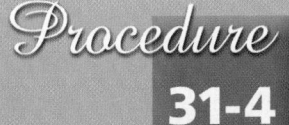

31-4 Dressing Change

STANDARD PRECAUTIONS:

 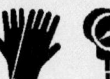

NOTE: After most minor surgical procedures have been completed, the wound is usually covered with a dry sterile dressing that may need to be removed periodically so that the wound can be checked for healing or for suture removal. Another dry sterile dressing may then be applied.

PURPOSE:
To remove a wound dressing and apply a dry sterile dressing.

EQUIPMENT/SUPPLIES:
Sterile field:
  Several sterile gauze sponges and other dressing material as needed
  Sterile bowl with Betadine solution
  Sterile dressing forceps
  Sponge forceps
Side area:
  Nonsterile gloves
  Sterile gloves
  Container of hydrogen peroxide or sterile water

Cotton-tipped applicators
Sterile adhesive strips
Antibacterial ointment/cream as ordered
Tape
Sponge forceps
Bandage scissors (2)
Waterproof waste bag
Biohazard waste container

PROCEDURE STEPS:
1. Wash hands.
2. Prepare sterile field. Add gauze sponges, bowl with solution, and forceps.
3. Position a waterproof bag away from sterile area.
4. Pour Betadine solution into sterile bowl.
5. Identify the patient and explain the procedure.
6. Reassure and comfort the patient as needed.
7. Loosen tape on dressing by pulling tape toward wound, or cut off bandage if necessary.
8. Put on nonsterile gloves or use forceps.
9. Carefully remove bandage, place in biohazard waste container. Do not pass over sterile field.
10. Remove dressing, taking care not to cause stress on the wound (Figure 31-26A).

(continues)

Procedure
31-4   (continued)

A. If stuck to the wound, pour small amounts of sterile water or hydrogen peroxide over dressing; allow to soak for a short time. Remove dressing when loose enough to remove without resistance. Note type and amount of drainage if present.

11. Place used dressing in waterproof bag without touching inside or outside of bag.

12. Assess wound and note any drainage or signs of infection. Remove and discard gloves in waterproof bag.

13. Wash hands.

14. Apply sterile gloves.

15. Clean the wound with Betadine solution (Figure 31-26B).

16. Dispose of used gauze in waterproof bag.

17. Using forceps, apply sterile gauze sponge(s) to wound (Figure 31-26C and D).

18. Remove gloves, dispose of in waterproof bag.

19. Secure dressing with adhesive tape (Figure 31-26E), roller bandage, or elastic bandage.

20. Dispose of waterproof bag in biohazard container.

21. Wash hands.

22. Document procedure and describe wound appearance (i.e., discharge, signs of infection, healing, etc.)

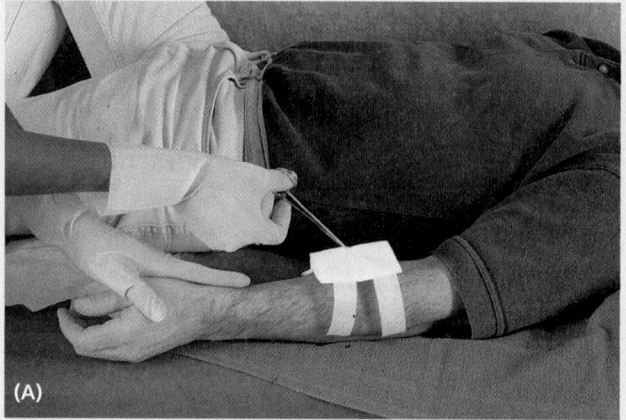
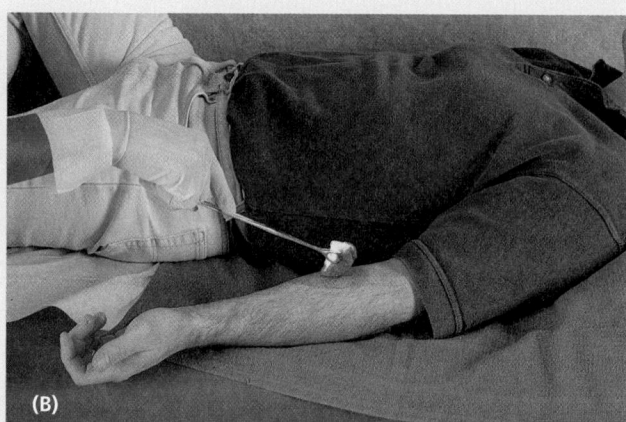
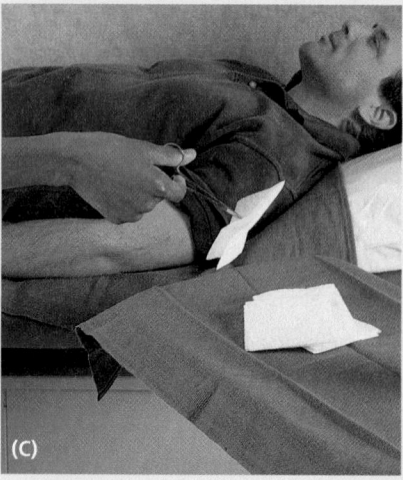
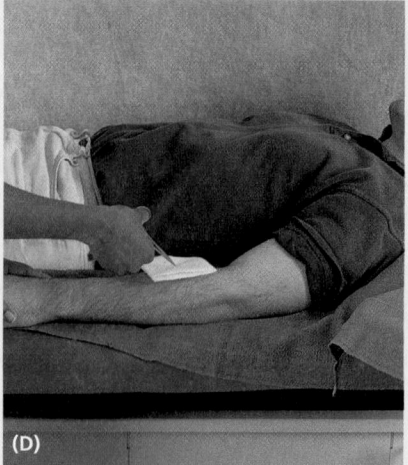
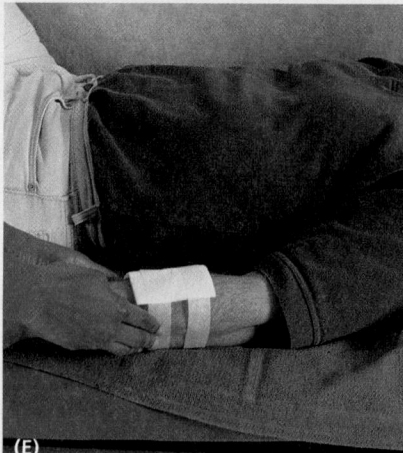

Figure 31-26 To change a dressing: (A) Gently remove dressing. Do not cause stress on wound. (B) Clean wound with Betadine solution. (C, D) Using dressing forceps, apply sterile gauze sponge(s) to wound. (E) Secure dressing with adhesive tape, roller bandage, or elastic bandage.

Procedure
31-5 Suture Removal

STANDARD PRECAUTIONS:

  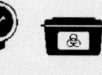

NOTE: Many minor surgical procedures require that suturing be done to approximate the skin edges to promote healing. Since these sutures are nonabsorbable, they must be removed when the wound has healed. The patient will return to the office or clinic to have the sutures removed. The medical assistant will remove the dressing and check the wound. The physician will also check the wound for degree of healing and determine that the sutures can be removed.

PURPOSE:
To remove sutures from a healed minor surgical wound (as per physician).

EQUIPMENT/SUPPLIES:
(See Figure 31-27.)
Gauze sponges
Bandage scissors
Biohazard waste container
Tape
Sponge forceps
Suture removal kit (suture scissors or staple remover, thumb forceps, and 4 × 4s)
Sterile latex gloves
Betadine solution or wash

PROCEDURE STEPS:
1. Identify patient.
2. Wash hands.
3. Open suture removal kit.
4. Apply sterile gloves.
5. Using thumb forceps, gently pick up one knot of a suture. Gently pull upward toward suture line. RATIONALE: Less pressure is exerted on suture line.
6. Using suture removal scissors, cut one side of the suture as close to skin as possible (Figure 31-28A and B). RATIONALE: Holding knot with forceps and cutting suture as close to skin as possible, the suture will be pulled out from under the skin, avoiding contamination of the wound.
7. Remove all sutures in the same manner, noting number of sutures removed. Dispose of the sutures on a sterile gauze sponge.
8. Examine the wound to be certain all sutures have been removed.
9. Apply Betadine solution to area.
10. Apply dry sterile dressing if ordered by the physician (see Procedure 31-4).
11. Remove gloves.
12. Dispose of used items per OSHA guidelines.
13. Wash hands.
14. Check patient's vital signs if indicated.
15. Explain wound care, provide written instructions to patient.
16. Arrange follow-up appointment if necessary.
17. Document the procedure.

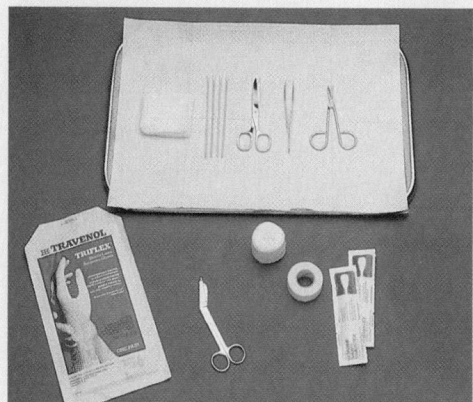

Figure 31-27 Equipment and supplies for suture removal.

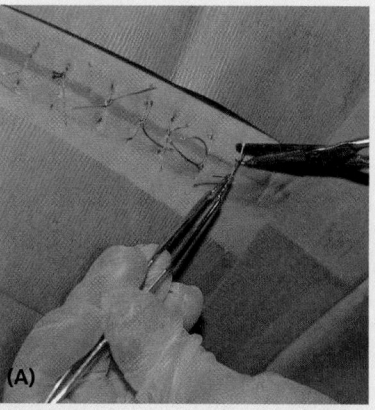 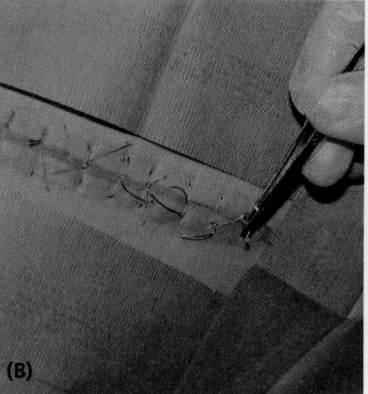

Figure 31-28 To move sutures: (A) Grasp suture knot with thumb forceps. Place curved tip of suture removal scissors just next to skin under the suture. Clip. (B) Gently pull the suture knot up and toward the incision with thumb forceps to remove.

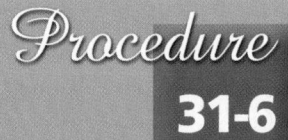

Application of Sterile Adhesive Skin Closure Strips

STANDARD PRECAUTIONS:

NOTE: On occasion, a superficial wound does not require sutures. However, the edges of the wound can be drawn together and sterile strips of adhesive are used to hold the edges of the wound together to facilitate healing.

PURPOSE:
To approximate the edges of a wound after the removal of sutures. Sometimes used in lieu of sutures or to give additional support along with sutures.

EQUIPMENT/SUPPLIES:
Sterile field:
  Suture removal instruments (as indicated)
  Sterile adhesive skin closure strips
  Iris scissors (straight)
  Tincture of benzoin (optional)
  Sterile cotton-tipped applicators (for tincture of benzoin)
Side area:
  Sterile gloves
  Dressings, bandages, and tape

PROCEDURE STEPS:
1. Identify the patient and explain the procedure.
2. Position patient comfortably.
3. Wash hands and apply gloves.
4. Remove bandages and dressings. See Procedure 31-4.
5. Clean and dry wound. See Procedure 31-4.
6. Assess the need for skin closure strips and alert the physician as indicated.
7. Remove gloves, wash hands, open container of tincture of benzoin, apply sterile gloves.

8. Apply tincture of benzoin to edges of wound if directed. Use sterile cotton-tipped applicator, taking care not to let it come into contact with the actual wound.
9. Remove strips from packaging one at a time. Apply one end of a skin closure strip to one side of the wound. Place the first strip over the center of the wound (Figure 31-29A).
10. Secure the end to the skin by carefully pressing.
11. Stretch the strip across the edge of the wound and secure on the other side in the same manner. This motion should bring the edges together without puckering the skin.
12. Apply the next two closure strips at halfway points between the first strip and each end of the wound (Figure 31-29B and C).
13. Continue in this manner until the edges are approximated. Keep wound edges in alignment.
Give postoperative care:
14. Dress and bandage if necessary.
15. Dispose of used items per OSHA guidelines.
16. Remove gloves and wash hands.
17. Check the patient's vital signs.
18. Explain wound care to the patient (and caregiver) and provide written instructions including symptoms of infection.
19. Assist the patient with any concerns or questions.
20. Arrange for follow-up appointment and medication as ordered.
21. Document the procedure.

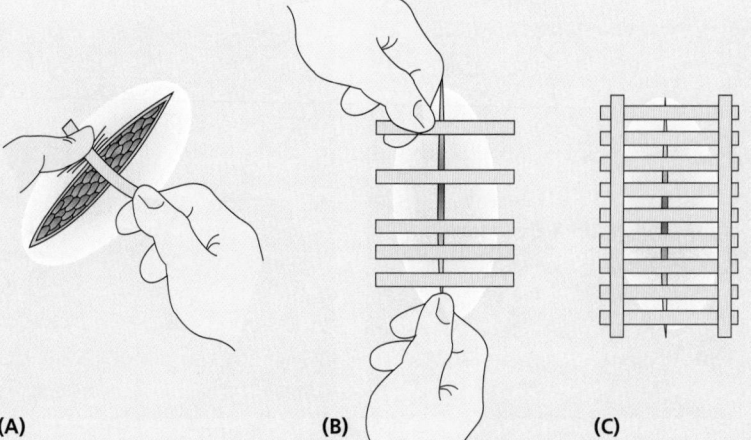

(A) (B) (C)

Figure 31-29 To apply skin closure strips: (A) Apply first strip in center of incision. (B) Apply closures to each side of center. (C) Apply closures parallel to incision.

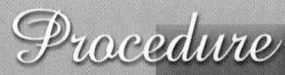

31-7 Sebaceous Cyst Excision

STANDARD PRECAUTIONS:

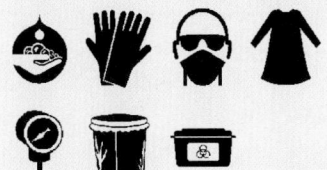

NOTE: A sebaceous cyst is a benign retention cyst, sometimes called a "wen." Sebaceous cysts are caused by an oil duct becoming "plugged" which causes the sebum (oil) to accumulate in the gland. Eventually the oil gland becomes distended. Sebaceous cysts that become inflamed or infected need to be removed. The patient may also elect to have a noninflamed sebaceous cyst removed if it is unsightly or located in a bothersome area. Incision and drainage of a sebaceous cyst is usually not the treatment of choice because they tend to recur if the entire cyst is not completely excised. Ideally, the entire cyst sac is removed intact, but occasionally the sac ruptures during removal and large amounts of foul-smelling biohazardous sebum can be expelled. In preparation for this occurrence, extra gauze sponges and gloves should be available.

PURPOSE:

To remove an inflamed or infected sebaceous cyst. To remove a sebaceous cyst that is not inflamed or infected but is located on an area of the body where the cyst is unsightly or where it may become irritated from rubbing.

EQUIPMENT/SUPPLIES:

Surgical tray:
Syringe/needle for anesthesia
Iris scissors (curved)
Mosquito hemostat (curved)
Scalpel blades and handle
Suture material with needle
Mayo scissors (curved)
Side area:
Skin prep supplies
Tissue forceps (2)
Gauze sponges (many)
Needle holder
Fenestrated drape (a drape with openings)
Antiseptic solution (Betadine)
Gloves (sterile and nonsterile)
Personal protective equipment
Anesthesia as directed

Dressing, bandages, tape
Specimen container/requisition (optional)
Biohazard waste container
Extra gauze sponges
Safety razor (optional)
Alcohol pledgets
Culturette (optional)

PROCEDURE STEPS:

1. Wash hands.
2. Identify the patient and explain the procedure.
3. Reassure and comfort the patient as needed.
4. Determine any known allergies and last tetanus booster.
5. Check for signed consent form.
6. Identify any health concerns to avoid possible complications.
7. Position the patient comfortably, lying down.
8. Perform the skin preparation as directed. (See Procedure 31-12.)
9. Wear appropriate PPE if cyst is infected. RATIONALE: Purulent material may drain out of the wound.
10. Assist physician to inject the anesthesia by holding the vial while the physician withdraws the appropriate amount of anesthesia. Continue to assist while the physician incises the cyst, removes it, and sutures the surgical incision. The physician will place the specimen in a container with a preservative to be sent to the pathology lab for analysis.
11. Support patient during surgery.

Give postoperative care:
12. Apply sterile gloves.
13. Clean area around the wound.
14. Dress and bandage as directed.
15. Dispose of items per OSHA guidelines. Remove gloves.
16. Wash hands.
17. Check the patient's vital signs.
18. Explain wound care to the patient (and caregiver) and provide written instructions including symptoms of infection.
19. Assist the patient with any concerns or questions.
20. Arrange for follow-up appointment and medication as ordered.
21. Document the procedure and that specimen sent to laboratory if appropriate.

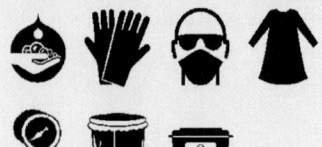

Procedure 31-8

Incision and Drainage of Localized Infections

STANDARD PRECAUTIONS:

NOTE: An abscess is a localized accumulation of pus surrounded by inflamed tissue. The body attempts to isolate pus into a pocket or abscess as a means of protecting itself by walling off the pathogens and preventing them from spreading throughout the body. Incision and drainage is the procedure of cutting into an area (often an abscess) for the purposes of draining the fluid/material. A culture of the exudate can be done to identify microorganisms. Rather than suturing or otherwise closing the wound, the physician may place a gauze wick or a penrose drain into the wound to facilitate continued drainage. The most commonly used type of wick is Iodoform. Iodoform is available in 5-yard lengths and widths of ¼ inch, ½ inch, and 1 inch. Iodoform is packaged sterile in glass bottles under the Johnson & Johnson brand name of Nu Gauze. Care must be taken when removing the desired length from the bottle to avoid contaminating the remaining gauze. To accomplish this, the medical assistant might hold the bottle and remove the lid to allow the physician to reach into the bottle with a sterile thumb forceps and pull out the desired length. Sterile scissors are then used to cut the strip without contaminating the remaining wick. The Iodoform is packed into the wound with a short length exposed. After several hours or days of continued draining, the wick may be removed, and the wound allowed to heal. The patient may be put on an appropriate antibiotic.

The medical assistant should exercise caution by wearing appropriate PPE when assisting with this procedure since the exudate can be heavy and contains pathogenic microorganisms.

PURPOSE:

To incise and drain an abscess or other localized infection.

EQUIPMENT/SUPPLIES:

Surgical tray:
  Syringe/needle for anesthesia
  Scalpel blades and handle
  Thumb forceps
  Mosquito hemostat (optional)
  Gauze sponges (many)
  Fenestrated drape
  Tissue forceps (2)
  Mayo scissors
  Iris scissors
  Antiseptic solution such as Betadine in sterile cup
Side area:
  Skin prep supplies
  Gloves (sterile and nonsterile)
  Personal protective equipment
  Anesthesia as directed
  Dressing, bandages, and tape
  Specimen container with preservative/requisition
    (optional)
  Biohazard waste container
  Extra gauze sponges
  Iodoform gauze wick or penrose drain
  Alcohol pledget
  Antiseptic solution
  Culturette (optional)

PROCEDURE STEPS:

1. Wash hands.
2. Identify the patient and explain the procedure.
3. Reassure and comfort the patient as needed.
4. Determine any known allergies and last tetanus booster.
5. Check for signed consent form.
6. Identify any health concerns to avoid possible complications.
7. Position the patient comfortably, lying down.
8. Put on PPE.
9. Perform the skin preparation as directed. (See Procedure 31-12.)
10. Assist the physician as needed to inject the anesthesia by holding the vial while the appropriate amount is aspirated for injection. The physician will incise the abscess and either Iodoform gauze or a penrose drain will be inserted into the wound to encourage drainage.
11. Support the patient as needed.

Give postoperative care:
12. Apply sterile gloves.
13. Clean area around the wound.

(continues)

Procedure 31-8 *(continued)*

14. Dress and bandage as directed. Several thicknesses of dressing material may be needed to absorb **exudate**, or the accumulated fluid in a cavity.
15. Dispose of items per OSHA guidelines. Remove gloves.
16. Wash hands.
17. Check the patient's vital signs.
18. Explain wound care to the patient (and caregiver) and provide written instructions such as to apply warm moist compresses to wound. Explain to watch for symptoms of infection.
19. Assist the patient with any concerns or questions.
20. Arrange for follow-up appointment and medication as ordered.
21. Document the procedure.

Procedure 31-9 Aspiration of Joint Fluid

STANDARD PRECAUTIONS:

 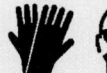

NOTE: The most common reason for aspirating fluid is to remove excess fluid from a joint, often the knee. A long sturdy needle is inserted into the joint capsule and fluid is removed. Often a long-acting anesthetic and cortisone are injected at the same time. The fluid can be diagnostically examined for blood, pus, and fatty substances and also cultured for infective pathogens. Postoperatively, the patient may be placed on anti-inflammatory medications to treat the inflammation and antibiotics if the culture is positive for pathogens.

PURPOSE:
To remove excess synovial fluid from a joint following injury.

EQUIPMENT/SUPPLIES:
Surgical tray:
  Syringe/needle for anesthesia
  Gauze sponges
  Sterile basin for aspirated fluid
  Fenestrated drape (optional)
  Syringe/needle for drainage

Side area:
  Skin prep supplies
  Gloves (sterile and nonsterile)
  Personal protective equipment
  Anesthesia as directed
  Cortisone medication as directed
  Culturette (optional)
  Pathology requisition
  Specimen container
  Biohazard waste container
  Extra gauze sponges (sterile, unopened)
  Alcohol pledgets
  Dressing and bandages

PROCEDURE STEPS:
1. Wash hands.
2. Identify the patient and explain the procedure.
3. Reassure and comfort the patient as needed.
4. Determine any known allergies and last tetanus booster.
5. Check for signed consent form.
6. Identify any health concerns to avoid possible complications.
7. Position the patient comfortably, lying down.
8. Put on PPE if needed.
9. Perform the skin preparation as directed. (See Procedure 31-12.)

(continues)

Procedure 31-9 *(continued)*

10. Assist the physician by holding the vial as anesthesia is aspirated. The physician will inject anesthesia and then insert a needle into the synovial sac and aspirate fluid with the syringe. The aspirated fluid will be put into a sterile bowl as the syringe fills with fluid. The process continues until excess fluid is removed.
11. Support the patient as needed.

Give postoperative care:

12. Apply sterile gloves.
13. Clean area around the wound.
14. Dress and bandage as directed.
15. Dispose of items per OSHA guidelines. Remove gloves.
16. Wash hands.
17. Check the patient's vital signs.
18. Explain wound care to the patient (and caregiver) and provide written instructions including symptoms of infection.
19. Assist the patient with any concerns or questions.
20. Arrange for follow-up appointment and medication as ordered.
21. Apply gloves and eye/mouth protection. Place aspirated fluid into a sterile container and cover tightly.
22. Send labeled specimen to the pathology lab if directed.
23. Document the procedure.

Procedure 31-10 Hemorrhoid Thrombectomy

STANDARD PRECAUTIONS:

NOTE: Hemorrhoids are dilated or varicose veins in the rectum, either internal or external. Sometimes a blood clot can form in a protruding portion of the hemorrhoid and the vessel can become inflamed. The hemorrhoid is incised with a scalpel blade and the clot removed with a hemostat forceps. Suturing is not usually necessary. Soaking the area in a sitz bath can aid in healing.

PURPOSE:
To excise inflamed hemorrhoids.

EQUIPMENT/SUPPLIES:
Surgical tray:
  Syringe/needle for anesthesia
  Mosquito hemostat (curved)
  Sterile basin
  Gauze sponges
  Fenestrated drape
Side area:
  Skin prep supplies
  Gloves (sterile and nonsterile)
  Personal protective equipment
  Anesthesia as directed
  Biohazard waste container
  Extra gauze sponges
  Soft absorbent pad, similar to sanitary napkin
  T-bandage (to hold pad in place)

PROCEDURE STEPS:
1. Wash hands.
2. Identify the patient and explain the procedure.
3. Reassure and comfort the patient as needed.
4. Determine any known allergies and last tetanus booster.
5. Check for signed consent form.
6. Identify any health concerns to avoid possible complications.
7. Position the patient comfortably, according to physician preference; usually lithotomy position is used.
8. Assist with adequate draping for patient comfort.

(continues)

31-10 (continued)

9. Apply PPE if necessary.
10. Perform the skin preparation as directed. (See Procedure 31-12.)
11. Assist the physician to aspirate the appropriate amount of local anesthesia. After administering the anesthesia, the physician will excise the hemorrhoids with a scalpel. Suturing is usually not necessary.
12. Support the patient as needed.

Give postoperative care:

13. Apply sterile gloves.
14. Assist the physician in placing the soft absorbent pad against the wound. It may be held in place with a T-shaped bandage.
15. Dispose of used items per OSHA guidelines. Remove gloves and wash hands.
16. Assist the patient as needed.
17. Check the patient's vital signs.
18. Explain wound care to the patient (and caregiver) per physician. Sitting in a tub of warm water is soothing and aids healing. Provide written instructions including signs of complications such as excessive bleeding or pain.
19. Assist the patient with any concerns or questions.
20. Arrange for follow-up appointment and medication as ordered.
21. Document the procedure.

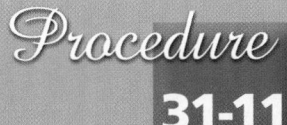

31-11 Chemical "Cold" Sterilization

STANDARD PRECAUTIONS:

PURPOSE:
To sterilize heat-sensitive items such as fiber-optic endoscopes and delicate cutting instruments using appropriate chemical solution.

EQUIPMENT/SUPPLIES:

Chemical solution	Timer
such as Cidex	Sterile water
Steris System®	Gloves—heavy duty
(Percacetic acid)	Sterile towel
Airtight container	Plastic-lined sterile drapes

PROCEDURE STEPS:

1. Sanitize items (see Chapter 22) that require chemical sterilization. Rinse and dry. RATIONALE: Recall that debris and body proteins must be scrubbed from items prior to sterilization.
2. Read manufactuer's instructions on original container of chemical sterilization solution. RATIONALE: Each brand of chemical sterilization solution has specific preparation instructions and germicidal properties; choose the solution that best fits the needs of the ambulatory care setting. Keep the solution in its original container to reduce chances of accidental poisoning.
3. Put on gloves. RATIONALE: Heavy-duty gloves help protect from sharp items puncturing the skin. Chemicals are harsh on the skin.
4. Prepare solution as indicated by manufacturer, place the date of opening or preparation on the container and initial it. RATIONALE: Following manufacturer's instructions ensures sterility. Note the expiration date of solution.
5. Pour solution into a container with an airtight lid, avoid splashing. RATIONALE: Chemicals should not be left exposed to open air in order to prevent evaporation and loss of potency, exposure to enviromental contaminants, accidental inhalation, or

(continues)

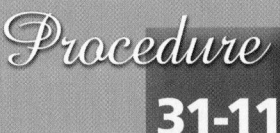

Procedure
31-11 *(continued)*

poisoning. Splashing may cause skin or mucous membrane contact and result in injury.

6. Place sanitized and dried items into the solution, completely submersing item(s). Avoid splashing when placing items into airtight container. RATIONALE: Total immersion is necessary for sterility to be achieved.

7. Close lid of container, label with name of solution, exposure time required per manufacturer, and initial. RATIONALE: Exposure time is the required time indicated by the manufacturer to achieve sterility. Initialing work ensures accountability and responsibility.

8. Do not open lid nor add additional items during the processing time. RATIONALE: Adding to the container interrupts the sterilization process and limits the effectiveness of the chemical.

9. Following the recommended processing time, lift item(s) from the container using sterile gloved hands or sterile transfer forceps. Carefully hold item above sterile basin and pour copious amounts of sterile water over it and through it (endoscopes) until adequately rinsed of chemical solution.

RATIONALE: Item(s) once processed are sterile and must be handled appropriately. Using sterile gloved hands or sterile transfer forceps ensures sterile-to-sterile contact and no contamination of the item(s). Sterile water is poured through the inner channels of endoscopes to rinse chemicals from the inside as well as the outside.

10. Hold item(s) upright for a few seconds to allow excess sterile water to drip off.

11. Place the sterile item on a sterile towel (which has been placed on a sterile field) and dry it with another sterile towel. The towel used for drying is removed from sterile field. The use of sterile drapes that have a plastic polylined barrier layer between two layers of paper is recommended for the sterile field. RATIONALE: Plastic-lined sterile drapes create a barrier to prevent moisture from drawing contaminants from the metal surgical instrument tray or countertop up into the sterile area.

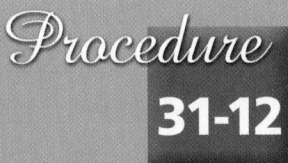

Procedure
31-12
Preparation of Patient Skin for Minor Surgery

STANDARD PRECAUTIONS:

NOTE: The skin contains many microorganisms and the patient's skin must be prepared prior to minor surgery to remove as many of the microorganisms as possible. Wound infection results when microorganisms enter the body. Since it is impossible to sterilize the skin, the operative site and an area surrounding it are scrubbed, shaved (hair harbors microorganisms), washed, and painted with an antiseptic such as Betadine solution.

PURPOSE:
To remove as many microorganisms as possible from patient's skin prior to surgery.

EQUIPMENT/SUPPLIES:
Absorbent pad
Drape
Disposable prep kit (includes: antiseptic soap, several sponges, razor, and a container for water)
Sterile water
Antiseptic solution
Sterile bowl

(continues)

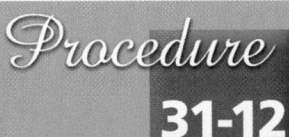

31-12 (continued)

Sterile gloves for medical assistant and physician
(2 pairs)
If kit is unavailable, equipment needed is:
Sterile bowls (2)
Antiseptic soap
Sterile gauze sponges
Sterile razor
Basin for soiled sponges

PROCEDURE STEPS:
1. Wash hands.
2. Assemble equipment.
3. Identify patient.
4. Explain procedure, provide privacy, and drape patient if appropriate.
5. Provide good light source.
6. Position patient for comfort and exposure of site.
7. Wash hands.
8. Protect area under preparation site with an absorbent pad.
9. Put on sterile gloves or use sterile transfer forceps.
10. Apply antiseptic soap (Betadine) with 4 × 4 sponges, beginning at operative site and moving outward in a circular motion from the center to away from center of prepared area. RATIONALE: Work from cleaner to least clean areas to prevent contamination.
11. Discard used sponges as necessary.

12. Using razor and holding skin taut, shave hair away from operative site, following hair growth pattern. RATIONALE: This prevents accidental nicks. Nicked skin can cause infection.
13. When hair has been removed, scrub again in a circular fashion as in step 10 for about 2 to 5 minutes.
14. Rinse shaved area with sterile water and dry with a sterile 4 × 4 gauze sponge.
15. Remove and appropriately discard absorbent pad, 4 × 4 sponges, disposable prep kit, and gloves. RATIONALE: This removes used supplies and equipment from prepped skin area and avoids contamination.
16. Wash hands.
17. Using sterile transfer forceps, remove a sterile towel to place under operative site. RATIONALE: Placing a sterile towel under the operative area keeps site free from contamination.
18. Cover with a sterile towel. Instruct patient not to touch the area.
19. Pour antiseptic solution (Betadine) into the sterile bowl. Physician will put on sterile gloves or will use sterile transfer forceps and using a sterile 4 × 4 gauze sponge will paint the operative site with the antiseptic solution. Let dry, drape patient with sterile drapes, and commence with the surgical procedure.

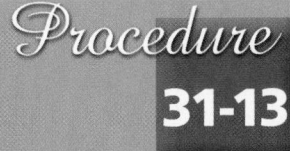

31-13 Setting Up and Covering a Sterile Field

STANDARD PRECAUTIONS:

PURPOSE:
Disposable sterile field drapes or sterile towels are used to isolate a sterile area or field as well as to cover the sterile field for use in minor surgery and sterile procedures. They are available in convenient peel-apart packages, fanfolded for ease of use, and often are two-tone in color to aid in differentiating one side from the other. Sterile towels are fanfolded and stored in canisters.

NOTE: A variety of materials, both disposable and nondisposable, can be used to set up and cover a sterile

(continues)

Procedure

31-13 *(continued)*

field. All material must contain certain criteria to be safe for use and all have advantages and disadvantages. For example, woven textile fabrics are moisture retardant and are effective barriers to microbial penetration. A combination of paper and plastic disposable drapes is an excellent barrier against microorganisms and moisture. Many times medical office preference is determined by financial consideration.

EQUIPMENT/SUPPLIES:

Disposable sterile field drapes (2) or sterile towels (2) (muslin or linen with water-repellent finish)
Mayo instrument tray/stand
Sterile transfer forceps (if needed)

PROCEDURE STEPS:

1. Wash hands.
2. Sanitize and disinfect a Mayo instrument tray.
3. Select an appropriate disposable sterile field drape and place the drape package on a clean, dry, flat surface, or remove a fanfolded sterile cloth towel from a canister using sterile transfer forceps.
4. If using disposable drape, peel open the package exposing the fanfolded drape. Assure that the cut corners of the drape are toward you; turn the package if necessary. Or: remove sterile towel from canister using sterile transfer forceps. RATIO-NALE: Sterile field drapes are fanfolded and positioned within the package to facilitate ease of use. Sterile towels are fanfolded and positioned within the canister for ease of use.
5. With thumb and forefinger of one hand, carefully grasp the top cut corner without touching the rest of the drape or towel and pick the drape or towel up high enough to assure that as it unfolds it does

not drag across a nonsterile area. RATIONALE: The drape or towel will naturally unfold as it is lifted, so care must be taken to assure that it is lifted quickly and allowed to unfold without touching a nonsterile surface.

6. Holding the drape or towel above waist level and away from the body, grasp the opposing corner so that both corners along the long edge of the drape are being held.
7. Keeping the drape or towel above waist level and away from the body, reach over the Mayo tray with the drape or towel. Take care that the lower edge of the drape or towel does not drag across the tray. RATIONALE: Sterile principles state that sterile items should be kept above the waist.
8. Gently pull the drape or towel toward you as it is laid onto the tray. If adjustment is needed to center the drape or towel, do not touch the center of the drape or towel, or reach over the sterile field. Walk around or reach underneath the tray to move it or make adjustments. RATIONALE: The edges that hang over the tray are no longer considered sterile.
9. To cover the sterile field with a second sterile drape or towel, follow steps 4 through 7; then instead of pulling the drape or towel toward you (as described in step 8), which would necessitate reaching over the sterile field, apply the covering drape or towel by holding it up in front of the field. Adjust the lower edge so it is even with the lower edge of the field drape or towel. With a forward motion, carefully lay the cover over the sterile field. RATIONALE: Reaching over the sterile field would contaminate the tray.

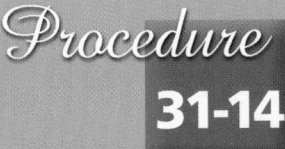

Procedure 31-14 Opening Sterile Packages of Instruments and Supplies and Applying Them to a Sterile Field

STANDARD PRECAUTIONS:

NOTE: Sterile instruments and supplies are packaged in a manner that allows them to be opened and accessed without compromising sterility. Refer to other sections of this chapter for the specific steps of wrapping techniques, sterile gloving, and setting up sterile fields. The "wrapping twice" method of double wrapping was used in preparing the surgical packs for the following procedure.

PURPOSE:

To open sterile packages of surgical instruments and supplies and place them onto a sterile field using sterile technique.

EQUIPMENT/SUPPLIES:

Mayo instrument tray
Sterile field drapes (2) or sterile towels (2)
Sterile gloves
Wrapped-twice sterile surgical instruments
Prepackaged sterile surgical supplies

PROCEDURE STEPS:

1. Assemble supplies.
2. Wash hands and set up sterile field.
3. Position package of surgical instruments on palm of nondominant hand with outer envelope flap on top. RATIONALE: This will facilitate opening the pack while protecting its sterile contents.
4. Grasping the taped end of the top flap, open the first flap away from you. Do not touch the inside of the flap (Figure 31-30A).
5. Grasping just the folded back tips of the side flaps, pull the right-sided flap to the right. Then pull the left-sided flap to the left, taking care not to reach over the package (Figure 31-30B and C). RATIONALE: Pulling the tips of the flaps toward each side allows the inner portion of the package to be exposed without contamination.
6. Pull the last flap toward you by grasping the folded-back tip taking care not to touch the inner contents of the package. RATIONALE: Pulling the last tip toward you allows you to avoid reaching over the inner contents of the package.
7. Gather all of the loose edges together to obtain a snug covering over your nondominant hand. Close your covered hand over the inner package and carefully apply the inner package to the sterile field (Figure 31-30D and E). RATIONALE: Gathering the loose edges prevents them from being dragged across the sterile field.

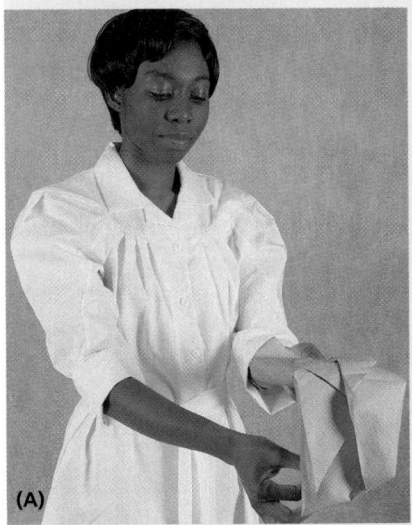
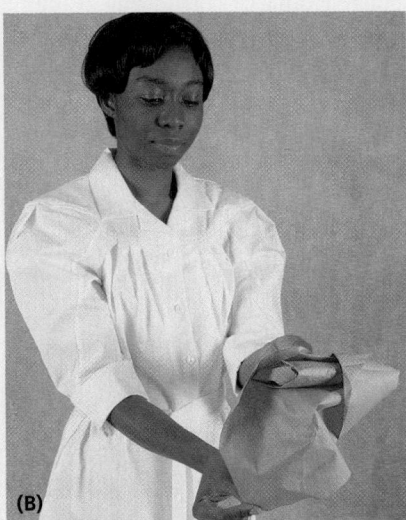
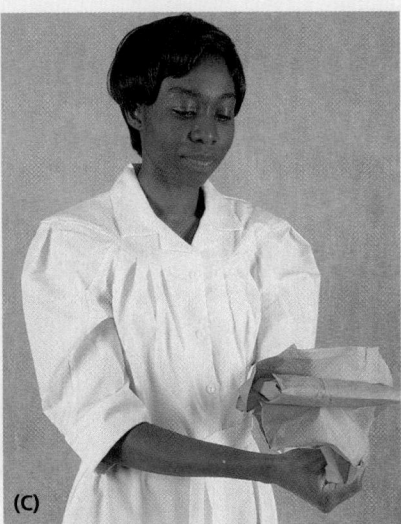

(A)   (B)   (C)

Figure 31-30 To open sterile packages: (A) Grasp the taped end of the top flap, and open the first flap away from you. Do not touch the inside of the flap. (B) Grasp just the folded back tips of the side flaps, and pull the right-sided flap to the right. (C) Now pull the left-sided flap to the left. Do not reach over the package.

(continues)

Procedure

31-14 *(continued)*

8. Open peel-apart packages using sterile technique by grasping both edges of the flaps and pulling them apart in a rolling down motion, keeping both hands together. The sterile item should be exposed gradually between the two peel-apart edges. The sterile inner contents may then be offered to the sterile-gloved physician or applied to the sterile field using a flipping motion (Figure 31-30F), taking care not to contaminate either the package contents or the field.

9. Apply sterile gloves. Arrange instruments and supplies in an organized and logical manner according to the physician's preference (Figure 31-30G and H). RATIONALE: Instruments should be arranged in the order of use. All handles should be pointed toward the user. Instruments should be

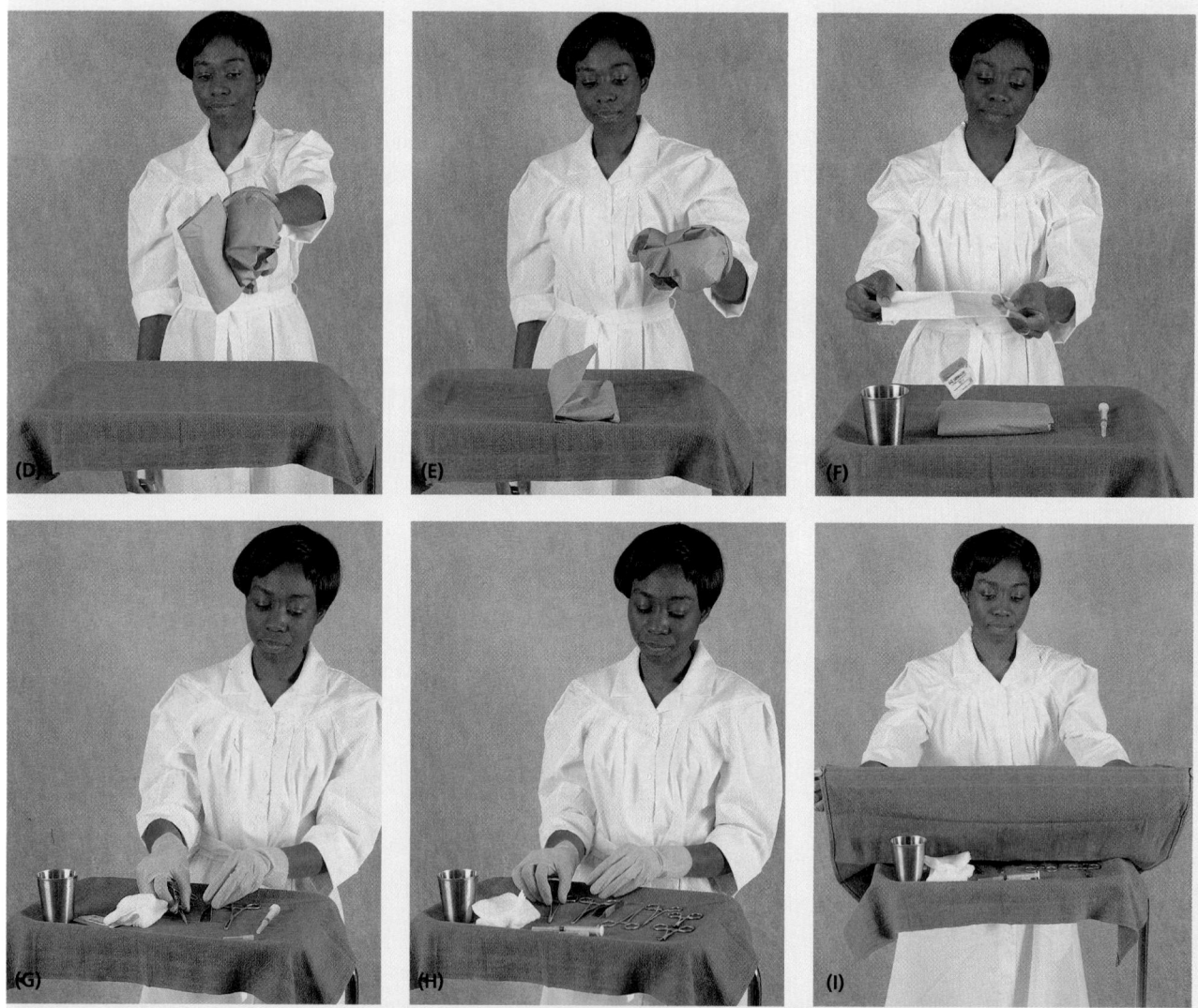

Figure 31-30 To open sterile packages: *(continued)* (D) Gather the loose edges together to obtain a snug covering over your nondominant hand. (E) Close the covered hand over the inner package, and apply the inner package to the sterile field. (F) Open peel-apart packages using sterile technique, exposing sterile item gradually. (G and H) Arrange instruments and supplies according to physician preference. (I and J) Apply the sterile field cover.

(continues)

Procedure 31-14 *(continued)*

separated as much as possible within the space of the field so entanglement of instruments is not a problem.

10. Apply the sterile field cover (Figure 24-30I and J). RATIONALE: A sterile cover will need to be applied if the surgical tray will not be used immediately, needs to be moved, or if the medical assistant leaves the tray unattended.

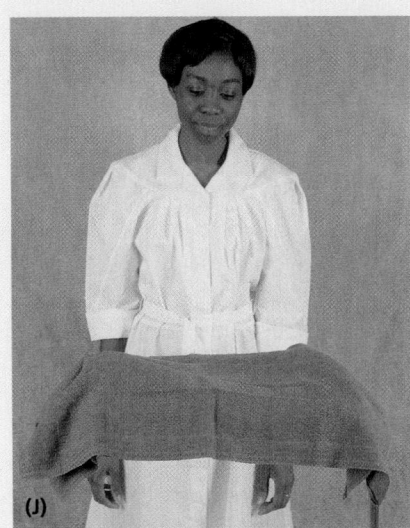

Figure 31-30
To open sterile packages: *(continued)*

Procedure 31-15 Pouring a Sterile Solution into a Cup on a Sterile Field

NOTE: Occasionally, sterile solutions will need to be poured into a sterile cup which has been placed onto the sterile tray. The solution is sterile, but the outside of the container is not; therefore special precautions need to be taken in order to pour the solution into the cup without contaminating the sterile field. The solution is always poured after the tray has been moved into the surgical area to avoid spilling during the movement.

STANDARD PRECAUTIONS:

PURPOSE:

To pour a sterile solution into a cup on a sterile tray in a sterile manner.

EQUIPMENT/SUPPLIES:

Covered sterile surgical tray with a sterile cup in upper right corner
Container of sterile solution

PROCEDURE STEPS:

1. Wash hands.
2. Transport the surgical tray into the surgical area before pouring the solution. Or: the surgical tray can be set up for immediate use in the surgical area. RATIONALE: The solution may tip and spill during transport.
3. Read the label of the solution container three times and check the expiration date. RATIONALE: To eliminate the possibility of pouring the wrong solution or an outdated solution.
4. Remove the cap from the solution container taking care not to touch the inner surface of the cap. Place the cap upside down on a nonsterile surface to avoid touching the inner surface of the cap with a nonsterile surface. When the cap is held in the hand, hold it right side up. RATIONALE: Touching the inside of the cap with either your hand or a nonsterile surface will contaminate the inside of an otherwise sterile container.

(continues)

Procedure
31-15   *(continued)*

5. Read the label again to assure accuracy. Place palm over the label to protect the label from stains. Pour a small amount of the solution into a bowl or cup that is outside the sterile field. RATIONALE: This action will cleanse the lip of the container. NOTE: If the surgical tray is set up in a surgical area, the solution can be poured prior to covering the surgical tray with a sterile drape or towel.

6. Carefully pull back the upper right corner of the tray cover to expose the cup. Take care to only touch the corner tip of the cover and not reach over the exposed field. RATIONALE: Touching the underside of the cover or reaching over the exposed sterile field will contaminate the sterile surgical tray.

7. Approaching from the corner of the tray, and using the cleansed side of the lip of the container, pour the needed amount of solution into the sterile cup (Figure 31-31). Precaution should be taken to avoid splashing, spilling, reaching over the field, or touching any of the sterile surfaces. RATIONALE: Splashing or spilling of the solution would cause the sterile field drape to become wet, which could cause contaminants to "wick" from the metal tray into the sterile field. Use of a

polylined sterile field drape will create a barrier.

8. Replace the cap of the solution container using sterile technique.

9. Replace the corner of the drape cover using sterile technique or cover with a sterile drape or towel.

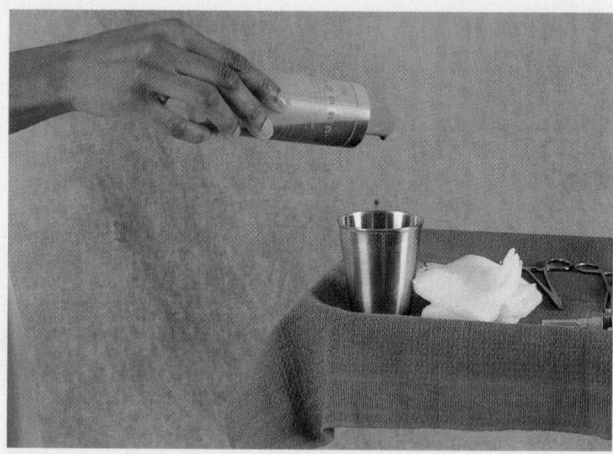

Figure 31-31   Approaching from the corner of the tray, pour the needed amount of solution into the sterile cup. Use the cleansed side of the container lip for pouring.

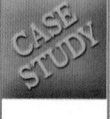

CASE STUDY 31-1

Cele Little, an eighty-something patient at Inner City Health Care, is having minor surgery performed on Thursday morning. Her sister, Dottie Tate, also a patient and also in her eighties, will come with Cele; a friend from the local senior citizen center has offered to drive them to the center and home again. Dottie is more nervous about the procedure, the removal of a bothersome cyst, than Cele. After talking with the sisters about the procedure, medical assistant Wanda Slawson, CMA, MLT, realizes this and wants to reassure Dottie but also wants her to be prepared to be caregiver to Cele.

CASE STUDY REVIEW

1. Where should Wanda begin in her communication with the two sisters?

2. What specific advice should Wanda give Cele and Dottie before the procedure?

3. What instructions should Wanda give the sisters to follow after the procedure?

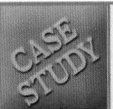

Letisha Brown has been scheduled to have a nevus excised from her upper back.

CASE STUDY REVIEW

31-2

1. Explain how you would prepare her for the surgery.
2. Explain how you would care for her postoperatively.
3. What will become of the excised nevus? Explain your actions.

SUMMARY

In assisting with minor surgery in the ambulatory care setting, the medical assistant needs to know sterile principles and understand the difference between medical and surgical asepsis. Knowledge of suture materials, instruments, and other supplies such as dressings and bandages is also critical. In preparing for minor surgical procedures, the medical assistant's communication skills will be needed, for patients can be apprehensive and will require both reassurance and education. In addition to understanding the basic process and preparations for assisting with minor surgery, the medical assistant should also be aware of the steps involved in some of the more common minor surgical procedures.

REVIEW QUESTIONS

Multiple Choice

1. Which of the following describes the primary purpose of surgical asepsis?
   a. to prevent microorganisms from collecting on the Mayo stand
   b. to prevent microorganisms from causing inflammation
   c. to prevent microorganisms from entering the body during an invasive procedure
   d. to prevent microorganisms from multiplying
2. A basic rule to follow to protect sterile items is:
   a. a sterile object may touch a nonsterile object under certain circumstances
   b. it is safe to turn your back on the sterile field if you leave plenty of room between you and the field
   c. provide the physician a separate container for contaminated instruments
   d. gloved hands are held at the same height as the hip bone
3. Which of the following is the smallest size suture material?
   a. 0
   b. 2-0
   c. 4-0
   d. 1

4. Which of the following is an example of absorbable suture material?
   a. gut
   b. chromium salts
   c. silk
   d. Dacron
5. What is the purpose of adding epinephrine to the local anesthetic?
   a. to prevent an allergic reaction
   b. to reduce blood flow in the operative site through vasoconstriction
   c. to reduce patient discomfort during the procedure
   d. to maintain patient vital signs
6. Which of the following actions might the physician take if a sebaceous cyst were infected?
   a. remove the cyst
   b. do a biopsy of the cyst
   c. perform cryosurgery on the cyst
   d. incise and drain the cyst

Critical Thinking

1. You have just removed a double-wrapped instrument pack from the autoclave and notice a small tear in the outermost wrap. The inner wrap appears to be intact. What would your action be? Why?

2. You are setting up a sterile surgical tray and have already applied your sterile gloves before you realize you forgot to place the suture package on the tray. You have several options. What are they and what are the advantages and disadvantages of each?

3. What would be the rationale behind leaving a wound open rather than suturing it? On what basis would this decision be made?

4. While you are preparing a patient for surgery, he confides in you that he doesn't have anyone to drive him home, but he only lives three miles away and plans to drive himself. How do you respond?

5. You have thoroughly explained the postoperative instructions to the patient and caregiver. Are written instructions also necessary? Why or why not?

6. While pouring a sterile solution into a bowl on the sterile field, you accidentally splash a very tiny amount of the solution onto the field. What is your next step? Explain your actions.

7. Dr. Woo asks you to assist him in repairing the laceration on Jaime Carrera's hand. Though you are un-sure, you think you may have noticed a tiny hole in the palm of your left glove. What is your next step?

8. While assisting during an incision and drainage of a localized infection on Abigail Johnson's left leg, you notice there is a large amount of exudate that discharges from the incisional site. What, if any, precautions should you take?

WEB ACTIVITIES

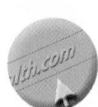

Search the Internet to explore the most current outpatient surgical procedures for hemorrhoids, cataracts, and cholelithiasis.

REFERENCES/BIBLIOGRAPHY

Bonewit-West, K. (2000). *Clinical procedures for medical assistants* (5th ed.). Philadelphia: W. B. Saunders Company.

Taber's cyclopedic medical dictionary (18th ed.). (1999). Philadelphia: F.A. Davis Company.

DIAGNOSTIC IMAGING

KEY TERMS

Claustrophobia
Dosimeter
Echocardiogram
Esophageal Varices
Fluoroscope
Ionizing Radiation
Noninvasive
Oscilloscope
Palliative
Radioactive
Radiograph
Radiolucent
Radionuclides
Radiopaque
Radiopharmaceuticals
Stomatitis
Transducer

OUTLINE

X-Ray Machine
Radiation Safety
Contrast Media
Patient Preparation
Positioning of the Patient
Fluoroscopy
Diagnostic Imaging
   Ultrasonography
   Positron Emission Tomography
    (PET)

Computerized Tomography
   (CT)
Magnetic Resonance Imaging
   (MRI)
Flat Plates
Filing Films and Reports
Radiation Therapy
Nuclear Medicine

OBJECTIVES

The student should strive to meet the following performance objectives and demonstrate an understanding of the facts and principles presented in this chapter through written and oral communication.

1. Define key terms as presented in the glossary.
2. Describe safety precautions for personnel and patients as they relate to ionizing radiation treatments.
3. Explain how fluoroscopy is used and explain its benefits.
4. Describe the various positions used during X-ray procedures.
5. Describe four X-ray procedures that require patient preparation.
6. Discuss the uses of ultrasonography, positron emission, tomography, computerized tomography, magnetic resonance, and flat plates.
7. Discuss how radiographs are stored.
8. Explain the differences among radiology, radiation therapy, and nuclear medicine.
9. Recall four side effects of radiation.

ADMINISTRATIVE

Administrative Procedures

- Schedule, coordinate, and monitor appointments
- Schedule inpatient and outpatient admissions and procedures

CLINICAL

Fundamental Principles

- Screen and follow up patient test results

Patient Care

- Prepare patients for examination, procedures, and treatments
- Coordinate patient care information with other health care providers

GENERAL (TRANSDISCIPLINARY)

Professionalism

- Project a professional manner and image
- Adhere to ethical principles

Communication Skills

- Adapt communication to individual's ability to understand

Legal Concepts

- Maintain confidentiality
- Practice within the scope of education, training, and personal capabilities
- Comply with established risk management and safety procedures

Instruction

- Instruct individuals according to their needs

In the radiology department of Inner City Hospital, there are several patients waiting to have their procedures performed. Wanda Shawson brings Don Waite to the department for an intravenous pyelogram. She is careful to make certain that Mr. Waite has been properly prepared for the procedure. She does not want the procedure to have to be repeated due to the inconvenience and anxiety it may cause Mr. Waite, nor does she want there to be additional expense and time spent repeating the procedure.

INTRODUCTION

X rays were named when a German physicist, Wilhelm Roentgen, discovered them in 1895. He noticed that the X rays were able to pass through human skin, paper, wood, and other solid materials. Because he did not know what they were, he called them X rays.

X rays or **radiographs** are a valuable diagnostic tool used to visualize internal organs and structures when searching for diseases and disorders. They are also a valuable therapeutic tool because they can be used to treat cancerous neoplasms.

Radiology uses X rays, radioactive substances, and ultraviolet rays. There are three specialties into which radiology can be classified: diagnostic radiology, radiation therapy, and nuclear medicine.

X rays are often not taken in an office setting; rather, they are taken in the radiology department of a hospital or a free-standing X-ray service outside of the hospital. Some X rays, such as those looking for a fractured bone, require no preparation, while others, such as an intravenous pyelogram, require special preparation.

In some states, medical assistants and other health care professionals who are not licensed to take radiographs are not allowed by law to assist with radiologic procedures. The medical assistants must have a basic understanding of radiology and radiology safety in order to instruct patients in proper preparation for radiologic procedures and to protect themselves from X-ray exposure.

X-RAY MACHINE

There are three main parts to an X-ray machine: the table, the X-ray tube, and the control panel. The tube is where the X rays are produced and then come out as a beam of X ray. Lead surrounds the tube except for the area where the beams of X ray are sent out. The table on which the patient lies is movable in several directions, even upright or angled. The control panel is positioned behind a lead wall especially designed for shielding the radiographer from X rays when an X ray is being taken (Figure 32-1).

RADIATION SAFETY

X rays, though invisible to the human eye, are extremely powerful and can be dangerous and harmful. Exposure to radiation can destroy tissue and permanently damage the eyes, bone marrow, and the skin. They are also harmful to the developing embryo and fetus, causing severe anomalies and death.

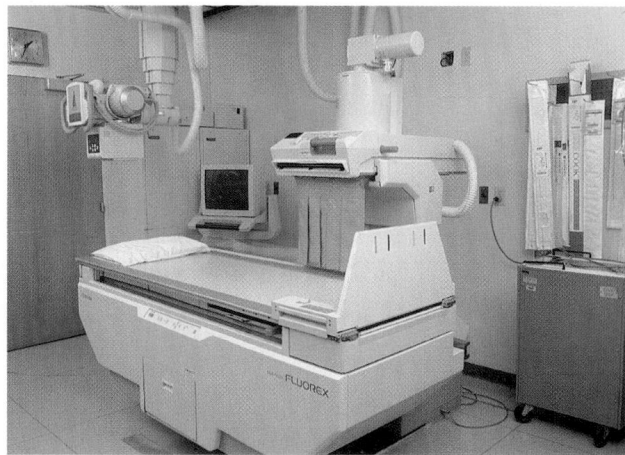

Figure 32-1   Radiographic room prepared for procedure.

Personnel in the X-ray department and others who are exposed to X rays must wear a **dosimeter**, a small badge-like device worn above the waist. The dosimeter contains a strip of film that measures the amount of X ray a person is exposed to. The dosimeter film is read on a regular basis and radiation exposure is reported to a supervisor. Exposure can come from the X-ray beam itself or from scattered rays that are produced when going through the patient's body.

Patients must wear lead aprons over the reproductive organs, and technicians must shield themselves with lead aprons and gloves if they are assisting, but shields are not necessary when standing behind the lead wall working the control panel. Additionally, walls in rooms where X rays are taken are lead-lined to absorb scattering rays.

CONTRAST MEDIA

Various body structures are of different densities. Bone is denser than skin and, therefore, can absorb more X rays leaving fewer to be picked up by the X-ray film. Thus, an X ray of bone will appear white. A lung is less dense, and the X rays can penetrate lung tissue. The lung appears black on the radiograph. If X rays do not penetrate a structure easily, it is termed **radiopaque**, if they penetrate readily, it is termed **radiolucent**. Contrast media are radiopaque and help to obtain a radiographic image of an internal organ or structure that ordinarily would be difficult to see because the contrast media cause the organs or structures of the body to absorb more radiation.

Some commonly used contrast media are barium sulfate, iodine compounds, air, and carbon dioxide. Barium is a chalky compound, and when mixed with water, can be swallowed by the patient or administered as an enema by a radiologic technician. It is used for upper and lower gastrointestinal series of X rays. The patient is told

to drink extra fluids to flush out barium. Iodine salts are radiopaque and are used for kidney, gallbladder, and thyroid exams. Some individuals are allergic to the iodine salts used as contrast media. Patients are asked whether they have any allergies, but in particular, allergies to foods that contain iodine, such as fish.

Air and carbon dioxide are used to visualize the spinal cord and joints, but have been replaced by use of the magnetic resonance imaging (MRI) machine.

PATIENT PREPARATION

By law, without special education and training about X rays, the medical assistant's role in X-ray procedures in most states will be limited to patient preparation information and explanations about what the patient can anticipate. A thorough knowledge of the procedure that the physician has ordered is essential, and the medical assistant must be certain that patients understand the preparation they are about to undertake. Verbal explanations should be followed up with written instructions. Many patients, fearful of what the ordered X ray will show, are anxious and frightened and can easily forget verbal instructions. Proper preparation is essential for the best results on the radiographs. Repeating a procedure because of inadequate preparation results in increased patient anxiety, time, expense, and inconvenience (Table 32-1).

TABLE 32-1   PATIENT PREPARATION AND PURPOSE OF X-RAY PROCEDURES

Test	Purpose	Patient Preparation	Procedure
Angiography	To visualize the inside of blood vessel walls. Helps to diagnose heart attacks, stroke, and aneurysm (Figure 32-2).	NPO 6–8 hours prior to exam.	1. Contrast medium (iodine) injected into an artery or vein. 2. Catheter threaded to the appropriate site. 3. Digital angiography can be done and stored on computer disk.
Barium swallow (upper GI series)	To study the esophagus, stomach, duodenum, and small intestine for disease (ulcers, tumors, hiatal hernia, esophageal varices) (Figure 32-3A).	Day prior: Light evening meal. NPO after midnight. Day of test: NPO. Postprocedural: Increase fluid intake. Take laxative as prescribed.	1. The patient is asked to drink a flavored barium mixture while standing in front of the fluoroscope. The radiologist observes the passage down the digestive tract. 2. The patient is turned to various positions to allow good visualization of the intestines. 3. X rays are taken.
Barium enema (lower GI series)	To study the colon for disease (polyps, tumors, lesions).	Prep kit (usually supplied by physician's office) to include bottle of magnesium citrate and Dulcolax tablet(s). Day prior: 1. Clear liquid allowed: carbonated beverages, clear gelatin, clear broth, coffee and tea with sugar. No milk or milk products. 2. 8 oz. of water every hour until bedtime. 3. Late afternoon, drink bottle of magnesium citrate. 4. Early evening, take Dulcolax tablet(s) as prescribed. 5. Light evening meal. NPO except water after dinner. Morning procedure: NPO, cleaning enema Postprocedural: 1. Increase fluid intake and dietary fiber. 2. Report to physician if no bowel movement within 24 hours of test.	1. The colon is filled with a barium sulfate mixture. 2. The patient is turned in various positions to allow the barium to fill the colon. Air is injected to move the barium along the colon. 3. When the colon is full, X rays are taken.
Cholangiography	To view the bile ducts for possible calculi or lesions.		Contrast medium injected and radiograph of bile ducts is taken.
Cholecystography	To study the gallbladder for disease (stones, duct obstruction), inflammation.	May have cleaning enema one hour before exam. Meal preceding exam is withheld. 1. Evening before test, fat-free dinner. 2. Patient takes dye tablets with 8 oz. of water. 3. Cathartic or cleansing enemas may be prescribed. 4. NPO after dinner and tablets.	1. A series of radiographs is taken. 2. A fatty meal may be given to stimulate the gallbladder to empty. 3. Other radiographs can then be taken to check gallbladder function.
Cystography	To view the urinary bladder for lesions, calculi.	Day prior: Light evening meal. Laxative in evening. NPO after midnight.	Contrast medium injected and radiograph of the urinary bladder is taken.
Hysterosalpin-gography	To view the uterus and fallopian tubes for blockage and lesions. To check for pelvic masses.	Laxative evening before. Cleansing enema day of exam. Meal prior to exam is withheld.	Contrast medium injected and radiographs taken of uterus and fallopian tubes. Carbon dioxide may also be used.
Intravenous Pyelography (IVP)	Visualization of kidneys, ureters, and bladder to detect kidney stones, lesions, strictures of urinary tract.	Eat a light evening meal and nothing after midnight. A laxative and enema are used to clean out the intestines to prevent a blocked view of the ureters behind the intestines.	A contrast medium of iodine salts is given intravenously after it has been determined that the patient is not allergic to iodine.
Mammography	To detect abnormalities in the breast, especially breast cancer.	Do not wear lotion, deodorant, or powders. Remove clothing from waist up. No contrast medium required.	Breast is positioned on the mammograph and compressed to flatten it. Two radiographs are taken of each breast, from the side and from above. (See Chapter 30.)
Retrograde Pyelography	To view the kidneys and urinary tract for abnormalities.	Drink 4–5 glasses of water prior to examination unless sedated, then NPO.	Contrast medium injected and radiographs taken of the kidneys and urinary bladder.

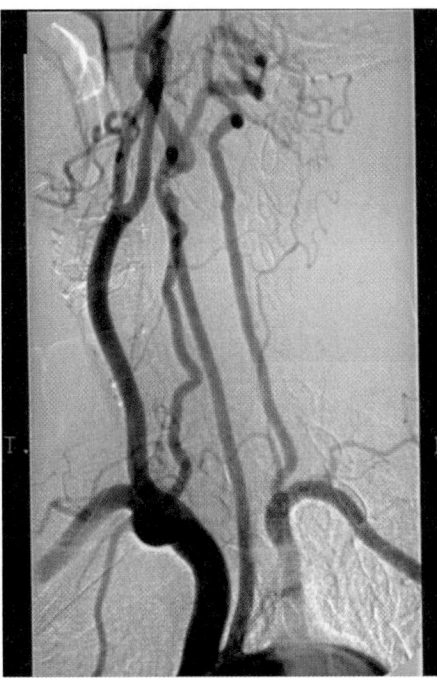

Figure 32-2 Carotid angiography.

POSITIONING THE PATIENT

The correct patient position is important for obtaining the best quality X ray and the type of examination that is necessary will determine patient position. Some basis views are:

- Anterioposterior view (AP)–the anterior surface of the body faces the X-ray tube and X rays are directed from the front toward the back of the body.

- Posteroanterior view (PA)–the posterior surface of the body faces the X-ray tube and X rays are directed from back to front (Figure 32-4A and 32-4B).

- Lateral view–X rays pass through the body from one side to the opposite side.

- Right lateral view (RL)–X rays are directed through the body from the left to the right side. The right side of the body is next to the film.

- Left lateral view (LL)–X rays are directed through the body from the right to the left side. The left side of the body is next to the film.

- Oblique view–the body is positioned at an angle.

- Supine view–the body is lying face up, on the back.

- Prone view–the body is lying face down, on the abdomen.

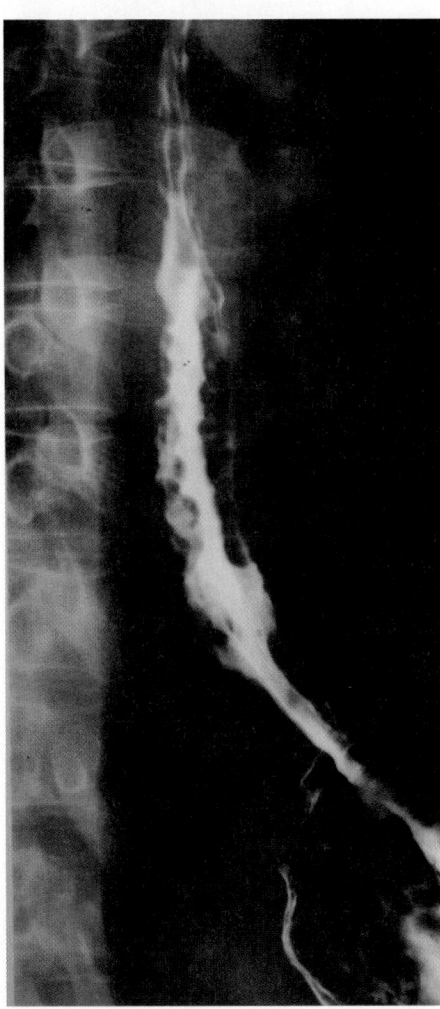

Figure 32-3A Esophageal varices.

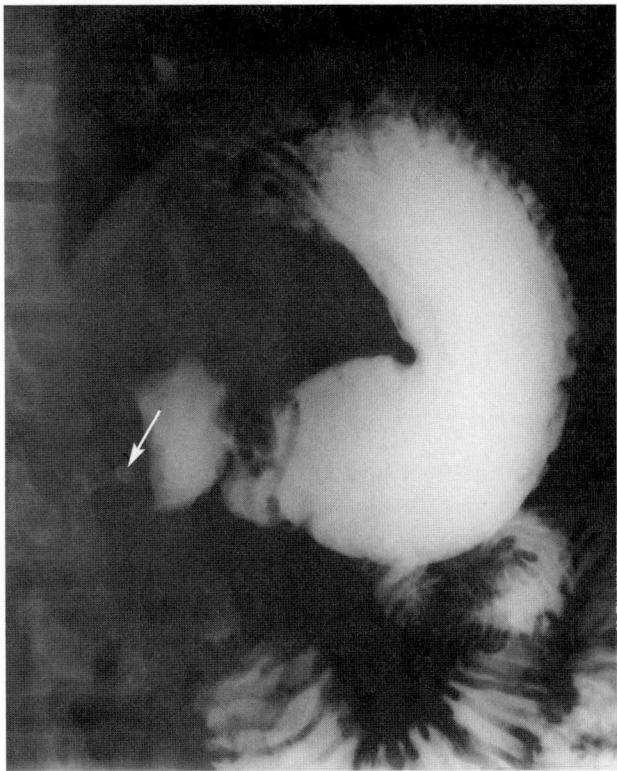

Figure 32-3B Duodenal ulcer.

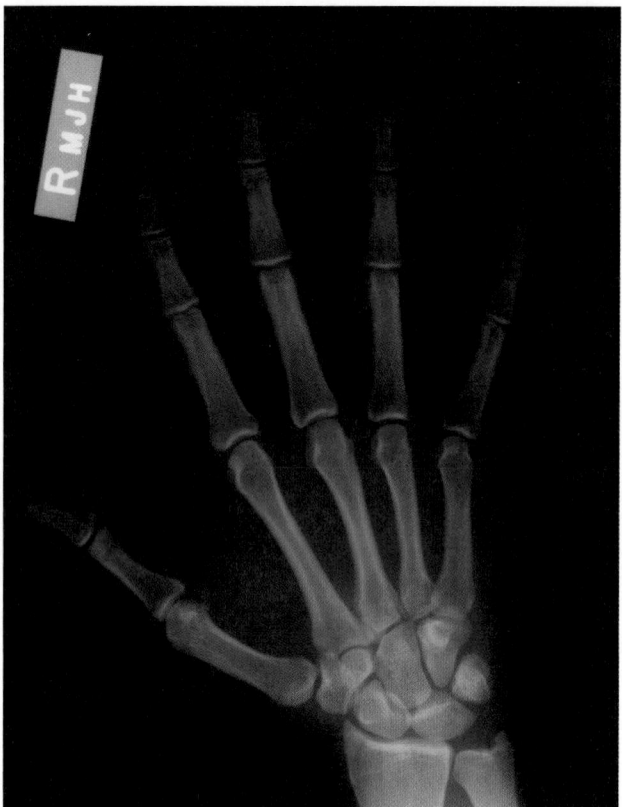

Figure 32-4A   PA hand.

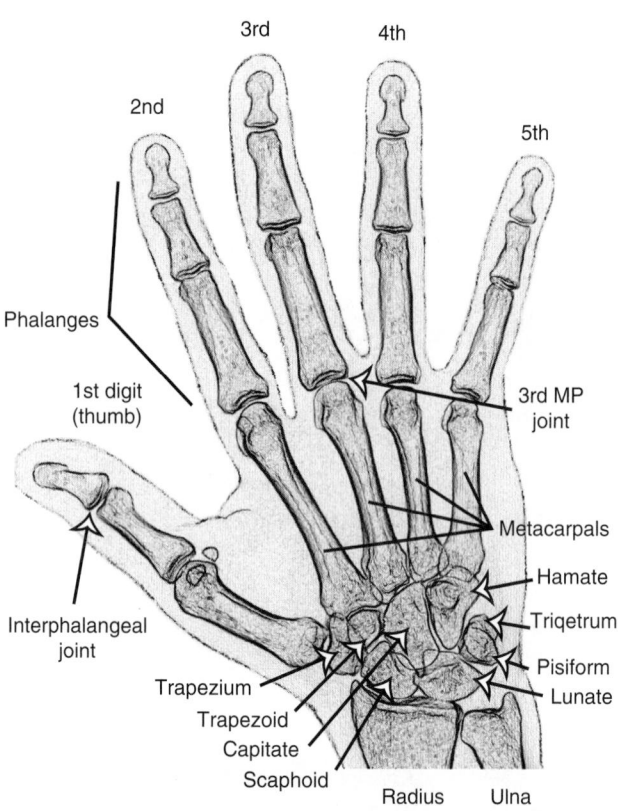

Figure 32-4B   PA hand.

FLUOROSCOPY

Fluoroscopy is the process of using a **fluoroscope** to view internal organs and structures of the body so that they may be seen in motion immediately by the radiologist. The patient is usually given a contrast medium and placed between the X-ray tube and the fluoroscope. Fluoroscopy is used for procedures such as cardiac catheterization and for viewing the function of the stomach and intestinal structures to detect any abnormalities (Figure 32-5).

DIAGNOSTIC IMAGING

Ultrasonography

Ultrasonography, computerized tomography, and magnetic resonance imaging allow for greater imaging detail than conventional radiographs. Ultrasonography, or ultrasound, has been available longer than the others. High-frequency sound waves (inaudible to the human ear) are used to image internal soft tissues. It can be used to help diagnose problems in the abdominal organs, the liver, and gallbladder. It cannot be used for skeletal structures or the lungs. An **echocardiogram**, an ultrasound of the heart, can view it and determine the size, shape, and position of the heart and the motion made by the valves

opening and closing. Ultrasound has advantages over other methods of viewing internal organs and structures in that it uses no X rays and allows for continuous viewing while organs and structures are in motion.

During ultrasound, a **transducer** is used with a coupling agent and sound waves are emitted from the head of the transducer. The transducer is placed firmly on the patient's body over the organ to be examined. The sound waves pass through the skin and bounce off the body's tissues and are reflected back to the transducer. These

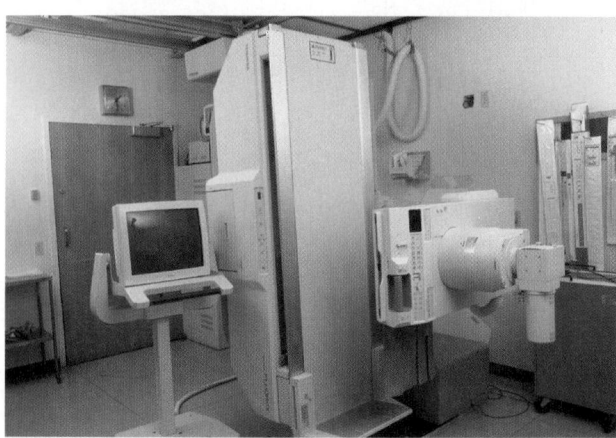

Figure 32-5   Fluoroscopic room ready for upper GI study.

echoes are displayed on an **oscilloscope**, showing a visual pattern or picture. The image or record produced is known as a sonogram or echogram. A permanent film for the patient's record and videotape can also be made.

Ultrasonography, because it is **noninvasive**, is widely accepted for obstetrical use. Gestational age can be determined, congenital anomalies detected, multiple fetuses noted, ectopic pregnancy diagnosed, and fetal size and position determined.

Ultrasound takes 15 to 45 minutes and the preparation depends on the body part being examined. An obstetrical ultrasound may require the patient to have a full bladder in order to push aside the intestines. An ultrasound of the gallbladder and liver require the patient to have had nothing to eat or drink for eight to 12 hours prior to the exam. The patient must remain still unless requested to change positions. Therapeutic ultrasonography is discussed in Chapter 33 (Figure 32-6).

Positron Emission Tomography (PET)

Positron emission tomography, or PET, is a radiographic procedure using a computer and a radioactive substance. The radioactive substance is injected into the patient's body and gives off charged particles. They combine with particles in the patient's body to produce color images that tell the amount of metabolic activity there is in an organ or structure.

PET imaging is primarily a diagnostic medical imaging modality. It makes use of specialized, intravenously injected **radiopharmaceuticals** that emit positrons, which can be detected out of the body due to high energy releases. Specialized detectors arranged around the patient sense the energy and map the location from which it originated inside the body. These radiopharmaceuticals can be chemically designed to localize in the heart, brain, or certain types of tumors throughout the body. A clinical image is formed by the accumulation of positron emissions in a target organ. The patient's emission pattern forms a clinical image. This image is compared to the normal distribution by the nuclear medicine physician.

Generally, low to moderate doses are used to diagnose disease in patients. Certain nuclear medicine treatment studies use specialized radiopharmaceuticals that will isolate in the area to be treated. These agents emit their energy locally, irradiate tissue, and usually do not leave the body, unlike diagnostic radiopharmaceuticals. The properties and intent of diagnostic radiopharmaceuticals are different from therapeutic radiopharmaceuticals (Figure 32-7).

Computerized Tomography (CT)

A computerized tomograph uses a small amount of radiation. The beams penetrate body tissues to produce a series of cross-sectional images of the body part being examined. It allows images of structures that cannot be seen with regular X rays. It is a noninvasive test that usually requires no preparation and uses the computer with a minimal amount of radiation. It rotates 360 degrees around the patient to obtain cross-sectional images that can be viewed on a monitor and on film. It is ideal for early detection of tissue tumors such as childhood cancers and abdominal tumors, and it helps in directing radiation therapy for tumor masses. On occasion, a contrast medium is injected for a better view of internal structures. If contrast medium is used, the patient must be NPO (have nothing by mouth) for four hours before the patient is placed onto a motorized table that moves the body part to be examined into a scanner that surrounds that part of the patient. In 15 to 20 minutes, an entire body can be scanned (Figures 32-8A, 32-8B and 32-8C).

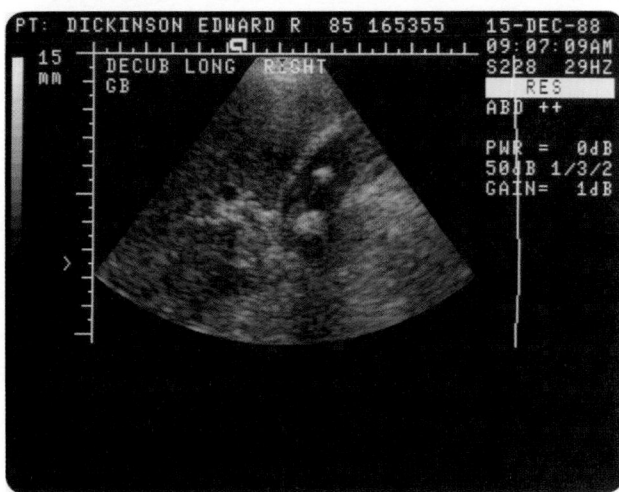

Figure 32-6 Sonogram of gallbladder with gallstones.

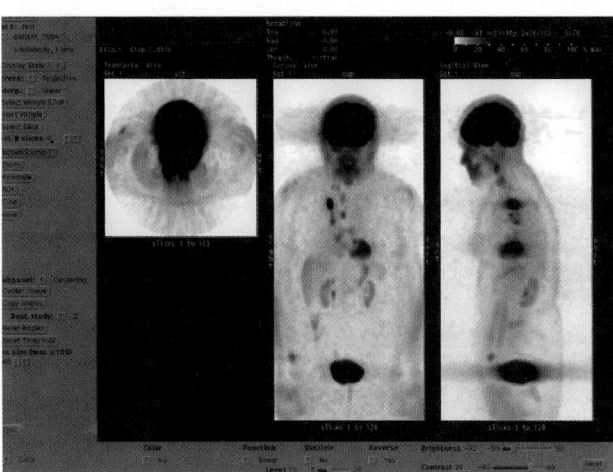

Figure 32-7 PET body scan demonstrates a tumor in the right lung.

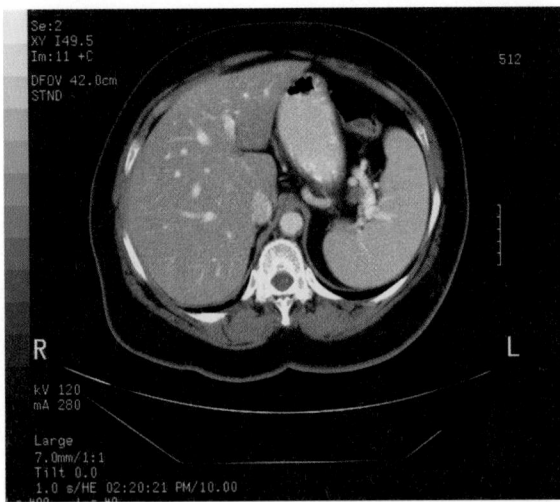

Figure 32-8A The positive contrast seen in the text and the highlighted hepatic vessels, inferior vena cava, aorta, and splenic artery denotes the administration of IV contrast media in this CT scan.

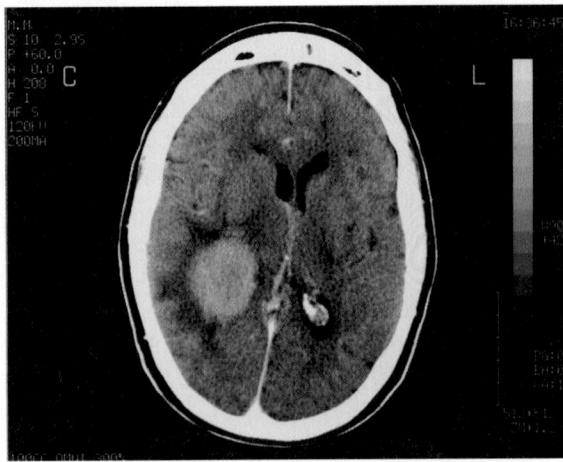

Figure 32-8B Axial CT scan demonstrates a meningioma surrounded by edema.

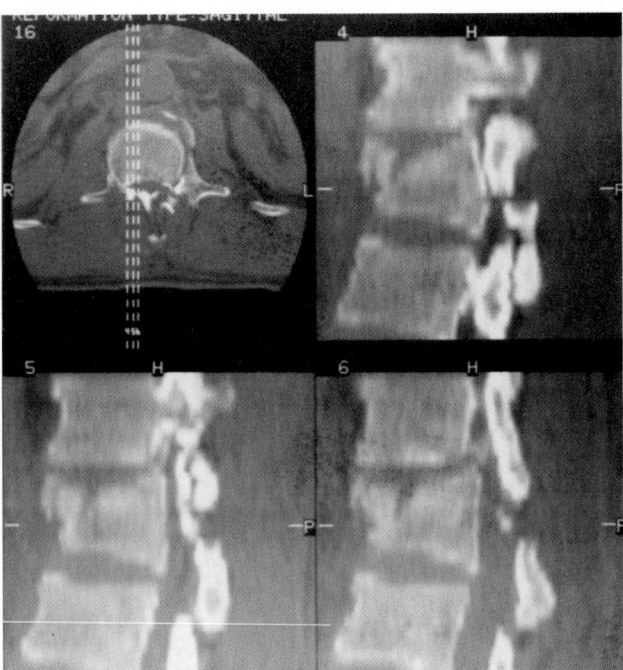

Figure 32-8C Axial scan showing a fractured thoracic vertebra. The three sagittally reconstructed images depict the area denoted by the dotted lines.

Magnetic Resonance Imaging (MRI)

Images produced by magnetic resonance imaging are of exceptionally high quality. No **ionizing radiation** is used, and it is noninvasive, safe, and painless procedure. All body areas can be viewed by the MRI, but it is especially helpful for soft tissues. It is very good for the spine, pelvis, and joints and is superior for visualizing the brain. The examiner can see through fluid-filled tissue with exceptional detail using an MRI machine. The computer forms the visual image.

The patient lies on a table inside a cylinder-shaped machine in which there is an electromagnet. The machine is sealed with the patient inside. Some patients who suffer from **claustrophobia** may need medication to help relieve symptoms of anxiety. Open MRI machines are now available and are particularly useful for those patients who are too apprehensive to be sealed in the traditional MRI machine.

Some drawbacks to the MRI are that it cannot be used for patients who have pacemakers or other metal clips left in place on internal structures or organs as part of a surgical procedure. An MRI is not as useful as conventional X rays or a CT scan for diagnosing fractured bones.

Patients are told to remove all objects that have metal: watches, belts, hairpins, rings, other metal jewelry, and credit cards because of the strong magnet in the MRI machine. Loose, comfortable clothing without zippers or snaps should be worn. The procedure takes about 45 minutes to an hour, during which time the patient must remain still. The technician, while not in the room with the patient, has a camera and microphone with which to communicate with the patient. An intermittent tapping sound can be heard throughout the procedure and earphones are available if the patient wants them (Figures 32-9 and 32-10).

Flat Plates

Flat plates are also known as "plain" films because they require no special technique or the use of contrast medium. This type of X ray is used on various parts of the body and is helpful in diagnosing problems in the skull, abdomen, chest, sinuses, and bone.

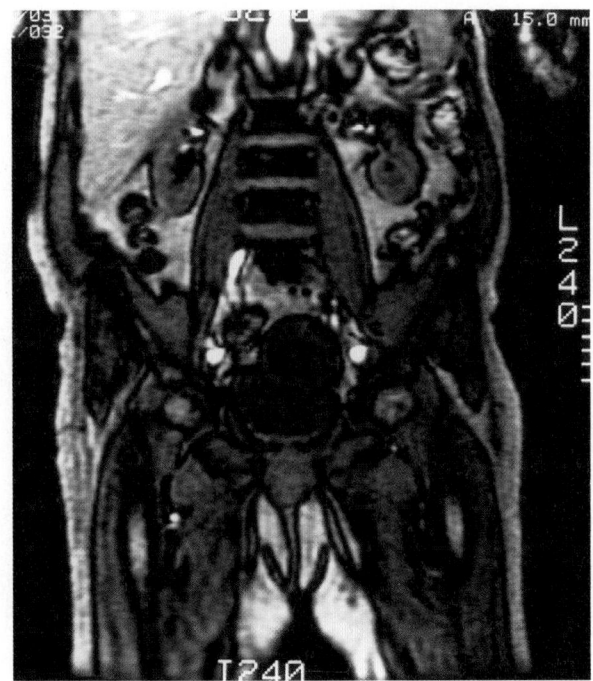

Figure 32-9 Coronal image of abdomen acquired during a breath hold in this MRI.

Filing Films and Reports

Because radiographs are part of the patient's permanent record, they must be safeguarded from the environment. Such conditions as heat, moisture, and light can damage them. Processed films are stored in special envelopes with the patient's name, date, and identification number marked on the outside. They are stored in a cool, dry place. The films are the property of the hospital or other facility where the films were taken and usually remain where they were taken. Storage on-site makes them accessible for future use for comparison purposes and eliminates the possibility of their being lost if they were allowed to be taken away from the facility where they were taken. Written reports of the findings are prepared by the radiologist and sent to the patient's physician(s) (Figure 32-11).

RADIATION THERAPY

Radiation therapy is generally used to treat tumors that cannot be surgically removed or are inaccessible for surgical removal, and for treatment of a malignant tumor that was surgically excised, but a portion of the tumor remains.

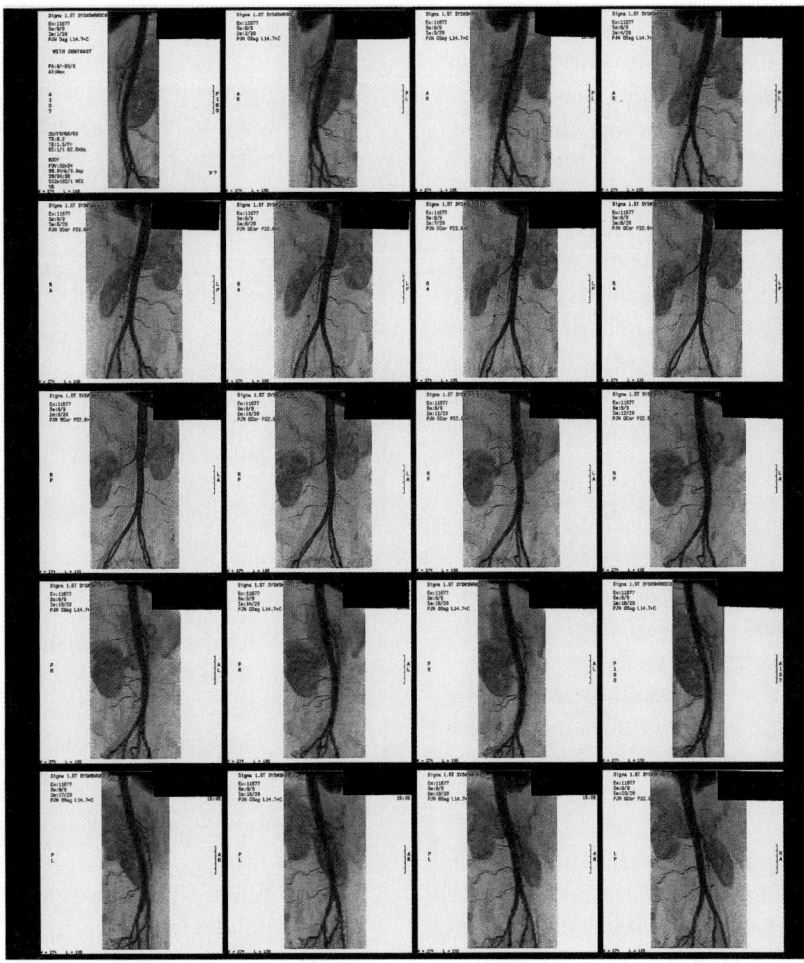

Figure 32-10 Magnetic resonance angiography.

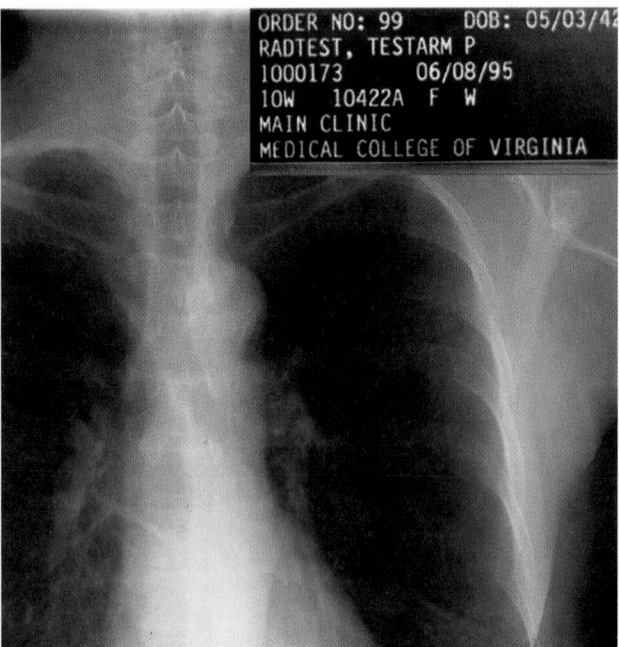

Figure 32-11A Radiograph showing patient identification information.

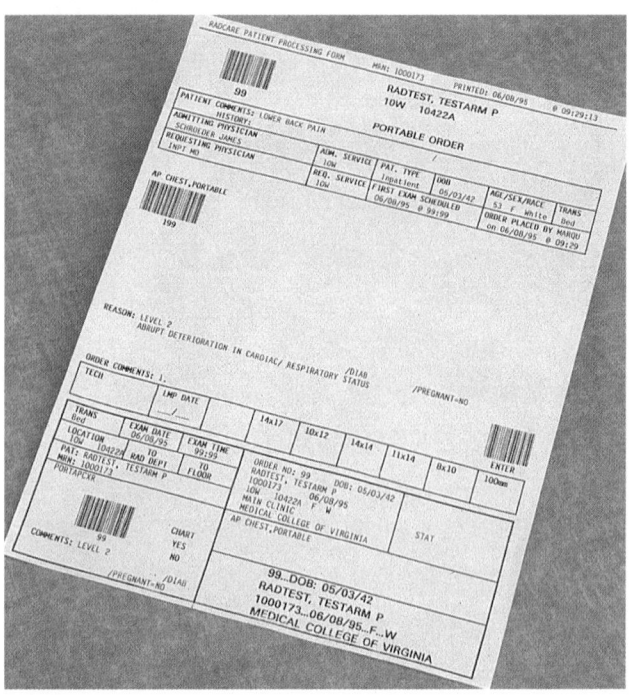

Figure 32-11B Sample requisition form.

When used to treat inaccessible or inoperable tumors, the treatment is considered **palliative** treatment. The treatments shrink the tumor, thereby lessening the symptoms. The treatments can be either external, with direct radiation aimed through the surface of the skin to an area within the body, or internal, using various applications of radioactivity such as seeds or beads that are planted inside the body and left there for a certain amount of time. The aim with radiation therapy is to interfere with cell growth and to disrupt the DNA. The object is to destroy as many of the malignant cells as possible without harming healthy cells surrounding the tumor. The side effects can be nausea, vomiting, hair loss, anorexia, bone marrow suppression, and **stomatitis**.

NUCLEAR MEDICINE

Nuclear medicine is the branch of medicine involved with the use of **radioactive** substances for diagnosis, therapy, and research. Specific training is necessary for this speciality.

Radioactive substances are administered to the patient either by mouth or by injection. The radioactive compounds, known as **radionuclides**, travel to an organ or area in the body that attracts them and creates an image of that area.

If the radionuclide is in an area that is abnormal, such as a tumor, it is referred to as "hot." If it does not concentrate in the abnormality, but surrounds it instead, this is known as a "cold" area. Both hot and cold areas are suggestive of abnormalities.

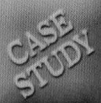

CASE STUDY 32-1

Gloria McDermott is scheduled to have a gastrointestinal (GI) series of X rays next week because of persistent complaints of stomach pain that is unrelieved by the prescription medication Dr. King has prescribed for her.

CASE STUDY REVIEW

1. How will you explain to her the purpose of the test?
2. How will you tell her about how to prepare for the exam?

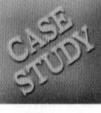

CASE STUDY 32-2

Raymond Brunnelle has had a series of X rays, a GI series, a cholecystogram, and an MRI of his abdomen. He has scheduled an appointment with a gastroenterologist and asks you to get all of the films for him.

CASE STUDY REVIEW

1. What is your response to his request?
2. Explain why they should be kept on-site.

SUMMARY

Radiology and diagnostic imaging are helpful in the diagnosis and treatment of diseases and conditions because procedures can be done to visualize internal structures and their functions. Radiation is not without its risks to personnel and patients, but by following specific safety precautions, the health and safety of all involved can be safeguarded.

The three specialty areas are radiology, radiation therapy, and nuclear medicine.

REVIEW QUESTIONS

Multiple Choice

1. Which of the following radiologic procedures does *not* require a contrast medium?
   a. hysterosalpingogram
   b. mammogram
   c. cholecystogram
   d. angiogram
2. A cholecystogram requires which type of contrast medium?
   a. air
   b. tablets
   c. carbon dioxide
   d. radionuclides
3. A cholangiogram will examine:
   a. upper GI tract
   b. lower GI tract
   c. bile ducts
   d. kidneys and ureters
4. In which of the following positions does the posterior aspect of the body face the X-ray tube and the anterior face the film?
   a. oblique
   b. anterioposterior
   c. posteroanterior
   d. prone
   e. supine
5. The radiologic procedure of choice for brain imaging is:
   a. computerized tomography
   b. positron emission tomography
   c. magnetic resonance imaging
   d. ultrasonogram
   e. thermography

Critical Thinking Questions

1. Describe the purpose of a lead apron and lead-lined walls in the radiology department.
2. For what is thermography used?
3. How are X rays used to diagnose?
4. How are X rays used to treat patient diseases or conditions?
5. Describe four types of contrast media.

6. What are the effects of radiation on an embryo or fetus?
7. To whom do X-ray films belong once they are taken and processed?
8. Describe how radiation therapy helps to destroy malignant neoplasms.
9. What special precautions should be taken when a patient is having an intravenous pyelogram, especially the initial time?
10. What do some state laws require of personnel who take X rays?

WEB ACTIVITIES

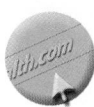

Access a web site regarding the radiologic technology profession to determine which states allow medical assistants to take and process X rays.

REFERENCES/BIBLIOGRAPHY

Bonewit-West, K. (2000). *Clinical procedures for medical assistants* (5th ed.). Philadelphia: W. B. Saunders Company.

Cornuelle, A., & Gronefeld, D. (1998). *Radiographic anatomy positioning: An integrated approach*. Stanford, CT: Appleton and Lange.

Cowling, C. (1998). *Radiographic positioning procedures, Volume II: Advanced imaging procedures*. Albany, NY: Delmar.

Early, P. J., & Sodee, D. B. (1995). *Principles and practice of nuclear medicine* (2nd ed.). St. Louis: Mosby-Year Book.

Fregmen, B. (1998). *Essentials of medical assisting administrative and clinical competencies*. Upper Saddle River, NJ: Brady-Prentice Hall.

Greathouse, J. (1998). *Radiographic positioning procedures, Volume I: Basic positioning and procedures*. Albany, NY: Delmar.

Kinn, M. E., & Woods, M. A. (1999). *The medical assistant: Administrative and clinical* (8th ed.). Philadelphia: W. B. Saunders Company.

Metler, F. A., Jr., & Guiberteau, M. J. (1997). *Essentials of nuclear medicine imaging* (4th ed.). Philadelphia: W. B. Saunders Company.

Taber's cylopedic medical dictionary. (18th ed.). (1999). Philadelphia: F. A. Davis Company.

Chapter 33

REHABILITATION AND THERAPEUTIC MODALITIES

KEY TERMS

Abduction
Activities of Daily Living (ADL)
Adduction
Ambulation
Assistive Device
Atrophy
Body Mechanics
Circumduction
Contracture
Cryotherapy
Dorsiflexion
Eversion
Extension
Flexion
Gait
Gait Belt
Goniometer
Goniometry
Hemiplegia
Hyperextension
Inversion
Modalities
Muscle Testing
Plantar Flexion
Pronation
Range of Motion (ROM)
Rehabilitation Medicine
Rotation
Supination
Thermotherapy
Ultrasound
Vasoconstriction
Vasodilation

OUTLINE

OBJECTIVES

The student should strive to meet the following performance objectives and demonstrate an understanding of the facts and principles presented in this chapter through written and oral communication.

1. Define the key terms as presented in the glossary.
2. Define rehabilitation medicine and explain its importance in patient care.
3. Discuss the importance of correct posture and body mechanics, and demonstrate how to safely transfer patients and lift or move heavy objects using proper body mechanics.
4. Describe safety precautions and techniques used when helping a patient to ambulate and demonstrate how to assist the patient to safely stand and walk.
5. Demonstrate how to safely care for the falling patient.
6. Describe assistive devices and the importance of each in helping patients to ambulate.

(continues)

OBJECTIVES (*continued*)

7. Demonstrate how to measure patients for a walker, crutches, and a cane and help them ambulate safely with each device.
8. Describe the ambulation gaits used with crutches.
9. Discuss the safety precautions and techniques used when pushing a wheelchair.
10. Explain the importance of joint range of motion and the method used to measure joint movement.
11. Explain the importance of therapeutic exercise and the types of therapeutic exercises used in patient rehabilitation.
12. Describe electromyography and its purpose.
13. Explain the purpose of the electrostimulation of muscle.
14. Identify by name the body movements used in range of motion (ROM) exercises.
15. Explain the body's physiological reactions to heat and cold therapeutic modalities.
16. Be able to identify and describe the various types of hot and cold modalities, and describe how ultrasound works.

ROLE DELINEATION COMPONENTS

CLINICAL
Patient Care
- **Prepare patient for examinations, procedures and treatments**
- **Assist with examinations, procedures and treatments**

GENERAL (TRANSDISCIPLINARY)
Legal Concepts
- **Document accurately**

Instruction
- **Instruct individuals according to their needs**
- **Teach methods of health promotion and disease prevention**

SCENARIO

In a large urgent care center like Inner City Health Care, a team of therapists is responsible for providing patients with a high level of rehabilitative care. However, the clinical medical assistants at Inner City also are involved on a daily basis in the care of patients who have suffered injuries such as fractures or severe back pain. Clinical medical assistant Wanda Slawson, CMA, MLT and clinical medical assistant Bruce Goldman, CMA are often responsible for transferring patients and getting them safely from the reception area to the examination room and from wheelchair to examination table. While being acutely aware of the needs and safety of the patient, Wanda and Bruce also make sure they protect themselves by using proper body mechanics, by observing good posture, by using their arm and leg muscles and not their back muscles, and by always bending from the hips and knees, not the waist. Wanda's and Bruce's observation of these important principles protects their health and ensures the safety of their patients.

INTRODUCTION

Physical disability affects millions of people in the United States, regardless of age, race, or socioeconomic status. Every year thousands of people survive strokes, head or spinal cord injury, or other debilitating illness or injury that leaves them unable to perform complete independent function. Some of these individuals recover completely. Others recover to their fullest ability, living the rest of their lives with some type of disability. Still other patients suffer from chronic conditions such as arthritis or severe back pain that incapacitates them to the extent they cannot work or completely care for themselves.

Rehabilitation medicine is a field of medical disciplines that uses physical and mechanical agents to aid in the diagnosis, treatment, and prevention of diseases or bodily injuries. Its goal is to aid in the restoration of those functions that have been affected by the patient's condition. For those who have suffered permanent loss of ability, it seeks to find practical substitutions for that loss while assisting patients to make the most of their remaining abilities.

Most rehabilitation services are prescribed by the physician in charge of a patient's care and, depending upon the patient's condition, can include a recommendation to one or several rehabilitation specialists. Most likely, that specialist will be a physical therapist, occupational therapist, speech therapist, or sports medicine specialist, although the field of rehabilitation medicine is certainly not limited to these four areas of specialty.

Professional rehabilitation therapists, in whichever field they practice, are specifically trained and licensed in their field of expertise to assess, plan, and execute the patient's treatment in an overall effort to restore that patient to the highest level of physical and social independence possible. The medical assistant, as a member of an interdisciplinary health team, can use medical assisting skills to enable patients to regain normal or near normal function after an illness or injury.

THE ROLE OF THE MEDICAL ASSISTANT IN REHABILITATION

As a medical assistant, you may find yourself working in one of the rehabilitation fields. Such opportunities might include an ambulatory care setting with a specialty in physical therapy or sports medicine, an orthopedic surgeon's practice, the occupational or speech therapy department of a large suburban hospital, or other outpatient clinic or medical office. For the more chronically ill, nursing homes and rehabilitation hospitals also focus on restoring patients to as much independence as possible.

Whatever the rehabilitation setting, you will most likely find that you are a member of an interdisciplinary team of health care professionals who bring a broad knowledge base to patient care (Table 33-1). However, the physician is responsible for prescribing any type of rehabilitative medicine.

It is important to remember that patients seeking rehabilitation treatment may have suffered a tremendous loss of physical ability, leaving them vulnerable to feelings of helplessness. They may be able to perform only limited activities of daily living (ADL) or normal daily self-care

TABLE 33-1	SOME OF THE SPECIALIZED FIELDS OF REHABILITATION MEDICINE
Physical Therapy/ Physiotherapy	The treatment of disorders with physical and mechanical agents and methods to restore normal function after injury or illness.
Occupational Therapy	The use of activities to help restore independent functioning after an injury or illness.
Speech Therapy	The diagnosis and treatment of speech disorders.
Sports Medicine	A branch of medicine that specializes in the treatment and prevention of injuries caused by athletic participation.

such as brushing their teeth, getting dressed, and eating. Perhaps they cannot even do the simple tasks we take for granted every day, leaving them completely dependent on another person for help.

Understanding and encouragement are vital to the recovery process of these patients. While working with disabled persons, remember that certain tasks may be very challenging to them. More than likely they are acutely aware of their impairment and feel frustrated at their loss of function and discouraged about the future. Some patients may also suffer some speech impairment, making communication difficult or impossible. Respect for their dignity will build their self-esteem and have a positive effect on their treatment.

PRINCIPLES OF BODY MECHANICS

Much of the medical assistant's work with disabled persons will require great physical effort, particularly if patients are incapable of lifting or moving themselves. Moving patients or heavy, awkward objects can be hazardous for the patient as well as the caregiver if not performed correctly.

Body mechanics is the practice of using certain key muscle groups together with good body alignment and proper body positioning to reduce the risk of injury to both patient and caregiver. Always be conscious of using proper body mechanics, not just on the job, but in everything that requires moving, lifting, pushing, or pulling heavy or awkward objects.

Posture

Practicing good body mechanics starts with good posture. Good posture protects the entire body, particularly the back, whether standing, sitting, or lying down.

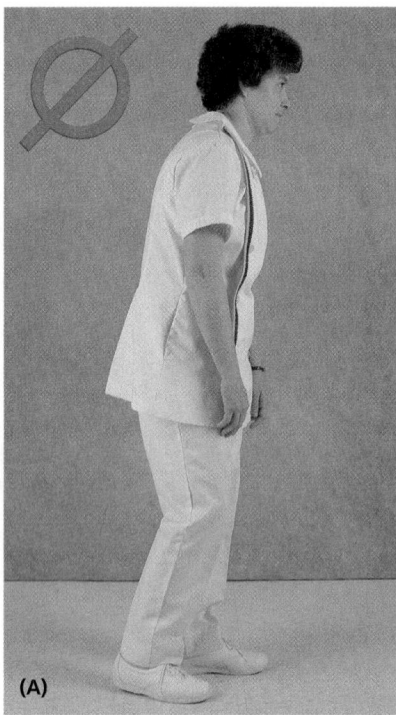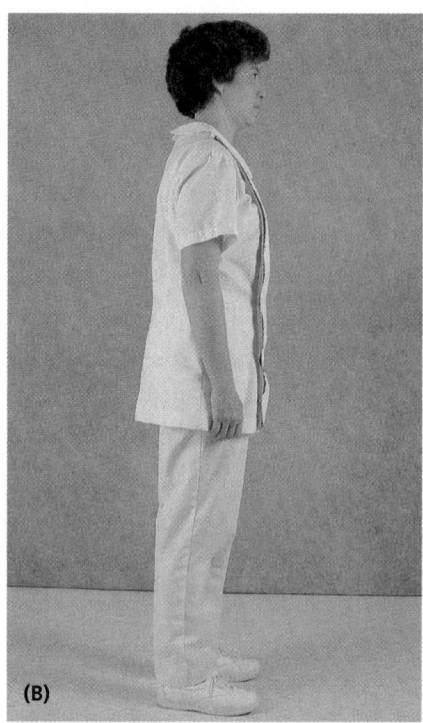

(A)   (B)

Figure 33-1 (A) A medical assistant demonstrating poor posture. (B) Good posture not only looks more professional but can prevent back injuries.

Glance at yourself sideways in a full-length mirror. When standing, does your posture most resemble that in Figure 33-1A or Figure 33-1B? When the body's muscle groups and body parts are in proper alignment, as shown in Figure 33-1B, the body is said to be in balance. Good balance is important for your body to function at its best. It enables you to lift, push, and pull easily and safely.

Frequently check your posture by reminding yourself to keep your chin and chest up, shoulders back, pelvis tilted slightly inward, feet straight and shoulder-width apart, and weight evenly distributed to both legs with a slight bend in your knees.

Using the Body Safely and Effectively

The spine is a flexible rod, designed to bend in many directions and hold the back steady. However, the muscles of the back are small and not meant for lifting heavy loads. They can be easily damaged if called upon to work beyond their natural ability. The muscles in the arms and legs, however, are large and were designed for heavy work. Rely on these muscles when lifting and carrying heavy objects, bending over or bending down, or moving patients.

It is important to keep several basic rules in mind whenever performing any task:

● Keep the back as straight as possible and feet shoulder-width apart to provide a good base of support (Figure 33-2).

● Always bend from the hips and knees, which enables the largest muscles of the legs to do the hard work, but *never* bend from the waist (Figure 33-3).

● Pivot the entire body instead of twisting it.

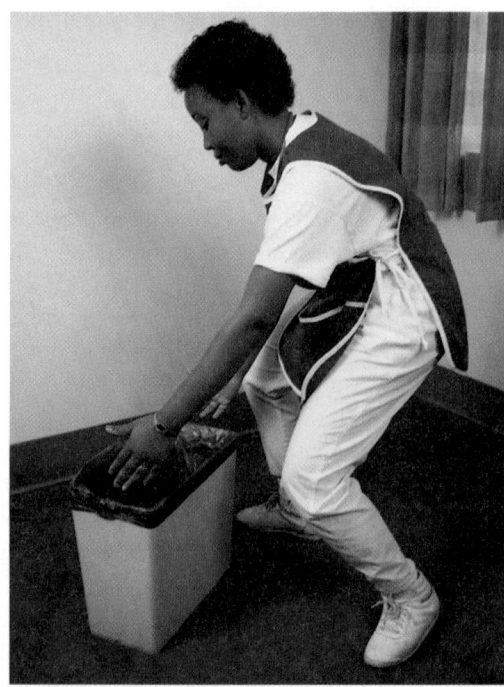

Figure 33-2 Provide a good base of support by keeping the back straight and feet apart.

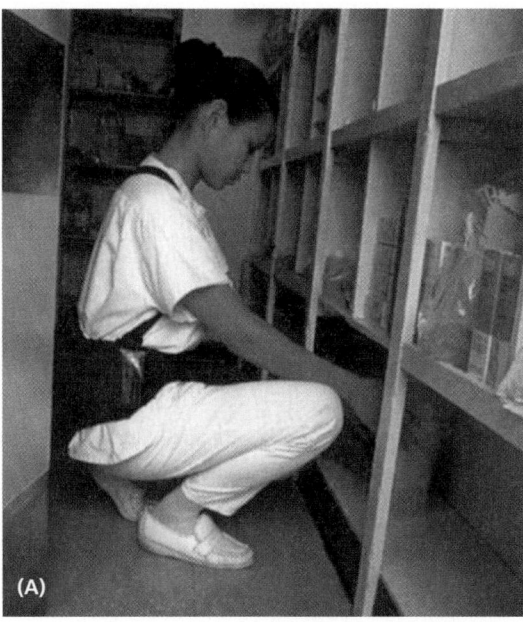
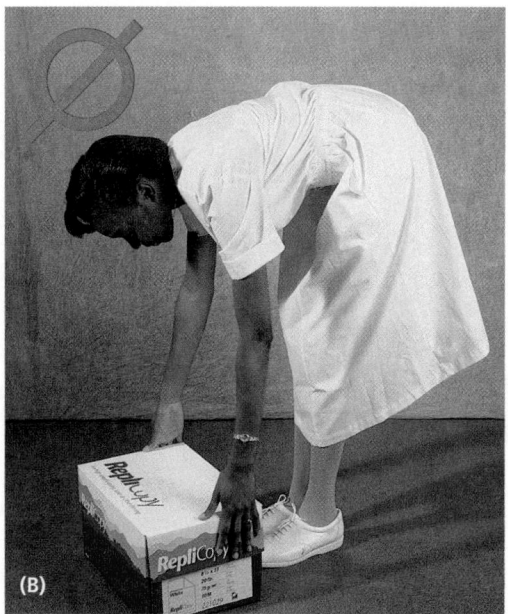

Figure 33-3 (A) Always bend from the hips and knees. (B) Never bend from the waist.

- Use the body's weight to push or pull any heavy object.
- Obtain help if unable to move a patient or object that is too heavy.

- Hold heavy objects close to the body (Figure 33-4).
- Make sure the path is clear and the area to receive the object is ready before lifting or moving it.
- Get into the habit of wearing a body support if a job includes much lifting (Figure 33-5).

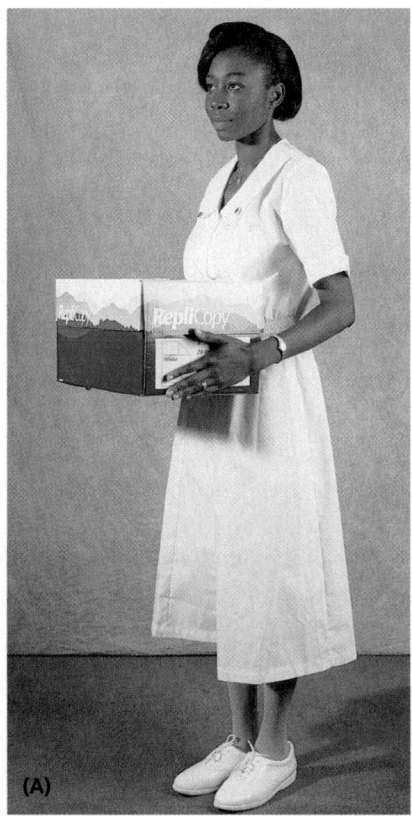
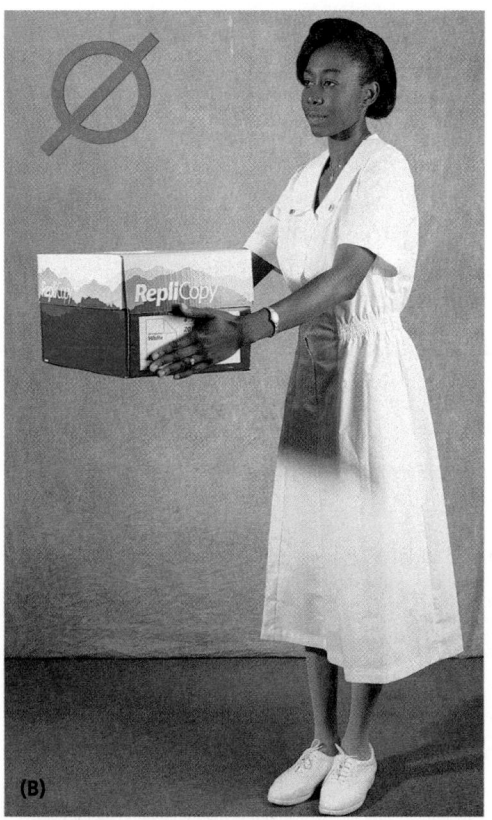

Figure 33-4 (A) When carrying heavy objects, hold them close to the body. (B) Never carry heavy objects out in front.

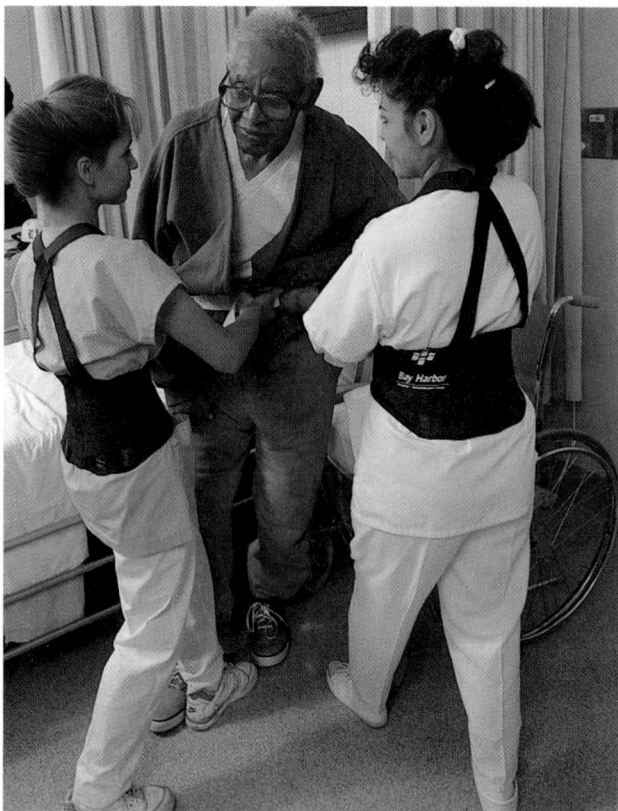

Figure 33-5 When a patient or object is too heavy, get help if necessary. Consider wearing a body support to protect the back if a job requires frequent lifting.

Lifting Techniques

When lifting patients or moving or lifting heavy objects, certain techniques should be used to prevent back injury:

- Get as close as possible to the object or person being lifted, since this allows the center of gravity to be maintained over the base of support.

- Keep the feet apart, one slightly in front of the other, and knees slightly bent.

- Use the large muscles of the legs and arms to lift, not back muscles.

- Keep the back straight to transfer the workload to larger arm and leg muscles.

- Bend from the hips and knees, squat down, and push up with leg muscles.

TRANSFERRING PATIENTS

It may be necessary to transfer patients if they cannot walk or lift themselves. Such patients may have a wide variety of disabilities, from severe back pain to **hemiplegia**, or paralysis of one side of the body resulting from a stroke, accident, or other condition. The frail elderly also require particular care when being transferred, as they are more prone to bruising and broken bones.

As a safety precaution, it is important to remember good body mechanics when transferring patients. The act of lifting and moving someone can throw off one's center of gravity and therefore the base of support. Provide a wider base of support by moving the feet further apart and bending slightly, using strong arm and leg muscles to lift.

Before beginning any transfer, observe certain precautions:

- Make sure the equipment is stable and firm. Lock the brakes of the wheelchair and make sure the exam table or other surface will not move during the transfer.

- Check that there are no obstructions to trip over when making the transfer.

- Take small shuffling steps, and avoid crossing the feet.

- It is best if the transfer surfaces being used are close to the same height. If possible, lower the examination table or bed to the height of the wheelchair.

- Position the equipment according to the patient's physical limitations or disability. If the patient is stronger on one side, make sure that is the side on which the transfer will take place. It not only makes the transfer easier, it gives the patient more confidence.

- Always use a **gait belt**, a safety belt worn around the patient's waist, when transferring a patient. Lift the patient by grasping the belt from underneath and lifting up. Never lift a patient by the arms, or under the armpits, as this could cause injury to you and the patient.

- Take advantage of any assistance the patient can provide in lifting and moving.

- Never have patients put their arms around your neck or on your shoulders as it could cause you to be injured.

- Make sure both you and the patient are wearing footwear that will not slip or hinder the transfer process in any way. If a prosthesis or brace is involved, make sure it is secure and will not present a problem.

- Thoroughly explain to the patient what you intend to do, and make sure the patient understands what to expect during the transfer. Instructions need to be simple and repeated when necessary.

- Practice good body mechanics. Get close enough to the patient so you can lift with your legs. Always bend at the hips instead of the waist.

- Ascertain beforehand whether or not assistance will be needed with the transfer.

- Finally, take sufficient time when completing each step. Many patients will want to help themselves. Respect their courage, but remember that safety is of the utmost importance.

See Procedure 33-1 for proper steps in transferring patients from a wheelchair to an examination table. Procedure 33-2 outlines steps for transfer from examination table to wheelchair.

ASSISTING PATIENTS TO AMBULATE

In spite of the great strides that have been made in recent years to provide access for disabled persons, ambulation, or walking, is a functional activity that still provides the ultimate level of independence and freedom. For many patients, being able to ambulate again gives them tremendous satisfaction because the act of walking more than anything else signifies their return to wellness. Some patients take months to walk again by undergoing exercises and treatment designed to strengthen specific muscles.

Before assisting with any type of ambulation, there are several safety issues to remember:

- Make sure the patient is ready to walk. If a patient has trouble sitting well, or cannot balance once standing up, walking should not be attempted.

- The patient should be wearing good shoes that are flat, supportive, and have a rubber sole.

- Check to be certain there are plenty of handholds or railings within easy reach should the patient become unstable during walking.

- A gait belt provides a firm hold on the patient should the patient require assistance with stability at any time. For the patient just starting to walk, this device should be used and held by the caregiver throughout the session.

- Monitor the patient when standing and throughout the ambulation session for signs of fatigue and vertigo.

- Ambulate only as long as the patient has strength. Never push the patient beyond endurance.

- Never hurry a patient.

- Be ready should a patient start to fall. Generally, patients will fall toward their weaker side, but sometimes their legs lose stability and they go straight down.

Procedures 33-3 and 33-4 detail the steps involved in assisting patients to stand and walk and caring for a falling patient.

ASSISTIVE DEVICES

For some patients, the extent of their physical disability may determine that ambulation is only possible with the help of an assistive device, or walking aid such as a walker, crutches, or cane. For others, their physical disability is such that mobility is not possible at all without the use of a wheelchair.

Some assistive devices provide stability and support, while others require more coordination. Depending upon the patient's condition, one assistive device may be used until the patient has gained enough strength and coordination to move on to another type of assistive device, with the ultimate goal of walking unaided. The device a patient needs depends both on the disability and the patient's recuperation curve and is prescribed after careful evaluation by the attending physician or other health professional (Table 33-2).

Whatever device a patient will be using, medical assistants may be called upon to measure the patient for the correct size and provide instruction in its proper use and care. Once the patient has become proficient on level surfaces, provide instruction on sitting, standing, turning around, and negotiating stairs, curbs, ramps, doors, and other obstacles. Additionally, patients should be taught how to protect themselves should they fall and how to get back up.

Walkers

Walkers are best used for patients who require maximum assistance with balance and coordination, as they provide stability and support when the patient is standing or walking. They provide patients with the ability to ambulate independently with confidence. In order to use one, patients must be strong enough to be able to hold themselves upright while leaning on the walker.

Various styles of walkers are available. The two most widely used walkers are those that have rubber tips on the legs (stationary walkers), and those with wheels on the bottom of the legs (rolling walkers). Walkers that have wheels can be easily pushed ahead by the patient while walking and are best for patients who primarily need a walker for balance.

Most walkers are made of aluminum and are lightweight; most can be easily folded for storage or transport. The major disadvantage is that they must be used on level ground and cannot be used on stairs. Walkers are also difficult to use when attempting to go through doorways and in small areas around the house.

TABLE 33-2 TYPES OF ASSISTIVE DEVICES

Assistive Device	Features	Patient Requirements
Walkers		
Standard	• Adjustable • Rubber tips	• Requires upper body strength • Provides maximum stability and support • Excellent for older persons
Rolling	• Legs have wheels • Otherwise same as regular walker	• Good for patients who need walker only for balance and not support
Crutches		
Axillary	• Wooden or steel • Worn under axillae	• Requires good upper body strength and balance • Not recommended for older persons • Best for younger persons with lower extremity or hip fractures that will heal in a short time • Provides greatest range of ambulation
Forearm (Lofstrand or Canadian)	• Shorter than axillary crutches • Has metal cuff worn around forearm	• Less stable than axillary crutches • Best for long-term crutch use • Reduces stress on axillary vessels and nerves • Requires upper body strength and more stability and coordination • Provides most maneuverability of all crutches
Platform	• Platform affixed to a crutch • Patient bears weight on forearm	• Best for patients with severe arthritis or poor use of hands • Does not require as much upper body strength • Requires good balance
Canes		
Standard	• Single leg • Curved handle • Rubber tip	• Good for patients with only one good arm, lateral instability, or balance conditions
Quad (four-point)	• Single cane resting on a platform with four legs • Rubber tips on legs	• Better for patients with more severe conditions • Does not require as much coordination, but still requires balance and upper body strength in one arm
Walkcane or Hemiwalker	• Has four legs that come all the way up to a handlebar • Rubber tips on all legs	• Provides most stability of all canes • Best for hemiplegic patients who require extra support on one side

Fitting a Walker. Most walkers can be adjusted for a proper fit. The height of the handgrip should be adjusted to the individual patient just below the patient's waist, or at the top of the femur so the elbow can be bent at a 30° angle when the patient is standing with hands on the handgrip (Figure 33-6).

Procedure 33-5 provides steps for assisting a patient to ambulate with a walker.

Crutches

Crutches provide the ambulating patient with a great deal more mobility and flexibility. They provide good stability and support, while allowing for a broad range of gait patterns and ambulating speeds.

Three basic types of crutches are prescribed, depending upon the patient's physical limitations and abilities: axillary crutches, forearm crutches (also called Lofstrand or Canadian crutches), and platform crutches (Figure 33-7).

Axillary crutches are made of wood or aluminum and are used primarily for persons who need crutches tem-

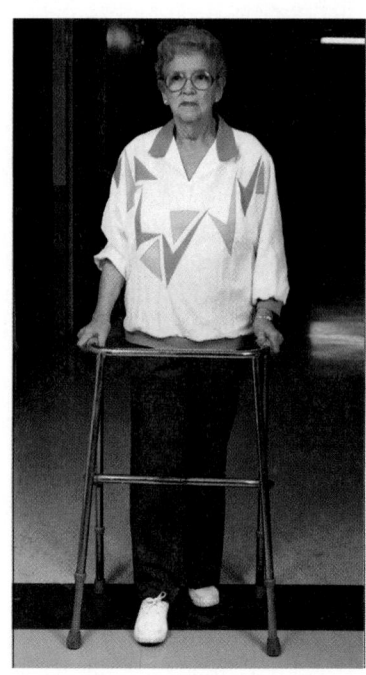

Figure 33-6 Proper fit for a walker. Note the patient's elbows are flexed at a 30° angle.

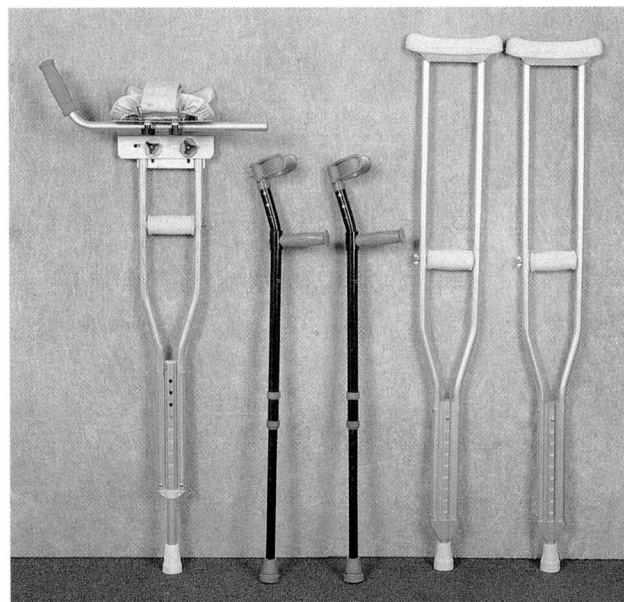

Figure 33-7 Types of crutches, from left to right: platform, forearm or Lofstrand, and axillary.

porarily while a lower extremity heals. Axillary crutches are ideal for stronger patients and pediatric patients who have minor injuries, but are not recommended for the frail elderly since upper body strength and balance are both required in order to use them (Figure 33-8). These crutches are easily transported and can be used to maneuver on stairs or in tight places.

Forearm crutches, or Lofstrand or Canadian crutches as they are also known, are shorter and provide less stability than axillary crutches. Forearm crutches are fixed with a metal or hard plastic cuff that fits around the patient's forearm. The weight is borne almost exclusively on the hand grip, requiring a great deal of upper body strength and coordination to use. This type of crutch is generally recommended for patients who will need crutches permanently or for a long period of time since they do not put any pressure on the axillary vessels and nerves (Figure 33-9).

The *platform crutch* is a third type of crutch that is recommended for patients who cannot grip the handles of other types of crutches or bear weight through their wrists or hands. The crutch has a platform attached to the top that includes a hand grip. It is high enough for the patient to use with the elbow bent at a right angle. The patient bears his weight completely on the forearm, which requires stability, strength, and coordination. The platform crutch is an ideal substitute for a cane when a patient only requires minimal weight transfer, but cannot bear weight on or grip with the hands (Figure 33-10).

Measuring a Patient for Axillary Crutches. To determine the right height of the crutches, have the patient stand tall. Be sure the patient is wearing good walking shoes. Adjust the height of the crutch so it is about two to three fingers, or two inches below the patient's axillae, or armpits (Figure 33-11). Adjust the

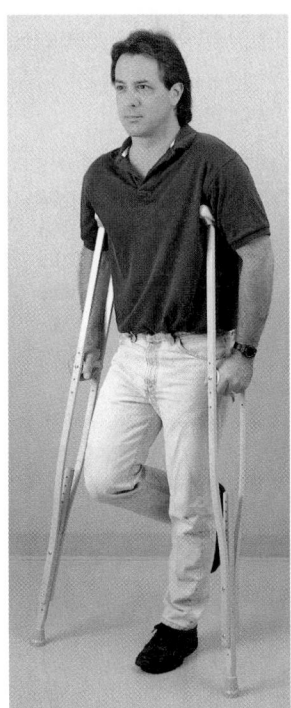

Figure 33-8 Patient using axillary crutches.

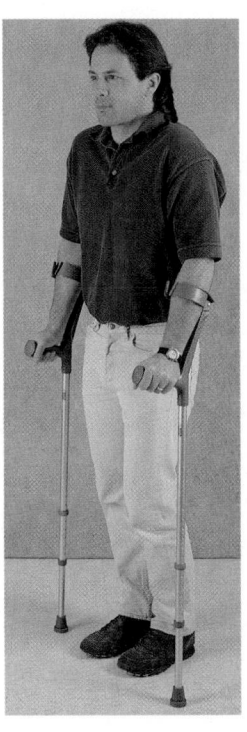

Figure 33-9 Patient using Lofstrand or forearm crutches.

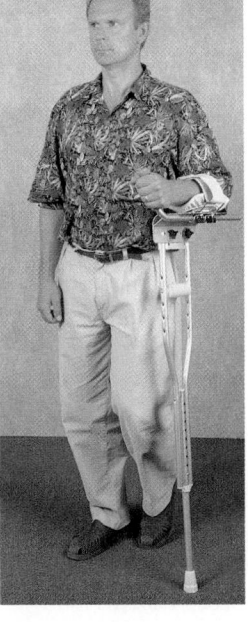

Figure 33-10 Patient using a platform crutch. This crutch is an ideal substitute for a cane if the patient cannot bear weight in his upper arm or on his hand.

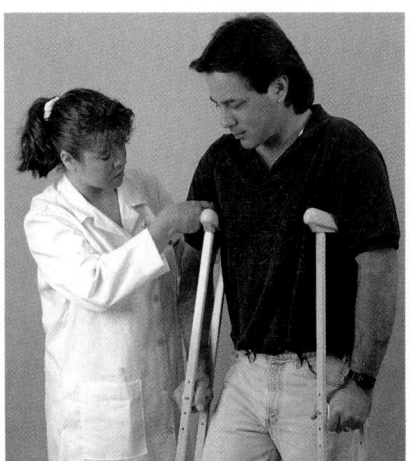

Figure 33-11 Measuring for axillary crutches. Note the height is about two to three fingers below the patient's armpit.

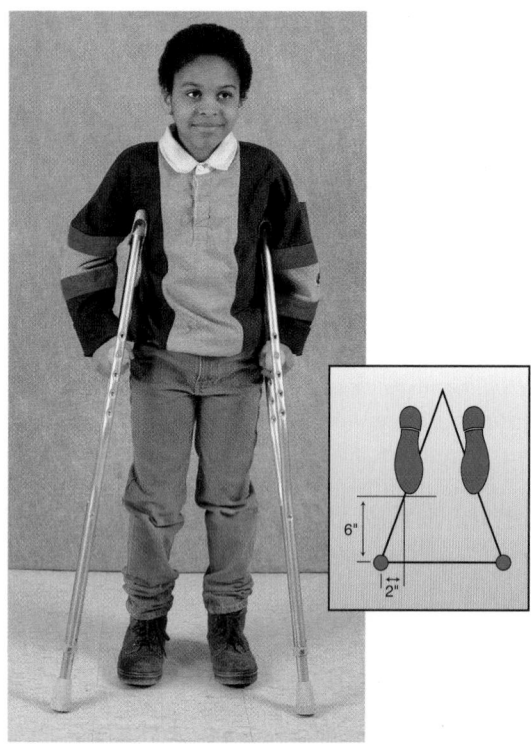

Figure 33-12   The distal end of the crutch should be 2 inches lateral and 6 inches anterior to the foot to form a triangle.

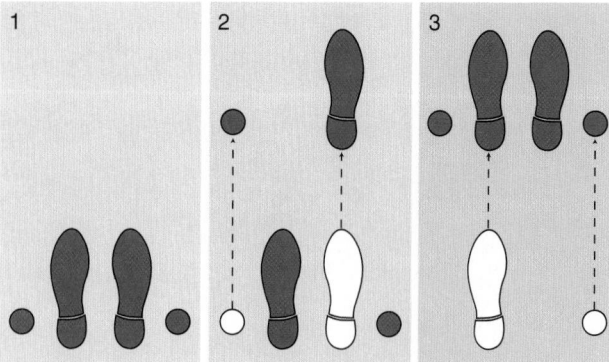

Figure 33-13   Two-point gait. The patient is bearing weight on both legs.

hand grips so the patient's elbows are bent at about a 20° to 30° angle. Position the crutch tips about 2 inches lateral and 6 inches anterior to the foot. When the patient is standing correctly, the crutch tips and patient's feet should form a triangle (Figure 33-12).

Procedure 33-6 indicates steps for teaching patients to ambulate with axillary crutches.

Crutch-Walking Gaits. The type of gait, or walk, a patient uses depends on the patient's injury and condition and is determined by the physician or licensed therapist. In crutch-walking gaits, each time the patient's foot or crutch touches the ground it is called a *point*. There are five gaits that are commonly used in crutch ambulation. The number of points in the gait relates to the number of feet and crutch tips that are on the ground at the same time.

Common crutch-walking gaits include two-point, three-point, four-point, swing-to, and swing-through gaits.

Two-Point Gait. There are two types of two-point gaits:

1. The first type is a nonweight-bearing gait. The patient places the crutch tips about 18 inches in front of him. He pushes off, taking the weight off his body and transferring it to his hands, then brings his strong leg forward past the crutches.
2. The second gait, called the two-point alternating gait, is used when the patient can bear weight on

both legs. The opposite foot and crutch are advanced forward at the same time (Figure 33-13). This gait is a more advanced gait, and is used after the four-point gait has been mastered.

Three-Point Gait. This gait is used when the patient can only bear partial weight on one leg, or just touch that foot to the floor. Both the crutches and the weak leg are advanced at the same time. The body weight is then transferred forward to the crutches, and the stronger leg is advanced and placed slightly in front of the crutches (Figure 33-14).

Four-Point Alternating Gait. This is a slower gait that is used for patients who can bear weight on both legs and

Patient Teaching Tip

When instructing patients in the use of axillary crutches, impress upon them the importance of putting all their weight on their hands, not on the armpits. Many patients using crutches for the first time mistakenly put the pressure on their armpits, which can damage the axillary nerve. Also reinforce the need for wearing flat, nonskid shoes when using crutches.

Throw rugs and other obstacles in the home or work area are a danger to patients on crutches. Remind them to have such hazards removed. Teach patients to check crutches daily for the following:

- Check that the wing nuts that adjust the crutches are tight.
- Check the crutch tips for wear and tear.
- Check the foam pads of the hand grips and armpit rests for tears.

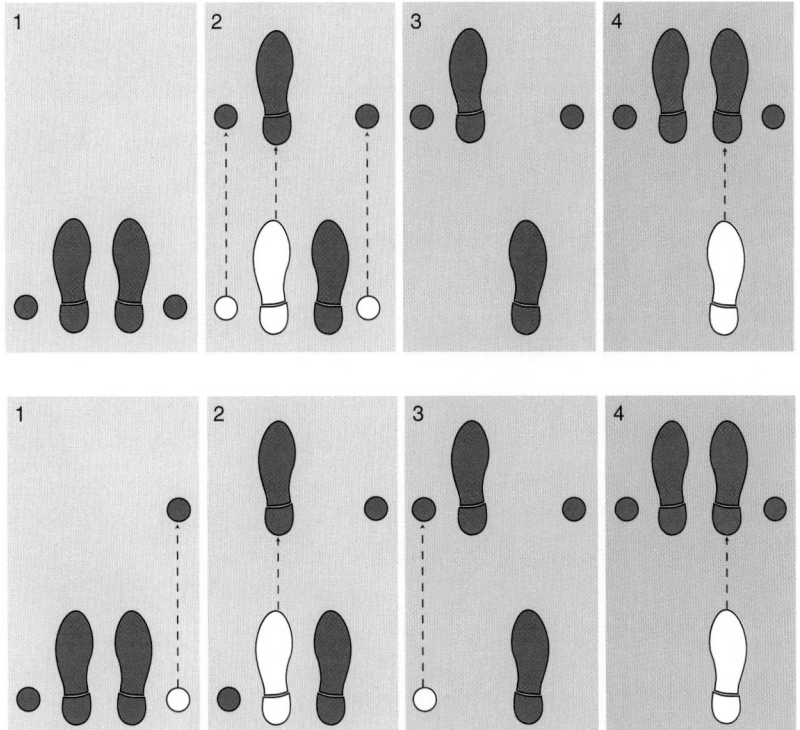

Figure 33-14   Three-point gait. The left leg is the weaker leg and bears no weight.

Figure 33-15   Four-point gait. The patient is bearing weight on both legs.

move each leg separately. The patient moves one crutch forward, then the opposite foot. The patient then moves the other crutch forward, then the opposite foot (Figure 33-15).

Swing-To Gait. The patient starts with the crutches at his side. He moves both crutches forward, transfers his weight forward, and swings both feet together up to the crutches.

Swing-Through Gait. Start with the crutches at the side. Move both crutches forward. Transfer the weight and swing both feet through the crutches, stopping slightly in front of the crutches.

Sitting. The patient backs into a straight chair with armrests until the seat of the chair touches the back of the legs. Crutches are held in the hand on the strong side and opposite the weak leg. With the other hand the patient can grasp the armrest of the chair and lower slowly into the chair.

Standing. The patient holds both crutches in the hand on the strong side, moves forward in the chair, grasps the armrest with the hand on the weaker side, then pushes up to a standing position.

Canes

A cane is used when the patient has one weak side and will need this assistive device for a longer period of time than crutches. It is also useful for patients who have a general but minor weakness on one side or those who have poor balance.

Canes come in three basic types, are made of either aluminum or wood, and have rubber tips. Some are adjustable and some are not (Figure 33-16). The first type of cane is called a *standard*, or single-tipped cane. It has a curved handle for gripping, and the newer canes have a hand grip attached. The standard cane is used for patients with less severe walking conditions and needs a small amount of support.

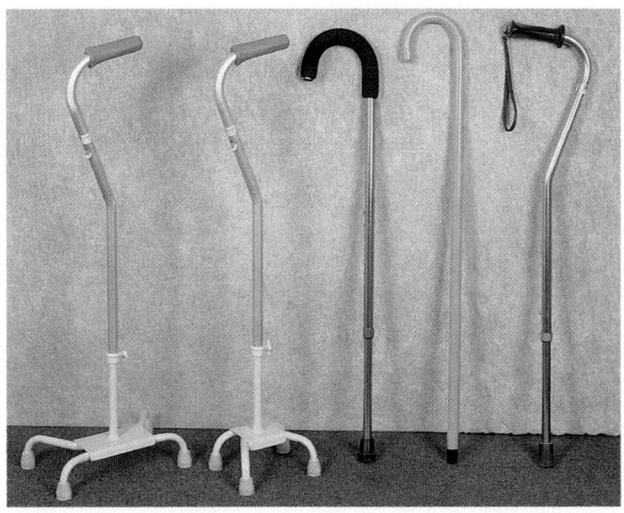

Figure 33-16   Types of standard canes: (A) Quad canes. (B) Single-tip canes.

The second type of cane is a four-legged, or *quad* cane. It is a single cane that rests on a four-legged platform, provides stability and a wide base of support, and is for patients with more severe walking difficulties.

The third type of cane is a *walkcane* (Figure 33-17). It has four legs and a handlebar for gripping, and provides the best support of all canes. This type of cane is also referred to as a Hemiwalker because it is ideal for hemiplegic patients who need the extra stability of this wide base. When the cane is the correct height, the elbow is flexed at a 20 to 30° angle.

Procedure 33-7 outlines the steps for teaching a patient how to walk safely with a cane.

Wheelchairs

Wheelchairs are mobile chairs that enable patients with severe ambulation conditions, or no ability to ambulate at all, to otherwise get around. Some must be moved manually, either by the patient or by someone else. Others are motorized and can be controlled completely by the patient (Figure 33-18).

Many advancements in wheelchair design over the years have enabled patients with chronic conditions to longer be restricted to a home or hospital environment. Today, all public buildings and many private ones have handicapped access ramps as an alternative to stairs, remote-controlled doors, elevators that can accommodate a wheelchair, and other amenities that enable wheel-

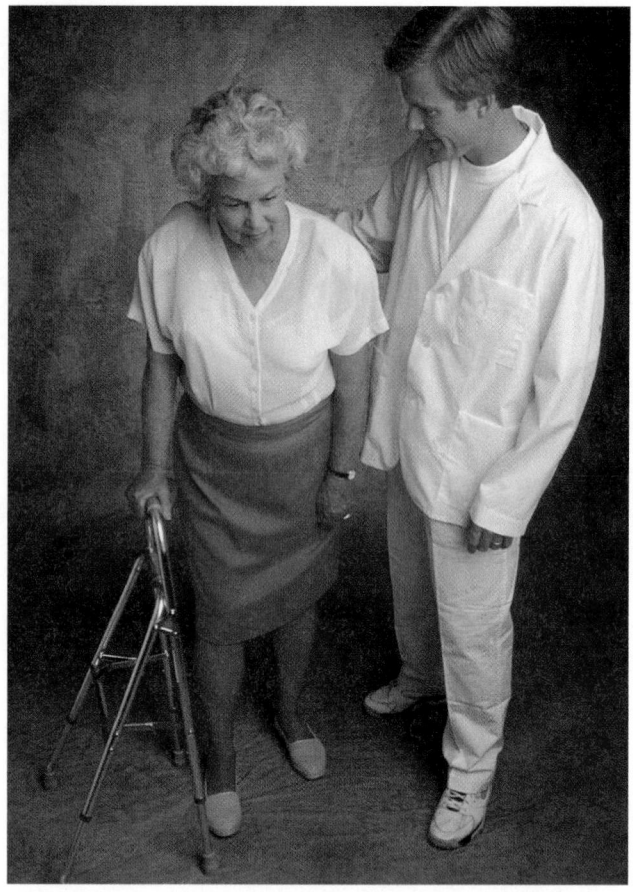

Figure 33-17   A walkcane being used by a hemiplegic patient. (Courtesy of Guardian Products)

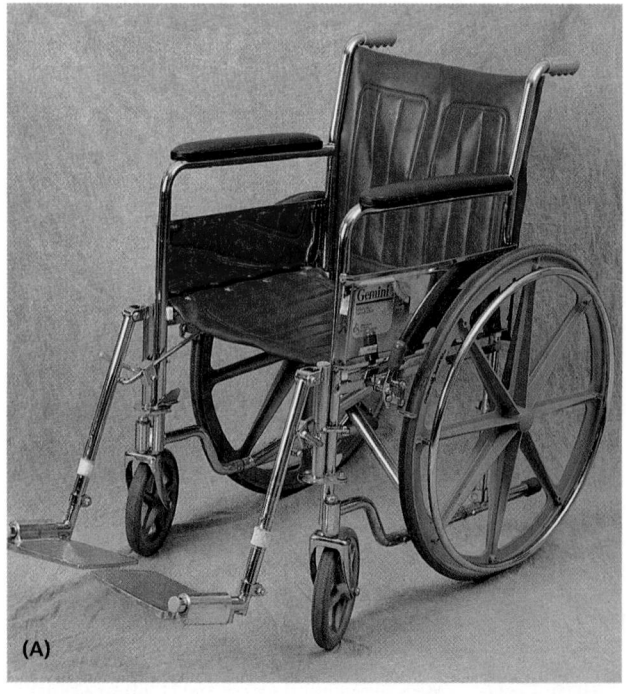

(A)

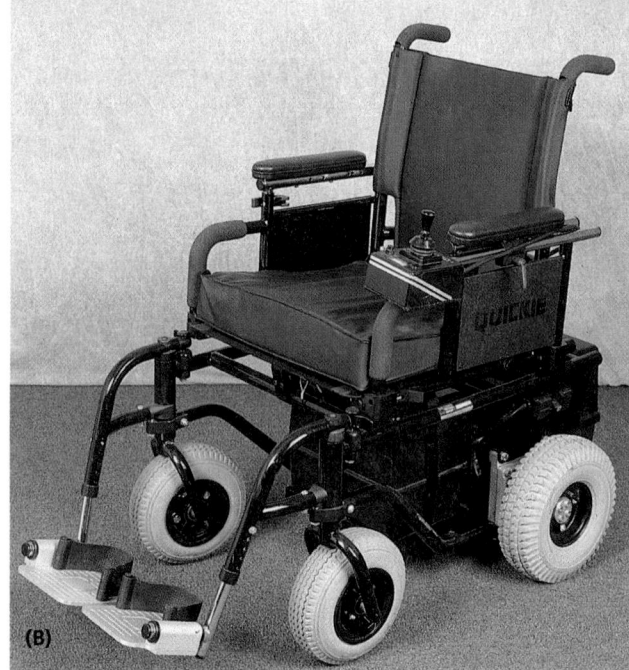

(B)

Figure 33-18   (A) A manual wheelchair. (B) A motorized wheelchair.

chair patients to get around almost as well as if they were ambulating.

There are many types of wheelchairs and modifications that can be tailored to suit a patient's particular disability and lifestyle. There are even wheelchairs that enable patients to take part in sports activities. Many car manufacturers can modify a van to accommodate a wheelchair, and some are equipped to allow wheelchair patients to drive.

Patients who will be using a wheelchair for a long time are taught how to maintain it. Depending upon their abilities, they check it regularly to make sure all the parts are working correctly, and, if they are able, to make any necessary repairs. Patients are taught to use the wheelchair safely and maneuver into and out of difficult spaces.

If a patient is being pushed by someone else, that individual must learn basic safety rules for transporting a patient:

- Make sure that the brakes are locked when transferring a patient into and out of a wheelchair and if a patient must be left alone in the wheelchair for any length of time, lock the brakes.
- Make sure the patient's feet are placed on the footrests when the wheelchair is in use.
- Guide the wheelchair from behind and use your weight to help push it (Figure 33-19).
- Always back into and out of elevators.
- Stay to the right in corridors.
- Back down slanted ramps.

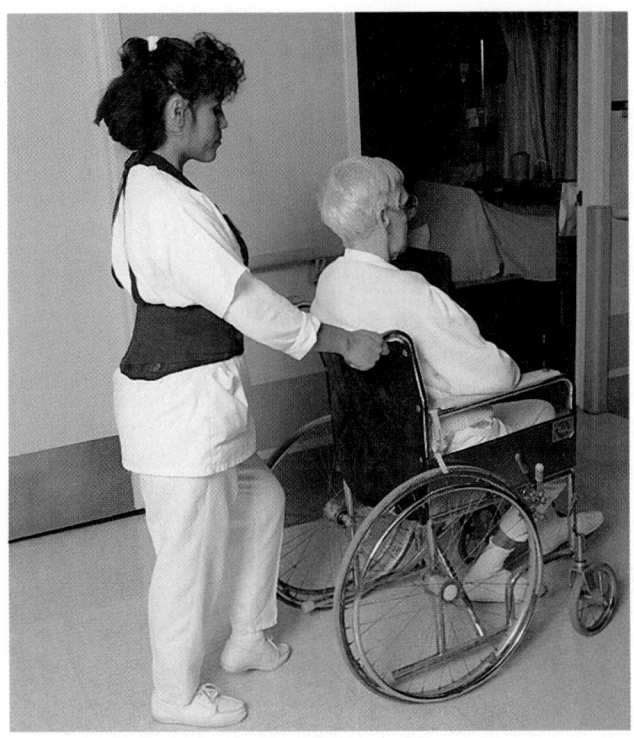

Figure 33-19 Guide the wheelchair from behind.

THERAPEUTIC EXERCISES

Range of Motion

The musculoskeletal system is a complex joining of bones, joints, ligaments, and tendons. Not only does it give structure to the body and protect the body's vital organs, it allows for movement so we can carry out a multitude of activities.

The bones of almost all the joints of the body are designed to move as well, each joint having its own **range of motion (ROM)**. Range of motion refers to the amount of movement that is present in a joint.

Normal ROM varies between people and depends upon several factors, such as age, gender, and whether the motion being performed is passive (assisted motion) or active (voluntary motion). There is a standard range of motion for all movable joints, and it is this standard that is used when evaluating the joint movement of a particular patient.

The measurement of joint motion is called **goniometry**. Joint movement is measured with an instrument called a **goniometer** and is always expressed in degrees. For example, the average person lying flat with arms to the sides can move the elbows from a 20° hyperextension (extending the arm beyond its normal limits) to 0° extension, through to 150° of flexion, or bending (Figure 33-20).

Range of motion evaluation is one of several tools used when developing a therapeutic program for a patient.

Muscle Testing

The other tool used for evaluating the movement abilities of a patient is muscle testing. While goniometry focuses on joint movement, **muscle testing** evaluates the motion,

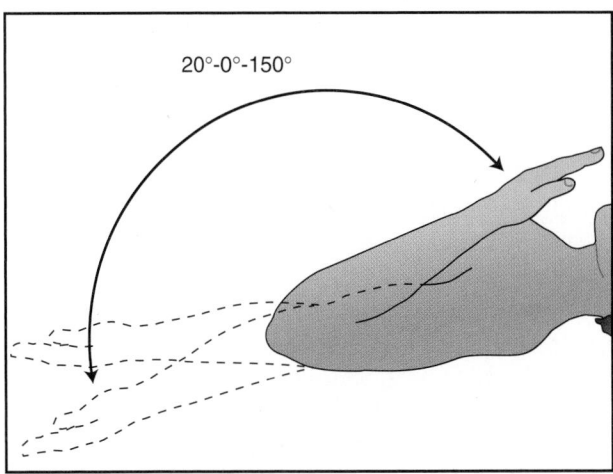

20°-0°-150°

Figure 33-20 Joint mobility is measured against standard ranges of motion (ROM) and is always expressed in degrees.

strength, and task potential of a given muscle. *Range of motion* testing for muscles determines how flexible and resilient a muscle may be. *Strength testing* shows how hard a muscle can work. *Task potential* of a muscle means how well a muscle can aid in accomplishing a given activity. As a medical assistant, you may assist with testing the patient for joint mobility, posture, and strength of muscles.

Types of Therapeutic Exercise

Without constant exercise, the musculoskeletal system would deteriorate. Joints would become stiff and contractures, or deformities, could develop. Muscles would atrophy, or shrink and lose strength. Bones would lose vital minerals such as calcium and phosphorus. And the body's overall circulation would decrease, which would in turn create a separate set of unhealthy conditions.

Like drugs, exercise has a powerful and systemic effect on the body. It involves the function of joints, bones, muscles, nerves, tendons, ligaments, as well as the circulatory and respiratory systems. Therapeutic exercises are prescribed after careful evaluation by a trained specialist and are tailored to each patient depending upon that patient's individual condition and rehabilitation goals. It is the role of the medical assistant to understand the goals and objectives of the therapeutic exercise program in order to better support and encourage patients to complete their program.

While an athlete uses exercise to build strength and endurance in order to attain a certain level of performance, therapeutic exercises are prescribed for a variety of therapeutic and preventive effects. They are used most commonly for therapeutic reasons to correct or prevent deformities, regain body movement after an accident or disease, restore joint motion after immobility, improve neuromuscular coordination, and improve or develop activities of daily living.

Exercise is also used for another important reason. It can prevent many common problems brought on by inactivity, such as those problems associated with respiration and circulation.

A variety of exercise programs are employed for therapeutic or preventive purposes.

1. *Active exercises*, which are self-directed and performed by the patient without assistance.
2. *Passive exercises*, which are performed by another person with no voluntary participation from the patient.
3. *Assisted exercises*, which help the patient voluntarily move weakened muscles with the use of an assistive device, such as a therapy pool.
4. *Active resistance exercises*, which provide voluntary movement against various types of manual or mechanical pressure to increase muscle strength.

Electromyography

Electrical activity of a muscle can be recorded on a graph or film to help to determine how well muscles contract. An electromyograph is the instrument used to test the electrical activity of a muscle. An electrode (using a small gauge needle) is inserted through skin into the muscle, and measurements can be made as to muscle strength.

Electrostimulation of Muscle

An electric current of low voltage can help to stimulate muscles to exercise by innervating the sensory and motor nerves for that muscle. It is helpful for a patient who has nerve damage to the muscle and cannot voluntarily move the muscle. The purpose is to prevent atrophy of the muscle and help to restore muscle function.

The low current of electricity passing through the patient's muscle acts similarly to the patient's own nerves causing the muscle to contract and relax. The stimulation is helpful to retrain a patient after suffering an injury to a muscle or muscle group.

Range of Motion Exercises

As a medical assistant, you may be called upon to perform range of motion exercises. Range of motion exercises are designed to maintain joint mobility and are either performed passively (someone else does the movement) or actively (the patient does the movement).

Joint movement has a special vocabulary. It will be helpful when learning range of motion exercises to consult the terms and their definitions, as shown in Table 33-3.

TABLE 33-3	TERMINOLOGY OF JOINT MOVEMENT
Abduction	Motion away from the midline of the body
Adduction	Motion toward the midline of the body
Circumduction	Circular motion of a body part
Dorsiflexion	Moving the foot upward at the ankle joint
Eversion	Moving a body part outward
Extension	Straightening of a body part
Flexion	Bending of a body part
Hyperextension	A position of maximum extension, or extending a body part beyond its normal limits
Inversion	Moving a body part inward
Plantar Flexion	Moving the foot downward at the ankle
Pronation	Moving the arm so the palm is down
Rotation	Turning a body part around its axis
Supination	Moving the arm so the palm is up

Before performing range of motion exercises on a patient, you will need to observe some general precautions:

- Always move the patient's limbs gently, within pain tolerance and the flexibility of the limb.

- Use slow, careful movements that allow the muscles time to adjust to the movement.

- Always support the limb above and below the joint.

- It is best to perform passive ROM with the patient in the supine position.

- ROM should never cause pain. If the patient reports pain at any time, the ROM exercises should be discontinued until a physician or other health care professional can determine the source of pain.

- Repeat each movement several times or as prescribed by the physician.

Procedure 33-8 provides ROM exercises for various parts of the upper body. Procedure 33-9 provides ROM exercises for lower extremities.

THERAPEUTIC MODALITIES

Sometimes, therapeutic exercise is not the best or only way to restore injured or painful joints and tissues. A patient's condition may respond equally well to certain physical agents, called **modalities**, which take advantage of the properties of heat, cold, electricity, light, and water to improve circulation, minimize pain, and correct or alleviate muscular and joint malfunction.

Many modalities have been around for centuries, and some can easily be performed by the patient or caregiver at home. Modalities can be used locally to treat a small area at a time or systemically to alter a patient's temperature or soothe many groups of painful muscles or joints. The patient's condition and rehabilitation program both influence the modality or combination of modalities used.

Heat and Cold

Heat, or **thermotherapy**, acts on the body by causing **vasodilation** (dilation of the blood vessels). The effect of heat increases circulation to an area and acts to speed up the repair process. Heat can be used to:

- Relax muscle spasms

- Relieve pain in a strained muscle or sprained joint

- Relieve localized congestion and swelling

- Increase drainage from an infected area

- Increase tissue metabolism and repair

However, because heat dilates the blood vessels and increases circulation, it also acts to speed up the inflam-

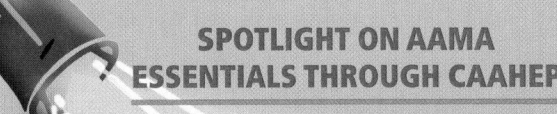

SPOTLIGHT ON AAMA ESSENTIALS THROUGH CAAHEP

- Understanding and encouragement are vital to the recovery process for those patients seeking rehabilitation treatment.

- Providing both physical and emotional support to a patient ambulating safely is an important part of the rehabilitation process following a period of sedentary recuperation.

- Being sensitive to the needs of a patient suffering from chronic pain is an important part of the medical assistant's responsibility in working with patients undergoing pain management treatment.

matory process, which can lead to more serious problems, such as increased bleeding and swelling. Heat should never be used on pregnant or menstruating women, as it can induce uterine contractions. Also, heat should not be used longer than its prescribed length of time.

Cold applications, or **cryotherapy**, are used to constrict blood vessels and slow or stop the flow of blood to an area. This process, also called **vasoconstriction**, slows down the inflammatory process, which can reduce or prevent swelling of inflamed tissues, reduce bleeding, numb the pain sensation by acting as a topical anesthetic, and reduce drainage to an area.

By understanding how heat and cold affects the body, it is easier to observe whether or not they are having the desired therapeutic effect. Heat and cold modalities can be extremely effective, which is why they are so widely used for treating certain physical conditions. However, the effects of heat and cold modalities depend on several conditions: the type of modality used, the length of time it is applied, the patient's condition, and the area or areas being treated.

 Precautions for Heat and Cold Applications. When applying either heat or cold modalities, you need to take certain precautions to avoid injury. If misused, any therapeutic modality can actually cause more damage to the site that is trying to heal. Prior to starting any treatment, keep the following precautions in mind:

- Infants and patients who cannot report a burning sensation should be watched carefully. Infants and the elderly are particularly susceptible to burns.

- Heat and cold sensitivity varies with the patient; check patients frequently and never leave them alone.

- Never have a patient lie on a heating pad, as severe burning can result. Place a rubber cover over the heating pad if using with moist dressings.

- Always wrap appliances with cloth before applying them to the skin.

- Only soak or immerse patients in water between 104°F to 113°F (40°C to 45°C). Temperatures of 116°F (47°C) or above can cause burning.

- Heat can cause uterine contractions in menstruating or pregnant women.

- Never use heat within the first 48 hours of an acute inflammatory process and never apply heat to newly burned skin.

- Watch carefully persons with impaired circulation, or cardiovascular, renal, sensorineural, or respiratory conditions, or osteoporosis.

- Lack of sensation to a therapy may mean impaired circulation to an area and the patient may be unable to report a burning sensation.

- As heat concentrates in metal materials, have patients remove all jewelry and other metal objects, and administer the treatment on nonmetal tables and chairs.

Moist and Dry Heat Modalities

Moist Heat Therapies. Moist heat refers to heat modalities that feel moist against the skin. Moist heat penetrates better than dry heat and aids in improving circulation, relaxation, and mobility.

Hot Soaks. Hot soaks are generally used for soaking the extremities and can easily be administered at home by the patient or caregiver. The patient's body part is gradually immersed in plain or medicated water no hotter than 110°F (44°C) for a short time, usually no more than about 15 minutes. The patient should be positioned to be comfortable. Observe the patient's skin for excessive redness and, if noticed, remove the limb at once. Always dry the skin carefully by patting, not rubbing it.

Total body immersion in hot water can be administered in a whirlpool bath or special Hubbard tank. This treatment is often prescribed to promote relaxation, circulation, and movement of limbs in preparation for exercise. The mechanical action of agitating water moving over the body in a whirlpool is called hydromassage and can

both relax muscles and stimulate circulation. The Hubbard tank is a bit larger and provides room for limited body exercise without the effects of gravity.

Hot Compresses and Packs. A hot compress is usually applied to a small area, and is prepared by soaking and wringing out either a square of gauze or other absorbent material (like a clean washcloth) and applying it for a limited time to the affected area (Figure 33-21). Hot compresses can easily be administered at home. A hot pack is used for a larger area and generally involves the use of a professional hot pack administered in the clinical setting. This type of hot pack is soaked in hot water, removed with tongs and drained, and placed over larger areas such as the back or shoulders.

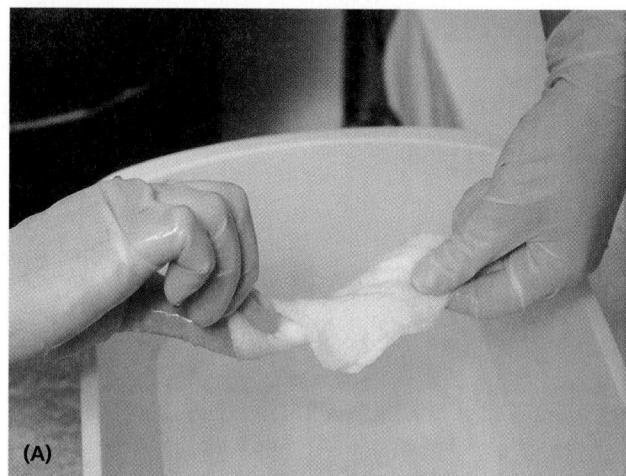
(A)

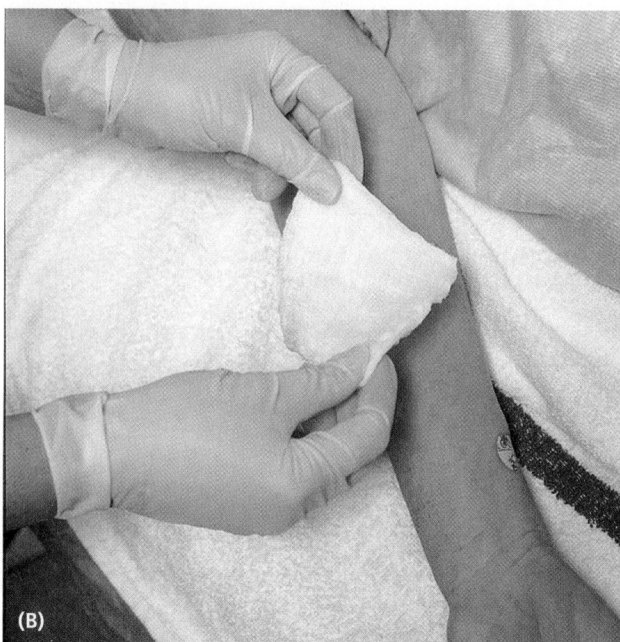
(B)

Figure 33-21 (A) Dip hot compresses frequently into a basin of hot water to keep them warm. (B) Apply compresses directly to the skin.

Paraffin Wax Bath. This type of treatment is most often used for chronic joint disease, such as rheumatoid arthritis. The bath mixture of seven parts paraffin to one part mineral oil is heated to melting (about 127°F) and the body part dipped in the mixture several times until a thick coat of wax builds up. The body part is then wrapped in foil, cloth, or plastic wrap to help insulate the heat, then left on for 30 minutes or less. Once peeled off, the circulatory effects of this treatment can last up to several hours. It is an excellent modality for warming up joints prior to range of motion or other exercises. This modality, ordered by a physician, will be carried out in the physical therapy department by a professional therapist.

Dry Heat Therapies.

Dry heat applications feel dry against the skin and do not penetrate like moist heat. They are used more to improve circulation for the purposes of relieving swelling and healing wounds, as well as to relax muscles and reduce muscle spasms. Most dry heat modalities can also be performed easily by the patient or caregiver at home.

Heating Pads and Packs. Heating pads and commercially prepared packs are used for smaller areas and should always be covered with a cloth prior to applying against the skin. Never let a patient lie directly on a heating pad, as burns can result. Set the switch on the heating pad to a low or medium setting and observe the proper time of exposure.

If you are using a hot water bottle, fill the bottle with water that does not exceed 125°F (52°C) (Figure 33-22) and expel the excess air so the bottle can be more pliable and fit to the contour of the body part being treated. Reduce the water temperature to

between 115°F and 125°F (46° to 52°C) for children over two and 105°F and 115°F (41° to 46°C) for children under two and elderly patients. Make sure the outside of the bottle is dry, and cover it with a cloth before applying it (Figure 33-23). Check the temperature often and refill it periodically to maintain the proper heat level.

An Aquamatic K-Pad® is a commercial pad that is safer to use than a heating pad or hot water bottle because you can maintain a constant temperature and regulate that temperature more carefully. It is a pad with tubes that are filled with distilled water and heated by a control unit (Figure 33-24). The pad must be covered and left on the patient for no more than about 30 minutes.

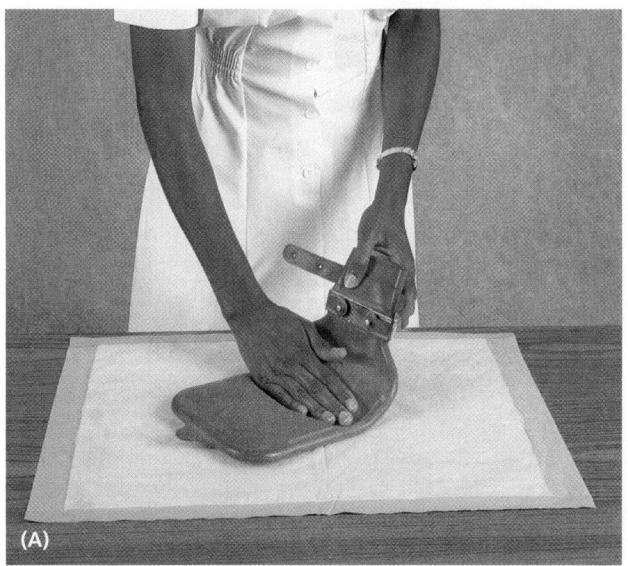

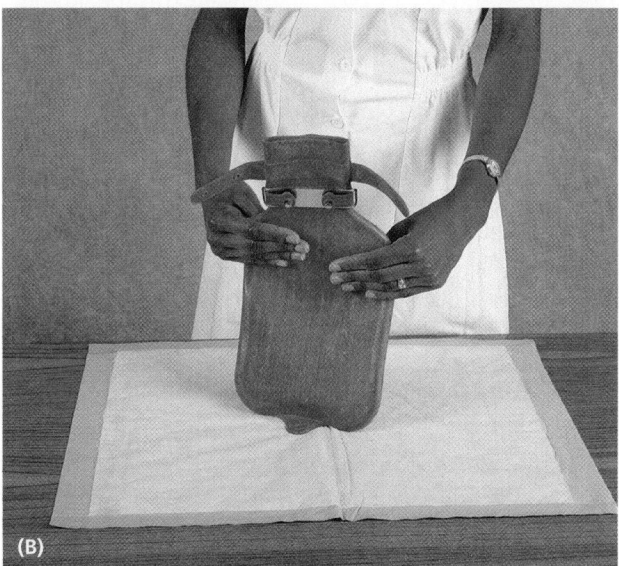

Figure 33-23 (A) Before filling it, expel the air from the hot water bottle by flattening it on the table. (B) After filling, hold the water bottle upright until the water reaches the neck to expel air. Dry the bag, and place in a protective cover.

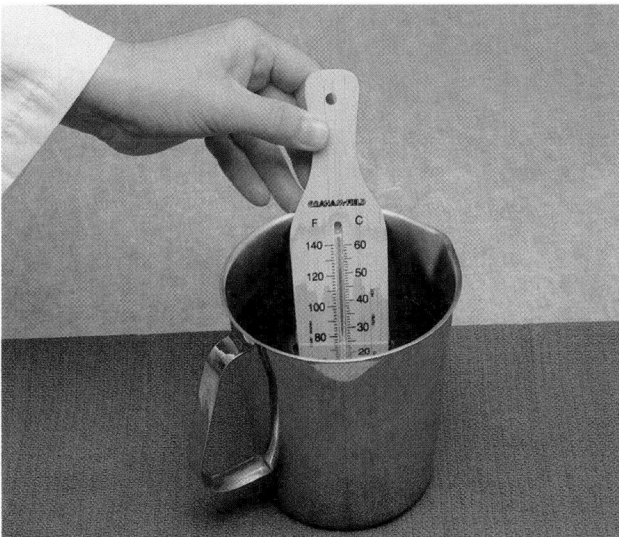

Figure 33-22 When using a water bottle, the water temperature should not exceed 125°F (52°C) or 115°F (46°C) for children under two and elderly patients.

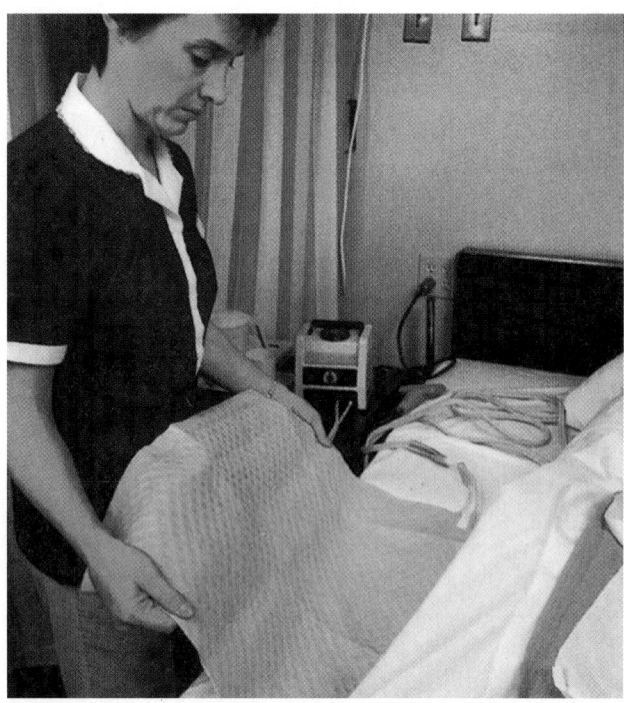

Figure 33-24 Use the Aquamatic K-Pad to maintain a constant temperature of heat.

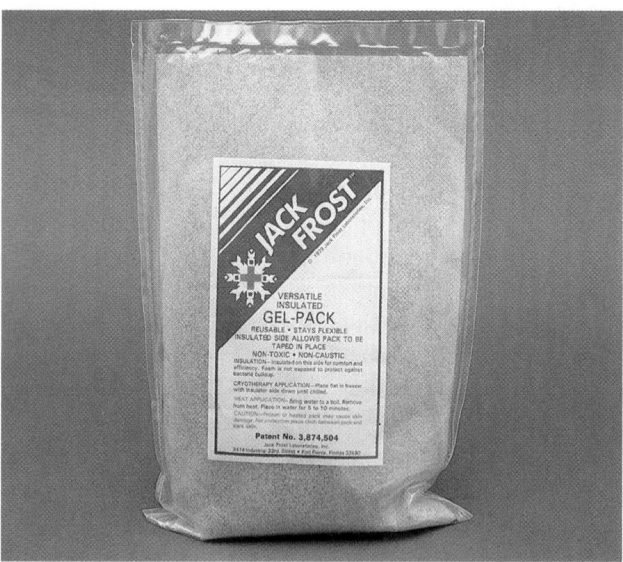

Figure 33-25 A chemical ice pack. These should be covered with a cloth before applying it to the skin.

Moist and Dry Cold Modalities

Moist Cold Therapies. Moist cold therapies refer to cold modalities that feel moist against the skin. Moist cold, as with moist heat, penetrates better than dry cold and is used to prevent swelling or edema, relieve pain or tenderness, and reduce body temperature. Most cold therapies can be performed easily at home by the patient or caregiver.

Cold Compresses and Packs. Cold compresses are used for smaller areas, and cold packs for larger areas. For a cold compress, immerse the cold cloth, gauze, or other clean material in a basin filled with ice and cold water. Wring out the cloth and apply it to the affected area. Keep the cloth cold by immersing it several times throughout the treatment. Cold or ice packs are administered in the same manner.

Dry Cold Therapies. Dry cold treatments are used for all the same reasons as a moist cold treatment, but are better for bleeding and acute injuries. Dry cold is also an excellent therapy for sprains, strains, burns, or bruises.

The temperature used depends on the area being treated and the method used, as well as the patient's tolerance for cold temperatures. In general, the colder the temperature, the shorter the duration of exposure.

Ice Packs. Dry cold treatments include ice packs and commercially prepared chemical ice packs. Always cover the pack with cloth before applying it to the skin (Figure 33-25). Generally, ice packs can be kept on the body longer than heat packs, about 30 minutes. See also Chapter 9. A commercial ice pack can be used for smaller areas and can usually be chilled in the freezer. Since they do not freeze and become solid, these ice packs are pliable, making them ideal for contouring to the body part being treated.

Deep Tissue Modalities

Ultrasound. Ultrasound is a high-frequency acoustic vibration that is part of the electromagnetic spectrum, and its frequencies are beyond the perception of the human ear. This type of treatment uses high-frequency

Patient Teaching Tip

Neither heat nor cold applications should be left on the skin for prolonged periods for both can have counterproductive effects if not monitored carefully. When applying heat or cold, periodically check the skin for signs of paleness or redness. If the patient experiences any tingling reaction, discontinue the application. Report the observations, and document.

sound waves that are converted to heat in the deeper tissues.

Ultrasound is an effective form of treatment for chronic pain or acute injuries such as sprains or strains. It relaxes muscle spasms, increases the elasticity of tissue such as tendons and ligaments, and stimulates circulation, which in turn speeds up the healing process.

 Ultrasound waves travel best in tissue that has a high concentration of water, such as muscles, but they cannot penetrate and move through tissue such as bone that has a low water content. In fact, ultrasound treatment must be used carefully near bones, particularly those near the surface, as their waves are capable of concentrating in one area and causing damage.

Since ultrasound waves cannot be conducted through air, a special gel is applied to the skin surface that acts as a conduit. The sound waves are generated through an applicator that is rubbed over the gel. This applicator must be kept moving to prevent any internal damage caused by too high a concentration of sound waves. The duration of treatment lasts anywhere from 5 to 15 minutes, depending upon the condition being treated and the recommendation of the physician or other health care provider. It is important to note that, because of its potential dangers, ultrasound treatment should only be administered if the medical assistant or other caregiver is specially trained in its safe and effective use.

Procedure 33-1 — Transferring Patient from Wheelchair to Examination Table

STANDARD PRECAUTIONS:

PURPOSE:
To move a patient safely from a wheelchair to the examination table.

EQUIPMENT/SUPPLIES:
Stool with rubber tips and a handle for gripping
Gait belt

PROCEDURE STEPS:
1. Wash hands.
2. Identify the patient and introduce yourself. Explain to the patient what you are going to do.
3. Place the wheelchair next to the examination table and lock the brakes. **CAUTION:** The side nearest the examination table should be the patient's stronger side to allow the patient to balance on that leg during the transfer.
4. Place the gait belt snugly around the patient's waist and tuck the excess end under the belt (Figure 33-26A).
5. Move the footrests up and out of the way. Have the patient place feet on the floor. Newer wheelchairs have removable footrests. Taking them off enables you to put the wheelchair closer to the examination table. There is also less chance of being bumped or bruised by the wheelchair.

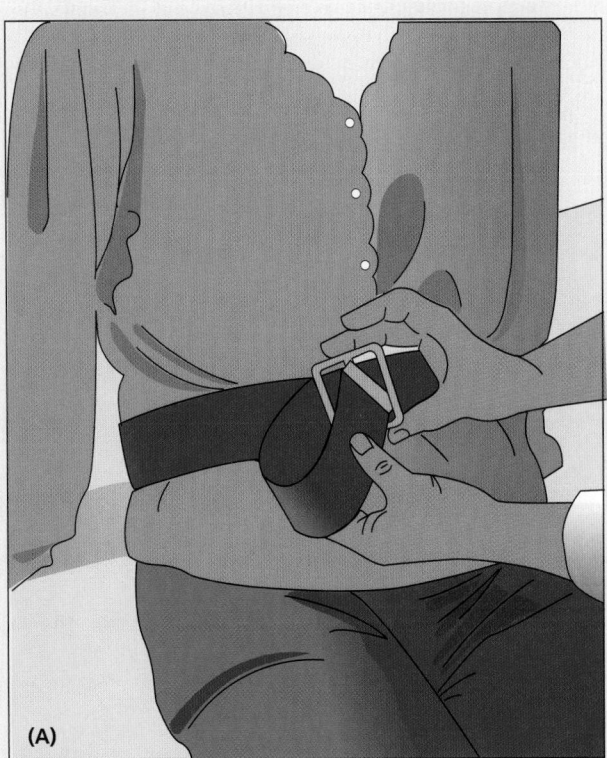

(A)

Figure 33-26 (A) A gait belt is always applied snugly around the patient's waist before attempting to move or ambulate with patients. *(continues)*

Procedure
33-1   *(continued)*

6. Position the stool in front of the examination table as close to the wheelchair as possible (Figure 33-26B).
7. Have the patient move to the edge of the wheelchair.
8. Stand directly in front of the patient with your feet slightly apart. Bending at the hips and knees, grasp the gait belt and have the patient place his hands on the armrests of the wheelchair so he can push up when you give the signal (Figure 33-26C). If the patient doesn't have the upper body strength to push off, simply let his arms rest in front of him.
9. Give a signal and lift the gait belt upward, pushing with your knees. If the patient has the strength in his good leg, he should push up with that leg in addition to pushing up with his arms.
10. Still grasping the gait belt, have the patient step onto the stool with the foot closest to the examination table, and pivot so his back is to the examination table (Figure 33-26D). Make sure the buttocks are lifted slightly higher than the bed. Support the patient's weaker, outer leg with your leg furthest from the examination table.

11. Have the patient grasp the stool handle and place his other hand on the examination table.
12. Gently ease the patient to a sitting position on the examination table.
13. Position the patient on the examination table as necessary.
14. Move the wheelchair and stool out of the way.

Modification: Two-Person Transfer
1. Place the gait belt snugly around the patient's waist and tuck the excess end under the belt.
2. Have one person stand in front of the patient and the other to the side, next to the examination table.
3. Both persons should grasp the gait belt from underneath. Have the patient place his hands on the armrests of the wheelchair.
4. On one person's signal, both persons pull the patient straight up. The patient should also push up with his hands, but if he doesn't have the upper body strength to push off, simply let his arms rest in front of him (Figure 33-27).

(continues)

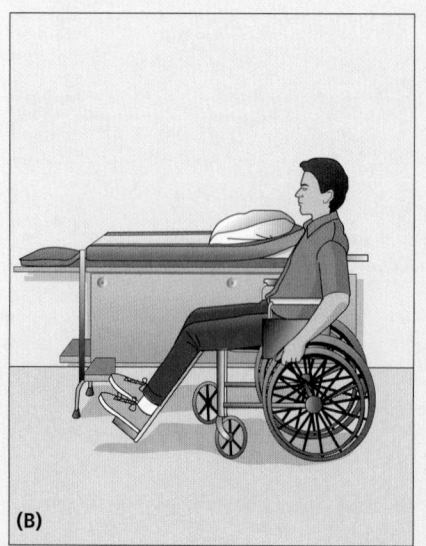
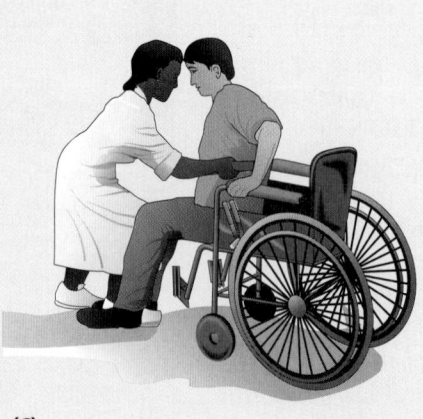
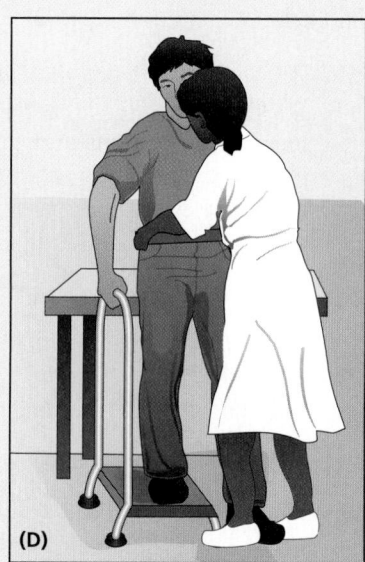

(B)   (C)   (D)

Figure 33-26   *(continued)* (B) Position the stool in front of the examination table and as close to the wheelchair as possible. (C) Before lifting, observe proper body mechanics to avoid injuring yourself or the patient. (D) Check that the patient's foot is firmly placed on the stool before completing the transfer.

Procedure

33-1 *(continued)*

5. The person nearest the examination table moves the wheelchair out of the way, while the other pivots the patient and has the patient place his stronger leg on the stool. If the patient has the upper body strength, he should also grasp the handle of the stool.
6. On one person's signal, both persons lift the patient onto the examination table.
7. Position the patient on the examination table as necessary.

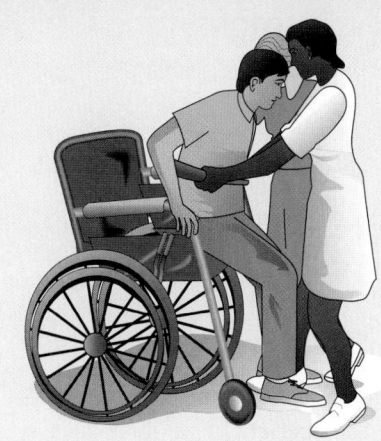

Figure 33-27 A two-person transfer when the patient does not have the upper-body strength to help move himself.

Procedure

33-2 Transferring Patient from Examination Table to Wheelchair

STANDARD PRECAUTIONS:

PURPOSE:
To move a patient safely from the examination table to a wheelchair.

EQUIPMENT/SUPPLIES:
Stool with rubber tips and a handle for gripping
Gait belt

PROCEDURE STEPS:
1. Wash hands.
2. Identify the patient and introduce yourself. Explain to the patient what you are going to do.
3. Position the wheelchair next to the examination table and lock the brakes. NOTE: Place the wheelchair so it is closest to the patient's stronger side so he can transfer his weight onto the stronger foot as he gets down.
4. Position the stool next to the wheelchair.
5. Assist the patient to rise to a sitting position. Place the gait belt snugly around the patient's waist and tuck the excess end under the belt.

6. Place your arm under the patient's arm and around his shoulders, and your other arm under his knees. Pivot the patient so his legs are dangling over the side of the examination table.
7. Keeping a hand on the patient, move so you are directly in front of him.
8. Grasp the patient by placing your hands under the gait belt. Plant your feet shoulder's width apart and bend your knees so you will have a strong base of support.
9. On your signal, pull the patient slightly toward you so his feet come down onto the stool. The patient should push off the examination table and grasp the stool handle for support.
10. Still grasping the gait belt, have the patient step onto the floor with his strong leg, and pivot at the same time so his back is to the wheelchair.
11. Have the patient grasp the armrests of the wheelchair.
12. Bending from your knees and hips, gently lower the patient into the wheelchair and make sure he is comfortably seated.
13. Lower the footrests and place his feet on them.

Procedure 33-3 Assisting the Patient to Stand and Walk

STANDARD PRECAUTIONS:

PURPOSE:
To help a patient ambulate safely.

EQUIPMENT/SUPPLIES:
Gait belt

PROCEDURE STEPS:
1. Wash hands.
2. Identify the patient and introduce yourself. Explain to the patient what you are going to do.
3. Lock the brakes on the wheelchair, if the patient is using one. Place the patient's feet on the floor and move the foot plates out of the way.
4. Instruct the patient to slide forward in the chair.
5. Place the gait belt around the patient's waist and tuck the excess end under the belt.
6. Standing directly in front of the patient, grasp the gait belt from underneath and assist her to stand on your signal. At the same time, have the patient push up on the armrests of the wheelchair.
7. Steady the patient momentarily and watch for balance, strength, and skin color. If necessary, take her pulse.
8. If the patient appears steady and has balance, strength, and good skin color, proceed by standing slightly behind and to the side of the patient's weaker side.
9. Grasp the gait belt with one hand and place the other hand on the patient's bent arm for support. Note the gait belt is grasped with your fingers under the belt, palm up and elbow bent (Figure 33-28).
10. Start with the same foot as the patient and keep in step with her.
11. Document the procedure including date, time, duration of ambulation, response of patient, and instructions given.

Modification: Two-Person Assist with Ambulation
1. Perform the preceding steps 1 through 5.
2. Have a person stand on either side of the patient. Grasp the gait belt from underneath with one hand, and place the other hand on the patient's back for support.
3. During ambulation, there should be a person on either side of the patient and slightly behind (Figure 33-29). Both persons should be grasping the gait belt throughout the ambulation session.
4. Document the procedure including date, time, duration of ambulation, response of patient, and instructions given.

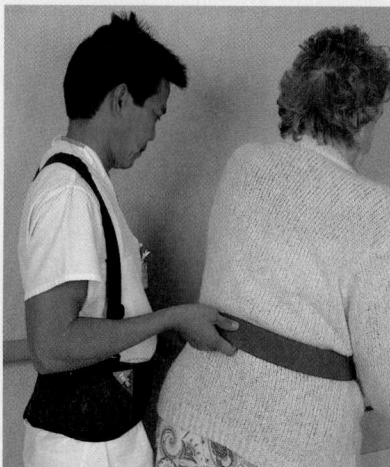

Figure 33-28 Firmly grasp the gait belt from underneath, with the palm up and elbow bent.

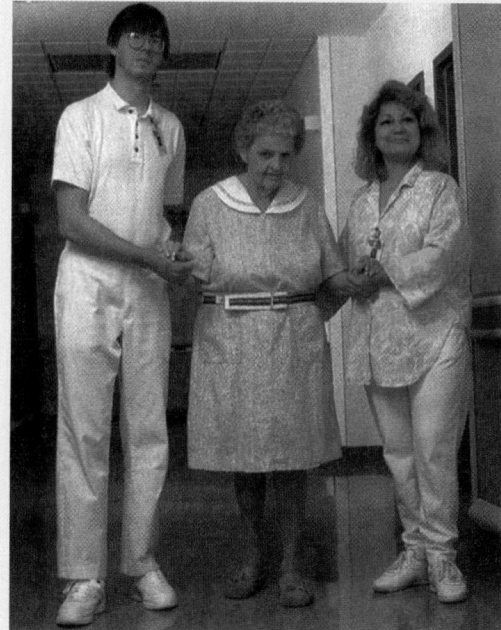

Figure 33-29 When two persons are assisting with ambulation, have them stand on either side of the patient.

33-4 Care of the Falling Patient

PURPOSE:
To help the patient fall safely to avoid injury.

EQUIPMENT/SUPPLIES:
Gait belt (should already be on patient)

PROCEDURE STEPS:

1. Keep a firm hand on the gait belt. **CAUTION:** Never grab clothing, as it can shift and become unstable.

2. If the patient falls backwards, widen your stance to become a more stable base of support for her to fall against (Figure 33-30). Gently guide the patient to the floor, call for assistance, and take her pulse.

3. If the patient falls to either side, steady her back onto her feet. To do this, you will need to move your foot in the direction she is falling. Inquire whether the patient would like to terminate the ambulation session and check for signs of fatigue. If necessary, call for assistance. Check blood pressure and pulse.

4. Should the patient fall forward, support her around the waist. Step forward with your outer leg and gently lower her to the floor, making sure to protect her from injury (Figure 33-31). Call for assistance and take blood pressure and pulse.

5. Have the patient examined by a nurse or doctor prior to moving her again.

6. Document the fall in an incident report.

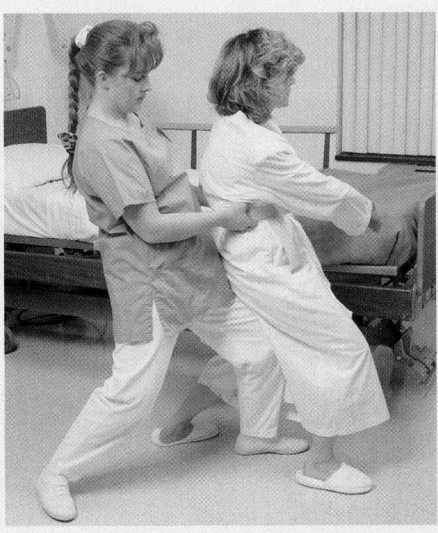

Figure 33-30 Support a falling patient with a wide base of support.

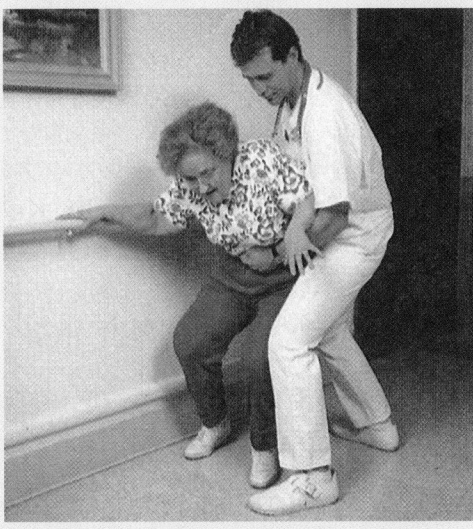

Figure 33-31 Ease the falling patient to the floor, and try to protect the head.

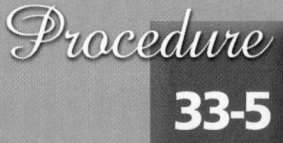

Assisting a Patient to Ambulate with a Walker

33-5

STANDARD PRECAUTIONS:

PURPOSE:
To allow a patient to ambulate independently and safely with a walker.

EQUIPMENT/SUPPLIES:
Walker
Gait belt

PROCEDURE STEPS:

1. Wash hands.
2. Identify the patient and introduce yourself. Explain to the patient what you are going to do.
3. Apply the gait belt snugly around the patient's waist and tuck the excess end under the belt.
4. Check the walker to be sure the rubber suction tips are secure on all the legs. Check the handrests for rough or damaged edges that could cut or pinch the patient. The adjustments should be tightened so they will not slip.
5. Be sure the patient is wearing good walking shoes with a rubber sole.
6. Check the height of the walker. The handrests should be level with the tip of the patient's femur, and the elbows should be flexed at a 30° angle.
7. Position the patient inside the walker, and instruct the patient to hold onto the handles while keeping the walker in front of him.
8. Position yourself behind and slightly to the side of the patient.
9. Have the patient lift the walker and place all four legs of the walker in front of him so the back legs are even with the patient's toes.
10. Instruct the patient to lean forward and transfer his weight so that he steps into the walker, first with his stronger leg, then the weaker leg. Make sure he brings his stronger leg past the weaker leg.
11. Monitor the patient carefully. Be alert for signs of fatigue and be ready to catch him if he should fall.
12. If the walker has rollers, the patient simply rolls the walker ahead a comfortable distance, then walks into it. The patient can also walk normally with a rolling walker by simply rolling it in front and leaning into the gait, using the walker for support.
13. Document the date, time, duration of ambulation, response of patient, and instructions given. Initial the report.

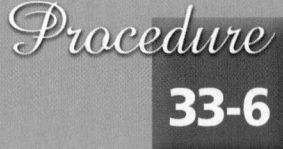

Teaching the Patient to Ambulate with Axillary Crutches

33-6

STANDARD PRECAUTIONS:

PURPOSE:
To teach the patient how to ambulate safely using axillary crutches.

EQUIPMENT/SUPPLIES:
Axillary crutches
Gait belt

PROCEDURE STEPS:

1. Wash hands.
2. Identify the patient and introduce yourself. Explain to the patient what you are going to do.
3. Assemble the axillary crutches and be sure they are in good working order. Make sure there are rubber suction tips on the bottom ends and that they are not worn or torn. Check the axillary bar and handrest to be sure they are covered with padding, and that the padding is not cracked or worn. Be sure the wing nuts are tight.

(continues)

Procedure 33-6 (continued)

4. Check the measurement of the crutches. Pediatric crutches must be used for pediatric patients.
5. Apply the gait belt and assist the patient to stand and place the crutches under the armpits.
6. Instruct the patient to carry his weight completely on his hands and not on his armpits.
7. Have the patient put all his weight on his good leg, and bend the weak leg slightly so it will not drag on the floor as he walks.
8. Assist the patient with the required gait.
9. Wash hands.
10. Document the date, time, duration of ambulation, and instructions given.

Procedure 33-7 Assisting a Patient to Ambulate with a Cane

STANDARD PRECAUTIONS:

PURPOSE:
To teach patients how to walk safely with a cane.

EQUIPMENT/SUPPLIES:
Appropriate cane for patient
Gait belt

PROCEDURE STEPS:
1. Wash hands.
2. Ascertain what type of cane the physician or therapist indicates your patient is to be using and assemble the equipment.
3. Identify the patient and introduce yourself. Explain to the patient what you are going to do.
4. Check the cane to be sure the bottom has a rubber suction tip. If a quad or walkcane is to be used, make sure all the legs have rubber suction tips.
5. Apply the gait belt snugly around the patient's waist if needed and tuck the excess end under the belt. Assist the patient to a standing position.
6. Place the cane relatively close to the body to the side of the foot of the strong leg. Adjust the cane so the handle is at the level of the patient's hip joint (Figure 33-32).
7. During weightbearing, the patient's elbow should be flexed 20° to 30°.
8. The cane and the involved leg are advanced simultaneously.
9. Have the patient move the weak leg forward while transferring the weight to the cane.
10. Have the patient move the strong leg forward past the cane.
11. Follow along behind and to the side of the patient's weak side.
12. Wash your hands.
13. Document the date, time, duration of ambulation, response of patient, and instructions given.

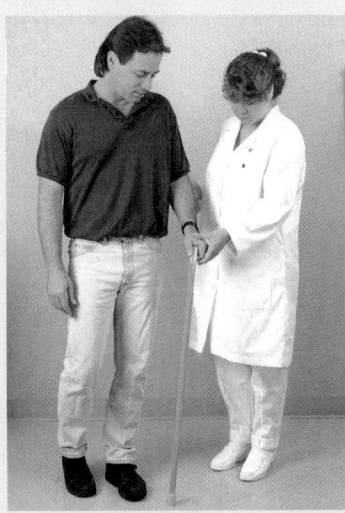

Figure 33-32 In placing the cane, be sure the handle comes to the top of the patient's hip and elbow is flexed 20 to 30°.

Procedure 33-8

Range of Motion Exercises, Upper Body

STANDARD PRECAUTIONS:

PURPOSE:

To maintain or increase joint mobility in the upper extremities and prevent contractures.

EQUIPMENT/SUPPLIES:

None

NOTE: This procedure is best done with the patient in the supine position (see Chapter 25). Repeat each movement several times.

PRE-PROCEDURE STEPS:

1. Wash hands.
2. Identify the patient and introduce yourself. Explain to the patient what you are going to do.

PROCEDURE STEPS:

Shoulder Flexion

1. Keep the patient's arm straight and hold the arm at the wrist and elbow.
2. Lift the patient's arm straight over his head until it rests flat on the bed or table above the patient's head (Figure 33-33).
3. Bend the patient's elbow if there is not enough room on the bed.
4. Bring the arm back to the patient's side.

Shoulder Abduction and Adduction

1. Keep the patient's arm straight by his side, with the palm of his hand facing up. Support the arm at the wrist and elbow.
2. Keeping the patient's arm straight, bring it out at a right angle to his body (Figure 33-34A).
3. Bring the arm back to the patient's side. Keeping the arm straight, bring it across the body (Figure 33-34B).
4. Return the patient's arm to a position parallel to the body. *(continues)*

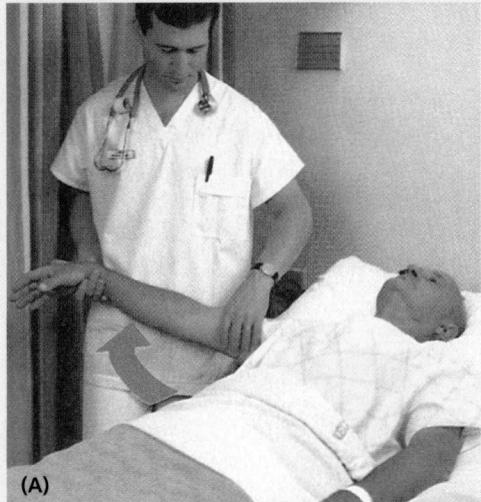

(A)

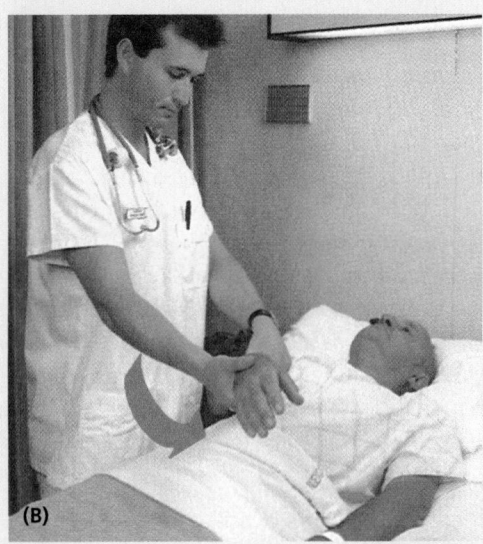

(B)

Figure 33-34 (A) Shoulder abduction. (B) Shoulder adduction.

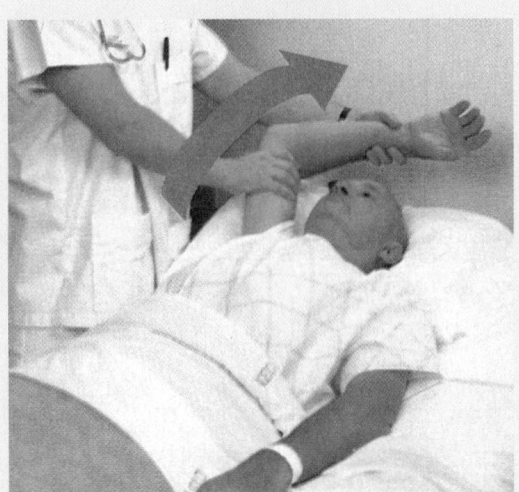

Figure 33-33 Shoulder flexion.

Procedure
33-8 (*continued*)

Internal and External Shoulder Rotation

1. Bring the arm out at a right angle from the body.
2. Bend the elbow at a right angle, keeping the upper arm on the bed.
3. Keeping the patient's arm at a right angle, gently press down on the shoulder with one hand while holding the patient's wrist with the other.
4. Move the hand gently back until it touches the bed next to the patient's head.
5. Bring the hand back down until the palm of the patient's hand touches the bed.

Elbow Flexion and Extension

1. With the patient's arm by his side and his palm up, flex and extend the elbow (Figure 33-35).

Wrist Extension and Flexion

1. Support the patient's arm above the wrist.

2. Holding the palm of the patient's hand, extend the wrist, then straighten it (Figure 33-36A).
3. Place your hand over the patient's hand while still supporting the wrist. Bend or flex the hand (Figure 33-36B).

Wrist Inversion and Eversion

1. Grasp the patient's wrist with one hand and grasp his hand with the other.
2. Slowly bend the patient's hand toward his body, then away from his body (Figure 33-37).

Wrist Supination and Pronation

1. Grasp the patient's wrist with one hand and his hand with the other.
2. Slowly turn the patient's hand toward his feet, then toward his face.   (*continues*)

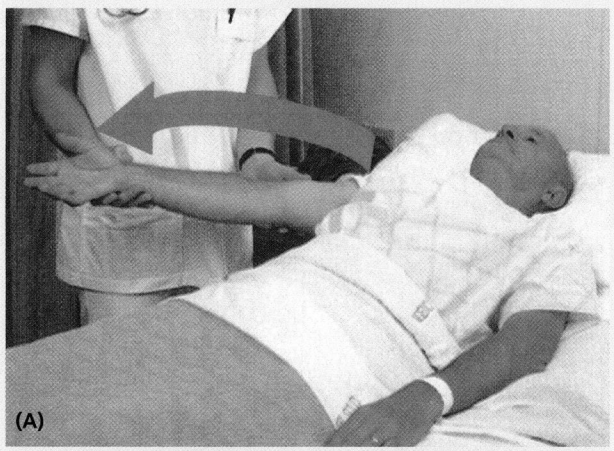

(A)

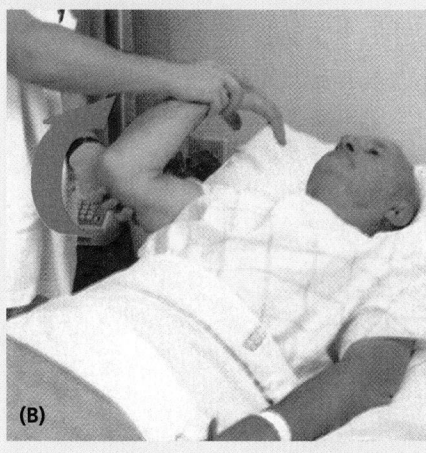

(B)

Figure 33-35   (A) Elbow extension. (B) Elbow flexion.

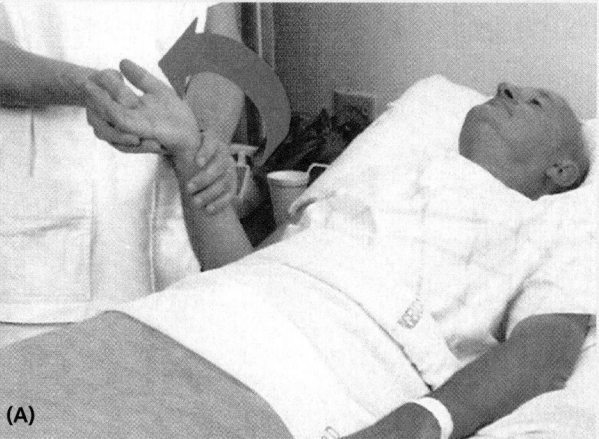

(A)

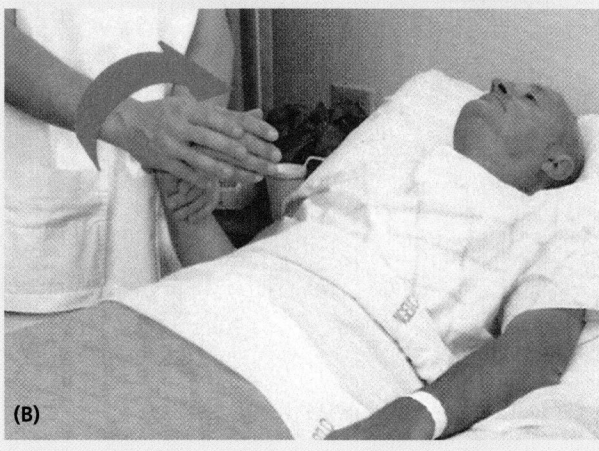

(B)

Figure 33-36   (A) Wrist extension. (B) Wrist flexion.

Procedure **33-8** *(continued)*

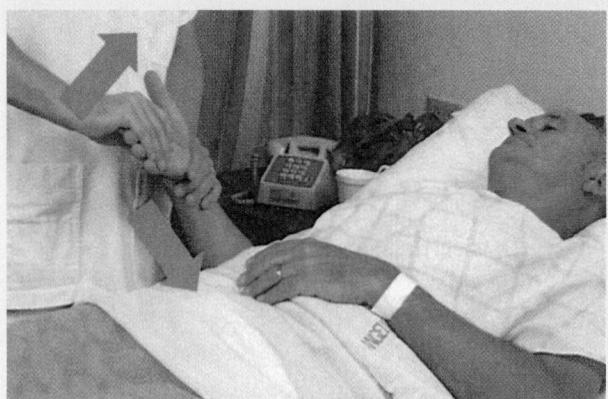

Figure 33-37   Wrist inversion and eversion.

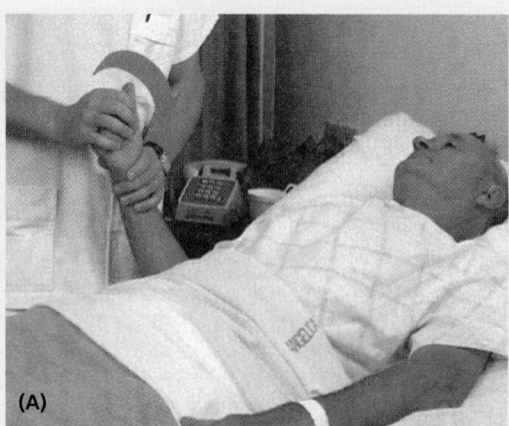

(A)

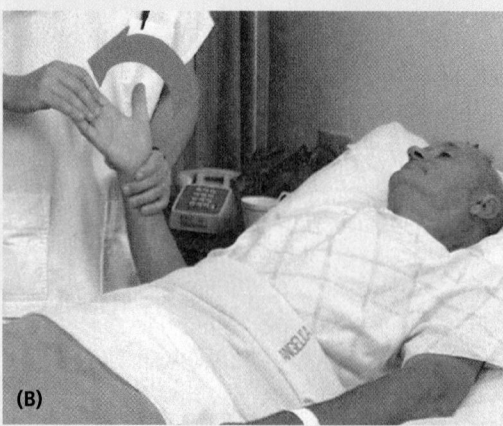

(B)

Figure 33-38   (A) Finger flexion. (B) Finger extension.

Finger Flexion and Extension
1. Support the patient's wrist with one hand. Cover his finger with the other hand and curl them over to make a fist (Figure 33-38A).
2. Uncurl the patient's fingers and straighten them (Figure 33-38B).

Finger and Thumb Abduction and Adduction
1. Hold the patient's hand flat. Slowly pull each finger away from the thumb (Figure 33-39A), then pull it back straight (Figure 33-39B).
2. Pull the thumb away from the rest of the fingers, then pull it back straight (Figure 33-40).

Thumb Opposition
1. Support the patient's hand.
2. Touch each finger with the thumb (Figure 33-41).

POST-PROCEDURE STEPS:
1. Wash hands.
2. Document the date, time, limbs given ROM, and response of patient. Initial the report.

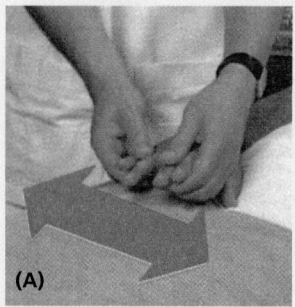
(A)

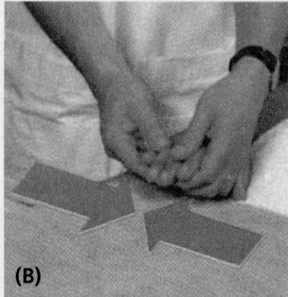
(B)

Figure 33-39   (A) Finger abduction. (B) Finger adduction.

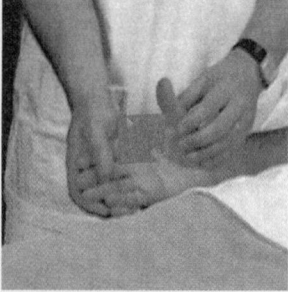

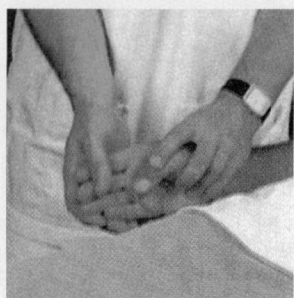

Figure 33-40   Abduction and adduction of the thumb and fingers.

Figure 33-41   Thumb opposition.

Procedure 33-9 Range of Motion Exercises, Lower Body

STANDARD PRECAUTIONS:

PURPOSE:
To maintain or increase joint mobility in the lower extremities and prevent contractures.

EQUIPMENT/SUPPLIES:
None
NOTE: This procedure is best done with the patient in the supine position. Repeat each movement several times.

PRE-PROCEDURE STEPS:
1. Wash hands.
2. Identify the patient and introduce yourself. Explain to the patient what you are going to do.

PROCEDURE STEPS:

Hip Abduction and Adduction
1. Support the patient's knee and ankle.
2. Keeping the patient's leg straight, move the entire leg away from the body (Figure 33-42A).

3. Move the patient's leg back, toward the midline of the body (Figure 33-42B).

Hip and Knee Flexion and Extension
1. Support the patient's knee and ankle.
2. Bend the patient's knee and raise it as far toward the patient's chest as his tolerance and comfort will allow (Figure 33-43A).
3. Lower and straighten the patient's leg (Figure 33-43B).

Hip Rotation
1. Support the patient's leg at the knee and ankle.
2. Roll the patient's leg in a circular motion, away from the body.
3. Roll the patient's leg in a circular motion, toward the body.

Ankle Dorsiflexion and Plantar Flexion
1. Keep the patient's leg flat on the bed. NOTE: It may be more comfortable if the patient's knee is slightly bent. Grasp his ankle with one hand and the heel of his foot with the other.

(continues)

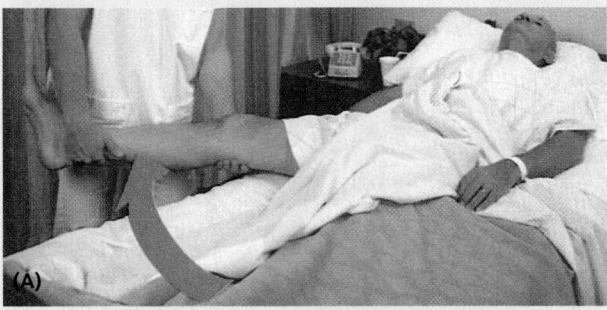

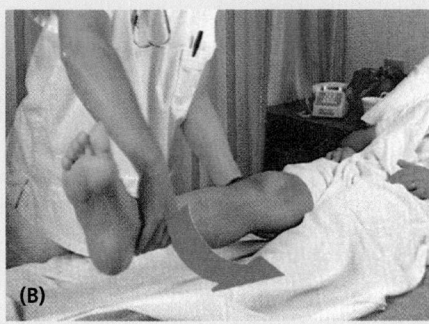

Figure 33-42   (A) Hip abduction. (B) Hip adduction.

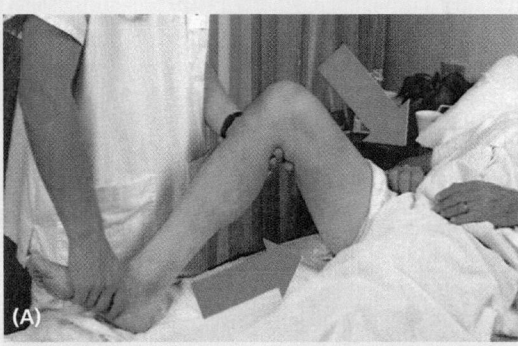

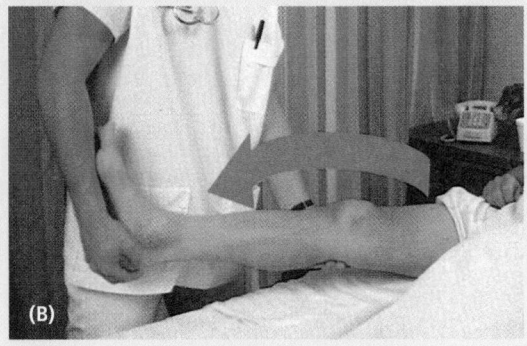

Figure 33-43   (A) Hip and knee flexion. (B) Knee extension.

Procedure

33-9   (continued)

2. With the hand holding the patient's heel, flex the patient's foot and rest the bottom of his foot against your forearm. Keep your elbow straight (Figure 33-44A).
3. Dorsiflex the ankle by pushing the foot toward the patient's knee with your arm.
4. Return the foot to its flexed position against your forearm.
5. Keeping your one hand on the patient's ankle, plantar flex the ankle by drawing the foot down toward the foot of the bed (Figure 33-44B).

Foot Inversion and Eversion
1. Grasp the patient's ankle with one hand and the arch of his foot with the other.
2. Gently turn the patient's foot inward (Figure 33-45A).
3. Return the patient's foot to the midline, then gently turn it outward (Figure 33-45B).

TOE FLEXION AND EXTENSION
1. Hold the patient's ankle in one hand and place your fingers over the patient's toes with the other hand.
2. Bend the toes, then straighten them.

TOE ABDUCTION AND ADDUCTION
1. Move each toe one at a time away from the second toe (Figure 33-46A).
2. Move each toe one at a time toward the second toe (Figure 33-46B).

POST-PROCEDURE STEP:
1. Wash hands.
2. Document the date, time, limbs given ROM, and response of patient. Initial the report.

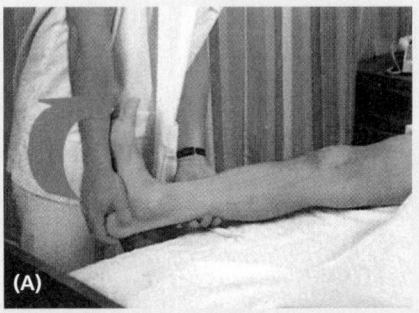
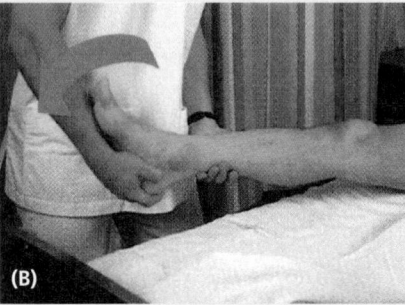

Figure 33-44   (A) Ankle dorsiflexion. (B) Plantar flexion.

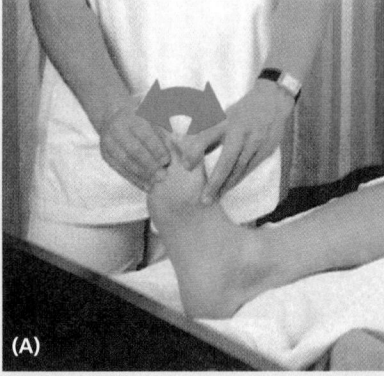

(A)

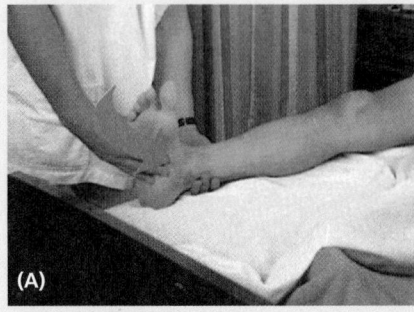
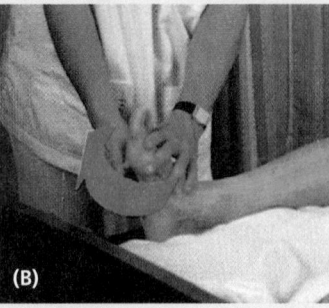

Figure 33-45   (A) Foot inversion. (B) Foot eversion.

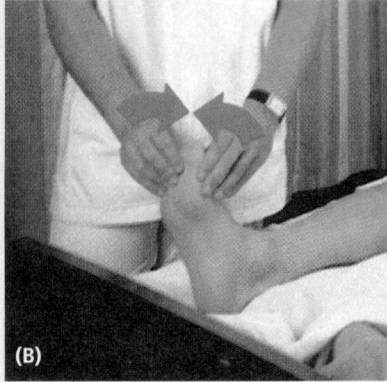

(B)

Figure 33-46   (A) Toe abduction. (B) Toe adduction.

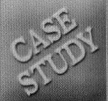

33-1

It is a mild summer afternoon in the city of Carlton, the home of Inner City Health Care. The softball season is in full swing, and Inner City has treated its share of players and spectators who have suffered minor injuries. On this particular Tuesday, Bill Schwarz, a regular patient, comes in late in the day in obvious pain. Bruce Goldman, the clinical medical assistant on duty, quickly gets the patient into a wheelchair. From the patient's description of the situation and the pain, Bruce suspects a sprained ankle. Dr. Woo is on call and available to examine the patient immediately and asks Bruce to transfer Bill from the wheelchair to the examination table.

CASE STUDY REVIEW

1. What are some of the general principles the medical assistant should observe during any transfer?
2. Summarize the steps involved in transferring the patient from the wheelchair to the examination table.
3. Summarize the steps involved in transferring the patient from the examination table to the wheelchair.

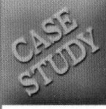

33-2

After diagnosing Mr. Schwarz with a sprained left ankle, Dr. Woo has prescribed an ace bandage to the ankle, crutches, and an ice pack to be applied to the ankle. He has also given Mr. Schwarz a prescription for pain relievers and has recommended that Mr. Schwarz stay off his feet as much as possible. He is to keep the leg elevated with an ice pack on it.

CASE STUDY REVIEW

1. Explain what you would tell Mr. Schwarz about applying the ice pack to his ankle at home.

SUMMARY

Rehabilitation medicine is a field of medical disciplines that specializes in both preventing disease or injury and restoring physical function. It uses a combination of physical and mechanical agents to aid in the diagnosis, treatment, and prevention of diseases or bodily injury, including exercise and a variety of treatment modalities.

Much of what a medical assistant might do on the job in this field involves some form of lifting or moving of heavy objects. It is important to remember to use good body mechanics in order to prevent back or other injury. When transferring patients, good body mechanics ensures the safety of both caregiver and patient. If necessary, get someone to help with the transfer.

Helping the patient to ambulate safely following a period of sedentary recuperation is an important part of a rehabilitation program. If they are not able to ambulate on their own, patients can be fitted for a variety of assistive walking devices, including walkers, crutches, and canes. Crutch walking, by far the most common use of an assistive device, can be done using one of several walking patterns, or gaits, depending

upon the patient's condition, strength, and stability. Whatever assistive device is used, it is important that the patient be measured correctly for that device and taught how to periodically check it for safety.

In addition to ambulation, there are a number of other types of therapeutic exercises. Depending upon the patient's condition, an exercise program can be prescribed after evaluating the patient's joint range of motion and muscle strength. Joints and muscles must be exercised regularly in order to avoid muscle atrophy or joint contractures, as well as improve circulation and maintain or improve overall health. Range of motion and other exercises can be performed either by the caregiver, the patient, or a combination of the two.

In addition to exercise, a variety of therapeutic modalities might also be used as part of the patient's rehabilitation program. The various properties of heat, cold, light, electricity, and water act on the body to improve circulation, minimize pain, or correct or alleviate joint and muscle malfunction. Heat dilates the blood vessels, thereby increasing circulation to an area and speeding up the repair process. Cold constricts the blood vessels, slowing circulation and therefore the inflammatory process. Ultrasound and other electrical diathermies use an electrical current to create heat in the deeper tissues of the body. It is important to understand how each modality affects the physiological functioning of the body and observe certain safety precautions to avoid injuring the patient.

REVIEW QUESTIONS

Multiple Choice

1. Brushing teeth, getting dressed, and eating are referred to as:
   a. rehabilitation medicine
   b. activities of daily living (ADL)
   c. body mechanics
   d. occupational therapy
2. Hemiplegia is defined as:
   a. inability of the patient to ambulate properly
   b. severe back pain
   c. paralysis of one side of the body
   d. confinement to a wheelchair
3. Ambulatory assistive devices include:
   a. gait belts
   b. walkers, canes, and crutches
   c. wheelchairs
   d. stools with handholds
4. Motion away from the midline of the body is called:
   a. adduction
   b. pronation
   c. extension
   d. abduction
5. Supination involves:
   a. placing the patient in the supine position
   b. moving the arm so the palm is up
   c. bending a body part
   d. straightening a body part

Critical Thinking

1. Define rehabilitation, and explain its importance in patient care.
2. If a patient should fall to the side, what action would you take to ensure safety?
3. Describe the procedure for measuring for axillary crutches.
4. What kind of patient would need a forearm crutch?
5. In crutch-walking gaits, what is a *point*?
6. Describe the five different types of crutch gaits.
7. List the six safety rules for transporting a patient in a wheelchair.
8. What is joint range of motion, how is it measured, and how is the measurement expressed?
9. How do heat and cold affect the body's physiology and for what conditions should each be used?
10. Describe how ultrasound works and identify the patient conditions for which it is an effective treatment.

WEB ACTIVITIES

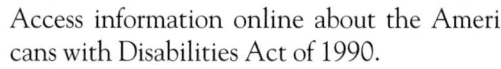

Access information online about the Americans with Disabilities Act of 1990.

1. To what group of people does the act apply?
2. What does the act provide for these individuals?
3. Does the act have any influence over access to physicians' offices and clinics? Explain.

REFERENCES/BIBLIOGRAPHY

Bonewit-West, K. (2000). *Clinical procedures for medical assistants* (5th ed.). Philadelphia: W. B. Saunders Company.

Frey, R., & Shearer Cooper, L. (1996). *Introduction to nursing assisting: Building language skills.* Albany, NY: Delmar.

Hegner, B., & Caldwell, E. (1999). *Nursing assistant: A nursing process approach* (8th ed.). Albany, NY: Delmar.

Keir, L., Wise, B. A., & Krebs, C. (1998). *Medical assisting: Administrative and clinical competencies* (4th ed.). Albany, NY: Delmar.

Medical assisting video series: Administrative and clinical procedures. (1997). Albany, NY: Delmar.

Norkin, C. C., & White, D. J. (1995). *Measurement of joint motion: A guide to goniometry* (2nd ed.). Philadelphia: F. A. Davis Company.

O'Sullivan, S. B., & Schmitz, T. (2000). *Physical rehabilitation: Assessment and treatment* (4th ed.). Philadelphia: F. A. Davis Co.

Simmers, L. (1998). *Diversified health occupations* (3rd ed.). Albany, NY: Delmar.

Taber's cyclopedic medical dictionary. (18th ed.). (1999). Philadelphia: F. A. Davis Company.

Weiss, R. C. (1999). *The physical therapy aide: A work text.* Albany, NY: Delmar.

Zakus, S. (1995). *Clinical procedures for medical assistants* (3rd ed.). St. Louis, MO: Mosby-Year Book, Inc.

Chapter 34

NUTRITION IN HEALTH AND DISEASE

KEY TERMS

Amino Acid
Antioxidant
Ascorbic Acid
Basal Metabolic Rate
Calorie
Carotene
Catalyst
Cellulose
Cholecalciferol
Cobalamin
Coenzyme
Digestion
Diuretic
Electrolytes
Extracellular
Fat-Soluble
Folic Acid
Glycogen
Homeostasis
Kwashiorkor
Major Mineral
Marasmus
Metabolism
Niacin
Nutrient
Nutrition
Oxidation
Preservative
Processed Food
Pyridoxine
Riboflavin
Saturated Fat
Thiamin
Tocopherol
Trace Mineral
Water-Soluble

OUTLINE

Nutrition and Digestion
Types of Nutrients
　Energy Nutrients
　Other Nutrients
Reading Food Labels
　Items on the Nutrition Label
　Comparing Labels
Nutrition at Various Stages of Life
　Pregnancy and Lactation
　Infancy
　Adolescence
　Elderly

Therapeutic Diets
　Weight Control
　Diabetes Mellitus
　Cardiovascular Disease
　Cancer
Diet and Culture

OBJECTIVES

The student should strive to meet the following performance objectives and demonstrate an understanding of the facts and principles presented in this chapter through written and oral communication.

1. Define the key terms as presented in the glossary.
2. Describe the relationship of nutrition to the functioning of the digestive system.
3. Identify the seven basic nutrient types.
4. Explain the relationship and balance between the three energy nutrients.
5. Distinguish between water-soluble and fat-soluble vitamins.
6. Explain the reason for nutrition labels on food packaging.
7. Read and interpret nutrition facts and ingredients on three food packages.
8. Discuss various therapeutic diets, and explain how each can help to control a particular disease state or accommodate a change in the life cycle.

**GENERAL
(TRANSDISCIPLINARY)**

Instruction

- **Instruct individuals according to their needs**
- **Teach methods of health promotion and disease prevention**
- **Locate community resources and disseminate information**

This morning at Inner City Health Care, clinical medical assistant Wanda Slawson, CMA, was conferring with Dr. Rice on three of the center's patients whose diets needed modification. With the help of Dr. Rice, Wanda was putting together dietary changes for patient Edith Leonard, who is in her early seventies and losing weight because she is not eating well enough or often enough; Corey Boyer, in the prime of adolescence and capable of eating large quantities of food with little nutritional value; and Annette Samuels, who recently discovered she was pregnant. All these patients have different nutritional requirements, and Wanda wants to encourage all to review and modify their diets.

INTRODUCTION

The human body is in a constant state of fluctuation. The outside environment is constantly changing, and the body requires **homeostasis**, or a continual internal environment, which, in turn, gives us a requirement for nutrients. The nutrients we take into our bodies replenish the materials we have used. In this way, homeostasis is maintained and our bodies have a relatively balanced internal environment. **Nutrition** is the study of the taking of nutrients into the body and how the body uses them.

The normal healthy individual will consume and use close to what the body needs in order to stay healthy. However, some individuals either do not consume enough nutrients or consume too much of a particular type of nutrient. These are poor diets that can cause particular disease states and the diet must be modified to return the patient to good health. In addition, specific disease states, such as diabetes mellitus, warrant a change from a normal diet in order to control the progress of the disease. The human body also goes through many changes in a lifetime and with these changes come new nutritional needs.

This chapter explores the balance of nutrients required for good health and examines therapeutic modifications to the diet that should take place at various life stages or in the presence of disease. The astute medical assistant will recognize the role of nutrition in maintaining health and use a knowledge of nutritional principles to encourage patients to adopt a healthy lifestyle.

NUTRITION AND DIGESTION

Nutrition includes ingestion, digestion, absorption, and metabolism of food. It is known that good nutrition has resulted in longer life spans and healthier individuals through the control of preventable diseases. The food eaten by an individual is used to build and repair cells and tissues of the body. Therefore, it is important to have knowledge and information about nutrition and to make appropriate food choices for optimum health. The well-nourished individual is less susceptible to infection and disease.

Patient education is important especially when the normal diet must be modified to treat the patient's illness. The medical assistant can answer questions only through a knowledge of good nutrition and what constitutes the therapeutic diets prescribed by the physician.

Digestion involves the physical and chemical changes that the body makes to food to make it absorbable. Absorption is the transfer of the nutrients from the gastrointestinal tract into the blood stream. Without absorption, the body would not receive the nutrients. Figure 34-1 shows the digestive system and its basic functions.

TYPES OF NUTRIENTS

Nutrients serve many purposes in the body. Some nutrients can provide energy in order for the body to perform activities such as the pumping of the heart, the division of cells, or the contraction of muscles. Nutrients also provide building blocks so that proteins or phospholipids can be made within the body or they can act as catalysts to help processes such as the clotting mechanism proceed at a

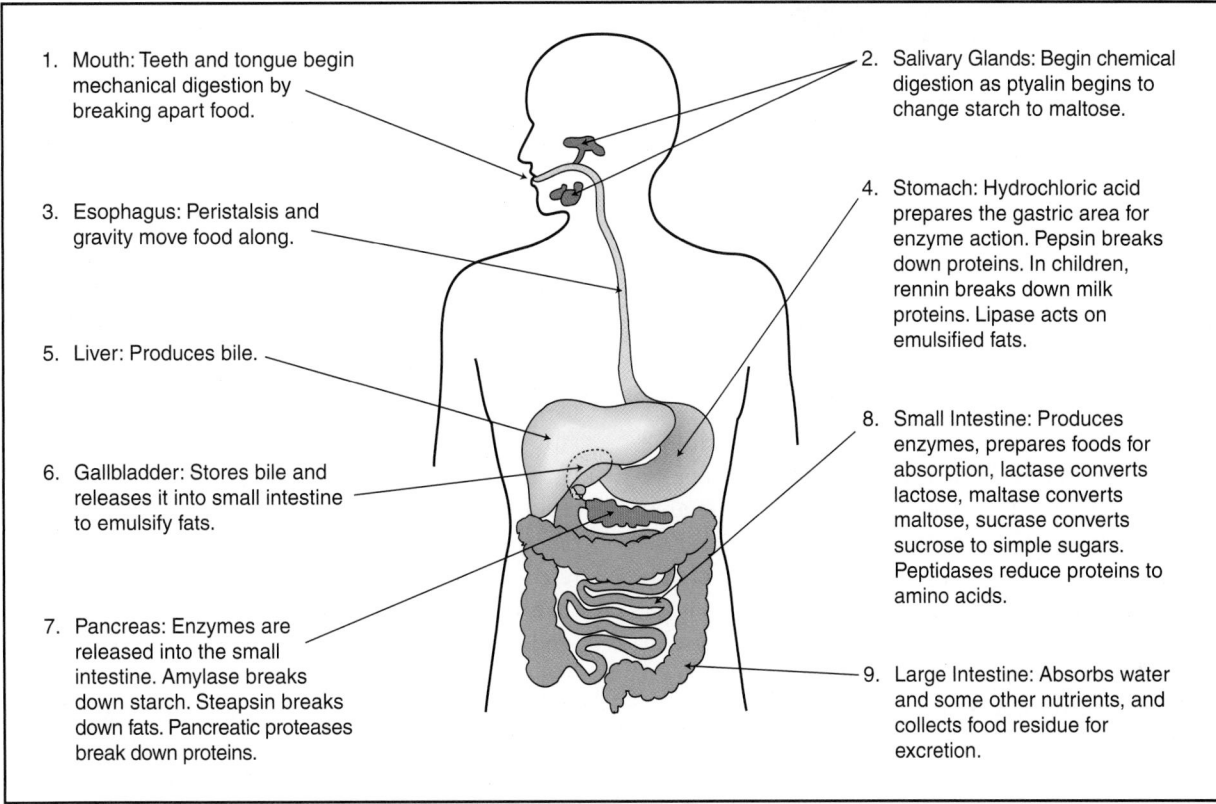

1. Mouth: Teeth and tongue begin mechanical digestion by breaking apart food.

2. Salivary Glands: Begin chemical digestion as ptyalin begins to change starch to maltose.

3. Esophagus: Peristalsis and gravity move food along.

4. Stomach: Hydrochloric acid prepares the gastric area for enzyme action. Pepsin breaks down proteins. In children, rennin breaks down milk proteins. Lipase acts on emulsified fats.

5. Liver: Produces bile.

6. Gallbladder: Stores bile and releases it into small intestine to emulsify fats.

8. Small Intestine: Produces enzymes, prepares foods for absorption, lactase converts lactose, maltase converts maltose, sucrase converts sucrose to simple sugars. Peptidases reduce proteins to amino acids.

7. Pancreas: Enzymes are released into the small intestine. Amylase breaks down starch. Steapsin breaks down fats. Pancreatic proteases break down proteins.

9. Large Intestine: Absorbs water and some other nutrients, and collects food residue for excretion.

Figure 34-1 The digestive system.

faster rate. Essentially, ingested substances that help the body stay in its homeostatic state can be called **nutrients**.

Nutrients can be divided into two groups: those that provide energy and those that do not. Table 34-1 shows examples of each of these two groups. Those that provide energy are comprised of three types: carbohydrates, fats (lipids), and proteins. Each of these three substances is used in ways other than making energy, but it is important to remember that these are the only substances from which the body can derive energy. Nutrients that do not provide energy are also important and perform other vital functions as described previously. These nutrients include vitamins, minerals, water, and fiber.

TABLE 34-1	TYPES OF NUTRIENTS

Nutrients are divided into two groups: those that provide energy and those that do not. Both groups are essential to good health

Energy Nutrients	Other Nutrients
Carbohydrates	Vitamins
Lipids (Fats)	Minerals
Proteins	Water
	Fiber

Energy Nutrients

The three energy nutrients, carbohydrates, fats, and proteins, have one thing in common: all can be converted into energy.

Carbohydrates. Carbohydrates are made up of carbon, hydrogen, and oxygen. Although many compounds are made up of these three elements, it is the ratio of these elements that is important. Carbohydrates are made up of units called sugars. The scientific term for sugar is saccharide, and carbohydrates can exist as monosaccharides, disaccharides, or polysaccharides.

A monosaccharide is composed of a single unit of sugar while disaccharides have two units of sugar. Together, monosaccharides and disaccharides are known as simple sugars. Examples of monosaccharides are glucose, fructose, and galactose. Glucose is the sugar that the body uses most efficiently, so most ingested sugar is broken down in the intestines and converted to glucose in the liver. Fructose is found largely in fruits, while galactose is a product of lactose digestion. Examples of disaccharides are lactose, maltose, and sucrose. Lactose is found primarily in milk or milk products. Maltose is a product of starch breakdown. Sucrose is one of the sweetest sugars and is what we commonly refer to as table sugar. It occurs naturally in many fruits and vegetables as well as sugar cane and the sugar beet, which are commercial sources of refined sugar.

Polysaccharides are also known as complex carbohydrates. They are made up of many units of sugar connected together. The most common polysaccharides are starches, glycogen, and fiber. Starches are the most important dietary complex carbohydrate. **Glycogen** is only ingested in small quantities, but is an important carbohydrate form for storage of glucose in the body. Fiber is a special polysaccharide because it cannot be digested.

Because the simple sugars are composed of only one or two units of sugar, their digestion takes little time and absorption occurs soon after ingestion. The body initially experiences a large increase in sugar concentration in the blood which is brought down to within a normal range by the release of insulin. The complex carbohydrates require more time to digest, and as a result there is a slow absorption of the single carbohydrate units as the larger starch molecule is broken down. This is demonstrated in Figure 34-2. In this case, there would be a moderate increase in the sugar levels in the blood and this would continue for a longer period of time. A continuous level of sugar in the bloodstream is necessary for a constant energy supply.

Fats. Fats, also called lipids, are also composed of carbon, hydrogen, and oxygen, but in a ratio different from carbo-

hydrates. They exist as triglycerides in the body. A triglyceride has three fatty acids attached to a glycerol molecule (Figure 34-3). The fatty acid component of a triglyceride has several important characteristics. The first is whether or not it is essential to the diet. The only true essential fatty acid in the human diet is linoleic acid, and all other fatty acids the body requires can be derived from this. Another important characteristic of fatty acids is saturation. When a fatty acid is saturated, every carbon molecule on the fatty acid holds as many hydrogens as possible. If it does not hold all the hydrogens possible, it is called unsaturated. The more unsaturated the fatty acid, the more liquid the fat. For example, lard has very saturated fatty acids and a thick consistency compared to corn oil, which has relatively unsaturated fatty acids and a thin consistency. If an **unsaturated fat** is hydrogenated, combined with hydrogen, it becomes more saturated. Saturated fats are more common in foods from animal sources than from plant sources. Generally, saturated fatty acids tend to raise the level of fats and cholesterol in the blood.

Proteins. While protein is also composed of carbon, hydrogen, and oxygen, it contains one more important element: nitrogen. The basic structural unit of protein is the **amino acid**. There are twenty-two amino acids in proteins. Eight of these are needed in the diet in order for the body to function normally. One more, histidine, is essential only during childhood. The rest of the amino acids can be synthesized from the eight, provided that they are present in adequate quantities. A complete protein is so named because it has all eight of the essential amino acids. An incomplete protein does not contain all of these. The best sources for complete proteins are meats and animal products such as milk and eggs. Most plants

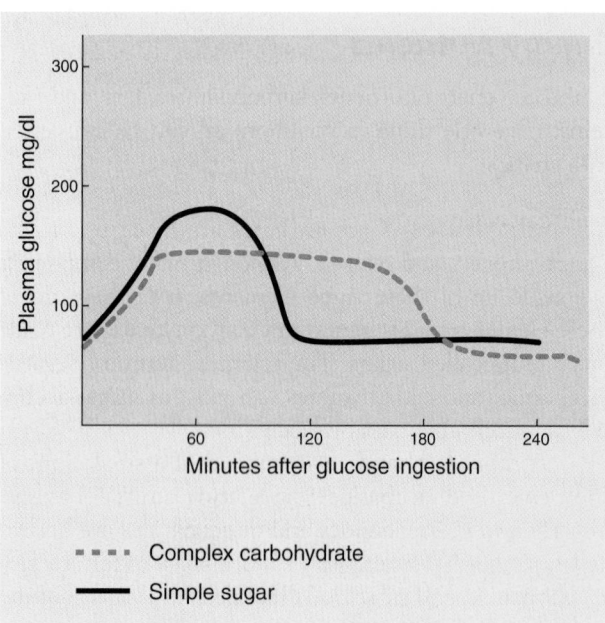

Figure 34-2 This graph shows how complex carbohydrates (red broken line) and simple sugar (black line) are used by the body (in minutes) after glucose ingestion. Simple sugar peaks to approximately 120–160 mg/dl in 60 minutes and returns to a normal level with 120 minutes. Complex carbohydrates (red broken line) never rise above approximately 130–140 mg/dl during a 60-minute period; that level is maintained for the next 120 minutes and then returns to normal.

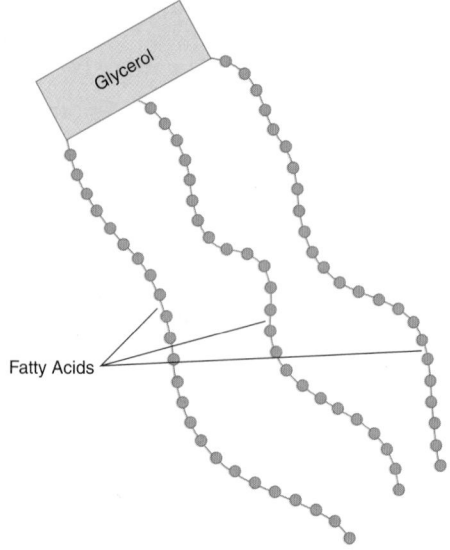

Figure 34-3 A triglyceride has three fatty acids attached to a glycerol molecule.

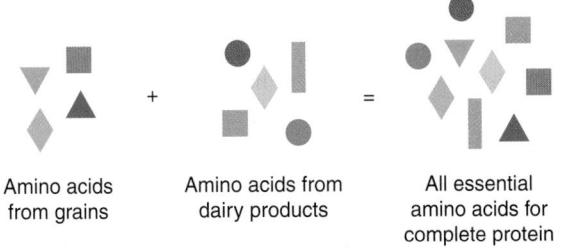

Amino acids from grains + Amino acids from dairy products = All essential amino acids for complete protein

Figure 34-4 Some foods, such as grains and dairy products, may not have all the essential amino acids when considered separately. Combined, however, these form a complete protein and therefore are considered complementary.

provide only incomplete proteins and must be combined with complementary incomplete proteins to obtain all eight amino acids (Figure 34-4).

Although protein is described as an energy nutrient, its main function is not to provide energy but to provide amino acids to be used as building components of body proteins, which can be used as enzymes, hormones, and as the basic structural unit in all body tissues and cells. The body uses carbohydrates and fats as its primary energy sources; however, when these are in short supply, the body diverts its use of protein for structural purposes to use it as an energy source. This has detrimental effects on the body.

Deficiencies in protein usually occur along with deficiencies in total Calories. The disease associated with these deficiencies is called protein-energy malnutrition (PEM). Another disease, **marasmus**, also includes deficiencies in minerals and vitamins but is often used interchangeably with PEM. The symptoms of marasmus include severe wasting, wrinkling of the skin, and growth failure. Another disease, **kwashiorkor**, was originally thought to be the result solely of protein deficiency, but now its cause is debated. The symptoms of kwashiorkor include edema, irritability, and growth failure. Both occur in infants and young children.

Energy Balance. While all of the energy nutrients are capable of supplying energy to the body, they do so in different ways and in varying amounts. The amount of energy that a substance is able to supply can be measured in large **Calories**. Nutrition is discussed in terms of the large Calorie, which is always capitalized to distinguish it from the small calorie. The large Calorie (abbreviation: C or Cal) is also expressed as a kilocalorie (abbreviation: kcal). One thousand small calories equal one large Calorie or one kilocalorie.

Carbohydrates and proteins both give four Calories for each respective gram. So, if ten grams of pure carbohydrate were ingested, it would yield forty Calories.

$$\text{10 grams of carbohydrate} \times \frac{\text{4 Calories}}{\text{gram of carbohydrate}} = \text{40 Calories}$$

Similarly, if ten grams of protein were used for energy, it would yield forty Calories.

$$\text{10 grams of protein} \times \frac{\text{4 Calories}}{\text{gram of protein}} = \text{40 Calories}$$

Fats, in comparison, yield nine Calories for every gram of fat. Fats, therefore, are a more energy-rich food source than carbohydrates or proteins because they give more Calories for every gram used. If ten grams of fat were used, it would yield ninety Calories.

$$\text{10 grams of fat} \times \frac{\text{9 Calories}}{\text{gram of fat}} = \text{90 Calories}$$

The total of all changes, chemical and physical, that take place in the body is called **metabolism**. The metabolic rate concerns itself with the changes in the body with respect to energy. It is the balance between the energy that is brought into the body and the energy used by the body. Energy is used during every action of the body, including voluntary activities such as walking or riding a bicycle and involuntary activities such as breathing and cellular repair.

The level of energy required for activities that occur when the body is at rest is called basal metabolism. The **basal metabolic rate (BMR)** will vary according to several factors. For example, the BMR will be higher in individuals with leaner body mass because it takes more energy to fuel the muscles than it does to store fat. BMR will also be higher for individuals in a period of high growth rate such as children and pregnant women.

Ideally, an individual will take in as many Calories as the body will use each day. When a person takes in more Calories than will be used, the body will store the excess energy in the form of fat. When a person uses more energy than is brought into the body, the body breaks down these stores. When the stores of fat are depleted, the body will start to break down its protein structures.

For an optimal energy balance in the body, the largest percentage of Calories in the diet should come from carbohydrates. Ideally, the percentage should be 50 to 60 percent of total calories consumed. The percentage of Calories attributable to fat should not be higher than 30 percent, with a percentage closer to 20 percent being preferred. Proteins should make up 10 to 20 percent of Calories in the diet.

Take note that these values are the percentage of the total Calories derived from each energy nutrient—not the percentage of grams. This distinction is important because of the difference in Calories derived from each energy nutrient. Figure 34-5 gives an example of these calculations.

The emphasis on carbohydrates was recently demonstrated with the U.S. Department of Agriculture's new

Label for Mystery Food:	Amount Per Serving
Calories	149
Total Fat	9g
Total Carbohydrate	14g
Total Protein	3g

The first calculation to make is one that converts grams to Calories.

$$9 \text{ grams of fat } \times \frac{9 \text{ Calories}}{\text{gram}} = 81 \text{ Calories due to fat}$$

$$14 \text{ grams of carbohydrate} \times \frac{4 \text{ Calories}}{\text{gram}} = 56 \text{ Calories due to carbohydrate}$$

$$3 \text{ grams of protein} \times \frac{4 \text{ Calories}}{\text{gram}} = 12 \text{ Calories due to protein}$$

The next calculation is to find the percentage of total Calories due to each of the energy nutrients.

$$\frac{81 \text{ Calories due to fat}}{149 \text{ total Calories}} = 54\%$$

$$\frac{56 \text{ Calories due to carbohydrate}}{149 \text{ total Calories}} = 38\%$$

$$\frac{12 \text{ Calories due to protein}}{149 \text{ total Calories}} = 8\%$$

Figure 34-5   Calculations of percentages of total calories due to fat, carbohydrate, or protein.

pyramid shape for the ideal diet, which has a base of foods from the breads, rice, and pasta groups (Figure 34-6).

 In many cultures outside of the United States, rice, bread, and noodles are the basis of the diet. In the United States, we have available great amounts of food from the dairy and meat groups. Unfortunately, dairy products and meats, while containing many good nutrients, also contain a great deal of fat. Studies have shown that many Americans are obese (as defined as weight being at least 20% greater than what their ideal weight should be). The American diet is too high in fat, has too many calories, salt, and cholesterol and insufficient amounts of complex carbohydrates and fiber. As a result, many illnesses and diseases occur, such as heart disease, high blood pressure, diabetes, and cancer. It is hoped that learning about nutrition by using this pyramid will help Americans make healthier food choices.

Other Nutrients

There are many other nutrients essential to maintaining good health. Although they do not provide the body with energy, they perform a variety of necessary functions. They include vitamins, minerals, water, and fiber.

Vitamins. Vitamins are a class of nutrient in which each specific vitamin has a function entirely its own. They are complex molecules and are required by the body in minute quantities. Vitamins were first named as letters of the alphabet. These names have been supplemented

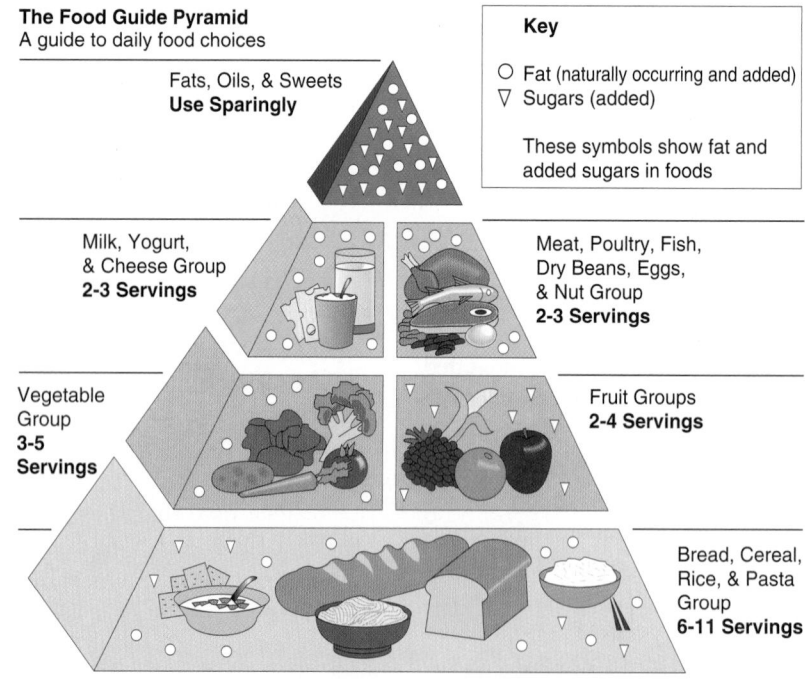

Figure 34-6   The U.S. Department of Agriculture's guide to a balanced diet takes the shape of a pyramid. The foundation of a good diet is made up of carbohydrate-rich foods; the fats, oils, and sugars represent the tip of the pyramid and should be used sparingly.
(Courtesy of U.S. Department of Agriculture)

with chemical names and both should be learned. Vitamins generally have one of two functions: to facilitate cellular metabolism by acting as a coenzyme with a catalyst, and to act as a component of tissue structure. A **catalyst** allows a chemical reaction to proceed at a much quicker rate and without as much energy input, and the **coenzyme** is the nonprotein part that acts with it. Neither a catalyst nor its coenzyme is used in the reaction and so each can be used again and again. Vitamins that work with catalysts are only needed in minute quantities.

Vitamins are divided into two classes based on water solubility. The vitamins that are not soluble in water are

said to be fat soluble. This is important because the **fat-soluble** vitamins are not carried into the bloodstream easily and are stored in fatty tissue, especially the liver. The **water-soluble** vitamins are not so easily stored and blood levels must be maintained by constant dietary intake. Toxicity can occur with high doses of either type of vitamin but is more likely to occur with the fat-soluble vitamins because they are stored in the body. The vitamins are listed in Table 34-2.

There are four fat-soluble vitamins, which include vitamin A, vitamin D, vitamin E and vitamin K. The first one, vitamin A, has two forms. The form that is used by

TABLE 34-2   VITAMIN SOURCES AND FUNCTIONS

Vitamins are divided into two classes based on water solubility: fat-soluble vitamins and water-soluble vitamins.

Name	Food Sources	Functions	Deficiency/Toxicity
Fat-Soluble Vitamins			
Vitamin A (carotene or retinol)	Animal Liver Whole milk Butter Cream Cod liver oil Plants Dark green leafy vegetables Deep yellow or orange fruit Fortified margarine	Dim light vision Maintenance of mucous membranes Growth and development of bones	Deficiency Night blindness Xerophthalmia Respiratory infections Bone growth ceases Toxicity Cessation of menstruation Joint pain Stunted growth Enlargement of liver
Vitamin D (cholecalciferol)	Animal Eggs Liver Fortified milk Plants None	Bone growth	Deficiency Rickets Osteomalacia Poorly developed teeth Muscle spasms Toxicity Kidney stones Calcification of soft tissues
Vitamin E (alphatocopherol)	Animal None Plant Margarines Salad dressing	Antioxidant	Deficiency Destruction of RBCs Toxicity Hypertension
Vitamin K (phytonadione)	Animal Egg yolk Liver Milk Plant Green leafy vegetables Cabbage	Blood clotting	Deficiency Prolonged blood clotting Toxicity Hemolytic anemia Jaundice
Water-Soluble Vitamins			
Thiamin (Vitamin B_1)	Animal Liver Eggs Fish Pork Beef Plants Whole and enriched grains Legumes	Coenzyme in oxidation of glucose	Deficiency Gastrointestinal tract, nervous and cardiovascular system problems Toxicity None

(continues)

TABLE 34-2 *(continued)*

Name	Food Sources	Functions	Deficiency/Toxicity

Riboflavin (Vitamin B_2)	Animal
	  Milk
	Plants
	  Green vegetables
	  Cereals
	  Enriched bread
		Aids release of energy from food	Deficiency
			  Cheilosis
			  Glossitis
			  Photophobia
			Toxicity
			  None

Pyridoxine (Vitamin B_6)	Animal
	  Pork
	  Milk
	  Eggs
	Plants
	  Whole grain cereals
	  Legumes
		Synthesis of nonessential amino acids
		Conversion of tryptophan to niacin
		Antibody production
			Deficiency
			  Cheilosis
			  Glossitis
			Toxicity
			  Liver disease

Vitamin B_{12} (cobalamin)	Animal
	  Seafood
	  Meat
	  Eggs
	  Milk
	Plants
	  None
		Synthesis of RBCs
		Maintenance of myelin sheaths
			Deficiency
			  Degeneration of myelin sheaths
			  Pernicious anemia
			Toxicity
			  None

Niacin (Vitamin B_3, nicotinic acid)	Animal
	  Milk
	  Eggs
	  Fish
	  Poultry
		Transfers hydrogen atoms for synthesis of ATP	Deficiency
			  Pellagra
			Toxicity
			  Vasodilation of blood vessels

Folacin	Animal
	  None
	Plants
	  Spinach
	  Asparagus
	  Broccoli
	  Kidney beans
		Synthesis of RBCs	Deficiency
			  Glossitis
			  Macrocytic anemia
			Toxicity
			  None

Biotin	Animal
	  Milk
	  Liver
	Plants
	  Legumes
	  Mushrooms
		Coenzyme in carbohydrate and amino acid metabolism
		Niacin synthesis from tryptophan
			Deficiency
			  None
			Toxicity
			  None

Pantothenic acid (Vitamin B_5)	Animal
	  Eggs
	  Liver
	  Salmon
	Plants
	  Mushrooms
	  Cauliflower
	  Peanuts
	  Yeast
		Metabolism of carbohydrates, lipids, and proteins
		Synthesis of acetylcholine
			Deficiency
			  None
			Toxicity
			  None

Vitamin C (ascorbic acid)	Fruits
	  All citrus
	Plants
	  Broccoli
	  Tomatoes
	  Brussel sprouts
	  Potatoes
		Prevention of scurvy
		Formation of collagen
		Healing of wounds
		Release of stress hormones
		Absorption of iron
			Deficiency
			  Scurvy
			  Muscle cramps
			  Ulcerated gums
			Toxicity
			  Raise uric acid level
			  Hemolytic anemia
			  Kidney stones
			  Rebound scurvy

the body is retinol, which is found in animal foods. The form found in plants is carotene. Carotene is converted into retinol in the body. Vitamin A is part of the pigment rhodopsin found in the eye and is responsible in part for vision, especially night vision. Vitamin A also gives strength to epithelial tissue and is required for healthy skin and mucous membranes. Sources of vitamin A include animal fats, butter, and cheese.

Vitamin D, also called cholecalciferol, is the fat-soluble vitamin involved in the metabolism of calcium in the body. It not only helps with absorption of this important mineral, but also with formation and maintenance of bone tissue. Vitamin D can be made in the body with exposure to sunlight. Rickets and osteomalacia are diseases caused by a deficiency in vitamin D. When deficiencies occur, especially during childhood, malformation of the skeleton is seen. Sources of vitamin D include milk, cod liver oil, and egg yolk.

Another fat-soluble vitamin is vitamin E, or tocopherol. It belongs to a group of compounds called antioxidants, which reduce the likelihood of oxidation of substances. This ability to reduce oxidation has recently led to suggestions that vitamin E may slow the aging process, but its true effectiveness is yet to be demonstrated. Vitamin E is found in lettuce and other green leafy vegetables, wheat germ, and rice.

Vitamin K is a fat-soluble vitamin required for the production of prothrombin. Prothrombin is one agent responsible for the clotting of blood. Deficiencies can result in prolonged blood clotting time and hemorrhage. Vitamin K is synthesized by intestinal bacteria, and bile is required for its absorption. About half of the body's requirement for vitamin K is fulfilled in this way. Sources of vitamin K include fats, fishmeal, oats, alfalfa, wheat, and rye.

Vitamin C, or ascorbic acid, is a water-soluble vitamin. Vitamin C is a constituent of connective tissue and acts to hold cells together. A deficiency of vitamin C causes scurvy, in which the walls of the capillaries become so weakened that they burst. Vitamin C also helps with wound healing and with the absorption of iron. Sources include most fresh fruits (especially citrus fruits) and vegetables (especially tomatoes).

The last group of water-soluble vitamins is the B-complex vitamin. It is important to remember that each vitamin in the B-complex is a separate vitamin with distinct functions. Vitamin B$_1$, or thiamin, helps in the conversion of glucose to energy. The disease beriberi is caused by thiamin deficiency and is characterized by neuritis edema, and cardiovascular changes. Sources include whole grain cereals, peas, beans, vegetables, and brewer's yeast. Vitamin B$_2$, or riboflavin, is also involved in energy production and is important in the production of proteins and necessary for normal growth. Sources include eggs, liver, milk, brewer's yeast, and green vegetables. A third B-complex vitamin, niacin, works with both thiamin and riboflavin in the production of energy. Lack of niacin results in gastrointestinal and central nervous system disturbances. All three of these vitamins are important throughout the body.

Vitamin B$_6$, or pyridoxine, has an important role in protein metabolism, especially the synthesis of proteins. It is also important in the metabolism of fats and carbohydrates. Vitamin B$_6$ is found in rice, beans, and yeast. Another B-complex vitamin, folic acid, is involved in the formation of DNA and the formation of red blood cells. Folic acid is found in liver, yeast, and green leafy vegetables. Vitamin B$_{12}$, or cobalamin, is another vitamin important to the functioning of red blood cells. This vitamin is responsible for the synthesis of the heme portion of hemoglobin, and deficiencies in vitamin B$_{12}$ result in the disease pernicious anemia. Because vitamin B$_{12}$ is only found in animal foods such as liver, kidney, and dairy products, pernicious anemia may be a problem for some vegetarians. Pernicious anemia may also occur when there is decreased production of a factor required for vitamin B$_{12}$ absorption. Other B-complex vitamins, pantothenic acid, vitamin B$_5$, and biotin, are generally responsible for energy metabolism.

Minerals. Minerals differ from vitamins in two distinct ways. While vitamins are complex molecules, minerals are singular elements. Another way that minerals differ from vitamins is that while vitamins are only required in minute quantities, some minerals are required in larger amounts. The foundation of the classification of minerals falls into two groups: major and trace minerals. No matter how small the quantity required of either a mineral or vitamin, all are vital to a healthy body. Some minerals are considered electrolytes, in that they become ionized and carry a positive or negative charge. The levels of these minerals in the bloodstream must be carefully balanced for the body to function in a healthy state.

There are seven major minerals (Table 34-3). They are calcium, phosphorus, sodium, potassium, magnesium, chlorine, and sulfur.

Calcium (Ca) is the mineral present in the largest quantity in the body because of its involvement in the structure of bone and teeth. It is also important in blood clotting, muscle contraction, and nerve conduction. Its levels in the blood must be kept at very narrow limits to ensure that the nervous and muscular tissues can function. This is especially important for the beating heart tissue. When there is a deficiency of calcium in the diet, calcium is taken from the bones to keep the blood calcium levels constant. The resulting deficient peak bone mass may put a person at risk for osteoporosis. This condition develops when there is not enough calcium in the bones and the bones become porous and easily broken.

TABLE 34-3	THE SEVEN MAJOR MINERALS AND THEIR FOOD SOURCES		
Name	**Food Sources**	**Functions**	**Deficiency/Toxicity**
Calcium (Ca)	Milk exchanges Milk, cheese Meat exchanges Sardines Salmon Vegetable exchanges Green vegetables	Development of bones and teeth Permeability of cell membranes Transmission of nerve impulses Blood clotting	Deficiency Osteoporosis Osteomalacia Rickets
Phosphorus (P)	Milk exchanges Milk, cheese Meat exchanges Lean meat	Development of bones and teeth Transfer of energy Component of phospholipids Buffer system	(Same as calcium)
Potassium (K)	Fruit exchanges Oranges, bananas Dried fruits	Contraction of muscles Maintaining water balance Transmission of nerve impulses Carbohydrate and protein metabolism	Deficiency Hypokalemia Toxicity Hyperkalemia
Sodium (Na)	Table salt Meat exchanges Beef, eggs Milk exchanges Milk, cheese	Maintaining fluid balance in blood Transmission of nerve impulses	Toxicity Increase in blood pressure
Chloride (Cl)	Table salt Meat exchanges	Gastric acidity Regulation of osmotic pressure Activation of salivary amylase	Deficiency Imbalance in gastric acidity Imbalance in blood pH
Magnesium (Mg)	Vegetable exchanges Green vegetables Bread exchanges Whole grains	Synthesis of ATP Transmission of nerve impulses Activator of metabolic enzymes Relaxation of skeletal muscles	
Sulfur (S)	Meat exchanges Eggs, poultry, fish	Maintaining protein structure Formation of high-energy compounds	

Phosphorus (P) is another mineral important in bone formation. Phosphorus also is involved in numerous activities associated with energy metabolism, as well as maintaining a proper pH balance in the blood.

Sodium (Na) and potassium (K) are two minerals that act as electrolytes. Together they work to maintain proper water balance. They also help in maintenance of proper pH balance and are involved in nerve and muscular conduction and excitability. In addition, potassium is involved in protein synthesis and release of insulin from the pancreas.

Magnesium (Mg) is another mineral that is involved with energy metabolism. It also functions in nerve and muscle excitability and is stored in bone.

Chloride (Cl) is very important in pH balance and is the major **extracellular** (outside the cell) anion. It is also a major component of gastric secretions in the form of hydrochloric acid.

The last major mineral is sulfur (S). It is a component of one of the amino acids and therefore is found in protein. It is also involved in energy metabolism.

The **trace minerals** are required in smaller quantities but are as important as the major minerals. Some of the more important trace minerals include iron, copper,

chromium, molybdenum, selenium, manganese, iodine, zinc, cobalt, and fluorine.

Iron is vital to life because of its role in the heme molecule, which carries oxygen to every cell in the body. Iron-deficiency anemia results when the diet is low in iron and is characterized by small, pale red blood cells. Iron is also part of the molecule myoglobin, found in muscle cells, and is involved in a number of metabolic reactions.

Copper, chromium, molybdenum, selenium, and manganese are trace minerals important as factors in a number of metabolic reactions. Selenium acts as an antioxidant and has been receiving much of the recent publicity that vitamin E has. Iodine is also involved in metabolism but is unique in that the only place that iodine is found is in the thyroid hormones. Without it, the thyroid gland would be unable to regulate the overall metabolism of the body.

Zinc is an important constituent of many parts of the body but most notable is its involvement with the immune system and growth of tissues. Deficiencies lead to decreased ability to heal and lower immune resistance. Cobalt is part of vitamin B_{12} and is therefore important for the functioning of red blood cells. Fluorine is involved in calcified tissues. Its involvement in strengthening teeth has led to the fluidation of most public water supplies. Its role in the prevention of osteoporosis has been suggested but is still under investigation.

Water. Water is the most important nutrient. The human body can go far longer without food than it can without water. Water has a multitude of functions in the body. It is the major solvent of the body and is the medium in which most biochemical reactions of the body take place. As a solvent, water also is essential for the removal of toxic waste from the body. In addition, it is an important component of many structures, the body being composed of 50 to 60 percent water. Being the major component of blood, water serves as a transporter. Another function of water is its lubricating role, especially in joints and in the digestive system. In addition, water helps control temperature within the body by eliminating excess heat through the evaporation of water secreted in the form of perspiration.

Because the body cannot store water, water that is lost daily must continually be replenished. Water is lost through perspiration, fecal material, urine, and respiration. Water can be replenished in part from foods that are ingested, but additional water should also be consumed. It is suggested that eight glasses of water be taken in per day. While other beverages are important sources of water, it should be considered that caffeine and alcohol are **diuretics** and will cause the body to lose water through increased urinary output. Beverages containing these substances should not be counted in the eight glasses of water.

Fiber. Although most fiber is carbohydrate in composition, it is included in its own section because of its special characteristics. Fiber comes only from plant sources. An adequate supply of fruits, vegetables, and grains is necessary to ensure enough fiber in the diet. Fiber cannot be digested and therefore is not absorbed into the body. Although fiber is not digested, it is important for the proper functioning of the gastrointestinal tract because it adds bulk to the fecal material as it is passed through the intestines; therefore, it gives the muscles of the tract something against which to work. Lack of fiber in the diet has been implicated in such gastrointestinal disorders as diverticulitis and colorectal cancer.

There are several types of fiber. Most are carbohydrates and include **cellulose**, gums, mucilages, algal polysaccharides, pectins, and hemicellulose. Another important fiber, lignin, is not a carbohydrate. It is suggested that the diet contain 15 to 20 grams of fiber per day. The American diet tends to be far below this suggestion, in part due to the consumption of processed foods. During processing, fiber is often removed. This is true with polished, or white, rice where the husk has been removed. Fiber levels should be increased gradually to prevent gastrointestinal distress, which can include diarrhea or flatulence.

READING FOOD LABELS

When assisting patients to change or modify their diets, the medical assistant must be knowledgeable not only about types of nutrients, but about how these nutrients are expressed in the foods we eat. The nutritional analysis presented on a package's food label is a helpful guide to understanding levels of fat, cholesterol, sodium, carbohydrate, protein, and vitamins contained in a particular food.

Many of the foods we eat are **processed foods**, which are cooked or packaged with parts removed or ingredients added. We rely on the labels on the cans, bottles, and boxes to tell us what nutrients are inside. The government wants to make it easier for people to understand the labels.

The government also wants to prevent food companies from fooling people into thinking something has good nutrition when it really does not. Food companies often put words on their labels to make people believe a product is healthy. Words like "healthy" and "light" or "lite" are not adequately descriptive. To discover what is in the package and if it is healthy, it is important to read the nutrition label (Figure 34-7).

Nutrition Facts
Serving Size: 1/2 Cup
Servings Per Container: 4

Amount Per Serving

Calories 100   Calories from Fat 30

	% Daily Value*
Total Fat 3g	5%
Saturated Fat 0g	0%
Cholesterol 0mg	0%
Sodium 340mg	14%
Total Carbohydrate 15g	5%
Dietary Fiber 1g	4%
Sugars 0g	
Protein 2g	

Vitamin A 0% • Vitamin C 0%
Calcium 0% • Iron 2%

*Percent Daily Values are based on a 2,000 calorie diet. Your daily values may be higher or lower depending on your calorie needs:

	Calories	2,000	2,500
Total Fat	Less than	65g	80g
Sat Fat	Less than	20g	25g
Cholesterol	Less than	300mg	300mg
Sodium	Less than	2,400mg	2,400mg
Total Carbohydrate		300g	375g
Dietary Fiber		25g	30g

Calories per gram:
Fat 9 • Carbohydrate 4 • Protein 4

Ingredients: Flour, Water, Yeast, Vegetable Oil, Salt, Artificial Flavor and Color.

Figure 34-7 Labels on food packages give facts about the ingredients and nutrition of the food in the package.

Items on the Nutrition Label

Serving Size. The nutrition information given is for one serving of the food. In this case, one serving is one-half cup of the food. This package contains four servings.

Calories. The label lists the number of calories per serving as well as the number of calories from fat per serving. This number should be less than 30 percent of the total calories. For example, if the total calories is 100, the calories from fat should be 30 or less.

The % Daily Value. The % daily value is the amount of a nutrient obtained by eating one serving of the product. The amount is given in a percentage based on a diet of 2,000 calories a day. For example, if the packaged food has 3 grams of fat, the total fat from eating one serving is 5% of the total fat that should be ingested in an entire day.

Fat and Cholesterol. Because it is important to eat a low-fat diet, the nutrition labels list both the total amount of fat and the amount of saturated fat per serving. Saturated fat comes from an animal source and contains more cholesterol than unsaturated fats, which come from vegetable sources. The cholesterol content is also listed.

Sodium. The amount of sodium per serving is listed. This category is especially important for patients on a sodium-restricted diet.

Carbohydrates. The total amount of carbohydrates per serving is listed along with the amount of carbohydrates that come from simple sugar. These two types of carbohydrates are separated for individuals who are trying to eat more complex carbohydrates and less simple sugar.

Other Information. The amount of fiber, protein, and only some vitamins and minerals are listed.

Ingredients. The ingredients contained in a packaged food are listed on the label. The item that is in the largest quantity is listed first. For example, if a product lists flour first and water second, there is more flour than water in the product. Preservatives, or chemicals added to food to keep it fresh longer, and artificial flavors and colors are often added to processed floods.

Comparing Labels

Look at some labels from snack foods that people eat when they want something crunchy and salty. Figure 34-8 (A), (B), and (C) show labels from potato chips, pretzels, and snack crackers. When comparing products, compare equal amounts. These products list the serving as 30 or 28 grams. That is close enough to compare the labels.

Patient Teaching Tip

Encourage patients to read and evaluate food labels. Typically, they should look for:

- No fat or the lowest amount of fat and saturated fat. Calories from fat should not be more than 30 percent of total calories.
- No cholesterol or low cholesterol. Total cholesterol should be less than 300 milligrams (mg) per day.
- Low sodium content. Total sodium should be less than 2,400 mg per day.
- High fiber. Fiber intake should be as high as possible.
- Vitamins and minerals. Some vitamins and minerals occur naturally and sometimes they are added to food during processing.

In reviewing these labels, note the amount of fat and saturated fat in each item. It might be assumed that potato chips, which are fried, would be high in fat. It may be surprising that the snack crackers have high fat content. Pretzels are the clear winner for a low-fat snack.

In terms of sodium, calories, and sugar, pretzels have the most sodium, but all three are high in sodium.

All three are low in sugar. Their calories are nearly the same as are the amounts of fiber and protein. The pretzels have the most carbohydrates and the crackers have the most artificial flavors, colors, and preservatives.

NUTRITION AT VARIOUS STAGES OF LIFE

As nutrients were discussed in the preceding sections, ranges of suggested normal requirements were offered. These ranges should be used as a guide, remembering that each individual is unique and there will be variations for requirements.

Pregnancy and Lactation

Pregnancy and lactation both cause marked changes in a woman's body and both require an increase in various nutrients. During pregnancy, not only does the growth of the fetus require additional nutrients, but the growth of the placenta, the increase in adipose tissue in the mother, the increased volume of blood, and the growth of breast tissue also require additional nutrients.

The increased demand for nutrients is not just a demand for Calories, but also for other specific nutrients to be increased, most notably protein. Protein require-

Potato Chips
Nutrition Facts
Serving Size: 1oz.
(28g/About 19 Chips)
Servings Per Container: 6

Amount Per Serving	
Calories 150	
Calories from Fat 90	

	% Daily Value*
Total Fat 10g	**15%**
Saturated Fat 2.5g	**13%**
Cholesterol 0mg	**0%**
Sodium 340mg	**14%**
Total Carbohydrate 15g	5%
Dietary Fiber 1g	**4%**
Sugars 1g	
Protein 2g	

Vitamin A 0% • Vitamin C 10%

Calcium   0% • Iron   2%

*Percent Daily Values are based on a 2,000 calorie diet. Your daily values may be higher or lower depending on your calorie needs:

	Calories	2,000	2,500
Total Fat	Less than	65g	80g
Sat Fat	Less than	20g	25g
Cholesterol	Less than	300mg	300mg
Sodium	Less than	2,400mg	2,400mg
Total Carbohydrate		300g	375g
Dietary Fiber		25g	30g

Calories per gram:

Fat 9 • Carbohydrate 4 • Protein 4

Ingredients: Potatoes, Vegetable Oil (Contains one or more of the following: Canola, Corn, Cottonseed, or Partially Hydrogenated Canola, Soybean or Sunflower Oil), Salt.

(A)

Pretzels
Nutrition Facts
Serving Size: 7 Pretzels
(30g)
Servings Per Container: 9.4

Amount Per Serving	
Calories 120	
Calories from Fat 10	

	% Daily Value*
Total Fat 1g	**2%**
Saturated Fat 0g	**0%**
Cholesterol 0g	**0%**
Sodium 360mg	**15%**
Total Carbohydrate 24g	8%
Dietary Fiber 1g	**4%**
Sugars 1g	
Protein 3g	

Vitamin A 0% • Vitamin C 0%

Calcium   0% • Iron   2%

*Percent Daily Values are based on a 2,000 calorie diet. Your daily values may be higher or lower depending on your calorie needs:

	Calories	2,000	2,500
Total Fat	Less than	65g	80g
Sat Fat	Less than	20g	25g
Cholesterol	Less than	300mg	300mg
Sodium	Less than	2,400mg	2,400mg
Total Carbohydrate		300g	375g
Dietary Fiber		25g	30g

Calories per gram:

Fat 9 • Carbohydrate 4 • Protein 4

Ingredients: Unbleached Wheat Flour, Water, Corn Syrup, Partially Hydrogenated Vegetable Oil (Soybean), Yeast, Salt, Bicarbonates and Carbonates of Sodium.

(B)

Wheat Snack Crackers
Nutrition Facts
Serving Size: 25 Cracker
(30g)
Servings Per Container: 7

Amount Per Serving	
Calories 150	
Calories from Fat 70	

	% Daily Value*
Total Fat 7g	**11%**
Saturated Fat 2g	**10%**
Cholesterol 0mg	**0%**
Sodium 310mg	**13%**
Total Carbohydrate 16g	5%
Dietary Fiber 1g	**4%**
Sugars 2g	
Protein 3g	

Vitamin A 0% • Vitamin C 0%

Calcium   0% • Iron   4%

*Percent Daily Values are based on a 2,000 calorie diet. Your daily values may be higher or lower depending on your calorie needs:

	Calories	2,000	2,500
Total Fat	Less than	65g	80g
Sat Fat	Less than	20g	25g
Cholesterol	Less than	300mg	300mg
Sodium	Less than	2,400mg	2,400mg
Total Carbohydrate		300g	375g
Dietary Fiber		25g	30g

Calories per gram:

Fat 9 • Carbohydrate 4 • Protein 4

Ingredients: Enriched Flour, Partially Hydrogenated Soybean and/or Cottonseed Oil, Dehydrated Potatoes, Steamed Crushed Wheat, Sugar, Salt, Natural and Artificial Flavors, Corn Syrup, Monosodium Glutamate, Dehydrated Cheddar Cheese, Dextrose, Nonfat Dry Milk, Artificial Color (Yellow 5, Yellow 6).

(C)

Figure 34-8   (A) An example of food label from potato chips. (B) An example of food label from pretzels. (C) An example of food label from snack crackers.

ments are nearly double during pregnancy. Because of the role vitamins play in metabolism and structure, they are needed in higher quantities than usual. In addition, calcium, phosphorus, and iron are needed in such high amounts that usually a vitamin supplement is prescribed. It is important that diet modifications are not simply an increase in Calories but include quality foods high in minerals, vitamins, and protein.

Pregnancy is an important time for both fetus and mother. It is normal and healthy for the mother to gain weight, and Calories should not be skimped at this time. During lactation there is still a requirement for higher levels of nutrients; however, overall, it is not as high as during pregnancy. A baby is more likely to be healthy and develop normally if the mother has good nutritional habits during pregnancy and breast-feeding.

Infancy

Infancy is a time of continuous growth, and many of the mother's nutritional requirements during pregnancy are still required by the baby after birth. In the first year of life, the baby will triple birth weight. The infant will need two to three times more Calories per kilogram (kg) of body weight than the normal adult. This is true for protein as well, and most of the vitamins and minerals are required at higher levels per kg. Most of these can be furnished with breast milk or formula; however, once iron stores have been used up, the infant will require an iron supplement, which is why pediatricians prescribe infant liquid iron supplement. Because of the high rate of growth, especially of the nervous system, infancy is a very important time to be sure nutritional requirements are met.

Adolescence

During adolescence, individuals experience the greatest levels of growth. The period of growth varies from person to person, but generally begins sooner with females. Except for times of pregnancy and lactation, the need for total nutrients is greatest at this stage of growth. At the end of the growth spurt, nutrient requirements decrease, and young adults must then also decrease the amount of food they consume.

Two particular nutrients that especially need to be altered during adolescence are iron and calcium. Iron requirements increase for the female as she begins menstruation. Calcium requirements increase for both males and females as bone development is occurring at a rapid rate.

Elderly

Aging is a natural process of the body. While aging occurs in different stages and at different rates for each individual, some generalities can be made. As we age, our cellular metabolism tends to slow. Coupled with a general decline in physical activity, this results in a decreased requirement for Calories. At the same time, there may be an increase in nutrient requirement in special circumstances. There is always an increased requirement for nutrients, vitamins, and protein in particular during illness, especially the prolonged illness that may occur in the elderly. With aging, there may be increased breakdown of cells, and as a result there is an increased requirement for nutrients that repair and builds cells and tissues. There is also a need to ingest more nutrients because of decreased absorption within the digestive tract. So while there is less need for Calories, there is more need for nutrient-rich foods.

This may become difficult for elderly individuals for several reasons. One may be an individual's psychological state. Loneliness and depression affect many elderly, especially after the loss of a spouse. Elderly may not like the idea of eating alone. The economic status of the individual also may present problems, as after retirement income will generally fall. Physiologically, taste tends to diminish with age and interest in food may decrease. In addition, problems with teeth and a decrease in salivary gland secretions may make eating painful. Many medications will cause a decrease in saliva production. Also, decreased motility in the gastrointestinal tract may lead to constipation, making eating uncomfortable. All these, as well as a general unwillingness to break old habits may make it difficult to change the diet to keep up with the body's aging process.

THERAPEUTIC DIETS

Thus far this chapter has examined the nutrient requirements of the body under normal conditions. There are times, however, when the body becomes diseased and nutrient requirements change. These changes may be due to disease states such as diabetes mellitus or conditions resulting from a poor diet such as obesity. Therapeutic diets are designed to overcome or control these conditions.

The diet can be modified in a number of ways. The number of overall Calories can be adjusted or one type of nutrient may be restricted or encouraged. The consistency, texture, and spiciness of food may be varied. The frequency of eating may be increased or decreased. When counseling patients, remember that habits are hard to change. The medical assistant should be supportive and encouraging.

Weight Control

Overweight and underweight are both weight disorders. The problem in defining overweight or underweight stems from the fact that there is no ideal weight for an entire population. There is only an ideal weight for the individual. Ideal weight can depend on many factors including age, gender, lean muscle mass, bone structure, and physical activity. Obesity is generally considered more than 20 percent overweight. Height-weight tables now generally give ranges that vary more than twenty pounds. The ratio of fat tissue to lean muscle mass is a better indicator of whether individuals are at their ideal weight than a specific weight.

Individuals will gain weight if they consume more Calories than they need. Conversely, individuals will lose weight if they use more Calories than they ingest. In either case, the individual must bring the amount of Calories ingested into balance with the amount used. For the overweight individual, this means either decreasing Calorie consumption, or increasing Calorie usage, or both. For the underweight individual, it usually entirely involves increasing Calorie consumption.

Weight loss has become a big business. However, individuals do not need to spend tremendous amounts of money to lose weight; patient education about low-Calorie, low-salt foods and a moderate exercise program are basic starting points for weight loss. Because losing more than 1 to 2 pounds a week can put an individual into nutritional deficiency, goals should not be set higher than this. Modifications made to the diet should then be maintained even after the weight is lost and should be continued throughout life. Losing weight takes much effort, and the patient needs constant encouragement and support from medical personnel and family.

Diabetes Mellitus

Diabetes mellitus is a disease in which there is either reduced or no production of insulin, or in which there is reduced or no response to insulin. Approximately 5 percent of the population has diabetes mellitus in some form. Most patients with this disease are not dependent on insulin and can control their condition by monitoring diet and weight.

Normally, after a meal, the body secretes the hormone insulin which makes its way to all cells of the body. Insulin signals the cells that the glucose is available and should be brought in so that it can be converted to energy. If the cells do not receive this signal, or do not respond to it, their ability to use glucose is markedly reduced. Because the body uses glucose as its main energy source, the ramifications of this affect almost every tissue of the body. In addition, the high levels of glucose that remain in the bloodstream put a tremendous strain on the kidney and other major body organs causing problems such as myocardial infarction, vascular diseases, neuropathy, and infections.

The effects of diabetes mellitus can be controlled with a general goal of maintaining a regular level of glucose in the bloodstream, avoiding large fluctuations between high and low levels. There are several ways suggested to accomplish this. Total Calories need not be altered, unless the diabetic patient is overweight. However, the ratio of carbohydrate, fat, and protein must be closely monitored. Total carbohydrates should be increased, but simple sugars should be avoided. Because of the longer rate of digestion and absorption of complex carbohydrates, these will be released over a longer period of time and prevent a sudden high level of glucose in the bloodstream, and are the type of carbohydrates diabetics need. Increasing fiber content also increases the time of absorption and decreases the likelihood of sudden increases in glucose levels in the bloodstream. Regular snacks may be added between meals to maintain levels of glucose. The trend is for patients to take charge of their own care. The role of educator for the medical assistant will be

an important one to facilitate patient self-management. See Chapter 36 for more information about diabetes and insulin.

Cardiovascular Disease

Cardiovascular disease is currently the leading cause of death in the United States. The unfortunate aspect is that much of it is preventable. Cardiovascular disease encompasses a variety of problems. Two of these problems, hypertension and atherosclerosis, often work hand in hand to perpetuate one another until a myocardial infarction occurs. It is important to remember that the conditions leading up to a myocardial infarction do not occur overnight. They have been developing slowly over many years, often asymptomatically. These conditions can be reduced or prevented with lifestyle modifications such as a healthy diet, moderate exercise, cessation of smoking, and weight management. The focus of this section will be on a healthy diet to prevent cardiovascular disease.

Hypertension, or elevated blood pressure, is often of unknown etiology. Sometimes it has a familial connection. When the blood pressure is only moderately increased, certain diet modifications can be used to lower it. If it is severe, drug therapy may be used in conjunction with diet therapy. The largest diet factor in controlling elevated blood pressure is restricting sodium because it plays such an important role in maintenance of water levels in the body. An increased volume of blood and water will increase the pressure on the blood vessel walls. Eliminating sodium includes more than simply eliminating use of table salt. Foods that are particularly high in sodium include smoked meats, luncheon meats, olives, pickles, chips, crackers, catsup, and cheese. In some cases, eliminating foods with only moderate salt levels may be indicated. These may include certain meats, breads containing baking powder or baking soda, shellfish, and some vegetables.

Atherosclerosis is another condition that can lead to a myocardial infarction. Atherosclerosis is hardening of the arteries due to deposits of fatty substance. It should not be confused with arteriosclerosis, which is a hardening of the arteries due to loss of the elasticity of the arterial wall. Atherosclerosis leads to arteriosclerosis which generally occurs because of a lack of exercise and elevated blood cholesterol levels. The elasticity can be regained by increasing activity, although it should be started slowly and under a physician's guidance. Atherosclerosis and arteriosclerosis often occur together. Smoking and hypertension will increase the likelihood of developing both of these conditions.

The conditions of atherosclerosis and arteriosclerosis facilitate each other. The fatty deposits associated with atherosclerosis tend to occur at points of damage to the inner walls of the artery. One of the causes of this damage is high pressure at points where there may be narrowing due to deposits that are already there, or due to the constriction of blood vessels due to nicotine. Carbon monoxide brought into the bloodstream during smoking also causes damage to the arterial walls. The deposits and hardening increase the blood pressure which in turn causes more damage and more deposits. It is a cycle that is difficult to stop. The best solution is prevention.

Fats and cholesterol in the diet have been strongly implicated in atherosclerosis. It is not only total fat that is important, but also types of fat ingested. The effect of high levels of fats and cholesterol in the diet will vary among individuals, and the factor in atherosclerosis is the levels of these substances in the bloodstream. Some individuals are able to ingest high amounts of fat and cholesterol without the body maintaining high levels of it in the blood. Unfortunately, this is not the case for everyone, and fat and cholesterol levels in the bloodstream must be closely monitored. Fat levels are measured by looking at triglycerides and lipoproteins. Lipoproteins are a complex made of fatty acids and proteins and are used to carry fat and cholesterol in the bloodstream. Low-density lipoproteins (LDL) are used by the body to transport fats and cholesterol to the body tissues. These are the lipoproteins more likely to deposit cholesterol and fat into the arterial wall. High-density lipoproteins (HDL) carry fats and cholesterol to the liver to be broken down and used. These lipoproteins are more likely to remove fats and cholesterol from the deposits in the arterial walls. HDL levels can be increased by exercise.

If total serum cholesterol and LDL levels are found to be elevated, the individual must modify the diet, and if severe enough, drug therapy may be indicated. The percentage of Calories from fat should be kept below 30 percent of total daily dietary intake, with less than a third of these coming from saturated fats. Cholesterol consumption should be less than 300 mg per day.

If a person suffers a myocardial infarction, it is important that the heart muscle be allowed to rest to facilitate proper healing. This includes bed rest, initially with a gradual progression to limited activity over about a two-week period. Then the patient is allowed to resume full activity. Rehabilitation consists of cessation of smoking, control of hypertension, weight reduction through a low-fat, low-calorie diet, and a program of exercise. All help to improve myocardial function.

Cancer

Cancer is a disease that comes in a variety of forms. It generally means that normal regulatory mechanisms within a cell have broken down. The result is that cells continue to grow in an unrestrained manner, diverting energy and nutrients from the patient's body to the cells' uncontrolled growth. There are many stages through which these cells may go, and they will go through them at varying rates. The ramifications of this new growth will vary depending on what types of cells are affected.

For these reasons, each cancer patient will have varying nutritional requirements. However, there are some generalities that can be made. First, there is definitely a need for increased Calories. Because the new growth has the ability to divert nutrients to itself, the result is the body receives fewer nutrients. It will then break down its own tissue. In addition, there is an increased need for nutrients to supply the immune system with energy and nutrients in its attempt to destroy the cancerous cells.

If the patient receives chemotherapy or radiation treatment, there is an even greater need for increased nutrients. These therapies are directed at killing cells that are rapidly dividing. This includes not only the cancerous cells, but also healthy cells such as those of the lining of the gastrointestinal tract and hair follicles. Increased nutrients are needed for repair and replacement of the lost cells, and protein levels in particular should be increased. Because of the disturbance of the gastrointestinal lining, digestion and absorption may also be decreased. It is important that the patient maintain as healthy a nutritional status as is possible rather than having to make up for nutritional deficiencies.

The patient will likely experience loss of appetite as well as nausea and vomiting. There are several ways to

SPOTLIGHT ON AAMA ESSENTIALS THROUGH CAAHEP

- In cases in which a patient does not want to eat, recommending that he or she share a meal with someone else may improve the appetite.

- Being aware of a patient's dietary needs, likes, and dislikes can help the medical assistant develop a nutritional plan that is both pleasant to the person's taste buds and appropriate for dietary needs.

- A medical assistant who has some knowledge of ethnic food choices can be reassuring to patients who may need to make some dietary changes but would like to make them within the parameters of their own cultures.

cope with this. First, food should be made as appealing as possible. Also, if the patient has difficulty swallowing, food can be liquefied in a food processor. Generally, food will be better tolerated if it is slightly chilled; extremes of temperature should be avoided. Several smaller meals may be easier to eat than three large meals.

DIET AND CULTURE

 Medical assistants are likely to come into contact with patients from many different ethnic groups. Many of these patients will have diets based upon traditional cultures, and some of the foods they eat, or the way they combine foods, may be unfamiliar to the medical assistant. Often, diets in other cultures are sensible ones, with foods chosen or combined to make up a complete protein. The medical assistant who has some knowledge of ethnic food choices can help reassure patients that the dietary changes they need to make are within the parameters of their own cultures. Table 34-4 presents some highlights of the food choices of different ethnic groups.

Vegetarian diets are also fairly common around the globe including the United States. With a good variety of

TABLE 34-4 SAMPLE FOOD CHOICES OF VARIOUS CULTURAL, RELIGIOUS, AND ETHNIC GROUPS	
Culture/Region/Group	**Diet and Food Choices**
Native American	It is thought that approximately half of the edible plants commonly eaten in the United States today originated with the Native Americans. Examples are corn, potatoes, squash, cranberries, pumpkins, peppers, beans, wild rice, and cocoa beans. In addition, they used wild fruits, game, and fish. Foods were commonly prepared as soups and stews, and dried. The original Native American diets were probably more nutritionally adequate than their current diets, which frequently consist of too high a proportion of sweet and salty, snack-type, empty calorie foods. Native American diets today may be deficient in calcium, vitamins A, C, and riboflavin.
U.S. Southern	Hot breads such as corn bread and baking powder biscuits are common in the U.S. South because the wheat grown in the area does not make good quality yeast breads. Grits and rice are also popular carbohydrate foods. Favorite vegetables include sweet potatoes, squash, green beans, and lima beans. Green beans cooked with pork are commonly served. Watermelon, oranges, and peaches are popular fruits. Fried fish is served often, as are barbecued and stewed meats and poultry. There is a great deal of carbohydrate and fat in these diets and limited amounts of protein in some cases. Iron, calcium, and vitamins A and C may sometimes be deficient.
Mexican	Mexican food is a combination of Spanish and Native American foods. Beans, rice, chili peppers, tomatoes, and corn meal are favorites. Meat is often cooked with the vegetable as in chili con carne. Corn meal is used in a variety of ways to make tortillas and tamales, which serve as bread. The combination of beans and corn makes a complete protein. While tortillas filled with cheese (called enchiladas) provide some calcium, the use of milk should be encouraged. Additional green and yellow vegetables and vitamin C-rich foods would also improve these diets.
Puerto Rican	Rice is the basic carbohydrate food in Puerto Rican diets. Vegetables commonly used include beans, plantains, tomatoes, and peppers. Bananas, pineapple, mangoes, and papayas are popular fruits. Favorite meats are chicken, beef, and pork. Milk is not used as much as would be desirable from the nutritional point of view.
Italian	Pastas with various tomato or fish sauces, and cheese are popular Italian foods. Fish and highly seasoned foods are common to Southern Italian cuisine while meat and root vegetables are common to northern Italy. The eggs, cheese, tomatoes, green vegetables, and fruits common to Italian diets provide excellent sources of many nutrients, but additional milk and meat would improve the diet.
Northern and Western European	Northern and Western European diets are similar to those of the U.S. Midwest, but with a greater use of dark breads, potatoes and fish, and fewer green vegetable salads. Beef and pork are popular as are various cooked vegetables, breads, cakes, and dairy products.
Central European	Citizens of Central Europe obtain the greatest portion of their calories from potatoes and grain, especially rye and buckwheat. Pork is a popular meat. Cabbage cooked in many ways is a popular vegetable as are carrots, onions, and turnips. Eggs and dairy products are used abundantly.
Middle Eastern	Grains, wheat, and rice provide energy in these diets. Chickpeas in the form of hummus are popular. Lamb and yogurt are commonly used as are cabbage, grape leaves, eggplant, tomatoes, dates, olives, and figs. Black, very sweet (Turkish) coffee is a popular beverage.
Chinese	The Chinese diet is varied. Rice is the primary energy food and is used in place of bread. Foods are generally cut into small pieces. Vegetables are lightly cooked and the cooking water is saved for future use. Soybeans are used in many ways, and eggs and pork are commonly served. Soy sauce is extensively used, but it is very salty and could present a problem with patients on low-salt diets. Tea is a common beverage, but milk is not. This diet may be low in fat.

(continues)

TABLE 34-4 *(continued)*

Culture/Region/Group	Diet and Food Choices
Japanese	Japanese diets include rice, soybean paste and curd, vegetables, fruits, and fish. Food is frequently served tempura style, which means fried. Soy sauce (shoyu) and tea are commonly used. Current Japanese diets have been greatly influenced by Western culture.
Southeast Asian	Many Indians are vegetarians who use eggs and dairy products. Rice, peas, and beans are frequently served. Spices, especially curry, are popular. Indian meals are not typically served in courses as Western meals are. They generally consist of one course with many dishes.
Thailand, Vietnam, Laos, and Cambodia	Rice, curries, vegetables, and fruit are popular in Thailand, Vietnam, Laos, and Cambodia. Meat, chicken, and fish are used in small amounts. The wok (a deep, round fry pan) is used for sautéing many foods. A salty sauce made from fermented fish is commonly used.
Jewish	Interpretations of the Jewish dietary laws vary. Those who adhere to the Orthodox view consider tradition important and always observe the dietary laws. Foods prepared according to these laws are called kosher. Conservative Jews are inclined to observe the rules only at home. Reform Jews consider their dietary laws to be essentially ceremonial and so minimize their significance. Essentially the laws require the following: • Slaughtering must be done by a qualified person, in a prescribed manner. The meat or poultry must be drained of blood, first by severing the jugular vein and carotid artery, then by soaking in brine before cooking. • Meat or meat products may not be prepared with milk or milk products. • The dishes used in the preparation and serving of meat dishes must be kept separate from those used for dairy foods. • A specified time, six hours, must elapse between consumption of meat and milk. • The mouth must be rinsed after eating fish and before eating meat. • There are prescribed fast days—Passover Week, Yom Kippur, and Feast of Purim. • No cooking is done on the Sabbath—from sundown Friday to sundown Saturday. These laws forbid the eating of: • the flesh of animals without cloven (split) hooves or that do not chew their cud • hind quarters of any animal • shellfish or fish without scales or fins • fowl that are birds of prey • creeping things and insects • leavened (contains ingredients that cause it to rise) bread during the Passover Generally, the food served is rich. Fresh smoked and salted fish, and chicken are popular, as are noodles, egg, and flour dishes. These diets can be deficient in fresh vegetables and milk.
Roman Catholic	Although the dietary restrictions of the Roman Catholic religion have been liberalized, meat is not allowed its adherents on Ash Wednesday and Fridays during Lent.
Eastern Orthodox	Followers of this religion include Christians from the Middle East, Russia, and Greece. Although interpretations of the dietary laws vary, meat, poultry, fish, and dairy products are restricted on Wednesdays and Fridays and during Lent and Advent.
Seventh Day Adventist	Generally, Seventh Day Adventists are ovolacto-vegetarians, which means they use milk products and eggs, but no meat, fish, or poultry. They may also use nuts, legumes, and meat analogues (substitutes) made from soybeans. They consider coffee, tea, and alcohol to be harmful.
Mormon (Latter Day Saints)	The only dietary restriction observed by Mormons is the prohibition of coffee, tea, and alcoholic beverages.
Islamic	Adherents of Islam are called Muslims. Their dietary laws prohibit the use of pork and alcohol, and other meats must be slaughtered according to specific laws. During the month of Ramadan, Muslims do not eat or drink during daylight hours.
Hindu	To the Hindus, all life is sacred and small animals contain the souls of ancestors. Consequently, Hindus are usually vegetarians. They do not use eggs as they represent life.
Vegetarians	There are several vegetarian diets. The common factor among them is that they do not include red meat. Some include eggs, some fish, some milk, and some even poultry. When carefully planned, these diets can be nutritious. They can contribute to a reduction of obesity, high blood pressure, heart disease, some cancers, and possibly diabetes. They must be carefully planned so they include all needed nutrients. Lacto-ovo vegetarians use dairy products and eggs but no meat, poultry, or fish. Lacto-vegetarians use dairy products but no meat, poultry, or eggs.

(continues)

TABLE 34-4 *(continued)*	
Culture/Region/Group	**Diet and Food Choices**
Vegans	Vegans avoid all animal foods. They use soybeans, chickpeas, and meat analogues made from soybeans. It is important that their meals be carefully planned to include appropriate combinations of the nonessential amino acids to provide the needed amino acids. For example, beans served with corn or rice, or peanuts eaten with wheat, are better in such combinations than any of them would be if eaten alone. Vegans can show deficiencies of calcium, zinc, vitamins A, D, and B$_{12}$ and, of course, proteins.
Zen Macrobiotic Diets	The macrobiotic diet is a system of ten diet plans developed from Zen Buddhism. Adherents progress from the lower number diet to the higher, gradually giving up foods in the following order: desserts, salads, fruits, animal foods, soups, and ultimately vegetables, until only cereals—usually brown rice—are consumed. Beverages are kept to a minimum and only organic foods are used. Foods are grouped as Yang (male) or Yin (female). A ratio of 5 : 1 Yang to Yin is considered important. Most macrobiotic diets are nutritionally inadequate. As the adherents give up foods according to plans, their diets become increasingly inadequate. These diets can be especially dangerous because avid adherents promise medical cures from the diets that cannot be attained, and so medical treatment may be delayed when needed.

grains, vegetables, fruits, and dairy products, a vegetarian diet can supply an individual with all the required nutrients. Pernicious anemia, a disease caused by lack of cobalamin (vitamin B$_{12}$), is sometimes associated with vegetarian diets that do not contain enough animal product (see the section on vitamins in this chapter). One type of vegetarian, vegan, does not eat any product associated with animals, including milk or eggs. This type of diet is particularly susceptible to nutritional deficiencies.

In speaking with patients about diet and dietary changes, it is important to remember that patients choose their diets for a variety of reasons, including cultural, religious, or ethical beliefs. The medical assistant should respect the patient's reasons for following a certain diet while encouraging any modifications.

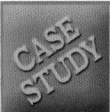

Anita Ferguson is a new patient at Inner City Health Care. She is a sixteen-year-old who is four months pregnant and came to the urgent care center only a couple of weeks ago. After Wanda Slawson, CMA, took Anita's medical history, and after Anita was examined by the physician, Wanda set aside time to answer any questions Anita might have about her pregnancy. Anita is obviously scared, wants the baby, but does not want her life to change. According to the history, Anita has lost a few pounds in the last two weeks.

34-1

CASE STUDY REVIEW

1. What patient education can Wanda provide to alert Anita to the importance of diet and weight gain during pregnancy?
2. What foods should Wanda encourage Anita to eat?
3. If Anita resists Wanda's suggestions and has not gained any weight by the next visit, how should Wanda proceed?

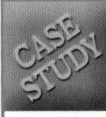

Dr. Lewis prescribed a diabetic diet for Mrs. Johnson.

CASE STUDY REVIEW

34-2

1. Describe what is included in a diabetic diet.
2. Describe the patient education you would employ to help Mrs. Lewis understand the diet and to help her reach her goal of improved health.

SUMMARY

Seven types of nutrients are required by the body for maintenance of good health. Carbohydrates, fats, and proteins provide energy for the body. Vitamins, minerals, fiber, and water cannot provide energy but are responsible for many vital processes within the body.

Nutritional needs change at various points in the life cycle. During pregnancy, lack of nutrients can be detrimental to the development of the fetus and the health of the expectant mother. The need for nutrients is great during infancy and childhood, with the greatest need for total nutrients occurring during adolescence. During adulthood, the requirement for Calories decreases. With the decrease in basal metab-

olism that occurs with aging, the requirement for Calories decreases even more.

At times of disease, the diet of the individual must be modified to help relieve stress put on the body by the disease, to give energy to fight the disease, and, in cases where the disease is diet-related, to lessen the severity of the disease.

It is important to have adequate nutritional intake during every stage of life. The healthier one is, the better one feels. Nutritional status should be examined and adjustments made if necessary with the goal of helping patients maintain a healthy body.

REVIEW QUESTIONS

Multiple Choice

1. The transfer of nutrients from the gastrointestinal tract into the bloodstream is:
   a. ingestion
   b. digestion
   c. absorption
   d. elimination
2. Fats are considered a(n):
   a. mineral
   b. vitamin
   c. energy nutrient
   d. fiber
3. The total of all chemical and physical changes that take place in the body is called:
   a. homeostatis
   b. metabolism
   c. a catalyst
   d. an antioxidant
4. According to the USDA food pyramid, you should:
   a. have 3 to 5 servings of vegetables a day
   b. severely limit the number of servings of pasta
   c. never use fats, oils, and sugars
   d. consider meat the foundation of the pyramid
5. Another name for vitamin E is:
   a. tocopherol
   b. caratene
   c. biotin
   d. pyridoxine

Critical Thinking

1. Evaluate your own diet. Write down every item you ingest for a day and find the values of the nutrients contained in the foods. A medical dictionary is a good source for listing the nutrient value of selected foods. If you are eating prepared foods, read the package food label. Remember, you are trying to get an idea of your average daily diet, so don't change your diet for your analysis unless you plan to maintain it. What is the balance of your energy nutrients? Are you getting enough vitamins and minerals? Are you getting adequate fiber? What modifications could be made?
2. For each of the following vitamins and minerals, suggest some symptoms that might appear if there were a deficiency.
   vitamin A
   vitamin K
   vitamin C
   thiamin
   riboflavin
   cobalamin (vitamin B_{12})
   calcium
3. Consider the functions of the various regions of the digestive system, and look up in a medical dictionary each of the following procedures. Describe the problems that might exist with the following procedures if diet modifications do not take place.
   colostomy
   gastroileostomy
   gastrectomy

4. Explain why a breakfast high in complex carbohydrates is an important goal.
5. Discuss why the new pyramid shape is an accurate portrayal of the ideal diet.
6. Write a response to a teenage woman who refuses to gain weight during her pregnancy.
7. What are some things to consider when assessing the diet of an elderly person?
8. Find five things a person can do to decrease the risk of heart disease. Compile a list from the class. How many of the items are associated with diet? How many of the items involve you?
9. Describe how the diet can be used to control diabetes mellitus. When a person becomes dependent on insulin, should the diet continue to be used?
10. Following is information from a label for peanut butter. Calculate the percentage of calories due to fat, protein, and carbohydrate.

Serving size	2 tbs.
Calories	204
Protein	9 grams
Carbohydrates	6 grams
Fat	16 grams

WEB ACTIVITIES

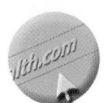 Search the Web for information about the U.S. Department of Agriculture's Food Guide Pyramid.

1. Is the pyramid appropriate for all ages?
2. Are the daily food choices the same for a child as for an adult?

Search community agencies on the Web for information about the following diseases and the role nutrition plays in prevention of the disease:

1. diabetes mellitus
2. arteriosclerotic heart disease
3. hypertension

REFERENCES/BIBLIOGRAPHY

Frey, R., & Shearer-Cooper, L. A. (1996). *Introduction to nursing assisting: Building language skills*. Albany, NY: Delmar.

Lankford, T. R. (1994). *Foundations of normal and therapeutic nutrition* (2nd ed.). Albany, NY: Delmar.

Mahan, L. K., & Arlin, M. (1999). *Krause's food, nutrition & diet therapy* (10th ed.). Philadelphia: W.B. Saunders.

Townsend, C. E. (2000). *Nutrition and diet therapy* (7th ed.). Albany, NY: Delmar.

Williams, S. R. (2001). *Basic nutrition and diet therapy* (11th ed.). St. Louis: Mosby-Year Book, Inc.

Chapter 35

BASIC PHARMACOLOGY

KEY TERMS

Abuse
Administer
Anaphylaxis
Contraindication
Dispense
Pharmacology
Prescribe
Pruritus
Urticaria

OUTLINE

OBJECTIVES

The student should strive to meet the following performance objectives and demonstrate an understanding of the facts and principles presented in this chapter through written and oral communication.

1. Define the key terms as presented in the glossary.
2. Recall five medical uses for drugs.
3. Describe three types of drug names and give an example, for one drug, of all three names.
4. List five sources of drugs.
5. Describe the Federal Foods, Drug, and Cosmetic Act and the Controlled Substance Act of 1970.
6. Name the five controlled substances schedules and describe appropriate storage of the substances. *(continues)*

OBJECTIVES (*continued*)

7. Define the law in terms of administering, prescribing, and dispensing drugs.
8. Describe the four most commonly used sections of the *Physician's Desk Reference* (PDR).
9. Describe the principal actions of drugs and three undesirable reactions.
10. Describe routes of drug administration and drug forms.
11. Describe handling and storing of drugs.
12. List emergency drugs and supplies.
13. Recall commonly abused drugs and describe their physical and emotional effects.
14. Critique the legal role and responsibilities of the medical assistant.

ROLE DELINEATION COMPONENTS

CLINICAL
Fundamental Principles
- Comply with quality assurance practices

Patient Care
- Maintain medication and immunization records

GENERAL (TRANSDISCIPLINARY)
Legal Concepts
- Document accurately
- Follow federal, state and local legal guidelines
- Maintain awareness of federal and state health care legislation and regulations
- Maintain and dispose of regulated substances in compliance with government guidelines
- Comply with established risk management and safety procedures

SCENARIO

Policy at Doctors Lewis & King dictates that a patient medication history is taken on the first appointment, routinely updated, and reviewed whenever medication is prescribed, dispensed, or administered. Both administrative and clinical medical assistants work together to ensure that this policy is carried out. When making a patient appointment, administrative medical assistants ask patients to bring with them any medications (keeping them in the labeled container) that they are currently using. When taking or updating a patient history, clinical medical assistants Audrey Jones and Joe Guerrero ask a number of questions of patients regarding medications and gently probe to assure that the patient includes all medications in the history and describes any allergy or hypersensitivity they may have to certain drugs.

INTRODUCTION

Pharmacology is the study of drugs, the science that is concerned with the history, origin, sources, physical and chemical properties, uses, and effects of drugs upon living organisms. Medical assistants in the ambulatory care setting need to understand basic pharmacology including the uses, sources, forms, and delivery routes of drugs; must know and be able to implement the intent of the law regarding controlled substances and other medications; and must have a knowledge of drug classifications and actions in order to be able to caution patients when taking prescription or nonprescription drugs. In addition, the medical assistant must be able to educate patients about a drug's intended purpose and the correct way to take the drug for maximum effectiveness. In this chapter, you will learn how to translate the doctor's prescription (℞) for the patient and calculate and administer drugs if this is legally allowed by the state in which you will practice as a medical assistant.

In this chapter, an overview of pharmacology is given; it is considered a review for medical assistants who have had a formal course in the subject. Information on dosage calculation and medication administration can be found in Chapter 36.

MEDICAL USES OF DRUGS

A drug is defined as a medicinal substance that may alter or modify the functions of a living organism. There are five medical uses for drugs.

- *Therapeutic*. Used in the treatment of a condition to relieve symptoms. An example is an antihistamine that may be used in the treatment of an allergy.

- *Diagnostic*. Used in conjunction with radiology and other diagnostic imaging procedures to allow the physician to pinpoint the location of a disease process. An example is dye tablets used in the X-ray study of the gallbladder.

- *Curative*. Used to kill or remove the causative agent of a disease. An example is an antibiotic.

- *Replacement*. Used to replace substances normally found in the body. Hormones and vitamins are examples of replacement drugs.

- *Preventive or Prophylactic*. Used to ward off or lessen the severity of a disease. Examples are immunizing agents such as vaccines.

DRUG NAMES

Most drugs have three types of names: chemical, generic, and trade or brand name.

- The chemical name describes the drug's molecular structure and identifies its chemical structure.

- The generic name is the drug's official name and is assigned to the drug by the United States Adopted Names Council. A generic drug can be manufactured by more than one pharmaceutical company. When this is the case, each company markets the drug under its own unique trade or brand name.

- A trade or brand name is registered by the U.S. Patent and Trademark Office and is approved by the U.S. Food and Drug Administration (FDA). The ® symbol following a drug's trade or brand name indicates that the name is registered and protected for 17 years. No other manufacturer can make or sell the drug during that time. Once the patent expires, any manufacturer can sell the drug under its generic name or a new trade name. The original trade name can not be reused.

Example:
Chemical name: 1, 4, 3, 6-dian hydrosorbitol-2, 5 dinitrate
Generic name: isosorbide dinitrate
Trade/Brand name: Sorbitrate®

When physicians prescribe a drug, they may use either the generic or trade name. It is not uncommon for physicians to prescribe the generic form of a drug because it is usually less costly for the patient. Sometimes physicians specify drugs by their trade names. Some states allow patients to request that their pharmacist dispense the generic drug equivalent unless the physician has specified that the drug be dispensed by its trade name. Also, in some states, a pharmacist may select a generic form of a drug if not specifically directed otherwise by the physician. Generic and trade name drugs have the same chemical composition and must adhere to identical FDA standards; therefore, according to most state laws, they can be used interchangeably. The drug label reflects the drug products dispensed.

HISTORY AND SOURCES OF DRUGS

Drugs prepared from roots, herbs, bark, and other forms of plant life are among the earliest known pharmaceuticals. Their origin can be traced back to primitive cultures where they were first used to evoke magical powers and to drive out evil spirits. Having discovered that certain plants were pharmacologically useful, a search was begun for sources of drugs.

Today this search continues. In addition to plants, drugs are derived from animals, minerals, and produced in laboratories utilizing chemical, biochemical, and biotechnological processes.

Plant Sources

The leaves, roots, stems, or fruit of certain plants may contain medicinal properties. For example, the dried leaf of the foxglove plant (*Digitalis purpurea*) is a source of digitalis, a cardiac glycoside used in the treatment of certain heart conditions.

Animal Sources

A number of essential extracts are obtained from tissues such as the pancreas and adrenal glands of animals. An example of a drug obtained from animals is insulin, a hormone that can be extracted from the pancreas of cows and hogs, though it is also made synthetically and by genetic engineering. Insulin is used in the treatment of diabetes mellitus. Two common compounds extracted from the adrenal glands of animals are adrenalin and cortisone.

Mineral Sources

Some naturally occurring mineral substances are used in medicine in a highly purified form. One such mineral is sulfur which has been used as a key ingredient in certain bacteriostatic drugs. It is now prepared synthetically and used in the treatment of urinary and intestinal tract infections.

Synthetic Drugs

These drugs are artificially prepared in pharmaceutical laboratories. By combining various chemicals, scientists can produce compounds that are identical to a natural drug or create entirely new substances. Thousands of drugs are now produced synthetically. Examples are Motrin® (ibuprofen) and Feldene® (piroxician).

Genetically Engineered Pharmaceuticals

Scientists are now capable of creating new strains of bacteria using a technique known as gene splicing. Through this process, hybrid forms of life have been created that benefit human beings by providing an alternative source of drugs, such as Humulin® (insulin) for the diabetic patient and interferon for use in treatment of cancer. These drugs can be manufactured in large quantities; thus, they are less expensive than natural substances.

DRUG REGULATIONS AND LEGAL CLASSIFICATIONS OF DRUGS

  Qualified medical practitioners who prescribe, dispense, or administer drugs must comply with federal and state laws. The laws govern the manufacture, sale, possession, administration, dispensing, and prescribing of drugs. All drugs available for legal use are controlled by the Federal Food, Drug, and Cosmetic Act. The law protects the public by ensuring the purity, strength, and composition of foods, drugs, and cosmetics. It also prohibits the movement in interstate commerce of altered and misbranded food, drugs, devices, and cosmetics. Enforcement of the act is the responsibility of the Food and Drug Administration (FDA), which is part of the Department of Health and Human Services (HHS).

Controlled Substance Act of 1970

One category of drugs—those with potential for abuse or addiction—is regulated by the Controlled Substance Act of 1970. It controls the manufacture, importation, compounding, selling, dealing in, and giving away of drugs that have the potential for abuse and addiction. The drugs are known as controlled substances and include heroin and cocaine and their derivatives and narcotics, stimulants, and depressants. The Drug Enforcement Agency (DEA) of the U.S. Justice Department monitors and enforces the act, which is also known as the Comprehen-sive Drug Abuse Prevention and Control Act. Under federal law, physicians who prescribe, administer, or dispense controlled substances must register with the DEA and renew their registration as required by state law.

Applications for registration are made directly to the DEA Registration Section, P.O. Box 28083, Central Station, Washington, DC 20038-8083. A licensed physician is issued a registration that must be renewed at regular intervals (Figure 35-1). The renewal form is sent approximately two months prior to the expiration date.

Controlled Substances Schedules. Controlled substances are classified according to five schedules:

- Schedule I specifies drugs that have a high potential for abuse and are not accepted for medical use within the United States. Examples are heroin and lysergic acid diethylamide (LSD).

- Schedule II drugs include those that also have a high abuse potential but that do have an accepted medical use within the United States. Examples are amphetamines and cocaine. Because of their high potential for abuse, a special DEA Form #222 must be used to order these drugs. The form is not necessary for Schedule III and IV drugs. A written prescription is required for Schedule II drugs and it can not be renewed.

- Schedule III drugs have a low-to-moderate potential for physical dependence, yet have a high potential for psychological dependency. Some examples are barbiturates and various drug combinations containing codeine and paregoric. Prescriptions for Schedule III drugs can be either written or oral. They can be refilled, but only five times within six months.

- Misuse or abuse of Schedule IV drugs can lead to limited physical or psychological dependency. Examples of these drugs include chloral hydrate and diazepam. Prescriptions for Schedule IV drugs may include refills, but refills are limited to five times within six months.

- Schedule V drugs have the lowest abuse potential of controlled substances. Some examples from this schedule are Lomotil® and Donnagel®. Some drugs from Schedule V may include refills, but refills are limited to five times within six months.

On occasion, the DEA will reclassify drugs and move them from one schedule to another.

So they can be readily identified, controlled substances are labeled with a large C with a Roman numeral inside it to indicate from which schedule the drug has come, for example, ⓒ.

Form DEA - 224 (Jun 1990) OMB No. 1117-0014

NAME

PROPOSED BUSINESS ADDRESS

CITY STATE ZIP CODE

RETAIN Copy 3. Mail Orig. and 1 copy with FEE to:

UNITED STATES DEPARTMENT OF JUSTICE
DRUG ENFORCEMENT ADMINISTRATION
CENTRAL STATION
P. O. Box 28083
WASHINGTON, D.C. 20038 - 8083
For INFORMATION, Call: (202) 307 7255

See "Privacy Act" Information on reverse

THIS BLOCK FOR DEA USE ONLY

APPLICATION FOR REGISTRATION
UNDER
CONTROLLED SUBSTANCES ACT OF 1970

Please PRINT or TYPE all entries.

No registration may be issued unless a completed application form has been received (21 CFR 1301.21).

REGISTRATION CLASSIFICATION: Submit Check or Money Order Payable to the **DRUG ENFORCEMENT ADMINISTRATION** in the Amount of **$ 60.00** (3 year registration period)

● **FEE MUST ACCOMPANY APPLICATION**

1. BUSINESS ACTIVITY: *(Check ☑ ONE only)*

A ☐ RETAIL PHARMACY B ☐ HOSPITAL/CLINIC C ☐ PRACTITIONER *(Specify Medical Degree, e.g., DDS, DO, DVM, MD, etc.)* D ☐ TEACHING INSTITUTION *(Instructional purposes only)*

2. SCHEDULES: *(Check ☑ all applicable schedules in which you intend to handle controlled substances. See Schedules on Reverse of Instruction Sheet.)*

SCHEDULE II ☐ NARCOTIC SCHEDULE II ☐ NONNARCOTIC SCHEDULE III ☐ NARCOTIC SCHEDULE III ☐ NONNARCOTIC SCHEDULE IV ☐ SCHEDULE V ☐

3. ☐ CHECK HERE IF YOU REQUIRE ORDER FORMS.

4. **ALL APPLICANTS MUST ANSWER THE FOLLOWING:**

(a) Are you currently authorized to prescribe, distribute, dispense, conduct research, or otherwise handle the controlled substances in the schedules for which you are applying, under the laws of the **State** or jurisdiction in which you are operating or propose to operate?

☐ YES - **State** License No. ______
☐ Not Applicable ☐ Pending

☐ YES - **State** Controlled Substance No. ______
☐ Not Applicable ☐ Pending

(b) Has the applicant ever been convicted of a crime in connection with controlled substances under State or Federal law, or ever surrendered or had a Federal controlled substance registration revoked, suspended, restricted or denied, or ever had a State professional license or controlled substance registration revoked, suspended, denied, restricted or placed on probation? ☐ YES ☐ NO

(c) If the applicant is a corporation (other than a corporation whose stock is owned and traded by the public), association, partnership, or pharmacy, has any officer, partner, stockholder or proprietor been convicted of a crime in connection with controlled substances under State or Federal law, or ever surrendered or had a Federal controlled substance registration revoked, suspended, restricted or denied, or ever had a State professional license or controlled substance registration revoked, suspended, denied, restricted or placed on probation? ☐ YES ☐ NO ☐ NOT APPLICABLE

IF THE ANSWER TO QUESTIONS 4(b) or (c) is YES, include a statement using the space provided on the **REVERSE** of this part.

● *ATTACH CHECK HERE* ●

Print or Type Name Here - Sign Below Applicant's Business Phone No.

SIGN HERE ▶ *Signature of applicant or authorized individual* *Date*

Title (If the applicant is a corporation, institution, or other entity, enter the TITLE of the person signing on behalf of the applicant ((e.g., President, Dean, Procurement Officer, etc....))

5. CERTIFICATION FOR FEE EXEMPTION

☐ CHECK THIS BLOCK IF INDIVIDUAL NAMED HEREON IS A FEDERAL, STATE, OR LOCAL OFFICIAL.

The Undersigned hereby certifies that the applicant herein is an officer or employee of a Federal, State or local agency who, in the course of such employment, is authorized to obtain, dispense, or prescribe controlled substances or is authorized to conduct research, instructional activity or chemical analysis with controlled substances, and is exempt from the payment of this application fee.

Signature of Certifying Official *Date*

Print or Type Name

Print or Type Title

Name of Institution or Agency

WARNING: SECTION 843(a)(4) OF TITLE 21, UNITED STATES CODE, STATES THAT ANY PERSON WHO KNOWINGLY OR INTENTIONALLY FURNISHES FALSE OR FRAUDULENT INFORMATION IN THIS APPLICATION IS SUBJECT TO IMPRISONMENT FOR NOT MORE THAN FOUR YEARS, A FINE OF NOT MORE THAN $30,000.00 OR BOTH.

Mail the Original and 1 copy with FEE to the above address. Retain 3rd copy for your records.

Figure 35-1 Licensed physicians who prescribe, administer, or dispense controlled substances must register with the Drug Enforcement Agency (DEA) of the U.S. Justice Department. The registration must be renewed at regular intervals.

The physician's DEA number must appear on each prescription for controlled substances.

A copy of the federal law and a complete list of controlled substances and their schedules are available from any DEA office.

Storage of Controlled Substances. Federal law requires that all controlled substances be kept separate from other drugs. They must be stored in a well-constructed metal box or compartment that has a double lock. Controlled substances must be protected from possible misuse and abuse, and persons who administer controlled substances must record them in a separate record book. The book must be maintained on a daily basis and kept for a minimum of two to three years, depending on state laws. Patient name, address, date of administration of the controlled substance, drug name, dose, and route and method of administration must be included in the record. Record keeping applies only to persons who administer or dispense controlled substances.

Controlled substances stored and used on the premises must be counted at the end of each workday, verified by two individuals for accuracy of count, and recorded on an audit sheet. An inventory record of Schedule II drugs must be submitted to the DEA every two years.

Due to the increase in office and clinic drug theft and substance abuse, as well as the stringent federal laws that apply to storing, dispensing, and administration of controlled substances, many offices and clinics do not keep controlled substances on the premises.

Medical Assistant Role and Responsibilities. Medical assistants are required to know the legalities that surround controlled substances. Medical assistant responsibilities may include:

1. Monitor the physician's DEA registration renewal date
2. Maintain legally designated records and inventories of drugs (Figure 35-2)
3. Provide security for all drugs, in particular controlled substances
4. Provide security for prescription pads
5. Properly destroy expired drugs and document
6. Know and understand federal and state laws that regulate drugs, including controlled substances

Prescription Drugs

State laws require that licensed practitioners who prescribe drugs must write and sign an order for the dispensing of drugs. This process is known as writing a prescription. Some examples of drugs that require a prescription are all of the controlled substances (except for

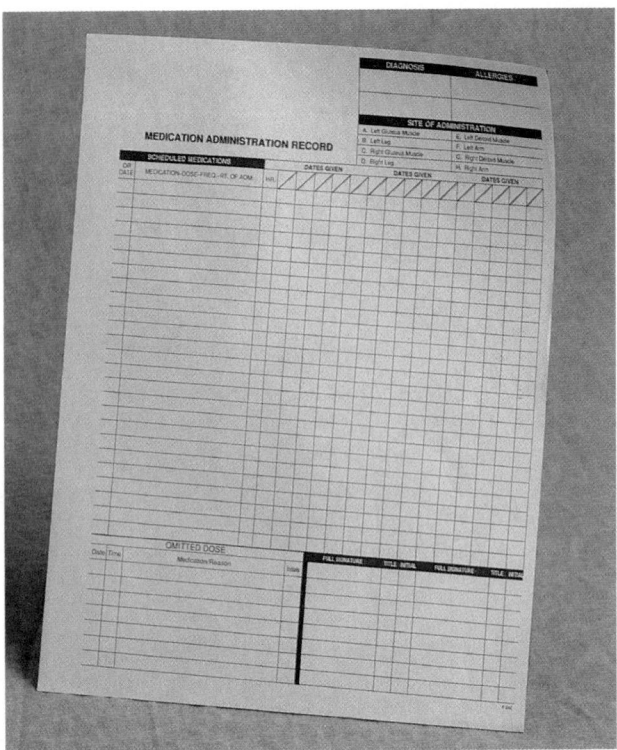

Figure 35-2 It is important to maintain patient medication records both for the safety of the patient and to protect the practice.

Schedule I) such as meperidine and pentobarbital, and other categories such as digoxin, a cardiac drug, and epinephrine, a vasoconstrictor.

Medical assistants need to advise patients after the physician prescribes a drug. See Figure 35-3 for a list of patient education considerations. Patients should also read warning labels on medication containers (Figure 35-4).

Guidelines for patients who take prescription medications include:

1. Take exactly as directed.
2. Inform the physician of unusual or adverse reactions.
3. Continue to take the medication for the duration of the prescribed number of days, weeks, etc.
4. If you want to discontinue the medication, inform your physician.
5. Do not take other medications or herbs concurrently without checking with your physician.
6. Do not take someone else's prescribed medication.
7. Store all medications away from children.
8. Discard unused medication properly.
9. Heed warning labels on medication containers.

Figure 35-3 Guidelines for patients when taking prescription medications.

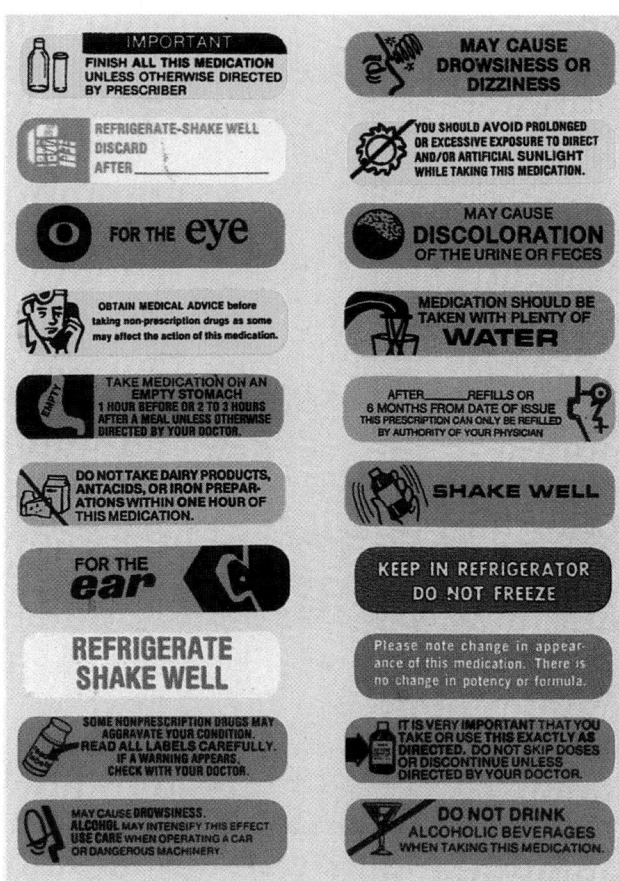

Figure 35-4 Warning labels are placed on prescription medication containers, and patients should be advised to read and adhere to the precautions or instructions.

Nonprescription Drugs

Drugs that are frequently referred to as over-the-counter (OTC) drugs fall into the category of nonprescription drugs. These drugs are readily accessible to the public. They do not require a prescription because the FDA considers them safe to use without a physician's advice. Examples of OTC drugs are aspirin, ibuprofen, and vitamins such as vitamin C. While over-the-counter drugs are considered safe, it is useful for the medical assistant to offer patients some guidelines (Figure 35-5).

Proper Disposal of Drugs

All drug labels contain an expiration date. When that date has been reached, the drug must be removed from the shelf and destroyed (Figure 35-6).

An expired drug cannot be dispensed nor administered because it could be harmful.

To destroy expired drugs, liquids and ointments can be rinsed down the drain and will be destroyed by the sewage system. Powdered drugs can be mixed with water and disposed of in the same manner. Pills and capsules can

Because patients are more aware and better informed about their health care needs, they are becoming more involved in making choices and decisions about their health care. When they choose to take over-the-counter (OTC) drugs, they need information and guidance. Over the past few years, some previous prescription drugs have been changed to OTC drugs. The safety of these drugs can only be assured if patients take them as directed.

Patients need to realize that OTC medications:

1. Can interact with other drugs (either prescribed or other OTCs) and cause undesirable or adverse reactions or complications
2. May be used in lieu of seeking professional help and thereby interfere with the need for medical care
3. Can mask symptoms and exacerbate an existing condition
4. May have several active ingredients, which may be found to be undesirable
5. Have a safe minimum dose, which may not have the desired therapeutic effect

Figure 35-5 Guidelines for patients when taking nonprescription (over-the-counter) medications.

be flushed down the toilet. Vials and ampules of liquid drugs are opened and their contents poured down the drain.

If a medication is removed from its original container, it should not be used (for example, the patient refused the medication); do not replace it in the container. Dispose of it as outlined earlier.

Outdated and expired controlled substances are handled differently. They must be returned to the pharmacy (as required by law). If a controlled substance has been either dropped onto the floor (and is thus unfit to be

Patient Teaching Tip

Many patients keep unused medications past their expiration date. This presents a potential health hazard, as some medications lose their potency after a period of time, while others become toxic. It is best to inform patients to discard any unused portion of medication by the stated date. Encourage patients to check their medicine cabinets at the same time every year so it becomes a routine practice.

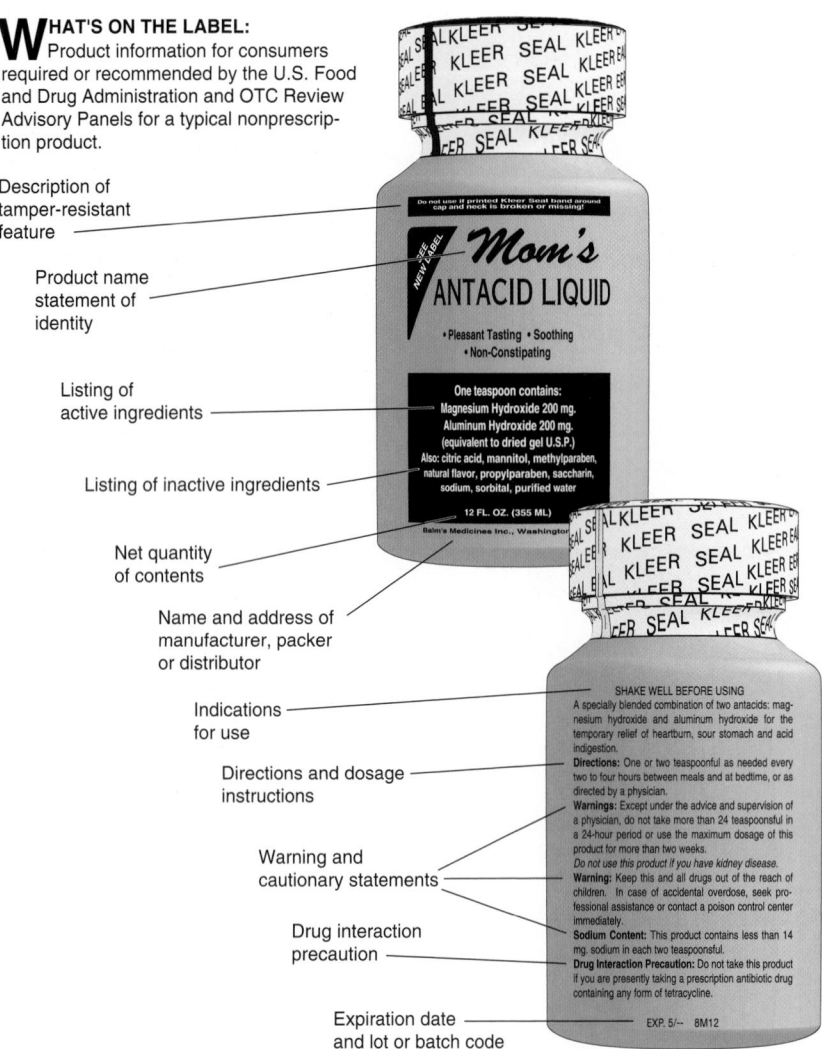

WHAT'S ON THE LABEL:
Product information for consumers required or recommended by the U.S. Food and Drug Administration and OTC Review Advisory Panels for a typical nonprescription product.

Description of tamper-resistant feature

Product name statement of identity

Listing of active ingredients

Listing of inactive ingredients

Net quantity of contents

Name and address of manufacturer, packer or distributor

Indications for use

Directions and dosage instructions

Warning and cautionary statements

Drug interaction precaution

Expiration date and lot or batch code

Figure 35-6 Medication labels contain valuable information essential to the safe and effective use of the drug.

SPOTLIGHT ON AAMA ESSENTIALS THROUGH CAAHEP

● Being aware of a patient's cultural or ethnic background will help in understanding his or her concerns about taking or refusing medications.

● Since patients may not have a complete understanding of the effects of over-the-counter drugs, it's important that the medical assistant be available to offer some guidelines.

● It's important to understand that older adults may need special assistance with their medications.

given to a patient) or has spilled (if in liquid form), a witness should verify the action and proper documentation must take place.

The local DEA office and local police must be notified and the appropriate paperwork completed if there has been a loss or theft of a controlled substance.

Administer, Prescribe, Dispense

There are three ways to handle drugs in the physician's office or clinic: by prescribing, dispensing, or administering them. To **prescribe** a drug means that the licensed practitioner (physician, physician assistant, or nurse practitioner) gives a written order to be taken to the pharmacist to be filled. To **dispense** a drug means to give the medication (either prescription or OTC) to the patient to be taken at another time. To **administer** a drug means to give it to the patient by mouth or injection or any other method of administration.

While state laws vary, some states allow certain professionals including medical assistants to prepare and administer medications under the licensed practitioner's supervision. Usually, it is the physician and pharmacist who dispense medications. However, medical assistants can also dispense samples of drugs under the physician's direction. Although medical assistants act as the physician's agent when they prepare and administer medication, they are ethically and legally responsible for their own actions and can be subject to legal action should harm come to a patient. The law requires that individuals who prepare and administer medications know the medications and their side effects.

DRUG REFERENCES AND STANDARDS

The strength, purity, and quality of drugs differ depending on how they are manufactured. To control the differences, standards have been set. By law, the various drug products must meet standards that are set forth by the U.S. Food and Drug Administration (FDA). A special reference book, *United States Pharmacopeia/National Formulary*, lists the drugs for which standards have been established. The book is recognized by the U.S. government as the official list of drug standards, which are enforced by the FDA. Every five years the book is updated in an attempt to include all drug products in the United States.

Other useful books used as references include the *Compendium of Drug Therapy* and *Desk Reference for Nonprescription Drugs*, and the *Physician's Desk Reference* (PDR), which is published annually by Medical Economics Company in cooperation with pharmaceutical companies. It is one of the most widely used reference books and is found in most offices and clinics. It is divided into seven sections of drug information, which are followed by other useful drug information such as a list of products, poison control 800 telephone numbers, conversion tables, and a guide to management of drug overdose (Figure 35-7).

How To Use the PDR

The four most commonly used sections of the PDR list drugs according to:

- Brand name and generic name (pink section), section 2
- Classification or category (blue section), section 3
- Product information (white section), section 5
- Alphabetical arrangement by manufacturers (white section), section 1

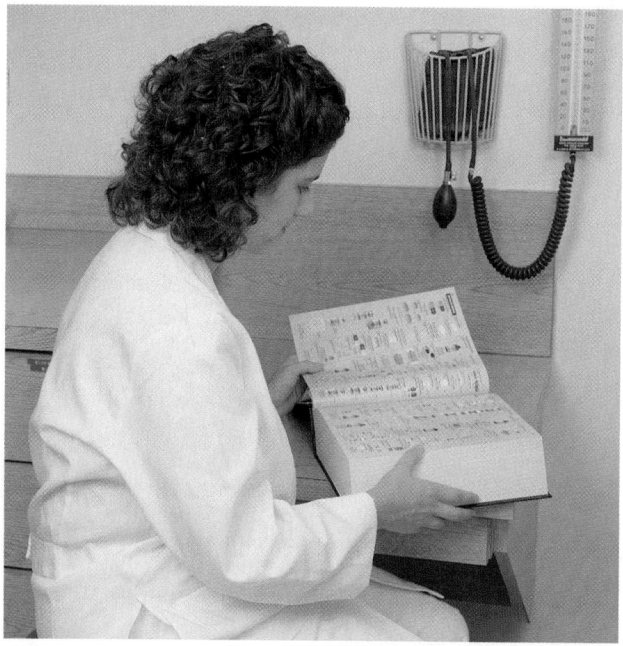

Figure 35-7 The *Physicians' Desk Reference* (PDR) is a valuable resource for the medical assistant who wishes to obtain information about a specific medication.

The following guidelines will assist you as you learn to use the PDR.

1. If you know the brand name of the drug, turn to the pink section and locate the drug in the alphabetical listing. The manufacturer's name will be in parentheses, followed by a page number or two page numbers. The first number is the product identification page number. The second number is the product information section (white).

Example: Look up Achromycin V capsules in a current PDR. This example is based on the 2000 edition.

Achromycin V®

[a-kro-mi-cin]

tetracycline HCl

for ORAL USE

Turn to page 1528 of the PDR (2000 edition) and note all the information provided about the drug.

- *Description.* Gives the origin and chemical composition of the drug.
- *Clinical Pharmacology.* Indicates the effect of the drug upon the body and the process by which the drug exerts this effect.
- *Indications.* States the various conditions, diseases, types of microorganisms, etc., for which the drug is used.

- *Contraindications.* States when the drug should not be given to a specified person.

- *Warnings.* Gives the potential dangers of the drug.

- *Precautions.* States the possible unfavorable effects that the drug may have upon a patient.

- *Adverse Reactions.* Lists the side effects of the drug.

- *Dosage and Administration.* States the amount (usual daily dose for adults and children) and time sequence of administration.

- *How Supplied.* Lists the various forms of the drug and their dosages.

2. If you know the classification of the drug, turn to the blue section and locate the category of the drug.

   Example: Antibiotics, systemic

   Tetracyclines

   Achromycin V® capsules (Lederle)
   p. 1528

NOTE: All controlled substances listed in the PDR are indicated with the symbol C with the Roman numeral II, III, IV, or V printed inside the C to designate the schedule in which the substance is classified.

   Example: Duramorph® Ⓒ, morphine sulfate USP.

Other Reference Sources

On occasion you may not find the drug that you are looking for listed in the PDR. When this happens:

- Refer to another drug reference book

- Ask a pharmacist about the drug

- Refer to the packet insert that comes in the drug package

The package insert that most manufacturers provide with their products is an important source of information about a particular drug. This is a brief description of the drug, its clinical pharmacology, indications and usage, contraindications (any symptom or circumstance that indicates that the use of a particular drug is inappropriate when it would otherwise be advisable), warnings, precautions, drug interactions, adverse reactions, overdose, dosage, and administration. The package insert can be a valuable source of information about drugs that might not be listed elsewhere.

Information about some older medications, such as digoxin, can be found in the package insert since they may have been deleted from the current PDR. The package insert also is a useful tool in the absence of a PDR.

CLASSIFICATION OF DRUGS

Drugs can be classified (arranged in groups) in a number of ways. Some examples are:

- Drugs used to treat or prevent disease (examples are hormones and vaccines)

- Drugs that have a principal action on the body (examples are analgesics and anti-inflammatory drugs)

- Drugs that act on specific body systems or organs (examples are respiratory and cardiovascular drugs)

- Drug preparation (examples are suppository, liquid)

Table 35-1 shows a list of common drug classifications. See the Appendix for the most widely prescribed generic and brand name medications.

PRINCIPLE ACTIONS OF DRUGS

In general, drugs may be grouped as follows: those that act directly upon one or more tissues of the body; those that act upon microorganisms; and those that replace body chemicals.

Certain drugs have selective action, such as stimulants, which increase cell activity, and depressants, which decrease cell activity.

Other drugs may have what is known as:

1. *Local action.* The drug acts on the area to which it is administered.
2. *Remote action.* A drug affects a part of the body that is distant from the site of administration.
3. *Systemic action.* The drug is carried via the bloodstream throughout the body.
4. *Synergistic action.* One drug increases the action of another.

Factors that Affect Drug Action

The four principal factors that affect drug action are: absorption, distribution, biotransformation, and elimination. These factors depend upon the individual patient, the form and chemical composition of the drug, and the method of administration.

1. *Absorption* is the process whereby the drug passes into the body fluids and tissues.
2. *Distribution* is the process whereby the drug is transported from the blood to the intended site of action, site of biotransformation, site of storage, and site of elimination.
3. *Biotransformation* is the chemical alteration that a drug undergoes in the body.
4. *Elimination* is the process whereby the drug is excreted from the body. Elimination occurs via the

TABLE 35-1 COMMON CLASSIFICATIONS OF DRUGS AND THEIR ACTIONS

Classification (with Phonetic Spelling)	Action	Examples of Drugs Commonly Used in Ambulatory Care Setting
Analgesic (an″al-je′sik)	An agent that relieves pain without causing loss of consciousness.	acetaminophen (Tylenol) acetylsalicylic acid (aspirin) ibuprofen (Advil, Motrin)
Anesthetic (an″es-thet′ik)	An agent that produces a lack of feeling. May be local or general depending upon the type and how administered.	lidocaine HCl (Xylocaine) procaine HCl (Novacaine)
Antacid (ant-as′id)	An agent that neutralizes acid.	Amphojel, Gelusil, Mylanta, Milk of Magnesia
Antianemic	An agent that replaces iron.	iron (imferon), ferrous sulfate
Antianxiety (an″ti-ang-zi′e-te)	An agent that relieves anxiety and muscle tension.	benzodiazepines: diazepam (Valium) chlordiazepoxide HCl (Librium) alprazolam (Xanax)
Antiarrhythmic (an″te-a-rith′mik)	An agent that controls cardiac arrhythmias.	lidocaine HCl (Xylocaine) propranolol HCl (Inderal)
Antibiotic (an″ti-bi-ot′ik)	An agent that is destructive to or inhibits growth of microorganisms.	penicillins (Pentids, Duracillin, Polycillin, Pipracil, Augmentin)
Anticholinergic (an″ti-ko″lin-er′jik)	An agent that blocks parasympathetic nerve impulses.	atropine, scopolamine, trihexyphenidyl HCl (Artane)
Anticoagulant (an″ti-ko-ag′u-lant)	An agent that prevents or delays blood clotting.	heparin sodium, Dicumarol, warfarin sodium (Coumadin)
Anticonvulsant (an″ti-kon-vul′sant)	An agent that prevents or relieves convulsions.	carbamazepine (Tegretol) phenytoin (Dilantin) ethosuximide (Zarontin)
Antidepressant (an″ti-dep-res′ant)	An agent that prevents or relieves the symptoms of depression.	monamine oxidase (MAO) inhibitors: isocarboxazid (Marplan), phenelzine sulfate (Nardil), amitriptyline HCl (Elavil), imipramine HCl (Tofranil), trazodone (Desyrel), fluoxentine (Prozac)
Antidiarrheal (an″ti-di-a-re′al)	An agent that prevents or relieves diarrhea.	Pepto-Bismol, Kaopectate, Diphenoxylate HCl (Lomotil)
Antidote (an-ti′dot)	An agent that counteracts poisons and their effects.	naloxone (Narcan)
Antiemetic (an″ti-e-met′ik)	An agent that prevents or relieves nausea and vomiting.	Tigan, Dramamine, Phenergan, Reglan, Marinol
Antihistamine (an″ti-his′ta-min)	An agent that acts to counteract histamine.	Dimetane, Benadryl, Seldane
Antihypertensive (an″ti-hi″per-ten′siv)	An agent that prevents or controls high blood pressure.	methyldopa (Aldomet) clonidine HCl (Catapres) metoprolol tartrate (Lopressor)
Anti-inflammatory (an″ti-in-flam′a-to-re)	An agent that counteracts inflammation.	naproxen (Naprosyn) aspirin, ibuprofen (Advil, Motrin)
Antimanic (an″ti-man′ik)	An agent used for the treatment of the manic episode of manic-depressive disorder.	lithium
Antineoplastic (an″ti-ne″o-plas′tik)	An agent that kills or destroys malignant cells.	busuflan (Myleran) cyclophosphamide (Cytoxan)
Antipsychotic	An agent that helps in schizophrenia and chronic brain syndrome.	haloperdol (Haldol) chlorpromazine (Thorazine)
Antipyretic (an″ti-pi-ret′ik)	An agent that reduces fever.	aspirin, acetaminophen (Tylenol)
Antitussive (an″ti-tus′iv)	An agent that prevents or relieves cough.	codeine, dextromethorphan (Pertussin, Romilar)
Antiulcer (an″ti-ul′ser)	An agent that relieves and heals ulcers.	cimetidine (Tagamet) ranitidine (Zantac)
Bronchodilator (brong″ko-dil-a′tor)	An agent that dilates the bronchi.	isoproterenol HCl (Isuprel) albuterol (Proventil)

(continues)

TABLE 35-1   *(continued)*

Classification (with Phonetic Spelling)	Action	Examples of Drugs Commonly Used in Ambulatory Care Setting
Contraceptive (kon"tra-sep'tiv)	Any device, method, or agent that prevents conception.	Envid-E 21, Ortho-Novum 10/11-21; 10/11-28 Triphasil-21
Decongestant (de"con-gest'ant)	An agent that reduces nasal congestion and/or swelling.	oxymetazoline (Afrin) phenylephrine HCl (Neo-Synephrine) pseudoephedrine HCl (Sudafed)
Diuretic (di"u-ret'ik)	An agent that increases the excretion of urine.	chlorothiazide (Diuril) furosemide (Lasix) mannitol (Osmitrol)
Expectorant (ek-spek'to-rant)	An agent that facilitates removal of secretion from broncho-pulmonary mucous membrane.	guaifenesin (Robitussin)
Hemostatic (he"mo-stat'ik)	An agent that controls or stops bleeding.	Humafac, Amicar, vitamin K
Hypnotic (hip-not'ik)	An agent that produces sleep or hypnosis.	secobarbital (Seconal); chloral hydrate; ethchlorvynol (Placidyl)
Hypoglycemic (hi"po-gli-se'mik)	An agent that lowers blood glucose level.	insulin; chlorpropamide (Diabinese)
Laxative (lak'sa-tiv)	An agent that loosens and promotes normal bowel elimination.	Metamucil powder, Dulcolax
Muscle relaxant (mus'el re-lak'sant)	An agent that produces relaxation of skeletal muscle.	Robaxin, Norflex, Paraflex, Skelaxin, Valium
Sedative (sed'a-tiv)	An agent that produces a calming effect without causing sleep.	amobarbital (amytal) butabarbital sodium (Buticaps) phenobarbital
Tranquilizer (tran"kwi-liz'er)	An agent that reduces mental tension and anxiety.	Thorazine, Mellaril, Haldol
Vasodilator (vas"o-di-la'tor)	An agent that produces relaxation of blood vessels; lowers blood pressure.	isorbide dinitrate (Isordil) nitroglycerin
vasopressor (vas"o-pres'or)	An agent that produces contraction of muscles of capillaries and arteries; elevates blood pressure.	metaraminol (Aramine) norepinephrine (Levophed)

gastrointestinal tract, respiratory tract, skin, mucous membranes, and mammary glands.

Undesirable Actions of Drugs

Most drugs have the potential for causing an action other than their intended action. For example:

1. *Side Effect.* An undesirable action of the drug that may limit the usefulness of the drug.
2. *Drug Interaction.* Occurs when one drug potentiates—increases—or diminishes the action of another drug. These actions may be desirable or undesirable. Drugs may also interact with various foods, alcohol, tobacco, and other substances.
3. *Adverse Reaction.* An unfavorable or harmful unintended action of a drug, such as an allergic reaction.

A patient may experience an allergic reaction to a drug after administration. It is often mild and may exhibit itself in the form of a rash, **urticaria**, or **pruritus**. On occasion, a severe reaction or **anaphylaxis** can occur, which is hypersensitivity to a drug or other foreign protein. It is the least common allergic reaction, but can become severe very quickly and result in dyspnea and shock. Loss of consciousness and death can result. To help prevent an allergic reaction or minimize its risk, the medical assistant should attempt to ascertain prior to administration of every drug whether the patient has any known allergies. The medical assistant should be aware of signs and symptoms of allergic reaction and notify the physician immediately so that appropriate emergency treatment can be given. One or two injections of epinephrine usually reverses the life-threatening symptoms of anaphylaxis and is followed by administration of an antihistamine such as Benadryl®.

DRUG ROUTES

Drugs are manufactured in a variety of forms and for various purposes. The route of a drug refers to how it is administered to the patient and thereby transported into the patient's body. Certain medications can be administered by more than one route, while others must be administered via a specific route.

The route of administration is determined by a number of factors. One factor is the action of the medication on the body, either local or systemic. Intravenous medication reaches the systemic circulation rapidly via the bloodstream and quickly becomes effective. Injections of medication and medications absorbed through mucous membranes are absorbed quickly. Oral medications take longer to act since they must be digested by the stomach and then be absorbed into the bloodstream.

Another factor in route selection is the physical and emotional state of the patient. The patient's consciousness level, emotional status, and physical restrictions are considered when selecting a route to administer medication.

A third factor to consider is the characteristics of the drug. An example is insulin. Insulin is destroyed by digestive enzymes; therefore, the route of administration must be by injection.

The most frequently utilized routes of administering medication to the patient are oral and parenteral routes: oral medications are taken by mouth; parenteral generally by injection. Other routes of administration include:

- Direct application to the skin (lotions, creams, liniments, ointments, and transdermal systems)
- Sublingual (tablets, liquid, drops)
- Buccal (tablets)
- Rectal (suppositories, ointments)
- Vaginal (suppositories, creams, tablets, applications)
- Inhalation (sprays, aerosols)
- Instillation (liquid, drops)

FORMS OF DRUGS

Drugs are compounded in three basic types of preparations: liquids, solids, and semisolids. The ease with which a drug's ingredients can be dissolved largely determines the variety of forms manufactured. Some drug agents are soluble in water, others in alcohol, and others in a mixture of several solvents.

The method for administering a drug depends upon its form, its properties, and the effects desired. When given orally, a drug may be in the form of a liquid, powder, tablet, capsule, or caplet. If it is to be injected, it must be in the form of a liquid. For topical use, the drug may be in the form of a liquid, powder, or semisolid. Oral and injectable medications are examples of preparations designed for internal use.

Liquid Preparations

Liquid preparations are those containing a drug that has been dissolved or suspended. Depending upon the solvent used, the drug may be further classified as an aqueous (water) or alcohol preparation. When prescribed for internal use, liquid preparations other than emulsions are rapidly absorbed through the stomach or intestinal walls.

Solid and Semisolid Preparations

Tablets, capsules, caplets, troches or lozenges, suppositories, and ointments are examples of solid and semisolid preparations. These products offer great flexibility as a means of dispensing different dosages of drugs (Figure 35-8).

Other Drug Delivery Systems

Technological advances have introduced new ways by which drugs can be introduced into the patient. In addition to the conventional preparations, the following miniature therapeutic systems offer special delivery of medication to targeted areas.

Transdermal System. The transdermal system of medication delivery consists of a small adhesive patch that may be applied to intact skin near the treatment site. For example, Transderm Scop® used for preventing motion sickness, may be applied behind the ear; Nitro-Dur® (Figure 35-9), used for preventing angina pectoris, may be applied to the chest; Estraderm®, used to treat menopausal symptoms, may be applied to the trunk, and Nicoderm®, used to relieve the body's craving for nicotine, may be applied to any area above the waist. A transdermal system generally consists of four layers (Figure 35-10):

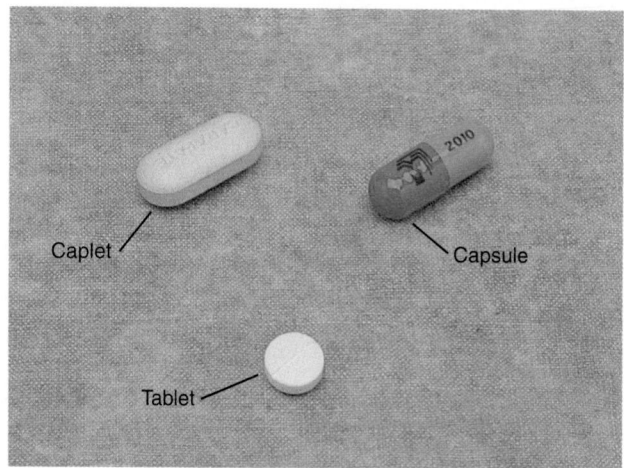

Figure 35-8 Drugs are manufactured in various forms, including solid preparations like this caplet, capsule, and tablet.

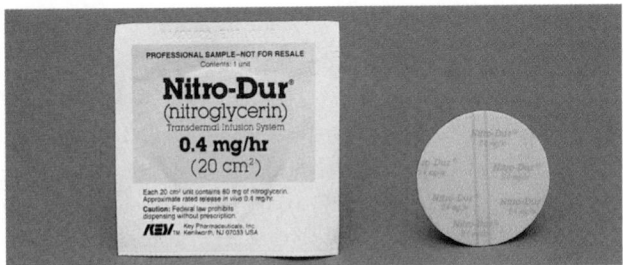

Figure 35-9   Nitro-Dur® is a transdermal system of delivering medication used for preventing and for long-term management of angina pectoris. It may be applied to the chest.

1. An impermeable backing that keeps the drug from leaking out of the system
2. A reservoir containing the drug
3. A membrane with tiny holes that controls the rate of drug release
4. An adhesive layer or gel that keeps the device in place

Eye-Curing Lens. Another innovative drug delivery system is one in which a drug, contained between two ultrathin plastic membranes, is placed inside the lower eyelid. It appears to cause little or no discomfort and provides a controlled release of the medication for an extended period of time. Pilocarpine, a miotic that causes contraction of the pupils, is being used in this method for the treatment of glaucoma.

Implantable Devices. These devices are available in several shapes and sizes and are positioned just beneath the skin near blood vessels that lead directly to the area to be medicated. For example, an infusion pump that is about the size of a hockey puck can be implanted below the skin near the waist to provide continuous delivery of chemotherapy to patients with liver cancer. This device, which has a refillable drug reservoir, is connected by an outlet catheter to the patient's blood vessel. In addition to providing a continuous supply of medication, these devices have the advantage of delivering higher doses with fewer side effects than can be realized through the systemic route.

STORAGE AND HANDLING OF MEDICATIONS

Certain precautions should be followed if the ambulatory care setting keeps medications on the premises. The goal should be to store all medications in their original containers in a separate room in a locked cabinet. Many medications require storage in a certain manner, such as a dark area or in a dark container (to keep light away from them) or in the refrigerator. Some must be kept in glass containers only because

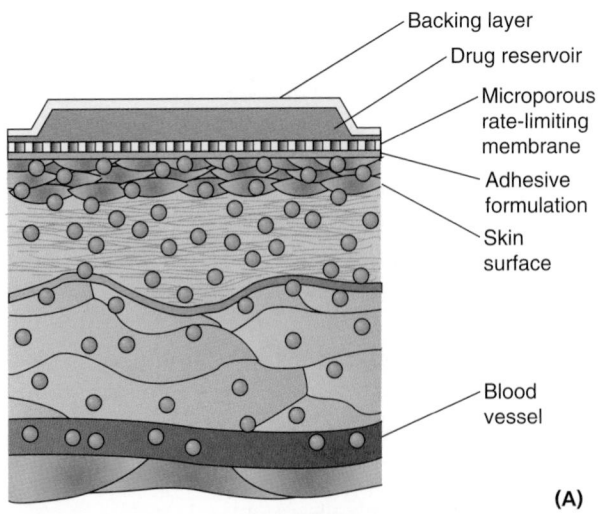

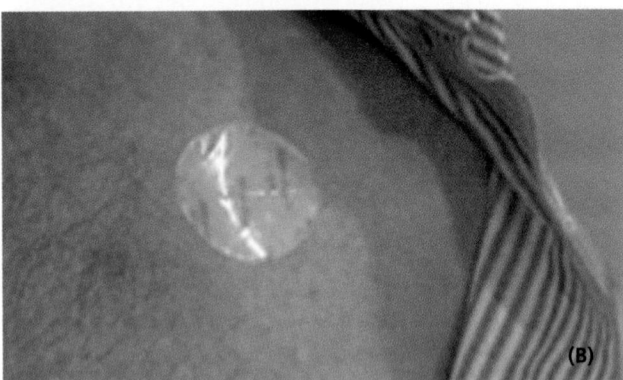

Figure 35-10   (A) The multilayer unit comprising Transderm-Nitro® delivers nitroglycerin into the bloodstream in a consistent, controlled manner for 24 hours. The very thin unit contains a backing layer, a reservoir of nitroglycerin, a unique rate-limiting membrane, and an adhesive layer that has a priming dose of nitroglycerin. (B) The patch is applied to the skin. (Courtesy of CIBA Pharmaceutical Company)

plastic may react with the medication's chemical composition. The drug label indicates proper storage and handling for each medication.

Keep medications that are for internal use separated from those intended for external use.

Access to medications is simplified if they are organized in the storage area either according to their classification (diuretic, hormones) or according to the alphabet.

EMERGENCY DRUGS AND SUPPLIES

The ambulatory care setting should maintain a tray, box, cabinet, or crash cart (see Chapter 9) especially and solely for drugs and supplies needed in an emergency such as anaphylaxis or other form of shock. The drugs listed in Table 35-2 are a sample of some general drugs to keep readily available for emergencies.

TABLE 35-2 EXAMPLES OF COMMON EMERGENCY DRUGS

Adrenalin (a-dren'a-lin) or **epinephrine** (ep-i-nef-rin)
A vasoconstrictor. Relieves anaphylactic shock.

Aminophylline (am-in-off'ilin)
A bronchodilator. Relaxes smooth muscle of the respiratory tract.

Benadryl (ben'a-dril)
An antihistamine that relieves allergic symptoms.

Compazine (com-pa'zeen)
An antiemetic. Relieves symptoms of nausea and vomiting.

Dextrose (deks'trose) 50%
Used for hypoglycemia to counteract hyperinsulinism.

Digoxin (di-jox'in)
Cardiac drug. Used for congestive heart failure, arryhthmias. Slows and strengthens heartbeat.

Diuril (di'ur-il)
Promotes excretion of urine.

Hydrocortisone (hi"dro-cort'i-zon)
An anti-inflammatory. Used to suppress swelling and shock.

Ipecac Syrup (i'pe-kak)
Emetic. Used to induce vomiting in certain types of poisonings.

Narcan (nar'can)
Antidote. Used in narcotic overdose.

Nitroglycerin (ni"tro-glis'er-in)
Vasodilator. Dilates coronary arteries. Used in treatment of angina pectoris.

Valium (val'e-um)
Antianxiety, muscle relaxant. Used to calm very anxious patients and to relax muscles. Valium is a Schedule IV drug and therefore must be kept in a locked cabinet.

Other supplies and equipment to keep along with the drugs on the emergency cart are:

- Intravenous materials such as IV fluids, needles, syringes, alcohol, swabs, constriction band, and tape
- Sphygmomanometer
- Stethoscope
- Oxygen and mask
- Airways
- Defibrillator
- Suction equipment (nasopharyngeal)

Check the tray on a regular basis (weekly, monthly, depending on use) according to need. Check the oxygen tank and gauge. Replace items that have been used as soon as possible and discard drugs and supplies that have reached their expiration dates. Document that the tray has been checked and updated. (See Chapter 9 for more information about emergencies in the office and other ambulatory areas.)

DRUG ABUSE

 There has been an enormous increase in the **abuse**, or misuse, of legal and illegal drugs. Any drug can be abused, whether it is penicillin, alcohol, or a controlled substance such as cocaine. Medical assistants, while caring for patients, may unexpectedly come in contact with patients who abuse or misuse drugs.

Medical assistants must be able to recognize the symptoms of drug abuse in a patient or coworker and report it to the physician. Health professionals including physicians are among the individuals who may have a problem with drug or alcohol abuse and this must be reported to the proper professional association. Refer to Chapter 7 for more information on drug abuse.

There are many programs available for treatment of drug abuse. Detoxification and rehabilitation are examples of treatment programs.

Following are examples of drug types most commonly abused:

- Marijuana, LSD ("acid"), Mescaline
- Narcotics: Cocaine, Heroin
- Amphetamines: Dexedrine®, Ritalin®
- Depressants: Valium®, alcohol
- Barbiturates ("barbs," "downers," "red devils") Nembutal®, Seconal®

Effects of Drug Abuse

When an individual is directly under the influence of a particular substance, acute effects of drug abuse are evident. For example, the acute effects of amphetamines may include symptoms that affect the central nervous system, such as euphoria, excitement, anorexia, or insomnia. Dilated pupils, nervousness, talkativeness, agitation, tachycardia, fever, and chills are other symptoms of amphetamine abuse.

As an abused substance, cocaine is usually sniffed or snorted into the nose or smoked in a form called crack or freebase. It is absorbed through the mucous membrane. Effects begin within a few minutes and then subside within an hour. Dilated pupils, elevated blood pressure, tachycardia, and increased body temperature are symptoms of the acute effects of cocaine. Euphoria and excitement are probable reasons for its high abuse potential. Death comes from respiratory and circulatory failure.

Barbiturates are used medically as sedatives to relieve anxiety. Abuse effects include slurred speech, confusion, poor motor coordination, and impaired judgment. Coma and death result from very high doses. Abrupt withdrawal can be fatal and symptoms include apprehension, weakness, tremors, delirium, and convulsions.

LSD (lyseric acid diethylamide) is a hallucinogenic agent with no medicinal benefit. It is an extremely potent drug causing altered perception and mood changes that range from euphoria to deep depression. Long-term use can cause chromosomal changes and prolonged adverse psychological effects such as suicide attempts.

Marijuana is usually used by smoking it in the form of a hand-rolled cigarette. Feelings of euphoria, relaxation, and drowsiness are the primary effects of the drug. Individuals lose inhibitions and may exhibit inappropriate behavior, poor coordination, and poor judgment. Hallucinations are possible. Tachycardia, increased appetite, and decreased pulmonary function are other symptoms that can occur and aggravate existing medical conditions such as heart disease or hypertension. Although marijuana has been shown to have some limited medicinal uses, in most states it remains classified as a Schedule I drug under the Federal Controlled Substance Act.

The same social pressures that influence young people to try alcohol are responsible for introducing people of all ages to the previously mentioned drugs and other chemical substances. Because it is easier to prevent drug abuse than it is to break an established habit, most efforts to combat drug abuse are directed at the young. However, people of all ages, including older people, may be or become abusers.

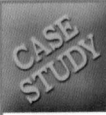

Maria Jover complains of vaginal discharge and discomfort. Dr. King confirms the diagnosis of a yeast infection by performing a smear and identifying the microorganism. Dr. King prescribes over-the-counter vaginal suppositories. After asking Maria if she has any questions, medical assistant Audrey Jones proceeds to help Maria understand the self-administration of this particular medication.

35-1

CASE STUDY REVIEW

1. The patient, Maria, asks Audrey Jones whether she can use some vaginal suppositories she bought last year. How should Audrey respond?

2. Maria tells Audrey that the last time she had a vaginal yeast infection she only used part of the recommended number of suppositories because the infection cleared up. How should Audrey respond?

3. Maria does not really like using suppositories. Should Audrey ask Dr. King to prescribe another form of medication for the yeast infection? What other forms might be available?

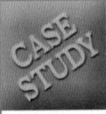

Dr. Lewis keeps a small quantity of various controlled substances on the premises for use in an emergency situation.

35-2

CASE STUDY REVIEW

1. What are the legalities that surround controlled substances in so far as Joe Guerrero, the medical assistant, is concerned?

2. What are his responsibilities?

SUMMARY

Medical assistants must know state and federal laws that govern the distribution and administration of medications and understand their role and responsibilities in light of these laws. Knowledge of drug regulations, the legal classifications of drugs including controlled substances, and prescribing, administering, and dispensing of drugs is essential to ensure compliance with the law.

Available resources and reference books will provide valuable information about pharmaceutical products, their classifications, routes, forms, storage and handling, and side effects.

Emergency drugs and supplies should be available on a crash cart or a tray or cabinet for the sole use in an office emergency.

With the increase of drug abuse and misuse, it is important for medical assistants to recognize the signs of drug abuse in patients and coworkers and to report abuse to the physician or supervisor.

REVIEW QUESTIONS

Multiple Choice

1. Which of the following drugs is commonly used in an emergency such as anaphylactic shock?
   a. lomotil
   b. interferon
   c. cytoxan
   d. epinephrine
2. Which of the following types of drugs do physicians prescribe most frequently?
   a. generic
   b. official
   c. chemical
   d. brand
3. An example of a drug that can be obtained from an animal is:
   a. digitalis
   b. insulin
   c. imferon
   d. sulfur
4. Which of the following is an example of a controlled substance?
   a. Nembutal
   b. Keflin
   c. Inderal
   d. Aldomet
5. After you have poured a medication and taken it to the patient, he refuses to take it. You should:
   a. give it to another patient who has the same medication prescribed
   b. return the refused medication to its original container
   c. save it for the next time the patient is due for another dose
   d. dispose of it down the sink and document

Critical Thinking

1. Drugs are derived from various sources. List five sources of drugs.
2. How does the Federal Food, Drug, and Cosmetic Act protect the public?
3. The _____ is recognized by the United States government as the official list of standardized drugs.
4. Describe the principal factors that affect drug action.
5. While preparing an injection of Demerol® (meperidine), you accidentally drop and break the ampule spilling its contents. Describe what actions you would take.

6. Name five emergency drugs that may be found on a crash cart or emergency tray. Describe the use and actions of each.
7. Under what circumstances can a medical assistant dispense stock medication?
8. Audrey Jones is considering taking a new position with a physician who is opening an office in another state. Audrey will be responsible for the clinical aspect of the practice. Where can Audrey find information about laws that apply to her in regard to administering medications? Where can she get information about the storage and handling on the premises of narcotics?
9. List several drug references and briefly describe the contents of the PDR.
10. After lunch, a newly hired medical assistant is helping you get Lenore McDonell back into her wheelchair following her physical examination. You strongly suspect that the medical assistant has been drinking alcohol because she is uncoordinated in her movements and there is a strong odor of what seems to be alcohol on her breath. Describe your next action.

WEB ACTIVITIES

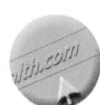

Explore on the Internet for information regarding the Drug Enforcement Agency.

1. Print a copy of Schedules I-V of the controlled substances.

REFERENCES/BIBLIOGRAPHY

Bonewit-West, K. (2000). *Clinical procedures for medical assistants* (5th ed.). Philadelphia: W. B. Saunders Company.

Physicians' desk reference. (2000). Montvale, NJ: Medical Economics.

Prickett-Ramutkowski, B., Barrie, A. T., Keller, C., Dazarow, L., & Abel, C. (1999). *Glencoe medical assisting: A patient-centered approach to administrative and clinical competencies.* New York: Glencoe/McGraw-Hill.

Rice, J. (1999). *Principles of pharmacology for medical assisting* (3rd ed.). Albany, NY: Delmar.

Taber's cyclopedic medical dictionary (18th ed.). (1999). Philadelphia: F. A. Davis Company.

Zakus, S. (2001). *Mosby's clinical skills for medical assistants* (4th ed.). St. Louis: Mosby-Year Book.

CALCULATION OF MEDICATION DOSAGE AND MEDICATION ADMINISTRATION

KEY TERMS

Administering
Apnea
BSA
Compounding
Dispensing
Hypoxemia
Meniscus
Nomogram
Parenteral
Precipitate
Retrolental Fibroplasia
Status Asthmaticus
Taut
Unit Dose

OUTLINE

OBJECTIVES

The student should strive to meet the following performance objectives and demonstrate an understanding of the facts and principles presented in this chapter through written and oral communication.

1. Define the key terms as presented in the glossary.
2. Discuss the legal and ethical implications of medication administration.
3. Describe the medication order.
4. Describe the parts of a prescription.
5. Define drug dosage.
6. State what information is found on a medication label.
7. Understand ratio and proportion.
8. Use the metric, household, and apothecary systems of measurement and convert between metric and apothecary systems.
9. Understand units of medication dosage.
10. Correctly calculate adult and children's dosages.
11. List the guidelines to follow when preparing and administering medications.
12. Describe safe disposal of syringes, needles, and biohazard materials.
13. Describe site selection for administration of injections.
14. Understand allergenic extracts.
15. Describe inhalation medication and its administration.

ROLE DELINEATION COMPONENTS

CLINICAL

Fundamental Principles

- Apply principles of aseptic technique and infection control
- Comply with quality assurance practices

Patient Care

- Prepare patient for examinations, procedures, and treatments
- Assist with examinations, procedures, and treatments
- Prepare and administer medications and immunizations
- Maintain medication and immunization records

(continues)

SCENARIO

At Doctors Lewis & King, office policy dictates that a medicine card must be written out prior to the administration of any medication to a patient. Clinical medical assistant Joe Guerrero, CMA, is very careful to check the physician's order, then prepare the medicine card before preparing and administering medication. He notes that the card contains the patient's name, the physician's order, and the date, time, and route the medication is to be administered. After giving the medication to the patient, Joe documents the fact in the patient file and then, according to procedure, tears up the medicine card.

INTRODUCTION

Despite the fact that many ambulatory care centers use what is known as the unit dose type of medication preparation, there remains a responsibility for medical assistants to know and understand how to calculate dosages of medication and to safely administer them to patients.

This chapter addresses calculation of adult and pediatric dosages of medication using the metric and apothecaries' systems. It also emphasizes the legal aspects of medication administration and discusses oral and parenteral medication administration.

ROLE DELINEATION
COMPONENTS (continued)

GENERAL
(TRANDISCIPLINARY)

Legal Concepts

- Document accurately
- Follow federal, state, and local legal guidelines
- Maintain awareness of federal and state health care legislation and regulations
- Maintain and dispose of regulated substances in compliance with government guidelines
- Comply with established risk management and safety procedures

LEGAL AND ETHICAL IMPLICATIONS OF MEDICATION ADMINISTRATION

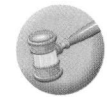

Members of the health care profession who prepare and administer medications are ethically and legally responsible for their own actions. Under law, these individuals are required to be licensed, registered, or otherwise authorized by a physician.

Each state has enacted laws governing the practice of medicine, nursing, and pharmacy. These laws vary from state to state; therefore, it is essential that medical assistants become familiar with the laws of the state in which they are employed before administering any medication. In some states, the only health professional authorized to give injections, other than a physician, is the registered nurse. In other states, legislation gives physicians broad authority to delegate responsibility for administering medication to other health care workers such as medical assistants. Laws have been passed in some states specifying which qualified and properly educated and trained persons may perform certain medical acts.

Regardless of the differences in state authorization laws, the courts will not permit the careless action of health care workers to go unpunished, especially when such actions result in harm or death to the patient. Under the law, those administering medications are expected to be knowledgeable about the drugs that they administer and the effects the drug(s) may and/or will have on the patient. Never administer a medication without thorough knowledge of

the drug. It is the medical assistant's responsibility to know the information about a medication listed in Figure 36-1 before administering it to a patient.

Ethical Considerations

Anyone who has access to medications may be tempted to use them for personal benefit. To do so is not only unethical, it is considered to be illegal. The conversion to personal use of medications intended for another is unethical and may cause harm to the patient. It is also unethical and illegal to take any

medication that belongs to your employer, even aspirin or drug samples, without proper authorization.

The Medication Order

The medication order is given by the physician. It is for a specific patient and denotes the drug to be given, the dosage, the form of the drug, the time for or frequency of administration, and the route by which the drug is to be given.

The Prescription

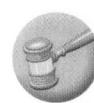

The prescription is a written legal document that gives directions for compounding, dispensing, and administering a medication to a patient. There are nine parts to a prescription (Figure 36-2).

The purpose of a prescription is to control the sale and use of drugs that can be safely and effectively used only under the supervision of a licensed physician. Federal law divides medicines into two main classes: prescription medicines and over-the-counter (OTC) medicines. The prescription is written by the physician and signed with an ink pen. The pharmacist fills the prescription according to the physician's order. Once the prescription has been filled, the assigned prescription number and all other information may be entered into a computer. The hard copy of the prescription is filed and kept for a minimum of seven years. Schedule II controlled substances prescriptions (see Chapter 35) are kept separate from other prescriptions and are

1. Drug name (generic and brand)
2. Action
3. Uses
4. Contraindications
5. Warnings when indicated
6. Adverse reactions
7. Dosage and route
8. Implications for patient care
9. Patient teaching
10. Special considerations

Figure 36-1 Medical assistants should have a thorough knowledge of any medication they administer to a patient and should consult references such as the *Physician's Desk Reference (PDR)*.

Parts of a Prescription

1. The physician's name, address, telephone number, and registration number. [1]
2. The patient's name, address, and the date on which the prescription is written.
3. The *superscription* that includes the symbol Rx ("take thou").
4. The *inscription* that states the names and quantities of ingredients to be included in the medication.
5. The *subscription* that gives directions to the pharmacist for filling the prescription.
6. The *signature* (Sig) that gives the directions for the patient.
7. The physician's signature blanks. Where signed, indicates if a generic substitute is allowed or if the medication is to be dispensed as written.
8. REPETATUR 0 1 2 3 p.r.n. This is where the physician indicates whether or not the prescription can be refilled.
9. □ LABEL Direction to the pharmacist to label the medication appropriately.

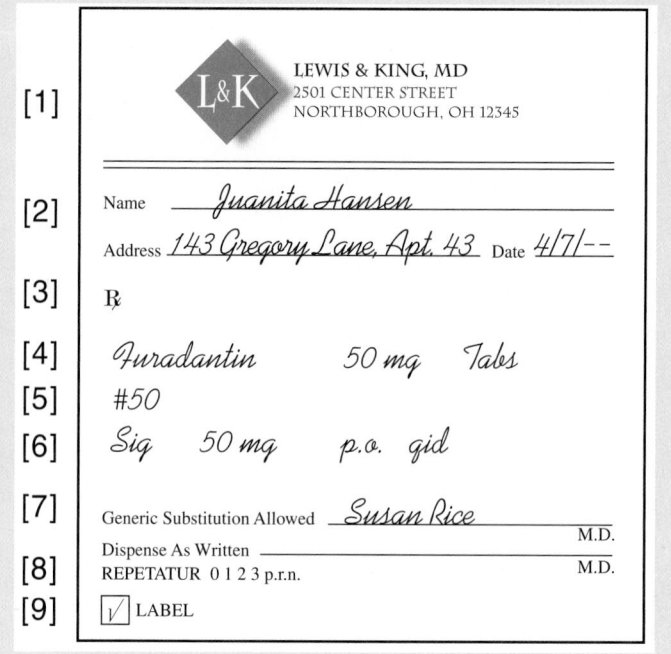

[1] LEWIS & KING, MD
2501 CENTER STREET
NORTHBOROUGH, OH 12345

[2] Name *Juanita Hansen*

Address *143 Gregory Lane, Apt. 43* Date *4/7/--*

[3] Rx

[4] *Furadantin   50 mg   Tabs*

[5] *#50*

[6] *Sig   50 mg   p.o.   qid*

[7] Generic Substitution Allowed *Susan Rice* M.D.

Dispense As Written _____ M.D.

[8] REPETATUR 0 1 2 3 p.r.n.

[9] ☑ LABEL

Figure 36-2 Prescriptions are written legal documents that give directions for compounding, dispensing, and administering a medication. Prescriptions have nine distinct elements.

stamped with a red C. Schedule III through V prescriptions are stamped with a red C and filed.

Prescriptions for Controlled Substances.

Federal laws require that specific procedures be followed by the physician when prescribing controlled substances. See Table 36-1.

All prescriptions for controlled substances must be dated and signed on the date issued, bearing the full name and address of the patient and the name, address, and DEA number (see Chapter 35) of the physician. The prescription must be written in ink or typewritten and signed by the physician's own hand.

TABLE 36-1	REQUIREMENTS FOR PRESCRIPTIONS FOR CONTROLLED SUBSTANCES		
	Verbal Order or Prescription	Written Prescription	Refills
Schedule I	NOT FOR MEDICINAL USE		
Schedule II	no	yes	no
Schedule III	yes	yes	5× or 6 months
Schedule IV	yes	yes	5× or 6 months
Schedule V	yes	yes	yes

Prescription Abbreviations and Symbols. It is important to be knowledgeable of the most common abbreviations used by the physician when an order for a prescription drug is given. The abbreviations are a clear and concise means of writing orders. This medical shorthand is an international language used by professional and nonprofessional people involved with patient care. All abbreviations in Table 36-2 should be memorized to enable medical assistants to prepare medications safely and accurately for administration.

DRUG DOSAGE

The dosage or dose is the amount of medicine that is prescribed for administration. It is determined by the physician or qualified practitioner who considers the following important factors: age, weight, gender, and other factors as well.

Age

The usual adult dose is generally suitable for the 20 to 60 age group. Infants, young children, adolescents, and the elderly require an individualized dosage regimen.

Weight

The average adult dosage is based upon 150 pounds (about 68 kilograms). Individuals who weigh less or more

TABLE 36-2	COMMON PRESCRIPTION ABBREVIATIONS AND SYMBOLS
Abbreviation or Symbol	**Meaning**
aa	of each
ac	before meals
AD	right ear
ad lib	as desired
AS	left ear
aq	water
AU	both ears
bid	twice a day
c	with
cc	cubic centimeter
caps	capsules
dil	dilute
ʒ	dram
elix	elixir
Gm	gram
gr	grain
gt or gtt	drop (drops)
h	hour
hs	at bedtime
IM	intramuscular
IU	international units
IV	intravenous
kg	kilogram
L	liter
liq	liquid
m or min	minim
mg	milligram
ml or ML	milliliter
mm	millimeter
NPO	nothing by mouth
non rep	do not repeat
OD	right eye
OS	left eye
OU	both eyes
℥	ounce
pc	after meals
per	by or with
po	by mouth
prn	as needed
pt	patient
q	every
qd	every day
qh	every hour
q (2, 3, 4) h	every (2, 3, 4) hours
qid	four times a day
qod	every other day
qs	of sufficient quantity
Rx	take
s	without
sc	subcutaneous
sol	solution
ss	one-half
stat	at once
tab	tablet
Tbs	tablespoon
tsp	teaspoon
tid	three times a day
tr	tincture
ung	ointment

than this should have the dosage based upon **BSA** (body surface area) or kilogram of body weight.

Gender

Many medications are contraindicated during pregnancy and breastfeeding. It is important that these two factors be known before any dose of medication is prescribed.

Other Factors

There are other factors that determine the dosage of a medication including:

1. Physical and emotional condition of patient
2. Disease process, especially kidney disease because of impaired excretion
3. Presence of more than one disease process
4. Causative microorganism(s) and the severity of the infection
5. Patient's past medical history, allergies, and idiosyncrasies
6. The safest method, route, time, and amount to effect the desired maximum result

THE MEDICATION LABEL

The medication label can be a source of valuable information to medical assistant and patient. Regardless of whether administering a prescription drug or taking a nonprescription product, an understanding of the information provided on the label is essential to the safe and effective use of any medicine. In addition to the name and address of the manufacturer, other important items of information on a medication label include:

- The trade or brand name for the medication
- The generic name (or listing of active and inactive ingredients)
- The National Drug Code (NDC) numbers that can be used to identify the manufacturer, the product, and the size of the container
- The dosage strength in a given amount of the medication
- The usual dosage and frequency of administration
- The route of administration
- Precautions and warnings
- The expiration date for the medication

Other information that may be on a medication label includes directions for storage and directions for mixing or reconstituting a powdered form of the drug. (See Figure 36-3.)

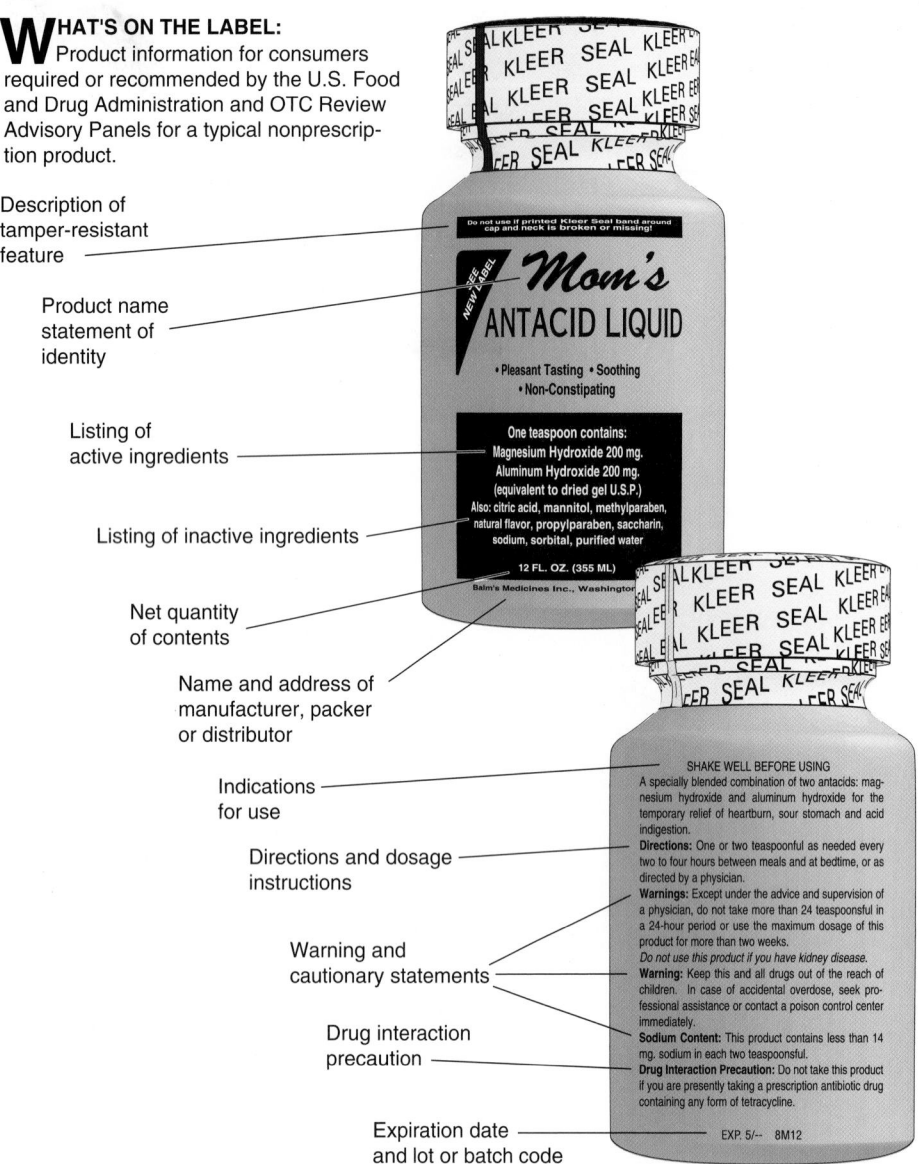

WHAT'S ON THE LABEL: Product information for consumers required or recommended by the U.S. Food and Drug Administration and OTC Review Advisory Panels for a typical nonprescription product.

Description of tamper-resistant feature

Product name statement of identity

Listing of active ingredients

Listing of inactive ingredients

Net quantity of contents

Name and address of manufacturer, packer or distributor

Indications for use

Directions and dosage instructions

Warning and cautionary statements

Drug interaction precaution

Expiration date and lot or batch code

Figure 36-3 Medication labels contain valuable information essential to the safe and effective use of the drug.

CALCULATION OF DRUG DOSAGES

The preparation and administration of medications is one of the most important and critical tasks that medical assistants perform. Today, drugs are more potent and more likely to cause physiological changes in the body; therefore, anyone who administers medications must do so with extreme care.

Incorrectly calculated or measured dosages are the leading cause of error in the administration of medications. A drug error is a violation of a patient's rights. It is important that medical assistants develop a working knowledge of mathematics in order to calculate or measure accurately a medication that is to be administered to a patient.

Understanding Ratio

Ratio is a method of expressing the relationship of a number, quantity, substance, or degree between two similar components. For example, the relationship of one to five is written 1:5. Note that numbers are side by side and separated by a colon.

In mathematics, a ratio may be expressed as a quotient, a fraction, or a decimal.

Ratio Expressed as a Quotient. A quotient is the number found when one number is divided by another number. The ratio one to five written as a quotient is $1 \div 5$.

Ratio Expressed as a Fraction. A fraction is the process of dividing or breaking a whole number into parts. The ratio one to five written as a fraction is ⅕.

Ratio Expressed as a Decimal. A decimal is a linear array of numbers based upon ten or any multiple of ten. To express the ratio one to five as a decimal, divide the denominator (5) into the numerator (1).

$$\text{(denominator)} \quad 5\overline{)1.0}^{\,0.2} \quad \text{(numerator)}$$

The ratio may be expressed as:

A *quotient*	A *fraction*	A *decimal*
$1 \div 5$	$\frac{1}{5}$	0.2

Understanding Proportion

Proportion is a process of expressing the comparative relationship between a part, share, or portion with regard to size, amount, or number. In mathematics, a proportion expresses the relationship between two ratios. In setting up a proportion, the ratios are separated by : or an = sign. In this text, the equal sign (=) is used to separate ratios.

Example: $3 : 4 = 1 : 2$
Read: Three is to four equals one is to two.

The four terms of a proportion are given special names. The *means* are the inner numbers or the second and third terms of the proportion.

Example: $3 : 4 = 1 : 2$ (4)   (1)
                       means

The *extremes* are the outer numbers or the first and fourth terms of the proportion.

Example: $3 : 4 = 1 : 2$ (3)   (2)
                       extremes

In a true proportion, the product of the means equals the product of the extremes.

Example: *means*   (16)   (1)
                  $8 : 16 = 1 : 2$

extremes   (8)   (2)
             $16 \times 1 = 16$ *(means)*
             $8 \times 2 = 16$ *(extremes)*

Solving for X. The proportion is a very useful mathematical tool. When a part, share, or portion of the problem is unknown, then x represents the unknown factor. You can determine the unknown by solving for x. The unknown factor x may appear any place in the proportion. [...] for x in the problem: $3 : 4 = x : 12$.

[...] that contain the x and place the [...] equal sign ($4x$).

2. Multiply the other terms and place the product to the right of the equal sign (36).
3. To find x, divide the product of x into the product of the other terms.

$$4x = 36$$
$$x = \frac{36}{4} \text{ or } 36 \div 4$$
$$x = 9$$

After finding the unknown factor, check your mathematical skills by determining if you have a true proportion. This technique is called proof or proving your answer. To prove your answer:

1. Place the answer you found for x back into the formula where x was.

$$3 : 4 = 9 : 12$$

2. Now multiply the means by the means, and the extremes by the extremes.
3. The results will equal each other.

Formula: $3 : 4 = x : 12$

Proof: $3 : 4 = 9 : 12$

$$4 \times 9 = 36$$
$$3 \times 12 = 36$$

Weights and Measures

There are three systems of measurement used in pharmacology to calculate dosage. These systems are metric, household, and apothecary. The metric system is used throughout the world as the official language of communication in scientific and technical fields. It is based upon the decimal system: the number 10 or multiples of 10.

Metric System Guidelines. The following guidelines are helpful when learning basic facts about the metric system:

1. Arabic numbers are used to designate whole numbers; e.g., 1, 250, 500, 1000.
2. Decimal fractions are used for quantities less than one; e.g., 0.1, 0.01, 0.001, 0.0001.
3. To ensure accuracy, place a zero before the decimal point; e.g., 0.1, 0.001, 0.0001.
4. The Arabic number precedes the metric unit of measurement; e.g., 10 grams, 2 millimeters, 5 liters.
5. The abbreviation for gram should be capitalized (Gm) or written as (g) to distinguish it from grain (gr).
6. The abbreviation for liter is capitalized (L).

7. Prefixes are written in lowercase letters; e.g., milli, centi, deci, deka.
8. Capitalize the measurement and symbol when it is named after a person; e.g., Celsius (C).
9. Periods are no longer used with most abbreviations or symbols.
10. Abbreviations for units are the same for singular and plural. An "s" is not added to an abbreviation to indicate a plural.

The Seven Common Metric Prefixes.

It is important to know common metric prefixes to have a solid foundation for determining metric equivalents. When a metric prefix is combined with a root of physical quantity, you arrive at multiples or submultiples of the metric system.

Example:

- **milli** (prefix): one-thousandth of a unit
  meter (root): a measure of length
  millimeter: one-thousandth of a meter

- **kilo** (prefix): one thousand units
  liter (root): a measure of volume
  kiloliter: one thousand liters

- **micro** (prefix): one-millionth of a unit
  gram (root): a measure of mass and/or weight
  microgram: one-millionth of a gram

Prefixes:

micro (mi'kro)	= one millionth of a unit written as 0.000001
milli (mil'i)	= one-thousandth of a unit written as 0.001
centi (sen'ti)	= one-hundredth of a unit written as 0.01
deci (des'i)	= one-tenth of a unit written as 0.1
deka (dek'a)	= ten units written as 10
hecto (hek'to)	= one hundred units written as 100
kilo (kil'o)	= one thousand units written as 1000

Fundamental Units:

Following are the fundamental units of the metric system:

meter (m)	length
liter (L)	volume
gram (Gm, g)	mass and/or weight

The meter is the fundamental unit of length in the metric system and originally formed the foundation for the entire system. A meter is equal to 39.37 inches, which is slightly more than a yard, or 3.28 feet.

A millimeter is about the width of the head of a pin. It takes approximately 2½ centimeters to make an inch; a decimeter is approximately 4 inches.

Meter (m)	=	Length
1 millimeter (mm)	=	0.001 meter
1 centimeter (cm)	=	0.01 meter
1 decimeter (dm)	=	0.1 meter
1 meter (m)	=	1 meter
1 dekameter (dam)	=	10 meters
1 hectometer (hm)	=	100 meters
1 kilometer (km)	=	1000 meters

The liter is the metric unit of volume. A liter is equal to 1.056 quarts, which is 0.26 gallon or 2.1 pints.

A milliliter is equivalent to one cubic centimeter (cc), because the amount of space occupied by a milliliter is equal to one cubic centimeter. The weight of one milliliter of water equals approximately one gram. It takes approximately 15 milliliters to make 1 tablespoon. It takes 15 or 16 minims to make one milliliter.

Liter (L)		Volume
1 milliliter (mL)	=	0.001 liter
1 centiliter (cL)	=	0.01 liter
1 deciliter (dL)	=	0.1 liter
1 liter (L)	=	1 liter
1 dekaliter (daL)	=	10 liters
1 hectoliter (hL)	=	100 liters
1 kiloliter (kL)	=	1000 liters

The gram is the metric unit of mass and/or weight. It equals approximately the weight of 1 cubic centimeter or 1 milliliter of water. A gram is equal to approximately 15 grains or 0.035 ounce.

Gram (Gm, g)		Mass and/or Weight
1 microgram (μg)	=	0.000001 gram
1 milligram (mg)	=	0.001 gram
1 centigram (cg)	=	0.01 gram
1 decigram (dg)	=	0.1 gram
1 gram (Gm, g)	=	1 gram
1 dekagram (dag)	=	10 grams
1 hectogram (hg)	=	100 grams
1 kilogram (kg)	=	1000 grams

The metric equivalents most frequently used in the medical field are:

Length	Volume
2½ centimeters (cm) = 1 inch	1000 milliliters (mL) or 1000 cubic centimeters (cc) = 1 liter (L)

Weight

1000 micrograms (μcg)	=	1 milligram (mg)
1000 milligrams (mg)	=	1 gram (Gm, g)
1000 grams (Gm, g)	=	1 kilogram (kg)
1 kilogram	=	2.2 pounds (lb)

TABLE 36-3 COMMON HOUSEHOLD MEASURES

Drop (gt) = approximate liquid measure depending on kind of liquid measured and the size of the opening from which it is dropped.

60 drops (gtt)	is equal to:	1 teaspoon (t or tsp)
1 dash	is equal to:	Less than ⅛ teaspoon
3 teaspoons (tsp)	is equal to:	1 tablespoon (T or tbsp)
2 tablespoons (tbsp)	is equal to:	1 ounce (oz)
4 ounces (oz)	is equal to:	1 juice glass
6 ounces (oz)	is equal to:	1 teacup
8 ounces (oz)	is equal to:	1 glass or cup
16 tablespoons or 8 ounces	is equal to:	1 measuring cup (c)
2 cups (c)	is equal to:	1 pint (pt)
2 pints (pt)	is equal to:	1 quart (qt)
4 quarts (qt)	is equal to:	1 gallon (gal)

Household Measurements.
Household measurements are approximate measurements. They are more frequently used in the home than in the medical field, but the medical assistant should be familiar with the common household measurements listed in Table 36-3.

Apothecary Measurements.
Apothecary measurements are rarely used today, but there are still some medications ordered in grains, drams, and minims; therefore, it is important that medical assistants learn some basic apothecary equivalents as listed in Table 36-4. Note that some of the apothecary measurements are also household measures. However, in the apothecary system, 12 ounces is equal to 1 pound; in the household system, 16 ounces is equal to 1 pound.

Because medications can be prescribed in either metric, apothecary, or household measurements, it is important

TABLE 36-4 BASIC APOTHECARY MEASUREMENTS

Apothecary Units of Weight

60 grains (gr)	is equal to	1 dram (dr)
8 drams (dr)	is equal to	1 ounce (oz)
12 ounces (oz)	is equal to	1 pound (lb)

Apothecary Units of Liquid Volume

60 minims (m)	is equal to	1 fluidram (fldr)
8 fluidrams (fldr)	is equal to	1 fluid ounce (fl oz)
16 fluid ounces (fl oz)	is equal to	1 pint
2 pints (pt)	is equal to	1 quart
4 quarts (qt)	is equal to	1 gallon (gal)

TABLE 36-5 APPROXIMATE EQUIVALENTS AMONG METRIC, APOTHECARY, AND HOUSEHOLD SYSTEMS

Metric	Apothecary	Household
DRY		
60 mg	1 gr	
1 Gm	15 gr	¼ tsp
15 Gm	4 dr	1 tbsp (3 tsp)
30 Gm	1 oz	1 oz (2 tbsp)
	12 oz	1 lb (16 oz)
1 kg		2.2 lb
LIQUID		
	1 m	1 gt
1 mL (1 cubic centimeter)	15 m	15 gtt
5 mL	1 fldr	1 tsp
15 mL	4 fldr	1 tbsp (3 tsp)
30 mL	1 oz (8 fldr)	1 fl oz (2 tbs)
500 mL	(1 pt)	(1 pt or 2 cups)
1000 mL	(1 qt or 2 pts)	4 cups (1 qt)
LENGTH		
2.5 cm		1 in
1 m		39.37 in

to know equivalents among all three in order to calculate the dose of prescribed medication. See Table 36-5.

Metric System Conversion.
The process of changing into another form, state, substance, or product is known as conversion. In the metric system, changing from one unit to another involves multiplying or dividing by 10, 100, 1000, and so forth. This can be done by the proportional method or by moving the decimal in the correct direction.

Proportional Method for Converting Metric Equivalents. There are six basic steps in the proportional method, plus an additional step to prove the answer. The following example will serve as a model for future applications of the proportional method of converting metric equivalents.

Example:
Convert 1500 milligrams to grams.

$$1500 \text{ mg} = \underline{\hspace{2cm}} \text{Gm, g}$$

Step 1. Since the unknown factor in the given formula is the number of grams contained in 1500 milligrams, substitute the symbol *x* for grams in the equation.

Step 2. Setting up the proportion requires that you know metric equivalents. For example, in this problem you have to know that 1000 milligrams (mg) = 1 gram (Gm, g).

Step 3. Since you know that 1000 mg is equal to 1 Gm, you can create one-half of the equation. Write the equivalent and place it on the left of the equal sign.

$$1000 \text{ mg} : 1 \text{ Gm} =$$

Step 4. Now that you have the left side of the equation, set up the right side by using the designated metric value 1500 mg : *x* Gm. Always write the smallest equivalent as to the largest equivalent, e.g., mg : Gm. By being consistent, it is less likely errors will occur.

$$1000 \text{ mg} : 1 \text{ Gm} = 1500 \text{ mg} : x \text{ Gm}$$

Step 5. Note that you have an equal equation:

$$\text{mg} : \text{Gm} = \text{mg} : \text{Gm}$$

The first values on either side of the equal sign are milligrams, and the second values on either side are grams.

Step 6. Now solve for the unknown (*x*) by multiplication and division. Multiply the means by the means and the extremes by the extremes. **NOTE:** Once the proportion is correctly set up, simply use the numbers as you multiply and divide.

$$1000 : 1 = 1500 : x$$

$$1000x = 1500$$
$$x = 1500 \div 1000$$
$$x = 1.5$$

$$\begin{array}{r} 1.5 \\ 1000\overline{)1500.0} \\ \underline{1000} \\ 500.0 \\ \underline{500} \end{array}$$

Step 7. To make sure the answer is correct, prove the work: Place the answer 1.5 Gm into the formula where *x* once was. Now multiply the means by the means and the extremes by the extremes.

$$1000 \text{ mg} : 1 \text{ Gm} = 1500 \text{ mg} : 1.5 \text{ Gm}$$
$$1500 = 1500$$

MEDICATIONS MEASURED IN UNITS

Medications such as insulin, heparin, some antibiotics, hormones, vitamins, and vaccines are measured in units (U). These medications are standardized in units based on their strengths. The strength varies from one medicine to another, depending upon the source, condition, and method by which it is obtained.

How to Calculate Unit Dosages

When calculating medications that are ordered in units, use either the proportional method or the formula method.

The Proportional Method

Example:
The physician orders 4000 USP units of heparin given deep subcutaneously. On hand is heparin 500 USP units per milliliter.

Step 1. Use the following proportion to calculate the dose:

Known unit on hand	:	Known dosage form	=	Dose ordered	:	Unknown amount to be given
5000 U	:	1 mL	=	4000 U	:	*x* mL

$$5000x = 4000$$
$$x = \tfrac{4}{5} = \tfrac{4}{5} \text{ mL or } 0.8 \text{ mL}$$

Use a tuberculin syringe to draw up 0.8 mL, or convert $\tfrac{4}{5}$ mL to minims.

Step 2. Convert $\tfrac{4}{5}$ mL to minims. **NOTE:** There are 15 or 16 minims per milliliter.
Multiply:

$$\frac{4}{\cancel{5}_1} \times \frac{\cancel{15}^3}{1} = \frac{4}{1} \times \frac{3}{1} = 12 \text{ minims}$$

Administer 12 minims (of 5000 U/ML for correct dose of 4000 units) to the patient.

The Formula Method

Example:
The physician orders 450,000 units of Bicillin 1M. On hand is Bicillin 600,000 units per milliliter.

Step 1. Use the following formula to calculate the dose:

$$\frac{\text{Dose ordered (desired)}}{\text{Dose on hand}} \times \text{Quantity} = \text{Amount to give}$$

$$\frac{450,000 \text{ U}}{600,000 \text{ U}} \times 1 \text{ mL} = \frac{45\cancel{0},\cancel{000}\text{U}^3}{6\cancel{00},\cancel{000}\text{U}_4} \times 1 \text{ mL} = \tfrac{3}{4} \text{ mL}$$

Step 2. You may convert to minims. If you do, multiply $\tfrac{3}{4}$ by 16.

$$\frac{3}{\cancel{4}_1} \times \frac{\cancel{16}^4}{1} = 12 \text{ minims}$$

The patient will receive 12 minims of Bicillin 600,000 U for the ordered dose of 450,000 U.

Insulin

Insulin is a chemical substance (hormone) secreted by the beta cells of the islets of Langerhans in the pancreas. Insulin is necessary for the proper metabolism of blood glucose and maintenance of the correct blood sugar level. Inadequate secretion of insulin, as in the disease diabetes mellitus, results in hyperglycemia and subsequent excessive production of ketone bodies. Eventual coma can ensue.

Patients' needs are individualized according to the severity of their disease; treatment includes taking insulin, controlling diet, and exercise. The diet is well-balanced and consists of the correct number of calories distributed among carbohydrates, fats, and proteins. Patients are taught to monitor blood and urine glucose levels at home throughout the day, for the dosage of insulin taken depends on the amounts of glucose detected. Uncontrolled diabetes mellitus can result in serious complications such as circulatory problems, especially in the feet and legs, bedsores, infection, and gangrene. Special care of the feet is essential. The mouth and teeth require excellent oral hygiene.

Diabetes

The National Diabetes Data Group of the National Institutes of Health organized the various forms of diabetes into the following categories:

Type I   Insulin-dependent diabetes mellitus (IDDM)
Type II   Noninsulin-dependent diabetes mellitus (NIDDM)
Type III Women who developed glucose intolerance in association with pregnancy

Patient Teaching Tip

Encourage patients with diabetes to enroll in diabetic education classes, which are offered at most local hospitals. Patients also need to realize that treatment of diabetes is a lifelong commitment and that they must abide by everything that the hospital teaches.

Type IV   Other types of diabetes associated with pancreatic disease, hormonal changes, adverse effects of drugs, or genetic or other anomalies.

Individuals with Type I diabetes must take insulin injections on a regular basis to maintain life. The dosage of insulin is expressed in units and is individualized by the physician for each patient. The amount of insulin that a person must take is based on blood and urine glucose levels, diet, exercise, and the individual's needs (Tables 36-6 and 36-7).

It is *extremely important* that the *exact dosage of insulin be taken by the patient*. Too little or too much insulin can cause serious problems ranging from a blood sugar level too low or too high, to coma, and even death. It may be the medical assistant's responsibility to administer insulin and/or to teach patients or their families how to administer insulin.

When administering insulin, the U-100 syringe (1 cc or LO-DOSE® ½ cc) is preferred. U-100 means there are 100 units of insulin per milliliter or cubic centimeter. Insulin dosage should always be expressed in units rather than in milliliters or cubic centimeters. For example, if the physician orders 30 units of U-100 NPH insulin, use a U-100 syringe and draw up 30 units of U-100 NPH insulin.

TABLE 36-6	RAPID-ACTING INSULIN: INSULIN PREPARATIONS U-100			
Rapid-Acting	**Onset of Action**	**Peak**	**Duration**	**Appearance**
Regular	½ hour	2½ to 5 hours	8 hours	Clear, colorless
Crystalline zinc	½ to 1 hour	2 to 4 hours	8 hours	Clear, colorless
Semilente	1½ hour	5 to 10 hours	16 hours	Cloudy
Humulin R	15 minutes	1 hour	6 to 8 hours	Clear, colorless
Mixtard	½ hour	4 to 8 hours	24 hours	Cloudy
Velosulin	½ hour	1 to 3 hours	8 hours	Clear
Novolin	½ hour	2½ to 5 hours	8 hours	Clear

TABLE 36-7   INTERMEDIATE-ACTING AND LONG-LASTING INSULIN: INSULIN PREPARATIONS U-100

	Onset of Action	Peak	Duration	Appearance
Intermediate-Acting				
NPH	½ hour	4 to 12 hours	24 hours	Cloudy
Lente	2½ hours	7 to 15 hours	24 hours	Cloudy
Insulatard NPH	½ hour	4 to 12 hours	24 hours	Cloudy
Novolin L	2½ hours	7 to 15 hours	22 hours	Cloudy
Novolin N	1½ hours	4 to 12 hours	24 hours	Cloudy
Humulin N	1 hour	4 hours	24 hours	Cloudy
Long-Acting				
Ultralente	4 hours	10 to 30 hours	36 hours	Cloudy
PZI (protamine zinc insulin)	4 to 8 hours	14 to 20 hours	36 hours	Cloudy

Precautions to Observe When Administering Insulin

- Be sure to use the proper insulin, the one ordered by the physician. Refer to Tables 36-6 and 36-7 for various insulin preparations.
- Do not substitute one insulin for another.
- Use the correct syringe, U-100.
- Dosage of insulin is always measured in units and is individualized for each patient.
- Check the label for the name and type of insulin, strength, and expiration date.
- Make sure the insulin has the proper appearance. Refer to Tables 36-6 and 36-7 for proper appearance of various insulins.

- When insulin is not in use, store it in a cool place and avoid freezing.
- When mixing insulins in one syringe, be certain they are compatible.
- Avoid shaking the insulin bottle. Roll gently in palms of hand to mix. This method prevents bubbles in the medication.
- Use a subcutaneous needle, but inject at a 90° angle.
- Use a site rotation system and select an appropriate site. Insulin injection sites must be rotated to prevent tissue damage. Record site used (Figure 36-4).
- Do not massage after injection.
- Always follow the physician's order and office policy when mixing insulins.

CALCULATING ADULT DOSAGES

Two measures, weight and volume, are used to determine the amount of medication that is to be administered. The weight of a medication may be expressed as any of the following:

- milliequivalent (mEq)
- microgram (mcg)
- milligram (mg)
- gram (Gm, g)
- grain (gr)
- unit (U)

The volume of a medication may be expressed as a:

- milliliter (ml)
- cubic centimeter (cc)

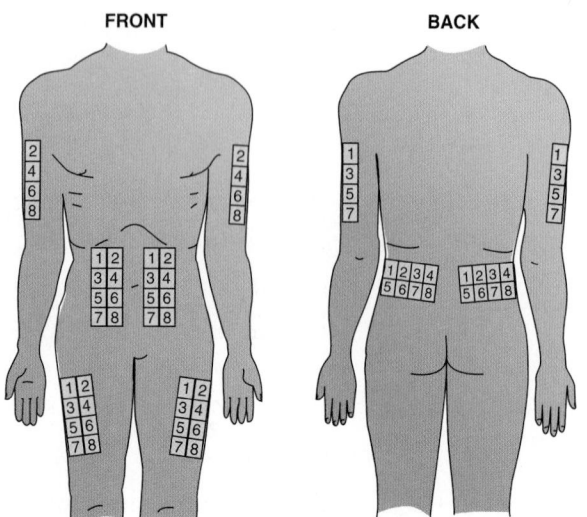

Figure 36-4   Sites and rotation for insulin administration.

- minim (m)
- dram (dr)
- ounce (oz)
- by a variety of household measures, such as the tea-spoon (tsp)

Many different methods can be used when calculating the dosage to be administered. Two of the most useful methods, the proportional method and the formula method, are described.

The Proportional Method

Example:
The physician orders 0.2 Gm of Equanil tabs. The dose on hand is 400 mg tabs.

Step 1. Determine whether the medication ordered and the medication on hand are available in the same unit of measure.

Step 2. If the medication ordered and the medication on hand are not in the same unit of measure, convert so that both measures are expressed using the same unit of measure.
Conversion: To change 0.2 Gm to mg

$$1000 \text{ mg} : 1 \text{ Gm} = x \text{ mg} : 0.2 \text{ Gm}$$
$$x = 200 \text{ mg}$$
$$\text{or}$$
$$\text{multiply } 0.2 \times 1000 = 200$$

Step 3. Now use the following proportion to calculate the dosage. Remember that 0.2 Gm was converted to 200 mg.

Known unit on hand	:	*Known dosage form*	=	*Dose ordered*	:	*Unknown amount to be given*
400 mg	:	1 tab	=	200 mg	:	*x* tab

$$400 : 1 = 200 : x$$

$$400x = 200$$

$$x = \frac{\overset{1}{\cancel{200}}}{\underset{2}{\cancel{400}}} \text{ (Reduce fraction to lowest terms)}$$

$$x = \tfrac{1}{2} \text{ tab of 400 mg.}$$

Step 4. Prove your answer. Place your answer in the original formula in the *x* position.

$$400 \text{ mg} : 1 \text{ tab} = 200 \text{ mg} : \tfrac{1}{2} \text{ tab}$$
$$200 = \tfrac{1}{2} \text{ of } 400$$
$$200 = 200$$

The Formula Method

Example:
The physician orders 0.2 Gm of Equanil tabs. The dose on hand is 400 mg tabs.

Step 1. Determine whether the medication ordered and the medication on hand are available in the same unit of measure.

Step 2. If the medication ordered and the medication on hand are not in the same unit of measure, convert so that both measures are expressed using the same unit of measure.
Conversion: To change 0.2 Gm to mg

$$1000 \text{ mg} : 1 \text{ Gm} = x \text{ mg} : 0.2 \text{ Gm}$$
$$x = 200 \text{ mg}$$
$$\text{or}$$
$$\text{multiply } 0.2 \times 1000 = 200$$

Step 3. Now use the following formula to calculate the dosage.

$$\frac{\text{Dose ordered (desired)}}{\text{Dose on hand}} \times \frac{\text{Quantity}}{1} = \begin{array}{c} \text{Amount to give} \\ \text{(form of drug)} \end{array}$$

$$\frac{\text{D}}{\text{H}} \times \text{Q} = \text{Amount to give}$$

The physician ordered 0.2 Gm of Equanil tabs (0.2 Gm converts to 200 mg). The dose on hand is 400 mg tabs.

$$\frac{200 \text{ mg}}{400 \text{ mg}} \times 1 \text{ tab} = \frac{200}{400} \text{ or } \tfrac{1}{2} \text{ tab}$$

Give ½ tab of 400 mg.

CALCULATING CHILDREN'S DOSAGES

Each child is an individual with differences in age, size, and weight. In the past, formulas such as Young's, Clark's, and Fried's rules were used to calculate pediatric dosages. These formulas determined what fraction of an adult dose was appropriate for a child. Since each child does not develop in the same way during a given time span, these formulas have been replaced by more exact methods of determining the correct dosage of medication for a child.

Today, there are two basic methods used to calculate children's dosages:

- According to kilogram of body weight
- According to body surface area (BSA)

The body weight method is generally the method of choice, since most medications are ordered in this way and it is easier to calculate. The body surface area (BSA) is an exact method, but one must use a formula and a nomogram (a device-graph that shows relationship among numerical values) to determine a correct dosage.

Body Surface Area

The body surface area (BSA) is considered to be one of the most accurate methods of calculating medication dosages for infants and children up to 12 years of age. This method requires the use of a nomogram that estimates the body surface area of the patient according to height and weight (Figure 36-5).

The body surface area is determined by drawing a straight line from the patient's height to the patient's weight. Intersection of the line with the surface area column is the estimated BSA. This figure is then placed in the following formula:

$$\frac{\text{BSA of child (m}^2)}{1.7 \text{ (m}^2)} \times \text{adult dose} = \text{child dose}$$

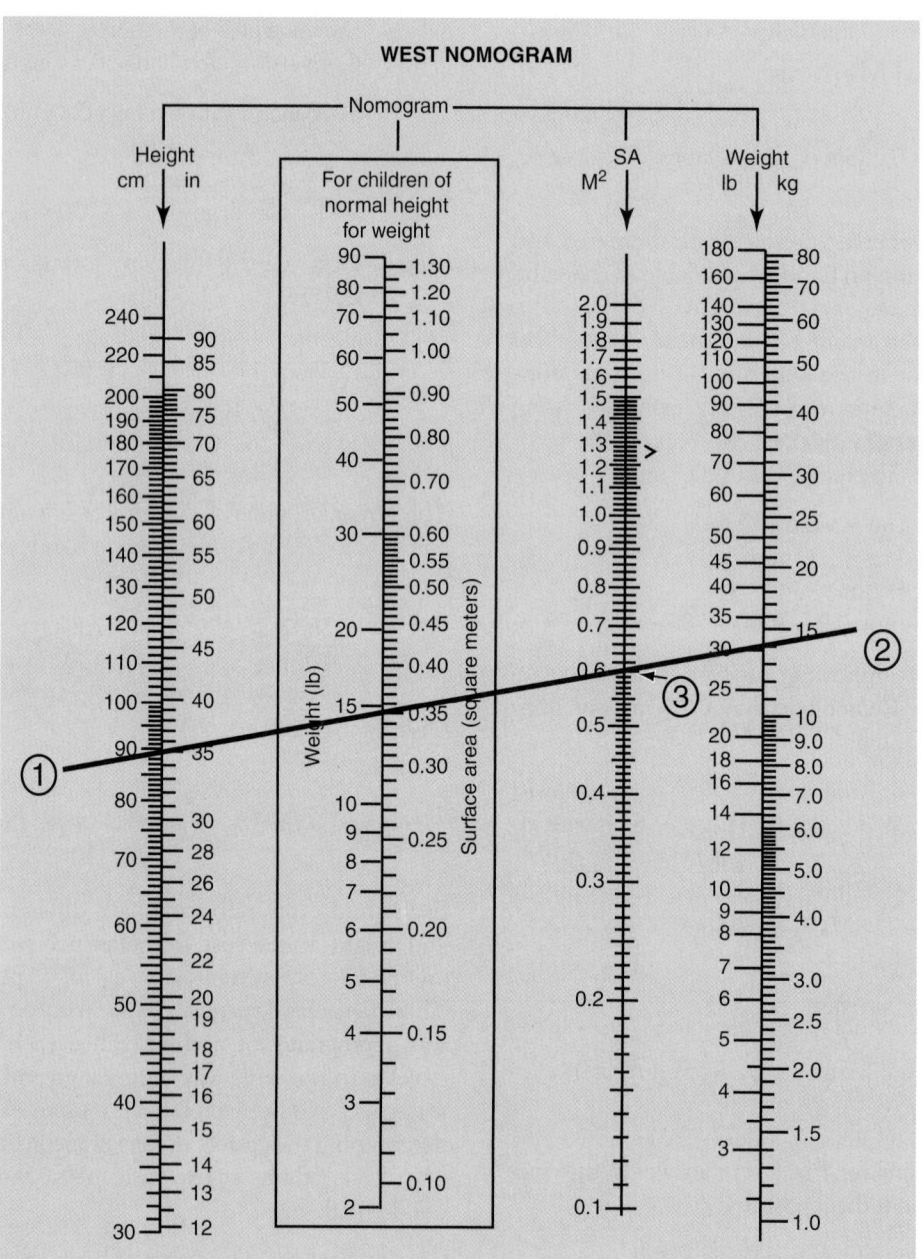

Figure 36-5   Body surface area (BSA) is determined by drawing a straight line from the patient's height (1) in the far left column to his or her weight (2) in the far right column. Intersection of the line with body surface area (BSA) column (3) is the estimated BSA (m²). For infants and children of normal height and weight BSA may be estimated from weight alone by referring to the enclosed area. (From *Nelson Textbook of Pediatrics* (15th ed.) by R. E. Behrman, R. M. Kleigman, & A. M. Arvin, 1996, Philadelphia: Saunders. Reprinted with permission.)

This formula is based on the average adult who weighs 140 pounds and has a body surface area of 1.7 square meters (1.7 m^2).

Example:

Marion Carrera is a 4-year-old child who is 40 inches tall and weighs 38 lbs. (BSA 0.7). The physician has ordered Demerol for pain. The average adult dose of Demerol is 50 mg per ml. What dosage will be given to Marion according to the BSA method?

$$\frac{0.7 \ (m^2)}{1.7 \ (m^2)} \times \frac{50 \ mg}{1} = \text{child's dose}$$

$$\frac{0.7 \ (m^2)}{1.7 \ (m^2)} \times \frac{50}{1} = \frac{35}{1.7} = 20.5 \ mg = 20.5 \ or \ 21 \ mg$$

Now use the formula $\dfrac{\text{Desired}}{\text{Have}} \times \text{Quantity}$ to convert mg to ml.

$$\frac{21 \ mg}{50 \ mg} \times 1 = x \ mL$$

$$\frac{21}{50} = 0.42 \ mL \text{ administered in a tuberculin syringe}$$

Kilogram of Body Weight

It may be the responsibility of the medical assistant to calculate the amount of dosage ordered by the physician according to the patient's body weight. Today, many medications are ordered in this manner; therefore, it is essential that you learn how to calculate dosage according to this method. The following example will guide you step by step through the mathematical process of calculating dosage according to kilogram of body weight.

There are 2.2 pounds in one kilogram.

Example:

The physician ordered an antiepileptic agent, Depakene (valproic acid) 15 mg/kg/day capsules for Clark Kipperley, who weighs 110 pounds. The medication is to be given in three divided doses.

Step 1. To express pounds in kilograms, divide the weight in pounds by 2.2. Convert the patient's weight to kilograms:

$$110 \div 2.2 = 50 \text{ kilograms}$$

Step 2. Now, calculate the prescribed dosage by placing 50 in the appropriate place:

$$15 \text{ mg/50/day}$$
$$15 \times 50 = 750 \text{ mg/day}$$

Step 3. To determine the amount of each dose, divide 750 by 3 (divided doses).

$$750 \text{ mg} \div 3 = 250 \text{ mg}$$

Depakene is available in 250 mg capsules and 250 mg/5 cc syrup. The physician ordered the medication in capsules, so Clark will receive a 250 mg capsule every 8 hours for a total of three doses a day.

In the same example, use the proportional method to calculate kilogram of body weight.

Step 1. To convert 110 pounds to kilograms, set up the proportion as follows:

$$2.2 \text{ 1b} : 1 \text{ kg} = 110 \text{ 1b} : x \text{ kg}$$

Step 2. Now, solve for x.

$$2.2 : 1 = 110 : x$$
$$2.2x = 110$$
$$x = 50$$

Step 3. Now, calculate the prescribed dosage by placing 50 in the appropriate place: mg/50 kg/day

$$15 \times 50 = 750 \text{ mg/day}$$

Step 4. To determine the amount of each dose, divide 750 by 3 (divided doses).

$$750 \div 3 = 250 \text{ mg per dose}$$

ADMINISTRATION OF MEDICATIONS

Regardless of a medication's form or the route by which it is administered, certain basic guidelines must be followed. These guidelines are:

1. Practice medical asepsis. (See Chapter 22.) Wash your hands before and after administering a medication. Remember OSHA guidelines and standard precautions (Chapter 22).
2. Work in a well-lighted area that is free from distractions.
3. Follow the "Six Rights" of proper drug administration (see following section).
4. Always check for allergies before administering any medication.
5. Give only drugs ordered by a licensed physician or practitioner who is authorized to prescribe medications.
6. Never give a medication if there is any question about the order.
7. Be completely familiar with the drug that you are administering before giving it to the patient. Look it up in the *PDR*.
8. Always check the expiration date on the medication label.
9. Never give a drug if its normal appearance has been altered in any way (color, structure, consistency, or odor).

10. Make out a medicine card (Figure 36-6) for medications, dose, route, and time exactly as ordered by the physician using the physician's order from the patient's record as a guide.

11. Give only those medications that you have actually prepared for administration.

12. Do not allow someone else to give a medication that you have prepared.

13. Once you have prepared a medication for administration, do not leave it unattended.

14. Be careful in transporting the medication to the patient.

15. When administering oral medications, stay with the patient until you are certain that the medication has been taken.

16. Shake (to mix) all liquid medications that contain a **precipitate** before pouring. A precipitate is a substance that separates from a solution if allowed to stand.

17. When pouring a liquid medication, hold the measuring device at eye level or place it on a flat surface and squat down so you can observe it at eye level. Read the correct amount at the lowest level of the **meniscus**, which is the top surface of the column of liquid.

18. Do not contaminate the cap of a bottle while pouring a medication. Place the cap with the rim pointed upward to prevent contamination of that portion that comes into contact with the medication.

19. Keep all drugs not being administered in a safe storage place.

20. Carefully follow the procedural steps for the type of medication that you are giving or the type of procedure you are performing.

21. Always keep safety precautions in mind. The United States Department of Health and Human Services, Public Health Service, and Centers for Disease and Prevention Control recommend following standard precautions for prevention of HBV, HIV, and other bloodborne diseases (refer to Chapter 22).

The "Six Rights" of Proper Drug Administration

The "Six Rights" have been developed as a checklist of activities to be followed by those who give medications. This easy-to-remember list should always be followed to ensure the proper administration of any drug:

1. *Right Drug*. To be sure that the correct drug has been selected, compare the medication order with the label on the medication. A frequent check of the medication label is a good way to avoid a medication error. One should make a practice of reading the label on each of the following three occasions:

   First: When the medication is taken from the storage area.

   Second: Just before removing it from its container.

   Third: Upon returning the medication container to storage or prior to discarding the empty container.

2. *Right Dose*. It is essential that the patient receive the right dose. If the dose ordered and the dose on hand are *not the same*, carefully determine the correct dose through mathematical calculation. When calculating dosage, it is advisable to have another qualified person verify the accuracy of your calculations before the medication is administered.

3. *Right Route*. Check the medication order to be sure that you have the right route of administration (Figure 36-7A).

A medicine card is written out prior to administration of any medication to the patient in the ambulatory care setting. The information is taken directly from the physician's order sheet of the patient's record. An example follows.

Information needed:

Patient name: Abigail Johnson

Physician's order: Cardizem (diltiazem hydrochloride) 180 mg po stat. Winston Lewis, MD.

The medicine card is then used to document the information on Mrs. Johnson's record. Following documentation, tear up the medicine card and discard.

Room 3

Johnson, Abigail

Cardizem

180 mg

po

stat

10/24/_ - 10 A.M.

Figure 36-6   A medicine card is used to prepare, administer, and record medications, dose, route, and time as ordered by the physician.

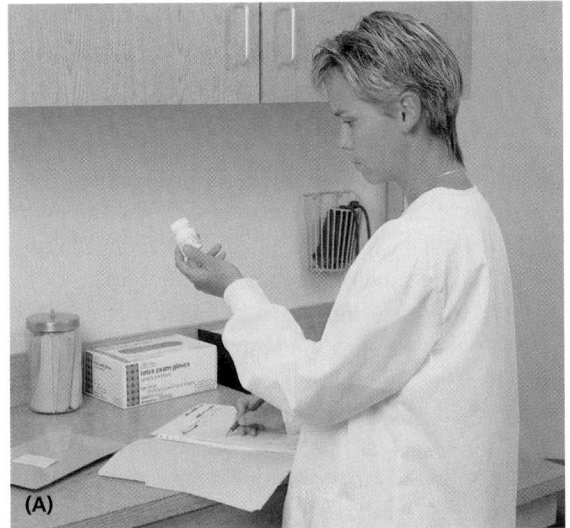

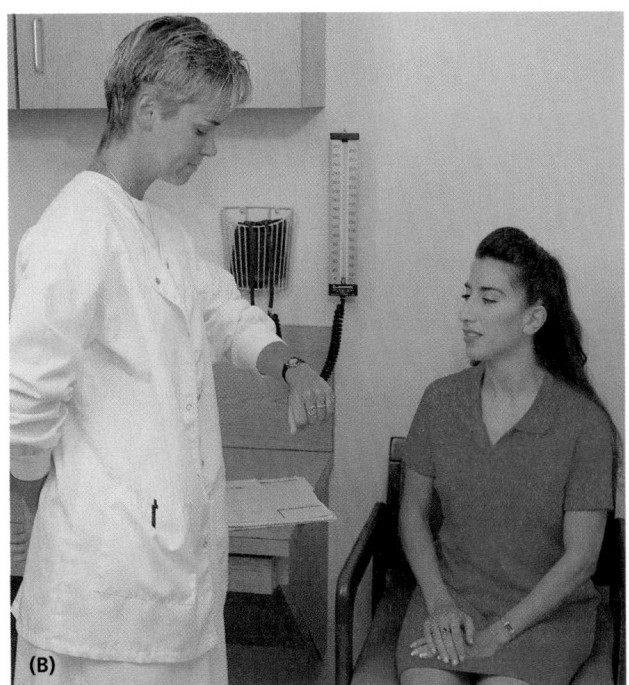

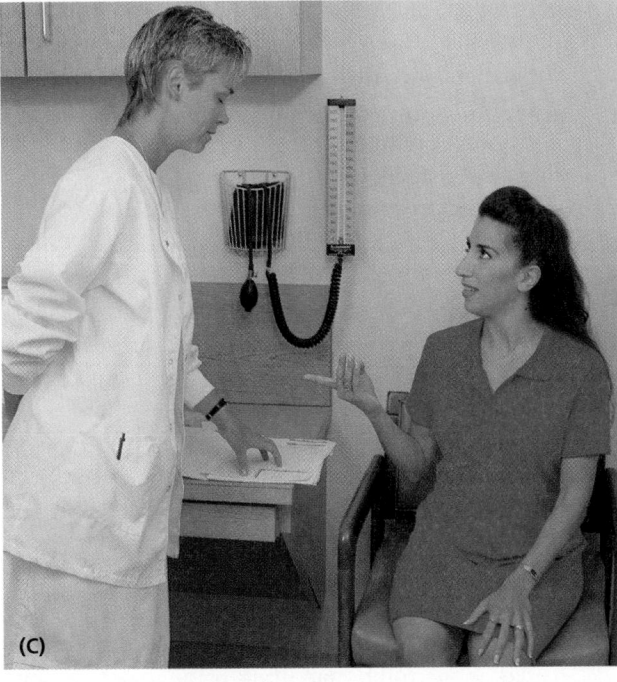

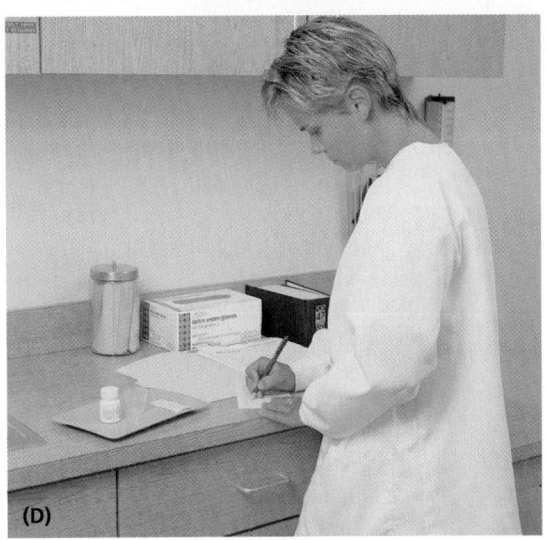

Figure 36-7 (A) Medical assistant checks the right drug, the right route, and the right dose of medication to administer. (B) Medical assistant checks for the right time to administer medication to the patient. (C) Medical assistant assesses patient before administering the medication. The medical assistant ascertains she has the right patient and asks the patient if she has any allergies. (D) Medical assistant documents administration of medication in patient's record.

4. *Right Time.* You are responsible for medicating the patient at the proper time. Check the medication order to ensure that a drug is administered according to the time interval prescribed. For a drug to be maintained at the proper blood level, care must be taken to administer it at the right time (Figure 36-7B).

5. *Right Patient.* Before administering any medication, always be sure that you have the right patient. A good safety practice is to correctly identify the

patient on each occasion when you administer a medication. In a hospital, always check the patient's identification bracelet. In the ambulatory care facility, call the patient by name or ask the patient to state her name (Figure 36-7C).

6. *Right Documentation.* The recording process is the vital link between physician, patient, and medical assistant. It is an account of the essential data that are collected and preserved. The patient's chart is a legal document; therefore, all data should be

recorded in ink or typed. The data should be accurate and clearly stated. It is important that certain data about drug administration be entered in the patient's chart (Figure 36-7D):

- Patient's name
- Date and time of administration
- Name of the medication and the amount (dosage) administered
- Route by which the medication was administered
- Any unusual reactions experienced by the patient
- Any complications in administering the drug (patient refusing to take the medication, difficulty in swallowing)
- If the medication was *not* given, state why and dispose of the medication according to agency policy
- Patient data, such as blood pressure, pulse, respirations, when appropriate
- Effectiveness of the drug (for example, a patient with Parkinson's disease shows improvement after three weeks of treatment with Levodopa)
- Your name or initials and title

Medication Error

Medication errors should not happen when personnel follow the "Six Rights" of proper drug administration and the essential medication guidelines; however, honest mistakes will be made periodically. A medication error occurs when any of the following happen:

1. A drug is given to the wrong patient.
2. The incorrect drug is given.
3. The drug is given via an incorrect route.
4. The drug is given at the incorrect time.
5. The incorrect dose is administered.
6. Incorrect data are entered on the patient's chart.

When a medication error occurs, follow standard procedure:

a. Recognize that an error has been made.
b. Stay calm. Assess the patient's condition and/or reactions to the medication.
c. Report the error immediately to the physician. Give the details of the mistake and the patient's reactions.
d. Follow the physician's order for correcting the error.
e. Document the error in the patient's record or the facility's record form.
   - Describe the type of error.
   - Describe the patient's reactions.
   - Describe the steps taken to correct the error.
   - State date, time, and your name.

Patient Assessment

Before administering any medication, carefully assess the patient's condition. An assessment should include, but is not limited to, the following conditions:

1. *Age.* Is the medication and route suitable for the patient at a particular stage in life? The stages of life include infancy, childhood, adolescence, adulthood, and old age. During infancy, early childhood, and old age, a smaller dose of medication may be required than would be appropriate for the other stages in life.

2. *Physical Conditions.* Potential problems associated with the patient's physical condition must be considered. Female patients during pregnancy or while breastfeeding should not be given certain contraindicated medications.

3. *Body Size.* The amount of medication given and size of the needle used are directly related to the size of the patient. Pediatric and geriatric patients usually have less subcutaneous and/or muscular tissue per body surface area than the average adult (see Body Surface Area, pages 730–731). Small, thin patients usually require less medication, and a shorter needle may be used to reach the appropriate tissue level. On the other hand, the large or obese patient may require more medication than the average adult and a longer needle to reach the appropriate tissue level.

4. *Gender.* Consider differences that are related to the gender of the patient.
   - *Muscular Build.* Male patients are generally more muscular than female patients. Always inspect and palpate muscle tissue with this in mind when determining the appropriate needle length to reach muscle tissue.
   - *Skin Texture.* Male patients usually have tougher skin than females. A young person's skin usually has more tone than that of an older person. Slightly more force is required to penetrate skin that is tough or lacking in tone.

5. *Injection Site.* Always inspect and palpate the skin before administering an injection. The following body areas should be avoided when choosing the site for an injection:
   - Any type of skin lesion
   - Burned areas
   - Inflamed areas
   - Previous injection sites
   - Any traumatized area
   - Scar tissue (vaccination, keloid)
   - Moles, warts, birthmarks, tumors, lumps, hard nodules
   - Nerves, large blood vessels, bones
   - Cyanotic areas

- Edematous areas
- Paralyzed areas
- Arm on same side as mastectomy

Correct injection sites are illustrated later in this chapter.

ADMINISTRATION OF ORAL MEDICATIONS

Oral medications are easily and economically administered with a high degree of safety. There are, however, several disadvantages associated with the oral route. For instance, the drug may:

- Have an objectionable odor
- Have an objectionable taste
- Cause discoloration of the teeth, mouth, and tongue
- Irritate the gastric mucosa
- Be altered by digestive enzymes
- Be poorly absorbed from the digestive system due to illness or nature of the medication
- Not be taken by the patient
- Have less predictable effects upon the body when given orally than when given by the parenteral route (by injection)
- Not be able to be swallowed if in tablet, capsule, or caplet form

Equipment and Supplies for Oral Medications

Three measuring devices commonly used in the administration of oral medications are the medicine cup, the water cup, and the medicine dropper. The medicine cup (Figure 36-8) comes in various sizes and shapes, depend-

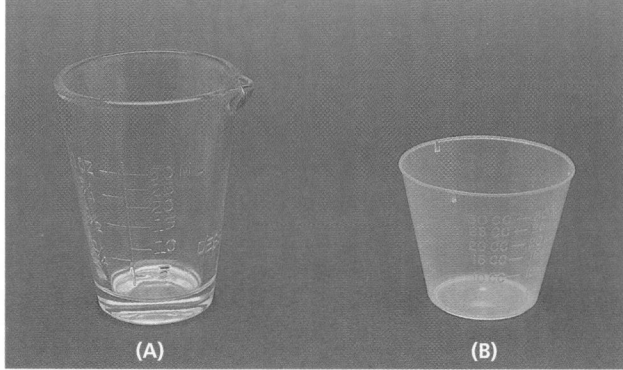

Figure 36-8 Medicine cups: (A) Glass. (B) Plastic.

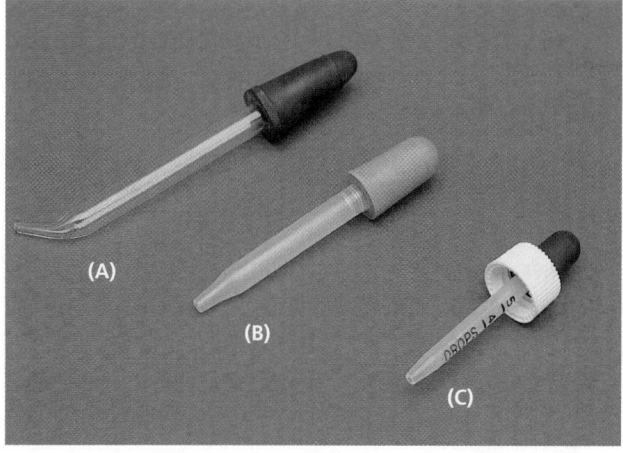

Figure 36-9 Various types of medicine droppers: (A) Glass. (B) Plastic. (C) Plastic calibrated.

ing upon its manufacturer and its intended use. Cups may be calibrated in fluid ounces, fluidrams, cubic centimeters (cc), milliliters (mL), and tablespoons.

The water cup is a small plastic or paper cup that is disposable. The average water cup holds 3 ounces of liquid.

The medicine dropper (Figure 36-9) may be calibrated in milliliters, minims, or drops. Medicine droppers are often included with the bottle of medication. Uncalibrated droppers may be provided when the medicine is administered only in drops. The size of the drop varies with the size of the dropper opening, the angle at which it is held, the force exerted on the rubber bulb, and the viscosity of the medication.

It is important that the appropriate measuring device be selected for a medication and the prescribed dosage accurately measured. The selection of the measuring device depends upon the physical structure of the medication (solid or liquid), the amount of medication prescribed, the size of the measuring device, and the calibrations on the container.

See Procedure 36-1 for administration of oral medications.

ADMINISTRATION OF PARENTERAL MEDICATIONS

The term **parenteral** is used to describe the injection of a liquid substance into the body via a route other than the alimentary canal. The most frequently used parenteral routes are:

Subcutaneous. Just below the surface of the skin. A subcutaneous injection is usually given at a 45-degree angle.

Intramuscular. Within the muscle. An intramuscular injection is given at a 90-degree angle, passing through the skin and subcutaneous tissue, and penetrating deep into muscle tissue.

Intradermal. Within the dermal layer of the skin. An intradermal injection is given at an angle between 10 degrees and 15 degrees.

Medications that have been prepared for use by injection are available in multiple dose form (vials) and in unit dose form (ampules and cartridge-needle units). (See Figure 36-10.) **Unit dose** forms are premeasured amounts, packaged on a per-dose basis.

Ampule. A small, sterile, prefilled container that usually holds a single dose of a hypodermic solution.

Cartridge-Needle Unit. A disposable sterile cartridge containing a premeasured amount of medication. This unit is designed for use in a nondisposable cartridge-holder syringe such as the Tubex® or Carpuject®.

Vial. A small, sterile, prefilled glass bottle containing a hypodermic solution.

Hazards Associated with Parenteral Medications

Injections of medications must be done with extreme care. Sterile technique must be used because the needle and medication are being introduced into the patient's body and microorganisms must not be transmitted. Appropriate site selection and proper technique assure effectiveness of the medication.

Additional dangers to be aware of when administering medications parenterally (by injection) include:

1. Allergic reaction (if present) will be swift
2. Injury to bone, nerve, or blood vessel
3. Breaking of needle in tissue (rare)
4. Injecting into a blood vessel instead of tissue. (This is avoided by checking for blood return, or aspiration.)

Reasons for Parenteral Route Selection

The parenteral route is selected because of:

1. Rapid response time to medication
2. Accuracy of dosage
3. Need to concentrate medication in a specific body part or area (joint or local anesthetic)
4. Inability to administer orally because the medication is destroyed by gastric juices or the patient is incapable of taking medication orally

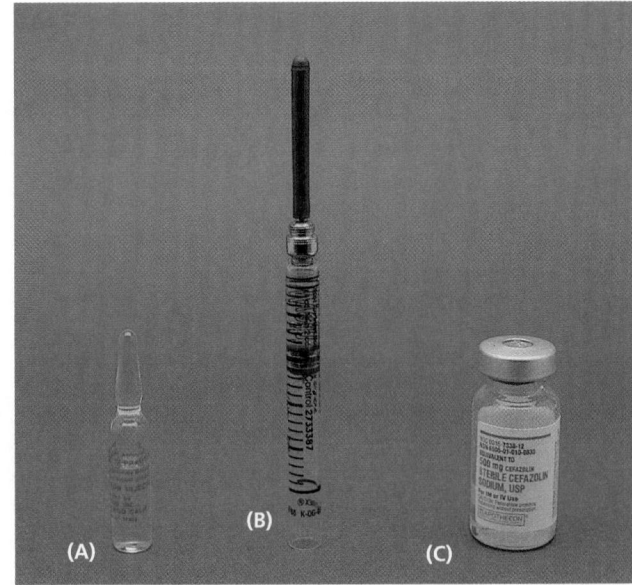

Figure 36-10 Medications given parenterally: (A) Ampule. (B) Sterile cartridge with premeasured medication. (C) Vial of powder for reconstitution.

Because parenteral medications are intended for use by injection, they must be supplied as liquids. Some medications are supplied in powder form and must be reconstituted to a liquid form for injection. See Procedure 36-8.

Because they must be in liquid form, the amount of parenteral medications is expressed in terms of volume (cubic centimeters, milliliters, minims, or ounces). The strength of the drug contained in the liquid is usually expressed in terms of its weight (milliequivalents, micrograms, milligrams, grams, grains, or units). Therefore, medications ordered for parenteral use are often ordered by both weight and volume.

Example:

Atropine sulfate injection (gr = weight; mL = volume)

$$0.4 \text{ mg (gr } \frac{1}{150}) \text{ per mL}$$

The parenteral route of drug administration offers an effective mode of delivering medication to a patient when a rapid and direct result is desired. Since the effect of a parenteral medication is faster than by the oral route, the accuracy of dosage calculation is very important.

Parenteral Equipment and Supplies

Syringes. Syringes are classified as disposable, nondisposable, and as combinations of these two types. They also may be classified according to their intended use. In addition to the standard hypodermic syringes that are in general use, there are special-purpose syringes for irrigations and/or oral feedings, tuberculin syringes, and insulin syringes.

Disposable Syringes. Disposable syringes are those that are sterilized, prepackaged, nontoxic, nonpyrogenic, and ready for use. They are available as a syringe-needle unit and are generally enclosed in individual peel-apart packages of durable paper or clear plastic. They are available in sizes from ½ cubic centimeter to 50 cubic centimeters. The 1-cc, 3-cc, and 5-cc syringes are the ones most often used when parenteral medications are administered.

A disposable syringe-needle unit consists of a syringe with an attached needle. The needle is covered by a hard plastic sheath to prevent it from accidentally penetrating the package or sticking the user. The unit may be sealed within a peel-apart package or encased in a rigid plastic container that has been heat-sealed to ensure sterility. Labeling usually includes the manufacturer's name, type and size of the syringe, gauge and length of the needle, and a reorder number. Packages are usually color-coded for ease of identification. Disposable syringes are generally preferred for the administration of parenteral medications because they ensure sterility and sharp needles. Also, disposable syringes eliminate the need for resterilizaton, which is costly, time-consuming, and possibly unsafe if not done properly.

Nondisposable Syringes. Nondisposable syringes are usually made of specially strengthened glass resistant to thermal shock. These units, consisting of round glass barrels with individually fitted plungers, are manufactured to exacting specifications.

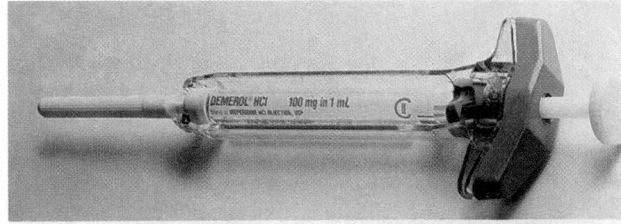

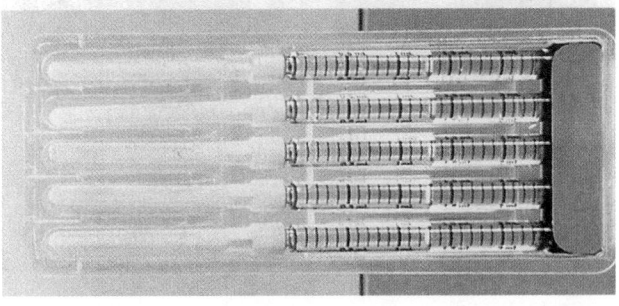

Figure 36-11   The Carpuject® is another kind of cartridge-injection system. This unit is shown with a package of prefilled cartridges. (Courtesy Sanofi Withrop Pharmaceuticals.)

Nondisposable glass syringes are available in sizes from 1 cubic centimeter to 50 cubic centimeters. These syringes are not often used for the administration of injections. They may be used by physicians to perform special procedures such as paracentesis, thoracentesis, thoracotomy, and tracheotomy.

Combination Disposable/Nondisposable Cartridge-Injection Syringes. A cartridge-injection system, such as the Carpuject® (Figure 36-11) or Tubex® (Figure 36-12A–E) consists of a disposable cartridge-needle unit and

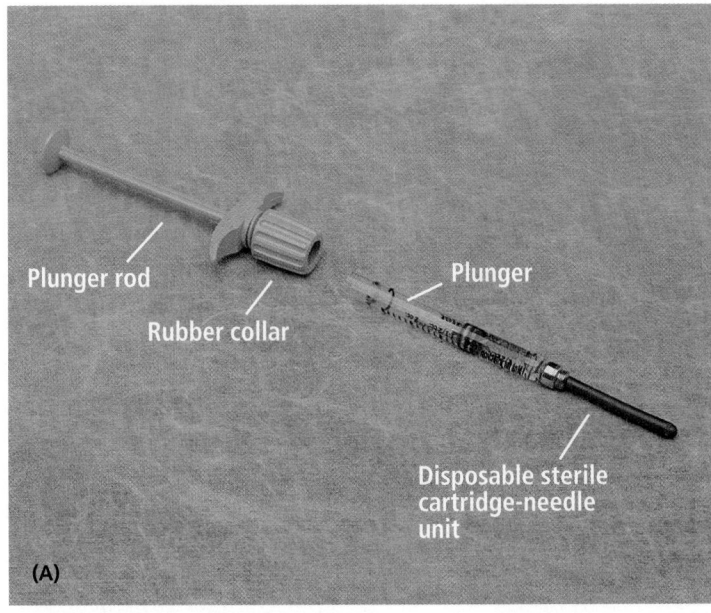

(A)

Plunger rod
Rubber collar
Plunger
Disposable sterile cartridge-needle unit

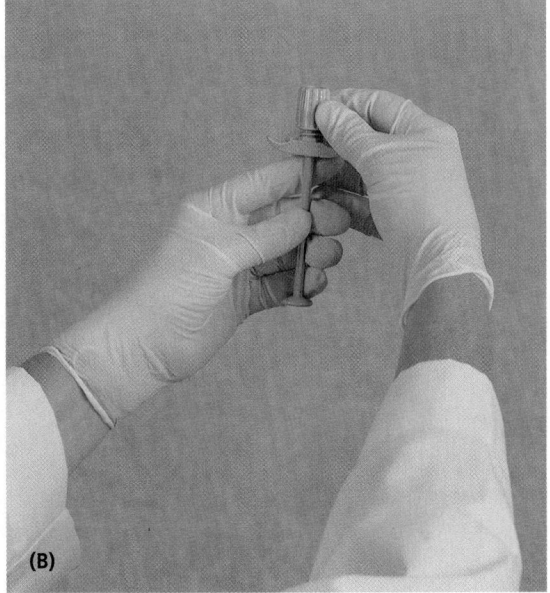

(B)

Figure 36-12   (A) Tubex® injector. Reusable cartridge holder with disposable sterile cartridge needle unit. (B) Turn ribbed collar to open position.

(continues)

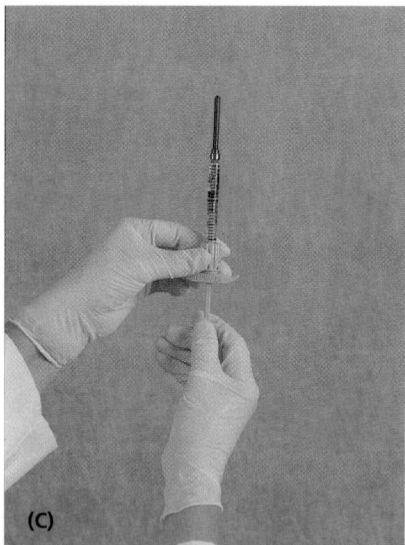
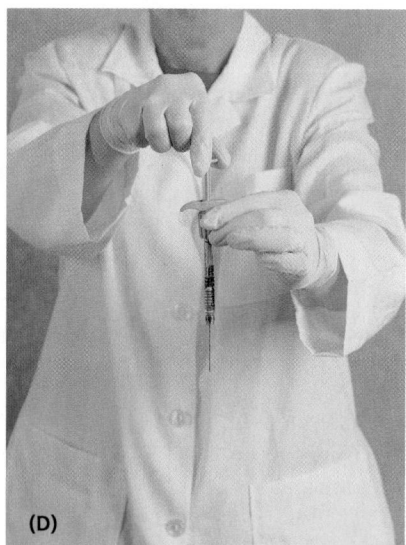
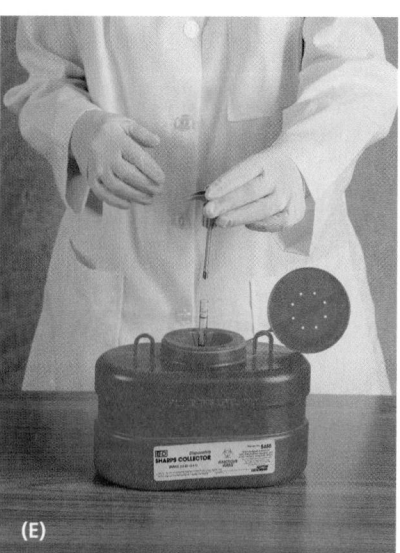

Figure 36-12 (*continued*) (C) Insert the sterile cartridge-needle unit into the open end of the injector. The ribbed collar is firmly tightened. The plunger of the injector and the plunger of the cartridge-needle unit are tightened and ready for use. (D) The medical assistant prepares to dispose of the cartridge-needle unit. The needle is not recapped. The plunger rod is disengaged by unscrewing. The ribbed collar is loosened. (E) The medical assistant holds the cartridge-needle unit over a sharps container and the unit drops into the container.

a nondisposable cartridge-holder syringe. The cartridge-needle unit is factory-sealed and sterile and contains a precisely measured unit dose of medicine. The cartridge-holder syringe may be made of durable chrome-plated brass or of plastic. These reusable syringes are designed for quick and safe loading and unloading of cartridge-needle units, which are manufactured in various sizes and dosage capacities, and contain a wide range of medications.

The combination of disposable/nondisposable syringe system is easy to use and convenient. When using this system, be careful to read the label and compare the medication order with the label. For example, the physician may order Demerol® 25 mg and the cartridge is 50 mg/cc. Give ½ cc and properly discard the other ½ cc according to office policy. Another person must witness the disposal of the Demerol®, which is a controlled substance.

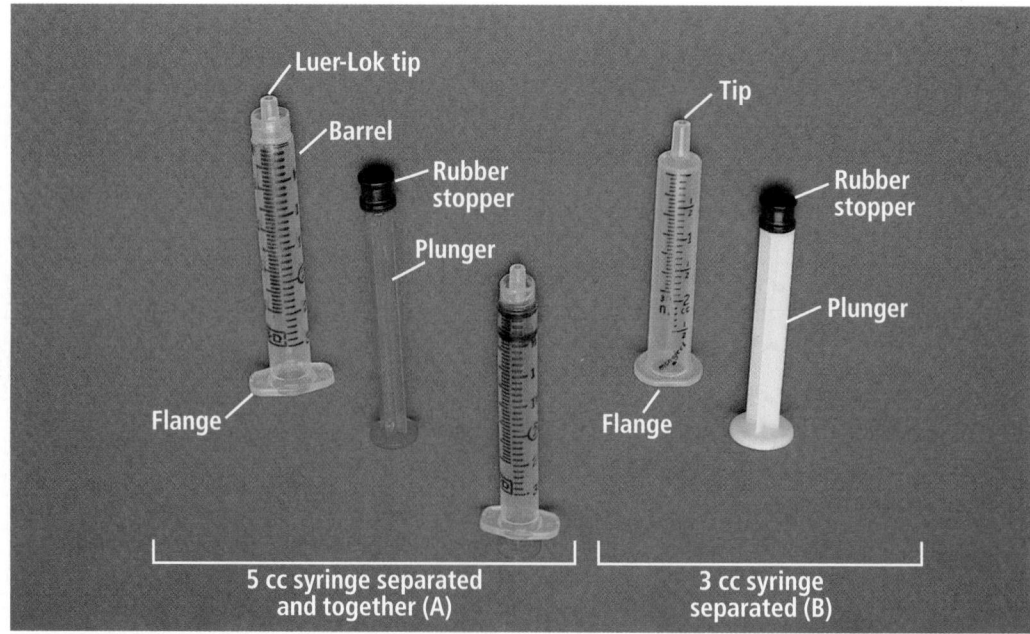

Figure 36-13 Parts of a syringe: (A) A 5-cc syringe separated and unseparated with Luer-Lok® tip. (B) A 3-cc syringe separated with plain tip.

TABLE 36-8	THE MOST FREQUENTLY USED SYRINGES FOR PARENTERAL MEDICATIONS	
Type of Syringes	**Size and Calibration**	**Typical Uses**
Hypodermic	3 cc Calibrated 0.1 15/16 minims/cc	Intramuscular and subcutaneous injections
Hypodermic	5 cc Calibrated 0.2	Venipuncture and intramuscular injections
Hypodermic	Larger sizes (10 cc, 30 cc, and 60 cc)	Medical/surgical treatments, aspirations, irrigations, venipunctures, gavage (tube-to-stomach) feedings
Tuberculin	1 cc Calibrated 0.1 and 0.01 16 minims/cc	To inject minute amounts for intradermal injections, allergy testing, allergy injections
Insulin	U-100 (0.5 cc) U-100 (1 cc)	Lo-Dose® administration of insulin Insulin administration

Parts of a Syringe. The component parts of a syringe consist of a barrel, plunger, flange, and tip (Figure 36-13).

The *barrel* is the part that holds the medication and has graduated markings (calibrations) on its surface for use in measuring medications.

The *plunger* is a movable cylinder designed for insertion within the barrel, and provides the mechanism by which a medication (or other substance) is drawn into or pushed out of the barrel.

The *flange* is at the end of the barrel where the plunger is inserted. It forms a rim around the end of the barrel where the plunger is inserted and has appendages against which one places the index and middle fingers when drawing up solution for injection. The flange also prevents the syringe from rolling when laid on a flat surface.

The *tip* is at the end of the barrel where the needle is attached.

The parts of a syringe that must remain sterile during the preparation and administration of a parenteral medication are the inside of the barrel, the section of the plunger that fits inside the barrel, and the syringe tip to which the needle is to be attached.

Types of Syringes and Uses. Syringes are named according to their sizes and uses. Table 36-8 lists the types, sizes, calibrations, and uses of syringes used in the administration of parenteral medications. Figure 36-14 shows various sizes of disposable syringes.

One should always choose a needle with sufficient length to reach the desired tissue level (see Table 36-9). A large person may require a longer needle to reach the correct body tissue than would be required for a smaller person. The delivery of medication to the proper tissue level is very important. A concentrated or irritating medication that is intended for deep intramuscular injection could be delivered instead into the subcutaneous tissue of an obese

patient if one selects a needle that is too short. Such an inappropriate injection may cause a sterile abscess. This unnecessary complication can be avoided by considering the size of the patient when choosing the length of the needle.

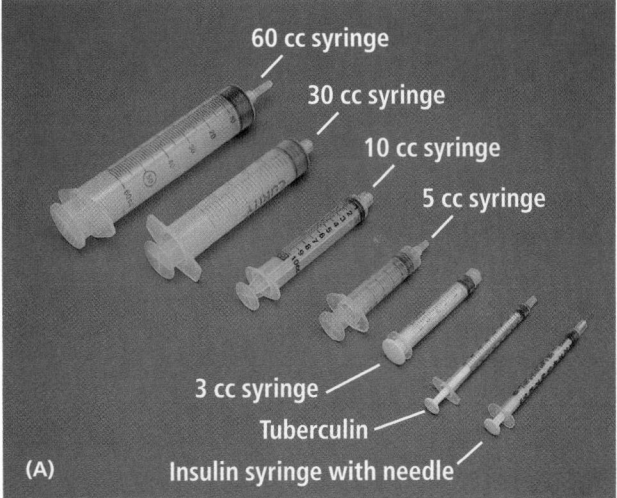

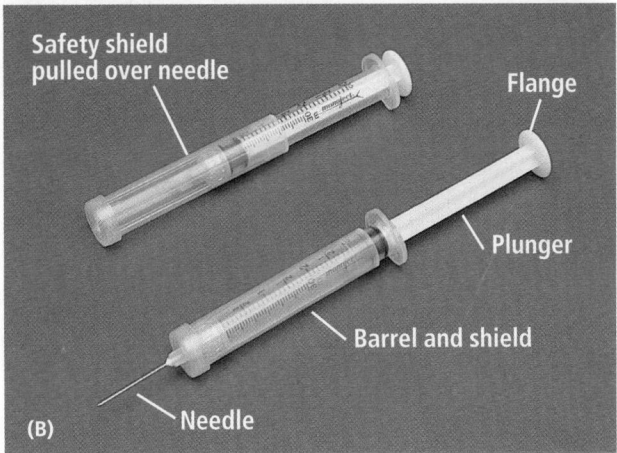

Figure 36-14 (A) Various sizes of disposable syringes. Note tuberculin and insulin syringes. (B) A type of safety syringe.

TABLE 36-9	SYRINGE-NEEDLE COMBINATIONS FOR VARIOUS PARENTERAL ROUTES	
Subcutaneous Injection	**Intramuscular Injection**	**Intradermal Injection**
3-cc syringe/25G, ⅝ inch needle	3-cc syringe/23G, 1 inch needle	1-cc syringe/25G, ⅝ inch needle
3-cc syringe/26G, ⅜ inch needle	3-cc syringe/22G, 1½ inch needle	1-cc syringe/26G, ⅜ inch needle
3-cc syringe/27G, ½ inch needle	3-cc syringe/21G, 1½ inch to 2 inch needle	1-cc syringe/27G, ½ inch needle
U-100 (1 cc)/26G, ½ inch needle		

Needles. Both disposable and nondisposable needles are available for use with syringes. Of these, the most frequently used are disposable needles, which are individually packaged in sterile paper or plastic containers. Disposable needles and syringe-needle units are available with a color-coded sheath. The sheath protects the needle and identifies its gauge and length. Needle gauges (G) range from 16 to 30, and their lengths vary from ⅜ inch to 2 inches. The needle's gauge is determined by the diameter of the lumen or opening at its beveled tip. The larger the gauge, the smaller the diameter of its lumen. For example, a 30-gauge needle is much smaller than a 16-gauge needle.

Nondisposable needles are made of high-quality stainless steel. They are equipped with a mounting hub that has a cylindrical opening designed to slip over the lock onto the tip of a syringe, such as a Luer-Lok®. See Figure 36-15 for various sizes and types of needles.

Parts of a Needle. Figure 36-16 shows the parts of a needle used to administer parenteral medications.

- The *point* is the sharpened end of the needle. The point is formed when the end of the shaft is ground away to form a flat, slanted surface called the *bevel*.
- The hollow core of the needle, when exposed at the beveled point, forms an oval-shaped opening called the *lumen*.
- The hollow steel tube through which the medication passes is the *shaft*.
- The other end of the shaft attaches to the *hub*, which is part of the needle unit that is designed to mount onto the syringe.
- The point at which the shaft attaches to the hub is called the *hilt*.

The Safe Disposal of Needles and Syringes. The careless disposal of used needles and syringes may present a health risk to any person coming into contact with the used equipment. An accidental stick by a contaminated needle could transmit diseases such as hepatitis B, syphilis, Rocky Mountain spotted fever, tuberculosis, malaria, varicella zoster, and acquired immunodeficiency syndrome (AIDS). Used needles and syringes should be discarded in a rigid, puncture-proof container (Figure 36-17). Do not recap the needle after giving the injection. Most needlesticks occur at this time. Refer to Chapter 22 for OSHA regulations.

Sharps Collectors. The B-D point-of-use Sharps Collector System eliminates the need to reshield the needle, thereby reducing the risk of an accidental needlestick.

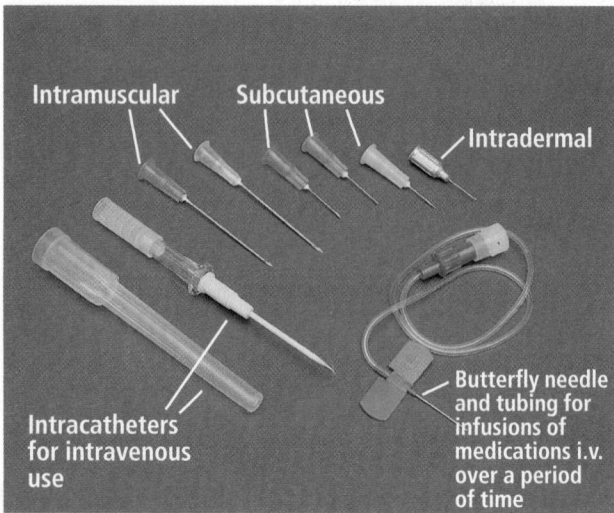

Figure 36-15 Various sizes and types of needles. Different colored hubs denote needle gauges.

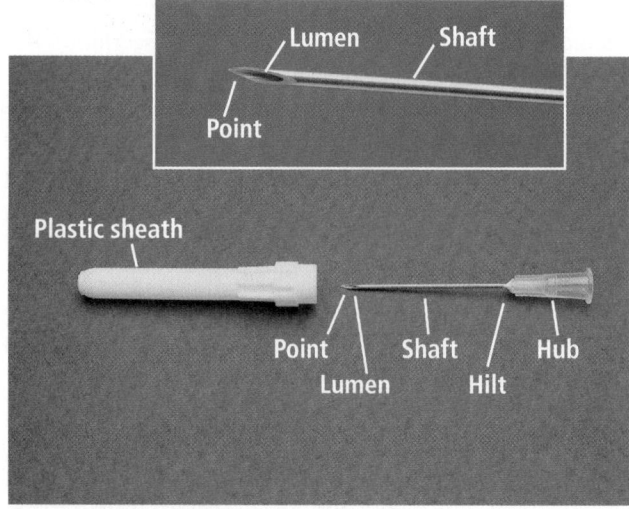

Figure 36-16 Parts of a needle and needle sheath. Inset shows point, lumen, and shaft.

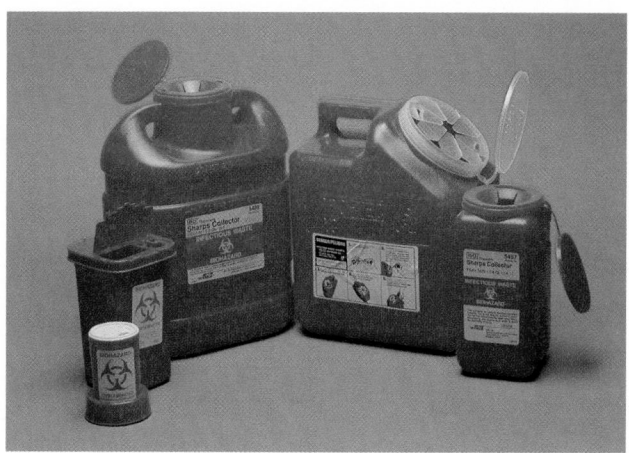

Figure 36-17   Place used needles, point down, in puncture-proof sharps containers.

Needles are placed point downward, away from the fingers. The disposable inner container is clearly marked and may be incinerated or autoclaved according to facility policy.

SITE SELECTION AND INJECTION ANGLE

The selection of a proper site for a subcutaneous, intramuscular, or intradermal injection and the correct angle of insertion for each will assure that the medication is delivered to the correct tissue type (see Figure 36-18).

A subcutaneous injection is given at an angle of 45 degrees just below the surface of the skin wherever there is

subcutaneous tissue. The shaded areas in Figure 36-19A are usually used for subcutaneous injections because they are located away from bones, joints, nerves, and large blood vessels.

An intramuscular injection is given at a 90-degree angle, passing through the skin and subcutaneous tissue and penetrating deep into muscle tissue. Body areas normally used for intramuscular injections are the dorsogluteal area, ventrogluteal area, deltoid muscle, and vastus lateralis.

Intradermal injections are given at an angle between 10 degrees and 15 degrees into the dermal layer of the skin. The body areas used for intradermal injections are the inner forearm and the middle of the back (Figure 36-19B). The reasons for the use of these two sites are that the skin is thin and there is very little hair.

Marking the Correct Site for Intramuscular Injection

To give a safe injection, it is necessary to become familiar with the anatomical structures associated with the injection site. With knowledge of where such structures are located, it is easier to mark injection sites that avoid bones, nerves, and large blood vessels.

Dorsogluteal Site. The dorsogluteal site is the traditional location for giving most (adult) deep intramuscular injections (Figure 36-20). Commonly referred to as the "upper outer quadrant of the buttocks," this description can be easily misinterpreted and result in an injection into the inappropriate area. To locate the correct site for a

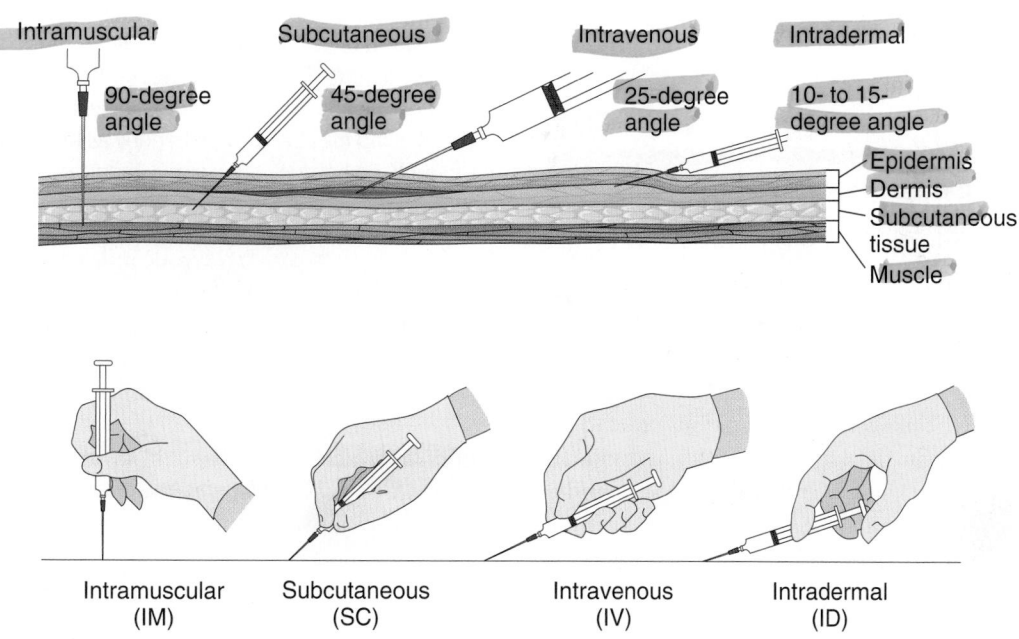

Figure 36-18   Angles of injection for intramuscular, subcutaneous, intravenous, and intradermal injections.

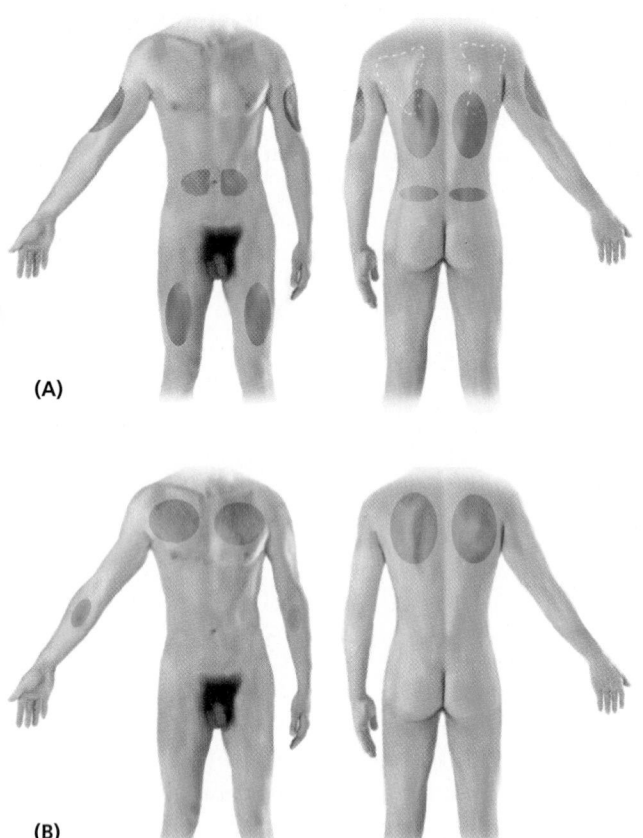

(A)

(B)

Figure 36-19   Injection sites: (A) Subcutaneous. (B) Intradermal.

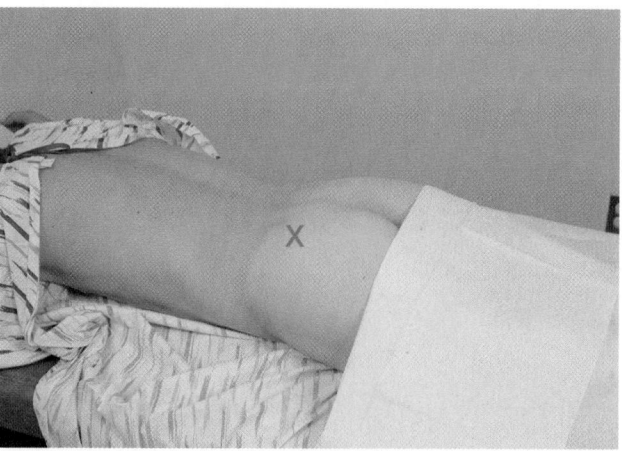

Figure 36-20   The dorsogluteal intramuscular injection site. Locate the posterior iliac spine and the greater trochanter. Draw an imaginary line between the two locations. The area above and outside this line is the injection site.

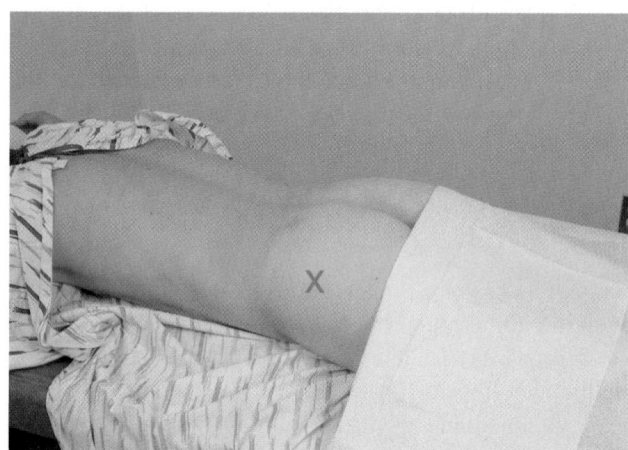

Figure 36-21   The ventrogluteal intramuscular injection site. Palpate the greater trochanter, iliac crest, and anterior superior iliac spine. If given into the patient's left buttock, the palm of the right hand is placed on the greater trochanter and the index finger on the anterior superior iliac spine. The middle finger is spread along the iliac crest posteriorly as far as possible. A "V" is formed. Give the injection in the middle of the V.

dorsogluteal injection, locate the posterior iliac spine and place a small x on this spot. Then locate the greater trochanter of the femur and mark this spot. Draw (or imagine) a diagonal line between the two locations. The area above and outside this line and about 3 inches below the iliac crest is the correct location of the dorsogluteal site.

Extreme caution should be used when giving intramuscular injections in the dorsogluteal area. Improper site selection can result in damage to the sciatic nerve or injection into the superior gluteal artery or vein. This site is contraindicated for infants and is used only as a site of last resort in children because of less muscle development. The muscle mass may be degenerated in the elderly, the nonwalking, or the emaciated patient.

Ventrogluteal Site. The ventrogluteal site can generally accommodate the majority of medications ordered for intramuscular injection. It may be used for individuals from infancy to adulthood. The ventrogluteal site is relatively free of major nerves and vessels, thereby making it a choice site for IM injections. To locate the ventrogluteal injection site, palpate to find the greater trochanter, the anterior superior iliac spine, and the bony ridge of the iliac crest (Figure 36-21). With these three locations identified, place the palm of your hand against the greater

trochanter with the tip of your index finger on the anterior superior iliac spine. Then spread your middle finger as far from the index finger as possible. Place an X in the center of the triangle formed by the middle and index fingers to mark the correct injection site.

Deltoid Muscle. The deltoid muscle is a small but adequate site for certain intramuscular injections. These IM preparations include vaccines, narcotics, sedatives, and vitamin preparations. The site should not be used for an infant. To locate the deltoid injection site, place your fingers on the shoulder and find the acromion (lateral triangular projection of the spine of the scapula forming the point of the shoulder) and the deltoid tuberosity that lies

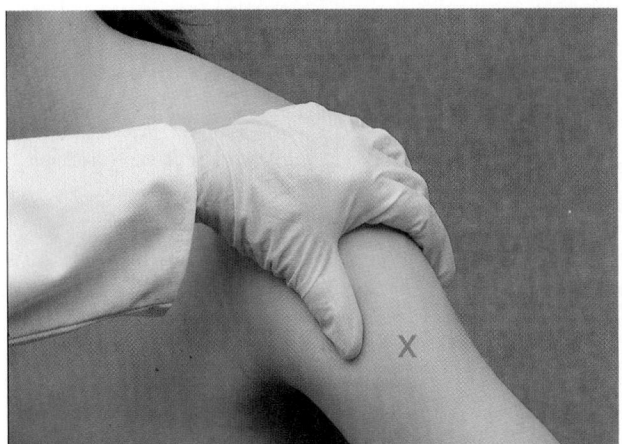

Figure 36-22 The deltoid intramuscular injection site is located on the upper outer aspect of the arm, below the lower edge of the acromion.

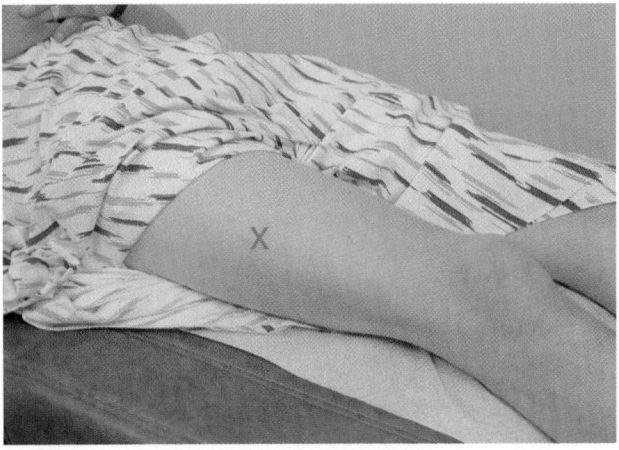

Figure 36-23 The vastus lateralis intramuscular injection site is located by dividing the leg into thirds by palpating the greater trochanter and the patella. The injection is given into the middle third of the area.

lateral to the side of the arm, opposite the axilla (Figure 36-22). The correct injection site is 1 to 2 inches (about the width of three fingers) below the acromion.

  CAUTION: Do not inject medicine into the upper and lower aspects of the deltoid muscle. Care should be taken to avoid brachial and axillary nerves and blood vessels, the radial nerve, acromion, and the humerus.

Vastus Lateralis Site. The vastus lateralis is the preferred site for intramuscular injections in infants and children. It is also used for IM injections in adults. This site generally accommodates the majority of IM injections

ordered and is a relatively safe site as the nerves and vessels supplying the area are not generally endangered. The vastus lateralis is a part of the quadriceps femoris. The muscle is located on the anterolateral aspect of the patient. For infants and children, the site lies below the greater trochanter of the femur and within the upper lateral quadrant of the thigh (Figure 36-23).

  For the adult patient, the correct injection site is within the middle third of the muscle.

  Figures 36-24A through 36-24E review the four injection sites.

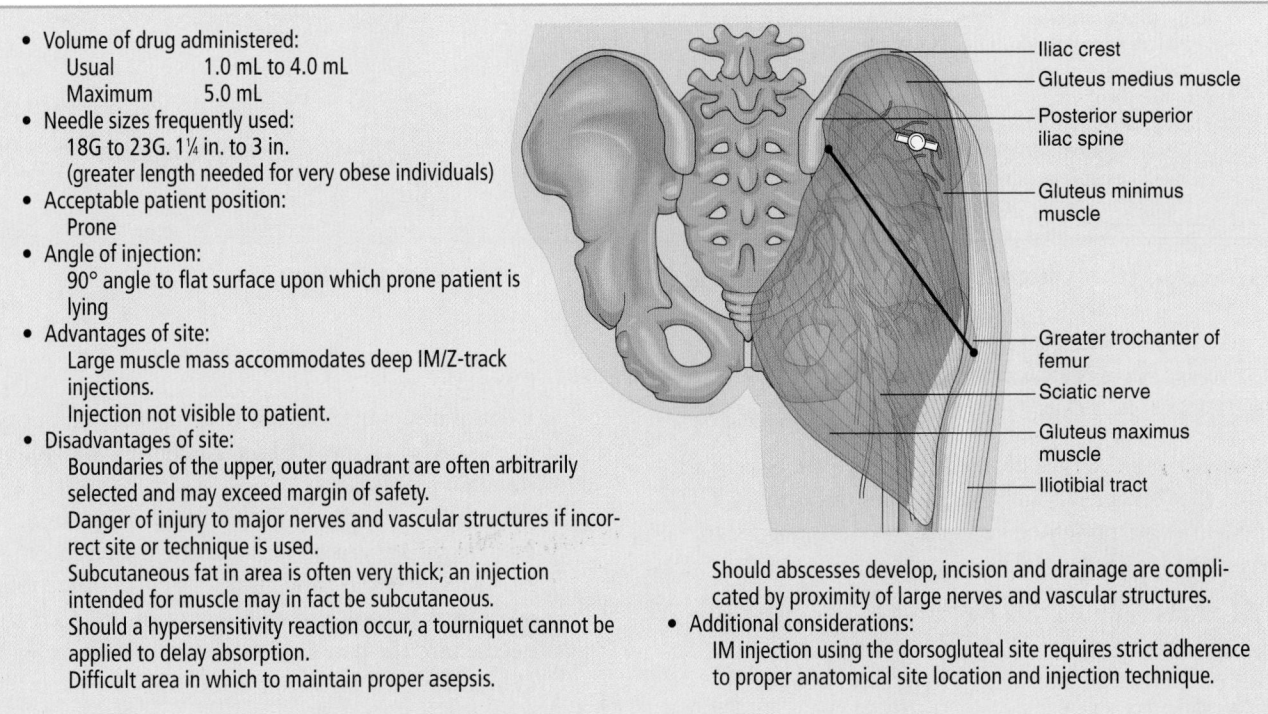

- Volume of drug administered:
   Usual   1.0 mL to 4.0 mL
   Maximum   5.0 mL
- Needle sizes frequently used:
   18G to 23G. 1¼ in. to 3 in.
   (greater length needed for very obese individuals)
- Acceptable patient position:
   Prone
- Angle of injection:
   90° angle to flat surface upon which prone patient is lying
- Advantages of site:
   Large muscle mass accommodates deep IM/Z-track injections.
   Injection not visible to patient.
- Disadvantages of site:
   Boundaries of the upper, outer quadrant are often arbitrarily selected and may exceed margin of safety.
   Danger of injury to major nerves and vascular structures if incorrect site or technique is used.
   Subcutaneous fat in area is often very thick; an injection intended for muscle may in fact be subcutaneous.
   Should a hypersensitivity reaction occur, a tourniquet cannot be applied to delay absorption.
   Difficult area in which to maintain proper asepsis.

Iliac crest
Gluteus medius muscle
Posterior superior iliac spine
Gluteus minimus muscle
Greater trochanter of femur
Sciatic nerve
Gluteus maximus muscle
Iliotibial tract

Should abscesses develop, incision and drainage are complicated by proximity of large nerves and vascular structures.
- Additional considerations:
   IM injection using the dorsogluteal site requires strict adherence to proper anatomical site location and injection technique.

Figure 36-24A Injection technique for dorsogluteal site, adult.

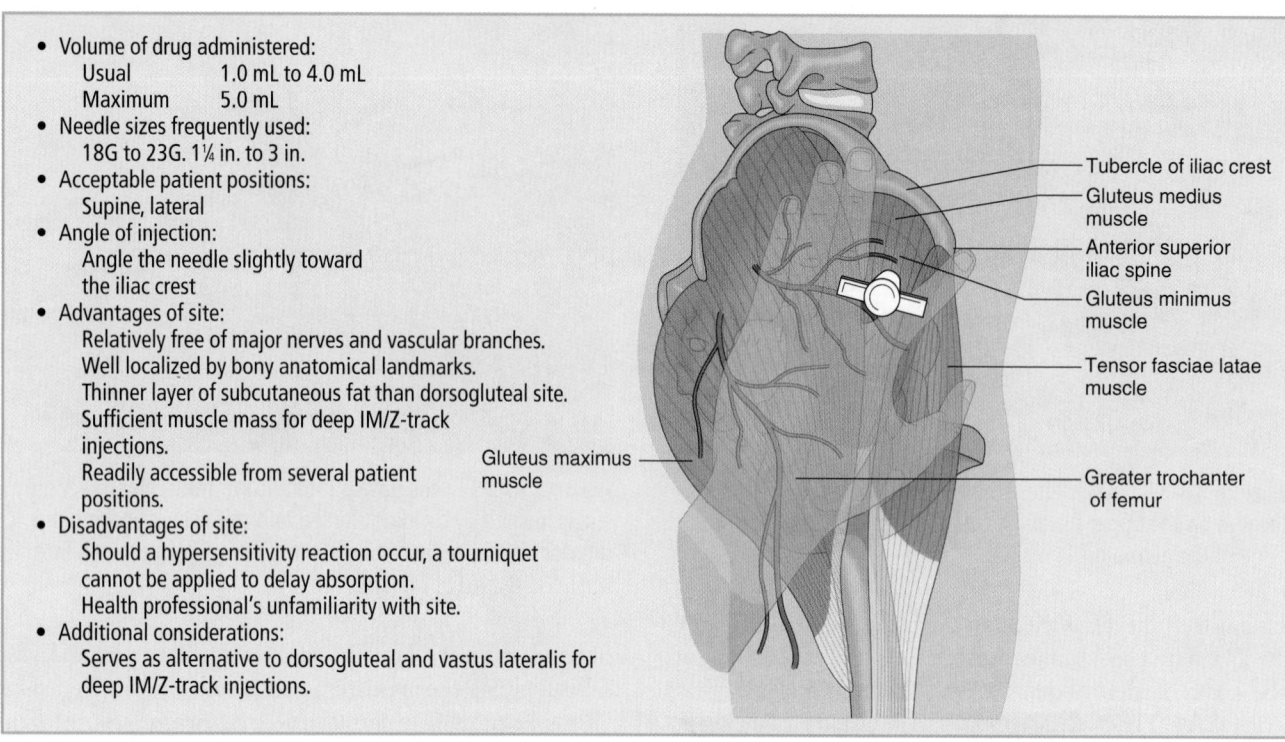

- Volume of drug administered:
    Usual   1.0 mL to 4.0 mL
    Maximum   5.0 mL
- Needle sizes frequently used:
    18G to 23G. 1¼ in. to 3 in.
- Acceptable patient positions:
    Supine, lateral
- Angle of injection:
    Angle the needle slightly toward
    the iliac crest
- Advantages of site:
    Relatively free of major nerves and vascular branches.
    Well localized by bony anatomical landmarks.
    Thinner layer of subcutaneous fat than dorsogluteal site.
    Sufficient muscle mass for deep IM/Z-track
    injections.
    Readily accessible from several patient
    positions.
- Disadvantages of site:
    Should a hypersensitivity reaction occur, a tourniquet
    cannot be applied to delay absorption.
    Health professional's unfamiliarity with site.
- Additional considerations:
    Serves as alternative to dorsogluteal and vastus lateralis for
    deep IM/Z-track injections.

Labels: Tubercle of iliac crest; Gluteus medius muscle; Anterior superior iliac spine; Gluteus minimus muscle; Tensor fasciae latae muscle; Gluteus maximus muscle; Greater trochanter of femur

Figure 36-24B   Injection technique for ventrogluteal site, adult.

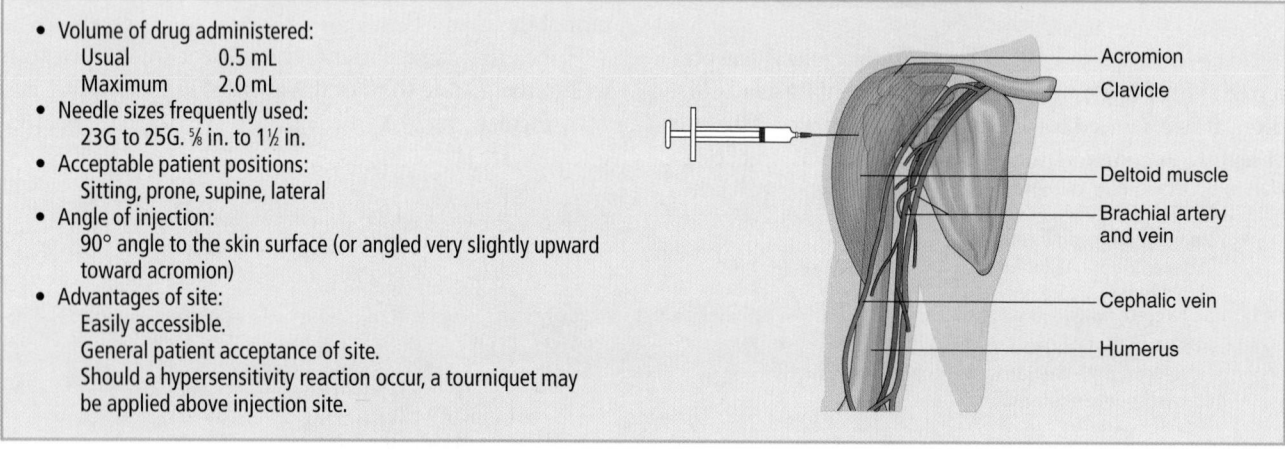

- Volume of drug administered:
    Usual   0.5 mL
    Maximum   2.0 mL
- Needle sizes frequently used:
    23G to 25G. ⅝ in. to 1½ in.
- Acceptable patient positions:
    Sitting, prone, supine, lateral
- Angle of injection:
    90° angle to the skin surface (or angled very slightly upward
    toward acromion)
- Advantages of site:
    Easily accessible.
    General patient acceptance of site.
    Should a hypersensitivity reaction occur, a tourniquet may
    be applied above injection site.

Labels: Acromion; Clavicle; Deltoid muscle; Brachial artery and vein; Cephalic vein; Humerus

Figure 36-24C   Injection technique for deltoid site, adult.

BASIC GUIDELINES FOR ADMINISTRATION OF INJECTIONS

Regardless of the type of injection, there are basic guidelines that one must follow to safeguard the patient. These guidelines are presented according to the sequence of the events to which they relate:

1. Adhere to the "Six Rights" of proper drug administration.
2. Always evaluate each patient as an individual.
3. Select a needle-syringe unit that is the appropriate size for the proper administration of a parenteral medication.
4. Correctly prepare the appropriate parenteral equipment and supplies for use. Wash hands and put on gloves. Always use OSHA guidelines and follow standard precautions.
5. Select the correct site for the intended injection.
6. Prepare the patient properly for the injection.
7. For subcutaneous and intramuscular injections, use a smooth, quick, dart-like motion to insert the needle into the patient's skin. Use the correct angle of insertion (45 degrees or 90 degrees) for the injection. Once the needle is inserted, gently pull back on the plunger (aspirate) to ensure that the needle is not in a blood vessel.

- Volume of drug administered:
    Usual   1.0 mL
    Maximum   5.0 mL
- Needle sizes frequently used:
    20G to 23G. 1¼ in. to 1½ in.
- Acceptable patient positions:
    Supine, sitting
- Angle of injection:
    90° angle to the skin surface (for small or thin adults the technique used for pediatric injections may be preferable)
- Advantages of site:
    Large muscle mass can tolerate relatively large quantities of medication.
    Surface area provides sufficient space for several injections.
    Free of major nerves and vascular branches.

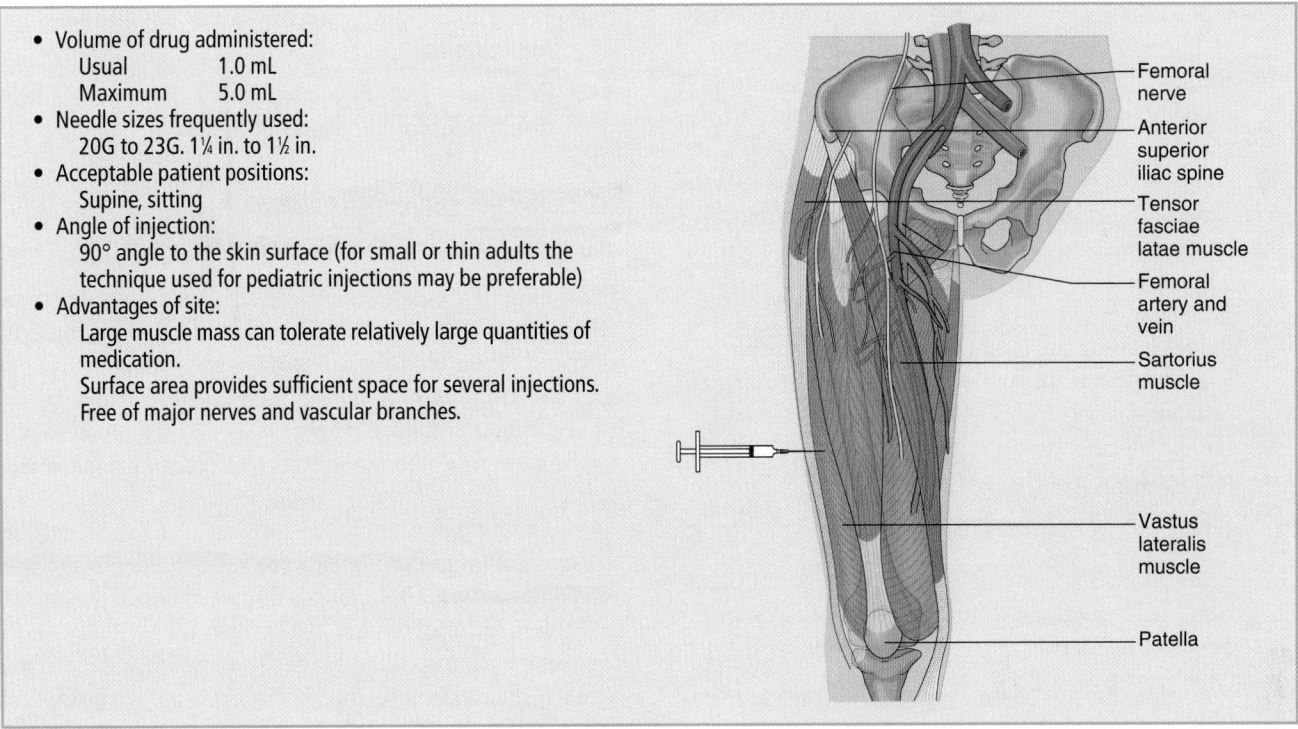

Figure 36-24D   Injection technique for vastus lateralis site, adult.

- Volume of drug administered:
    Usual   < 0.5 mL (infants);
                     1.0 mL (pediatric)
    Maximum   1.0 mL (infants);
                     2.0 mL (pediatric)
- Needle sizes frequently used:
    22G to 25G. ⅝ in.
- Acceptable patient positions:
    Supine, sitting
- Angle of injection:
    45° angle to the frontal, sagittal, and horizontal planes of the thigh (directed toward the knee)
- Advantages of site:
    Relatively large muscle mass at birth.
    Suitable site for infants.
    Surface area provides sufficient space for several injections.
    Free of major nerves and vascular branches.

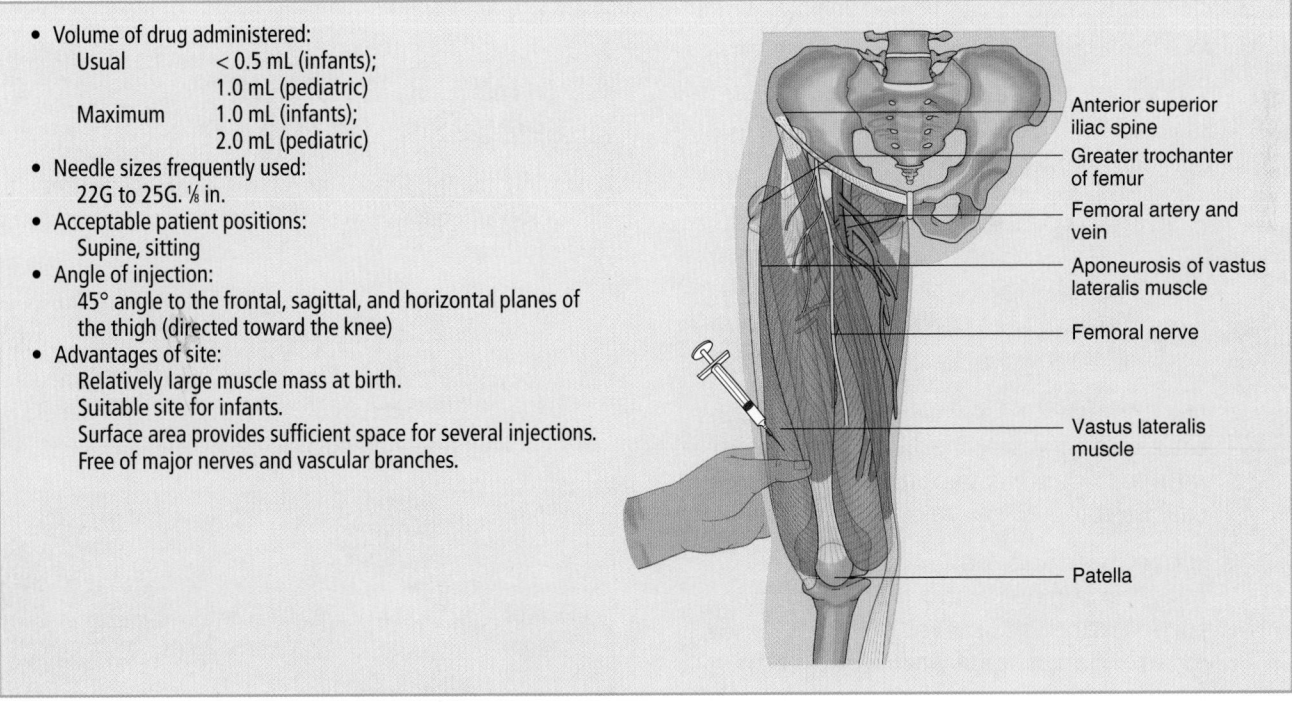

Figure 36-24E   Injection technique for vastus lateralis site, pediatric.

CAUTION: If blood appears in the syringe upon aspiration, smoothly withdraw the needle, properly discard the used unit, and prepare another injection for administration. Repeat the preceding steps.

8. Slowly inject the medication into the patient.

9. With a quick, smooth motion, remove the needle from the injection site. Discard the syringe needle unit in a puncture-proof container. Cover the injection site with a dry, sterile cotton swab and gently massage the site.

CAUTION: Do not massage the site when administering insulin, Imferon, or heparin.

10. Remove the cotton swab and check for bleeding. If bleeding occurs, apply a sterile Band-Aid® to the injection site. Remove gloves.

11. Observe the patient for any signs of hypersensitivity.

12. Take precautions to ensure the patient's safety.

13. Properly discard the used equipment and supplies. This should be done as soon as possible.

14. Wash hands.

15. Before leaving the room, make sure that the patient is given proper instructions and is experiencing no unusual effects.

16. Follow documentation procedures to record the administration of the medication.

Procedures 36-2 through 36-8 include:

- Procedure 36-2 General Procedure for Administration of Subcutaneous, Intramuscular, and/or Intradermal Injections

- Procedure 36-3 Withdrawing (Aspirating) Medication from a Vial

- Procedure 36-4 Withdrawing (Aspirating) Medication from an Ampule

- Procedure 36-5 Administering a Subcutaneous Injection

- Procedure 36-6 Administering an Intramuscular Injection

- Procedure 36-7 Administering an Intradermal Injection

- Procedure 36-8 Reconstituting a Powder Medication for Administration Equipment

Z-TRACK METHOD OF INTRAMUSCULAR INJECTION

Imferon is an example of a medication that must be administered by using the Z-track method. This medication and others that are irritating to the subcutaneous tissues and may discolor the skin are given in this manner. (The *Physician's Desk Reference* is a good reference source for help in determining the correct technique for injections.)

The Z-track technique is similar to an intramuscular injection, except that the skin is pulled to the side prior to needle insertion. This causes a displacement of the tissues and the medication enters in a manner that will not allow it to seep back into the subcutaneous tissues and up to the skin's surface. Because the medications are irritating, for the comfort of the patient, change the needle on the syringe after aspirating the medication from the ampule or vial before injecting the patient with the medication. See Procedure 36-9.

ADMINISTRATION OF ALLERGENIC EXTRACTS

It may be the responsibility of the medical assistant to administer allergenic extracts. It is important to observe the following:

- Allergic extracts are *always* given in subcutaneous tissue, *never* in the muscle.

- Use a tuberculin syringe with a 25G, ⅝ inch needle, or a 26G, ⅜ inch needle, or a 27G, ½ inch needle or ICC allergist syringes (Figure 36-25).

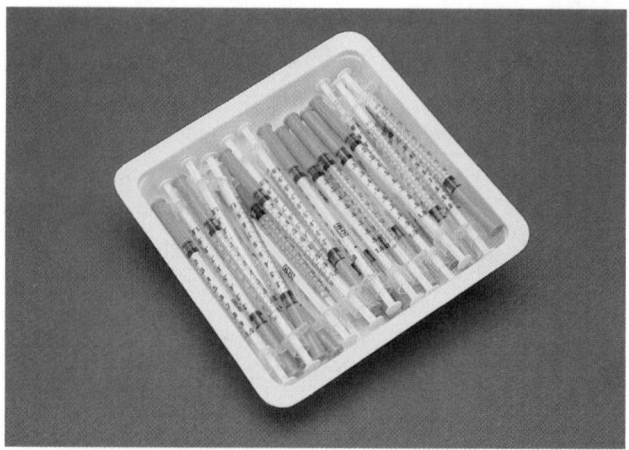

Figure 36-25   Allergist syringes.

- Use a site rotation system for each injected extract.

- Correctly document the procedure.

- Allergenic extracts should be refrigerated; they should retain potency for 10 to 12 weeks.

- Adverse reactions such as itching, swelling, and redness should be reported immediately to the physician.

- Severe reactions such as anaphylactic shock have occurred; therefore, emergency equipment and supplies must be available for use (see Chapter 35 for emergency supplies).

- Allergy testing can only be done when physician is present.

Example:
Patient's Name:

Date	Dose	Site
6/24/__	1st 0.05 cc s.c.	Lt. arm
6/27/__	2nd 0.10 cc s.c.	Rt. arm
6/30/__	3rd 0.15 cc s.c.	Lt. arm

 CAUTION: The patient should be observed for 15 to 30 minutes following the injection of an allergenic extract.

Susceptible individuals can develop allergic reactions to many foreign substances. It is prudent that the allergic person be totally aware of those substances and/or things that are known allergens.

INHALATION METHODS OF MEDICATION ADMINISTRATION

The act of drawing breath, vapor, or gas into the lungs is known as inhalation. Inhalation therapy may involve the administration of medicines, water vapor, and such gases as oxygen, carbon dioxide, and helium.

An inhaler may be used to deliver medications to the lungs. Medications that utilize an inhaler include bronchodilators, mucolytic agents, and steroids. Inhalers are useful in the delivery of treatment for chronic obstructive pulmonary disease (COPD) and/or reversible obstructive airway disease. An inhaler is a small, handheld apparatus, usually an aerosol unit, that contains a microcrystalline suspension of medication. When activated, it produces a fine mist or spray containing the medication. This suspension is then drawn into the respiratory tract, settling deep into the lungs and alveoli.

Implications for Patient Care

- Patients should be instructed to follow the prescribed medication regimen. The prescribed medicine and the type of inhaler to be used will

Patient Teaching Tip

- Patients should be advised to avoid overuse of the inhaler. Tolerance, rebound bronchospasm, and adverse cardiac effects can occur from overuse. Instruct the patient to notify the physician should the prescribed dose of medication fail to produce the desired effect.
- Instruct the patient to perform good oral hygiene, including rinsing of the mouth and mouthpiece of equipment, after the inhalation treatment (to prevent the possible growth of fungi).
- Caution the patient against the continued use of a metered-dose canister after the stated number of actuations. If the medication contains adrenaline, fatalities can occur if heart rate increases and blood pressure rises.

determine the method of administration. A handheld inhaler may be utilized for oral or nasal inhalation, depending on the type ordered by the physician.

Inhalation therapy may be contraindicated in patients with delicate fluid balance, cardiac arrhythmias, **status asthmaticus**, and hypersensitivity to the medication. As with any medication, the physician will determine the treatment regimen for each patient.

Administration of Oxygen

Oxygen is a colorless, odorless, tasteless gas that is essential for life. When the body does not have an adequate supply of oxygen, a state of **hypoxemia** (lack of oxygen in the blood) develops, and the irreversible damage to vital organs is possible. When a lack of oxygen threatens a person's survival, supplemental oxygen must be prescribed and administered immediately, and arterial blood gas analysis will have to be made after oxygen administration has been started. If it is not an emergency or life-threatening situation, an arterial blood gas analysis will be made before the physician prescribes the dosage and method of administration. The normal range for oxygen in the arterial blood is 80 to 100 mm Hg (millimeters mercury). Oxygen is supplied in tanks (Figure 36-26) for use in the ambulatory care setting, but in a hospital setting oxygen is piped in through a wall pipe system.

Dosage. When oxygen is to be administered, dosage is based on individual needs. Since oxygen is a drug, the

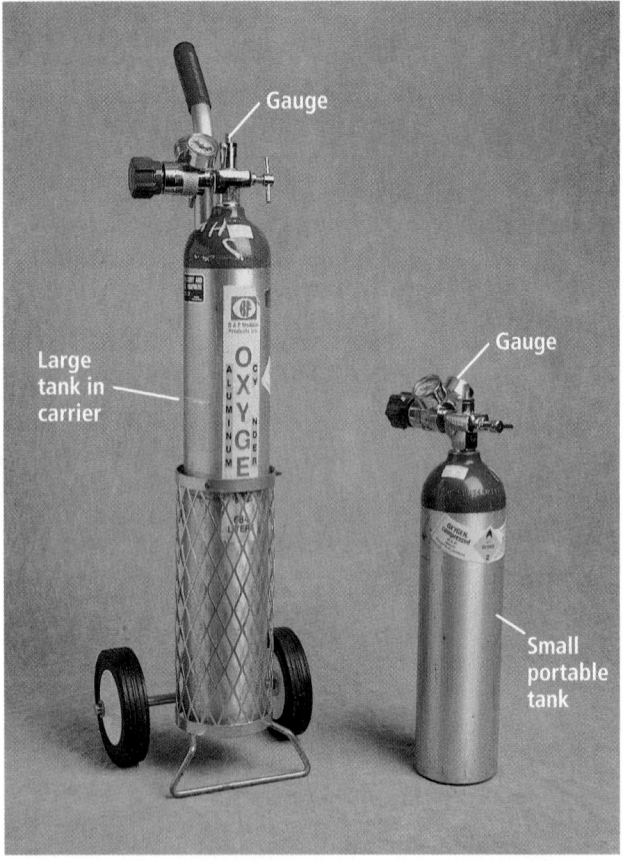

Figure 36-26   Oxygen tanks. Note gauge at top of tanks.

physician will prescribe the flow rate, concentration, method of delivery, and length of time for administration. Oxygen is ordered as liters per minute (LPM) or L/min and as percentage of oxygen concentration (%).

It is the medical assistant's responsibility to follow physician orders and adhere to the guidelines for proper drug administration. Always assess the patient as an individual, explain the procedure, and carefully observe the patient for signs of improvement or symptoms of oxygen toxicity.

CAUTION: Oxygen toxicity may develop when 100 percent oxygen is breathed for a prolonged period. As with any other drug, toxicity depends upon dose, time, and the patient's response. The higher the dose, the shorter the time required to develop toxicity. Symptoms of oxygen toxicity are substernal pain, nausea, vomiting, malaise, fatigue, numbness, and a tingling of the extremities.

High concentrations of inhaled oxygen cause alveolar collapse, intra-alveolar hemorrhage, hyaline membrane formation, disturbance of the central nervous system, and **retrolental fibroplasia** in newborns.

NOTE: **Apnea** (absence of breathing) can result when giving oxygen at a flow-rate greater than 2 liters per minute to COPD patients, especially those with emphysema.

Methods of Oxygen Delivery. Many methods are available today for the delivery of oxygen. The more commonly prescribed methods include the use of nasal cannulas, nasal catheters, and masks. Other methods of delivery involve the use of isolettes, hoods, and tents.

Nasal Cannula. When a low concentration of oxygen is desired, the nasal cannula (Figure 36-27) is the simplest and most convenient method for the administration of oxygen. Made of plastic, the nasal cannula consists of two hollow prongs through which oxygen passes, and a strap or other device to secure it to the patient's head (Figure 36-28). Do not place the direct flow of O_2 against the patient's nasal mucosa, as this causes tissue dehydration.

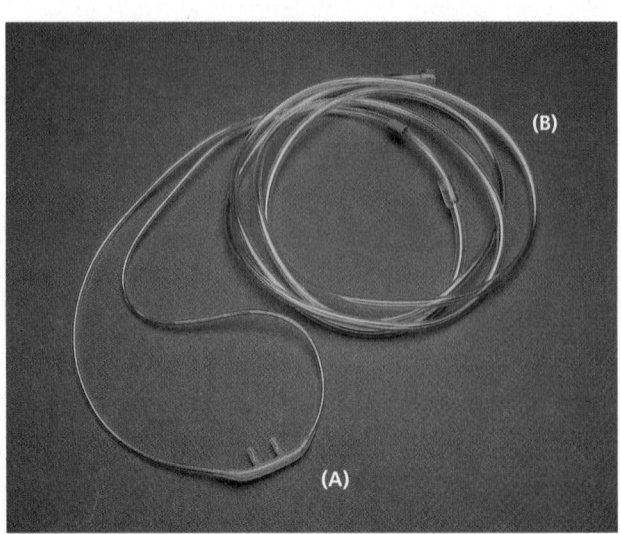

Figure 36-27   (A) Oxygen cannula. (B) Tubing.

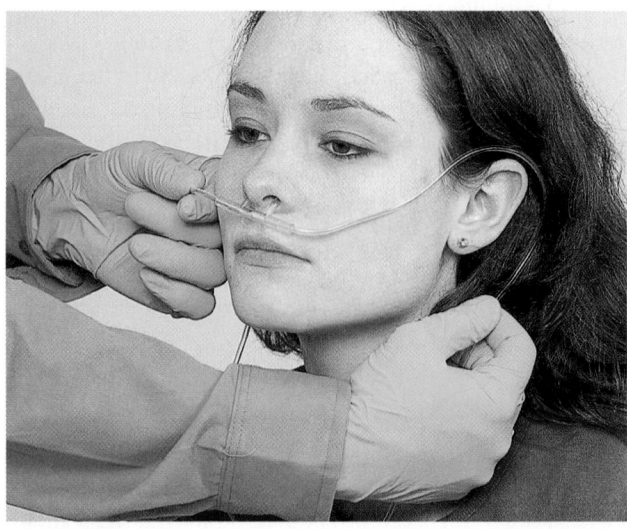

Figure 36-28   Medical assistant adjusts nasal cannula around patient's head for oxygen administration.

Flow rates greater than 2 to 4 liters per minute require humidification.

Nasal Catheter. The nasal catheter is a disposable plastic tube that has small holes at the inserted end. These holes diffuse the flow of oxygen for better distribution to lung tissue with minimum dehydration. The nasal catheter is seldom used today, because it causes mucus membrane irritation and has to be changed every 8 hours. Due to the discomfort caused to the patient by the catheter, the nasal cannula is the preferred method for the delivery of oxygen.

Mask. The common types of masks used for inhalation therapy include plastic disposable, partial rebreather, non-rebreather, and Venturi (Figure 36-29). These devices are employed when the patient requires high humidity and a precise amount of oxygen. To be effective, the mask must be fitted snugly to the patient (Figure 36-30).

    CAUTION: Oxygen must be humidified before delivery to the patient in order to prevent drying of the respiratory mucosa.

Oxygen Safety Precautions. Oxygen supports combustion; thus, there is the danger of a fire being started when oxygen is in use. Extreme caution should be exercised because ignition can be caused by friction, static electricity, or a lighted cigar or cigarette when O_2 is being administered. In the physician's office, oxygen is generally stored in tanks. These tanks must be checked on a regular basis and replaced as necessary.

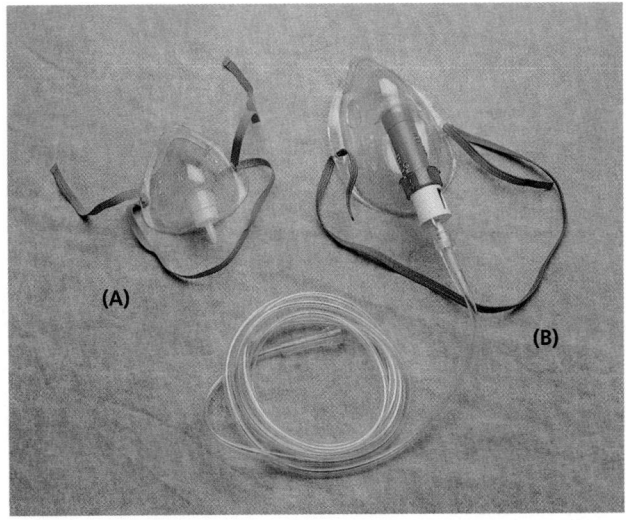

Figure 36-29 Oxygen masks: (A) Without tubing. (B) With tubing.

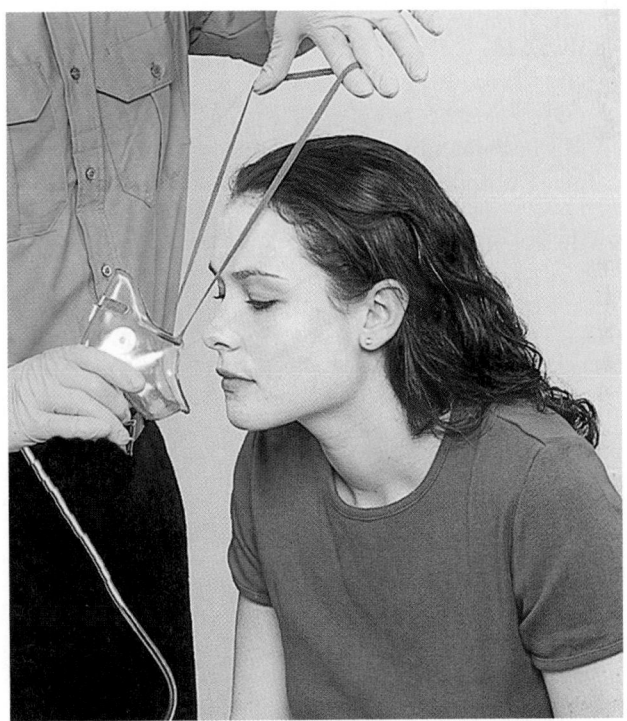

Figure 36-30 Medical assistant adjusts oxygen mask around patient's head.

Patient Teaching Tip

Explain safety measures to the patient who uses oxygen at home. Cigarettes, lighters, candles, and other smoking materials should not be used in the room where oxygen is used. Instruct the patient to wear nonstatic-producing clothing, such as cotton.

Procedure

36-1 **Administration of Oral Medications**

STANDARD PRECAUTIONS:

PURPOSE:
Correctly administer an oral medication after receiving a physician's order and assembling the necessary equipment and supplies.

EQUIPMENT/SUPPLIES:
Proper medication
Medicine card
Water, milk, or juice for patient

PROCEDURE STEPS:
1. Verify the physician's order.
2. Follow the "Six Rights" (Figure 36-31A).
3. Perform medical asepsis handwash.
4. Work in a well-lighted, quiet, clean area.
5. Assemble equipment and supplies.
6. Obtain the correct medication using the medicine card.
7. Compare the medication label with the medicine card (first time).
8. Check the expiration date.
9. Calculate dosage if necessary.
10. Correctly prepare (a, b, or c) (Figure 36-31B).
    a. Multiple dose solid medication
    b. Unit dose medication
    c. Liquid medication
11. Compare medicine label with medicine card (second time).
12. Return medication to shelf and check label (third time).
13. Properly transport the medicine.
14. Identify the patient. Explain the procedure.
15. Assess patient. Take vital signs if indicated.
16. Assist patient to a comfortable position.
17. Provide water, milk, or juice (unless contraindicated).
18. Administer the medication. Be certain that the patient takes the medicine (Figure 36-31C).
19. Provide for the patient's safety: Observe the patient for any adverse reactions.
20. Care for equipment and supplies according to OSHA guidelines.
21. Wash hands.
22. Document the procedure in the patient chart using the medicine card (Figure 36-31D).

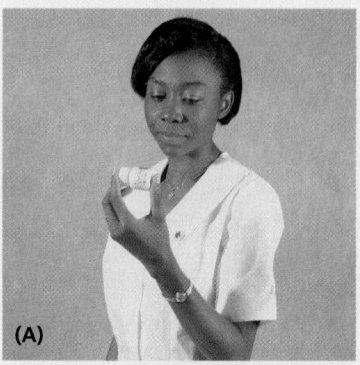

(A)

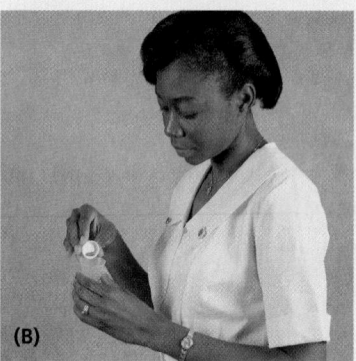

(B)

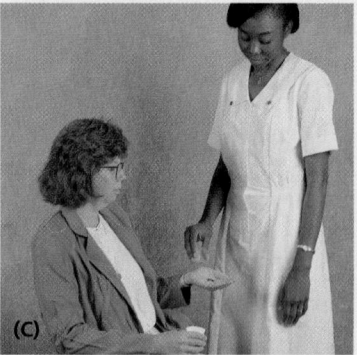

(C)

Figure 36-31   (A) Medical assistant checks for right drug, right dose, right route, and expiration date before pouring medication. (B) Medical assistant pours capsules from the cover of the medicine container into a medicine cup prior to administering medicine to the patient. The medication is poured into cover to avoid contamination of medicine. (C) Medical assistant administers the medication, being certain that patient takes the medicine.   *(continues)*

Procedure

36-1 *(continued)*

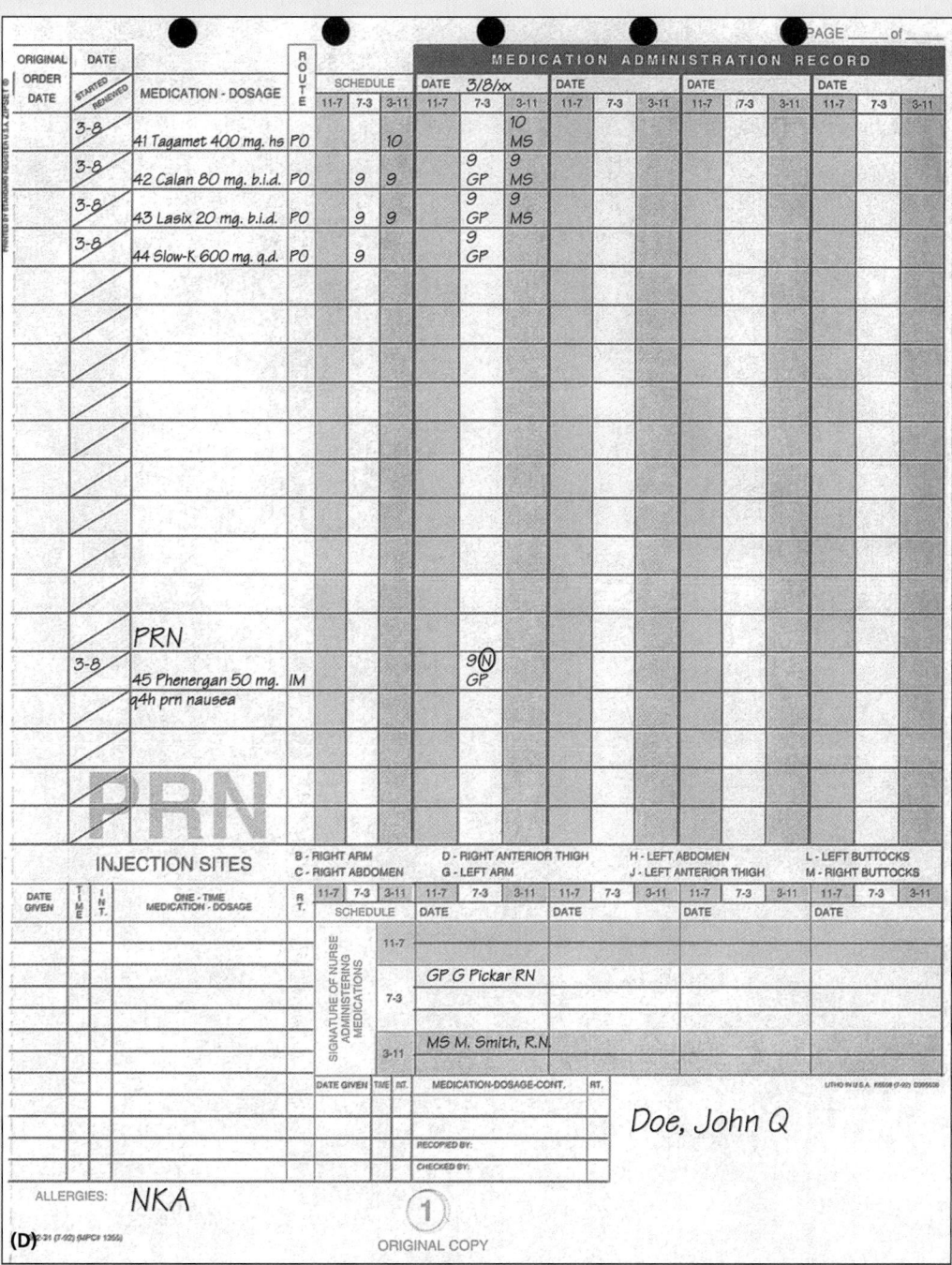

Figure 36-31 *(continued)* (D) Example of a medication administration record for patient's chart.

Administration of Subcutaneous, Intramuscular, and Intradermal Injections

STANDARD PRECAUTIONS:

PURPOSE:
To properly administer subcutaneous, intramuscular, and intradermal injections.

EQUIPMENT/SUPPLIES:
Medication as ordered by the physician and medicine card
Appropriately sized needle-syringe unit
Alcohol wipes
Disposable gloves
Sharps container

PROCEDURE STEPS:
1. Verify the physician's order. Make out medicine card taking information from physician's order sheet from patient record.
2. Follow the "Six Rights."
3. Perform medical asepsis handwash. Adhere to OSHA guidelines.
4. Work in a well-lighted, quiet, clean area.
5. Obtain the appropriate syringe-needle unit and alcohol wipe.
6. Obtain the correct medication.
7. Compare the medication label with the medicine card (first time).
8. Check expiration date on medicine.
9. Calculate dosage, if necessary.
10. Prepare syringe-needle unit for use (Figure 36-32A–E).
11. Withdraw medication from container.
12. Compare medicine label with the medicine card (second time).
13. Place filled syringe-needle unit on the medicine tray with medicine card. Check the medication label with the medicine card (third time).
14. Correctly transport the medicine to the patient.
15. Identify the patient. Explain the procedure.
16. Assess the patient. Put on gloves.
17. Prepare the patient for the injection (drape, position, allay apprehension).

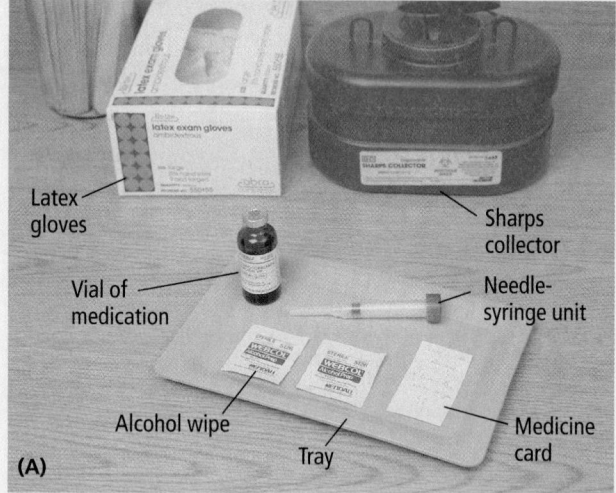

(A)

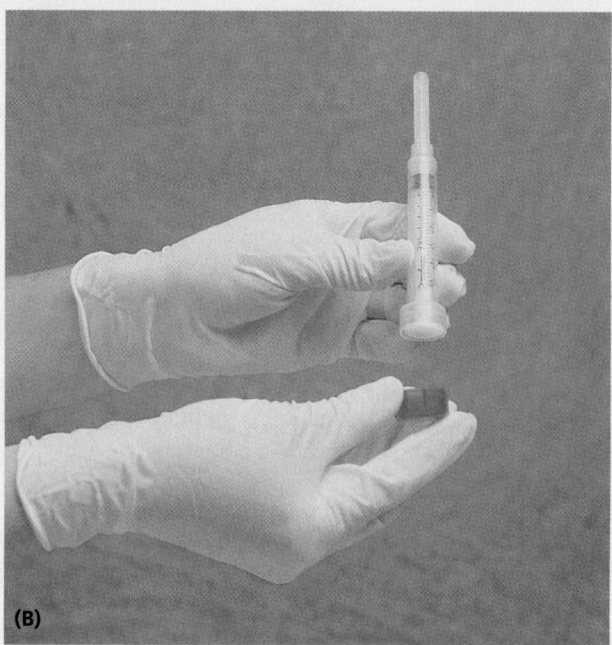

(B)

Figure 36-32 Preparing the syringe-needle unit for use: (A) Assemble the equipment and supplies needed to draw up medication from a vial. (B) Remove the cap from the cover of the sterile syringe-needle unit. *(continues)*

Procedure

36-2   *(continued)*

18. Select an appropriate injection site. Follow a rotating schedule if appropriate.
19. Cleanse the injection site with a sterile alcohol wipe. Use a circular motion, working from the center out to about 2 inches beyond the planned injection site.
20. Allow the skin to dry.
21. Administer the injection. Aspirate to be certain needle is not in a blood vessel (except for intradermal injection). Immediately dispose of syringe-needle unit in a puncture-proof container.
22. Massage injection site unless contraindicated (insulin, Imferon, heparin).
23. Observe the patient for signs of difficulty.
24. Inspect the injection site for bleeding, apply Band-Aid if necessary.

25. Properly dispose of used equipment and supplies. Remove gloves.
26. Perform medical asepsis handwash.
27. Correctly document the procedure.

Procedure to follow should the medical assistant sustain an accidental needlestick after the injection:

- Thoroughly wash the site where the stick occurred.
- Cleanse the skin with an antiseptic.
- Report the incident.
- Document the incident and retain a copy for yourself.
- Obtain medical attention. Be tested for HBV and HIV.
- Fill out appropriate OSHA paperwork (200 form).

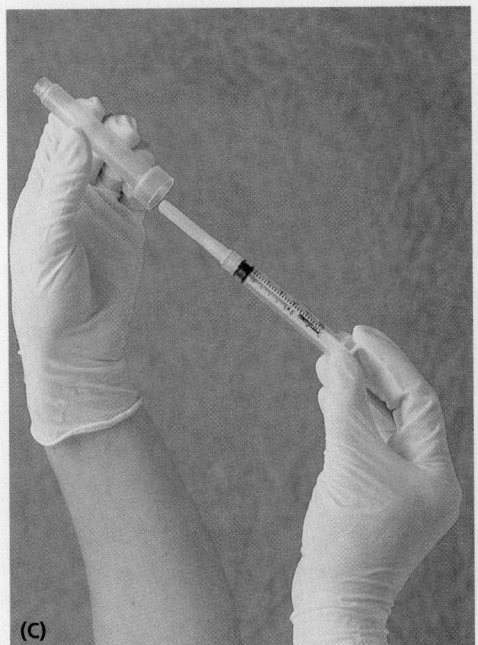
(C)

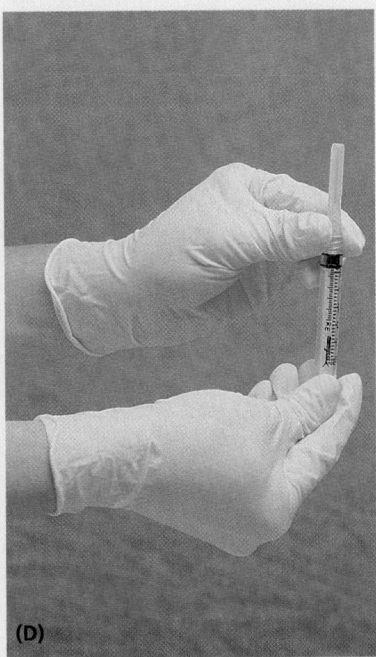
(D)

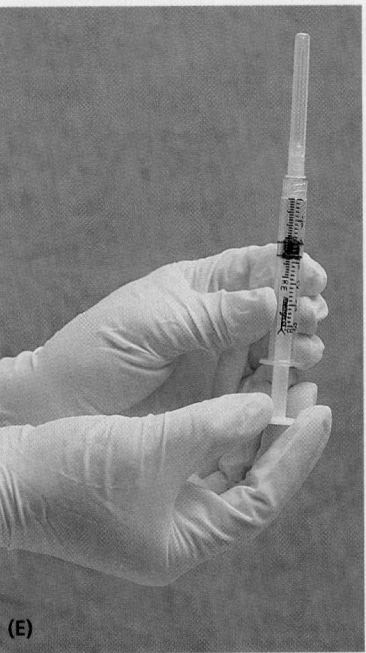
(E)

Figure 36-32   *(continued)* (C) Pull the sleeve of the cover off and remove the syringe-needle unit. (D) Secure the needle by twisting it clockwise. (E) Pull the plunger to check for ease of gliding operation.

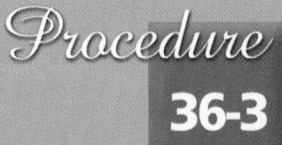

Withdrawing (Aspirating) Medication from a Vial

Procedure 36-3

STANDARD PRECAUTIONS:

PURPOSE:
Medication is supplied in a variety of packaging. Medication from a vial must be aspirated into a syringe for parenteral injection.

EQUIPMENT/SUPPLIES:

Medication order	Vial of medication
Medicine card	Alcohol wipes
Appropriate syringe and needle with cover	Disposable gloves
	Sharps container

PROCEDURE STEPS:

1. Read the medication order and assemble equipment. Check for the "Six Rights." Read the vial label by holding it next to the medicine card (first time).
2. Wash hands. Apply gloves.
3. Select the proper size needle and syringe for the medication and the route (e.g., for subcutaneous injection of insulin, 100-U insulin syringe and 25G, ⅝ inch needle). If necessary, attach the needle to the syringe.
4. Check the vial label against the medicine card (second time).
5. Remove the metal or plastic cap from the vial. If the vial has been opened previously, clean the rubber stopper by applying an alcohol wipe in a circular motion (Figure 36-33A).
6. Remove the needle cover—pull it straight off.
7. Inject air into the vial as follows:
   a. Hold the syringe pointed upward at eye level. Pull back the plunger to take in a quantity of air that is equal to the ordered dose of medication.
   b. Hold the vial upright (inverted) according to personal preference. Take care not to touch the rubber stopper.
   c. Insert the needle through the rubber stopper of the vial. Inject the air by pushing in the plunger (Figure 36-33B).
8. Withdraw the medication: Hold the vial and the syringe steady. Pull back on the plunger to with-

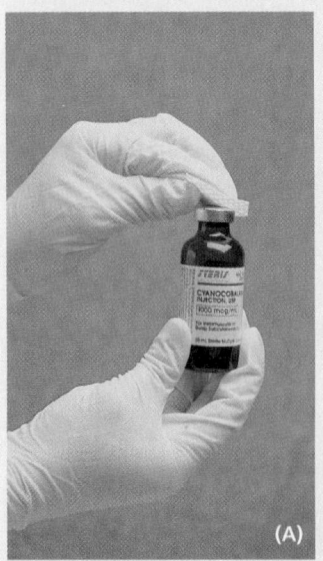
(A)

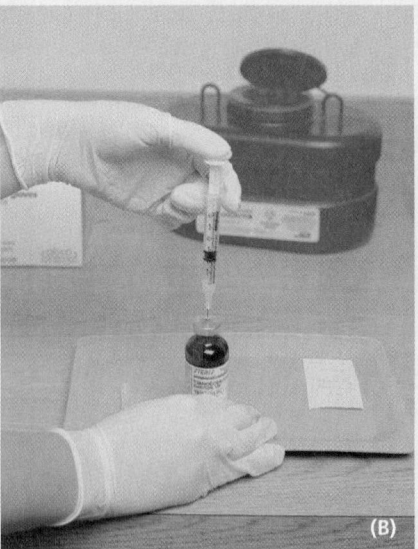
(B)

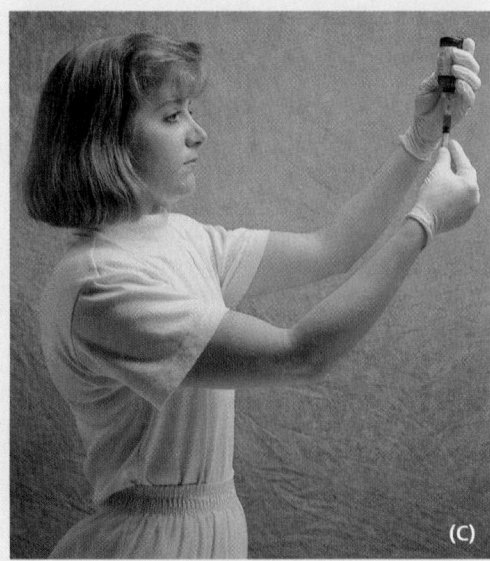
(C)

Figure 36-33 (A) Disinfect the rubber stopper on the medication vial with an alcohol wipe. (B) Keeping the bevel of the needle above the fluid level, inject an amount of air equal to medication quantity to be withdrawn. (C) Hold syringe pointed upward at eye level and with the bevel of the needle in the medication. Pull back plunger and aspirate the quantity of medication ordered.

(continues)

draw the measured dose of medication. Measure accurately. Keep the tip of the needle below the surface of the liquid; otherwise, air will enter the syringe. Keep syringe at eye level (Figure 36-33C).

9. Check the syringe for air bubbles. Remove them by tapping sharply on the syringe (Figure 36-33D). Check measurement for accuracy.

10. Remove the needle from the vial. Replace the sterile needle cover (Figure 36-33E).

11. Check the vial label against the medicine card (third time).

12. Place the filled needle and syringe on a medicine tray or cart with an alcohol wipe and the medicine card. The dose is now ready for injection.

13. Return multiple-dose vials to the proper storage area (cabinet or refrigerator). Dispose of unused

medication in a single-dose vial according to facility procedure. (Remember, disposal of a controlled substance must be witnessed and the proper forms signed.)

14. If medication is a tissue irritant, change to another sterile needle. RATIONALE: Tissue irritants can cause tissue necrosis.

15. Discard used syringe-needle unit immediately after use in a sharps container.

16. Remove gloves and dispose in biohazard waste container.

17. Wash hands.

18. Document the procedure.

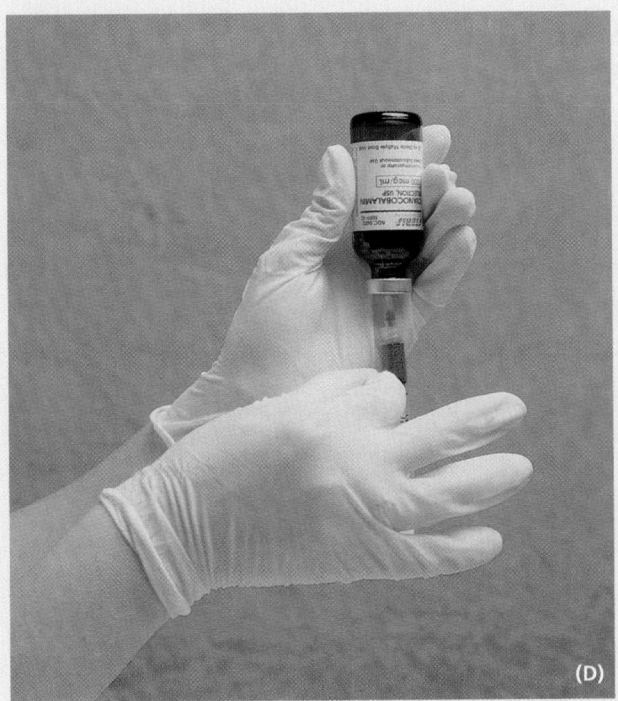
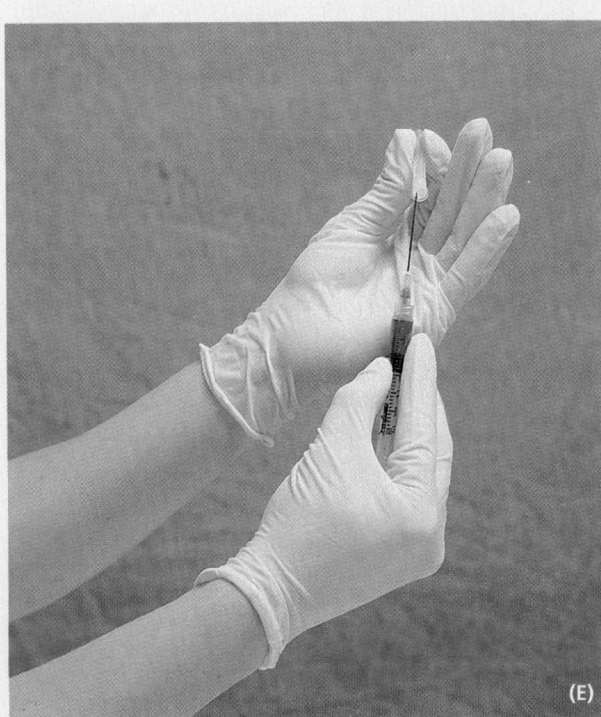

Figure 36-33 *(continued)* (D) Tap syringe to eliminate air bubbles. Hand should hold syringe while tapping it. (E) After the correct dose has been withdrawn, recover the sterile needle. Place medication on a tray along with medication card and an alcohol wipe and safely transport to the patient.

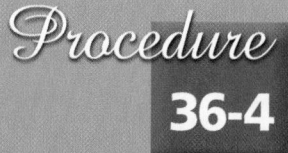

Procedure 36-4

Withdrawing (Aspirating) Medication from an Ampule

STANDARD PRECAUTIONS:

PURPOSE:

Medication is supplied in a variety of packaging. An ampule is a sterile, glass, single-dose container of liquid medication. It is aspirated into a syringe for parenteral injection.

EQUIPMENT/SUPPLIES:

Medicine tray and medicine card
Ampule of medication
Alcohol wipes
Sterile gauze sponges
Sharps container
Sterile needle-syringe unit
Gloves

PROCEDURE STEPS:

1. Check the physician's order. Write out medicine card.
2. Wash hands and gather equipment. Put on gloves.
3. Obtain ampule of medication. Read label and check medicine card for correct medication, dose, route, and time (first time). Check medication expiration date.
4. Flick ampule of medication (medication will often get "trapped" above the neck of the ampule). A sharp flick of the wrist will help force all of the medication down below the neck of the ampule into the body of the ampule (Figure 36-34A). RATIONALE: This is important to ensure all medication is available in the body of the ampule in order to calculate the correct dose. If some of the medication remains trapped above the neck in the top of the ampule, some medication will not be available for use and it is possible to give an incorrect dose, especially if the patient is to receive the entire contents of the ampule.
5. Thoroughly disinfect the neck with an alcohol swab. Check label (second time). RATIONALE: The needle will enter the opening of the ampule and wiping the neck of the ampule prior to removal of the top ensures disinfection of the neck or opening of the ampule.
6. With a sterile gauze, wipe dry the neck of the ampule. Completely surround the ampule with the gauze and forcefully snap off the top of the ampule by pushing the top away from you (Figure 36-34B). RATIONALE: Ensure medical assistant safety from possible injury from broken glass. Discard top in sharps container.
7. Place opened ampule down on medicine tray. Check label (third time).
8. With a prepared sterile syringe-needle unit that has a filter on the needle, aspirate the required dose into the syringe (Figure 36-34C). Cover needle with sheath and transport to patient on the medicine tray. RATIONALE: Filtered needles prevent glass particles from being aspirated with medication.
9. Identify the patient.

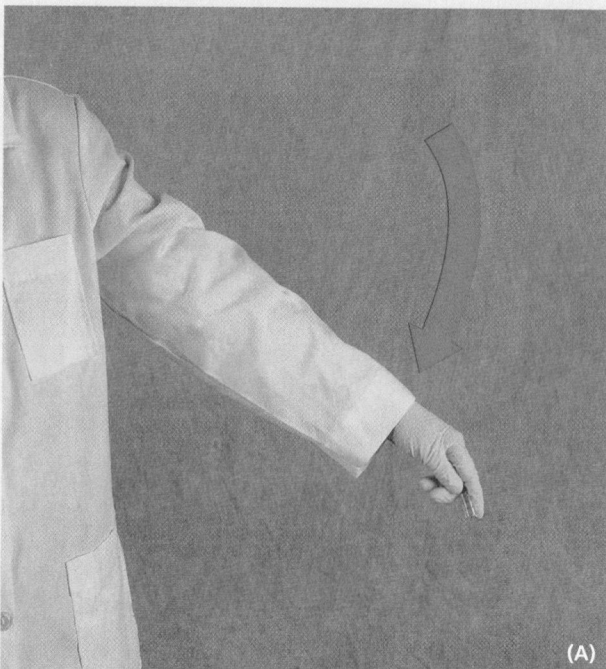

Figure 36-34 (A) Hold ampule by the top and force all the medication into the bottom of the ampule by a snap of the arm and wrist.

(continues)

Procedure

36-4   *(continued)*

10. Administer medication.
11. Discard syringe-needle unit into sharps container. Alcohol wipes and gauze are discarded in biohazard waste container.

12. Remove gloves and dispose in biohazard waste container.
13. Wash hands.
14. Document the procedure.

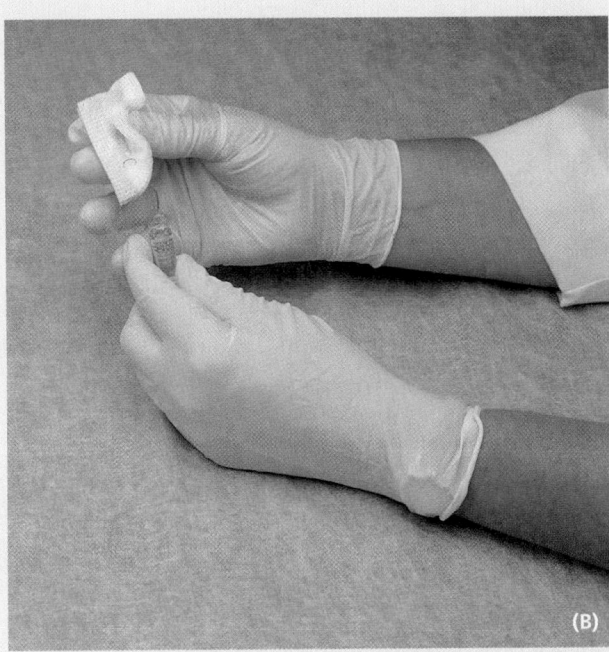

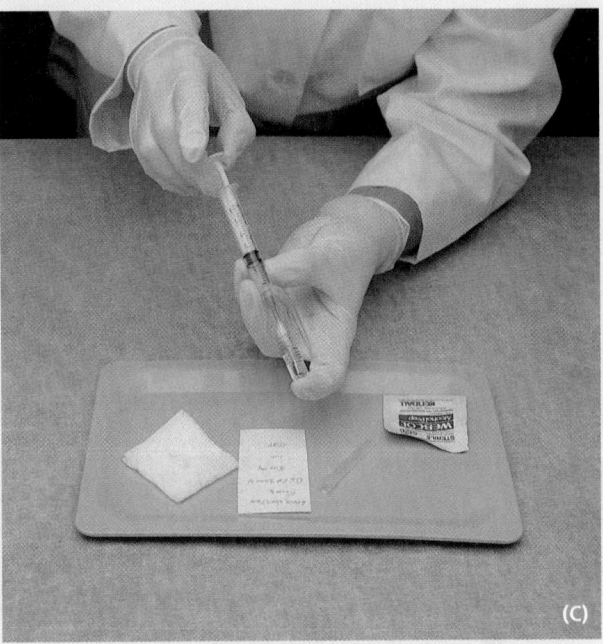

Figure 36-34   *(continued)* (B) Remove top from ampule. Turn hand up and out simultaneously. (C) Aspirate required dose into syringe.

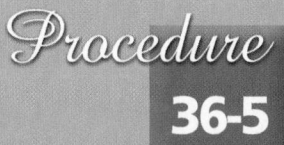 **36-5** **Administering a Subcutaneous Injection**

STANDARD PRECAUTIONS:

PURPOSE:

Correctly administer a subcutaneous injection after receiving a physician's order and assembling the necessary equipment and supplies.

EQUIPMENT/SUPPLIES:

Medication ordered   Alcohol wipes
  by physician   Disposable gloves
Medicine card   Sharps container
Appropriately sized
  needle-syringe unit

PROCEDURE STEPS:

1. Verify the physician's order. Make out a medicine card.
2. Follow the "Six Rights."
3. Perform medical asepsis handwash. Adhere to OSHA guidelines.
4. Work in a well-lighted, quiet, clean area.
5. Obtain the appropriate equipment and supplies.
6. Obtain the correct medication.
7. Compare the medication label with the medicine card (first time).
8. Check expiration date on medicine.
9. Calculate dosage, if necessary.
10. Correctly prepare the parenteral medication.
11. Compare medication label with the medicine card (second time).
12. Replace medication in appropriate area (shelf, refrigerator). Compare the medication label (third time).
13. Correctly transport the medicine to the patient.
14. Identify the patient. Explain the procedure.
15. Assess the patient. Put on gloves.
16. Prepare the patient for the injection (drape, position, allay apprehension).

17. Select an appropriate injection site.
18. Correctly cleanse the site using a circular motion starting with the injection site and moving outward to a 2-inch diameter. Allow skin to dry.
29. Remove needle guard.
20. Grasp skin to form a 1-inch fold.
21. Insert needle quickly at a 45-degree angle (Figure 36-35).
22. Aspirate to be certain needle is not in a blood vessel.
23. Slowly inject the medicine.
24. Correctly remove the needle and syringe.
25. Immediately dispose of needle and syringe in a sharps container.
26. Cover site. Massage (unless contraindicated as with insulin, Imferon, and heparin).
27. Provide for patient's safety.
28. Remove gloves and wash hands.
29. Document the procedure. Example: 12/16/2001 10 AM NPH insulin 8 units S.C. (L) deltoid area. S. Jones, CMA.

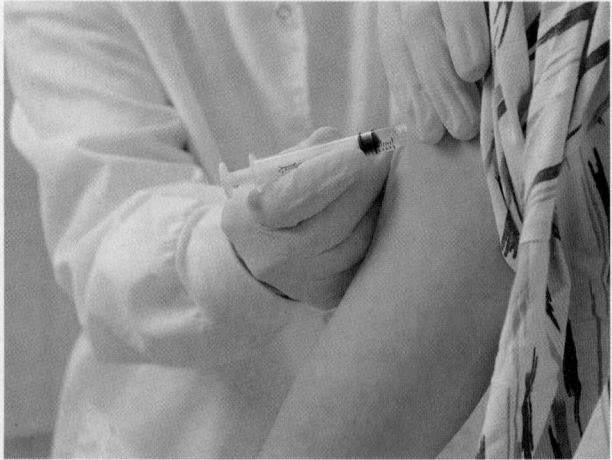

Figure 36-35   Insert needle at 45-degree angle into upper arm.

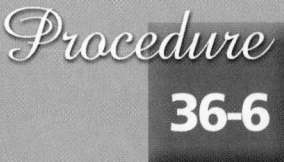

Administering an Intramuscular Injection

STANDARD PRECAUTIONS:

PURPOSE:

Correctly administer an intramuscular injection after receiving a physician's order and assembling the necessary equipment and supplies.

EQUIPMENT/SUPPLIES:

Medication ordered by physician with medication card
Appropriately sized needle-syringe unit
Alcohol wipes
Disposable gloves
Sharps container

PROCEDURE STEPS:

1. Verify the physician's order. Make out a medicine card.
2. Follow the "Six Rights."
3. Perform medical asepsis handwash. Adhere to OSHA guidelines.
4. Work in a well-lighted, quiet, clean area.
5. Obtain the appropriate equipment and supplies.
6. Obtain the correct medication.
7. Compare the medication label with the medicine card (first time).
8. Check expiration date.
9. Calculate dosage, if necessary.
10. Correctly prepare the parenteral medication.
11. Compare medicine label with the medicine card (second time).
12. Replace medication on appropriate shelf and compare medication label with medicine card (third time).
13. Correctly transport the medicine to the patient.
14. Identify the patient. Explain the procedure.
15. Assess the patient. Put on gloves.
16. Prepare the patient for the injection (drape, position, allay apprehension).
17. Select an appropriate injection site.
18. Correctly cleanse the site using a circular motion and covering a 2-inch diameter. Allow the skin to dry.
19. Remove needle guard.
20. Stretch the skin **taut**, pulling it tight.
21. Using a dart-like motion, insert needle to the hub at a 90-degree angle (Figure 36-36).
22. Release the skin.
23. Aspirate to check for blood.
24. Slowly inject the medicine.
25. Correctly remove the needle and syringe.
26. Immediately dispose of needle and syringe in a sharps container.
27. Cover site. Massage (unless contraindicated as with insulin, Imferon, and heparin).
28. Dispose of equipment. Remove gloves.
29. Wash hands.
30. Observe the patient for signs of difficulty.
31. Provide for patient's safety.
32. Document the procedure. Example: 12/16/2001 10 AM Demerol 75 mg I.M. (L) deltoid area. S. Jones, CMA.

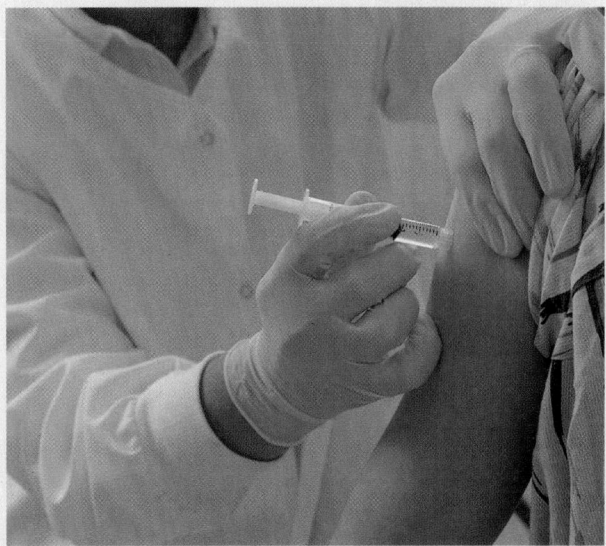

Figure 36-36 Using deltoid area of upper arm, insert needle to the hub at a 90-degree angle.

Procedure 36-7
Administering an Intradermal Injection

STANDARD PRECAUTIONS:

PURPOSE:

Correctly administer an intradermal injection after receiving a physician's order and assembling the necessary equipment and supplies.

EQUIPMENT/SUPPLIES:

Medication as ordered by physician with medication card
Appropriately sized needle-syringe unit
Alcohol wipes
Disposable gloves
Sharps container

PROCEDURE STEPS:

1. Verify the physician's order. Make out a medicine card.
2. Follow the "Six Rights."
3. Perform medical asepsis handwash. Adhere to OSHA guidelines.
4. Work in a well-lighted, quiet, clean area.
5. Obtain the appropriate equipment and supplies.
6. Obtain the correct medication.
7. Compare the medication label with the medicine card (first time).
8. Check expiration date.
9. Calculate dosage, if necessary.
10. Correctly prepare the parenteral medication.
11. Compare medication label with the medicine card (second time).
12. Replace medication on appropriate shelf and compare medication label with medicine card (third time).
13. Correctly transport the medicine to the patient.
14. Identify the patient. Explain the procedure.
15. Assess the patient. Put on gloves.
16. Prepare the patient for the injection (drape, position, allay apprehension).
17. Select an appropriate injection site (Figure 36-37A). For other sites, refer back to Figure 36-19B.

18. Correctly cleanse the site using a circular motion and covering a 2-inch diameter. Allow the skin to dry.
19. Remove needle guard.
20. Pull the skin tissue taut.
21. Carefully insert the needle at a 10- to 15-degree angle, bevel upward to about ⅛ inch. Do not aspirate.
22. Steadily inject purified protein derivative (PPD) (Figure 36-37B). Within 24 to 72 hours, a bleb, or slight elevation of the skin, will be produced at the injection site.
23. Correctly remove the needle after a brief delay. RATIONALE: Minimizes leakage.
24. Immediately dispose of needle and syringe in a sharps container.

(continues)

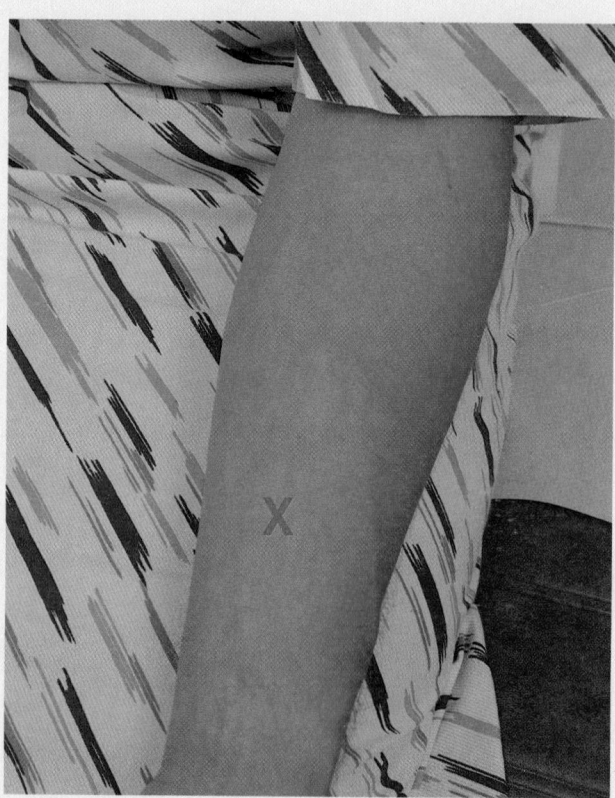

Figure 36-37A   One site for administering an intradermal injection is near the center of the forearm.

Procedure 36-7 *(continued)*

25. Blot site. Do not massage. Dispose of equipment. Remove gloves.
26. Wash hands.
27. Observe the patient for signs of difficulty.
28. Provide for patient's safety.
29. Document the procedure. Example: 10/14/2001 10 AM 0.1 ml PPD I.D. (L) forearm. S. Jones, CMA.
30. The injected area should be read for the amount of induration (hardness) or reaction to the PPD to determine active or inactive tuberculosis exposure.
31. If injection area is hardened and elevated, make follow-up appointment for patient.

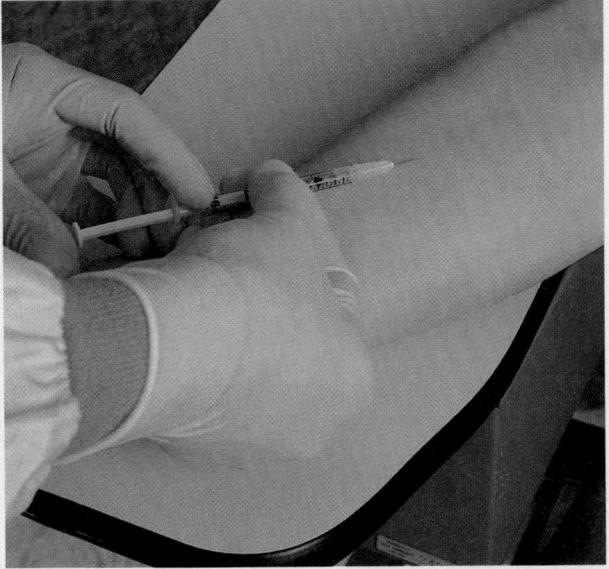

Figure 36-37B Steadily inject the medicine.

Procedure 36-8 Reconstituting a Powder Medication for Administration

STANDARD PRECAUTIONS:

PURPOSE:
Drugs for injection may be supplied in a powdered (dry) form and must be reconstituted to a liquid for injection. A diluent (usually sterile water) is added to the powder, mixed well, and the appropriate dose is drawn up to be administered.

EQUIPMENT/SUPPLIES:
Medication as ordered by the physician and medicine card
Diluent
2 appropriately sized needles and syringe units
Alcohol wipes
Disposable gloves
Sharps container

PROCEDURE STEPS:
1. Medical assistant prepares the needle-syringe unit in preparation for reconstituting powder medication (Figure 36-38A).
2. Remove tops from diluent and powder medication containers and wipe with alcohol swabs (Figure 36-38B).
3. Insert the needle of a sterile needle-syringe unit through the rubber stopper on the vial of diluent that has been cleansed with an alcohol wipe. The needle-syringe unit should have an amount of air in it equal to the amount of diluent to be withdrawn (Figures 36-38C and D).
4. Withdraw the appropriate amount of diluent to be added to the powder medication (Figures 36-38E and F). Cover the sterile needle on the syringe containing appropriate amount of diluent.

(continues)

Procedure

36-8 *(continued)*

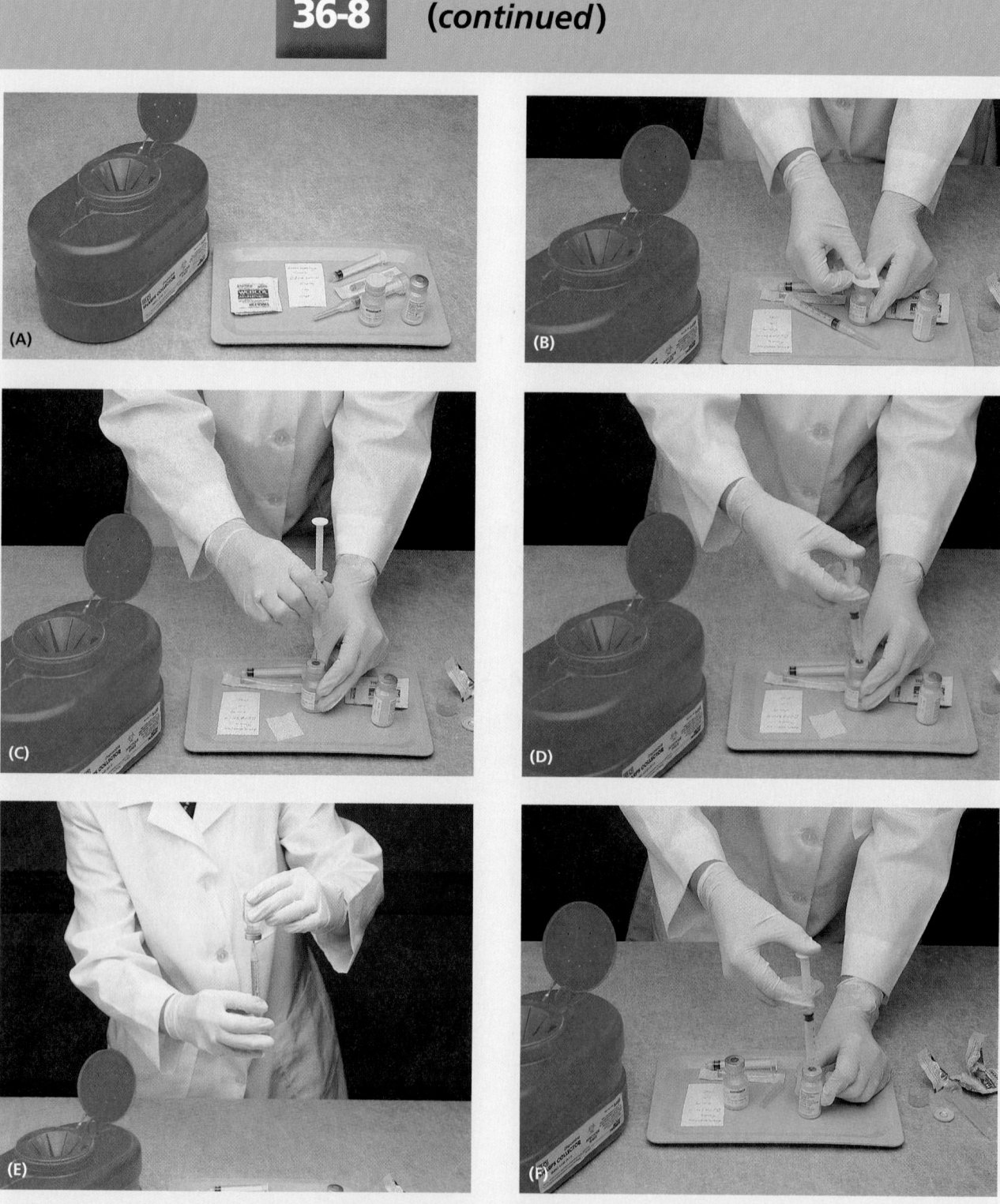

Figure 36-38 (A) Supplies for reconstituting powder medication. (B) Remove top from diluent and powdered medication. Wipe top of each with an alcohol wipe. (C) Prepare to inject air in an equal amount to diluent being removed from the vial. (D) Inject air into the vial. (E) Prepare to separate vial from needle-syringe unit after withdrawing diluent. (F) Inject diluent into vial containing powdered medication. Top of vial should be cleansed again with an alcohol wipe.

(continues)

Procedure
36-8   *(continued)*

5. Add this liquid to the powder medication that has been cleansed with an alcohol wipe (Figure 36-38G).
6. Remove needle and syringe from vial with powder medication and diluent and discard into sharps container (Figure 36-38H).
7. Roll the vial between the palms of the hands to completely mix together the powder and diluent (Figure 36-38I). Label the multiple dose vial with the dilution or strength of the medication prepared, the date and time, your initials, and the expiration date.

8. With a second sterile needle and syringe, withdraw the desired amount of medication (Figure 36-38J).
9. Flick away any air bubbles that cling to side of syringe (Figure 36-38K).
10. The medicine tray with reconstituted medication is ready for transport to the patient (Figure 36-38L).
11. Proceed as in steps 11–32 of Procedure 36-6, Administering an Intramuscular Injection.

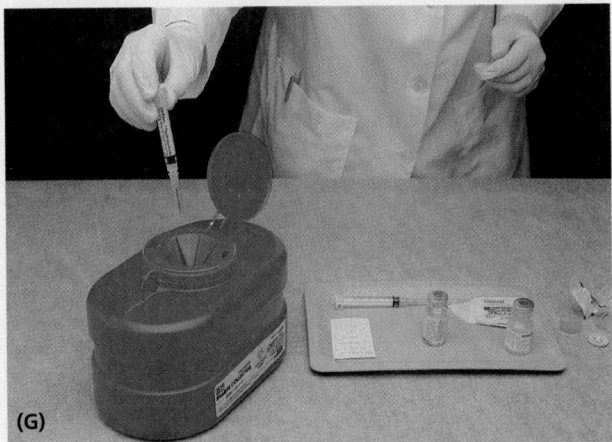
(G)

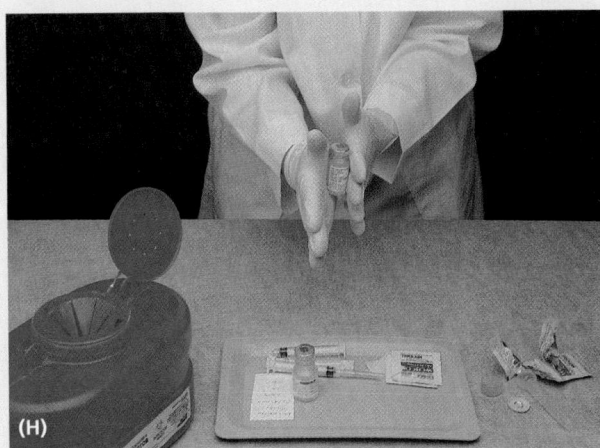
(H)

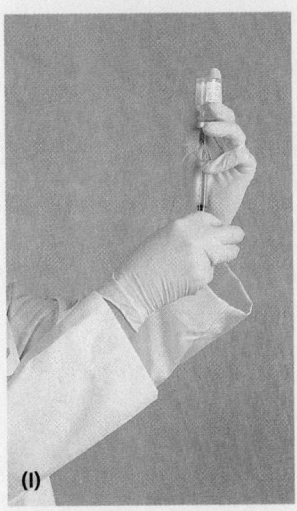
(I)

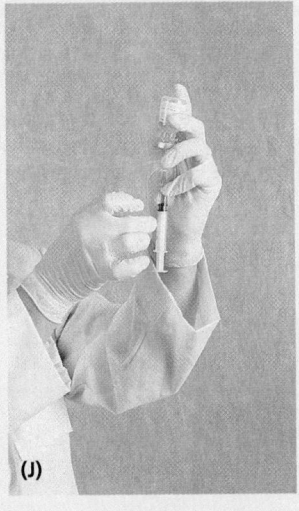
(J)

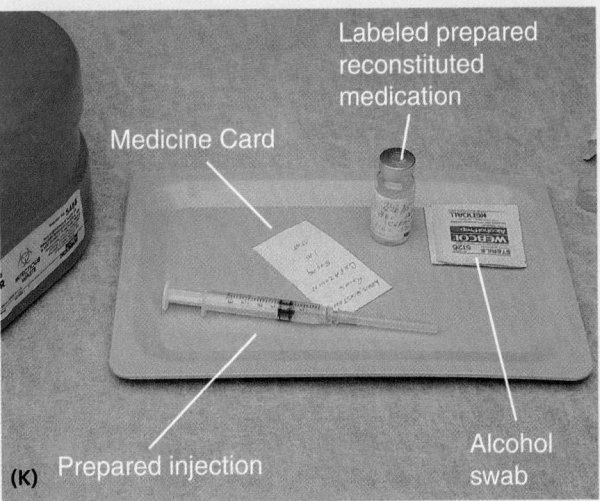
(K)

Figure 36-38 *(continues)* (G) Discard recapped needle-syringe unit after mixing. (H) Roll vial of powdered medication between palms of hands with the diluent to mix well. Label vial with date, amount of diluent added, strength of dilution, time mixed, and your initials. (I) Use a second sterile needle-syringe unit to draw the prescribed dose of medication ordered by the physician. (J) Flick away any air bubbles that cling to the side of the syringe. (K) Medicine tray shows prepared injection ready for transport to patient. Labeled, reconstituted medication will be placed on the shelf or in the refrigerator according to the manufacturer's instructions.

Procedure 36-9   Z-Track Intramuscular Injection Technique

STANDARD PRECAUTIONS:

PURPOSE:

Correctly administer a Z-track intramuscular injection after receiving a physician's order and assembling the necessary equipment and supplies.

EQUIPMENT/SUPPLIES:

Medication ordered by physician and medicine card
Appropriately sized needle-syringe unit
Alcohol wipes
Disposable gloves
Sharps container

PROCEDURE STEPS:

1. Verify the physician's order. Make out a medicine card.
2. Follow the "Six Rights."
3. Perform medical asepsis handwash. Adhere to OSHA guidelines.
4. Work in a well-lighted, quiet, clean area.
5. Obtain the appropriate equipment and supplies.
6. Obtain the correct medication.
7. Compare the medication label with the medicine card (first time).
8. Check expiration date.
9. Calculate dosage, if necessary.
10. Correctly prepare the parenteral medication.
11. Compare medicine label with the medicine card (second time).
12. Replace medication on shelf and compare medication label with medicine card (third time).
13. Correctly transport the medicine to the patient.
14. Identify the patient. Explain the procedure.
15. Assess the patient. Put on gloves.
16. Prepare the patient for the injection (drape, position, allay apprehension).
17. Select an appropriate injection site.
18. Correctly cleanse the site using a circular motion and covering a 2-inch diameter. Allow the skin to dry.
19. Remove needle guard.
20. Pull the skin laterally 1½ inch away from the injection site.
21. Insert needle quickly, using a dart-like motion at a 90-degree angle. Maintain Z position (Figure 36-39).
22. Aspirate to check for blood.
23. Slowly inject medication.
24. Wait 10 seconds before removing needle to allow medication to begin to be absorbed.
25. Remove needle and syringe at same angle of insertion.
26. Release traction of the Z position in order to seal off the needle track. This prevents medication from reaching the subcutaneous tissues and the surface of the skin.
27. Immediately dispose of needle-syringe unit in a sharps container.
28. Cover site. Do not massage.
29. Remove gloves.
30. Wash hands.
31. Observe patient for signs of difficulty.
32. Provide for patient safety.
33. Document the procedure.

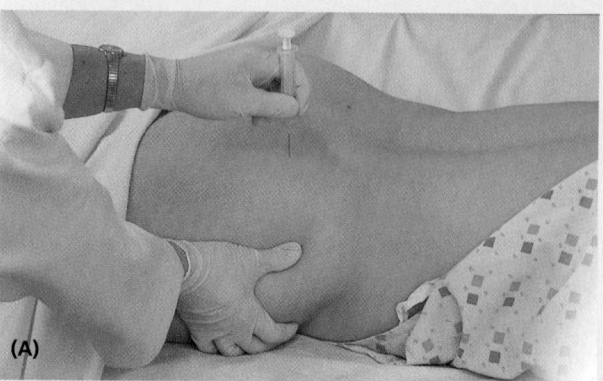

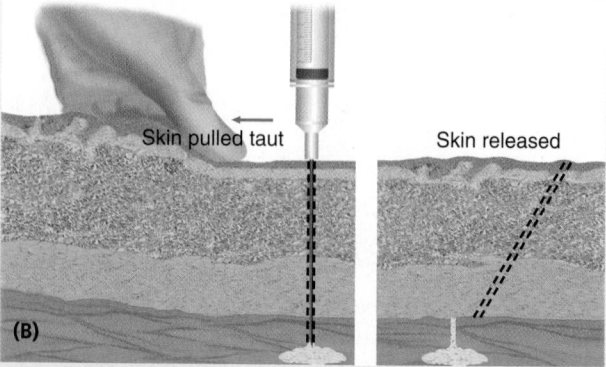

Skin pulled taut   Skin released

Figure 36-39   Z-track technique for IM injection: (A) With client supine, grasp and pull the muscle laterally before injecting medication. (B) Inject medication. Keep skin pulled taut for 10 seconds. Quickly withdraw the needle and release the skin to seal the site.

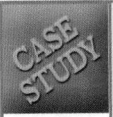

CASE STUDY 36-1

Abigail Johnson, a patient of Dr. Lewis, has been unable to keep her Type II noninsulin-dependent diabetes mellitus under control with oral hypoglycemics, and Dr. Lewis has decided that Abigail needs to begin to take insulin injections. Today in the clinic her fasting blood glucose level is 190 mg/mL. Dr. Lewis prescribes Humulin® insulin 10 units subcutaneously stat.

CASE STUDY REVIEW

1. What size insulin syringe should be used?
2. What does the medication label state are the number of units per milliliter? Show how to calculate the correct dosage.
3. Discuss the route of administration and the specifics about insulin administration that require it to be given slightly differently from other s.c. injections.
4. Describe several topics of discussion in which you would engage Abigail to help her learn how to better control her disease.

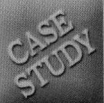

CASE STUDY 36-2

Alice Chambers weighs 28 pounds and is 33 inches tall. The adult dose is erythromycin 400 mg every 6 hours by mouth.

CASE STUDY REVIEW

1. Calculate the dose of erythromycin Alice needs.
2. If the physician ordered erythromycin by injection rather than by mouth, how would the dose be calculated if the erythromycin adult dose is 400 mg per milliliter?
3. What size needle and syringe is appropriate for giving Alice the injection?

SUMMARY

Administering medications is one of the most important and essential responsibilities that the medical assistant performs. In this chapter, a review of some of the fundamental elements of pharmacology, dosage calculations, and medication administration have been presented.

Each state has enacted laws governing the practice of medicine, nursing, and pharmacy. These laws vary from state to state; therefore, it is essential that one become familiar with the laws of the state in which one is employed before administering any medication.

Under the law, those administering medications are expected to be knowledgeable about the drugs that they administer and the effects the drug may and/or will have on the patient. They are responsible for their own actions.

REVIEW QUESTIONS

Multiple Choice

1. A written legal document that gives directions for compounding, dispensing, and administering medication to a patient is a:
   a. medicine card
   b. prescription
   c. medication order
   d. subscription

2. An abbreviation symbol that means nothing by mouth is:
   a. non rep
   b. NPO
   c. IM
   d. mm

3. Insulin-dependent diabetes mellitus is:
   a. Type I
   b. Type II

c. Type III
d. Type IV
4. Body surface area is used:
   a. when calculating children's dosages
   b. when calculating adult dosages
   c. when determining an injection site
   d. when selecting an appropriately sized needle
5. An injection given just below the surface of the skin is called a(n):
   a. intramuscular injection
   b. intradermal injection
   c. subcutaneous injection
   d. parenteral injection

Critical Thinking

1. Describe the process to follow to determine the state law regarding a medical assistant administering medications.
2. What is a medication order? Describe its purpose.
3. List nine parts of a prescription and define each part.
4. Name and describe factors that can affect medication dosage. Explain why and how the dosage is affected.
5. List the fundamental units of the metric system.
6. Name two methods used to calculate children's dosages of medication.
7. List and describe the "Six Rights."
8. A fellow student tells you that she accidentally gave a patient the incorrect dose of medication. Explain in detail what should be done.
9. You accidentally stick yourself with a used needle. What are the steps to take?
10. Discuss allergenic extracts. What are they? What safeguards are needed following administration?
11. List two reasons for the physician to prescribe oxygen for a patient. Describe how oxygen is administered and oxygen safety.

Calculation Problems

1. Calculate the following dosages according to body surface area (BSA):
   If the adult dose of E.E.S. tabs is 400 mg every 6 hours, what is the dosage for a child who is 35 inches tall and weighs 28 pounds (BSA 0.57)?
   If the adult dose of penicillin V potassium, USP, is 250 mg every 6 to 8 hours, what is the dosage for a child who is 24 inches tall and weighs 35 pounds (BSA 0.56)?

2. Calculate the following dosages according to kilogram of body weight:
   The physician orders Augmentin 20 mg/kg/day for Sally Whitney, who weighs 72 pounds. The dose is to be divided and given every 8 hours. What is the total dose? What is the amount to be given every 8 hours?
   The physician orders Cefadyl 40 mg/kg for George Kipperley, who weighs 78 pounds. The dose is to be divided into 4 equal doses. What is the total dose? What is the amount to be given in four equal doses?
   The physician orders Garamycin 2.0 mg/kg every 8 hours for a child who weighs 86 pounds. What is the correct dosage?
3. The physician ordered 64 units of U-100 Humulin insulin. Shade the correct dosage on the U-100 syringe pictured.

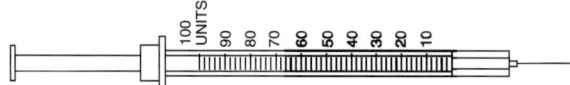

Using the proportional or formula method, calculate the following dosages.
4. The physician orders 125 mg of Diamox. On hand you have 250 mg tablets. You will give _____ tablets to your patient.
5. The physician orders 250 mg of Tagamet liquid. On hand you have 300 mg/5 mL. How many milliliters will you give?

WEB ACTIVITIES

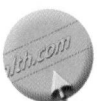

1. Search for a website to explore the various types of safety needles available for injection and venipuncture. What is the most recent ruling by OSHA in regard to these types of needles?

REFERENCES/BIBLIOGRAPHY

Pickar, G. D. (1999). *Dosage calculations* (6th ed.). Albany, NY: Delmar.
Rice, J. (1999). *Principles of pharmacology for medical assisting* (3rd ed.). Albany, NY: Delmar.
Taber's cyclopedic medical dictionary. (18th ed.). (1999). Philadelphia: F. A. Davis Company.

Chapter 37

ELECTROCARDIOGRAPHY

KEY TERMS

Amplified
Amplitude
Angiogram
Arrhythmia
Artifact
Augment
Baseline
Bipolar
Bradycardia, Sinus
Calibration
Cardiac Catheterization
Cardiac Cycle
Cardioversion
Countershock
Defibrillation
Defibrillator
Deoxygenated
Depolarize
Diastole
Electrocardiogram
Electrocardiograph
Electrocardiography
Electrodes
Electrolyte
Galvanometer
Infarction
Ischemia
Isoelectric
Lead
Mounting
Noninvasive
Normal Sinus Rhythm
Oscilloscope

(continues)

OUTLINE

Anatomy of the Heart
Electrical Conduction System of the Heart
The Cardiac Cycle and the ECG Cycle
    Calculation of Heart Rate on ECG Graph Paper
Types of Electrocardiographs
    Single-Channel ECG
    Multichannel ECG
    Automatic ECG Machines
    ECG Telephone Transmissions
    Facsimile Electrocardiograph
    Interpretive Electrocardiograph
ECG Equipment
    Electrocardiograph Paper
    Electrolyte
    Sensors or Electrodes
    Care of Equipment
Lead Coding
The Electrocardiograph and Lead Placement
    Standard Limb or Bipolar Leads
    Augmented Leads
    Chest Leads or Precordial Leads

Standardization of the Electrocardiograph
Standard Resting Electrocardiography
Mounting the ECG Tracing
Interference or Artifacts
    Somatic Tremor Artifacts
    Alternating Current (AC) Interference
    Wandering Baseline Artifacts
    Interrupted Baseline Artifacts
Cardiac Conditions and Diseases
    Myocardial Infarctions (Heart Attacks)
Cardiac Arrhythmias
    Atrial Arrhythmias
    Ventricular Arrhythmias
Defibrillation
Other Cardiac Diagnostic Tests
    Holter Monitor (Portable Ambulatory Electrocardiograph)
    Treadmill Stress Test or Exercise Tolerance ECG
    Echocardiography

OBJECTIVES

The student should strive to meet the following performance objectives and demonstrate an understanding of the facts and principles presented in this chapter through written and oral communication.

1. Define the key terms as presented in the glossary.
2. Follow the circulation of blood through the heart starting at the vena cavae.

(continues)

767

OBJECTIVES (*continued*)

3. Describe the electrical conduction system of the heart.

4. State three reasons why patients may need an electrocardiogram.

5. Identify the various positive and negative deflections and describe what each represents in the cardiac cycle.

6. Explain the purpose of standardization of the electrocardiograph.

7. Identify the twelve leads of an ECG and describe what area of the heart each lead represents.

8. State the function of ECG graph paper, electrodes (sensors), and electrolyte.

9. Describe various types of ECGs and describe their capabilities.

10. Explain each type of artifact and explain how each can be eliminated.

11. Name and describe the purposes of the various cardiac diagnostic tests as outlined in this chapter.

12. Identify the placement of Holter monitor electrodes.

13. Describe the reason for a patient activity diary during ambulatory electrocardiography.

14. Identify six arrhythmias and explain the cause of each.

15. Explain how to calculate heart rates from an ECG tracing.

16. Identify a common coding system used to code each lead on an ECG tracing.

17. Describe the procedure for mounting and ECG tracing.

ROLE DELINEATION COMPONENTS

CLINICAL

Fundamental Principles

- Apply principles of aseptic technique and infection control
- Comply with quality assurance practices
- Screen and follow up patient test results

Diagnostic Orders

- Perform diagnostic tests

Patient Care

- Obtain patient history and vital signs
- Prepare and maintain examination and treatment areas

(*continues*)

SCENARIO

Wanda Slawson, CMA, clinical medical assistant at Inner City Health Care, recently had her own physical examination which included her first electrocardiogram. This is now Wanda's baseline ECG which provides a basis for future ECG readings to be compared. Since Wanda currently has no heart problems, future tests will indicate differences from her normal baseline ECG. It was very different for Wanda to be the patient versus the person performing the ECG. Having the test performed on her, Wanda can now relate to feelings many of her patients must have felt when having an ECG. These included feelings of fear that the test may be abnormal; a cold feeling because even though the room temperature was normal, she was uncovered and the electrolyte gel was cold when applied; and anxiousness because she found it difficult to stay completely still through the entire tracing. Wanda could empathize much more with her patients after she had the test than she did before her test. Wanda now makes a more concerted effort to allay patient fears and make patients comfortable during electrocardiograms.

INTRODUCTION

Many physicians include an **electrocardiogram** (ECG or EKG) as part of a complete physical examination, especially for patients who are 40 years or

● **Prepare patient for examinations, procedures, and treatments**

● **Assist with examinations, procedures, and treatments**

**GENERAL
(TRANSDISCIPLINARY)**

Legal Concepts

● **Document accurately**

Instruction

● **Instruct individuals according to their needs.**

more of age, for patients with a family history of cardiac disease, or for patients who have experienced chest pain. It is a noninvasive, safe, and painless procedure that can provide the physician with valuable information about the health of the patient's heart. A graphic representation of the heart's electrical activity, an electrocardiogram measures the amount of the electrical activity produced by the heart and the time necessary for the electrical impulses to travel through the heart during each heartbeat.

Some reasons for **electrocardiography** are to: (1) detect myocardial **ischemia**, (2) estimate damage to the myocardium caused by a myocardial **infarction**, (3) detect and evaluate cardiac **arrhythmia**, (4) assess effects of cardiac medication on the heart, and (5) determine if electrolyte imbalance is present. The ECG is used in conjunction with other laboratory and diagnostic tests to assess total cardiac health.

In a medical office or ambulatory care setting, it is the medical assistant who records the ECG; therefore, special knowledge and skills are necessary and include these aspects of the correct electrocardiography procedures: patient preparation, operation of the **electrocardiograph**, elimination of **artifacts**, **mounting** and/or labeling the ECG, and maintenance and care of the instrument.

ANATOMY OF THE HEART

The heart has four chambers: two upper chambers known as atria, and two lower chambers known as ventricles. **Deoxygenated** blood enters the right atrium from the superior and inferior vena cavae and passes through the tricuspid valve into the right ventricle. In a healthy heart, the blood between right and left sides cannot mix together. It then travels to the lungs via the pulmonary arteries. The deoxygenated blood gives off the carbon dioxide and picks up oxygen in the capillary bed of the lungs. Oxygenated blood is pumped through the pulmonary vein into the left atrium, through the mitral valve, into the left ventricle. The oxygenated blood then passes through the aortic valve into the aorta and from the aorta to all cells, tissues, and organs of the body (Figure 37-1). The cycle begins with each heartbeat.

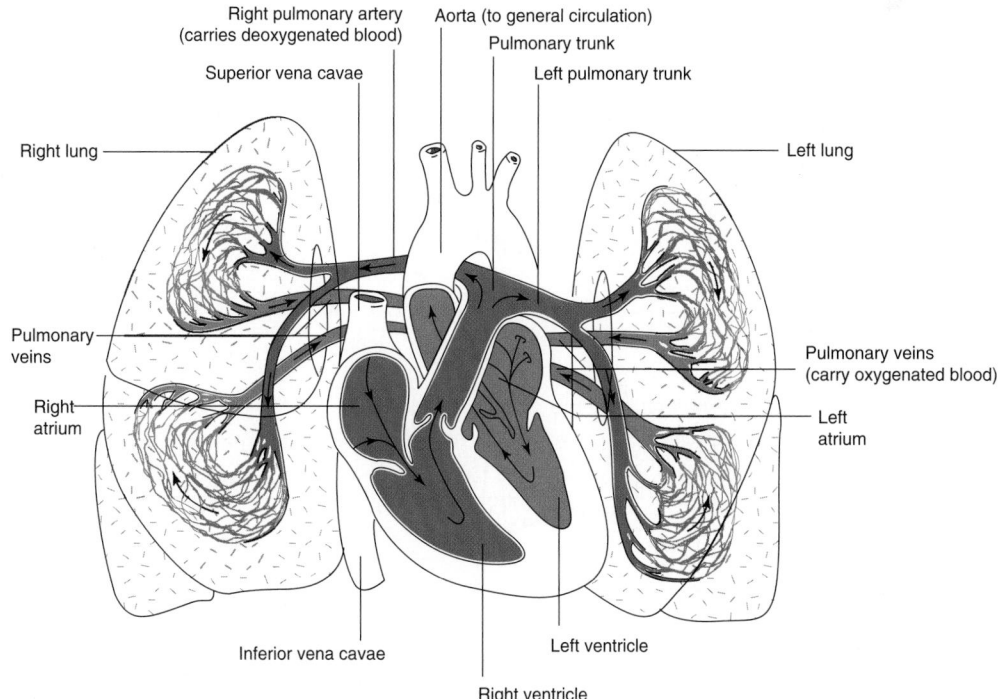

Figure 37-1   Oxygenated blood passing through the heart and onto the rest of the body.

On its external surface, the heart is surrounded by coronary arteries that supply the myocardium with its blood supply from which oxygen and nutrients are obtained. (See Chapter 30, Circulatory System.)

ELECTRICAL CONDUCTION SYSTEM OF THE HEART

The body's natural pacemaker, the sinoatrial (SA) node, is located in the upper part of the right atrium. It sends out an electrical impulse that begins and regulates the heartbeat. When the electrical impulses are dispersed through the atria, it causes them to **depolarize** or contract. From the atria, the electrical impulses travel toward the ventricles, to the atrioventricular (AV) node, located at the base of the right atrium. From here, the electrical impulses are transmitted to the bundles of His. The bundle of His divides into right and left bundle branches which continue the electrical impulses on to the Purkinje fibers. These fibers disperse the electrical impulses to the right and left ventricles causing them to contract. The heart relaxes very briefly (**repolarization**), then a new electrical impulse is begun by the SA node and the cycle begins again (Figure 37-2). This cycle is known as the **cardiac**

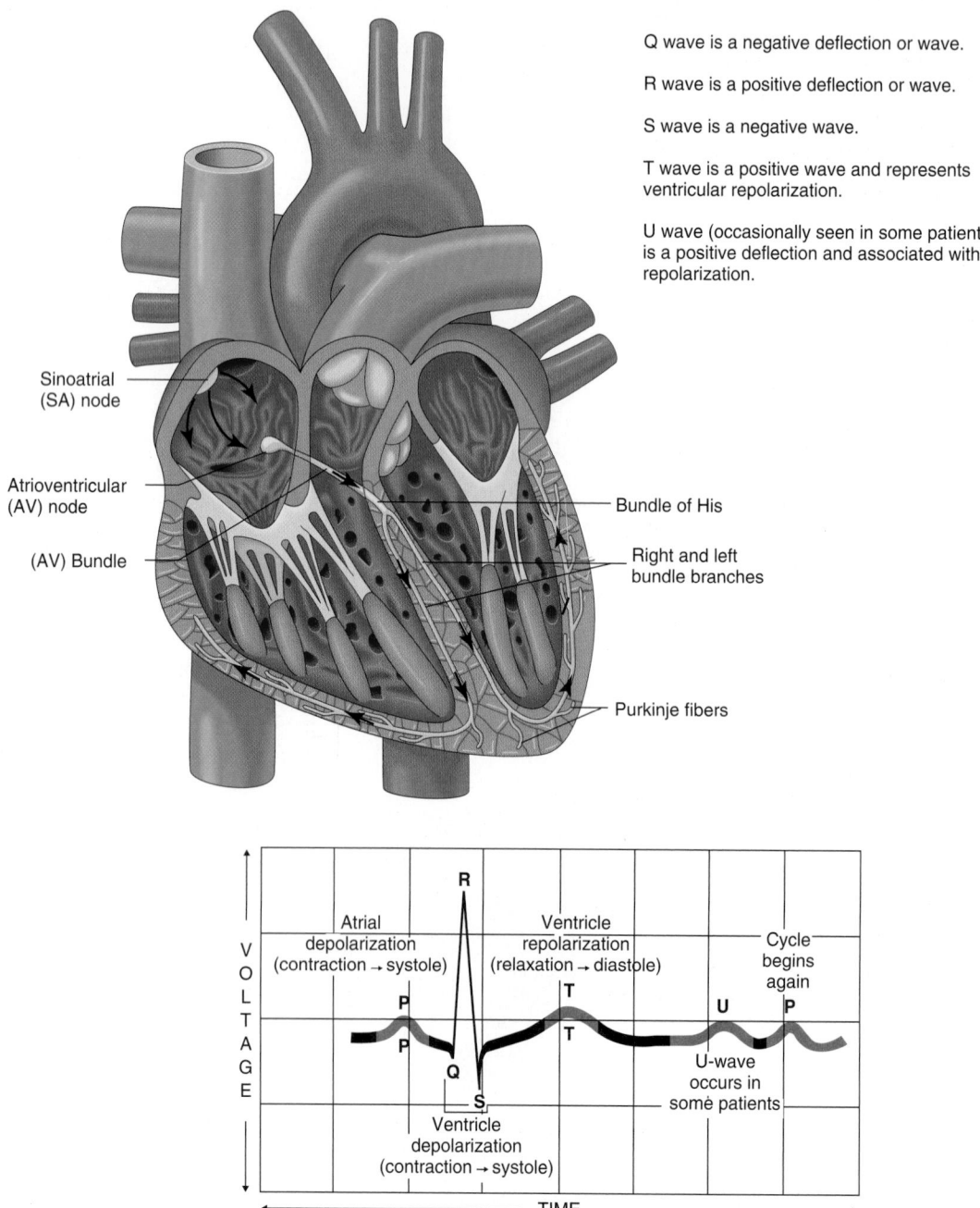

Q wave is a negative deflection or wave.

R wave is a positive deflection or wave.

S wave is a negative wave.

T wave is a positive wave and represents ventricular repolarization.

U wave (occasionally seen in some patients) is a positive deflection and associated with repolarization.

Figure 37-2 The heartbeat is controlled by electrical impulses which comprise the continuous cardiac cycle.

cycle and it represents one heartbeat. The electrocardiograph records the electrical activity that causes the contraction (**systole**) and the relaxation (**diastole**) of the atria and ventricles. The ECG cycle is the recording or the graphic representation of the cardiac cycle. These electrical impulses can be recorded on special ECG paper or displayed on an **oscilloscope**.

THE CARDIAC CYCLE AND THE ECG CYCLE

The **baseline**, or **isoelectric**, line is the flat line that separates the various waves. It is present when there is no current flowing in the heart. The waves are either deflecting upward, known as positive deflection, or deflecting downward, known as negative deflection from the baseline.

The P, QRS, and T waves, recorded during the ECG, represent the depolarization (contraction) and repolarization (relaxation) of the myocardial cells. The P wave represents atrial depolarization and is recorded as a positive deflection. The QRS complex represents ventricular depolarization and is measured from the beginning of the first wave of the QRS to the end of the last wave of the QRS (refer back to Figure 37-2).

Each complete cardiac cycle takes about 0.8 seconds with each wave taking an appropriate amount of time if the heart is healthy. By observing and measuring the size, shape, and location of each wave on an ECG recording, the physician can analyze and interpret the conduction of electricity through the cardiac cells, the heart's rhythm and rate, and the health of the heart in general.

Calculation of Heart Rate on ECG Graph Paper

ECG graph paper is divided into 1-mm squares (small squares) and 5-mm squares (large squares). Each large square is 25 small squares and is 5 mm high and 5 mm wide. On the horizontal line, one small square represents 0.04 second. On the vertical line, one small square represents 1 mm of voltage. Because a large square is five small squares wide and five deep, each small square represents 0.2 second horizontal and 5 mm vertical. **NOTE:** Every fifth line, both horizontally and vertically, is darker than the other lines, making squares that are 5 mm × 5 mm (Figure 37-3). These measurements are accepted worldwide and enable the physician to interpret the time of each deflection on the horizontal line and cardiac electrical

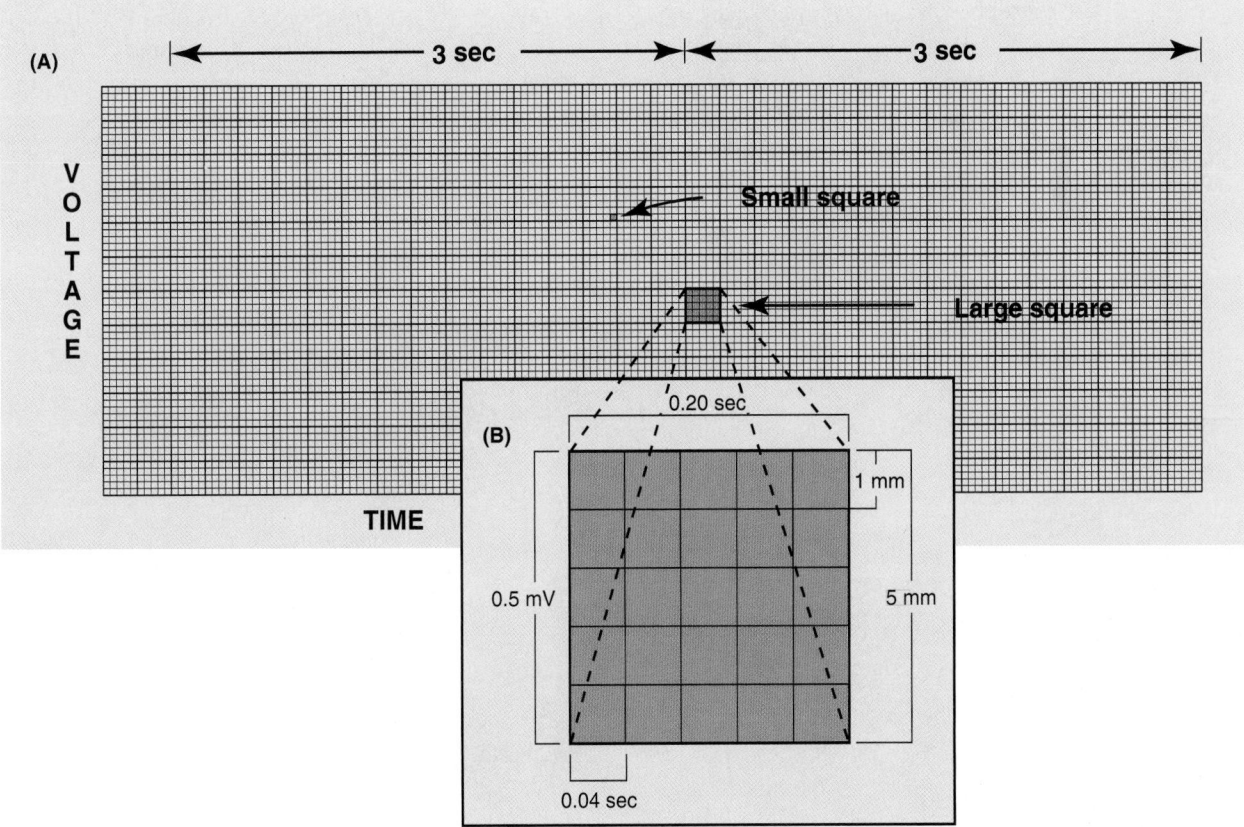

Figure 37-3 ECG graph paper measurements allow medical professionals to determine the time and voltage of heartbeats. (A) The small square is 1 mm wide and 1 mm high. One small square = 0.04 second. (B) The large square consists of 25 small squares and measures 5 mm wide and 5 mm high. One large square = 0.04 × 5 or 0.2 second.

activity (voltage) on the vertical line to help determine cardiac health.

Because all cardiac complexes consist of P, QRS, and T, and the electrocardiograph paper measures time on the horizontal line, it is possible to calculate heart rate. Count the number of 5-mm boxes (number within the dark lines) between two R waves. Divide this number into 300. The result will be the heart rate per minute.

Example: One small square (1 mm) = 0.04 second in time
One large square (5 mm) = 0.04 × 5 = 0.2 second
Divide 60 seconds (one minute) by 0.2 second
60 ÷ 0.2 = 300

Example: There are 3 large squares between two R waves.
300 ÷ 3 = 100
The heartbeat is 100 beats per minute.

TYPES OF ELECTROCARDIOGRAPHS

Single-Channel ECG

A conventional twelve-lead single channel electrocardiograph can be used in either manual mode or automatic mode. When using automatic mode, the twelve-lead ECG tracing is complete in less than 40 seconds. With a single channel machine, only one lead can be recorded at a time. If not automatic, the single-channel ECG requires manually turning the lead selector on and off between each of the twelve leads. It may also require the leads to be coded so that they can be identified later and properly mounted. Lead coding and mounting are explained more fully later in this chapter. The ECG tracing from a single-channel machine will need to be cut and mounted onto special forms, if available, or onto an 8½ × 11 inch plain piece of paper for filing into the patient record. See Figure 37-4 for a sample of a single-channel ECG machine and tracing.

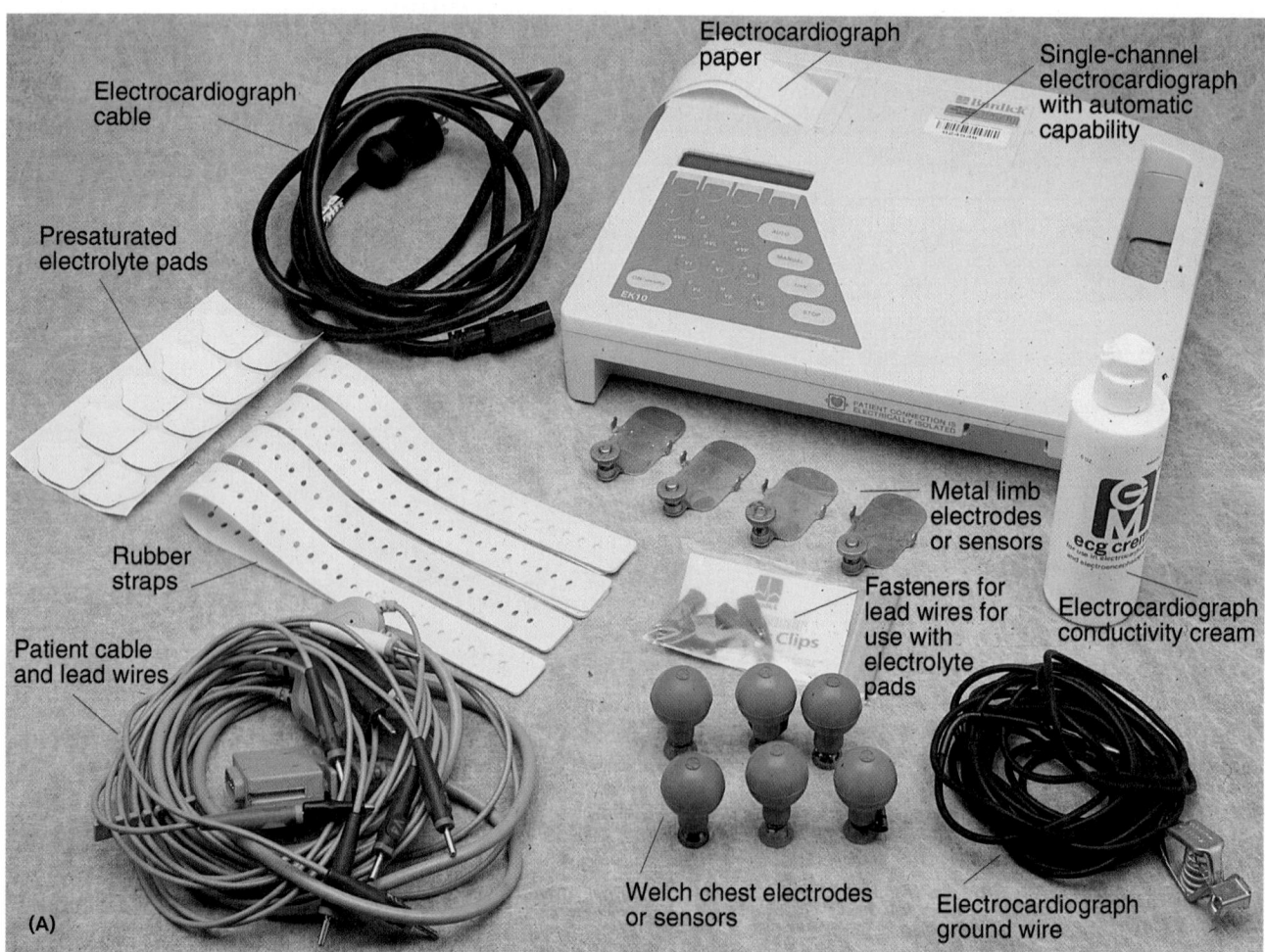

Figure 37-4 (A) Single-channel electrocardiograph and supplies needed for ECG.

(continues)

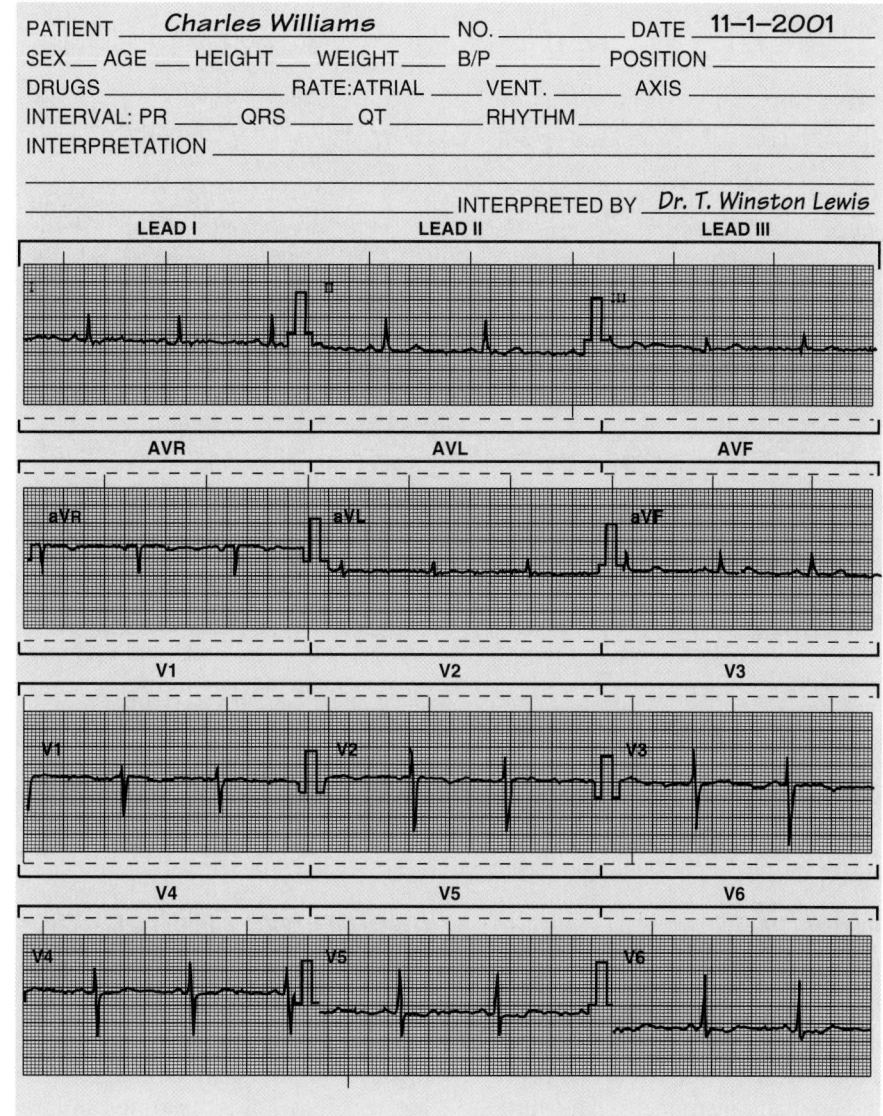

PATIENT ___Charles Williams___ NO. _____ DATE _11-1-2001_
SEX __ AGE __ HEIGHT __ WEIGHT __ B/P _____ POSITION _____
DRUGS _____ RATE:ATRIAL ____ VENT. ____ AXIS _____
INTERVAL: PR ____ QRS ____ QT _____ RHYTHM _____
INTERPRETATION _____
_____ INTERPRETED BY _Dr. T. Winston Lewis_

Figure 37-4 (*continued*) (B) Mounted single-channel ECG tracing or recording.

Multichannel ECG

An electrocardiograph that can simultaneously record several different leads is known as a multichannel electrocardiograph. The conventional electrocardiograph records one lead at a time. A three-channel machine, one type of multichannel ECG, records three channels at one time. It records Lead I, II, and III, followed by aVR, aVL, and aVF, followed by V_1, V_2, and V_3, followed by V_4, V_5, and V_6. The advantage of the multichannel machine is its speed. The most common multichannel machine used in the physician's office is the three-channel machine. This type of machine requires three-channel recording paper which is 8½ × 11 inches and fits into the patient record with no cutting or mounting. Refer to Figure 37-5 for an example of a multichannel machine and tracing.

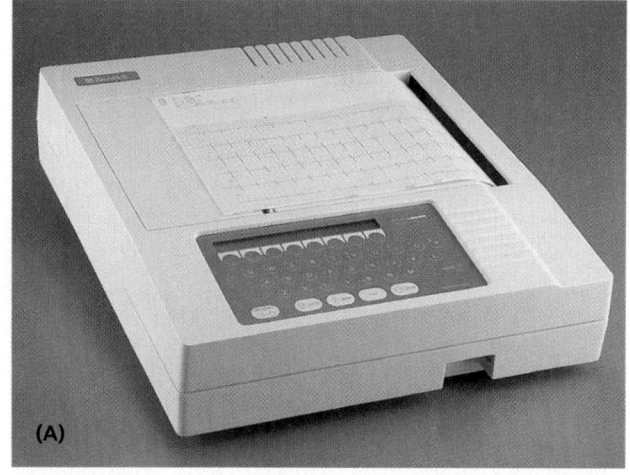

Figure 37-5 (A) Multichannel (three-channel) Burdick E350 ECG Machine. (*continues*)

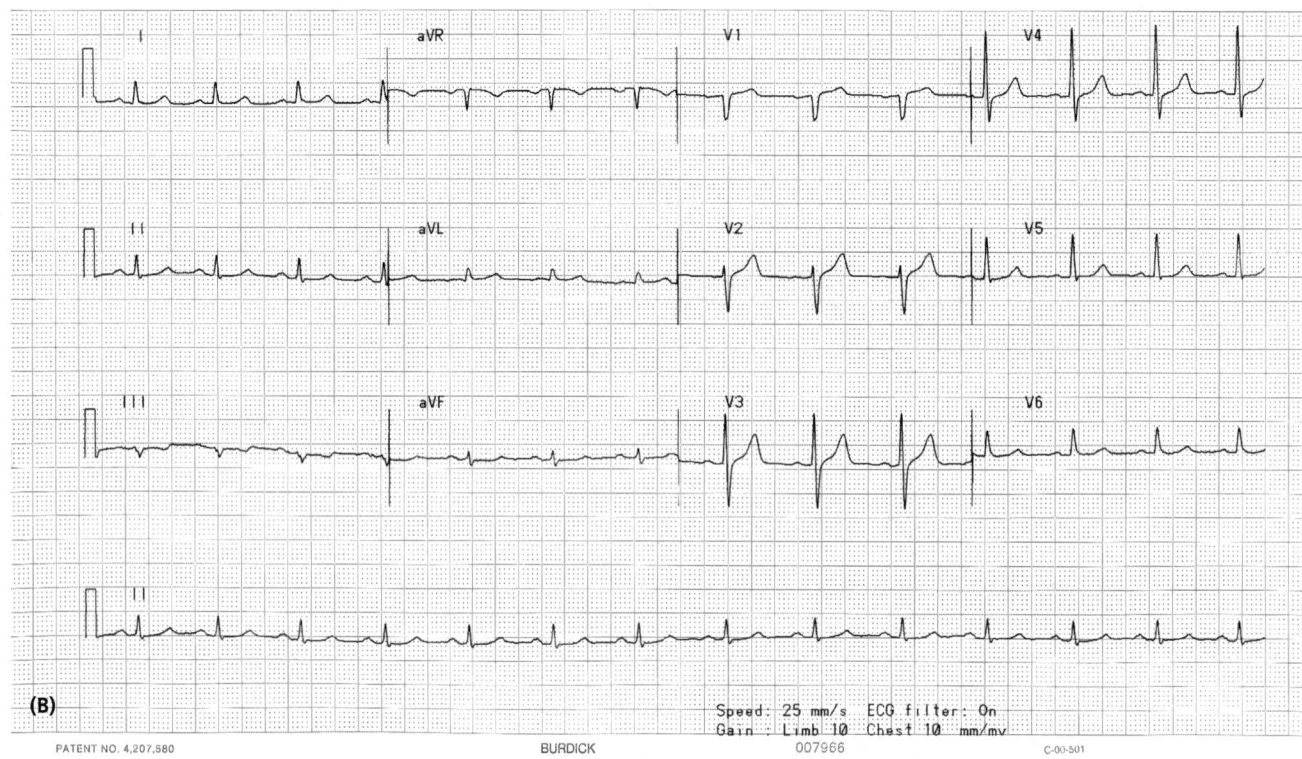

Figure 37-5 (*continued*) (B) Example of three-channel ECG recording where three leads are recorded simultaneously. (Courtesy of Siemens Burdick, Inc.)

Automatic ECG Machines

When using an automatic electrocardiograph, the lead length and switching of leads are done automatically by the electrocardiograph and there is no need to advance the control knob. For these reasons, both time and paper can be saved with the automatic instrument. The automatic instrument also comes equipped with a manual control that can be used if a longer tracing is necessary.

ECG Telephone Transmissions

An electrocardiogram can be transmitted via the telephone line to an ECG interpretation site when using an electrocardiograph with such capabilities. A recording printout and interpretation (many times interpretation is done by a cardiologist and/or by a computer) are transmitted automatically on the electrocardiograph. Results of the ECG can be verbally transmitted as well.

Facsimile Electrocardiograph

The physician may need a rapid, expert ECG interpretation from an off-site diagnostician. Direct ECG fax transmits from the electrocardiograph to a fax machine and a high-quality facsimile is produced. This saves time by eliminating the step of copying the report and sending it via the fax machine.

Interpretive Electrocardiograph

The interpretive electrocardiograph has a built-in computer program that interprets the ECG tracing while it is being recorded allowing for faster diagnosis and treatment. The physician in charge will review the tracing before a diagnosis is confirmed and treatment is begun.

ECG EQUIPMENT

Electrocardiograph Paper

ECG paper can be either black or dark blue and is wax or plastic coated with a white or pink background and color lines. The paper is heat and pressure sensitive so as the heated stylus of the electrocardiograph moves across the paper, the background coating is melted away revealing the black or blue color of the paper and the ECG cycles are recorded or traced. The heat of the stylus can be adjusted to obtain a sharp, clear recording, or tracing. Medical assistants should learn how to adjust the proper control using the specific manual or instructions that accompany the instrument in their facility.

Electrolyte

Because the skin is a poor conductor of electricity, there are various types of electrolyte applied with each elec-

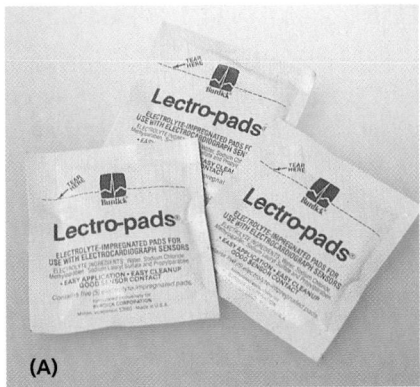 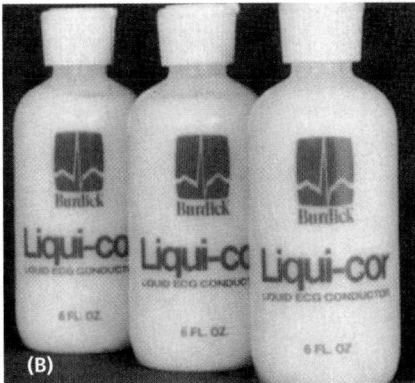 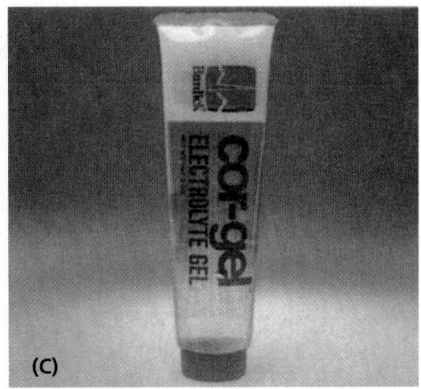

Figure 37-6 Various types of electrolyte: (A) Presaturated electrolyte pads. (B) Electrolyte lotion. (C) Electrolyte gel usually used with defibrillator. (Courtesy of Siemens Burdick, Inc.)

trode to help pick up the electrical current produced by the contraction and relaxation of the heart. The impulses are transmitted to the electrocardiograph by metal tips on the patient lead wires or cables that are attached to the electrodes. Electrolyte is manufactured in the form of a gel, lotion, or paste, or may be presaturated pads (Figure 37-6A-C).

Sensors or Electrodes

There are various types of sensors or **electrodes** made of metal or other conductive material used in taking an ECG. The sensors detect the electrical impulses on the body surface and relay them through cables, or leads, that are attached to the electrodes on one end to the ECG machine attached to the other end of the cables. Welch cups and metal sensors are found on some older model ECG machines and are still being used in some agencies. Other agencies have converted the Welch cups and metal sensors through the use of disposable electrodes and

reusable clips. The clips replace the metal sensors and are attached to the lead wires. The clips grasp hold of the disposable electrodes that have been applied to the limbs and chest.

Metal Sensors or Electrodes. Small metal sensors are secured to the fleshy parts of a patient's arms and legs using stretchable rubber straps. Electrolyte is applied to the side of the electrode touching the skin (Figure 37-7A).

Welch Sensors or Electrodes. A type of chest electrode, the Welch electrode consists of a rubber bulb with a metal suction cup. The electrolyte is placed onto the metal suction cup before it is applied to the chest wall (Figure 37-7B).

Disposable Electrodes. Disposable electrodes are permeated with electrolyte and can be used on both the limbs and chest (Figure 37-7C). They are made of a self-adhesive

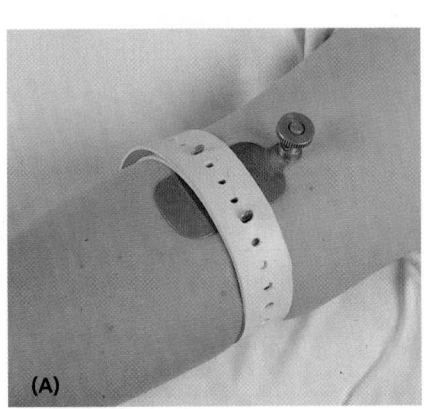 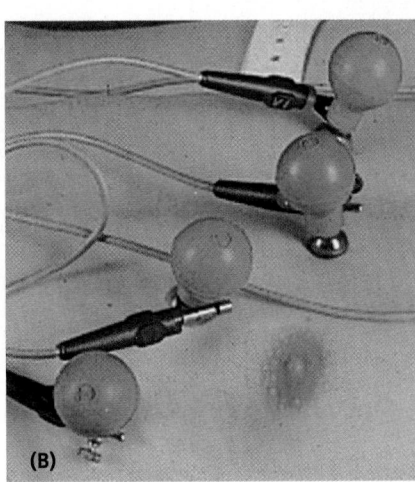 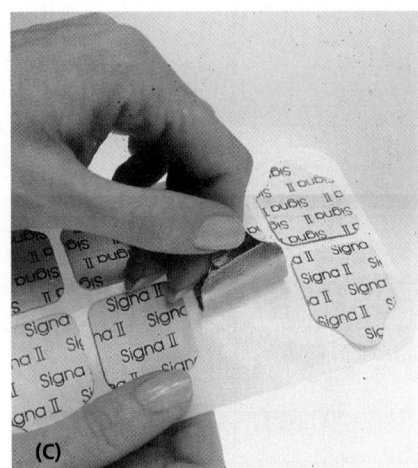

Figure 37-7 Various types of electrodes or sensors: (A) Metal limb electrode and strap. (B) Welch electrodes. (C) Signa II disposable sensors. (Courtesy of Siemens Burdick, Inc.)

conductive material that requires no additional electrolyte. These sensors are applied to the skin of the limbs and chest and held in place by the adhesive backing. The self-adhesive electrodes are discarded after use.

Care of Equipment

Many offices and ambulatory care areas use the standard electrocardiograph with metal electrodes and rubber limb straps. The newer computerized electrocardiographs require disposable electrodes and presaturated electrolyte pads.

It is important to note that clean electrodes will help ensure a good tracing. Metal electrodes should be cleaned with a mild detergent and occasionally scrubbed with a cleaner such as Soft Scrub®, rinsed, and dried. The rubber straps used to attach the electrodes to the patient's limbs should be washed in a mild detergent, rinsed, and dried. Use a cotton-tipped applicator to clean the holes in the rubber straps and inside the suction-type Welch chest electrode.

LEAD CODING

There are a number of codes that are used to identify each lead recorded on the ECG reading. These codes are necessary for later identification and for mounting purposes. Newer electrocardiographs will automatically mark (code) each lead in the upper margin of the ECG paper during the recording. Older electrocardiographs must be manually coded by depressing the lead marker button. See Figure 37-8 for an example of a common coding system.

THE ELECTROCARDIOGRAPH AND LEAD PLACEMENT

The standard electrocardiogram consists of twelve leads that record the heart's electrical activity from different angles, allowing for a thorough three-dimensional interpretation of its activity. The electrical impulses given off by the heart can be picked up by electrodes and then conducted into the instrument through **lead** wires. Electrodes consist of materials that are good conductors of electricity. Since the electrical activity that comes from the body is

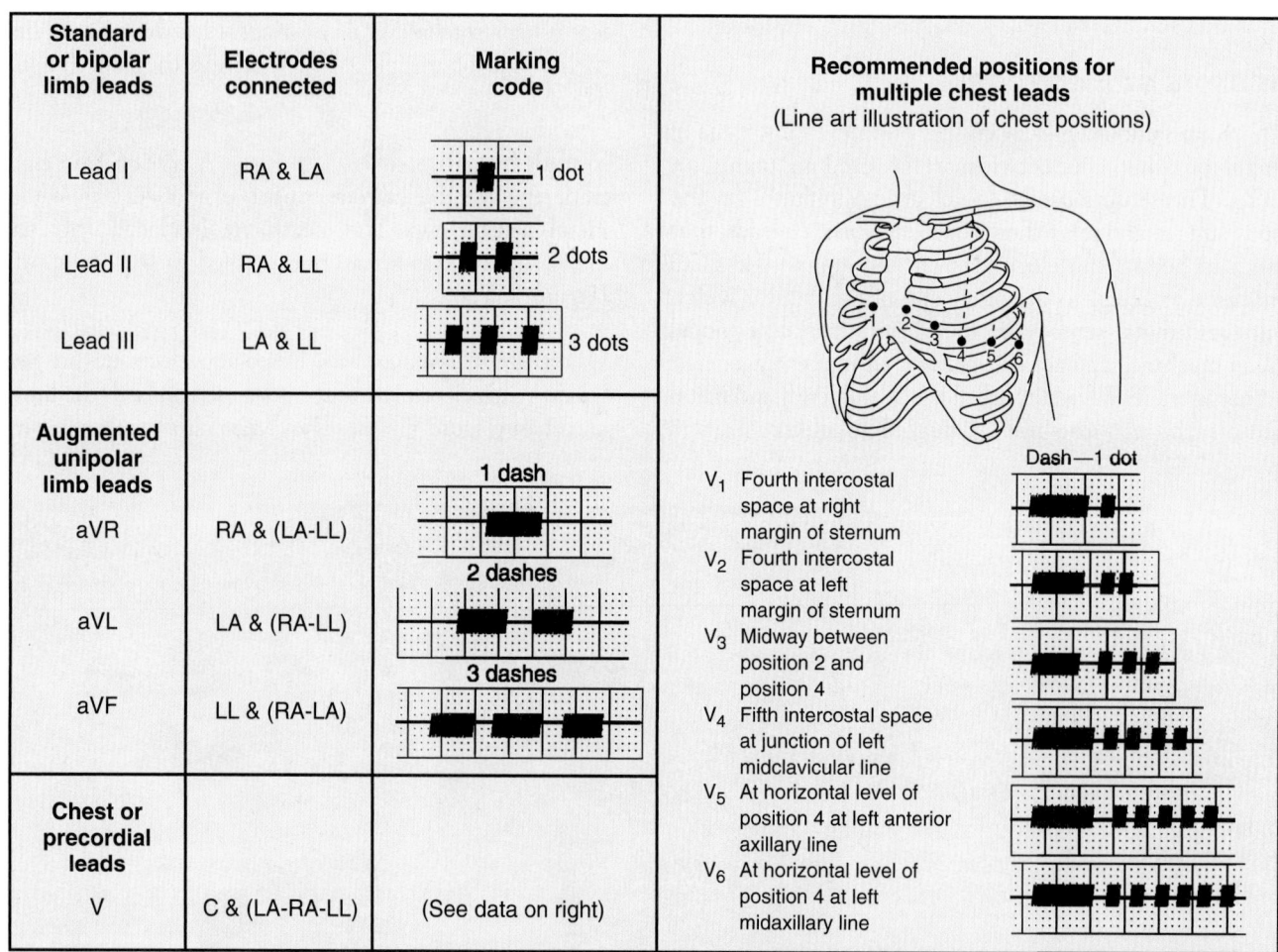

Figure 37-8 Example of a common coding system for ECG leads that must be manually coded on older electrocardiographs. Accurate coding is accomplished by pressing the lead marker button appropriately. (Courtesy of Siemens Burdick, Inc.)

small, it is made larger, or **amplified**, by the amplifier of the instrument. The voltage is changed into a mechanical motion by the **galvanometer** and recorded on the electrocardiograph by the stylus.

The electrodes are placed on the patient's four limbs and chest. The four limb leads are right arm (RA), left arm (LA), right leg (RL), and left leg (LL). The right leg electrode is not used as part of the recording. It is an electrical reference point only. The limb leads are placed on the fleshy area of upper arms and lower legs. The chest leads are known as precordial leads, V leads, or C leads, and use an electrode for each of six areas on the chest wall or one electrode that is moved to six different positions on the chest wall. (This depends upon the type of electrocardiograph being used.)

Standard Limb or Bipolar Leads

The first three leads that are recorded on a standard ECG are called Lead I, Lead II, and Lead III (Figure 37-9A).

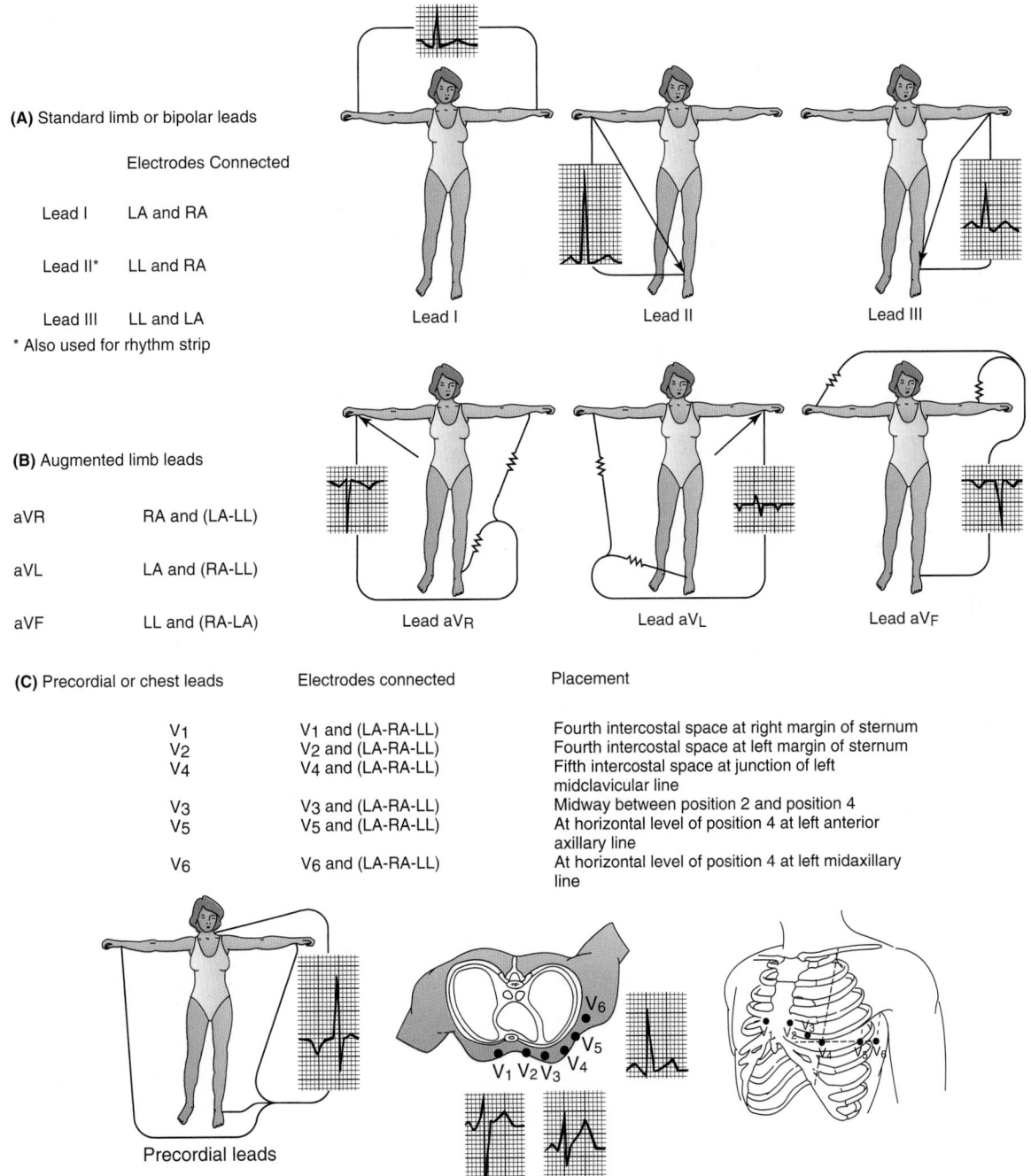

(A) Standard limb or bipolar leads

	Electrodes Connected
Lead I	LA and RA
Lead II*	LL and RA
Lead III	LL and LA

* Also used for rhythm strip

(B) Augmented limb leads

aVR	RA and (LA-LL)
aVL	LA and (RA-LL)
aVF	LL and (RA-LA)

(C) Precordial or chest leads

	Electrodes connected	Placement
V1	V1 and (LA-RA-LL)	Fourth intercostal space at right margin of sternum
V2	V2 and (LA-RA-LL)	Fourth intercostal space at left margin of sternum
V4	V4 and (LA-RA-LL)	Fifth intercostal space at junction of left midclavicular line
V3	V3 and (LA-RA-LL)	Midway between position 2 and position 4
V5	V5 and (LA-RA-LL)	At horizontal level of position 4 at left anterior axillary line
V6	V6 and (LA-RA-LL)	At horizontal level of position 4 at left midaxillary line

Figure 37-9 Lead types, connections, and placement: (A) Standard limb or bipolar leads. (B) Augmented limb leads. (C) Precordial or chest leads.

These are known as **bipolar** leads because each of them uses two limb electrodes that record simultaneously. Lead I records electrical activity between the right arm (RA) and left arm (LA); lead II records electrical activity between the right arm (RA) and left leg (LL); lead III records activity between the left arm (LA) and left leg (LL). Lead II is used as a **rhythm strip** because it portrays the heart's rhythm better than the other leads. The rhythm strip is usually a separate longer recording approximately 6 to 12 inches.

Augmented Leads

The next three leads are **augmented** leads and are designated aVR, aVL, and aVF (Figure 37-9B). The aV stands for augmented voltage; the R, L, and F stand for right, left, and foot (or leg). These are **unipolar** leads. Lead aVR records electrical activity from the midpoint between the left arm and left leg to the right arm. Lead aVL records electrical activity from the midpoint between the right arm and the left leg to the left arm. Lead aVF records electrical activity from the midpoint between the right arm and left arm to the left leg. Because these three leads produce such small electrical impulses, the ECG machine augments, or increases, their size in order to record them.

Chest Leads or Precordial Leads

The remaining six leads of the standard twelve-lead ECG are the chest leads or **precordial** leads (Figure 37-9C). These too are unipolar leads and are designated V_1, V_2, V_3, V_4, V_5, and V_6. These leads record the heart's electrical impulse from a central point within the heart to one of six predesignated positions on the chest wall where an electrode is attached. The correct position must be used for each lead recording.

The anatomical positions for placement of the chest or precordial leads are:

V_1—fourth intercostal space at right margin of sternum
V_2—fourth intercostal space at left margin of sternum
V_4—fifth intercostal space on left midclavicular line
V_3—midway between V2 and V4 (**NOTE:** This is correct order, V3 after V4.)
V_5—horizontal to V4 at left anterior axillary line
V_6—horizontal to V4 at left midaxillary line

When using a conventional electrocardiograph, the chest electrode must be moved manually one by one to each of the six chest lead positions. This necessitates stopping the instrument between each chest lead in order to move the electrode to the next appropriate position on the chest wall. Some electrocardiographs allow for all six chest leads to be applied at one time; therefore, there is no interruption between chest lead recordings. (See Figure 37-23 in Procedure 37-1).

STANDARDIZATION OF THE ELECTROCARDIOGRAPH

The value of an ECG recording depends on its being performed accurately. To ensure a precise and reliable recording, the ECG instrument must be standardized before an ECG is performed. The standardization of the instrument is a quality assurance check to determine if the machine is set and working properly. Standardization measurements have been adopted internationally as a means of accurate **calibration** according to universal measurements. The universal standard is that one millivolt of cardiac electrical activity will deflect the stylus exactly 10 mm high. This is the equivalent of 10 small squares on the ECG paper. Figure 37-10 shows an example of the 10-mm standardization and an electrocardiogram with all twelve leads recorded in minutes simultaneously with no interruption.

On occasion, R waves may be very large and go off the paper. Repositioning the stylus may not correct the situation. In such instances, the medical assistant can record the lead(s) in which the R wave is very large at one-half standard. This action will record all ECG cycles at half their normal **amplitude**.

Conversely, the waves of the ECG cycles may be very small, making it difficult to interpret. In this circumstance, the medical assistant can record the ECG cycles at twice the normal standard. This action will record ECG cycles at twice their normal amplitude. Whenever a change is made from a normal standardization mark (10 mm high) to either a one-half standardization mark (5 mm high) or a double standardization mark (20 mm high), the medical assistant must include the adjusted standardization mark with the particular lead to alert the physician to the change in standard. The instrument must be returned to normal standard to prevent accidentally running the next lead at a standard other than normal. The tracing paper is usually run at 25 mm per second. If cycles are too close together, speed can be adjusted to 50 mm per second. Make a note on the ECG paper if speed is changed.

STANDARD RESTING ELECTROCARDIOGRAPHY

Regardless of the type of electrocardiograph used, the basic components of the standard electrocardiography procedure remain the same. Patient preparation, placement of limb and chest leads, attachment of lead wires, and elimination of artifacts vary little from one electrocardiograph to another. Procedure 37-1 explains a twelve-lead ECG using a conventional single-channel electrocardiograph with reusable metal sensors for the limbs and six chest electrodes. Procedure 37-2 explains a

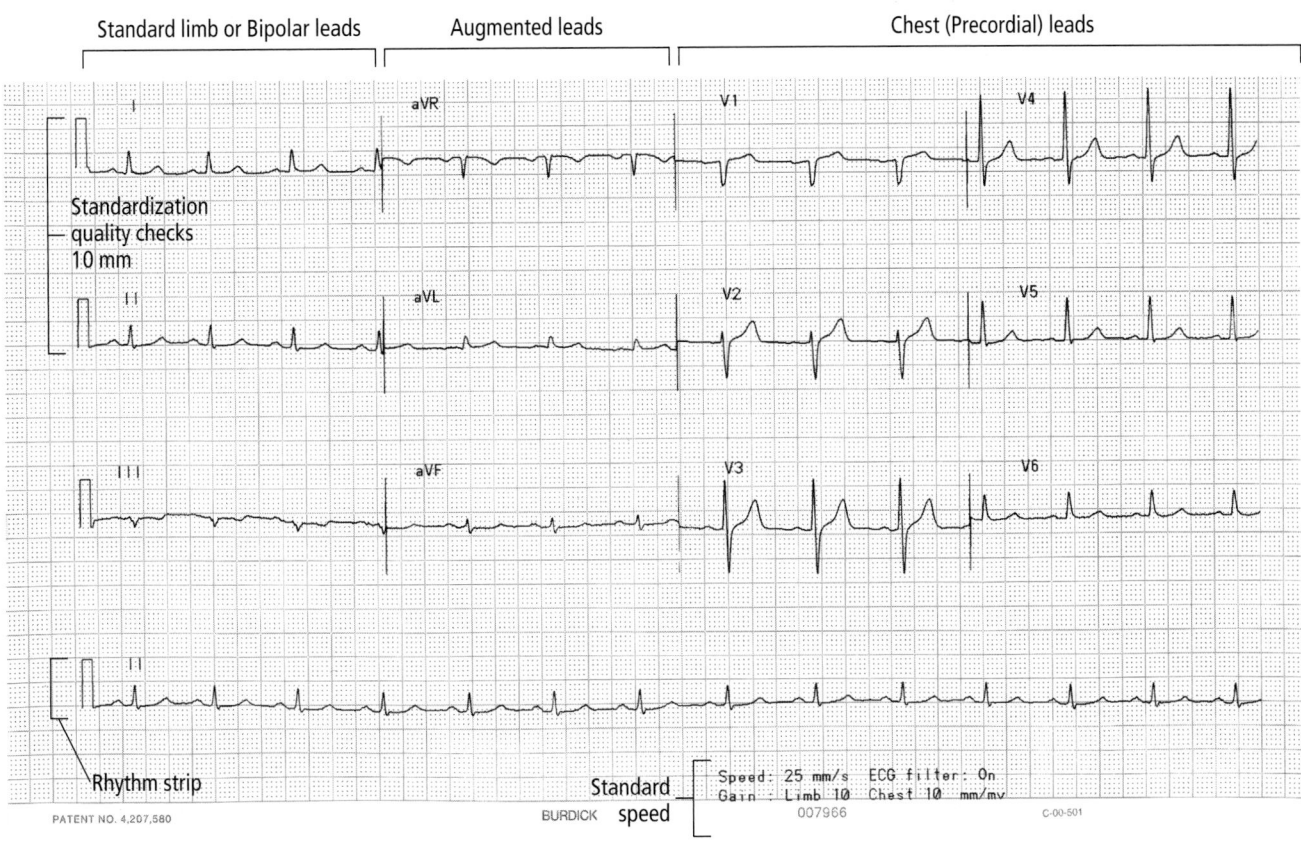

Standard limb or Bipolar leads   Augmented leads   Chest (Precordial) leads

Standardization
quality checks
10 mm

Rhythm strip

PATENT NO. 4,207,580   BURDICK   Standard speed

Speed: 25 mm/s   ECG filter: On
Gain : Limb 10   Chest 10   mm/mv
007966   C-00-501

Figure 37-10   An electrocardiogram showing all twelve leads recorded in minutes at one time with no interruption.

twelve-lead ECG using a three-channel machine with disposable electrodes. Medical assistants must be familiar with the electrocardiograph machine in their facility and should thoroughly review the manufacturer's instruction manual that accompanies the machine prior to performing the procedure. Knowledge of the basic procedures included here can be adapted for all other electrocardiographs.

MOUNTING THE ECG TRACING

Commercially prepared mounting forms are available and the medical assistant should mount the completed tracing after the physician has reviewed the entire recording (Figure 37-11). It is important that each lead be individually cut, mounted, and identified. Include the patient's name, date, address, age, gender, blood pressure, height and weight, and cardiac medications on the mounting form.

INTERFERENCE OR ARTIFACTS

The ECG is a valuable diagnostic aid to the physician and must be performed accurately. The medical assistant is responsible for obtaining a recording that can be easily read and interpreted by the physician.

There can be unusual and unwanted activity in the tracing not caused by the electrical activity of the heart. These defects in the ECG tracing are known as artifacts and their appearance can make the ECG tracing difficult to read and interpret. Four of the more common artifacts are somatic tremor, alternating current interference, wandering baseline, and interrupted baseline. The medical

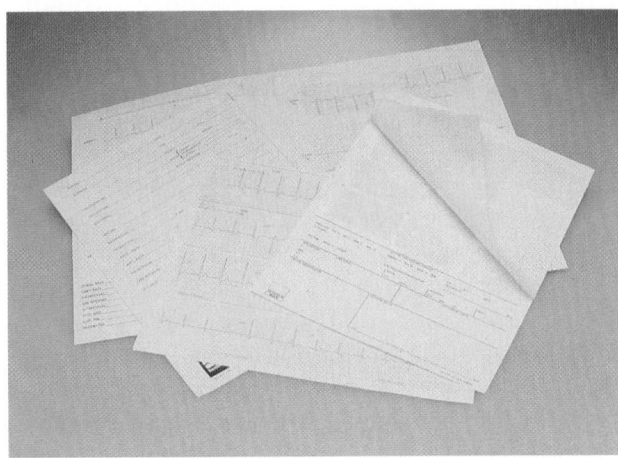

Figure 37-11   Various types of mounts for ECG tracing paper for patient's permanent record. (Courtesy of Siemens Burdick, Inc.)

assistant should understand the causes of each type of artifact and know how to eliminate them.

Somatic Tremor Artifacts

This type of artifact is also known as muscle tremor. It is characterized by unnatural baseline deflections such as jagged peaks or irregularity of spacing and height. The tracing appears fuzzy (Figure 37-12A). Somatic tremor occurs when the patient is apprehensive or uncomfortable and can result in involuntary muscle movement. Voluntary muscle movement occurs when the patient moves, talks, coughs, and so on. Parkinson's disease, a nervous system disorder, is an example of involuntary somatic tremor. It is not possible for the patient to control the muscle tremors. (Often, involuntary somatic tremor can be minimized somewhat by having the patient slide the hands under the buttocks during the recording.)

It is natural for the patient to feel apprehensive prior to and during the ECG tracing. Reassurance and an explanation of the procedure will allay apprehension and relax muscles. Be certain the patient is comfortable. Use pillows for the head and under the knees; be sure the temperature of the room is comfortable. These simple techniques will help to minimize somatic tremor.

Alternating Current (AC) Interference

This type of artifact is caused by electrical interference and appears as a series of small regular peaks (Figure 37-12B). Electricity present in medical equipment or wires in the area can leak a small amount of energy into the room in which the ECG is being recorded. The current can be picked up by the patient's body and it will be detected by the ECG tracing as an alternating current (AC) artifact.

Common Causes of AC Interference Artifacts. Some common causes of AC interferences are:

1. Improper grounding of electrocardiograph. There are three-pronged plugs in the newer electrocardiographs that are inserted into a properly grounded three-receptacle outlet. This reduces AC interference. Older instruments may have only a two-pronged plug necessitating the use of a separate ground wire attached to the unit and connected to a ground such as a cold water pipe.
2. Presence of other electrical equipment in the room. Unplug other electrical equipment in the room (electrical examination tables, lamps, autoclaves, and so on).
3. Electrical wiring in the floor, ceiling, or walls. Move the ECG table away from walls.

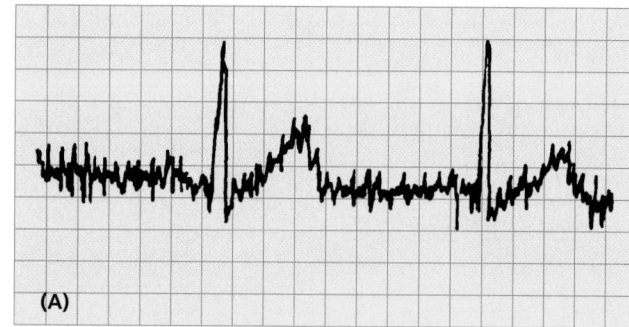

(A)

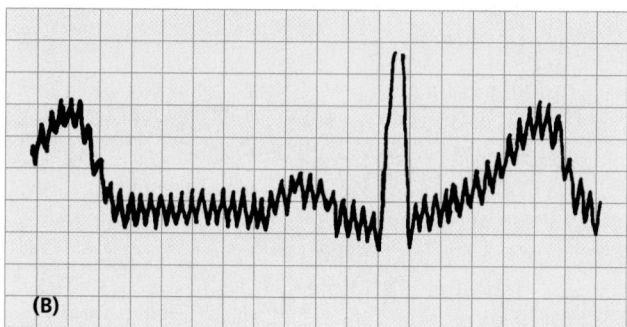

(B)

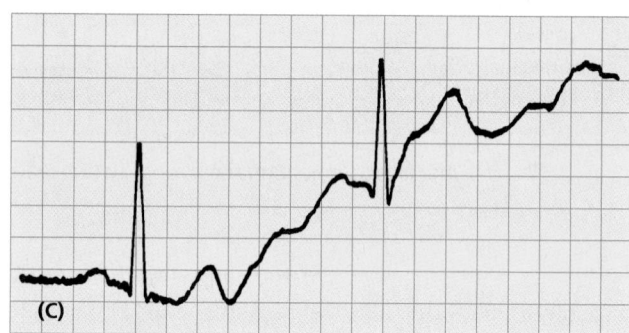

(C)

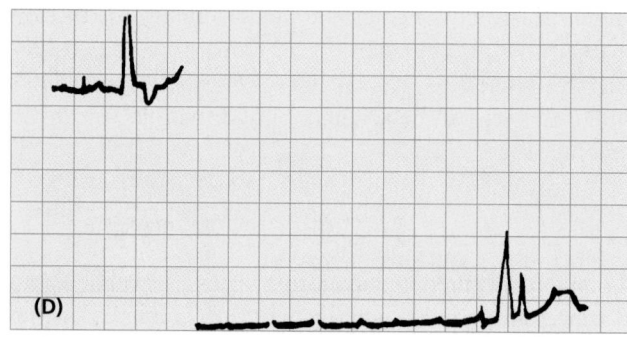

(D)

Figure 37-12   ECG artifacts. (A) Somatic tremor. (B) Alternating current (AC). (C) Wandering baseline. (D) Interrupted baseline. (Courtesy of Siemens Burdick, Inc.)

4. Crossed lead wires and lead wires not following body contour. Straighten lead wires and be sure they are positioned to follow the patient's body contour.
5. Corroded or dirty electrodes and/or metal tips of the lead wires. Reusable electrodes and tips of lead wires must be cleaned and rinsed completely after each use.

Wandering Baseline Artifacts

A wandering baseline occurs when the stylus suddenly moves from the center of the ECG paper resulting in the complexes "wandering" across the ECG paper; for example, from the top of the paper to the bottom, or bottom to top (Figure 37-12C). This makes it difficult to follow the complexes when the physician reads the recording and interprets it.

Common Causes of Wandering Baseline Artifacts. Wandering baseline artifacts can be caused by the following conditions:

1. Electrodes applied too loosely or too tightly. There should be equal tension on all four limb leads, metal tips should be firmly attached to the electrodes, and the patient cable should not have tension on it nor be dangling to cause pulling on the electrode.
2. Corroded or dirty electrodes and/or metal tips of the lead wires (refer to number 5 in AC interference).
3. Inappropriate amount or poor-quality electrolyte gel or paste. Each electrode should have the same amount of electrolyte gel or paste on it.
4. Lotions, oils, or creams on the patient's skin. Remove any of these substances before applying the electrode by vigorously rubbing the area with rubbing alcohol.

Interrupted Baseline Artifacts

On occasion, the baseline will become interrupted and there will be a break between complexes (Figure 37-12D). A probable cause could be a broken patient cable or a lead wire that may have become detached from an electrode.

CARDIAC CONDITIONS AND DISEASES

Myocardial Infarctions (Heart Attacks)

Myocardial infarctions (heart attacks) are the number one cause of death in the United States today. With the approval of your employer physician, medical assistants are in an excellent position to offer healthy tips and suggestions from which patients can benefit. For instance, they can offer patient health tips regarding diet and exercise while applying the ECG equipment (Table 37-1).

CARDIAC ARRHYTHMIAS

The medical assistant should recognize cardiac arrhythmias that occur during the ECG recording and make the physician aware of them as soon as they are noticed. The normal, healthy ECG cycle consists of P, QRS, and T in a regularly appearing sequence or pattern. The term **normal**

Patient Teaching Tip

Atherosclerosis is the build-up of fatty deposits on the lining of coronary arteries causing narrowing and obstruction of the arteries. Blood flow to the heart muscle is diminished particularly when the heart is called upon to work harder; e.g., during increased physical activity, emotional stress, exposure to cold temperatures, and after a heavy meal. The heart's muscle tissue responds to these conditions by symptoms of pain or discomfort beneath the sternum, into the neck, jaw, left arm and shoulder, and throat. Rest usually relieves the pain. This condition is known as angina pectoris.

Treatment for angina consists of rest and medication. Nitroglycerin may be prescribed in tablet or patch form. Change in lifestyle and other suggestions as noted in Table 37-1 may be recommended. Tests that the physician may order include a twelve-lead ECG, a stress ECG (stress test), blood tests, chest X ray, and coronary angiogram.

Pain that does not subside following rest may indicate a more serious condition: a complete obstruction of the coronary arteries and no blood flow to the heart muscle, a myocardial infarction, or heart attack. Seek immediate medical attention if pain persists.

sinus rhythm refers to an ECG that is within normal limits (WNL). The normal adult heart rate is 60 to 100 beats per minute. A rate less than 60 beats per minute is known as **sinus bradycardia** (Figure 37-13A); a rate greater than 100 beats per minute is known as **sinus tachycardia** (Figure 37-13B). These two heart rates, while regular in rhythm, are still considered to be cardiac arrhythmias.

TABLE 37-1	HEALTHY BEHAVIORS TO ADOPT FOR A HEALTHY HEART

The physician may want the medical assistant to remind patients of the following healthy behaviors:

1. Avoid tobacco.
2. Take medications as prescribed.
3. Report any unusual symptoms or problems to the physician.
4. Eat a low-fat, low-cholesterol, low-sodium diet.
5. Exercise regularly with physician's permission.
6. Get adequate rest.
7. Keep weight under control and at an acceptable level.
8. Practice stress reduction behaviors.

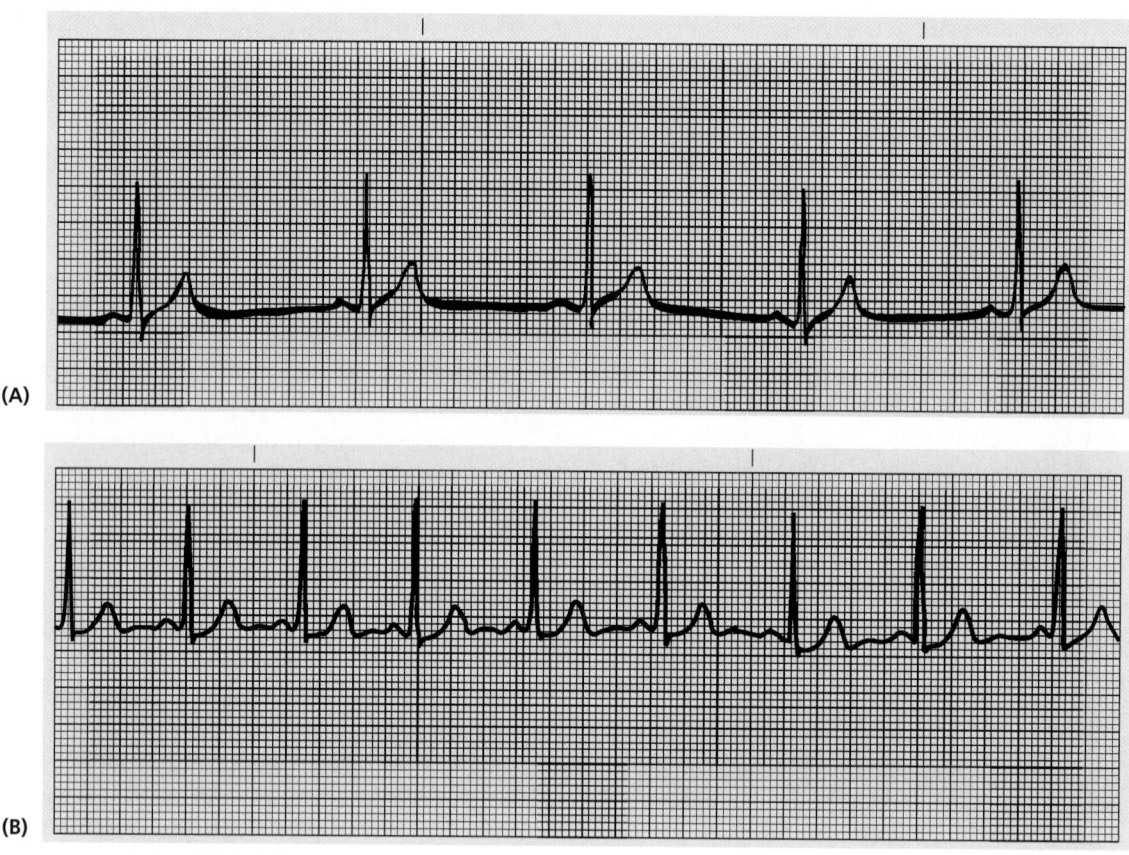

Figure 37-13 (A) Heart rate shown is 50 bpm, known as sinus bradycardia since it is less than 60 bpm. One large square = 0.2 second; one minute (60 seconds) ÷ 0.2 = 300. There are 6 large squares between R waves: 300 ÷ 6 = 50 bpm. (B) Sinus tachycardia is a heart rate faster than 100 bpm.

Atrial Arrhythmias

Premature Atrial Contractions (PAC). Healthy persons can experience premature atrial contractions. They are seen in patients who use tobacco and stimulants such as caffeine, but can forewarn of more serious cardiac problems. This type of arrhythmia is characterized by a cardiac cycle that occurs before the next cycle is due. The P wave is shaped differently from the P wave of the normal cycle (Figure 37-14A).

Paroxysmal Atrial Tachycardia (PAT). This arrhythmia also can be seen in healthy individuals; however, it can appear in persons with cardiac disease. PAT is characterized by its unprovoked sudden onset and abrupt termination. The heart rate is regular and ranges between 160 to 250 beats per minute. The episode usually lasts only a few seconds and the heart rate then returns to its original rate (Figure 37-14B). The patient may describe a fluttering in the chest, apprehension, shortness of breath, and on occasion, dizziness.

Atrial Fibrillation. This arrhythmia can be seen in healthy patients or those with cardiac disease. In younger patients, common causes can be congenital heart disease and mitral valve damage due to rheumatic heart disease. In older patients, the arrhythmia can be due to hypertension, coronary artery disease, or mitral valve prolapse. It is characterized by extremely rapid, incomplete contractions 400 to 500 bpm (beats per minute) resulting in small, irregular, and uncoordinated complexes that are difficult to measure accurately because the P waves cannot be distinguished (Figure 37-14C).

Ventricular Arrhythmias

Premature Ventricular Contractions (PVCs). This arrhythmia can be seen in healthy patients and patients with hypertension, coronary artery disease, and lung disease. In healthy patients, PVCs can be caused by tobacco, anxiety, alcohol, and medications that contain epinephrine (Figure 37-15A). PVCs are seen on ECG

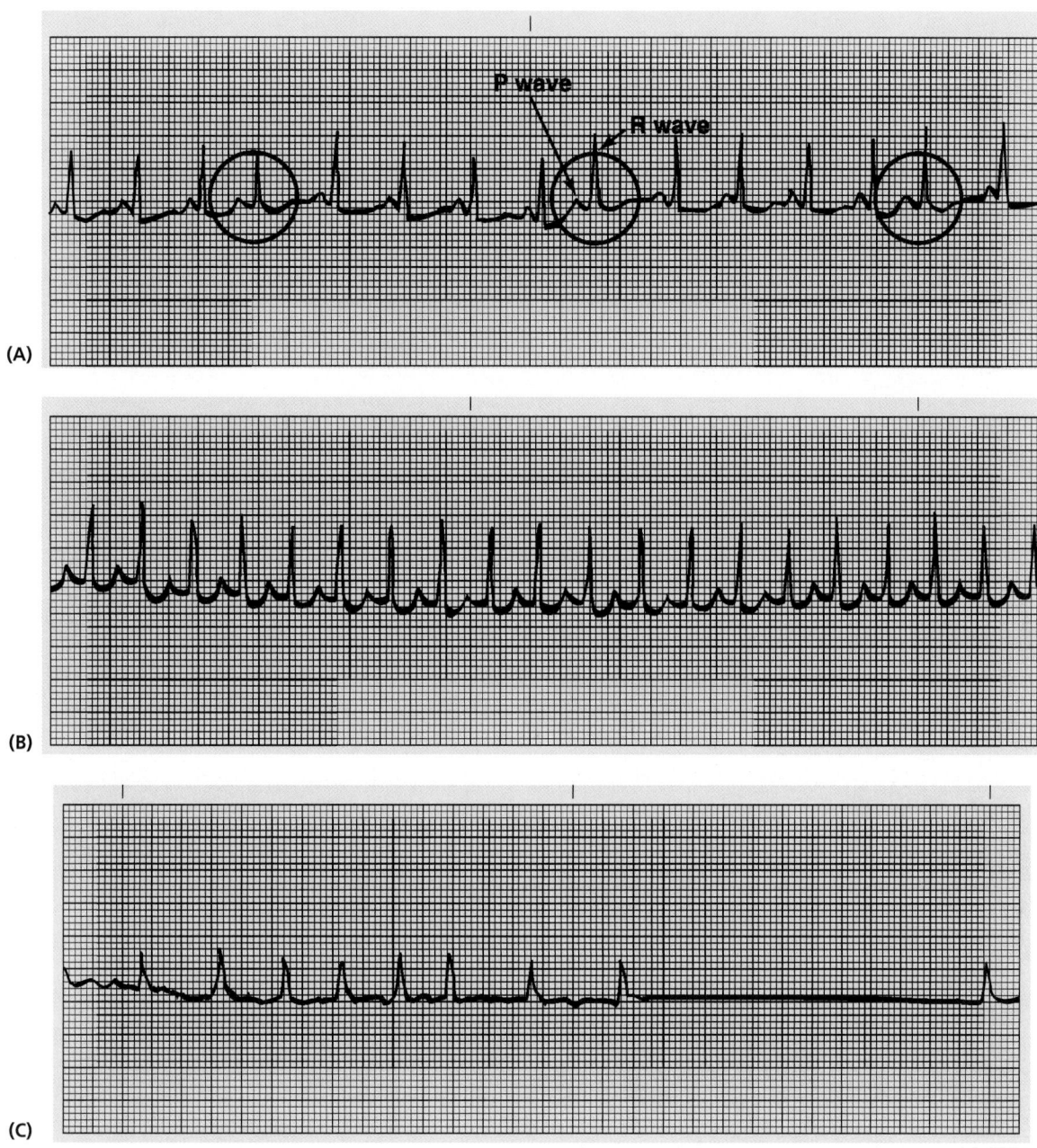

Figure 37-14 Atrial arrhythmias: (A) Premature atrial contractions (PAC). (B) Paroxysmal atrial tachycardia (PAT). (C) Atrial fibrillation.

tracings fairly frequently and are considered common disturbances in the rhythm. They are characterized by a beat that comes early in the cycle, has no P wave, a wide QRS complex, and a different T wave. The PVC is followed by a pause before the occurrence of the next normal cycle.

Ventricular Tachycardia. This arrhythmia is seen in patients with cardiac disease, both acute and chronic. It is common in coronary artery disease and frequently the patient experiencing a myocardial infarction will have ventricular tachycardia as a result of the infarction (Figure 37-15B). The arrhythmia is manifested by three or more

PVCs that occur at a rate ranging from 150 to 250 beats per minute. There are no P waves and the QRS complexes are distorted. Ventricular tachycardia is life threatening and can rapidly deteriorate into fibrillation and cardiac standstill.

Ventricular Fibrillation. This arrhythmia is seen in patients experiencing a myocardial infarction or in patients with existing cardiac disease. It may be preceded by PVCs or ventricular tachycardia or may begin as ventricular fibrillation. It is a life-threatening arrhythmia (Figure 37-15C).

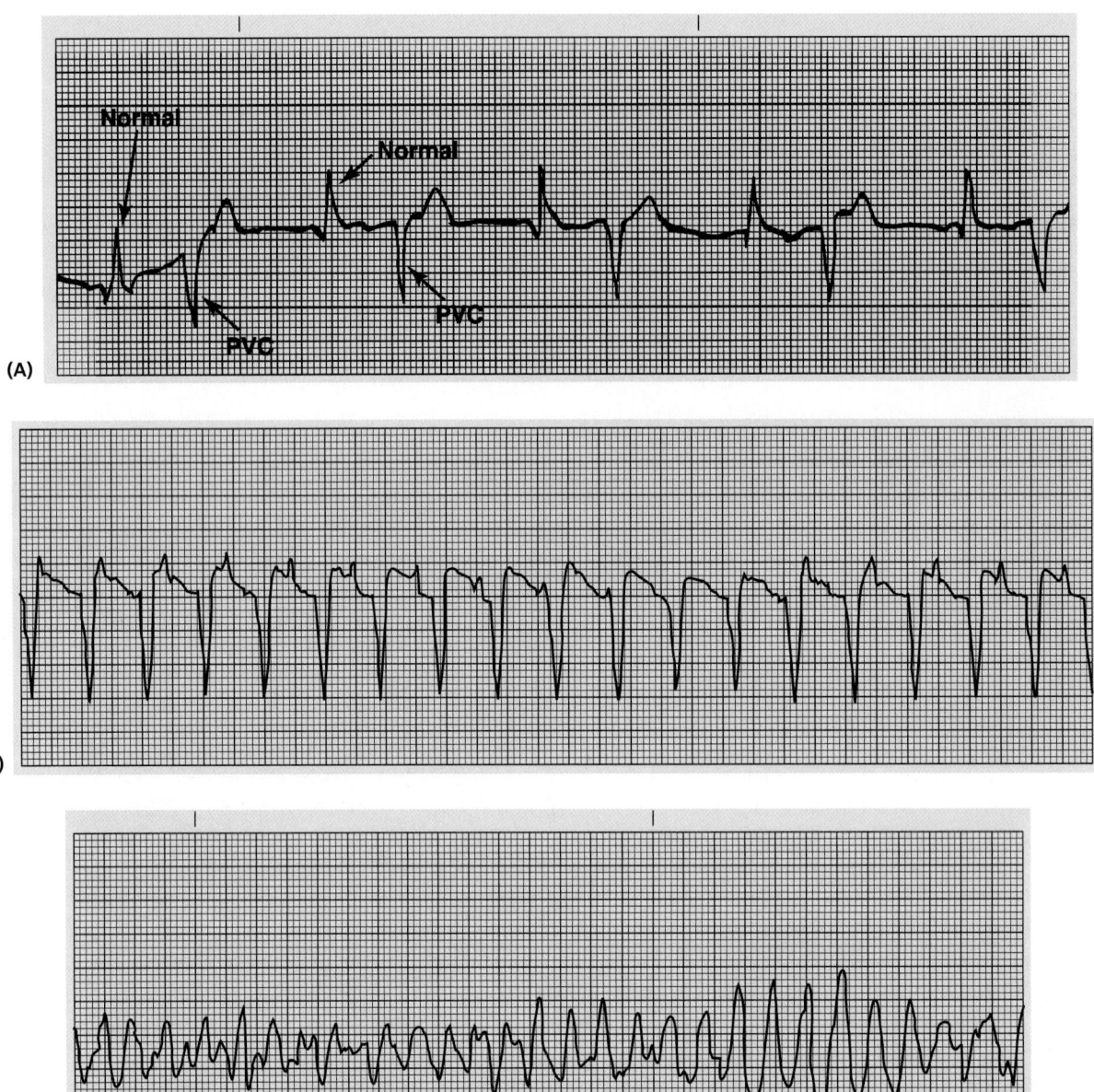

Figure 37-15   Ventricular arrhythmias: (A) Premature ventricular contractions (PVCs). (B) Ventricular tachycardia. (C) Ventricular fibrillation.

DEFIBRILLATION

A defibrillator is an electrical device that applies countershocks to the heart through electrodes or pads placed on the chest wall (Figure 37-16). The purpose is to convert cardiac arrhythmia into normal sinus rhythm. This is known as defibrillation or cardioversion. In some offices and clinics, a defibrillator is kept on a crash cart for quick access in emergency situations. The medical assistant should regularly check the equipment for proper operation and preparedness, and assist the physician as needed. See Chapter 9.

OTHER CARDIAC DIAGNOSTIC TESTS

Holter Monitor (Portable Ambulatory Electrocardiograph)

The Holter monitor is a portable continuous recording of cardiac activity for a 24-hour period (Figure 37-17). The patient is monitored while going about the usual daily activities with no restrictions. This noninvasive test helps to diagnose cardiac arrhythmias by correlating them

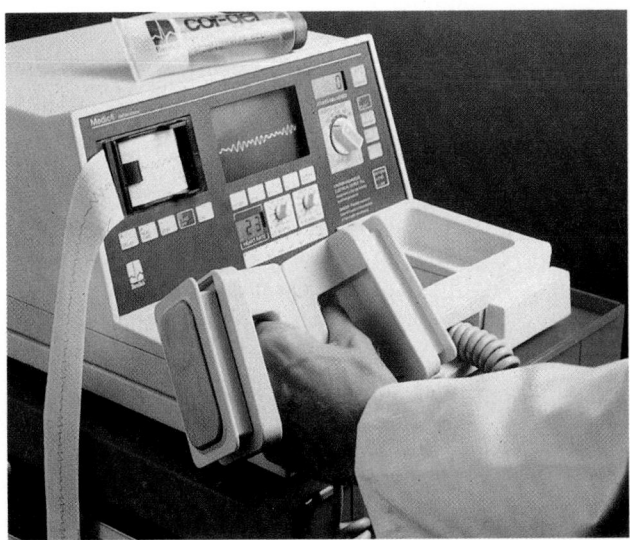

Figure 37-16 The Medic IV defibrillator. (Courtesy of Siemens Burdick, Inc.)

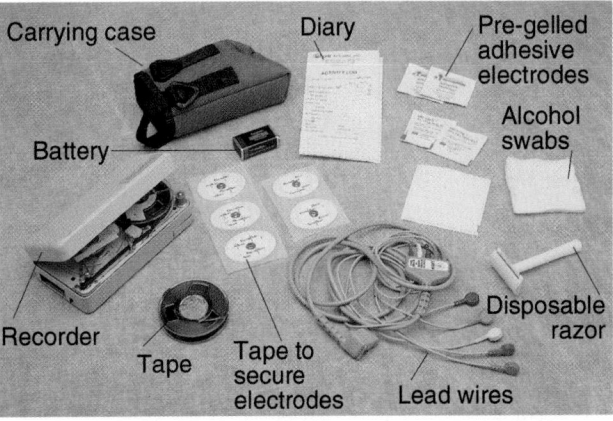

Figure 37-17 Holter monitor and supplies needed for application.

with the patient's symptoms. Some symptoms are **syncope**, fatigue, chest pain, and vertigo. This type of monitoring is useful for patients whose arrhythmias are sporadic in nature and whose arrhythmia is not able to be found on a twelve-lead ECG tracing. Also, ambulatory monitoring helps assess the function of an artificial pacemaker and the effectiveness of antiarrhythmic medications.

Special electrodes are placed in the appropriate areas of the patient's chest and lead wires are then attached to the electrodes. A special portable tape recorder, computer or magnetic, will continually record the heart's electrical activity for a 24-hour period. The monitor is a battery-operated recorder that is placed in a leather pouch or bag and is worn by the patient either on a belt around the waist or by a strap over the patient's shoulder.

Medical Assistant's Role. The medical assistant is responsible for preparing the patient, instructing the patient, and applying and removing the monitor.

Following are examples of some of the daily activities that should be recorded by the patient in the patient activity diary:

- Eating meals
- Ascending and descending stairs
- Sexual activity
- Medications taken
- Times of sleep
- Smoking
- Bowel movements
- Physical exercise

Holter Monitor Attachment. Once the Holter monitor has been attached to the patient, the monitor should be checked for effectiveness by attaching the **test cable** to the monitor and the other end to an ECG instrument. A baseline strip can be recorded to verify the correct wave activity and lack of artifact. If there are inaccurate readings, the monitor may not have been applied properly. The medical assistant can reconnect the leads to the electrodes or reposition the electrodes and reconnect the leads (see Procedure 37-3).

Holter Monitor Electrode Placement. Special disposable electrodes, which are round plastic and have an adhesive back, are available for the Holter monitor. These

Patient Teaching Tip

When preparing patients to wear a Holter monitor instruct them to:
1. Keep a diary of daily activities, symptoms, and emotions, and note the time of occurrence.
2. Do not shower, bathe, or swim while wearing the monitor because the recording could be interrupted or the monitor could be damaged.
3. Do not handle the electrodes. Doing so could cause artifacts.
4. Do not remove the recorder from its case.
5. Do not use an electric blanket. This can cause interference.
6. Depress the event marker only briefly and when experiencing a significant symptom. Overuse of the marker can mask the ECG tracing.

TABLE 37-2	HOLTER MONITOR ELECTRODE PLACEMENT	
Electrode	**Lead**	**Location**
A (black)	mV_1	Fourth intercostal space at right of the sternal edge
B (white)	mV_5	Right clavicle, just lateral to sternum
C (brown)	mV_1	Left clavicle, just lateral to the sternum
D (red)	mV_5	Fifth intercostal space at left axillary line
E (green)	Ground	Lower right chest wall

electrodes contain an electrolyte gel and are discarded once used. There may be either four or five electrodes depending on whether or not the monitor has a built-in ground. Notice that the leads for the Holter monitor are applied to different locations than the electrodes of a resting ECG. Table 37-2 explains the lead placement.

Patient Activity Diary. The patient activity diary is an important component of the monitoring procedures. As noted in the Patient Teaching Tip, all activities and emotional states, and the time of their occurrence, should be noted during the 24-hour monitoring time. Symptoms such as chest pain, shortness of breath, dizziness, palpitations, and so on, and the time the event occurred should also be noted. Patient symptoms recorded while being monitored can be compared to the patient's notations in the activity diary and correlated to the heart's activity. Symptoms can be further noted by the patient briefly depressing an event marker button located at one end of the monitor. This places an electronic "tag" on the tape. This signal can alert the person interpreting the ECG to look for a significant event or abnormality on the tape.

Holter Monitor Removal. The patient is instructed to return to the office or ambulatory care center 24 hours later to have the monitor removed. The tape is analyzed by a Holter monitor scanner or by a computer. This is usually done in the ECG department of a nearby hospital. The physician will receive a written report with samples of any abnormalities that were picked up during the monitoring period.

Treadmill Stress Test or Exercise Tolerance ECG

On occasion patients have symptoms of cardiac problems that do not appear as abnormalities on a resting ECG.

SPOTLIGHT ON AAMA ESSENTIALS THROUGH CAAHEP

● Take the time to talk with the patient when instructing him or her on keeping a daily activity record while wearing a Holter monitor. This will assist the patient to cut down on undue stresses and thus make the monitoring much more accurate and reliable.

● When preparing a patient for electrocardiography, it is important that the medical assistant be understanding and sensitive to the patient's fears and concerns about a possible heart problem.

● By explaining the electrocardiogram before performing the procedure, the medical assistant encourages the patient to be better informed and generally more cooperative and less anxious.

The physician may prescribe a treadmill stress test or exercise tolerance test to aid in the determination of the patient's diagnosis and prognosis. The test is done to diagnose heart disorders, to diagnose the probable cause of the patient's chest pain, and to assess the patient's cardiac ability following cardiac surgery. The treadmill stress test is a noninvasive ECG tracing taken under controlled conditions while the patient is closely monitored by the physician. Frequent blood pressure readings are done. The patient wears comfortable clothing and flat shoes such as sneakers with rubber soles and exercises on a treadmill at prescribed rates of speed (Figure 37-18). Electrodes are applied to the chest only.

The myocardium requires extra oxygen during exercise and in the presence of narrowed or obstructed coronary arteries. The additional workload on the myocardium will often be demonstrated as an abnormality on the ECG recording. There should be no pain, shortness of breath, or excess fatigue. If any of these or other unusual symptoms occur, the physician will terminate the test as this could indicate cardiac disease.

At the conclusion of the test, the patient is told to rest. Monitoring continues until the vital signs and heart rate return to normal. Prior to the patient leaving the office, the patient should be instructed to rest, refrain from a hot bath or shower, avoid stimulants such as caf-

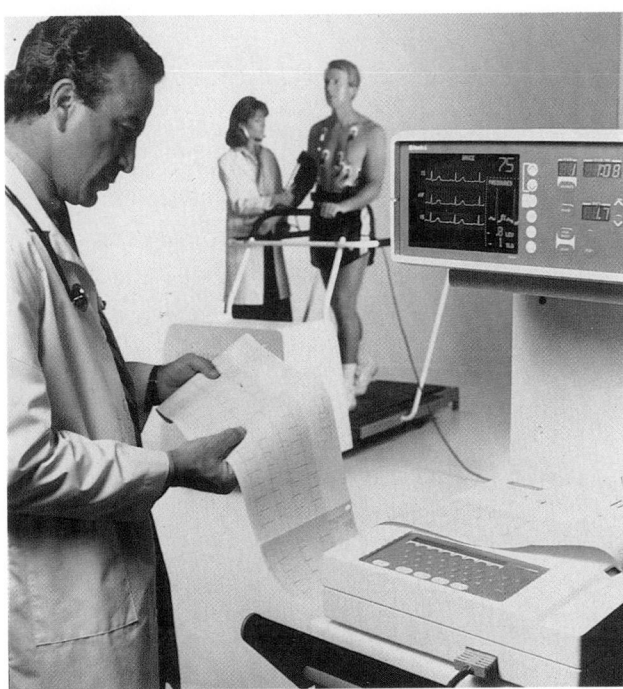

Figure 37-18 **The EXTOL 350 ST Stress System.** (Courtesy of Siemens Burdick, Inc.)

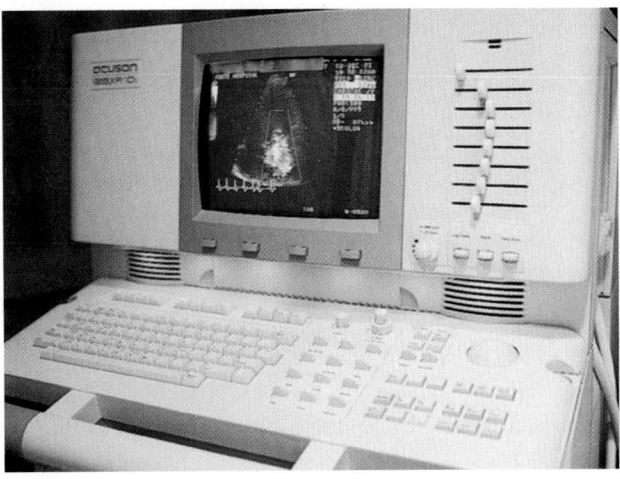

Figure 37-19 **Echocardiograph.** (Photo by Marcia Butterfield, Courtesy of W. A. Foote Memorial Hospital, Jackson, MI)

feine, and avoid extreme temperature changes for several hours.

Complications such as a myocardial infarction or a serious arrhythmia can occur during testing. While these events are unusual, appropriate emergency equipment must be readily available and checked frequently for proper functioning. Some equipment to have on hand for cardiac emergencies include oxygen, antiarrhythmic drugs, an Ambu-bag™, a defibrillator, an airway, an endotracheal tube, and a laryngoscope.

Further diagnostic tests such as **cardiac catheterization** may be necessary to diagnose the extent of the atheroscleratic buildup and obstruction of the coronary arteries.

Echocardiography

Echocardiography is a noninvasive, diagnostic test that uses ultrasound (ultrahigh-frequency sound waves) to image the internal structures of the heart (Figure 37-19). X rays are not used. General anatomy, myocardial function, valve function, and heart chamber size can be evaluated.

During **ultrasonography**, a handheld **transducer** acts as a transmitter and receiver of the high-frequency sound waves as it is held against the chest wall and moved over the heart area. As the sound waves go through the skin and hit internal structures, echoes are sent back to the transducer. A machine converts the images when the various structures provide different echoes. The images can then be examined by a computer and converted into photographs and films of structures and blood flow.

There is little patient preparation other than to have the patient lie on the examination table with the four-limb leads of a twelve-lead electrocardiograph attached. The test is usually performed by a **sonographer**.

Procedure 37-1

Perform Twelve-Lead Electro-cardiogram, Single-Channel

STANDARD PRECAUTIONS:

PURPOSE:

To obtain an accurate, graphic, artifact-free reading of the electrical activity of the patient's heart to identify arrhythmias, estimate damage caused by MI, assess effects of cardiac medication, determine if electrolyte imbalance is present, identify cardiac ischemia, and determine the effects of hypertension or other disorders on the heart.

EQUIPMENT/SUPPLIES:

Examination or ECG table with pillow and sheet or blanket
Patient gown
Single-channel electrocardiograph with patient cable wires
Electrolyte (gel, lotion, paste, or presaturated pads)
ECG tracing paper
Metal electrodes (sensors)
Rubber straps
Gauze squares
Mounting form

PROCEDURE STEPS:

1. Perform tracing in a quiet, warm, and comfortable room away from electrical equipment that may cause artifacts. RATIONALE: Patient is less apprehensive in a quiet atmosphere. Alternating current (AC) interference is minimized when ECG is performed away from electrical equipment.

2. Wash hands, gather equipment, identify the patient, and explain the procedure to the patient. RATIONALE: Following these universal steps minimizes transmission of microorganisms and reassures patient.

3. Have the patient remove clothing from the waist up and uncover lower legs; Nylon stockings must be removed; socks can be worn. RATIONALE: Electrodes must be placed on bare skin for optimum conductivity of electricity. Provide a sheet or blanket for privacy and warmth. Place the patient in supine position on the examination table with arms and legs supported. Pillows may be used under the knees and head. RATIONALE: All four limbs and chest must be uncovered for proper electrode placement.

4. Explain that the procedure is painless and why it is necessary not to move or talk during the procedure. RATIONALE: Patient cooperation ensures good quality tracing.

5. Place the electrocardiograph with the power cord pointing away from the patient. Do not allow the cable to go underneath the table. RATIONALE: This helps reduce AC interference.

6. Apply the limb electrodes by first connecting the rubber straps to the tabs on the electrodes. Apply a pea-size dab of electrolyte to the electrode; either paste or gel can be used (Figure 37-20).

(continues)

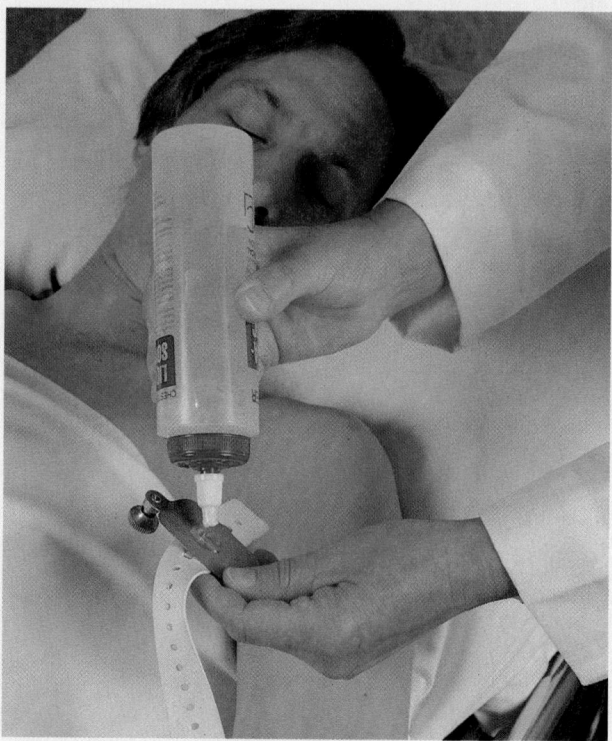

Figure 37-20   The rubber strap is attached to the metal electrode and a small amount of electrolyte gel is placed on the side of the electrode applied to the patient's skin.

Procedure

37-1 (continued)

Apply the electrodes to the fleshy parts of the four limbs. Rub the electrolyte into the patient's skin. Lead connectors of the electrodes should be pointing toward the feet. Pull the rubber strap around the limb until it just meets, then pull tighter one more hole and secure (Figures 37-21 and 37-22). RATIONALE: A more stable connection with the lead wires is possible when the lead connectors point to the feet. Electrolyte rubbed into the patient's skin helps ensure good contact between the electrode and the skin. Straps applied too tightly or too loosely can cause artifacts. By applying electrodes to the fleshy part of the limbs, artifacts are minimized.

7. If using a Welch cup chest electrode, apply electrolyte to chest position, rub the edge of each cup in the electrolyte, and secure it in position by squeezing the bulb end of the cup to create suction on the skin of the chest wall (Figure 37-23). When using the Welch cup electrode with a single channel non-automatic machine, only one chest lead can be recorded at a time because there is only one chest lead wire. Therefore, chest lead V_1 should be placed in position and be ready to be recorded. The first seven leads, I,

II, III, aVR, aVL, aVF, and V_1, can be recorded before it is necessary to temporarily stop recording while the Welch cup is moved to each successive chest lead. It is necessary to turn the machine to AMP OFF between each V lead because the medical assistant will manually remove the V lead and place it on the next

(continues)

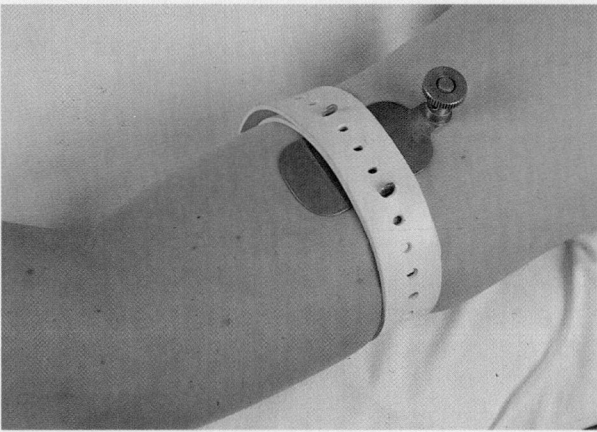

Figure 37-22 Electrode held in place on upper arm by rubber strap. Pull the rubber strap around until the holes line up with the protrusions on the electrode with no tension, then pull the strap one hole tighter and secure.

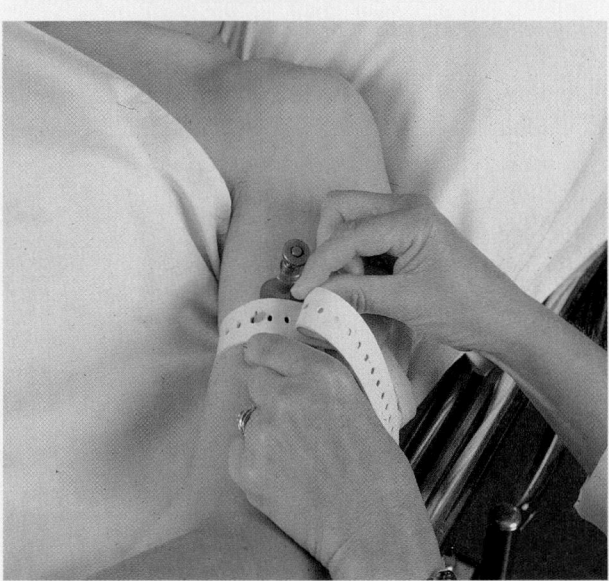

Figure 37-21 Application of rubber strap and electrode to patient's upper arm. Placing electrode on upper arm minimizes somatic tremor.

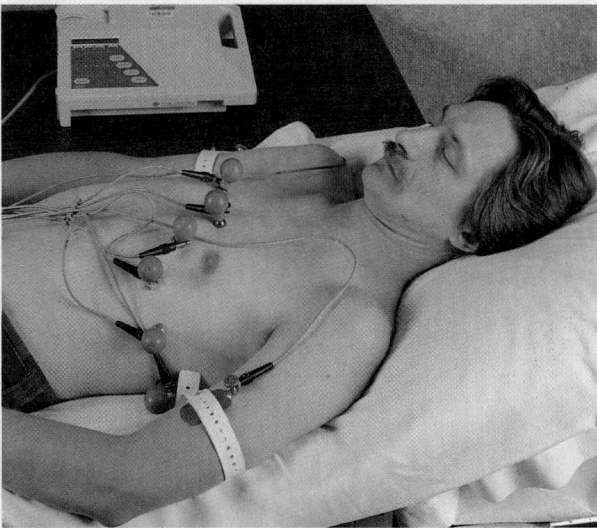

Figure 37-23 An automatic electrocardiograph with all six chest leads applied simultaneously using Welch electrodes allows all chest leads to be recorded at one time.

Procedure

37-1 (continued)

appropriate V lead position. If the machine were not turned to AMP OFF between each V lead as the medical assistant moves the Welch cup, this would interrupt the tracing, cause the stylus to become erratic, and distort the tracing. After the Welch cup has been moved to the next appropriate V lead, the stylus is adjusted, the machine is turned to AMP ON, and six to eight inches of the V lead is recorded.

8. Tightly connect the lead wires to the electrodes. Be sure to connect the correct lead wires to the correct electrodes. The lead wires are labeled with abbreviations (RA, LA, RL, LL, and V or C). The lead wires are color-coded as follows: RA=white, LA=black, RL=green, LL=red, V or chest=brown or multi-colored depending on model of machine. The lead wires should follow the patient's body contour. RATIONALE: Following body contour minimizes artifacts.

9. The patient cable is supported either on the table or the patient's abdomen. Plug the patient cable into the electrocardiograph.

10. Turn instrument to ON.

11. The lead selector switch should be on STD (standard). Center the stylus. The record switch should be on Run (25 mm/sec). Check the standardization for the instrument by quickly pressing the standardization button. The standardization mark should be 10 mm or 10 small squares high. If it is more or less than this, adjust the instrument appropriately. RATIONALE: Standardization ensures a dependable and accurate tracing.

12. Center the stylus and run about 4 to 5 complexes of each lead I, II, and III by placing the record switch on Run (25 mm/sec) and turning the lead selector switch appropriately.

a. While recording, be sure the stylus and recording are near the center of the paper. If not, use the position control knob to move up or down to adjust as needed. None of the waves should fall off the graph paper.

b. Watch for artifacts and correct if present.

c. Determine if a change in standard or stylus position is needed by observing the amplitude of the R wave.

13. Continue with leads aVR, aVL, aVF, and record about 4 to 5 complexes of each lead by turning the lead selector to the appropriate position.

14. Record 6 to 8 complexes of each of the V leads by turning the lead selector control to the appropriate position.

15. Place another standardization at the end of the tracing by putting the lead selector on STD and depressing the button. Run the tracing through the instrument and turn the machine to OFF. Remove the tracing from the instrument and immediately label with patient's name, date, and time of day. Sign your initials. Unplug the power cord.

16. Disconnect the lead wires and remove the rubber straps and electrodes from the patient. Cleanse or wipe patient's skin to remove paste or gel electrolyte.

17. Assist patient as needed.

18. Provide physician with uncut tracing.

19. Clean and return equipment per OSHA guidelines.

20. Wash hands.

21. Document procedure.

22. Cut and mount the tracing, remembering to handle carefully. Label appropriately and place in patient's record.

Procedure 37-2

Perform Twelve-Lead Electrocardiogram, Three Channel

STANDARD PRECAUTIONS:

PURPOSE:

To obtain an accurate, graphic, artifact-free reading of the electrical activity of the patient's heart to identify arrhythmias, estimate damage caused by MI, assess effects of cardiac medication, determine if electrolyte imbalance is present, identify cardiac ischemia, and determine the effects of hypertension or other disorders on the heart.

EQUIPMENT/SUPPLIES:

Examination or ECG table with pillow and sheet or blanket
Patient gown
Three-channel automatic electrocardiograph with patient cable wires
Disposable electrodes
ECG tracing paper
Gauze squares
Mounting form

PROCEDURE STEPS:

1. Follow steps 1 through 5 of Procedure 37-1 for ECG with single-channel machine.
2. Prepare patient's skin for disposable electrode attachment. If patient's skin is oily, wipe electrode area with alcohol and let dry.
3. Apply electrodes firmly to fleshy parts of limbs. Point tabs of electrodes attached to arms in a downward position, place electrodes attached to legs in an upward position. RATIONALE: Tab position allows for better connection and keeps pulling on lead wires to a minimum.
4. Locate chest sites and apply electrodes with tabs pointing in a downward position.
5. Connect lead wires to the electrodes. An alligator clip (a special clip applied to the end of the lead wires) will grasp the tab on the electrode.
6. Plug patient cable into machine. Support patient cable to avoid pulling or tangling of it.
7. Turn on the ECG. Enter patient data by keying it into machine. Notice the data on the LCD screen (patient data includes: patient's name, age, height, weight, gender, ID number, and cardiac medications).
8. Press AUTO for automatic and run the ECG to obtain the tracing. The standardization is automatically inserted at the beginning and the twelve leads follow in the three-channel mode. Watch for artifacts and take the appropriate steps to eliminate them should they occur.
9. Disconnect the lead wires and remove the electrodes from the patient. Dispose of the electrodes.
10. Assist patient as needed.
11. Provide physician with uncut tracing.
12. Clean and return equipment per OSHA guidelines.
13. Wash hands.
14. Document procedure.
15. Cut and mount the tracing, remembering to handle carefully. Label appropriately and place in patient's record.

Procedure

37-3 Perform Holter Monitor Application

STANDARD PRECAUTIONS:

PURPOSE:
To detect sporadic cardiac arrhythmias, to determine correlation of symptoms with activity, to evaluate chest pain and cardiac status following pacemaker implantation or after acute myocardial infarction.

EQUIPMENT/SUPPLIES:

Holter monitor	Alcohol swabs
Patient activity diary	Gauze
Blank magnetic tape	Tape
Disposable electrodes	Carrying case
Razor	Belt or shoulder strap

PROCEDURE STEPS:

1. Wash hands and assemble equipment.
2. Prepare the equipment by removing old (used) battery from the monitor and replacing it with a new battery. Insert a blank magnetic tape into the monitor. RATIONALE: Installing a new battery each 24-hour period will ensure the monitor will function because it will have sufficient power.
3. Wash hands.
4. Identify the patient and explain the procedure. RATIONALE: Adherence to patient guidelines helps ensure an accurate tracing.
5. Have patient remove clothing from the waist up.
6. Have patient sit on the examination table or chair. RATIONALE: This allows for patient comfort and relaxation and for the medical assistant to place the electrodes appropriately.
7. Locate the correct electrode placement on the chest wall. The skin must be prepared in the following way:
   a. Dry shave patient's chest at each electrode site if chest is hairy.
   b. Rub the shaved area with an alcohol swab. Let area dry (Figure 37-24).
   c. Abrade the skin slightly with a dry 4 × 4 gauze. Areas should be red. RATIONALE: Shaved site and abraded skin help the electrodes to adhere better to the skin and facilitate easier removal.

8. Take the electrodes from the package and peel away the backing from one of them (electrode should be moist). Continue to remove electrodes one by one and attach as in step 9.
9. Apply adhesive-backed electrode to the appropriate sites by applying firm pressure at the center of the electrode and moving outward toward the edges. Starting at the center of the electrode, apply pressure firmly and move outward on the electrode. Run your fingers along the outer rim to ensure firm attachment. Avoid moving from one side of electrode to the other. Gel could be forced out and could cause interference. RATIONALE: Firmly attached electrodes ensure a good quality tracing.
10. Attach the lead wires to the electrodes. Connect them to the patient cable.
11. Secure each electrode with adhesive tape. RATIONALE: The tape secures the electrodes by reducing the tugging and pulling on them.

(continues)

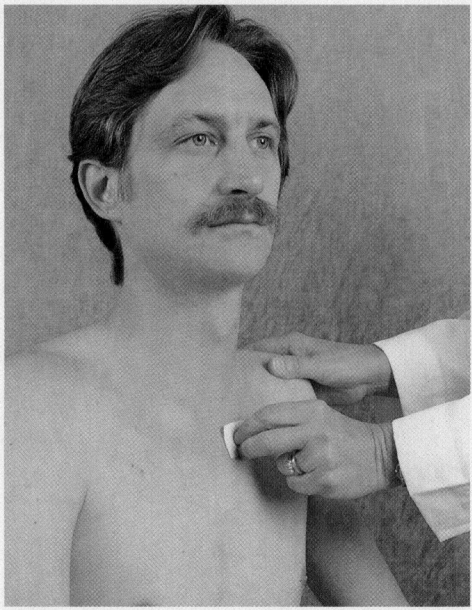

Figure 37-24 Preparation of patient skin with alcohol prior to placement of electrodes for Holter monitor.

Procedure
37-3 *(continued)*

12. Plug the monitor into an electrocardiograph with the test cable. Run a baseline tracing. RATIONALE: Running a baseline tracing will validate proper setup of electrodes and confirm there is no malfunction of the leads or cable.

13. Place the electrode cable so that it extends from between the buttons of the patient's shirt or from below the bottom of the shirt.

14. Place the recorder into its carrying case and either attach it to the patient's belt or over the patient's shoulder. Be certain there is no pulling on the lead wires (Figure 37-25). RATIONALE: Pulling on electrodes could cause them to become detached.

15. Plug the electrode cable into the monitor. Record the starting time in the patient activity log (diary). RATIONALE: The beginning time is noted in order to correlate cardiac activity with the patient activity log.

16. Give the activity log to the patient, being certain that the patient information is completed. RATIONALE: The activity log helps correlate cardiac activity with patient symptoms.

17. Inform patient what time the following day the monitor will be removed. Remind the patient to bring along the activity log.

18. Wash hands.

19. Document procedure in the patient's record.

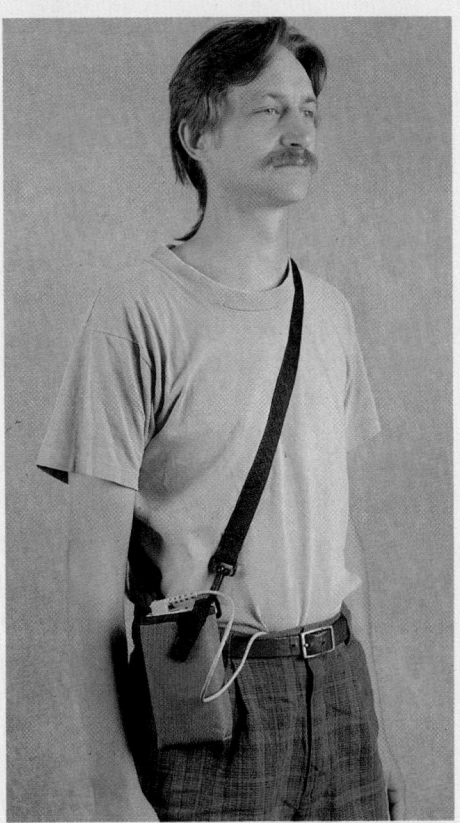

Figure 37-25 Holter monitor in its carrying case and secured by a shoulder strap. The monitor can also be applied on a belt and worn around the patient's waist.

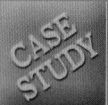

Abigail Johnson, in her mid-seventies, arrives at the urgent care center complaining of chest pains. She has been seen on two other occasions for similar pain and has a history of diabetes, hypertension, arteriosclerotic heart disease, and angina pectoris. Medical assistant Wanda Slawson immediately alerts Dr. Rice of Mrs. Johnson's chest pain and then takes her into the cardiac examination and treatment room. Dr. Rice tells Wanda to have Mrs. Johnson take one of her nitroglycerin tablets and to perform an ECG on her. Mrs. Johnson is restless and anxious as Wanda prepares for the ECG and while the tracing is in progress. There is significant somatic tremor. Wanda attempts to allay Mrs. Johnson's apprehension in order to obtain a good quality ECG. The patient's pain subsides within a few minutes and she begins to feel better.

CASE STUDY REVIEW

1. What immediate action could Wanda have taken if Mrs. Johnson's pain had not subsided?

2. Mrs. Johnson tells Wanda that Dr. Rice explained arteriosclerotic heart disease and angina pectoris to her, but that she was nervous and understood little and that she is embarrassed to admit that to Dr. Rice. How can Wanda explain, in language that the patient can comprehend, what causes arteriosclerotic heart disease and angina, and what Mrs. Johnson experiences during an attack of angina? What strategies can Wanda teach Mrs. Johnson to promote healthier habits and prevent more serious heart problems?

3. Research community resources that are available for persons with Mrs. Johnson's heart condition. Explain how Mrs. Johnson could benefit from them.

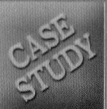

George Matthews, 79-year-old patient of Dr. Abbott, has a history of cardiovascular heart disease. He tells Dr. Abbott that today he has been experiencing "palpitations and slow and fast heartbeats and sometimes dizziness." Dr. Abbott orders a resting ECG that shows no evidence of arrhythmia and decides that a Holter monitor electrocardiograph for Mr. Matthews might be helpful in diagnosing a cardiac arrhythmia.

CASE STUDY REVIEW

1. Describe why Dr. Abbott ordered a Holter monitor electrocardiography for Mr. Matthews.

2. What instructions will you give to Mr. Matthews about wearing the monitor?

3. Mr. Matthews says he isn't certain what activities should be recorded in the patient activity diary. Explain what they are and the reason for their importance.

SUMMARY

Electrocardiography is a noninvasive painless procedure that is helpful in diagnosing heart disease. Cables with sensors are attached to the patient's arms, legs, and chest. The electrocardiograph amplifies the electrical currents generated when the myocardium contracts and relaxes with each heartbeat. A series of deflections (waves) is recorded on special ECG paper when a heated stylus on the electrocardiograph moves across the paper. The cardiac cycles that appear are then interpreted by the physician. The recording or tracing, known as an electrocardiogram, represents the heart's rate, rhythm, and other myocardial actions. Each of the twelve leads of the recording becomes part of the patient's permanent record.

In addition to a resting ECG, other types of electrocardiography can be done. Cardiac stress testing is done while the patient is physically challenged to perform increasingly strenuous exercises. The heart's tolerance to the increased demands placed on it during exercise can be observed and recorded while the patient is being closely monitored. This type of electrocardiography helps diagnose heart disease that would not be evident if a resting ECG were done.

Holter electrocardiography or ambulatory cardiac monitoring is an ECG test done as the patient goes about normal daily activities. The patient wears chest leads and carries a small recording device on a belt or on a strap over the shoulder for a period of 24 hours and documents activities in the patient activity diary. This type of electrocardiography helps diagnose cardiac arrhythmias that occur sporadically and may be difficult to capture on a resting ECG because of their unpredictability. Echocardiography is a diagnostic test that uses ultrasound to image the internal structures of the heart. Myocardial function, valvular function or defects, and chamber size can be determined.

In most instances, the medical assistant is responsible for patient preparation, patient education, operation of the electrocardiograph, elimination of artifacts, mounting, labeling, and placing ECG readings into the patient's file, and maintenance and care of the equipment. The diagnostic value of the test depends on the medical assistant's accuracy and skill.

REVIEW QUESTIONS

Multiple Choice

1. Which of the following is the most common type of artifact?
   a. somatic tremor
   b. AC interference
   c. wandering baseline
   d. interrupted baseline
2. Which of the following causes somatic tremor?
   a. too much electrolyte
   b. cable across patient's lap
   c. corroded sensors
   d. Parkinson's disease
3. One cardiac cycle (heartbeat) takes approximately how long?
   a. 0.2 second
   b. 0.4 second
   c. 0.6 second
   d. 0.8 second
4. Which of the following indicates ventricular depolarization?
   a. QRS complex
   b. P wave
   c. T wave
   d. S-T segment
5. Another name for V leads is:
   a. precordial
   b. augmented
   c. standard
   d. limb

Critical Thinking

1. The physician wants you to explain to Mrs. Johnson what behaviors she can adopt to have a healthy heart. With a partner, role-play medical assistant and patient and explain to the patient what she can do to improve her heart's health.
2. Mr. Williams has a diagnosis of Parkinson's disease. The physician requests an ECG. What strategies can you use to ensure an adequate tracing?
3. During the electrocardiogram, the equipment malfunctions. What options are available to the medical assistant?
4. Name four cardiac abnormalities that can be detected on an ECG.
5. Explain the significance of the small and large boxes on ECG paper. There are 2½ large boxes between each cardiac cycle. What is the heartbeat per minute?
6. Identify the placement of the twelve leads of the ECG.
7. The patient coughs and moves during the ECG. How can this affect the ECG tracing?
8. Explain standardization and why it is important.
9. What causes AC interference, wandering baseline, and interrupted baseline and how can they be eliminated?
10. State three purposes for a Holter monitor to be used and give the instructions that the patient will need to know while wearing the monitor.

WEB ACTIVITY

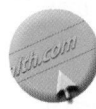

Search on the web for a national organization that focuses on heart and blood vessel disorders.

1. Print information about risk factors for cardiovascular heart disease.
2. What is the mortality rate for first-time myocardial infarctions for men versus women? Is there any difference in the mortality rate?
3. Are the symptoms identical in males and females when they are experiencing a myocardial infarction? Explain the similarities/differences between them.

REFERENCES/BIBLIOGRAPHY

Bonewit-West, K. (2000). *Clinical procedures for medical assistants* (5th ed.). Philadelphia: W. B. Saunders Company.

Keir, L., Wise, B., & Krebs, C. (1998). *Medical assisting. Administrative and clinical competencies* (8th ed.). Albany, NY: Delmar.

Krebs, C., & Heller, M. (1997). *Delmar's clinical handbook for healthcare professionals*. Albany, NY: Delmar.

Krebs, C., & Wise, B. (1998). *Medical assisting: Clinical competencies* (4th ed.). Albany, NY: Delmar.

Shea, D., & Carter-Ward, A. (1996). *Medical assisting: Clinical skills manual*. Albany, NY: Delmar.

Taber's cyclopedic medical dictionary. (18th ed.). (1999). Philadelphia: F. A. Davis Company.

Zakus, S. (1995). *Clinical procedures for medical assistants* (3rd ed.). St. Louis: Mosby-Year Book, Inc.

Unit

9

LABORATORY PROCEDURES

SAFETY AND REGULATORY GUIDELINES IN THE MEDICAL LABORATORY

KEY TERMS

Acetone
Aegis
Body Fluid
Calibration
Chemotherapeutic Agents
Communicable
Ethyl Alcohol
Excretion
Federal Register
Forensic
Formaldehyde
Fume Hood
Kit
Mandate
Medical Asepsis
Microscopy
Proficiency Testing
Pulmonary Edema
Quality Assurance
Quality Control
Reimbursement
Requisition
Secretion
Standard
Suppressed Immune System
Waived

OUTLINE

Clinical Laboratory Improvement Amendments of 1988 (CLIA '88)
  The Intention of CLIA '88
  General Program Description
  Categories of Testing
  Contents of the Law
  CLIA '88 Regulation for Quality Control in Automated Hematology
  Aftermath of CLIA '88
  Impact of CLIA on Medical Assistants

  Where to Find More Information Regarding CLIA '88
Occupational Safety and Health Administration (OSHA) Regulations
  The Standard for Occupational Exposure to Hazardous Chemicals in the Laboratory
  Chemical Hygiene Plan
OSHA Regulations and Students
  Avoiding Exposure to Chemicals
Cumulative Trauma Disorders

OBJECTIVES

The student should strive to meet the following performance objectives and demonstrate an understanding of the facts and principles presented in this chapter through written and oral communication.

1. Define the key terms as presented in the glossary.
2. Identify the governmental agency that regulates procedures performed on patients and describe the agency's main concerns.
3. List the types of human specimens that CLIA regulates.
4. Name two performance requirements CLIA imposes on all laboratories.
5. Describe how CLIA '88 regulates the use of quality control in automated hematology instruments.
6. Recall the three categories of testing and list several from the waived category.
7. Discuss the importance of CLIA to the medical assistant.
8. Identify and discuss the contents of the law of CLIA '88.
9. Describe HCFA form 116 and explain its purpose.
10. Identify two OSHA standards that seek to safeguard employees.
11. Describe MSDS manuals and their purpose. Differentiate among the four colors and five numbers of the National Fire Protection Association.

ROLE DELINEATION COMPONENTS

CLINICAL
Fundamental Principles
- Apply principles of aseptic technique and infection control
- Comply with quality assurance practices

GENERAL (TRANSDISCIPLINARY)
Legal Concepts
- Follow federal, state, and local legal guidelines
- Maintain awareness of federal and state health care legislation and regulations
- Comply with established risk management and safety procedures

INTRODUCTION

Laboratory safety is a concern for all: management, staff, and patients. An unsafe work environment and/or work practices can threaten the emotional and physical health of the health care worker as well as the patient. Injuries are costly on many levels: personally to the injured individual, lost work days, workers' compensation, medical treatment, potential legal action, and potential fines from regulatory agencies. These situations have a direct effect on the individuals involved, but also have an indirect effect by lowering staff morale, ultimately resulting in less productivity. Management's response to safety is the key. Appropriate orientation, annual reviews, periodic drills, and consistent enforcement of staff adherence to policy are all part of a successful laboratory safety program.

All health care providers continually come into contact with patients who are ill. Some patients have **communicable** or contagious diseases; others may have a **suppressed immune system** that does not protect them from infection. In the course of performing your duties as a medical assistant, you will be in contact with blood and **body fluids** that may be highly infectious. It is of extreme importance that your health and safety as well as the health and safety of your patients be protected.

There are a number of infection control measures that can be used to reduce the transmission of bloodborne and other pathogens. **Medical asepsis**, also known as infection control, consists of procedures and practices that health care professionals use to prevent the spread of infection (see Chapter 22: Medical Asepsis, Disease, and Infection Control). State and federal agencies also have established policies, procedures, and guidelines for health care providers and employers to follow in order to reduce the risk of transmission of infectious diseases. This chapter as well as Chapter 22 will examine the major guidelines.

The Centers for Disease Control and Prevention (CDC) in Atlanta, Georgia, a division of the United States Public Health Department, is an agency that investigates various diseases in an attempt to control them and makes recommendations on how to prevent the spread of disease. The CDC issued the system of seven isolation categories for patients with infectious diseases; it recommended the guidelines known as universal precautions; and, in 1996, it released standard precautions, which represent the most current and comprehensive approach to infection control.

The Clinical Laboratory Improvement Amendments of 1988 (CLIA '88) and the Occupational Safety and Health Administration (OSHA) also regulate the safety of patients and health care workers. CLIA '88 comes under the **aegis**, or protection, of the Health Care Financing Administration (HCFA) of the United States Department of Health and Human Services (HHS) of the federal government. OSHA comes under the United States Department of Labor. Both agencies require that health care settings, including clinical laboratories, adhere to the strict regulations that they set forth.

The purpose of CLIA '88 is to safeguard the public by regulating all testing of specimens taken from the human body. The purpose of OSHA is to require employers to ensure employee safety in regard to occupational exposure to potentially harmful substances.

CLIA '88 and OSHA guidelines will be examined independently. Table 38-1 summarizes both guidelines.

CLINICAL LABORATORY IMPROVEMENT AMENDMENTS OF 1988 (CLIA '88)

The Clinical Laboratory Improvement Amendments of 1988 (CLIA '88) were designed to set safety policies and procedures that protect patients.

In 1988 there was a public outcry as a result of articles published in the *Washington Post* and the *Wall Street Journal* and televised reports of deaths that were attributed to misread Pap smears. The public wanted action taken to ensure its safety, particularly in regard to laboratory testing. The outcry prompted the federal government to become more involved in regulating laboratories.

Although CLIA had been enacted into law in 1967, the issue of the misread Pap smears caused Congress to

TABLE 38-1 FEDERAL HEALTH AND SAFETY GUIDELINES

Guidelines	Issuing Agency	Purpose
Standard Precautions	Centers for Disease Control and Prevention (CDC), United States Public Health Department, Atlanta, Georgia	Issued in 1996 to augment and synthesize universal precautions and techniques known as body substance isolation (BSI). Standard precautions contain measures intended to protect all health care providers, patients, and visitors from infectious diseases.
Transmission-based Precautions	CDC	Designed to reduce the risk of airborne, droplet, and contact transmission of pathogens. These are used in addition to standard precautions and are intended for specific categories of patients.
Universal Blood and Body Fluid Precautions (Universal Precautions)	CDC	Released in 1985 to assist health care providers to greatly reduce the risk of contracting or transmitting infectious diseases, particularly AIDS and hepatitis B.
Clinical Laboratory Improvement Amendments of 1988 (CLIA '88)	Health Care Financing Administration (HCFA), United States Department of Health and Human Services (HHS)	Safeguards the public by regulating all testing of specimens taken from the body
Occupational Safety and Health Administration (OSHA) Guidelines	OSHA, United States Department of Labor	Requires employers to ensure employee safety in regard to occupational exposure to potentially harmful substances

reexamine the regulations it had set forth in 1967. Thus, CLIA '88 was passed and included amendments to the original law. The amended regulations took effect on September 1, 1992.

States can seek exemptions from the CLIA standards if they have regulations that are comparable to those imposed by CLIA. If the federal government grants the state an exemption, laboratories in these states are under the control of state standards and applicable fees, not federal standards and fees. As of October, 1999, the states of California, New York, Oregon, and Washington have achieved state-exempt status.

Some accrediting bodies have revised their rules in an effort to meet HCFA's CLIA '88 requirements. HCFA can then give deemed status (equivalency) to these accrediting bodies. Laboratories accredited by these "deemed status" bodies are considered to meet HCFA's requirements. To date, HCFA has granted deemed status to the organizations listed in Table 38-2.

The Intention of CLIA '88

The intent of CLIA '88 is to protect the public by regulating all laboratory tests performed on specimens taken from the human body; i.e., blood and body secretions and excretions. The specimens are those used in the diagnosis, treatment, and prevention of disease. Previous regulations (Medicare, Medicaid, and CLIA '67) were based on the site and scope of the laboratory testing. CLIA '88 regulates laboratory testing irrespective of site, scope, volume, or frequency. As of July, 2000, registered CLIA laboratories total over 145,000 with physicians' office laboratories making up over 65 percent of the total. The regulations require that all laboratories in the United States and its territories meet performance requirements that are based on how complex a test is and the risk factors that are associated with incorrect test results. Laboratories must comply with the requirements in order to be certified by the United States Department

TABLE 38-2 APPROVED ACCREDITING ORGANIZATIONS UNDER CLIA '88

American Association of Blood Banks
8101 Glenbrook Road
Bethesda, MD 20814-2749
Government Relations
(301) 907-6977

American Osteopathic Association
142 East Ontario Street
Chicago, IL 60611
(312) 202-8070

American Society of Histocompatibility and Immunogenetics
P.O. Box 15804
Lenexa, KS 66285-5804
(913) 541-0009

College of American Pathologists
325 Waukegan Road
Northfield, IL 60093-2750
Laboratory Accreditation Program
(800) 323-4040

Commission on Office Laboratory Accreditation
9881 Broken Land Parkway, Suite 200
Columbia, MD 21046-1158
(410) 381-6581

Joint Commission on Accreditation of Healthcare Organizations
One Renaissance Boulevard
Oakbrook Terrace, IL 60181
(630) 792-5783

of Health and Human Services (HHS). The following laboratories are exempt from the regulations: labs that perform only tests for **forensic**, or legal, purposes; research laboratories that do not produce results used in patient treatment; facilities certified by the National Institute on Drug Abuse to perform only urine drug testing; and states, territories, and municipalities with licensure. (Currently, California, Florida, Georgia, Hawaii, Nevada, North Dakota, Rhode Island, Tennessee, Virginia, the Commonwealth of Puerto Rico, and the municipality of New York City are licensed.)

It is necessary to understand what the CLIA '88 regulations encompass and how they impact medical assistants and other health care workers who participate in testing human specimens. It is important because all laboratories, including laboratories in ambulatory care physicians' office laboratories (POL), must abide by the CLIA law.

CLIA '88 regulations are based on the complexity of tests performed and they affect all aspects of the laboratory. They specify the type of test performed, personnel involved in testing, and **quality control.**

General Program Description

Congress passed CLIA in 1988, establishing quality standards for all laboratory testing to ensure the accuracy, reliability, and timeliness of patient test results regardless of where the test was performed. A laboratory is defined as any facility that performs laboratory testing on specimens derived from humans for the purpose of providing information for the diagnosis, prevention, or treatment of disease, or impairment or assessment of health. CLIA is user-fee funded; therefore, all costs of administering the program must be covered by the regulated facilities.

The final CLIA regulations were published on February 28, 1992 and are based on the complexity of the test method; thus, the more complicated the test, the more stringent the requirements. Three categories of tests have been established: waived complexity; moderate complexity, including the subcategory of provider-performed **microscopy** (PPM); and high complexity. CLIA specifies quality standards for proficiency testing (PT), patient test management, quality control, personnel qualifications, and quality assurance as applicable. Because problems in cytology laboratories were the impetus for CLIA, there are also specific cytology requirements.

The Health Care Financing Administration (HCFA) is charged with the implementation of CLIA, including laboratory registration, fee collection, surveys, surveyor guidelines and training, enforcement, approvals of PT providers, accrediting organizations, and exempt states. The Centers for Disease Control and Prevention (CDC) is responsible for test categorization and CLIA studies.

To enroll in the CLIA program, laboratories must first register by completing an application, pay fees, be surveyed if applicable, and become certified. CLIA fees are based on the certificate requested by the laboratory (i.e., waived, PPM, accreditation, or compliance) and the annual volume and types of testing performed. Waived and PPM laboratories may apply directly for their certificate because they are not subject to routine inspections. Those laboratories that must be surveyed routinely, i.e., those performing moderate and/or high complexity testing, can choose whether they wish to be surveyed by HCFA or by a private accrediting organization. The HCFA survey process is outcome-oriented and utilizes a quality assurance focus and an educational approach to assess compliance.

Data indicates that CLIA has helped to improve the quality of testing in the United States. The total number of quality deficiencies has decreased approximately 40 percent from the first laboratory survey to the second. Similar findings were demonstrated in the review of PT data. The educational value of PT in laboratories was known before CLIA existed. Initial PT failures are also addressed with an educational, rather than punitive, approach by CLIA.

Work is currently in progress with the CDC and HCFA to develop a final CLIA rule that will reflect all comments received and new technologies.

Categories of Testing

CLIA '88 is under the aegis of the Health Care Financing Administration (HCFA) of the HHS. HCFA has designated three categories of testing:

1. Waived tests
2. Moderate-complexity tests, including PPM
3. High-complexity tests

Each of these categories has different requirements for personnel and quality control.

Waived tests are simple, unvarying, and require a minimum of judgment and interpretation. Test error carries minimal hazard to the patient. Waived tests represent the lowest percentage of the total number of tests performed (Table 38-3).

Provider-performed microscopy tests are moderate-complexity tests but represent a subcategory which was added at the request of physicians.

To categorize moderate- and high-complexity tests, the following criteria are used:

- The degree of operator intervention needed

- The necessary knowledge and experience the operator possesses

- The degree of maintenance and troubleshooting needed to perform the tests

TABLE 38-3 LIST OF ANALYTES CURRENTLY ON THE CLIA '88 WAIVED LIST			
Amines	Gastric occult blood	Nicotine and/or metabolites	Urine qualitative dipstick glucose
Amphetamines	Glucose or glucose monitoring device	Opiates	Urine qualitative dipstick ketone
Bladder tumor-associated antigen	Glycosylated hemoglobin (HbA1C)	Ovulation test by visual color comparison	Urine qualitative dipstick leukocytes
Cannabinoids (THC)	hCG, urine	Phencyclidine (PCP)	Urine qualitative dipstick nitrite
Catalase, urine	Helicobacter pylori antibodies	Prothrombin time	Urine qualitative dipstick pH
Cholesterol, HDL	Helicobacter pylori (bacteriology)	Spun microhematocrit	Urine qualitative dipstick protein
Cholesterol, total		Streptococcus group A	
Cocaine metabolites	Hematocrit	Triglyceride	Urine qualitative dipstick specific gravity
Creatinine	Hemoglobin	Urine dipstick or tablet analytes, nonautomated	Urine qualitative dipstick urobilinogen
Erythrocyte sedimentation rate	Infectious mononucleosis antibodies	Urine qualitative dipstick bilirubin	
Ethanol	Ketones, blood	Urine qualitative dipstick blood	Vaginal pH
Fecal occult blood	Methamphetamines		
Fructosamine	Microalbumin		

Source: Clara Sliva, Acting CLIA Coordinator

Note: Tests waived by FDA from January 31–July 26, 2000; CDC through March, 2000. There are over 500 Test Systems (products) approved for the analytes listed above. For an up-to-date list, visit the CDC website at www.phppo.cdc.gov.

Approximately 75 percent of all tests are of moderate complexity and 24 percent are of high complexity. Physicians' office laboratories are not restricted to tests in the waived category.

Thus far, over 5,000 tests have been categorized by CLIA '88 and, except those listed in Table 38-3, fall into either the moderate- or high-complexity category. It is important to realize that tests can be moved between or among categories and that revisions have been made since CLIA '88 went into effect in 1992. The best way to remain informed is by calling the manufacturer and asking whether your particular instrument or **kit** is in the moderate-complexity category. You can also obtain a list of categories as well as the complete CLIA '88 guidelines from the **Federal Register**. (Information on toll-free phone numbers, addresses, and order numbers are provided in the appendices.)

Contents of the Law

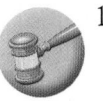

1. All laboratories are required to register with CLIA '88 even if just one test is performed and regardless of whether there is Medicare and Medicaid **reimbursement** and regardless in which of the categories the test is found.
2. The regulations apply to all laboratories. Previously unregulated laboratories could enroll until January 1, 1994.
3. The regulations are specific to the complexity of the test. Standards become more stringent as the complexity of the test increases.

4. A laboratory must obtain a certificate to perform tests. An initial filing for a certificate is made on form 116 with HCFA of the Department of Health and Human Services. One of five certificates can be obtained. (There can be a state exemption as previously mentioned.)
   a. *Certificate of Waiver.* This certificate is issued to a laboratory to perform only waived tests.
   b. *Certificate for Provider-Performed Microscopy (PPM) Procedures.* This certificate is issued to a laboratory in which a physician, midlevel practitioner, or dentist performs no tests other than the PPM procedures (Table 38-4). This certificate permits the laboratory to also perform waived tests.

TABLE 38-4   PROVIDER-PERFORMED MICROSCOPY (PPM) PROCEDURES
• All direct wet-mount preparations for the presence or absence of bacteria, fungi, parasites, and human cellular elements
• All potassium hydroxide (KOH) preparations
• Pinworm examinations
• Fern tests
• Postcoital direct, qualitative examinations of vaginal or cervical mucus
• Urine sediment examinations
• Nasal smears for granulocytes
• Fecal leukocyte examinations
• Qualitative semen analysis (limited to the presence or absence of sperm and detection of motility)

c. *Certificate of Registration*. This certificate enables the entity to conduct moderate and/or high complexity laboratory testing until the entity is determined by survey to be in compliance with the CLIA regulations.
d. *Certificate of Compliance*. This certificate is issued to a laboratory after an inspection finds the laboratory to be in compliance with all applicable CLIA requirements.
e. *Certificate of Accreditation*. This is a certificate that is issued to a laboratory on the basis of the laboratory's accreditation by an organization approved by HCFA.

As of July, 2000, over 145,000 CLIA certificates have been issued. Of certificates granted, 53 percent have been Certificates of Waiver, 22 percent have been Certificates for Provider-Performed Microscopy (PPM) Procedures, 15 percent have been Certificates of Registration or Compliance, and 10 percent have been Certificates of Accreditation.

All five certification categories must be renewed every two years and be accompanied by a fee ranging from $100 to $600.

HCFA Form 116

HCFA form 116 (Figures 38-1 and 38-2) for the clinical laboratory application for CLIA, HCFA-116 must be completed and returned to the Health Care Financing Administration of the United States Department of Health and Human Services within thirty days of receipt. The form collects information regarding a laboratory's operation and is needed to evaluate fees, to determine baseline data, to update existing data, and to fulfill legal requirements. The information obtained from the application will give the surveyor of the laboratory a perspective of the laboratory's operation and if it will be subject to an on-site inspection.

After a laboratory has been certified, it must notify HCFA within six months if it changes the types of tests it performs. This could alter the laboratory's classification.

5. Some examples of sanctions or penalties imposed by HCFA for noncompliance with the CLIA law follow:

DEPARTMENT OF HEALTH AND HUMAN SERVICES
HEALTH CARE FINANCING ADMINISTRATION

FORM APPROVED
OMB NO. 0938-0581

CLINICAL LABORATORY IMPROVEMENT AMENDMENTS OF 1988 (CLIA)
APPLICATION FOR CERTIFICATION

According to the Paperwork Reduction Act of 1995, no persons are required to respond to a collection of information unless it displays a valid OMB control number. The valid OMB control number for this information collection is 0938-0581. The time required to complete this information collection is estimated to average 30 minutes to 2 hours per response, including the time to review instructions, search existing data resources, gather the data needed, and complete and review the information collection. If you have any comments concerning the accuracy of the time estimate(s) or suggestions for improving this form, please write to: HCFA ,7500 Security Boulevard, N2-14-26, Baltimore, Maryland 21244-1850 and to the Office of the Information and Regulatory Affairs, Office of Management and Budget, Washington, D.C. 20503.

I. GENERAL INFORMATION

☐ Initial Application ☐ Change in Certification Type	CLIA IDENTIFICATION NUMBER ____D________ *(If an initial application leave blank, a number will be assigned)*
Facility Name	Federal Tax Identification Number Telephone No. *(include area code)* Fax No. *(include area code)* ( ) ( )
Facility Address-*Physical Location of Laboratory (Building, Floor, Suite if applicable.)*	Mailing/Billing address *(If different from street address, include attention line and/or Building, Floor, Suite)*
Number, Street *(No. P.O. Boxes)*	Number, Street
City State Zip Code	City State Zip Code
Name of Director *last first middle initial*	

II. TYPE OF CERTIFICATE REQUESTED (Check One)

☐ Certificate of Waiver (*Complete Sections I - VI and VIII - X*)

☐ Certificate for Provider Performed Microscopy Procedures (PPMP) (*Complete Sections I - X*)

☐ Certificate of Compliance (*Complete Sections I- X*)

☐ Certificate of Accreditation (*Complete Sections I through X*) **and** indicate which of the following organization(s) your laboratory is accredited by for CLIA purposes, or for which you have applied for accreditation for CLIA purposes

☐ JCAHO ☐ AOA ☐ AABB
☐ CAP ☐ COLA ☐ ASHI

FORM HCFA-116 (11/98) Page 1 of 4

III. TYPE OF LABORATORY ***(check the one most descriptive of facility type)***

__ 01 Ambulatory Surgery Center	__ 09 Hospice	__ 17 School/Student Health Service
__ 02 Community Clinic	__ 10 Hospital	__ 18 Skilled Nursing Facility/Nursing Facility
__ 03 Comp. Outpatient Rehab. Facility	__ 11 Independent	__ 19 Physician Office
__ 04 Ancillary Testing Site in Health Care Facility	__ 12 Industrial	__ 20 Other Practitioner *(specify)* ____
	__ 13 Insurance	__ 21 Tissue Bank/Repositories
__ 05 End Stage Renal Disease Dialysis Facility	__ 14 Intermediate Care Fac. for Mentally Retarded	__ 22 Blood Banks
__ 06 Health Fair		__ 23 Rural Health Clinic/Federally Qualified Health Center
__ 07 Health Main. Organization	__ 15 Mobile Laboratory	
__ 08 Home Health Agency	__ 16 Pharmacy	__ 24 Ambulance
		__ 25 Other *(specify)* ____

Is this a Medicare/Medicaid certified facility? ☐ Yes ☐ No
If yes, indicate Medicare provider number____ Medicaid number____

IV. HOURS OF LABORATORY TESTING (list times during which **laboratory testing** is performed)

	SUNDAY	MONDAY	TUESDAY	WEDNESDAY	THURSDAY	FRIDAY	SATURDAY
FROM: AM							
PM							
TO: AM							
PM							

(For multiple sites attach the additional information using the same format)

V. MULTIPLE SITES (Must meet one of the regulatory exceptions to apply for this provision)

Are you applying for the multiple site exception?

☐ No **If no,** go to section VI. ☐ Yes **If yes,** provide total number of sites under this certificate____ and complete remainder of this section .

Indicate which of the following regulatory exceptions applies to your facility's operation.

Is this a not-for-profit or Federal, State or local government laboratory engaged in limited (not more than a combination of 15 moderate complexity or waived tests per certificate) public health testing and filing for a single certificate for multiple sites? ☐ Yes ☐ No
If yes, list name, address and tests performed for each site below.

Is this a hospital with several laboratories located at contiguous buildings on the same campus within the same physical location or street address and under common direction that is filing for a single certificate for these locations? ☐ Yes ☐ No
If yes, list name or department, location within hospital and specialty/subspecialty areas performed at each site below.

If additional space is needed, check here ____ and attach the additional information using the same format.

NAME AND ADDRESS / LOCATION		TESTS PERFORMED / SPECIALTY / SUBSPECIALTY
Name of laboratory or hospital department		
Address/location (number, street, location if applicable)		
City, State, ZIP	Telephone No. ( )	
Name of laboratory or hospital department		
Address/location (number, street, location if applicable)		
City, State, ZIP	Telephone No. ( )	
Name of laboratory or hospital department		
Address/location (number, street, location if applicable)		
City, State, ZIP	Telephone No. ( )	

FORM HCFA-116 (11/98) Page 2 of 4

Figure 38-1 Form HCFA-116.

Infraction	*Penalty*
Failure to enroll with HCFA	Denial or revocation of certificate
Nonparticipation in proficiency testing	A score of zero (a score of 80 percent is required)
Failure to return the proficiency testing result	A score of zero

In addition, Medicare and Medicaid payments may be suspended or terminated and civil penalties of up to a $10,000 fine per violation or per day of noncompliance may be imposed.

For CLIA '88 conditions other than proficiency testing, newly regulated laboratories will not be subjected to penalties during the first inspection cycle unless it is determined that the laboratories' inadequacies pose immediate patient danger.

6. The law **mandates quality assurance** for nonwaived tests. Laboratories are required to establish policies and procedures through programs that assess test quality; identify problems and correct them; assure precise, dependable, and punctual reporting of test results; and guarantee sufficient competent staff. In addition, laboratories must assure that all quality control data are studied, and if there is a complaint, an investigation must be undertaken and appropriate action taken and recorded. It is a requirement that quality assurance records be maintained.
7. The law mandates quality control for nonwaived tests. Laboratories are required to have an adequate supply of equipment to perform the number and types of tests that they offer. A procedures manual must be available in the testing area and must include complete testing instructions. Documentation of maintenance programs for instruments, equipment, and test systems must be evident.
8. The law establishes requirements for the correct collection, transportation, and storage of specimens and the reporting of results. (See No. 14, Patient Test Management.)
9. The law mandates maintenance of records, equipment, and facilities of labs performing nonwaived tests. (See No. 15, Documentation.)
10. The law mandates personnel standards. There are requirements for personnel who perform nonwaived tests and they spell out the necessary qualifications and responsibilities required of them. Each person

VI. WAIVED TESTING

Indicate the **estimated TOTAL ANNUAL TEST** volume for **all waived tests** performed. ________

VII. NONWAIVED TESTING (Including PPMP testing)

If you perform testing other than or in addition to waived tests, complete the information below. If applying for one certificate for multiple sites, the total volume should include testing for ALL sites.

Place a check (√) in the box preceding each specialty/subspecialty in which the laboratory performs testing. Enter the estimated annual test volume for each specialty. **Do not include testing not subject to CLIA, waived tests, or tests run for quality control, calculations, quality assurance or proficiency testing when calculating test volume.** (For additional guidance on counting test volume, see the information included with the application package.)

If applying for certificate of accreditation, indicate the name of the accreditation organization beside the applicable specialty/subspecialty for which you are accredited for CLIA compliance. (JCAHO, AOA, AABB, CAP, COLA or ASHI)

SPECIALTY / SUBSPECIALTY	ACCREDITING ORGANIZATION	ANNUAL TEST VOLUME	SPECIALTY / SUBSPECIALTY	ACCREDITING ORGANIZATION	ANNUAL TEST VOLUME
Histocompatibility		____	☐ **Hematology**	____	____
☐ Transplant	____		**Immunohematology**		____
☐ Nontransplant	____		☐ ABO Group & Rh Group	____	
Microbiology		____	☐ Antibody Detection (transfusion)	____	
☐ Bacteriology	____		☐ Antibody Detection (nontransfusion)	____	
☐ Mycobacteriology	____		☐ Antibody Identification	____	
☐ Mycology	____		☐ Compatibility Testing	____	
☐ Parasitology	____		**Pathology**		____
☐ Virology	____		☐ Histopathology	____	
Diagnostic Immunology		____	☐ Oral Pathology	____	
☐ Syphilis Serology	____		☐ Cytology	____	
☐ General Immunology	____		☐ **Radiobioassay**	____	____
Chemistry		____	☐ **Clinical Cytogenetics**	____	____
☐ Routine	____				
☐ Urinalysis	____				
☐ Endocrinology	____				
☐ Toxicology	____				

TOTAL ESTIMATED ANNUAL TEST VOLUME ________

FORM HCFA-116 (11/98) Page 3 of 4

VIII. TYPE OF CONTROL

Enter the appropriate two digit code from the list below ____ ____ (enter only one code)

Voluntary Nonprofit	**For Profit**	**Government**	
01 Religious Affiliation	04 Proprietary	05 City	08 Federal
02 Private		06 County	09 Other Government ________ (Specify)
03 Other ________ (Specify)		07 State	

IX. DIRECTOR AFFILIATION WITH OTHER LABORATORIES

If the director of this laboratory serves as director for additional laboratories that are separately certified, please complete the following:

NAME OF LABORATORY	ADDRESS	CLIA IDENTIFICATION NUMBER

X. INDIVIDUALS INVOLVED IN LABORATORY TESTING

Indicate the total number of individuals involved in laboratory testing (directing, supervising, consulting or testing). Do not include individuals who only collect specimens or perform clerical duties. For nonwaived testing, only count an individual one time, at the **highest** laboratory position in which they function. (Example Pathologist serves as director, technical supervisor and general supervisor. This individual would only be counted once (under director)).

A. WAIVED TESTING
Total No. of Individuals ____

B. NONWAIVED TESTING(INCLUDING PPMP)
Total No. of Individuals ____
Director ______ **Technical supervisor** ______
Clinical consultant ______ **General supervisor** ______
Technical consultant ______ **Testing personnel** ______
Cytotechnologist ______

ANY PERSON WHO INTENTIONALLY VIOLATES ANY REQUIREMENT OF SECTION 353 OF THE PUBLIC HEALTH SERVICE ACT AS AMENDED OR ANY REGULATION PROMULGATED THEREUNDER SHALL BE IMPRISONED FOR NOT MORE THAN ONE YEAR OR FINED UNDER TITLE 18, UNITED STATES CODE OR BOTH, EXCEPT THAT IF THE CONVICTION IS FOR A SECOND OR SUBSEQUENT VIOLATION OF SUCH A REQUIREMENT SUCH PERSON SHALL BE IMPRISONED FOR NOT MORE THAN 3 YEARS OR FINED IN ACCORDANCE WITH TITLE 18, UNITED STATES CODE OR BOTH.

CONSENT: THE APPLICANT HEREBY AGREES THAT SUCH LABORATORY IDENTIFIED HEREIN WILL BE OPERATED IN ACCORDANCE WITH APPLICABLE STANDARDS FOUND NECESSARY BY THE SECRETARY OF HEALTH AND HUMAN SERVICES TO CARRY OUT THE PURPOSES OF SECTION 353 OF THE PUBLIC HEALTH SERVICE ACT AS AMENDED. THE APPLICANT FURTHER AGREES TO PERMIT THE SECRETARY, OR ANY FEDERAL OFFICER OR EMPLOYEE DULY DESIGNATED BY THE SECRETARY, TO INSPECT THE LABORATORY AND ITS OPERATIONS AND ITS PERTINENT RECORDS AT ANY REASONABLE TIME AND TO FURNISH ANY REQUESTED INFORMATION OR MATERIALS NECESSARY TO DETERMINE THE LABORATORY'S ELIGIBILITY OR CONTINUED ELIGIBILITY FOR ITS CERTIFICATE OR CONTINUED COMPLIANCE WITH CLIA REQUIRMENTS.

SIGNATURE OF OWNER/DIRECTOR OF LABORATORY *(sign in ink)*	DATE

FORM HCFA-116 (11/98) Page 4 of 4

Figure 38-2 Form HCFA-116.

who does the tests must be licensed by the state if required, have a high school diploma or equivalent, have adequate training, and be able to demonstrate an understanding of laboratory procedures, **calibration**, or standardization of instruments, specimen collection, and quality control. Personnel must report test results accurately and with dependability. All high-complexity tests must be done by technologists and technicians except for cytology, which requires more stringent qualifications.

11. The law mandates **proficiency testing** for non-waived tests. The procedures and tests found in the waived category are exempt from proficiency testing, regardless of the type of laboratory in which the tests are performed. Moderate- and high-complexity test laboratories must enroll in proficiency testing programs that are approved by the United States Department of Health and Human Services. The proficiency testing samples are checked in the same manner as patient specimens. Unsatisfactory performance on a proficiency testing check can result in various penalties ranging from termination of the laboratory's license to operate to the termination of reimbursement from Medicare and Medicaid. January, 1994 was the phase-in date for previously unregulated laboratories to enroll in proficiency testing, but proficiency testing will continue to be required for laboratories that were regulated by March 4, 1990.

12. The law mandates unannounced on-site inspection. All laboratories in the moderate- and high-complexity category are subject to unannounced inspections by HHS or an agency assigned to the task by HHS. Laboratories that perform only waived tests must prove that tests are being done according to the manufacturer's directions. Inspections can involve interviewing employees, observation of employees performing tests, analysis of data, and documentation of results. Violations of requirements by any laboratory can result in penalties. The cost of inspection will be billed to the laboratory.

13. The law mandates an annual listing of laboratories that have had action taken against them.

14. The law mandates patient test management. All laboratories must have a strategy for properly receiving and processing specimens and for the precise reporting of the results. Written instructions regarding collection, safeguarding of specimens, and labeling of specimens must be available for patients. There must be a specific procedure for the reporting of life-threatening results and a follow-through to the person requesting the test. Test records must be kept for two years following the reporting of results.

15. The law mandates documentation. The following documentation must be done and be available:
    - Specimen
      Patient preparation
      Specimen collection procedure
      Proper labeling technique
      Preservation of specimen if applicable
    - Proficiency testing
      Corrective action taken
    - Quality control and quality assurance
      Any corrective action taken
    - Problem and complaint log
    - **Requisitions** or written requests
      Patient name
      Name and address of laboratory
      Date and time of collection
      Name of test requested
      Diagnosis
    - Results
      Name and address of laboratory where test is done
      Test name
      Test results, including normal ranges listed on test results
      Disposition of unacceptable specimens must be released to authorized person
    - Log of Results
      Printouts from instruments report must be kept
      Identification of person performing test
      Patient identification number
      Specimen identification
      Date
      Time specimen is received in laboratory
      Specimen rejection log maintained
      Records and dates of all tests done

Criteria. To be categorized as a PPM procedure, the procedure must meet the following criteria:

1. The examination must be personally performed by one of the following practitioners:
   a. A physician during the patient's visit on a specimen obtained from his or her own patient or from a patient of a group medical practice of which the physician is a member or an employee
   b. A midlevel practitioner, under the supervision of a physician or in independent practice only if authorized by the state, during the patient's visit on a specimen obtained from his or her own patient or from a patient of a clinic, group medical practice, or other health care provider of which the midlevel practitioner is a member or an employee
   c. A dentist during the patient's visit on a specimen obtained from his or her own patient or from a

patient of a group dental practice of which the dentist is a member or an employee

2. The procedure must be categorized as moderately complex.
3. The primary instrument for performing the test is the microscope, limited to bright-field or phase-contrast microscopy.
4. The specimen is labile, or a delay in performing the test could compromise the accuracy of the test result.
5. Control materials are not available to monitor the entire testing process.
6. Limited specimen handling or processing is required.

CLIA '88 Regulation for Quality Control in Automated Hematology

CLIA '88 regulations require that three different procedures be performed in the quality control protocol for automated hematology instruments. The procedures include calibration, control samples, and proficiency testing. CLIA's regulations require that the automated hematology instrument be calibrated at regularly scheduled intervals with either a calibrator sample or a normal control sample. Many manufacturers of automated hematology instruments recommend or may require that the instrument be recalibrated at shorter intervals than are required by CLIA '88. CLIA '88 mandates that two levels of control samples be tested first each day on any parameter that will be performed on a patient's sample. These quality control checks must be performed before the patient's sample is tested. The results for quality control samples must fall within two standard deviations of the expected mean value for that sample. Standard deviations and Levy-Jennings charts were discussed in the quality control chapter. One of the two levels of control samples must be in the normal range; the other may be either an abnormal high or low sample.

In addition to calibrations and control sample testing, an ambulatory care setting that utilizes automated hematology instruments must enroll in a proficiency testing program with a reference laboratory that is CLIA '88 approved.

Aftermath of CLIA '88

There are many individuals who have serious concerns about whether CLIA has led to improved testing as was intended, or if the law has just produced an overload of paperwork and problems. Some question if the law will be fully implemented or even eliminated altogether.

 Important developments help to put the law into perspective. HCFA has postponed the date that Medicare payments would be cut off for failure to register. The deadline has been postponed at least three times. The American Medical Association (AMA) complained that unannounced inspections of physicians' office laboratories (POL) would disrupt patient office visits. As a result, the Secretary of Health and Human Services declared that POL inspections would be announced.

The category of Provider-Performed Microscopy (PPM) was added as another certificate and testing category because physicians argued that the microscopic tests were essential to their practice. Already the PPM has expanded to include midlevel practitioners such as nurse practitioners, nurse midwives, and physician assistants.

The law states that CLIA must be self-supporting. There are far fewer laboratories registered than was originally anticipated, and the result is a significantly lower amount of revenue than had been expected.

It is interesting to note that the CDC has proposed easing CLIA regulations by adding another category of testing. It would fall between the waived tests and the moderately complex tests. The tests within this new category would be subject to minimal regulation. This proposal is under consideration. Many question whether CLIA will have any value if this event occurs.

Impact of CLIA on Medical Assistants

CLIA '88 requires every facility that tests human specimens for diagnosis, treatment, and prevention of disease to meet specific federal requirements. The law applies to any facility that performs tests for the preceding purposes. This includes any physicians' office laboratories and ambulatory care setting, two typical areas where medical assistants have found employment. The law covers all facilities even if only one test or a few basic tests are done and even if there is no charge for the testing.

Medical assistants may be responsible not only for performing the tests, but also for maintaining personnel records including such information as workers' college diplomas, state licenses, national certifications, employees' continuing education, and recredentialing. Employee hepatitis B status must also be on file. Medical assistants may be involved with compiling a procedures manual on how to perform every test done; these must be reviewed every year. An instrument log must be available on each piece of equipment. Systems must be in place for calibration, quality control, quality assurance test recording, and proficiency testing (if higher than waived category tests are performed). Documentation by medical assistants is of utmost importance; for instance, there may be a quality control plan in action, but it may not be written down in detail.

Due to the fact that HCFA has received only a fraction of the money that they expected to collect from application fees, there is very little money to carry the

CLIA '88 program forward. Medical assistants must realize that CLIA '88 is the law even though a number of laboratories have not seen inspectors nor felt any impact from the CLIA '88 regulations. Some laboratories are delaying concern about CLIA '88 rules and do not understand the law and, therefore, have not fully implemented the regulations. Medical assistants must know and comply with the law and be prepared for a CLIA inspection. Penalties are imposed on laboratories that are not in compliance with the law.

Medical assistants who perform clinical laboratory procedures need to be aware that they must keep up with government changes.

Where to Find More Information Regarding CLIA '88

The original CLIA '88 guidelines and updates are available from the Federal Register for a fee. See the appendices for ordering information or visit HCFA at www.HCFA.gov and click on the *Laboratory Testing* (CLIA) icon.

OCCUPATIONAL SAFETY AND HEALTH ADMINISTRATION (OSHA) REGULATIONS

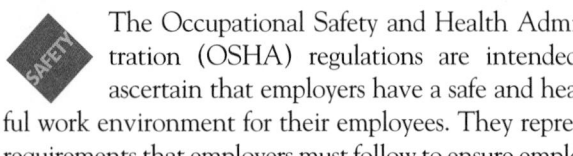 The Occupational Safety and Health Administration (OSHA) regulations are intended to ascertain that employers have a safe and healthful work environment for their employees. They represent requirements that employers must follow to ensure employee safety and health.

There are two standards that comprise the regulations that have the primary impact on a clinical laboratory, *The Occupational Exposure to Hazardous Chemicals in the Laboratory*, an amended version of the original standard *The Hazard Communication Standard*, and *The Bloodborne Pathogen Standard*. Each **standard** will be described independently. See Chapter 22 for *The Bloodborne Pathogen Standard*.

The Standard for Occupational Exposure to Hazardous Chemicals in the Laboratory

In an effort to reduce the number of chemically related illnesses and injuries in the workplace, OSHA published its *Hazard Communications Standard* in 1983. This led many states to develop *right-to-know* laws. In 1992, OSHA expanded the *Hazard Communications Standard*, and published *The Occupational Exposure to Hazardous Chemicals in the Laboratory Standard* which specifically addressed clinical laboratories.

The intention of this law is to heighten employee awareness of risks linked with chemical dangers. It serves

to improve work practices through employee training and identification of hazardous chemicals that exist in the workplace. The use of protective equipment is utilized to protect employees from harmful chemicals.

Chemical Hygiene Plan

The Chemical Hygiene Plan (CHP) on hazardous chemicals is the core of the OSHA safety standard on hazardous chemicals. A written plan must specify the training and information requirements of the standard. Certain specific control measures such as **fume hoods** and glove boxes must be included in the plan. A designated employee is the chemical hygiene or safety officer. Provisions for housekeeping and maintenance of the facility are included. OSHA standards are not optional and penalties are imposed for noncompliance with the standard. Employers must take the time to meet the requirements not only in order to be in compliance with the law, but to protect employees as well.

All laboratories and ambulatory care settings, including physicians' offices must comply with a chemical hygiene plan in order to meet the OSHA regulations. The only laboratories exempt from compliance are those that exclusively use methods that do not place employees at risk for exposure to chemicals that are hazardous. For example, there may be physicians' office laboratories (POLs) that perform only dipstick tests or use other commercially prepared kits in which reagents are not exposed and as a result they are exempt from compliance. The primary component of the OSHA standard is that a written chemical hygiene plan and program must be operational if chemicals are stored in a facility and handled by employees. Some examples of chemicals include, but are not limited to: stains, **ethyl alcohol**, sodium hypochlorite (household bleach), **formaldehyde**, fixatives, preservatives, injectables such as **chemotherapeutic agents**, **acetone**, and so on. Many laboratory accidents result in chemical-related illnesses ranging from eye irritations to **pulmonary edema**.

There are three primary goals that an employer must accomplish to be in compliance with the OSHA standard for chemical exposure. The first is that there must be an inventory undertaken and a list compiled of all chemicals considered hazardous. The following information must be documented (Figure 38-3): the quantity of chemical stored per month or year; whether the substance is gas, liquid, or solid; the manufacturer's name and address; and the chemical hazard classification.

Second, a material safety data sheet (MSDS) (Figure 38-4) manual must be assembled. MSDS manuals are often supplied by the manufacturer when the chemicals are ordered and will give information regarding whether or not a chemical is hazardous. All other MSDS information must be requested from the manufacturer. The MSDS sheets must be alphabetized and indexed and be reviewed on a regular basis and modifications made. The manual must be available to all employees. The various chemicals are labeled using the National Fire Protection Association's color and number method (Figure 38-5).

SAMPLE
CHEMICAL INVENTORY FORM

Office of _____

Date _____

Chemical Name	Catalog #	Quantity Stores L./gm. (monthly)	Physical State	Hazard Class				Manufacturer	Comments
				H	F	R	P		

(H) Health
0 - Minimal
1 - Slightly
2 - Moderate
3 - Serious
4 - Extreme

(F) Fire Hazard
0 - Will not burn
1 - Slight
2 - Moderate
3 - Serious
4 - Extreme

(R) Reactivity
0 - Stable is not reactive
    with water
1 - Slight
2 - Moderate
3 - Serious
4 - Extreme

(P) Protection
A. - Goggles
B. - Goggles/Gloves
C. - Goggles/Gloves/Apron
D. - Face Shield/Gloves/Apron
E. - Goggles/Gloves/Mask
F. - Goggles/Gloves/Apron/Mask
X. - Gloves

Figure 38-3   Sample chemical inventory form for listing chemicals on the premises, including quantity, physical state, hazard class, manufacturer, and comments. (Courtesy of POL Consultants)

MATERIAL SAFETY DATA SHEET

I – PRODUCT IDENTIFICATION

COMPANY NAME: We Wash Inc.

ADDRESS: 5035 Manchester Avenue	Tel No: (314) 621-1818
Freedom, Texas 79430	Nights: (314) 621-1399
	CHEMTREC: (800) 424-9343

PRODUCT NAME: Spotfree

Product No.: 2190

Synonyms: Warewashing Detergent

II – HAZARDOUS INGREDIENTS OF MIXTURES

MATERIAL:	(CAS#)	% By Wt.	TLV	PEL
According to the OSHA Hazard Communication Standard, 29CFR 1910.1200, this product contains no hazardous ingredients.		N/A	N/A	NA

III – PHYSICAL DATA

Vapor Pressure, mm Hg: N/A   Vapor Density (Air=1) 60–90F: N/A
Evaporation Rate (ether=1): N/A   % Volatile by wt N/A
Solubility in H_2O: Complete   pH @ 1%   Solution 9.3–9.8
Freezing Point F: N/A   pH as Distributed: N/A
Boiling Point F: N/A   Appearance: Off-White granular powder
Specific Gravity H_2O=1 @25C: N/A   Odor: Mild Chemical Odor

IV – FIRE AND EXPLOSION

Flash Point F: N/AV   Flammable Limits: N/A

Extinguishing Media: The product is not flammable or combustible. Use media appropriate for the primary source of fire.

Special Fire Fighting Procedures: Use caution when fighting any fire involving chemicals. A self-contained breathing apparatus is essential.

Unusual Fire and Explosion Hazards: None Known

V – REACTIVITY DATA

Stability - Conditions to avoid: None Known

Incompatibility: Contact of carbonates or bicarbonates with acids can release large quantities of carbon dioxide and heat.

Hazardous Decomposition Products: In fire situations heat decomposition may result in the release of sulfur oxides.

Conditions Contributing to Hazardous Polymerization: N/A

(continues)

Figure 38-4   Example of a Material Safety Data Sheet (MSDS) listing product name, hazardous ingredients, physical data, fire, explosion, reactivity, health hazard data, emergency and first aid procedures, spill or leak procedures, protection/control measures, and special precautions. (Courtesy of POL Consultants)

Spotfree
VI – HEALTH HAZARD DATA

EFFECTS OF OVEREXPOSURE (Medical Conditions Aggravated/Target Organ Effects)
A. ACUTE (Primary Route of Exposure)   EYES: Product granules may cause mechanical irritation to eyes.
    SKIN (Primary Route of Exposure): Prolonged repeated contact with skin may result in drying of skin.
    INGESTION: Not expected to be toxic if swallowed, however, gastrointestinal discomfort may occur.
B. SUBCHRONIC, CHRONIC, OTHER: None known.

VII – EMERGENCY AND FIRST AID PROCEDURES

EYES: In case of contact, flush thoroughly with water for 15 minutes. Get medical attention if irritation persists.
SKIN: Flush any dry Spotfree from skin with flowing water. Always wash hands after use.
INGESTION: If swallowed, drink large quantities of water and call a physician.

VIII – SPILL OR LEAK PROCEDURES

Spill Management: Sweep up material and repackage if possible.
    Spill residue may be flushed to the sewer with water.

Waste Disposal Methods: Dispose of in accordance with federal, state and local regulations.

IX – PROTECTION INFORMATION/CONTROL MEASURES

Respiratory: None needed   Eye: Safety   Glove: Not
                                                                 glasses   required

Other Clothing and Equipment: None required

Ventilation: Normal

X – SPECIAL PRECAUTIONS

Precautions to be taken in Handling and Storing: Avoid contact with eyes. Avoid prolonged or repeated contact with skin.
    Wash thoroughly after handling. Keep container closed when not in use.
Additional Information: Store away from acids.

Prepared by: D. Martinez   Revision Date: 04/11/_ _

Seller makes no warranty, expressed or implied, concerning the use of this product other than indicated on the label. Buyer assumes all risk of use and/or handling of this material when such use and/or handling is contrary to label instructions.

While Seller believes that the information contained herein is accurate, such information is offered solely for its customers' consideration and verification under their specific use conditions. This information is not to be deemed a warranty or representation of any kind for which Seller assumes legal responsibility.

Figure 38-4   (*continued*)

CHEMICAL WARNING LABEL DETERMINATION

The Hazard Communication Act contains specific labeling requirements. Labels must be on all hazardous chemicals that are shipped to and used in the workplace. Labels must not be removed. Material safety data sheets for all chemicals will be available to employees.

Manufacturer Requirements: Chemical manufacturers are required to evaluate chemicals, determine status as hazards, provide material safety data sheets (MSDS), and label all shipped chemicals properly. Manufacturer labels must never be removed. The best way to determine the hazards of the chemical is to read the MSDS, obtain an OSHA designated list or State Hazardous Substance list. For most mixed chemicals, it is necessary to contact the manufacturer for MSDS.

Office Chemicals: Search through your office and write down all chemicals you have in the office. Most pharmaceuticals and common household products do not come under this standard. Ingredients can then be compared to a list of regulated substances or MSDS sheets will provide necessary information.

Employer's Responsibility: Any hazardous chemical used in the workplace that is not in its original container *must* be labeled with the identity of the chemical and hazards. "Target Organ" chemical labels may be used. The label must include the chemical and common name, warnings about physical and health hazards, and the name and address of the manufacturer. The employer is to compile a chemical inventory list that is to be updated as needed. MSDS information should be located in a place where it is accessible to all employees. Label and MSDS information should be provided during the safety training program.

Identity: The term *identity* can refer to any chemical or common name designation for the individual chemical or mixture, as long as the term used is also used on the list of hazardous chemicals and the MSDS.

NOTE: If a chemical is poured into another container for immediate use, it does not need to be labeled.

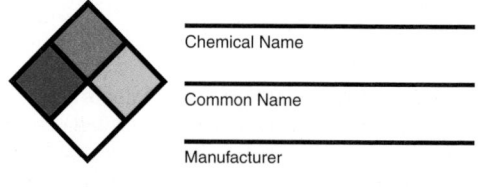

Figure 38-5   Chemical warning label determination indicates necessary information for labels, including manufacturer's requirements, office chemicals, employer's responsibility, and identity of chemical or its common name. (Courtesy of POL Consultants)

There are four colors, each signifying a warning to the person handling the chemical(s). They are:

- Blue signifies a health hazard

- Red signifies a fire hazard

- Yellow signifies an instability hazard

- White signifies use of personal protective equipment (PPE)

The numbers 0–4 are used in conjunction with the colors to indicate the level of risk for each product and are assigned by the manufacturer using the rating system. The numbers can be found on the MSDS. See Figure 38-6.

Third, the employer is required to provide a hazard communication educational program to the employee

RED: FIRE HAZARD

4 = Danger: Flammable gas or extremely flammable liquid
3 = Warning: Flammable liquid
2 = Caution: Combustible liquid
1 = Caution: Combustible if heated
0 = Noncombustible

YELLOW: REACTIVITY

4 = Danger: Explosive at room temperature
3 = Danger: May be explosive if spark occurs or if heated under confinement
2 = Warning: Unstable or may react if mixed with water
1 = Caution: May react if heated or mixed with water
0 = Stable: Nonreactive when mixed with water

BLUE: HEALTH HAZARD

4 = Danger: May be fatal
3 = Warning: Corrosive or toxic
2 = Warning: Harmful if inhaled
1 = Caution: May cause irritation
0 = No unusual hazard

WHITE: PPE

A   Goggles
B   Goggles, gloves
C   Goggles, gloves, apron
D   Face shields, gloves, apron
E   Goggles, gloves, mask
F   Goggles, gloves, apron, mask
X   Gloves

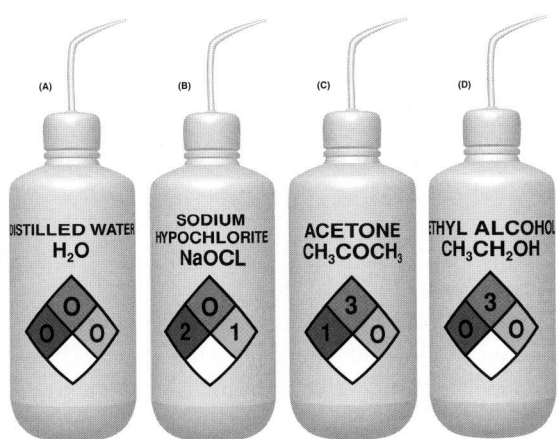

Figure 38-6 Four containers are marked using the National Fire Association's color and number method for identifying and warning of chemical hazards: (A) distilled water: presents no health, fire, or reactivity hazard and requires no PPE when used (all areas represented by zeros); (B) sodium hypochlorite: does not promote a fire hazard (red/0); is harmful if inhaled (blue/2); and it may react if heated or mixed with water (yellow/1); (C) acetone: a flammable liquid (red/3); may cause irritation (blue/1); stable and nonreactive when mixed with water (yellow/0); (D) ethyl alcohol: a flammable liquid (red/3); no unusual health hazard (blue/0); stable and nonreactive when mixed with water (yellow/0). (Courtesy of POL Consultants)

within thirty days of employment and before the employee handles any hazardous chemicals (Figure 38-7A). The training program should consist of the location and identification of hazardous chemicals, how to read and understand the labels on the chemicals, where the MSDS manual is kept, when to use personal protective equipment, and procedures to follow for chemical spills. The training sessions must be documented, signed by the employer, and permanently retained in the employee record (Figure 38-7B).

January, 1991 was the deadline for laboratories (including POLs) to have a chemical hygiene plan (CHP) in place.

Requirements of Chemical Hygiene Plan. The requirements for a CHP include:

- Employers must have an operational written plan (a manual) relevant to the safety and health of employees.
- Written instructions on the use of personal protection equipment must be available.
- Fume hoods or biohazard hoods must be checked regularly.
- Training sessions must be held for employees regarding their right to know what hazardous chemicals are in their work environment.

SAFETY TRAINING FORM

Safety training will be offered to all employees within 30 days of employment or before the employee assumes responsibilities that involve exposure to body fluids or chemicals.

Items to be covered in training session:

- General explanation of OSHA laws
- General explanation of the epidemiology and symptoms of HBV and HIV
- Who is at risk in office
- Modes of transmission of HBV and HIV
- Method of control in workplace
- Universal precautions
- Handwashing
- Personal protective equipment
- How to clean up spills
- What to do after a needlestick injury
- Medical follow-up after an exposure
- Cleaning protocol for office
- Hazardous Communication Standard
- Types of chemical labels
- How to read MSDS and NFPA signs
- Warning signs
- How to get MSDS
- Location of MSDS
- How to store chemicals
- How to record chemical inventory
- Hazardous Waste laws
- How to comply with laws
- How to use and label bio-bins and sharps containers
- How to keep records
- Who keeps the records
- Medical consent forms
- HBV forms
- Safety training certificate
- Engineering control records

Figure 38-7A Safety Training Form is an example of items to be covered by employer during training session regarding OSHA laws and exposure to chemicals, blood, body fluids, or OPIM. (Courtesy of POL Consultants)

- It is the employer's legal responsibility to provide medical attention for an employee should an accidental chemical spill occur.
- The responsibility for executing training sessions, keeping manuals current, and documentation is designated to an employer.
- Instruction must be provided regarding disposal of hazardous waste produced in the workplace.

SAMPLE

CERTIFICATE OF TRAINING

_____
First Name   Middle Initial   Last Name

has completed the

OSHA HAZARD COMMUNICATION
INFORMATION TRAINING PROGRAM

This certificate indicates your successful participation in a program instructing you of your rights as a worker and the proper handling of hazardous substances in the workplace.

_____
Date

_____
Employee Signature

_____
Instructor's Signature

_____
Employer's Signature

Figure 38-7B Sample Certificate of Training shows employee has completed OSHA hazard communication information training program. (Courtesy of POL Consultants)

(Usually a hazardous waste company is contracted by the employer.)

- Each employee's record must have a written statement, signed by the employer, stating the employer's responsibility to arrange for employee training and a safe work environment.

Importance of Chemical Standard to Medical Assistants. Meeting the requirements set forth by OSHA is not optional. All must comply or face penalties. All employees, including medical assistants, have the right to know and be given information and be educated regarding chemical hazards that they are exposed to in their place of employment. Medical assistants can be exposed to hazardous chemicals through skin contact, injection, or inhalation. Since many laboratory accidents result in chemical-related illnesses, it is important for medical assistants to understand how the law affects them, their place of employment, and

their employer. Medical assistants and other health care providers should know what hazards they face, and know the proper technique for handling, storing, and disposing of hazardous chemicals.

OSHA REGULATIONS AND STUDENTS

With the passage of the OSHA laws, all students with potential exposure to chemicals and bloodborne pathogens should follow all safety procedures as outlined by OSHA. Because students are not considered employees of a health care facility and are attending an educational institution, they do not fall under the OSHA guidelines. They should, however, take precautions to avoid contact with potentially infectious materials and toxic chemicals wherever learning is taking place.

Avoiding Exposure to Chemicals

Students may come into contact with harmful chemicals when doing procedures that can cause such problems as burns to the skin and eyes. Students will be made aware of these through information packaged with kits and the MSDS. As a general rule, if the chemical comes in contact with the skin, it must be flushed with water immediately and continued for five minutes. Chemicals that get into the eye must be flushed for fifteen minutes (unless contradicted on the label). Refer to the MSDS for specific postexposure procotol. Eyewash stations and showers should be available in case of accidental exposure to hazardous chemicals with a follow-up in the emergency room.

Chemical spills should be carefully cleaned following the procedure for the particular chemical. Spill cleanup kits that consist of various items such as a shovel, cardboard, PPE, neutralizing agent, and/or absorbent material should be available.

Toxic fumes can occur with certain chemicals and certain tests can cause lung irritation and damage. This type of chemical should be handled under a fume hood that will take the fumes away by means of a ventilation mechanism.

A student safety laboratory manual outlining an exposure control plan with emphasis on standard precautions, PPE, work practice controls, lists of hazardous chemicals, and MSDS should be compiled and accessible. Students should be thoroughly familiar with its contents. Additionally, students should be educated as to the location and identification of hazardous chemicals just as employees are.

It is of utmost importance that students learn about and understand the OSHA standards and comply with them. In so doing, they will safeguard themselves from harmful chemicals and bloodborne pathogens.

CUMULATIVE TRAUMA DISORDERS

Recently OHSA has been focusing its attention on a new threat to the workplace, ergonomic hazards. Ergonomics is the study of the workplace. OSHA published its first standard, *Ergonomic Hazards,* in 1991. At the heart of these guidelines is the prevention of cumulative trauma disorders. Cumulative trauma disorders are injuries involving the musculoskeletal and/or nervous system, such as carpal tunnel syndrome and trigger finger. They are the result of long-term, repetitive work actions, such as gripping, keyboard use, pipetting, and microscopy. Limiting or preventing repetitive work actions is the key to minimizing cumulative trauma disorders. Use of ergonomically correct equipment and supplies, proper work site design, staff training, and job rotation are essential in creating an ergonomically sound workplace.

SUMMARY

Infectious diseases and accidents occur through lack of education and carelessness. Medical assistants must understand the importance of the regulations and guidelines set forth by the federal government and follow through by helping employers implement them. In doing so, the health and safety of patients and health care workers will be protected, the spread of infectious diseases can be kept under control, and the risk of contracting an infectious disease such as AIDS or hepatitis B will be greatly minimized.

Every medical office and ambulatory care setting must, by law, have clearly written and readily available manuals containing information about standard precautions, CLIA '88, and OSHA for the safe handling, storage, and disposal of blood, body fluids, and chemicals.

Through consistent use of standard precautions and adherence to the CLIA and OSHA laws, health care providers can acquire the behaviors and techniques needed to safeguard themselves and their patients.

Because of frequent changes in the laws, it is necessary for medical assistants and all other health care providers to keep abreast of the government mandates.

REVIEW QUESTIONS

Multiple Choice

1. Standard precautions were issued by:
   a. HHS
   b. CDC
   c. HCFA
   d. OSHA
2. CLIA '88 was made law in order to regulate:
   a. the disposal of infectious waste
   b. the use of chemicals in the workplace
   c. laboratory tests performed on specimens taken from the human body
   d. the transmission of the HIV virus
3. The core of the OSHA safety standard for chemical exposure is:
   a. the dipstick test
   b. the Chemical Hygiene Plan
   c. the quantity of chemical stored per month
   d. the MSDS manual
4. The agency that requires employers to ensure employee safety concerning occupational exposure to potentially harmful substances is:
   a. CDC
   b. United States Public Health Department
   c. HCFA
   d. OSHA
5. Successful laboratory safety programs include:
   a. threats to the emotional and physical health of health care workers
   b. lost work days and increased workers' compensation claims
   c. orientation, periodic drills, and consistent enforcement of policy
   d. potential fines from regulatory agencies
6. CLIA regulations specify all the following except:
   a. the type of test performed
   b. the personnel involved in testing
   c. quality control
   d. the methods used in testing
7. The agency charged with implementing CLIA is:
   a. CDC
   b. United States Public Health Department
   c. HCFA
   d. OSHA
8. Which is not an approved provider for PPM procedures?
   a. a physician
   b. a nurse practitioner

c. a dentist

d. a medical assistant

9. The standard published by OSHA to prevent cumulative trauma disorders is:

a. Workplace Standard

b. Standard for Prevention of Cumulative Trauma

c. Ergonomic Hazards

d. Ergonomic Standard

Match the chemical warning color with the hazard represented.

10. Blue	a. Reactivity or instability
11. Red	b. Use PPE
12. Yellow	c. Health
13. White	d. Fire
	e. Disaster

Critical Thinking

1. Explain the purpose of CLIA '88 and tell why the law was amended.
2. Name three categories of testing and explain each category.
3. Discuss the fifteen major components of CLIA '88.
4. Describe quality control and quality assurance. Why are they important?
5. What is HCFA form 116? Explain its use.

6. You have been asked to develop a manual for your physician/employer. The manual is to detail a Chemical Hygiene Plan (CHP) for all employees in the office. How would you proceed? What should be included in the plan? In the CHP include three major goals that will ensure the physician/employer's compliance with the hazard standard. You have been asked to compile a manual of the Material Safety Data Sheets. What must be included in the manual and from where does the information come?

REFERENCES/BIBLIOGRAPHY

Medical Economics Inc. (1993). *Medical laboratory observer*. Montvale, NJ: Medical Economics Inc.

Occupational Exposure to Hazardous Chemicals in Laboratories Federal Register 55:1450, 1990.

Occupational Safety and Health Administration Hazard Communication; final rule part III Federal Register 31852-31886, 1987.

U.S. Department of Health and Human Services, Health Care Financing Administration. (1992, February 28). *Clinical laboratory improvement amendments 1988*. (Federal Register No. 069-001-00042-4). Washington, DC: U.S. Government Printing Office.

INTRODUCTION TO THE MEDICAL LABORATORY

KEY TERMS

Assay
Asymptomatic
Baseline Values
Biopsy
Clinical Chemistry
Clinical Diagnosis
Condenser
Control Test
Cytology
Diagnosis
Diaphragm
Differential Diagnosis
Electrolyte
Glucose
Hematology
Histology
Hospital-Based Laboratories
Immunohematology
Immunology
Invasive
Microbiology
Mycology
Objective
Parasitology
Patient Service Centers
Physicians' Office Laboratories (POL)
Profile
Qualitative Test
Quantitative Test
Reagent
Reference Laboratories
Reference Values
Requisition
Serum
Urinalysis
Virology

OUTLINE

The Laboratory
  Purposes of Laboratory Testing
  Types of Laboratories
  Laboratory Personnel
  Laboratory Departments
Quality Controls/Assurances in the Laboratory
  Control Tests
  Proficiency Testing
  Preventative Maintenance
  Instrument Validations
  The Medical Assistant's Role

Laboratory Requisitions and Reports
Specimen Collection
  Proper Procurement, Storage, and Handling
  Processing and Sending Specimens to a Laboratory
Microscopes
  Types of Microscopes
  How to Use a Microscope
  How to Care for a Microscope

OBJECTIVES

The student should strive to meet the following performance objectives and demonstrate an understanding of the facts and principles presented in this chapter through written and oral communication.

1. Define the key terms as presented in the glossary.

2. Explain eight purposes of laboratory testing.

3. Describe the main similarities and differences between independent laboratories and physicians' office laboratories (POLs).

4. Explain the levels of laboratory personnel in relation to their education, skills, and duties.

5. List eight different departments within the medical laboratory and list at least two types of testing performed within each of those departments.

6. Name nine of the most common laboratory profiles and explain the body system or function being surveyed.

7. Explain the concepts of quality control and quality assurance in the medical laboratory.

8. Describe at least three methods of assuring quality in the medical laboratory.

(continues)

OBJECTIVES (*continued*)

9. Demonstrate how to correctly complete a laboratory requisition.
10. List ten pieces of information required on a written laboratory requisition.
11. Explain the rationale behind proper patient preparation prior to laboratory testing.
12. Explain where accurate and reliable information might be obtained about proper procurement, storage, and handling of laboratory specimens.
13. On a diagram, label the parts of a compound microscope.
14. Explain the function of a compound microscope.
15. Demonstrate the proper use of a compound microscope.
16. List six rules to assure proper care of a compound microscope.

ROLE DELINEATION COMPONENTS

CLINICAL
Diagnostic Orders
- Collect and process specimens
- Perform diagnostic tests

Patient Care
- Coordinate patient care information with other health care providers

GENERAL (TRANSDISCIPLINARY)
Legal Concepts
- Document accurately
- Comply with established risk management and safety procedures
- Participate in the development and maintenance of personnel, policy, and procedure manuals
- Develop and maintain personnel, policy, and procedure manuals (adv)

Instruction
- Instruct patients according to their needs

SCENARIO

At Inner City Health Care, Dr. Susan Rice has ordered urine tests for Annette Samuels, who came to the clinic complaining of stomach cramps. Certified medical assistant Wanda Slawson will obtain the necessary specimen and send it to an independent laboratory for testing. Wanda gives Annette specific instructions on how to prepare for the urine test and on how to collect the urine. She asks Annette if she has any questions and she has Annette repeat the instructions to be sure she understands them. When Annette returns with the specimen, Wanda immediately labels it and prepares it to be sent to the laboratory. With a reassuring smile, she tells Annette when to call the clinic for the results.

INTRODUCTION

Physicians use laboratory tests to diagnose illnesses, assess patients' health, and manage chronic diseases such as diabetes and arthritis. Medical assistants in physicians' offices, clinics, and laboratories may be responsible for patient preparation, obtaining specimens, and testing or sending specimens to an independent laboratory. It is important for medical assistants to be aware of laboratory procedures to ensure accurate testing.

THE LABORATORY

The current health care environment offers numerous options in the methods used to process laboratory tests. The specimen may be obtained and the test performed within the physician's office laboratory (POL) or the specimen may be procured and packaged for transport to a separate lab. Another option is to refer the patient to a separate laboratory for collection and testing of the specimen.

 Each laboratory setting has specific requirements for the training and qualifications of the health care personnel who work in that setting. The equipment, supplies, and paperwork as well as the instructions given to the patient are also determined by the type of laboratory. Whichever laboratory setting is selected, the focus should be on the safety of the public, the patient, and the health care personnel, while always maintaining quality testing to ensure accurate results.

Purposes of Laboratory Testing

Physicians (and other health care providers) depend on the ability of medical laboratories to help in determining a patient's state of health and/or disease in some of the following ways:

To Record an Individual's State of Health. Blood tests may be performed periodically, usually during a routine physical examination, to be assured of healthy normal ranges, also known as **reference values**. Then in the future, if illness occurs, the **baseline values** are available for comparison. Sometimes, places of employment or life insurance companies request laboratory tests to be assured that their employees or clients are free of illegal or dangerous drugs. Employment-required drug and alcohol testing is a classic example of this reason for testing.

To Detect Asymptomatic Conditions or Diseases. Occasionally a patient will have no complaints of illness and will be **asymptomatic**, exhibit no symptoms that might be associated with a disease process, but during routine screening or testing in another, perhaps unrelated, area, a disorder may be discovered. An example is a young man presenting at the office for an athletic physical. During routine urinalysis, it is discovered he is harboring a mild bladder infection.

To Confirm a Clinical Diagnosis. When a patient complains of specific symptoms and describes a particular condition (subjective information), and data is compiled through a clinical examination (objective information), the physician may be able to determine a **diagnosis** without the aid of laboratory tests. This is referred to as a **clinical diagnosis**. To confirm a clinical diagnosis, the physician will order laboratory tests. For example, a child has symptoms of a strep throat infection such as sudden onset of sore throat, fever, headache, and upset stomach. Upon visual examination, the physician discovers small abscesses on the child's tonsils. The physician is almost certain that the diagnosis will be strep throat, but a quick and simple strep test is performed to confirm the clinical diagnosis.

To Differentiate Between Two or More Diseases. Sometimes a patient presents with a combination of symptoms that can be related to more than one condition. In order for the physician to diagnose accurately, a laboratory test is performed. In situations like these, the physician chooses to perform the simplest and least **invasive** laboratory test in order to rule out a particular disease before requiring more extensive testing. This is known as a **differential diagnosis**. For example, if the child in the preceding case had a negative strep test but perhaps exhibited other more systemic symptoms, a blood test might confirm mononucleosis or another condition. The physician is then able to differentiate between the two diagnoses—strep throat and mononeucleosis.

To Diagnose. If symptoms are vague, thereby making the clinical diagnosis difficult for the physician, a series of laboratory tests may be required. Sometimes a **profile**, or group of related tests, is ordered. This helps narrow the field for diagnosis. An example is if a patient presents with complaints of severe fatigue, but preliminary testing does not reveal a diagnosis. Further testing will eventually either lead the physician in a specific direction or at least eliminate a wide variety of conditions.

To Determine the Effectiveness of Treatments. After a patient has been diagnosed and has begun treatment, the physician monitors the patient's health to be sure that the treatment is therapeutic. For example, a patient diagnosed with epilepsy must take an effective amount of antiseizure medication. A blood test is used to check the level of medication in the patient's system. A periodic blood test can also be used to determine the effectiveness of dietary and lifestyle changes in lowering blood cholesterol levels.

To Prevent Diseases/Disorders. Protection of the public, families, and coworkers can warrant laboratory tests. An example is protecting an unborn child from contracting genital herpes through the birthing process. A culture of the mother's cervical and vaginal mucosa helps to determine if the child is at risk. If the culture is positive, performing a caesarean section is the treatment of choice to protect the newborn from contracting herpes.

To Prevent the Exacerbation of Diseases. Patients with chronic conditions require regular blood tests to prevent exacerbation of the disease. When the results of the blood test are obtained, the physician or patient determines whether it is necessary to adjust the diet and/or medication. For example, a patient with diabetes tests her blood regularly to measure the blood sugar, or **glucose**, level. If the blood sugar level is too high or too low, the patient may adjust her insulin dosage or have something to eat to return her blood sugar level to normal.

Types of Laboratories

There are many different types and locations of medical laboratories. They are identified by their size, capabilities, and affiliations. Independent laboratories may be located within medical centers or large clinics. They often have small satellite patient service centers located near more isolated medical facilities or in areas of convenience to patients. Satellite laboratories facilitate patients' specimens being obtained closer to their neighborhoods and/or ambulatory care settings. The specimens are usually couriered back to the independent central laboratory for processing.

Hospital-based laboratories perform most of the tests required by that hospital area, but even large hospitals utilize reference laboratories for specialized testing. Reference laboratories are independent, regionally located laboratories that service larger areas. Reference laboratories are used by hospitals and physicians for complex, expensive, or specialized tests.

In a business sense, medical laboratories are quickly becoming more and more competitive. Growth and profitability depend on community relations and service, convenience, efficiency, cost, location, and even reputation. Competition often places the medical assistant and other medical personnel in a position of being asked to recommend a particular medical laboratory over another. Unless the physician-employer has a strong preference for utilizing a particular laboratory, or not referring to a particular laboratory, the patient should choose the laboratory. The patient's insurance plan may also be a factor in determining which laboratory is used. Many insurance plans require the patient to use a particular laboratory or to choose a laboratory from those participating in the plan in order to guarantee payment for the tests. The medical assistant is then a resource for options rather than a referral service. The law is very clear that a physician may not have a financial interest in the laboratory to which he or she refers patients.

Point-of-Care Testing (POCT).
With the many changes in health care delivery and managed care, the clinical laboratory is also experiencing changes to improve clinical services in the laboratory area. On the forefront of change in the laboratory is point-of-care testing (POCT), also referred to as near-patient testing or bedside testing. Medical conditions, location of the patient, and treatment methods often require laboratory results as quickly as possible so proper medical care can be administered without delay. POCT uses small instruments that provide rapid, accurate results when used correctly.

Medical personnel can be trained to do laboratory tests of moderate complexity (as defined by CLIA '88) during POCT. The laboratory staff, because of their education, knowledge, and experience in this area, are responsible for advice and management of the quality control and various aspects of this new area of testing. The extension of this laboratory service demands cooperation and cross-departmental efforts from all nontraditional personnel in the health care facility. POCT also has provided new career tracks for the laboratorian, along with multiple skills for several disciplines of health care providers.

Physicians' Office Laboratories.
Physicians' office laboratories (POLs) are those laboratories physically set within the office. Some of the more commonly performed medical laboratory tests can easily and inexpensively be performed in the office by the medical assistant. With a simple fingerstick and a few readily available medical supplies, a patient's hematocrit and hemoglobin levels can be determined. Another commonly performed test in the ambulatory care setting is the urinalysis in which urine is physically, chemically, and microscopically examined for irregularities. With the availability of the many varieties of self-contained kits, tests for strep throat, pregnancy, blood sugar (serum glucose) levels, and hidden (occult) blood in stool can be performed quickly. Other kits are being developed daily. Patients may utilize a kit that can be purchased without a prescription at home. Some of the home kits available to the general public are "just as accurate" as the kits used in medical offices. The major difference is that the person performing the test may not be trained, which may affect the accuracy of the test results. More training, education, and credentialing are required as the complexity of the testing and equipment increases. If the results are not within normal limits (in some cases, positive), the physician needs to be consulted for confirmation and diagnosis/treatment. (See CLIA '88 in Chapter 38 for specific testing parameters.)

Laboratory Personnel

All independent medical laboratories must be managed by a pathologist, a physician who specializes in disease processes. Additional staffing consists of clinical laboratory scientists, technicians, clinical laboratory assistants, phlebotomists, and medical assistants. Many agencies certify laboratory personnel.

Clinical Laboratory Scientist.
Certified clinical laboratory scientists are qualified to perform analysis testing in all departments of the laboratory. They often are department supervisors and have leadership roles within the laboratory personnel structure. Clinical laboratory scientists have earned a bachelor's degree and completed a minimum of one year of internship training. Certification is then obtained by passing a national certification examination issued by one of the following agencies:

MT (ASCP)—Medical Technologist
American Society of Clinical Pathologists
MT (AMT)—Medical Technologist
American Medical Technologists
CLS (NCA)—Clinical Laboratory Scientist
National Certification Agency for Medical
Laboratory Personnel
RMT (ISCLT)—Registered Medical Technologist
International Society for Clinical Laboratory
Technology
CLT (HHS)—Clinical Laboratory Technologist
Department of Health and Human Services

Clinical Laboratory Technician (CLT)/Medical Laboratory Technician (MLT).

Certified clinical laboratory technicians are qualified to perform qualitative and quantitative testing under supervision. Clinical laboratory technicians have completed two years of formal education and training. Certification is then obtained by passing a national certification examination issued by one of the following agencies:

MLT (ASCP)—Medical Laboratory Technician
American Society of Clinical Pathologists
MLT (AMT)—Medical Laboratory Technician
American Medical Technologists
CLT (NCA)—Clinical Laboratory Technician
National Certification Agency for Medical
Laboratory Personnel

RLT (ISCLT)—Registered Laboratory Technician
International Society for Clinical Laboratory
Technology

Medical Assistant. Medical assistants are multi-skilled professionals dedicated to assisting in patient-care management. Medical assistants work in medical offices, clinics, and ambulatory care centers. They perform administrative duties and clinical procedures, including basic waived laboratory tests. Formal education, training, and externship are obtained through community colleges, vocational-technical schools, and proprietary (private) institutions. Certification is obtained through a national certification examination issued by the following organizations (see Chapter 1 for additional information regarding certification):

CMA—Certified Medical Assistant
American Association of Medical Assistants and
the National Board of Medical Examiners
RMA—Registered Medical Assistant
American Medical Technologists

Laboratory Departments

Laboratories are usually divided into departments and may even be subdivided, depending on the size and specialties within the laboratory (Figure 39-1). The various departments perform special tests within their expertise (Table 39-1). Categorization becomes evident when test results are requested over the telephone or whenever

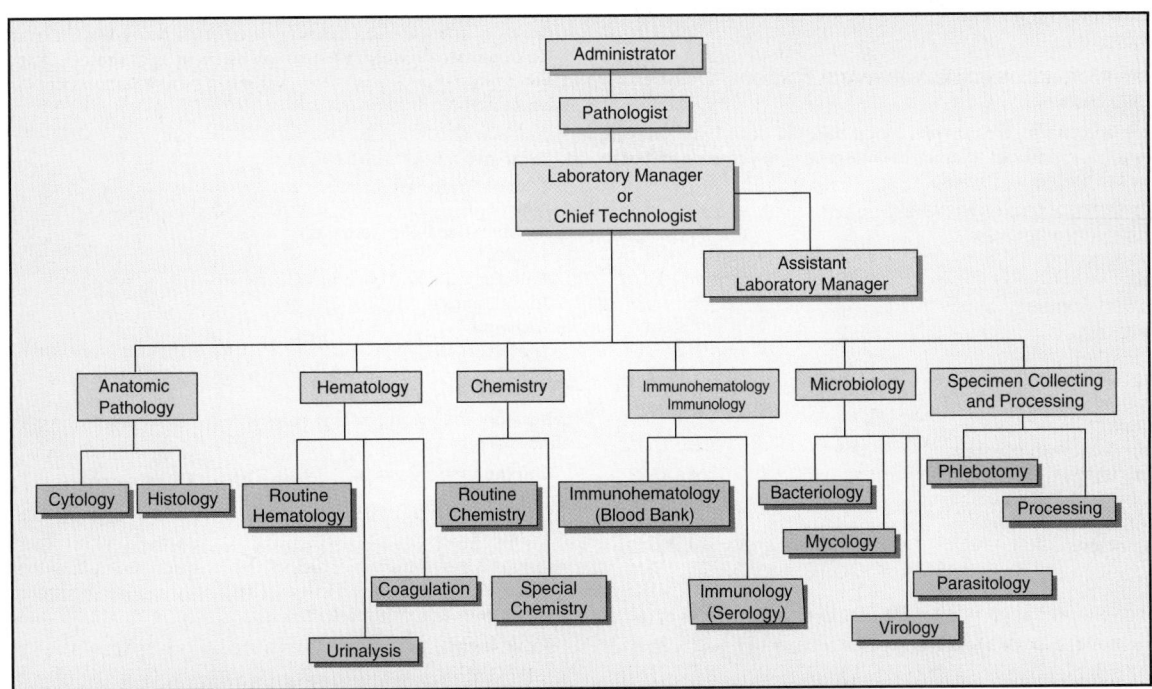

Figure 39-1 Departments in a typical medical laboratory.

TABLE 39-1 CATEGORIES OF LABORATORY TESTS

Categories of laboratory tests are listed, including the definition of each and commonly performed tests or pathologic condition in each category. Those tests that are commonly known by their abbreviations are listed as such.

HEMATOLOGY

Hematology is the science dealing with the study of blood and the blood-forming tissues. Laboratory analysis in hematology deals with the examination of blood for the detection of pathologic conditions and includes areas such as blood cell counts, cellular morphology, the clotting ability of the blood, and identification of cell types.

> White blood cell count (WBC)
> Red blood cell count (RBC)
> Differential white blood cell count (Diff)
> Hemoglobin (Hgb)
> Hematocrit (Hct)
> Prothrombin time (PT)
> Erythrocyte sedimentation rate (ESR)
> Platelet count

CLINICAL CHEMISTRY

Laboratory analysis in clinical chemistry involves detecting the presence of chemical substances or determining the amount of substances present in body fluids, excreta, and tissues (e.g., blood, urine, cerebrospinal fluid). The largest area in clinical chemistry is blood chemistry.

> Glucose
> Blood urea nitrogen (BUN)
> Creatinine
> Total protein
> Albumin
> Globulin
> Calcium
> Inorganic phosphorus
> Chloride
> Sodium
> Potassium
> Bilirubin
> Cholesterol
> Triglycerides
> Uric acid
> Lactate dehydrogenase, LD (LDH)
> Aspartate aminotransferase, AST (SGOT)
> Alanine aminotransferase, ALT (SGPT)
> Alkaline phosphatase
> Phospholipids

SEROLOGY (IMMUNOLOGY/IMMUNOHEMATOLOGY) AND BLOOD BANKING

Laboratory analysis in serology and blood banking deals with studying antigen-antibody reactions to assess the presence of a substance and/or to determine the presence of disease.

> Syphilis detection tests (VDRL, RPR)
> C-reactive protein test (CRP)
> ABO blood typing
> Rh typing
> Rh antibody titer test
> Cross-match
> Direct Coombs' test
> Cold agglutinins
> Rheumatoid factor (RA factor)
> Mono test
> Heterophil antibody titer test
> Hepatitis tests
> HIV tests: ELISA and Western blot
> Antistreptolysin O (ASO) titer
> Pregnancy tests

URINALYSIS

Urinalysis involves the physical, chemical, and microscopic analysis of urine.

> A. Tests included in the physical analysis of urine:
>   Color
>   Clarity
>   Specific gravity

B. Tests included in the chemical analysis of urine:
>   pH
>   Glucose
>   Protein
>   Ketones
>   Blood
>   Bilirubin
>   Urobilinogen
>   Nitrite
>   Leukocytes

C. Tests included in the microscopic analysis of urine:
>   Red blood cells
>   White blood cells
>   Epithelial cells
>   Casts
>   Crystals

MICROBIOLOGY

Microbiology is the scientific study of microorganisms and their activities. Laboratory analysis in microbiology deals with the identification of pathogens present in specimens taken from the body (i.e., urine, blood, throat, sputum, wound, urethra and vagina, cerebrospinal fluid). Examples of infectious diseases diagnosed through identification of the pathogen present in the specimen include

> Candidiasis
> Chlamydia
> Diphtheria
> Gonorrhea
> Meningitis
> Pertussis
> Pharyngitis
> Pneumonia
> Streptococcal sore throat
> Tetanus
> Tonsillitis
> Tuberculosis
> Urinary tract infection

PARASITOLOGY

Laboratory analysis in parasitology deals with the detection of the presence of disease-producing human parasites or eggs present in specimens taken from the body (e.g., stool, vagina, blood). Examples of human diseases caused by parasites include

> Amebiasis
> Ascariasis
> Hookworm disease
> Malaria
> Pinworm disease (enterobiasis)
> Scabies
> Tapeworm disease (cestodiasis)
> Toxoplasmosis
> Trichinosis
> Trichomoniasis

CYTOLOGY

Laboratory analysis in cytology deals with the detection of the presence of abnormal cells.

> Chromosome studies
> Pap test

HISTOLOGY

Histology is the microscopic study of the form and structure of the various tissues making up living organisms. Laboratory analysis in histology deals with the detection of diseased tissues.

> Tissue analysis
> Biopsy studies

(Adapted from *Clinical Procedures for Medical Assistants* (3rd ed.) by K. Bonewit-West, 1995, Philadelphia: W. B. Saunders Company. Adapted with permission.)

there is a need to converse with laboratory personnel. Through knowledge of the various departments within the laboratory, information can be more readily obtained.

Hematology Department. The hematology department tests the formed (cellular) elements of the blood. These tests may be quantitative or qualitative. The quantitative tests involve actual number counts such as counting the number of white blood cells (WBC), red blood cells (RBC), or platelets. The qualitative tests focus on the quality or characteristics of the components, such as the size, shape, and maturity of the cells. In addition, the hematology department tests the ability of the blood components to perform their individual tasks correctly. An example of this is testing the coagulation ability of clotting factors in blood.

Urinalysis Department. Urinalysis is the physical, chemical, and microscopic examination of urine. Required cultures are sent to the microbiology or bacteriology department (Figure 39-2).

Clinical Chemistry Department. The clinical chemistry department analyzes the chemical composition of blood, cerebrospinal fluid, and joint fluid. Some of the procedures within this department include assay of enzymes in the serum, serum glucose, or electrolyte levels. Toxicology, including therapeutic drug monitoring (TDM) and identification of drugs of abuse, is also performed in this department.

Immunohematology (Blood Bank) Department. Immunohematology is a special area that deals with blood typing procedures, cross-matching, and the separation and storage of blood components for transfusion as well as antibody-antigen reactions.

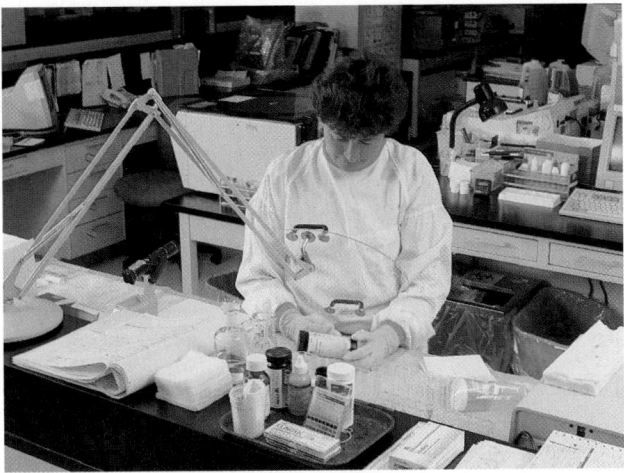

Figure 39-2 Clinical reference laboratories may have a separate urinalysis department where the laboratory professional tests urine for physical, chemical, or microbiological properties.

Serology (Immunology) Department. The serology (immunology) department is the area of the laboratory that performs tests to evaluate the body's immune response, both production of antibodies and the cellular immune response. Procedures in this area include the detection of antibodies to bacteria and viruses, as well as antibodies produced against one's own body (autoimmune), as in rheumatic diseases such as rheumatoid arthritis and lupus erythematosus. Diseases such as AIDS have helped move laboratory evaluation of the cellular immune system out of the research setting and into the diagnostic setting of the medical laboratory. Molecular biology and flow cytometry are becoming commonplace in today's medical laboratory. Traditionally serology has been an area within the microbiology department, but with the introduction of many new immunologic techniques, most medical laboratories now include a separate immunology department.

Microbiology Department. The microbiology department is the area in the laboratory where microorganisms such as bacteria and fungi are grown in an appropriate medium and then identified. Sensitivity tests are then performed to identify which antibiotics can effectively eradicate the pathogenic organisms. Mycology is an area within the microbiology department where fungi are studied. Virology is an area within the microbiology department where viruses are studied.

Parasitology Department. Parasitology is a subdivision of the microbiology department where ova and parasite (O & P) tests are performed on specimens such as feces. The specimens are examined for the presence of parasites and/or their eggs.

Cytology Department. The cytology department is the area in which microscopic examinations of cells are performed to detect early signs of cancer and other diseases. The Papanicolaou test, known as the pap smear, for irregular cervical cells is an example of a test performed in the cytology department.

Histology Department. Histology is the study of biopsied tissue samples for the determination of disease. Frozen samples or biopsies are sliced/stained and then microscopically examined for cancer and other anomalies.

Profiles of Laboratory Tests. Laboratory tests are often categorized into related groups to provide information about a particular body system or related bodily function. The groups are usually referred to as profiles (Figure 39-3). Additionally, laboratory tests are organized into panels for ease of ordering. For a current list of HCFA-approved organ- and disease-oriented panels, refer to Table 39-2.

TABLE 39-2	HCFA-APPROVED ORGAN- AND DISEASE-ORIENTED PANELS (WITH CPT CODES) EFFECTIVE APRIL 1, 2000

Basic Metabolic Panel (CPT code 80048)

BUN (84520)

Calcium, total (82310)

Carbon dioxide (82374)

Chloride (82435)

Creatinine (82565)

Glucose (82947)

Potassium (84132)

Sodium (84295)

General Health Panel (CPT code 80050)

Comprehensive metabolic panel (CPT code 80053)

CBC w/manual differential (80054) or CBC w/automated differential (85025)

TSH (84443)

Electrolyte Panel (CPT code 80051)

Carbon dioxide (82374)

Chloride (82435)

Potassium (84132)

Sodium (84295)

Comprehensive Metabolic Panel (CPT code 80053)

Albumin (82040)

Alkaline phosphatase (84075)

Bilirubin, total (82247)

BUN (84520)

Calcium, total (82310)

Carbon dioxide (82374)

Chloride (82435)

Creatinine (82565)

Glucose (82947)

Potassium (84132)

Protein, total (84155)

Sodium (84295)

SGOT (AST) (84450)

SGPT (ALT) (84460)

Obstetric Panel (CPT code 80055)

CBC w/manual differential (80054) or CBC w/automated differential (85025)

Hepatitis B surface antigen (87340)

Rubella antibody (86762)

Syphilis test, qualitative (e.g., VDRL, RPR) (86592)

Antibody screen, RBC (86850)

Blood typing, ABO (86900) and Rh (D) (86901)

Lipid Panel (CPT code 80061)

Cholesterol (82465)

HDL cholesterol (83718) and LDL cholesterol, calculated

Triglyceride (84478)

Renal Function Panel (CPT code 80069)

Albumin (82040)

BUN (84520)

Calcium, total (82310)

Carbon dioxide (82374)

Chloride (82435)

Creatinine (82565)

Glucose (82947)

Phosphorous (84100)

Potassium (84132)

Sodium (84295)

Arthritis Panel (CPT code 80072)

Uric acid (84550)

ESR, erythrocyte sedimentation rate (85651)

Fluorescent noninfectious agent, screen (86255)

Rheumatoid factor, qualitative (86430)

Acute Hepatitis Panel (CPT code 80074)

Hepatitis A antibody, IgM (86709)

Hepatitis B core antibody, IgM (86705)

Hepatitis B surface antigen (87340)

Hepatitis C antibody (86803)

Hepatic Function Panel (CPT code 80076)

Albumin (82040)

Alkaline phosphatase (84075)

Bilirubin, direct (82248)

Bilirubin, total (82247)

Protein, total (84155)

SGOT (AST) (84450)

SGPT (ALT) (84460)

TORCH Antibody Panel (CPT code 80090)

Cytomegalovirus antibody, IgG (86644)

Herpes simplex (1 & 2) antibody, IgG (86694/86695)

Rubella antibody, IgG (86762)

Toxoplasmosis antibody (86677)

CHEMISTRY 1 PROFILE
28060 (2-87)

X PROFILE NAME

Profile 1 (general)

Glucose	Alkaline Phos.
BUN	SGOT
Bilirubin,Total	LDH
Protein,Total	Cholesterol
Albumin	A/G Ratio
Calcium	Globulin
Phosphorus	T₄
Uric Acid	

Profile 2 (thyroid)

T₃ (22%-35%) _____
T₄ (4.5-12.0 ug/ml) _____
T₇ (1.10-4.55) _____

Profile 3 (renal)

Sodium (135-148mlEq/L.) _____
Potassium (3.5-5.0Eq/L.) _____
CO₂ (24-32mmol/L) _____
Chloride (98-110mEq/L.) _____
Glucose (70-110mg/dl) _____
BUN (7-22mg/dl) _____
Creatinine (0.6-1.3mg/dl) _____

Profile 4 (hepatic)

Bilirubin,Total	Alkaline Phosphatase
Bilirubin, Direct	SGOT
Protein, Total	LDH
Albumin	A/G Ratio
	Globulin

SGPT (3.36 U/L) _____
Gamma GT (5-85 U/L) _____
Liver LDH (0-20 U/L) _____

54248

Profile 5 (lipid)

Cholesterol (140-300 mg/dl) _____
Triglyceride (30-200 mg/dl) _____
HDL Cholesterol (32-96 mg/dl) _____

Profile 6 (cardiac)

SGOT (22-47 U/L) _____
LDH (100-190 U/L) _____
CPK* (21-232 U/L) _____
*CPK Isoenzymes done
only if CPK is elevated

Ordering Physician

Nurse/Ward Clerk

Date Ordered

Profile 7 (iron)

Total Iron
Total Iron Binding
  Capacity (TIBC)
Unsaturated Iron Binding
  Capacity (UIBC)

TO BE DONE
☐ STAT
☐ ROUTINE
☐ TIME _____ AM PM
COMMENTS

Profile 8 (coagulation)

Protime PT. _____ sec
   Control _____ sec
APTT (23-33 sec) _____
Fibrinogen (177-375mg/dl) _____
Antithrombin III _____
Plasminogen _____

CHEM LOG #   AT5-7

Profile 9 (dementia)

PROFILE I (GENERAL)
B12
FOLATE
CALLED TO
CALLED BY
DATE
TIME
☐ AM ☐ PM

Collected By	Reported
Tech/Nurse	Tech
Date	Date
Time	Time
☐ AM ☐ PM	☐ AM ☐ PM

CHEMISTRY 1 PROFILE

Figure 39-3 Example of a chemistry profile of laboratory tests.

QUALITY CONTROLS/ASSURANCES IN THE LABORATORY

The accuracy of any laboratory test result depends on all safeguards being followed. These standards ensure the quality of the testing equipment, supplies, personnel, and the accuracy of the test results. There are many factors that can compromise the accuracy of laboratory test results. Among these factors are collection of specimen, temperature, amount or age of specimen, time limits of test, and using chemicals or reagents past their expiration dates. Even when laboratory guidelines are strictly followed, inaccurate results may be obtained by using test kits that have been exposed to extreme heat or cold, or using chemicals or reagents after their expiration. It is important to follow all laboratory guidelines, but the medical assistant must also confirm that the specimen, chemicals, and test kits are handled and processed properly.

Control Tests

To further ensure accurate test results, **control test** samples are tested along with the patient's sample. The control samples have a known value, negative or positive result, or abnormal or normal result, which is compared with the results of the patient's test. One of the purposes of this control measure is to minimize human error. By being able to compare a sample of known value or positive (or negative) test result with the patient's test, the health care worker performing the test can accurately determine the result. An error in the testing method may be discovered if the control sample does not test accurately.

Another purpose of the control test is to check the **reagents** or chemicals. If the control sample is not showing accurate results, it may be determined that the chemicals (reagents) are faulty or have expired.

Proficiency Testing

CLIA '88 requires laboratories to participate in an accredited proficiency program for certain identified tests (see Chapter 38 for CLIA '88 requirements). Proficiency testing is similar to quality control in that "known" proficiency samples are tested the same as patient samples. The difference is an approved outside agency evaluates the accuracy of the testing and submits the performance records to HCFA for CLIA '88 compliance.

Preventative Maintenance

Preventative maintenance helps identify potential problems before they actually occur. Procedures include manufacturer-recommended maintenance on equipment; daily temperature checks on refrigerators, freezers, and incubators; daily checks on expiration dates of reagents and supplies; and instrument log and centrifuge checks.

Instrument Validations

The quality of test results can be ensured by consistently checking the calibration and linear range of the instruments and machines. If the equipment is not maintained or is functioning improperly, accurate test results cannot be assured.

The Medical Assistant's Role

Medical assistants are educated to perform administrative office duties, prepare patients, collect specimens, and perform tests in such a manner that patients and health care personnel are safe from contamination, the patient is not harmed, the sample is reliable, and the test is accurate. These four aspects of quality laboratory testing are critical for accuracy. When the patient is prepared properly, the specimen is obtained as expertly as possible, the reagents and equipment are in the best condition and calibration possible, and the test is performed by a trained professional, the test results will be accurate.

LABORATORY REQUISITIONS AND REPORTS

A written **requisition** for laboratory work must be sent to the laboratory with the patient or with the specimen (Figure 39-4). These forms are preprinted with the most commonly requested tests separated into logical categories. Additional space is provided for writing special requests. The laboratories that patients use will be happy to provide your medical agency with these forms. Laboratory requisi-

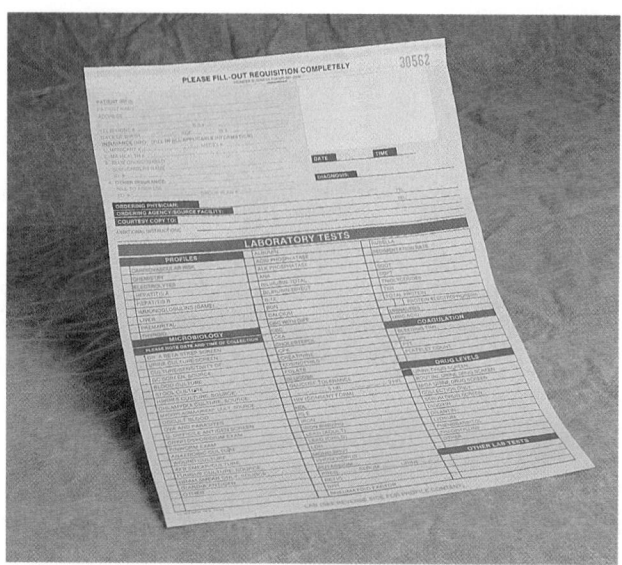

Figure 39-4 Sample laboratory requisition form.

SPOTLIGHT ON AAMA ESSENTIALS THROUGH CAAHEP

- Always try to explain a procedure to the patient in a clear and nonthreatening manner.

- Maintaining a well-run and highly efficient medical office laboratory assists all employees to function in a professional and positive manner.

- Presenting a sensitive and professional demeanor when assisting patients to obtain specimens will help the patient to take part in his or her treatment and the collection process.

tion forms are now computer-generated, and the physician-employer's name, address, and other information necessary for proper reporting and recordkeeping are often preprinted on the forms. If the requisitions are not preprinted, spaces are provided for the information to be written in. Patient information must be complete, accurate, and clearly legible. A properly completed requisition contains the following data:

- Physician's name, account number, address, and telephone number. This information is necessary in order to contact the office for any clarification or further information, and to report the results.

- Patient's name, address, and telephone number. Be sure the name is complete and spelled correctly. Avoid using alternate versions of the patient's name without also including the proper, legal name. Make certain to include apartment numbers and zip codes. This information will be used for billing purposes as well as medical records. Social Security numbers and middle initials are very helpful when it is necessary to differentiate between patients.

- Patient's billing information, insurance, and identification number. Since the patient is often not the person who is the subscriber to the insurance, the subscriber's name, address, telephone number, and insurance identification numbers are extremely important, especially if the patient does not live with the subscriber. Some patients have secondary insurance coverage. Be sure to include that data also. The laboratory would prefer to receive an additional sheet of information than to have incomplete insurance records in its business office.

- Unique patient identifier. This can be an identification number that is hospital- or laboratory-generated. In the outpatient setting this can be the patient's Social Security number or date of birth.

- Patient's age/date of birth and sex. Age and sex both influence the results of some tests and should not be assumed.

- Source of specimen. This information is especially important when dealing with tests such as cultures and biopsies. In the case of cultures, knowing the source of the specimen aids the laboratory in determining whether the specimen contains normal flora or is abnormal for that area of the body.

- Time and date of the specimen collection. Some tests require that the specimen be tested fairly quickly after leaving the body; other tests must be performed after a period of time has elapsed. The time and date of the specimen collection are important because accuracy can be compromised if the specimen is not sent to the laboratory in a reasonable amount of time.

- Test requested. This is usually a matter of putting a check mark in the appropriate box on the requisition, but it is surprising how often labs receive specimens with nicely completed requisitions and no indication of the test desired.

- Medications the patient is taking. Since medication can influence some test results, it is important that the laboratory be provided this information. Patients are often asked to refrain from taking certain medications prior to testing. Be sure to consult with the physician to verify orders.

- Clinical diagnosis. The physician's tentative diagnosis is very useful to the laboratory in helping to differentiate between diagnoses or confirm a diagnosis. The clinical diagnosis may also alert the laboratory personnel to any possible special considerations of which to be aware. For example, if diabetes is suspected, the laboratory will give special consideration to the glucose value. The diagnosis or preferably the ICD-9 code is also necessary for billing.

- Urgency of results. Sometimes the physician needs a test to be performed immediately (STAT) or would like a result as soon as possible (ASAP). The physician's orders need to be clearly stated on the requisition. Additional space is also provided for other special instructions if necessary.

- Special collection/patient instructions. Examples include fasting specimens, timed collections, and do not collect from a specific area.

The laboratory will send back a written report (Figure 39-5) that will contain the following information:

- Name, address, and telephone number of the laboratory

- Referring physician's name, address, and identification numbers

- Patient's name, identification number, age, and sex

- Date the specimen was received by the laboratory

- Date and time the specimen was collected

- Date the laboratory reported the results

- The test name, results, and normal reference ranges if applicable

When the results are received, the medical assistant should attach them to the patient's chart for the physician to review and initial before filing them. The physician should be alerted to any abnormal test results as soon as possible. Labs often send results via computer-generated reports directly to the physician's office or hospital (Figure 39-6).

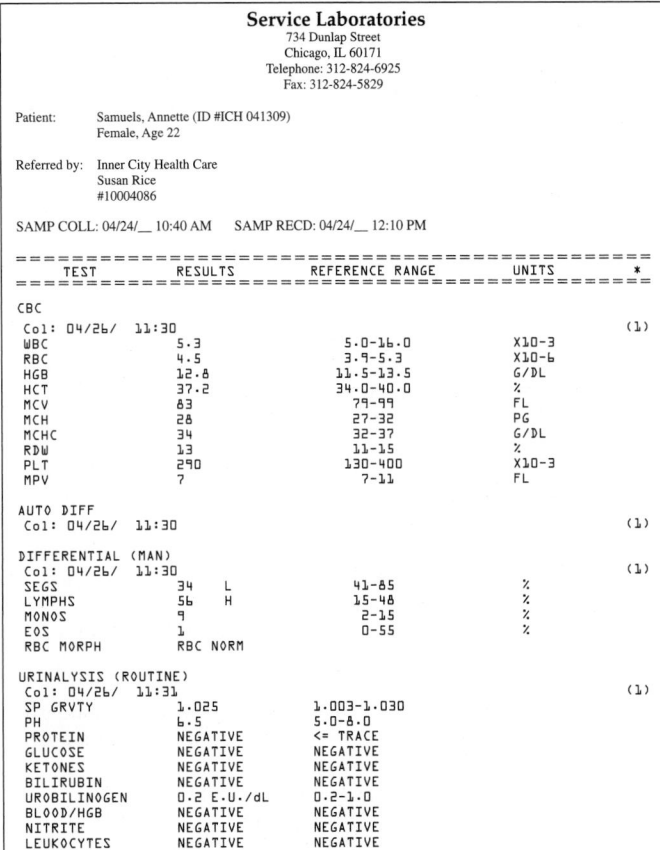

Figure 39-5 Sample computerized laboratory report.

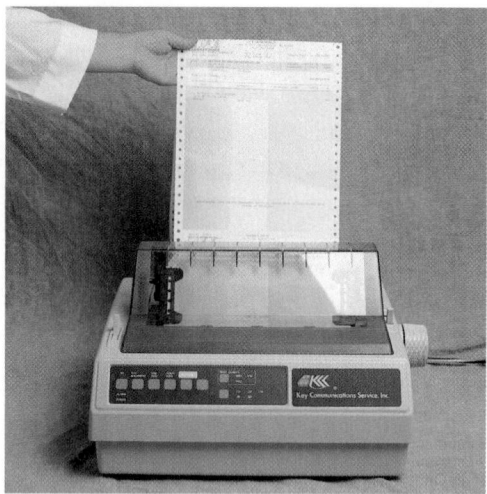

Figure 39-6 Computerized laboratory report transmitted directly from the reference lab to the physician's office.

SPECIMEN COLLECTION

Proper Procurement, Storage, and Handling

Instructions for procuring, storing, and handling and transporting laboratory specimens properly may be obtained from the independent laboratories. Most labs will provide the office/clinic with a step-by-step instruction manual (Figure 39-7) and will also be available to answer any additional questions by telephone.

Obtaining the specimen in the proper manner and using the right equipment will assure that a high-quality specimen is submitted to the laboratory. Some guidelines for specimen collection follow:

● Check the physician's orders and identify the patient.

PHLEBOTOMY GUIDELINES
(Labeling, Specimens, Patient ID, Etc.)

I. PRINCIPLE

The following sections concerning patient identification, patient information, venipuncture versus fingerstick, performing venipunctures and/or fingersticks, and potential problems are intended to establish basic guidelines. If any problems or unusual circumstances arise which are not covered, contact the main laboratory for assistance.

It must be stressed that the phlebotomists serve as laboratory representatives to the patients. A friendly, cooperative, cheerful attitude is mandatory. Please consult the Laboratory Manual, Compendium, or Central Laboratory before collecting the specimens for nonroutine procedures.

II. PHLEBOTOMY SAFETY

1. Smoking is prohibited in the patient drawing area and specimen processing area. Smoking is annoying to some patients, the burning cigarette is an ignition source to flammable liquids (such as alcohol), and the handling of cigarettes from bench to mouth is a route of exposure for potentially hazardous or infectious materials.
2. Laboratory coats are provided and must be worn when drawing or processing patient specimens.
3. Disposable laboratory gloves must be worn for patient contact or specimen handling. Gloves should be changed between patients or when they become soiled or damaged. They should be disposed of in the biohazard bag. If skin lesions are present on the hands (cuts, abrasions, punctures, burns, eczema, blisters, sores, etc.), the lesions should be covered with a bacteriostatic ointment such as Neosporin, and bandaged before putting on gloves.
4. Protective eye goggles/face shields should be worn when popping open specimen stoppers because of aerosols which may result. A piece of gauze wrapped over the specimen stopper as it is removed will also decrease aerosols. Standard eyeglasses do not provide the necessary protection and are not to be used in place of goggles/face shields.
5. Specimen spills are to be cleaned up immediately with a dilute bleach solution. If specimens spill on your lab coat, clean the area with soap and water, and then disinfect with bleach solution. If a spill soaks through to your street clothes, they should be removed and the area affected washed imme-

diately. Spills on countertops or centrifuges should be cleaned immediately with dilute bleach. All processing countertops should be wiped down routinely with dilute bleach at the end of each day.

A dilute bleach solution is prepared by adding one (1) part of household bleach (e.g., Clorox®) to nine (9) parts of water.
6. Needles should be used for phlebotomy only, and should never be recapped, cut, or bent. After use, they should be placed in a labeled, puncture-resistant container. When full, the container should be sealed and discarded into the biohazardous waste container. Never discard needles directly into the biohazardous waste container or empty full needle containers into the waste.
7. All contaminated waste (gloves, test tubes, bandages, cotton, towels, etc.) should be discarded in clearly labeled biohazard bags. When the bag becomes approximately two-thirds full, it should be securely tied to prevent spillage. All bags are picked up by a licensed waste disposal company for proper disposal. When the waste disposal company removes the waste, they will leave a paper called a "Hazardous Waste Manifest." All manifests must be kept on file at the drawstation.
8. Do not centrifuge uncapped tubes. Always make sure a centrifuge is on a level surface and properly balanced before turning it on.

III. PROCEDURE

A. Patient Identification
All patients must be identified on the test tube label.

B. Patient Information
It is the physician's responsibility to inform the patient of the necessity for the laboratory tests ordered. If questioned, the phlebotomist should refer any and all questions to the physician.

C. Requisition Information
A properly completed requisition should contain the following information:
  a. Name of patient
  b. Sex and age of patient
  c. Requesting physician
  d. Type of test(s) to be performed
  e. Time and date of collection

Figure 39-7 Sample laboratory manual page. (Courtesy of Whatcom Pathology Laboratory, Bellingham, WA)

- Refer to the laboratory instruction manual or consult the laboratory for specific collection instructions.
- Instruct the patient in any necessary dietary restriction.
- Instruct the patient to ingest special food or take other substances if required.
- Select or provide to the patient appropriate containers with the proper preservatives in them, if required.
- Be certain to label the specimen with the patient's name, identification number, date, type of specimen, time of collection, and physician's name. Label the container, not the lid, since the lid will be removed during testing. Label the container, not the wrapping, since the wrapping will be separated from the container when testing is performed, e.g., throat swabs.
- Obtain the specimen or instruct the patient to provide the specimen according to the directions given by the laboratory.
- Follow applicable OSHA blood-borne pathogens guidelines (refer to Chapter 22) when packaging the specimen for transport so it will not leak or contaminate the courier or other office staff and so that it will safely arrive at the laboratory without being damaged or destroyed (Figure 39-8).

Processing and Sending Specimens to a Laboratory

Specimens collected by the medical assistant are often sent from the office to a laboratory many miles away or are picked up by a courier representing the outside laboratory. These are often large commercial laboratories that are not associated with a local hospital laboratory. The patient's

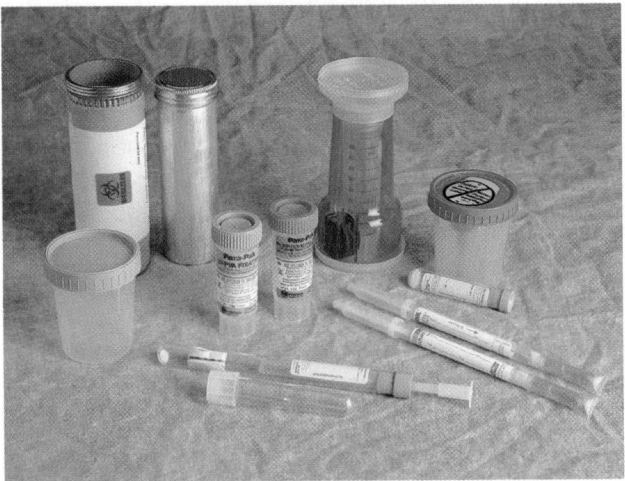

Figure 39-8 Various types of collection and transport containers used for laboratory specimens.

insurance often dictates the laboratory contracted to perform the patient's testing. It is not unusual for several different laboratories to pick up at one location. A situation could be that the blood work from patient Jones would go to laboratory A, the blood work from patient Smith would go to laboratory B, and a urine sample from patient Doe would be tested in the laboratory within the building. It sometimes can be confusing as to where to send the specimen.

All these laboratory test results are dependent on the quality of the specimen submitted. The quality of the specimen depends on the patient preparation, proper collection, correct patient identification, and transportation of the specimen. If there is any doubt or question regarding the type of specimen to be collected, it is imperative that the appropriate laboratory be called to clarify the specimen needed. There are often differences between laboratories; the type of specimen acceptable for one laboratory is not necessarily the acceptable specimen for another laboratory.

Serum Blood Collection. Most laboratory tests are performed on serum, plasma, or whole blood. Generally, when a serum sample is needed, a serum separator tube is used. There will be certain restrictions in some cases. When using a serum separator tube, several steps must be followed:

1. Perform venipuncture by the preferred method (refer to Chapter 40).
2. Invert the tube 5 times to activate the clotting.
3. Allow the tube to clot upright in a rack for at least 30 minutes but no longer than an hour.

4. Centrifuge the tube at 2,500 rpm for 15 minutes.
5. Store the tube upright or transfer the serum to a plastic transport vial for pickup by the laboratory. There will be different requirements for different laboratories.

NOTE: Do not use serum separator tubes for therapeutic drug monitoring or for toxicological studies. The gel has a tendency to lower the levels of constituents being tested. Collect the sample in a plain, red-top, evacuated tube. Remove the serum immediately after centrifugation and place the serum in a plastic transport vial.

Plasma and Whole Blood Collection. Tubes containing an anticoagulant are used to collect plasma and whole blood samples. There are a variety of different anticoagulant tubes that can be used. The anticoagulant needed in the tube will be specified by the laboratory that will be testing the specimen. The anticoagulant is denoted by the color of the stopper of the tube. Preparing the plasma specimen for transport or testing is similar to specimen serum preparation.

1. Perform venipuncture by the preferred method (refer to Chapter 40).
2. Invert the tube 8–10 times to mix the blood with the anticoagulant.
3. Centrifuge the tube at 2,500 rpm for 10 minutes.
4. Transfer the plasma to a plastic transport vial for pickup by the laboratory. Do not allow any blood cells to mix with the plasma specimen. Indicate the specimen is a plasma specimen and what type of anticoagulant tube was used. There will be different requirements for different laboratories.

To prepare the whole blood specimen for transport or testing:

1. Perform venipuncture by the preferred method (refer to Chapter 40).
2. Invert the tube 8–10 times to mix the blood with the anticoagulant.
3. Maintain the tube at room temperature unless otherwise instructed. Never freeze a whole blood sample unless specifically instructed to do so.

Urine Collection. For routine analysis and microscopic examination, a clean-catch midstream random urine is usually collected. The specimen is usually collected at the time of the patient's office visit.

1. With an antiseptic wipe, have the patient clean the glans (tip) of the penis for a male, or the labia for a female.
2. Following cleansing, rinse using a second antiseptic wipe to the area.
3. Void a small amount of urine in the toilet bowl.

4. Continue to void and collect the urine in a sterile urine collection cup. Instruct the patient not to touch the specimen cup on the inside or touch their body or clothing to the cup.
5. Carefully place the lid onto the specimen container. Screw the lid tightly to prevent leakage.
6. Give the urine to the medical assistant.

A 24-hour urine may also need to be collected. It is essential that the patient be thoroughly instructed in the proper method of collection to ensure the most accurate results. Some 24-hour urines require the addition of hydrochloric acid to the collection container before the start of the collection. Have the patient collect the urine in a smaller collection container and then pour the urine into the larger container to avoid acid burns to the patient. The collection procedure follows:

1. The patient should maintain the same amount of fluid intake as normal.
2. During collection, the urine should be kept in a refrigerator or a cool place.
3. At the start of the 24-hour collection, have the patient empty his or her bladder with the first morning void but do not include this urine in the 24-hour collection.
4. Collect the next voiding and all other urine voids for the next 24-hour period.
5. The last sample should be the following first morning void.
6. The total volume of urine is measured by the medical assistant. An aliquot of the urine is then poured into a transport container and sent to the laboratory with the total 24-hour volume noted. It is important to note the dates and times of collection. Some 24-hour urine tests require a corresponding blood test, e.g., creatinine clearance, to be collected during the collection period. Verify specific collection requirements with the testing laboratory.

Feces Collection. Fecal specimens are required for a variety of laboratory tests. Various collection containers are provided by the laboratory depending on the specific test. Sterile urine collection cups can be used to collect random specimens for culture and examination for cells. Special collection cups containing formalin are used for ova and parasite testing. Mailing kits for the detection of occult blood are available to patients for ease of collection. As with all patient self-collections, detailed written instructions need to be reviewed with the patient. A special preweighed container is used for timed feces collection. As with the 24-hour urine collection, an aliquot of the feces is sent to the laboratory with the total weight recorded.

MICROSCOPES

One of the most used pieces of equipment in the medical laboratory is the microscope. Consisting of a light source, eyepieces, objectives, condenser, and diaphragm, the microscope enables us to see bacteria and other microorganisms that are much too small to be seen without magnification.

Types of Microscopes

The most commonly used microscope in the clinic is the compound microscope (Figure 39-9). As the name indicates, the image is compounded by the use of two different lenses. One lens compounds or increases the magnification produced by the other lens. The first lens system is located in the objectives and the second lens system is in the eyepiece (ocular). The light source is a bulb in the base. The light is directed up through the specimen on the slide and into the objective lenses. The light, or image, is then reflected by the condenser onto the specimen to the ocular lenses for visualization.

The eyepiece may have a single (monocular) lens, or there may be two (binocular) lenses. This lens is not adjustable or changeable. The magnification in the eyepiece is usually ten times (10X) the normal size of the object being viewed.

The objective lenses are adjustable between low power, high power, and oil immersion. The low-power objective lens allows the item being viewed to be magnified ten times larger than life. This magnification combined with the ten times magnification of the ocular lens allows us to see microscopically one hundred times the normal size (10X × 10X = 100X).

By combining the ten-power (10X) ocular lens with the high-power objective lens, which has the magnification power of forty-four times life (44X), we are able to increase our magnification vision to four hundred and forty times the normal size (10X × 44X = 440X). This is enough magnification to see large microorganisms, but it is still not enough to see smaller organisms, such as bacteria, clearly. An oil-immersion lens is needed to view bacteria closely.

The oil-immersion lens enables us to multiply the ocular lens magnification (10X) by one hundred (100X) to reach a possible total magnification of one thousand times normal life size (10X × 100X = 1,000X). Because more light is needed to actually see this amount of magnification, the lens is immersed in oil. This prevents the scattering and loss of light rays, which naturally occurs when light travels through air, consequently increasing the efficiency of the magnification.

Other types of microscopes have been developed especially for specific uses. One is the phase contrast microscope specifically designed for viewing specimens that are transparent and unstained. Some microscopic specimens must be stained with a fluorescent dye in order to be examined in detail (for example, when detecting specific bacteria). A fluorescent microscope is the instrument best suited for viewing those specimens. In dark-field microscopy, the light is reflected from an angle, which causes the specimen to appear as a bright object on a dark field.

Another type of microscope is the electron microscope (Figure 39-10). Special training is required to operate this very sophisticated instrument. The electron microscope is very large (several feet tall) and expensive; therefore, it is only found in larger regional and hospital laboratories. An electronic beam, rather than light, is passed through the specimen. The image is projected onto a fluorescent screen and may then be photographed and enlarged. Using the electron microscope enables us to view extremely small organisms, such as viruses, in great detail and in three dimensions. Figure 39-11 illustrates blood cells seen using an electron microscope.

How to Use a Microscope

Besides being able to adjust a microscope's magnification, it may be necessary to adjust focus. The microscope contains a coarse adjustment and a fine adjustment. The coarse adjustment is to be used with the low-power (short) objective only. The coarse adjustment is used to bring the object into view. The fine adjustment may then be used to sharpen the image. Depending on the individual microscope, the coarse and fine adjustments may raise and lower the nosepiece, which houses the objectives, or they may raise and lower the stage, or platform, on which the slide rests.

It is important always to remember to raise the platform of the lower objectives using the coarse adjustment and the low-power objective *while viewing the slide from the side*. This allows the lens to come close to the slide without

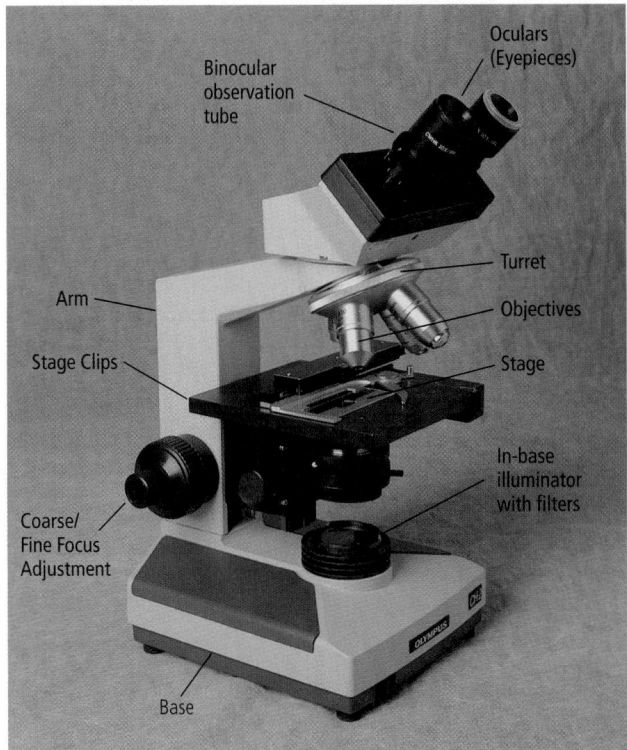

Figure 39-9 Compound microscope.

(image labels: Oculars (Eyepieces); Binocular observation tube; Turret; Objectives; Stage; In-base illuminator with filters; Arm; Stage Clips; Coarse/Fine Focus Adjustment; Base)

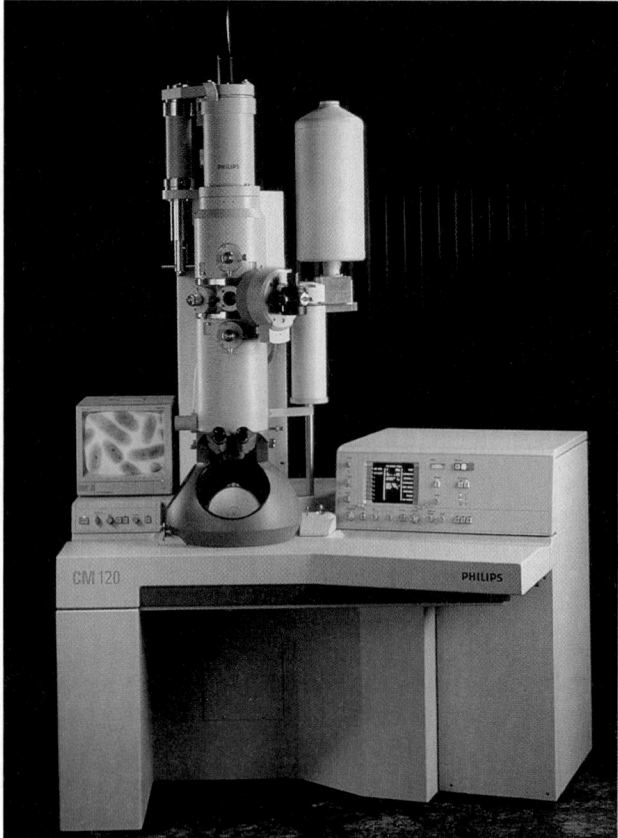

Figure 39-10   S440 scanning electron microscope. (Courtesy of Philips Electronic Instruments Co.)

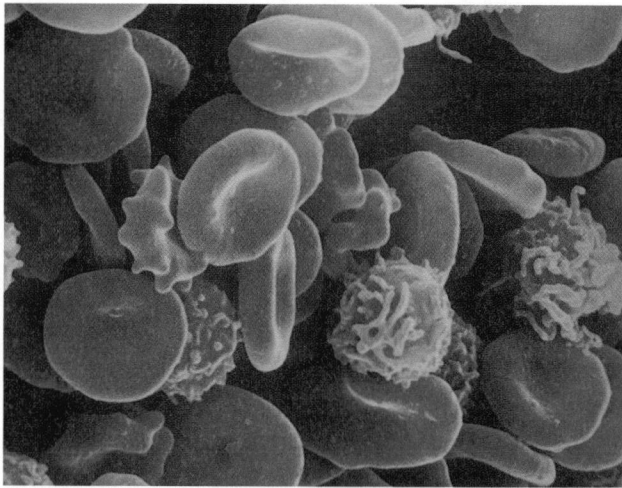

Figure 39-11   Blood cells as seen under an electron microscope. (Courtesy of Philips Electronic Instruments Co.)

- Always follow the manufacturer's and clinic's rules for the care and maintenance of the microscopes.
- Carry the microscope with one hand securely supporting the base and the other hand holding the arm (Figure 39-12).
- Keep the microscope covered when it is not being used.
- Clean the lenses with special lens paper and lens cleaner after each use. Using standard tissue can scratch the lenses.
- Always focus away from the lens to prevent the lens from coming into contact with the slide.
- Use oil only with the oil-immersion lens.

actually touching it. If the slide is not viewed from the side for the coarse adjustment, there is the possibility of running the objective through the slide and seriously damaging the lens and the microscope. After bringing the slide and objective together, the adjustments may be made through the ocular, always moving away from the slide. Once the item is in view, the fine adjustment may be used for clarity.

The bulb in the base, which directs light through the slide, first goes through a condenser and then through an iris diaphragm. The condenser is used to control the intensity of the light and the iris diaphragm may be adjusted to control the amount of light.

To use the oil-immersion lens, place a drop of cedar or mineral oil on top of the cover slip directly over the specimen on the slide. Then carefully lower the oil-immersion lens into the oil, making sure that the lens never actually touches the slide.

How to Care for a Microscope

Microscopes can be very expensive and, like any precision instrument, should be treated with care. Some practices that will extend the life of a microscope and maintain the quality of its performance are:

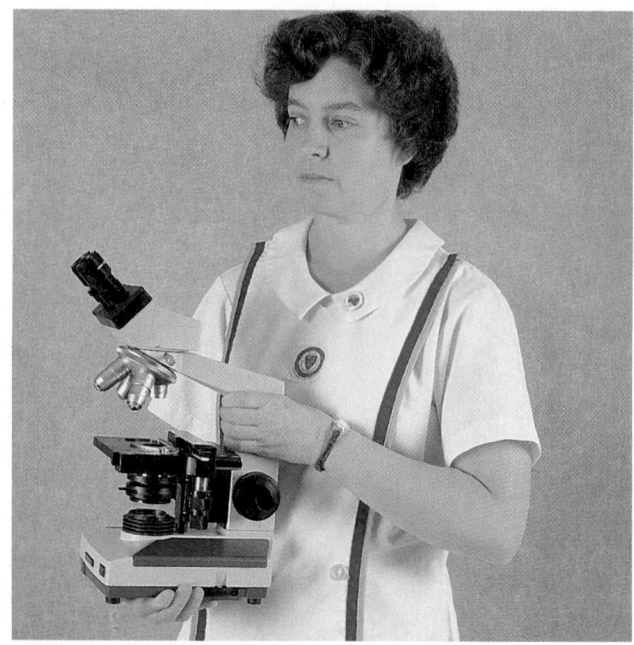

Figure 39-12   Proper way to carry a microscope.

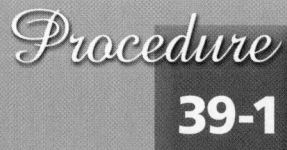

39-1 Using the Microscope

STANDARD PRECAUTIONS:

PURPOSE:

To properly use a microscope to view microscopic organisms using the coarse and fine adjustments as well as the low- and high-power objectives.

EQUIPMENT/SUPPLIES:

Hand disinfectant
Microscope (monocular or binocular)
Lens paper
Lens cleaner
Prepared slides (commercially available)
Immersion oil
Surface disinfectant
Note: Procedure will vary slightly according to microscope design. Consult the operating procedure in the microscope manual for specific instructions.

PROCEDURE STEPS:

1. Wash hands.
2. Assemble equipment and materials.
3. Clean the ocular(s) and objectives with lens paper.
4. Use the coarse adjustment to raise the nosepiece unit.
5. Raise the condenser as far as possible by turning the condenser knob.
6. Rotate the 10X, or low-power, objective into position, so that it is directly over the opening in the stage.
7. Turn on the microscope light.
8. Open the diaphragm until maximum light comes up through the condenser.
9. Place the slide on the stage (specimen side up) and secure with clips. The condenser should be positioned so that it is almost touching the bottom of the slide.
10. Locate the coarse adjustment.
11. Look directly at the stage and 10X objective and turn the coarse adjustment until the objective is as close to the slide as it will go. Stop turning when the objective no longer moves.
    Note: Do not lower any objective toward a slide while looking through the ocular(s).

12. Look into the ocular(s) and slowly turn the coarse adjustment in the opposite direction (as in step 11) to raise the objective (or lower the stage) until the object on the slide comes into view.
13. Locate the fine adjustment.
14. Turn the fine adjustment to sharpen the image.
    Note: If a binocular microscope is used, the oculars must be adjusted for each individual's eyes.
    a. Adjust the distance between the oculars so that one image is seen (as when using binoculars).
    b. Use the coarse and fine adjustments to bring the object into focus while looking through the right ocular with the right eye.
    c. Close the right eye, look into the left ocular with the left eye, and *use the knurled collar on the left ocular* to bring the object into sharp focus. (Do not turn the coarse or fine adjustment at this time.)
    d. Look into the oculars with both eyes to observe that the object is in clear focus. If it is not, repeat the procedure.
15. Scan the slide by either method:
    a. Use the stage knobs to move the slide left and right and backward and forward while looking through the ocular(s),
    or
    b. Move the slide with the fingers while looking through the ocular(s) (for microscope without movable stage).
16. Rotate the high-power (40X) objective into position while observing the objective and the slide to see that the objective does not strike the slide.
17. Look through the ocular(s) to view the object on the slide; it should be almost in focus.
18. Locate the fine adjustment.
19. Look through the ocular(s) and turn the fine adjustment until the object is in focus. Do not use the coarse adjustment.
20. Adjust the amount of light. This can be done by closing the diaphragm, lowering the condenser, or adjusting the light at the source.
21. Scan the slide as in step 15, using the fine adjustment if necessary to keep the object in focus.
22. Rotate the oil-immersion objective to the side slightly (so that no objective is in position).

(continues)

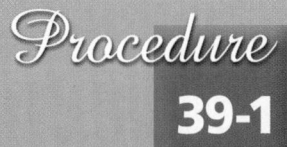

Procedure 39-1 *(continued)*

23. Place one drop of immersion oil on the portion of the slide that is directly over the condenser.
24. Rotate the oil-immersion objective into position, being careful not to rotate the 40X objective through the oil.
25. Look to see that the oil-immersion objective is touching the drop of oil.
26. Look through the ocular(s) and slowly turn the fine adjustment until the image is clear. Use only the fine adjustment to focus the oil-immersion objective.
27. Adjust the amount of light using the procedure in step 20.
28. Scan the slide using the procedure in step 15.
29. Rotate the 10X objective into position (do not allow the 40X objective to touch the oil).
30. Remove the slide from the microscope stage and gently clean the oil from the slide with lens paper.

A copeland jar containing a solvent cleaner, such as xylene, can be used to remove excess oil from the slide.

31. Clean the oculars, 10X objective, and 40X objective with clean lens paper and lens cleaner.
32. Clean the 100X objective with lens paper and lens cleaner to remove all oil.
33. Clean any oil from the microscope stage and condenser.
34. Turn off the microscope light and disconnect.
35. Position the nosepiece in the lowest position using the coarse adjustment.
36. Center the stage so that it does not project from either side of the microscope.
37. Cover the microscope and return it to storage.
38. Clean the work area; return slides to storage.
39. Wash hands.

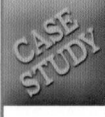

CASE STUDY

39-1

Edith Leonard came to Inner City Health Care because she was experiencing sight failure, constant thirst, and fainting spells. After examining Edith, Dr. Ray Reynolds ordered a glucose tolerance test. Certified medical assistant Wanda Slawson gave Edith a special diet that she was to follow for the three days preceding the test and instructions regarding fasting before the test.

Edith has returned to the clinic to have the test. "Did you follow the diet I gave you, Mrs. Leonard?" Wanda asks. "Yes, I did." "Did you have anything to eat this morning?" "No, but I did have a cup of coffee. I thought it would be all right because I drink it black. I can't start the day without my coffee."

CASE STUDY REVIEW

1. Should Wanda perform the test? Explain your answer.
2. How can Wanda emphasize the importance of following the diet, fasting, and test instructions?
3. What can Wanda do to try to ensure Edith's cooperation?

SUMMARY

If disease did not exist, we would have little need for clinical laboratories. If we were not susceptible to viral illnesses, if bacteria never infected our bodies, if our bodies always operated in their healthiest state regardless of what we did to them, and, perhaps most important of all, if we chose our parents wisely, there would be little that a clinical laboratory would be asked to do. The fact that our bodies are susceptible to disease necessitates the existence of clinical laboratories.

Along with clinical laboratory personnel, medical assistants play an important role in laboratory testing. They prepare patients for tests, obtain specimens, and perform simple, routine tests or send specimens to the appropriate laboratory. Medical assistants are educated to perform these tasks in a manner that ensures the accuracy of the test and safeguards the health of patients and health care personnel.

REVIEW QUESTIONS

Multiple Choice

1. All of the following statements concerning point-of-care testing (POCT) are true *except:*
   a. performed at the patient's bedside
   b. must be performed by certified laboratory professionals
   c. provides for rapid, accurate results
   d. the medical laboratory's role includes training and management of quality control
2. Independent medical laboratories must be managed by a:
   a. clinical laboratory technologist
   b. pathologist
   c. clinical laboratory technician
   d. medical assistant
3. The hematology department of a laboratory:
   a. studies microorganisms and their activities
   b. studies blood and blood-forming tissues
   c. detects the presence of disease-producing human parasites or eggs present in specimens taken from the body
   d. detects the presence of abnormal cells
4. The quality of patient test results is maintained by:
   a. instrument calibration procedures
   b. preventative maintenance procedures
   c. quality control testing
   d. all of the above
5. When a patient or specimen is sent to a laboratory for testing, the medical assistant also sends:
   a. a written requisition
   b. a report
   c. the patient's file
   d. an insurance form
6. The most commonly used microscope in the clinic is the:
   a. fluorescent microscope
   b. electron microscope
   c. phase contrast microscope
   d. compound microscope

Critical Thinking

1. A patient asks you to recommend a laboratory for the tests ordered by the physician. How will you respond to the request? What are some factors that will influence your response?
2. A patient performed a pregnancy test at home, but the physician has requested a pregnancy test in the office. Explain to the patient why the home test may not be as accurate as the test performed in the office.
3. Discuss the differences in education between a clinical laboratory technologist, a clinical laboratory technician, and a medical assistant.
4. The physician has ordered a chemistry profile for a patient. What is a profile and how will it help the physician to diagnose the patient's condition?
5. Explain why it is important to handle and process specimens, test kits, and chemicals properly.
6. Discuss the medical assistant's role in laboratory testing and how it affects the accuracy of test results.
7. The time and date of specimen collection were not included on the requisition form. Why is this data always important to the laboratory?
8. You have been asked to collect a plasma sample for testing at an independent laboratory. Describe how you will collect the sample. How will you determine which anticoagulant is needed in the tube?
9. Describe how to use a microscope to observe microscopic organisms.
10. Explain how a compound microscope is able to magnify.

WEB ACTIVITIES

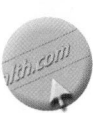

1. For each group of laboratory personnel discussed in this chapter, search the Internet for a web site that pertains to it. What kind of information does it offer?
2. Locate a local hospital's web site. Does it outline all the specialty departments described in this chapter? What unique services do they offer?
3. Visit your insurance company's web site. Does it specify which labs must be used?

REFERENCES/BIBLIOGRAPHY

Bonewit-West, K. (1995). *Clinical procedures for medical assistants* (4th ed.). Philadephia: W. B. Saunders Company.

Henry, J. B. (1996). *Clinical diagnosis and management by laboratory methods* (19th ed.). Philadelphia: W. B. Saunders Company.

Lane, K. (1993). *Saunders manual of medical assisting practice.* Philadelphia: W. B. Saunders Company.

Marshall, J. (1993). *Fundamental skills for the clinical laboratory professional.* Albany, NY: Delmar.

Walters, N. J., Estridge, B. H., & Reynolds, A. P. (2000). *Basic medical laboratory techniques* (4th ed.). Albany, NY: Delmar.

Wedding, M. E., & Toenjes, S. A. (1998). *Medical laboratory procedures* (2nd ed.). Philadelphia: F. A. Davis Company.

Chapter 40

PHLEBOTOMY: VENIPUNCTURE AND CAPILLARY PUNCTURE

KEY TERMS

Additive
Aliquot
Anticoagulant
Buffy Coat
Cannula
Centrifuge
Constrict
Dilate
Edematous
Erythrocyte
Hematoma
Hemoconcentration
Hemolysis
Hypoglycemia
Integrity
Leukocyte
Luer
Lipemia
Oxygenated
Palpate
Phlebotomy
Plasma
Primary Container
Serum
Thixotrophic Separator Gel
Thrombocyte
Tourniquet
Venipuncture
Viscosity

OUTLINE

OBJECTIVES

The student should strive to meet the following performance objectives and demonstrate an understanding of the facts and principles presented in this chapter through written and oral communication.

1. Define the key terms as presented in the glossary.

2. Explain the medical assistant's responsibility to the patient in terms of quality of care and respect of the patient as a human being.

3. Explain why the medical assistant has a special responsibility to present a neat, pleasant, and competent demeanor.

4. Differentiate between serum and plasma.   (*continues*)

5. State the relationship between diameter and the gauge of the needle.
6. Explain the principle of the evacuated tube system.
7. State the manner in which anticoagulants prevent coagulation.
8. Name the anticoagulant associated with the various color-coded evacuated tubes.
9. State the purpose of additives to evacuated tubes.
10. Explain the three skills used in collecting blood specimen.
11. Explain the importance of correct patient identification, complete specimen labeling, and proper handling, storage and delivery.
12. Explain how a tourniquet makes the veins more prominent.
13. Describe the step-by-step procedure for drawing blood with a syringe, evacuated tube system, butterfly, or capillary puncture.
14. Explain how to handle the various reactions a patient might have to venipuncture.

ROLE DELINEATION COMPONENTS

CLINICAL

Fundamental Principles

- Apply principles of aseptic technique and infection control
- Comply with quality assurance practices
- Screen and follow up patient test results

Diagnostic Orders

- Collect and process specimens
- Perform diagnostic tests

GENERAL (TRANSDISCIPLINARY)

Legal Concepts

- Document accurately
- Comply with established risk management and safety procedures

SCENARIO

At Inner City Health Care, medical assistant Bruce Goldman often performs venipunctures. Bruce is personable and has an easy-going manner that makes patients feel comfortable with him. He takes time to talk to patients before performing a venipuncture to determine their feelings about the procedure and to learn about their previous experiences. Bruce is confident and professional in his interactions with patients. He is always well-groomed and he treats patients with respect. Using his social, technical, and administrative skills, Bruce is usually able to collect the necessary blood samples while providing a positive experience for patients.

INTRODUCTION

The task of collecting blood samples from patients for diagnostic testing is known as phlebotomy. The health care professional who performs this duty varies at each health care setting. The task of phlebotomy is not restricted to one individual. A variety of individuals are cross trained to do phlebotomy and other tasks. Many health care settings do not have enough patients to justify having a phlebotomist available at all times. Therefore, the medical assistant may be designated to perform phlebotomies.

WHY COLLECT BLOOD?

Phlebotomy is the process of collecting blood or bloodletting as a therapeutic measure. The history of bloodletting dates back to the early Egyptians and continues into modern times. Phlebotomy in the past was a method to cure individuals with "bad" blood. The blood was drained out of individuals as a treatment, thereby alleviating the patient's symptoms. Phlebotomy is now used to help determine the disease process taking place and to determine the method of treatment. Without the collection of blood samples, physicians would have few means available to assist them in making diagnoses.

THE MEDICAL ASSISTANT'S ROLE IN PHLEBOTOMY

A phlebotomist is a person trained to obtain blood specimens by venipuncture and capillary puncture techniques. The phlebotomist's primary role is to collect blood as efficiently as possible for accurate and reliable test results. How the medical assistant will be involved in phlebotomy will vary greatly from one health care environment to another. The medical assistant performing venipuncture will directly contact the patient, and perform tasks that are critical to the patient's diagnosis and care. During the direct contact with the patient, the medical assistant will leave an impression with the patient. It can be positive or negative depending on the skill with which the medical assistant performs the venipuncture.

It is the medical assistant's responsibility to provide high-quality care to patients. The medical assistant must act professionally when working with patients. Professionalism is displayed by performing tasks in an efficient, competent manner, wearing clean, neat attire, and showing concern for patients and their feelings.

Patients will not tell family and friends that their blood was run through expensive state-of-the-art instruments but rather that the person drawing their blood sample was friendly and skilled. A smile and a kind word can allay a patient's fear and do a lot to win a permanent customer and patient to the physician's office.

ANATOMY AND PHYSIOLOGY OF THE CIRCULATORY SYSTEM

To be prepared to collect blood, the medical assistant must understand the system that carries the blood and the composition of the blood. The system in which the blood is transported is the circulatory system. Blood forms in the organs of the body. The bone marrow is the primary factory for production of blood cells. The lymph nodes, thymus, and spleen are also sites for the production of blood cells. The function of blood is to carry oxygen to body tissues and to remove the waste product carbon dioxide. The blood also carries nutrients to all parts of the body and moves the waste products to the lungs, kidneys, liver, and skin for elimination.

The circulatory system consists of the heart, which pumps blood through the body by way of tubing called arteries, veins, and capillaries. When blood flows away from the heart, it flows in arteries. Blood flowing back to the heart flows through the veins. Connecting most of the arteries and veins are the capillaries (Figure 40-1).

ARTERIES VERSUS VEINS	
Arteries	**Veins**
1. Carry blood from the heart, carry oxygenated blood (except pulmonary artery)	1. Carry blood to the heart, carry deoxygenated blood (except pulmonary vein)
2. Normally bright red in color	2. Normally dark red in color
3. Elastic walls that expand with surge of blood	3. Thin walls/less elastic
4. No valves	4. Valves
5. Can feel a pulse	5. No pulse

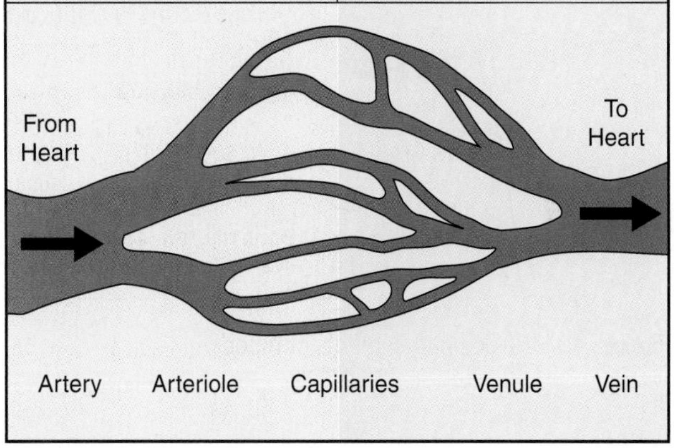

Figure 40-1 Blood flows from the heart through the arteries and back to the heart through the veins.

Arteries have a thick wall that helps them withstand the pressure of the pumping action of the heart. The arteries branch to form arterioles, which branch again to become capillaries. The capillaries then begin coming together to form venules and the venules then become veins. As blood flows through the body, it follows this path of artery-arteriole-capillary-venule-vein. **Oxygenated** arterial blood, which contains a high level of oxygen, leaves the heart and carries the oxygen to the tissue by releasing the oxygen through the cell walls of the capillaries. At the same time, carbon dioxide is being absorbed by the blood and then transported to the lungs to be exhaled as a waste product. The flow of the blood also regulates body temperature. When the body gets warm, the capillaries in the extremities **dilate** and let off heat. This process then cools the body. If the body becomes cold, the capillaries **constrict** and less blood flows through, thereby conserving heat for the rest of the body.

The body contains approximately 6 liters (l) of blood, 45 percent of which is formed elements. The formed cellular elements consist of **erythrocytes, leukocytes,** and **thrombocytes** (Figure 40-2). The remaining

	White Blood Cell (Leukocyte)	Red Blood Cells (Erythrocyte)	Platelet (Thrombocyte)
Function	Body defense (extravascular)	Transport of oxygen and carbon dioxide (intravascular)	Stoppage of bleeding
Formation	Bone marrow, lymphatic tissue	Bone marrow	Bone marrow
Size/shape	9–16 micrometers; different size, shape, color, nucleus (core)	6–7 micrometers; bioconcave disc. Normally no nucleus in circulatory blood	1–4 micrometers; fragments of megakaryocytes
Life cycle	Varies, 24 hours–years	100–120 days	9–12 days
Numbers	5–10,000/ cubic millimeter	4.5–5.5 million/ cubic millimeter	250–450,000/ cubic millimeter
Removal	Bone marrow, liver, spleen	Bone marrow, spleen	Spleen

Figure 40-2   Cellular elements of blood.

55 percent of the blood is liquid. Generally 2 milliliters (ml) of blood will yield about 1 milliliter of fluid. The liquid portion of uncoagulated blood is known as plasma. Blood flowing through the body contains a substance called fibrinogen. The clotting process converts the fibrinogen into fibrin. The fibrin is like a sticky spider web that traps the formed elements into the fibrin mass called a clot. The clot then contracts and the liquid (serum) portion is extracted. The serum is a clear straw-colored liquid that is used for many of the tests done in the laboratory. The main difference between serum and plasma is that plasma contains fibrinogen, serum does not.

The formed elements and the liquid portion of the blood are often separated for laboratory testing. To speed the removal of the serum from a tube of blood, an instrument called a **centrifuge** spins the blood. A carrier holds the tubes of blood and when the centrifuge is activated, the carrier spins. The spinning action of the carrier pushes the blood cells to the bottom of the tube. The blood separates according to weight. The clot goes to the bottom of the tube and the serum goes to the top.

To produce a plasma specimen, the blood must be prevented from clotting by the use of a chemical anticoagulant. Blood collected in a tube containing an anticoagulant can be centrifuged to separate the formed elements (cells) from the plasma. The bottom layer will contain the erythrocytes, then there will be a thin layer called the buffy coat. The buffy coat contains a mixture of leukocytes and thrombocytes. On top of all these layers is the plasma layer. The plasma will contain fibrinogen and usually is slightly hazy (Figure 40-3).

Collection of Blood Samples

The most commonly used method for blood collection is venipuncture. To obtain a blood sample, the medical

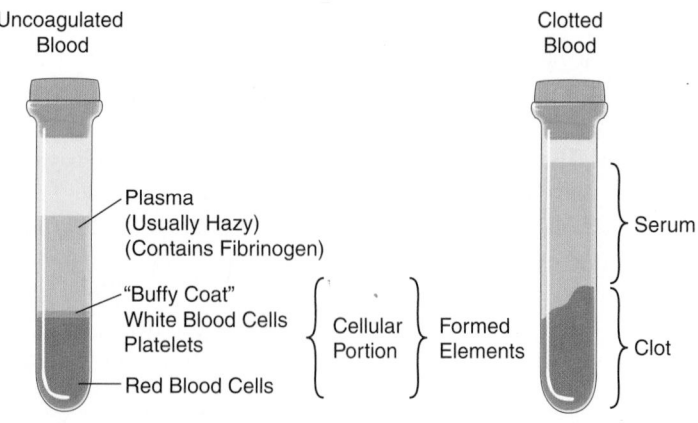

Figure 40-3   Blood tubes.

assistant must locate a vein that is acceptable for blood collection. The preferred site for venipuncture is the antecubital fossa, which is located anterior to the elbow on the inside of the arm. The veins are near the surface and are large enough to give access to the blood (Figure 40-4). The median cubital vein is the vein that is used the majority of the time. When this vein is not available, any of the other veins that can be felt may be used. These veins include the basilic, cephalic, and median veins. When necessary, veins on the dorsal surface of the hand or wrist may be used for venipuncture, but they are more painful for the patient and may require a smaller needle or the use of a butterfly apparatus.

The veins of the feet are an alternative when the arms are not available. A physician's permission is needed before drawing blood from the veins of the legs and feet.

The physician may not want the patient's leg or foot veins punctured because the act of drawing blood may cause clots to form. These clots then have the possibility of dislodging and causing a blockage elsewhere in the body. It would be extremely rare for a medical assistant to use this location. A phlebotomist or registered nurse in the physician's office should be consulted before a foot puncture is considered.

The arteries in the arm consist of the brachial artery in the brachial region of the arm and the radial and ulnar arteries in the wrist (Figure 40-5). Special techniques are necessary to puncture arteries to obtain a blood specimen for the examination of gases absorbed by the blood. Arterial punctures and the techniques used to draw blood from these locations for blood gas testing are not generally done by a medical assistant.

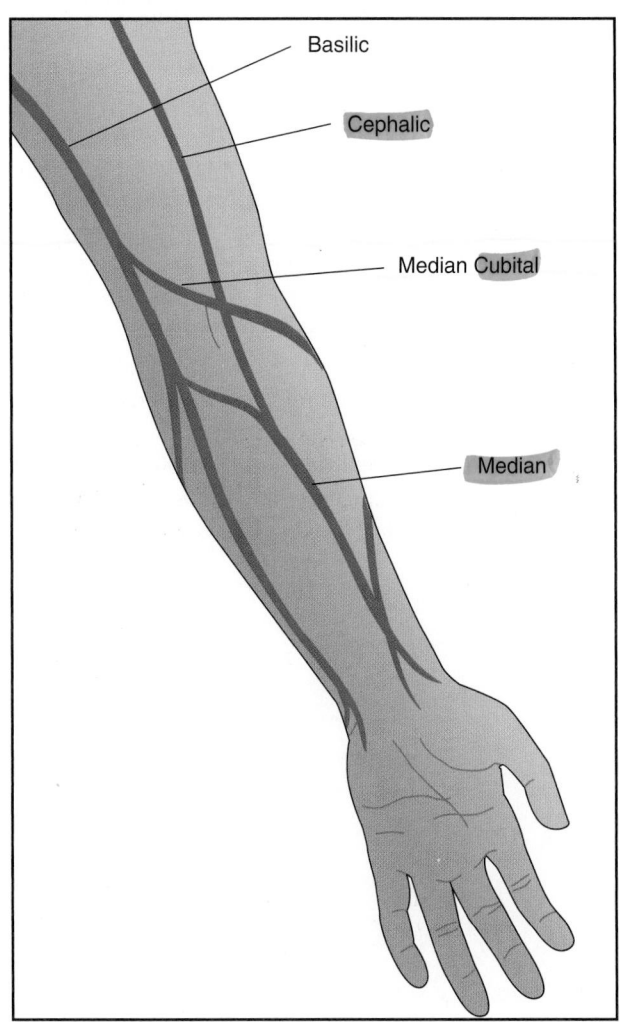

Figure 40-4   Superficial veins of the arm.

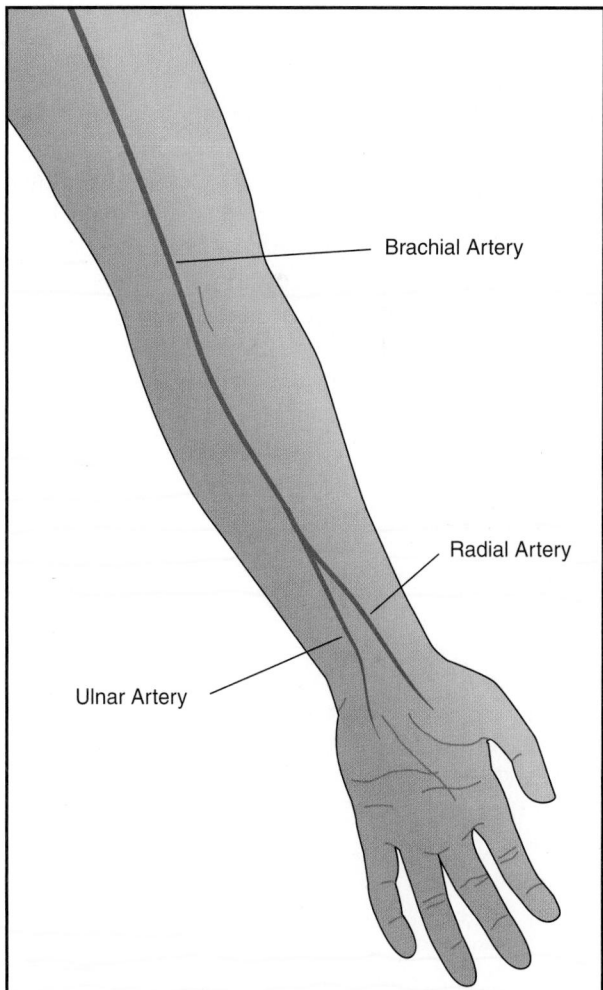

Figure 40-5   Arteries of the arm.

VENIPUNCTURE EQUIPMENT

All methods of venipuncture require the invasive procedure of opening a vein to obtain a blood sample.

Syringes and Needles

The syringe and needle method is one of the oldest methods known and does not destroy the **integrity** of the vein. Syringes are made of either glass or plastic. Most of the syringes currently being used are manufactured from plastic and are disposable (Figure 40-6). Syringes vary in volume from 1 milliliter to 50 milliliters.

Pulling on the plunger of a syringe creates a vacuum within the barrel. The larger the syringe, the greater the amount of vacuum that can be obtained. Too large a vacuum will have the tendency to pull too hard on the vein and may cause the vein to collapse. Vein collapse can be avoided by pulling the plunger slowly and by resting between pulls to allow the vein time to refill. Patients that have fragile, thin, or "rolling" veins that collapse when using an evacuated tube system are typical examples of patients that may be better venipunctured with a syringe. Pediatric or geriatric patients typically have these types of veins. The use of a syringe and needle is limited by the capacity of the syringe. The use of a syringe larger than 10–15 milliliters is not recommended. If a large amount of blood is needed, a butterfly collection set should be used. Syringes are also used in special procedures when the blood must be drawn and then transferred to a different container.

The recommended length of the needle is 1 to 1½ inches in length. The most common gauges of needles that are used in health care are 25, 23, 22, 21, 20, 18, and 16, with the smallest diameter needle being a 25 gauge and the largest being a 16 gauge (Table 40-1).

Safety Needle

 A new safety blood collection needle now available virtually eliminates risks associated with accidental needlesticks through an effective

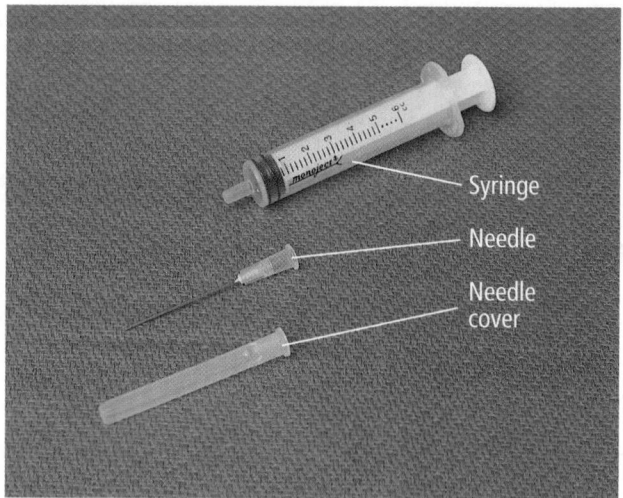

Figure 40-6 Needle and syringe components.

means of passive protection. The Bio-Plexus Punctur-Guard® needle is similar in appearance, size, performance, and general operation to the standard needles used in venipuncture. The unique feature of the needle assembly is a blunt **cannula**, called a blunting member, placed within an otherwise standard needle.

When the Punctur-Guard® needle assembly is inserted into the patient, the blunting member is in its retracted position. When the operator applies additional pressure to the blood collection tube, the blunting member locks into place beyond the needle's tip. The blunting member helps to prevent the needle from accidentally sticking anyone after it is removed from the patient (Figure 40-7). Since the blunting member is hollow, fluids flow normally through the Punctur-Guard® needle, similar to standard needles currently in use. However, because the Punctur-Guard® needle is blunted before it is removed from the patient, the danger of an accidental needlestick is virtually eliminated.

TABLE 40-1	NEEDLE GAUGES
Size	**Purpose**
25	Smallest gauge needle, often causes hemolysis of blood
23	Used with butterfly system, or syringes 0–5 ml in capacity
22	
21	Used with evacuated tube systems
20	
18	Large size, not often used for venipuncture
16	

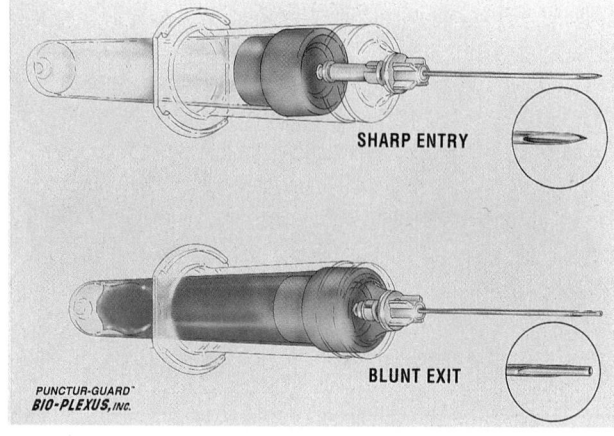

Figure 40-7 Safety blood-collection needle. (Courtesy of Bio-Plexus, Inc., Tolland, CT.)

Evacuated Tube System

The evacuated tube system is often called the Vacutainer system. Vacutainer can be a misnomer because the term *Vacutainer*® is a brand name for the evacuated tube system manufactured by Becton Dickinson and Company, Rutherford, NJ. Medical assistants often say Vacutainer when they are using another company's product.

The principle of the evacuated tube blood collection system is the same principle as a syringe creating a vacuum when the plunger is pulled. A difference is the evacuated tube system is a closed system, adding an element of safety. In the evacuated tube system, a tube with a vacuum already in it attaches to the needle and the tube's vacuum is replaced by blood. The tubes can be glass or plastic. The total system consists of a double-pointed needle, a plastic holder or adapter, and a series of vacuum tubes with rubber stoppers (Figure 40-8).

The key to the evacuated tube system is the needle. The needle is a double-pointed needle with a different length needle on each end and a screw hub near the center. The longer needle has a bevel that enters the vein. The shorter needle pierces the rubber stopper in the blood collection tube. The needle that pierces the rubber stopper of the tube has a sleeve that functions as a valve to stop the flow of blood when the tube is removed (Figure 40-9). Pushing the tube into the holder compresses the sleeve and exposes the needle as it enters the tube. As the tube is removed, the sleeve slides back over the needle and stops the flow of blood.

The needle is thought of as a pipeline that is going to deliver blood from the patient to the tube. The blood is pulled out of the patient due to the vacuum inside the tube.

The patient will experience the least pain if the bevel of the needle is facing upward when the needle is inserted into the vein. The bevel of the needle is upward when the opening in the needle is visible when you look straight down on the needle as it is inserted into the skin. The needle should be inserted at a 15-degree angle to the surface of the skin (Figure 40-10). This technique allows the point of the needle to enter the skin first with little drag or bunching up of the skin, thereby reducing the pain of the puncture.

The holder for the needle makes the task of collecting the blood sample easier. The holder is held in the same manner as you would hold the barrel of a syringe. The holders come in two sizes, one size for adult venipuncture and one size for small diameter tubes used on pediatric patients (Figure 40-11). The holders have

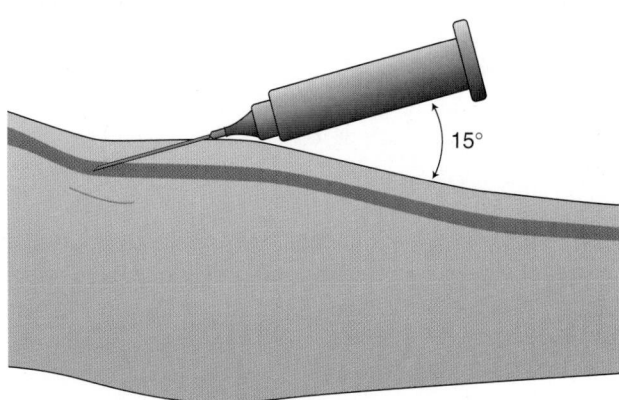

Figure 40-10 Proper angle of needle insertion for venipuncture.

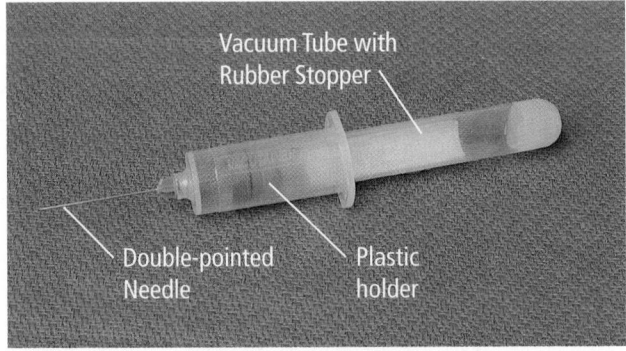

Figure 40-8 Evacuated tube blood-collection system.

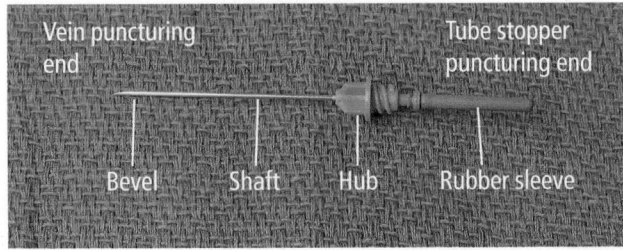

Figure 40-9 Needle for evacuated-tube system.

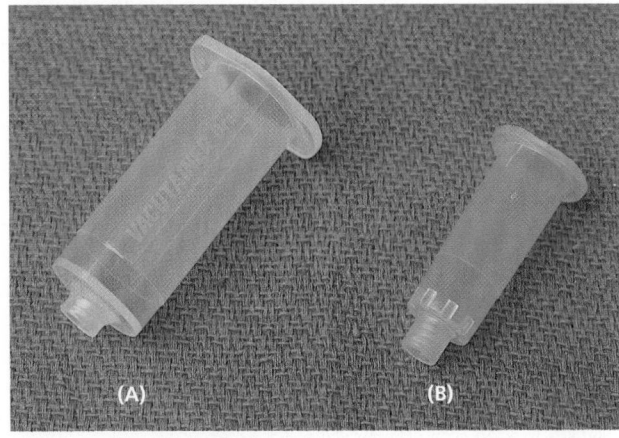

Figure 40-11 Holders for evacuated-tube system: (A) Adult holder. (B) Pediatric holder.

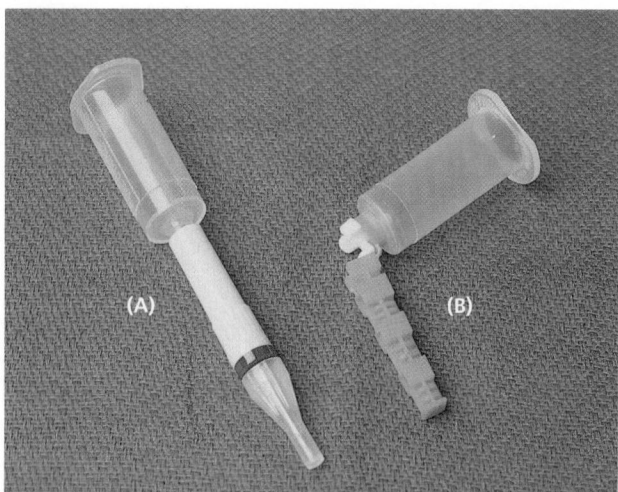

Figure 40-12   Safety tube holders: (A) Safety needle and holder. (B) Locking cover.

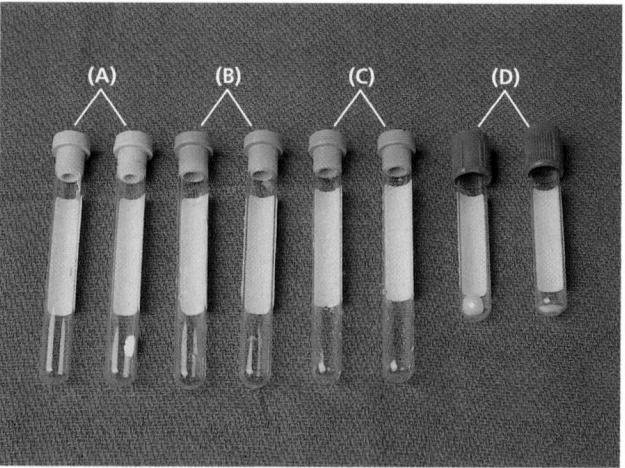

Figure 40-13   Basic anticoagulant tubes: (A) Gray: anti-glycocytic agent. (B) Light blue: citrate. (C) Lavender: EDTA. (D) Green: heparin. (A), (B), and (C) are B-D Vacutainer tubes with conventional stoppers. (D) is a B-D Vacutainer tube with Hemogard closure.

changed in recent years from the basic holders to include safety holders with outer sleeves that slide over the contaminated needle or covers that snap closed over the contaminated needle. The outer sleeve or locking cover protects the medical assistant from needlesticks until the needle and holder can be discarded into a puncture-proof container (Figure 40-12).

Anticoagulants

Different tests require different types of blood specimens. Some specimens require a serum sample and need to be drawn in a tube that allows the blood to clot. Others require a whole blood or plasma specimen and need to be drawn in a tube that does not allow the blood to clot. To prevent the clotting of the blood, the tube contains an anticoagulant. An anticoagulant is a chemical substance that prevents the clotting by removing calcium in the form of calcium salts or by inhibiting the conversion of prothrombin to thrombin. Coagulation occurs naturally according to the steps in Table 40-2. If a step is prevented, the blood does not clot.

The process of clotting can be prevented in the sample tube. A tube containing an anticoagulant removes one of the steps in the process, preventing the blood from clotting. The step removed depends on the anticoagulant

TABLE 40-2   STEPS TO BLOOD CLOTTING
1. Uncoagulated blood
2. Calcium utilized
3. Prothrombin converts to thrombin
4. Fibrinogen converts to fibrin
5. Clot forms

used. The basic anticoagulants used consist of oxalates, citrates, ethylenediaminetetraacetic acid (EDTA), or heparin (Figure 40-13). Anticoagulants are identified by tube color. It is important to use the correct anticoagulant for the test because the improper anticoagulant can alter test results (Table 40-3).

Various **additives** are used to improve the quality of the specimen. These additives are not anticoagulants or preservatives but are used to improve specimen quality or accelerate specimen processing. Some serum tubes have a clot activator that speeds the clotting process. The clot activator consists of silica (small glass) particles on the sides of the tubes that initiate the clotting process. The silica particles work as a catalyst for the clotting process by helping the clotting process to start.

A type of clot activator that is used for STAT (emergency) testing is thrombin. The thrombin is in the tube to chemically increase the speed of the clotting process and to hasten the complete formation of the clot.

Serum and plasma tubes can also be purchased with a **thixotrophic separator gel** (Figure 40-14). The gel is an inert material that undergoes a temporary change in **viscosity** during centrifugation. When centrifuged, the gel changes to a liquid and moves up the sides of the tube to engulf the cells or clot. The gel forms a solid plug and separates the cells/clot from the plasma/serum (Figure 40-15).

Tourniquets

The **tourniquet,** when applied to the arm, constricts the flow of blood in the arm and makes the veins more prominent. The tourniquet is a soft, pliable, rubber or elastic strip approximately 1 inch wide by 15 to 18 inches long.

TABLE 40-3 TUBE GUIDE

Tube stopper color*	Additive	Additive Action	Laboratory Use
Gray (1,2)	Potassium oxalate	Binds calcium	Glucose test/Alcohol levels
	Fluoride	Inhibits glycolysis	
	Iodoacetate	Inhibits glycolysis	
	Lithium heparin	Inhibits prothrombin to thrombin	
Light Blue (1,2)	Sodium citrate	Binds calcium	Used for coagulation studies. Tubes must be filled to the proper level
Lavender (1,2)	Ethylenediamine-tetraacetic acid (EDTA)	Binds calcium	Hematology testing—Complete blood count
Green (1,2)	Lithium heparin	Inhibits prothrombin to thrombin	Plasma determinations in chemistry
	Sodium heparin		
Royal Blue (1,2)	Sodium heparin	Inhibits prothrombin to thrombin	Plasma toxicology/Trace elements
	No additive	Clot forms	Serum toxicology/Trace elements
Yellow/Gray (1) Orange (2)	Thrombin	Fast clot formation	STAT serum determinations
Red (1,2)	No additive	Clot forms	Serum testing
Yellow (1,2)	SPS (sodium polyanetholesulfonate)	Binds calcium / Aids in recovery of microorganisms	Blood cultures
Red/gray (1) Gold (2)	Clot activator and thixotropic gel	Serum separator	Serum determination in chemistry
Brown (1,2)	Sodium heparin	Inhibits prothrombin to thrombin	Lead determination

*Tube stopper colors on Becton-Dickinson Vacutainer® brand tubes. (1) Color of conventional stopper, (2) Color of Hemogard closure.

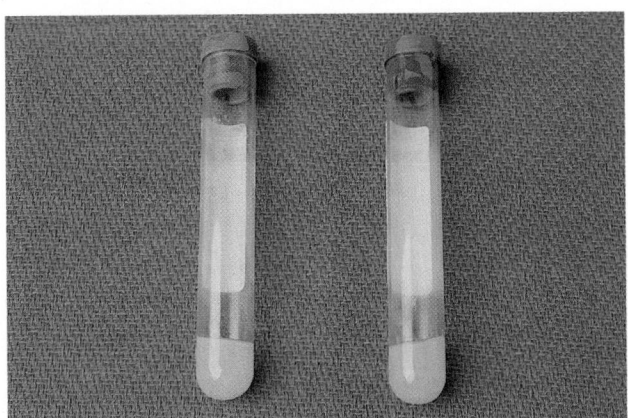

Figure 40-14 Thixotrophic gel tubes.

The rubber strip serves as the best tourniquet for all conditions. Velcro strips are also available. The Velcro strip cannot be cleaned easily and is too expensive to dispose of after each use. The rubber strip can easily be released with one hand. Being about 1 inch wide, it does not cut into the patient's arm but distributes the pressure. The tourniquet can easily be wiped off with alcohol to prevent spreading of infection and is inexpensive enough that it can be replaced often (Figure 40-16). If a patient has been identified as having a latex hypersensitivity, you must use a nonlatex tourniquet.

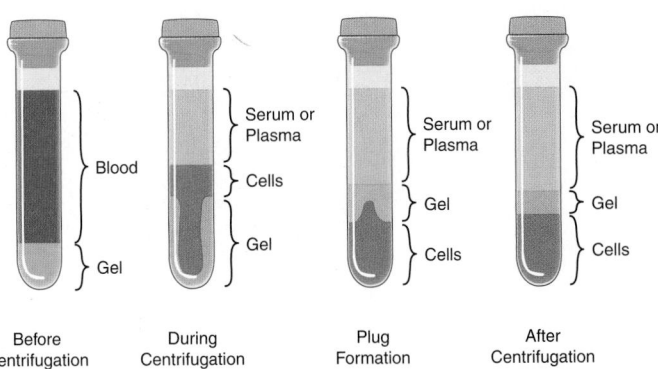

Figure 40-15 Separator gel tube: centrifugation process.

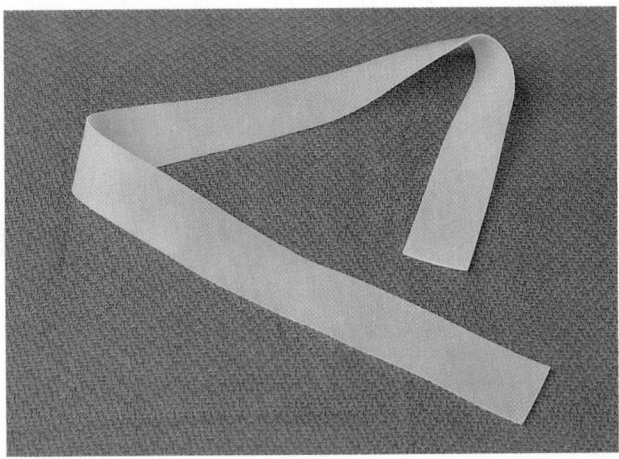

Figure 40-16 Soft rubber tourniquet.

A blood pressure cuff can also be used as a tourniquet. Its use is primarily for veins that are difficult to locate using a standard tourniquet. The blood pressure should be taken first and then the cuff should be maintained slightly below the diastolic pressure.

Specimen Collection Trays

The medical assistant may need a specimen collection tray to hold all the equipment necessary for proper specimen collection. The tray can be taken to the patient in the examination room so that whatever procedure is performed the phlebotomy can be conducted without searching for the proper equipment. The trays vary depending on the type of collections done. Since the tray is also used to transport blood specimens, the OSHA Bloodborne Pathogen Standard requires the tray be all red in color or prominently labeled with an approved biohazard symbol. In some cases, a tray will not be adequate and there will be the need for a stocked cart to roll from exam room to exam room. The tray is usually preferred because it is more portable and can easily be taken to the patient. The trays come in a variety of sizes and shapes to better fit the preference and needs of the individual collecting the blood sample (Figure 40-17). Most medical assistants will not need a tray or cart. The equipment will be in a special drawer for venipuncture equipment in each examination room or in a central lab area.

VENIPUNCTURE TECHNIQUE

Venipuncture is a detailed process that consists of many steps (Table 40-4).

TABLE 40-4   STEPS IN VENIPUNCTURE
1. Identify the patient.
2. Verify diet/drug restrictions; e.g., fasting vs. nonfasting.
3. Wash hands. Put on gloves, as well as safety glasses and mask if there is a potential for blood splatter.
4. Assemble supplies and inspect equipment.
5. Reassure the patient.
6. Position the patient.
7. Verify paperwork and tubes.
8. Perform venipuncture.
9. Fill the tubes (if syringe and needle are used).
10. Bandage the patient's arm.
11. Dispose of sharps in the proper container.
12. Label the tubes.
13. Remove gloves, safety glasses, and mask, and wash hands.
14. Chill specimen (only for certain tests).
15. Eliminate diet restrictions.
16. Process paperwork.
17. Send correctly labeled tubes to the office laboratory or prepare them to be sent to a reference laboratory.

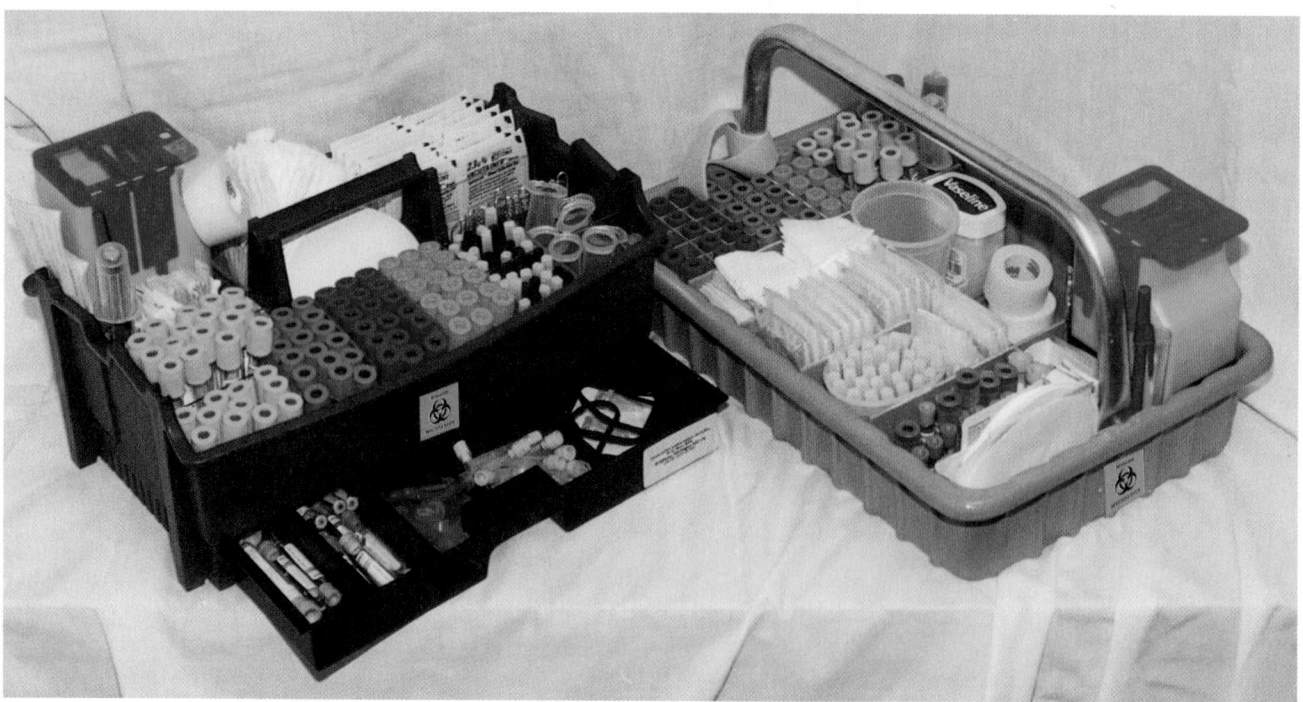

Figure 40-17   Two types of stocked phlebotomy trays.

Approaching the Patient

The medical assistant uses many skills when interacting with patients during phlebotomy. Three of the skills used are:

1. Social skills
2. Technical skills
3. Administrative skills

Social skills are used by the medical assistant to obtain cooperation from the patient. Some patients will be calm while others may be extremely frightened. The nicest patient may be irritable and may even become physically and/or emotionally abusive when placed in the unfamiliar health care setting. The medical assistant uses social skills to put the patient at ease, allay the patient's fears, and persuade the patient to allow blood to be drawn.

After calming the patient and explaining the procedure, the medical assistant uses technical skills to perform the phlebotomy with a minimum of pain to the patient. As important as it is to obtain a good specimen, it is equally important to treat the patient with empathy. Using social and technical skills, the medical assistant can provide a positive experience for the patient. A patient who has had a positive experience will talk with friends and neighbors about that experience, which could result in new patients for the physician's office, the clinic, or the laboratory.

For the medical assistant, administrative skills involve drawing the correct patient's blood and correctly labeling the specimen. Incorrect labeling constitutes the greatest number of errors in phlebotomy. All patient specimens must be positively identified on the **primary container**, the container that holds the specimen, to avoid any errors in reporting of results, thereby affecting patient diagnosis or treatment.

Preparing Supplies and Greeting the Patient

Prepare all supplies and equipment prior to the venipuncture. Place all tubes within easy reach in order to avoid crossing over the patient and possibly moving the needle after it is in the patient. Remember that occasionally a tube will not fill completely; therefore, it is best to keep a few spare tubes or have the phlebotomy tray within reach. The first step to a successful venipuncture is to put the patient at ease.

Patient and Specimen Identification

Proper patient and specimen identification is essential to accurate patient testing. The results of specimen testing will be incorrect if the specimen is not accurately identified. When entering the room, do not say, "Mr. Jones, I'm

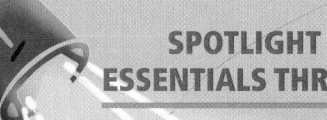

SPOTLIGHT ON AAMA ESSENTIALS THROUGH CAAHEP

- Maintaining a smile and offering a kind word can allay a patient's fear and do a lot toward winning a long-term patient for the physician's office.

- When performing a venipuncture, the medical assistant should be friendly, outgoing, and explain the procedure to the patient.

- Genuine concern for patients generally results in happier patients who choose the same physician for care in the future.

here to draw your blood," assuming if the patient says "Yes" this is Mr. Jones. The patient may not have been paying attention and may answer yes even if it is not his name. Ask the patient to state his full name. If the patient is in the hospital, a check of the patient's wristband is essential.

Greeting the Patient

1. Reassure the patient that the procedure is going to be simple and there will only be a slight inconvenience.
2. Be friendly, outgoing, and talk to the patient, explaining the procedure. Polite conversation with all patients gives them the feeling someone cares about them.
3. Do not tell the patient that the procedure will not be painful.
4. Exhibit concern for patients, as this will result in happier patients who will return in the future for care from the same physician.

Once the medical assistant has identified the patient and the blood is drawn, the specimen needs proper identification. The patient's first and last name, any assigned identification number, the date, the time, and the initials of the person collecting the specimen must be written on the tube immediately after drawing the patient's blood. Label the tubes before leaving the patient's presence. By doing so, if the tubes are taken to the physician's office laboratory or an outside reference laboratory, the specimens will be properly identified. Any paperwork or forms accompanying the specimens must be

[handwritten annotation: if hit aretry, spurts Dark blood.]

checked with the blood tubes to verify that names and numbers match.

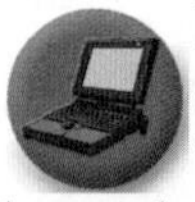

Many offices are using various types of computer systems for test ordering and result reporting. The computer label has several advantages in that it lists the specific tests that are ordered and the required specimen and specimen requirements. The label can also be adhesive so it can be attached directly to the tube. Smaller labels can also be printed at the same time for smaller aliquot specimens. An **aliquot** specimen is a portion of a specimen that has been taken for use or storage. The computer has multiple advantages in timing the printing of orders, sorting lists of orders for one patient at one time, and speeding entry of draw times and test results. The computer labels print off in a roll with one label following the other. Two attached labels (Figure 40-18) require special attention. One label must be checked carefully with the other to assure that each label is for the same person, date, and time. Labels may also contain bar codes to assist in electronic patient and specimen identification. With computerized systems, the medical assistant will verify by entering information into the computer when the blood is drawn.

Positioning the Patient

The position of the patient is critical for proper patient blood collection. The best position is the position that is comfortable for the patient and the health care professional. Proper positioning of the patient will make the patient feel more at ease and facilitate the performance of the venipuncture.

Figure 40-18   Adhesive computer labels for identifying specimen tubes from one patient.

Positioning the Patient

Before a patient's blood is drawn, discuss with the patient any previous problems with blood being taken. Usually one of two situations must be addressed:

1. Patient that does not have a problem with having blood drawn.
   a. The patient must be in a seated or reclining position before any attempt is made to draw blood.
   b. Do not allow the patient to sit on a tall stool or stand while drawing blood. There is always the possibility that the patient will faint (syncope) and be injured.
   c. The sitting position requires a chair with adequate arm supports that are adjustable for the best venipuncture position.
2. Patient who will faint (syncope).
   a. Apprehensive patients and patients who indicate they have fainted in the past when having blood drawn should be instructed to lie down.
   b. The reclining position is the ideal position from which to draw a blood sample from the patient.
   c. A pillow may be required to help support the patient's arm by keeping it straight for easier venous access.

Selecting the Appropriate Venipuncture Site

The appropriate venipuncture site can vary depending on the patient. The usual site that is first checked is the antecubital region of the arm. The primary vein used in the antecubital region of the arm is the median cubital vein. This is usually the prominent vein in the middle of the bend of the arm. Refer back to Figure 40-4. The basilic, cephalic, or median vein can be used as an alternative. These veins may not be accessible or may not be prominent enough to obtain a blood sample. The next step is to go to the back of the hand to determine other possibilities. The veins in the back of the hand have the tendency to "roll" more than the arm veins because they are not supported by as much tissue and are closer to the surface. To avoid this, the vein will have to be held in place by the index finger and the thumb while a smaller gauge needle or a butterfly is used. The hand veins are ideal for a 3–5 cc syringe with a 22 gauge needle. Careful, slow pulling on the syringe will obtain the blood sample without collapsing the vein or hemolyzing the blood. The veins at the back of the wrist are also an alternative, but they are generally much more painful than the other sites. The foot and ankle veins may also be used if the patient's physician gives permission to use them. The veins in the foot or ankle will also have the tendency to "roll." The medical assistant will in all likelihood never draw from the foot or ankle, but this is an area that will give an acceptable blood sample when all other attempts have failed.

The order for checking for the best available site is (1) antecubital region of the arm, (2) back of hand, (3) back of wrist, and (4) ankle or foot. The next alternative is to have a more experienced medical assistant check. If venous access is not possible, draw the sample by capillary puncture.

A tourniquet must be used to assist the medical assistant in feeling a vein. The tourniquet is applied 3–4 inches above the intended puncture site. It is applied tightly enough to stop the flow of blood in the veins but not so tightly as to prevent the flow of blood in the arteries (Figures 40-19A–D). This is similar to damming a small stream. When a stream is dammed, the water forms a pond in front of the dam. With the tourniquet applied, the veins fill with blood, pooling in the veins below the tourniquet. This pooling of blood makes the veins more prominent. The veins can then be **palpated** (examined with the fingertips) to determine their direction, depth, and size. The tourniquet should be on the arm no longer than one minute. A stream will become stagnant when it no longer flows. A tourniquet that is left on too long will cause **hemoconcentration** of the blood, an increased concentration of constituents in the blood sample that may lead to inaccurate test results. If the patient has very sensitive skin or a skin problem, the tourniquet should be applied over the patient's upper arm clothing or a piece of gauze pad. This will minimize the discomfort felt by the patient.

The tourniquet often causes greater discomfort for patients than the venipuncture itself. The tourniquet should ideally be removed as soon as blood flow is established. This is not practical for the novice medical assistant. The act of removing the tourniquet may move the needle and/or vein just enough so that no more blood can be obtained and a second venipuncture must be performed. It is recommended to wait until just before the needle is removed from the patient to remove the tourniquet. If the tourniquet is not removed before the needle is removed, the patient will bleed heavily. Blood will be forced out of the needle hole and into the surrounding tissue, resulting in a **hematoma** (an accumulation of blood around the venipuncture site).

Performing a Safe Venipuncture

The first step in collecting a venous blood specimen is to find the site that will give the best blood return. The vein

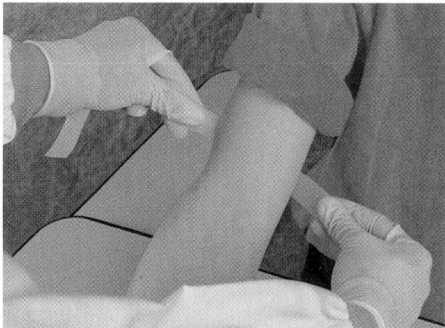

Figure 40-19A Wrap the tourniquet around the arm 3 to 4 inches above the venipuncture site. Keeping the tourniquet flat to the skin will help minimize the discomfort felt by the patient.

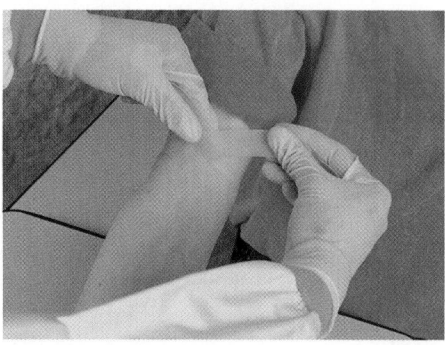

Figure 40-19B Stretch the tourniquet tight and cross the ends.

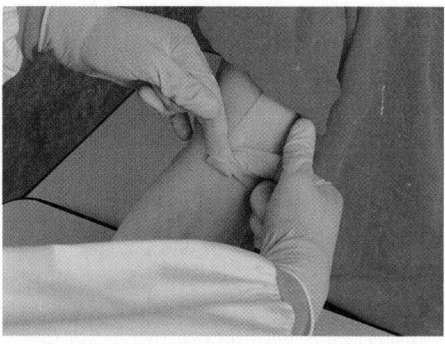

Figure 40-19C While holding the ends tight, tuck one portion of the tourniquet under the other.

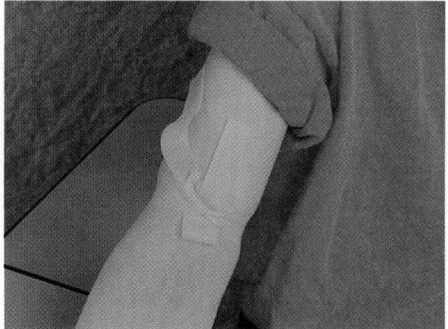

Figure 40-19D Check that the tourniquet will not come loose. The ends of the tourniquet should be pointed upward and not hang into the intended venipuncture site.

must be palpated with the tip of the index finger. Feel for and trace the path of the vein several times. Avoid using the thumb because it has a pulse and is not as sensitive as the rest of the fingers. The vein will feel soft and bouncy to the touch. The roundness of the vein and the direction it follows may be determined. All veins are not straight up and down the arm. If no veins become prominent, retie the tourniquet tighter but not so tightly as to stop the flow of arterial blood into the arm. If the tourniquet is tied tightly enough to stop arterial blood flow, the patient will no longer have a pulse in the wrist. If this occurs, immediately remove the tourniquet as this indicates that blood has ceased flowing below the tourniquet.

If the "vein" that is felt has a pulsing action to it, it is an artery, not a vein, and the vessel should not be punctured. Tendons can be deceptive and give the appearance of veins. They do not have the soft, bouncy feel and will be hard to the touch. Puncturing a tendon will give no blood return and will be painful to the patient. Nerves also run the length of the arm. The nerves cannot be seen or felt, but by avoiding deep probing venipunctures, the chance of puncturing a nerve will be diminished. If the patient complains that the venipuncture is extremely painful, it is best to stop and try another site.

Veins of **edematous** arms, which are swollen due to fluid in the tissue, will not be prominent and the tourniquet will not be effective because of the swelling. Using the tourniquet in this instance may cause tissue damage. It leaves a temporary indentation in the arm. Areas of scarring should also be avoided due to possible injury or excessive pain to the patient. Specimens collected from an area of a hematoma may cause erroneous test results. If another vein site is not available, the specimen is collected distal from the hematoma. Because of the potential for harm to the patient due to lymphostasis (the stoppage of the flow of lymph), the arm on the side of a mastectomy should be avoided. If the patient has had a double mastectomy, a physician should be consulted prior to drawing the blood.

Syringe Specimen Collection

The patient has been identified, paperwork and tubes have been verified, equipment has been assembled, and the patient is in a comfortable position. Handwashing is the most critical step to preventing the spread of infection. Before touching the patient, medical assistants should wash their hands. It is good practice to wash your hands in view of the patient to give the patient confidence in your technique. The next step is to tie the tourniquet. Have the patient close the hand and then select a vein. If possible, place the patient's arm in a downward position. After locating an acceptable vein, mentally map the location. Set mental sites on the vein by visualizing the puncture site as the target for an accu-

rate puncture. Cleanse the site with a gauze pad wet with 70 percent isopropyl alcohol solution. A commercially prepared alcohol pad or one with 0.5 percent chlorhexidine in alcohol may also be used. Clean the skin in a circular motion from the center of the intended puncture site to the outside. Allow the area to air dry to prevent hemolysis of the specimen and to prevent the patient from feeling a burning sensation from the puncture.

Some authorities suggest putting on gloves first and then palpating for the vein. This technique is required for the patient who is isolated due to a communicable disease and is good practice for all patients. Standard precautions require that personal protective equipment be worn when there is a chance of coming in contact with blood and body fluid. If the patient has veins that are difficult to palpate, the gloves may be put on after the site has been palpated and before the cleansing. To avoid forgetting where the collection site is, palpate the vein 1–2 inches above and below the intended puncture site. It helps the medical assistant feel that the vein is located in a straight line and these points can be used to "reset" the mental crosshairs without contaminating the venipuncture site. Safety glasses and a mask must be worn if there is a potential for blood spatter.

The syringe technique is used less often than the evacuated tube system. The techniques developed in the syringe method are building blocks for the evacuated tube technique and all other techniques that the medical assistant uses for obtaining a blood specimen.

The syringe is ideal for collecting small volumes of blood from fragile surface veins such as veins in the back

Correct Hand Position to Hold a Syringe

1. The needle is attached to the syringe.
2. Hold the syringe and needle system in your dominant hand, cradling it on your four fingers. A right-handed person would hold the syringe in the right hand, leaving the left hand to pull on the plunger. A left-handed person would do the opposite.
3. Place the thumb on top of the syringe (Figure 40-20).
4. With the syringe held in this position, turn it slightly so the bevel of the needle is facing up.
5. Hold the hand in such a position that by tilting the point of the needle down slightly the needle will enter the skin at a 15 degree angle and about 0.5 cm below the point where the vein was felt.

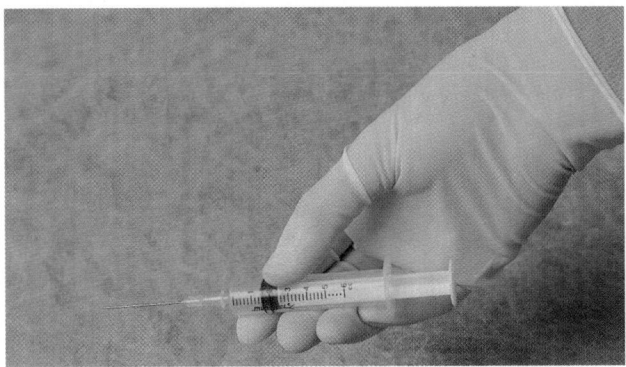

Figure 40-20   Proper hand position to hold a syringe.

of the hand. Procedure 40-2 gives detailed instructions for venipuncture with syringe.

When a syringe is used, the blood obtained must be placed in appropriate containers. To place the blood in empty evacuated tubes, puncture the stopper with the syringe needle and allow blood to enter the tube until the flow stops. Do not remove the rubber stoppers. Running blood down the side of the tube after removing the stopper is not recommended because aerosols and splattering of blood can occur. This is why masks and goggles are recommended for this type of venipuncture. Do not hold the tube in your hand as you puncture the stopper. There is the potential for missing the stopper or slipping off the stopper and puncturing yourself. The best method is to place the tubes in a test tube rack and then puncture the tubes using only one hand. The tube will fill itself; do not force the blood into the tube. This technique will maintain the proper ratio of blood to anticoagulant. Immediately upon filling, mix any tubes containing additives. The order of filling the tubes is important.

Fill sterile collection tubes first to prevent microorganism contamination. The additive tubes are filled before the nonadditive tubes to avoid contamination with microscopic clots. The blood that is last to come out of the syringe was the first blood to go in and has the poten-

tial to have started to clot. The empty syringe and needle are immediately placed into a sharps container without recapping the needle.

Evacuated Tube Specimen Collection

The evacuated tube system is an improvement over the syringe method yet maintains many similarities. When the syringe method is used, a vacuum is created as the medical assistant pulls on the syringe plunger. The evacuated tube method has the vacuum already in the tube. Another advantage of the evacuated tube system is that with multiple blood samples, syringes do not need to be changed; only the tubes need to be changed.

The similarity between the evacuated tube system and the syringe system is that the holder and needle are held in the same manner (Figure 40-21). The syringe is held in a manner that allows the medical assistant access to pull on the plunger. Access must be left in the evacuated tube system for one tube to be pulled out and another inserted. The hand that pulled on the plunger of the syringe is the hand that changes tubes with the evacuated tube system.

The procedure for venipuncture with the evacuated tube system follows the same steps as the syringe method with only slight variations.

With multiple tube draws, the order of drawing the tubes is important. Check with the tube manufacturer for the recommended order of draw. The National Committee for Clinical Laboratory Standards (NCCLS) recommends the following order of draw from a single venipuncture using the evacuated tube system.

Order of Filling Tubes from a Syringe

1. Blood culture tubes or bottles (sterile procedures)
2. Coagulation "citrate" tube (blue tube)
3. Heparin tube (green tube)
4. EDTA tube (lavender tube)
5. Oxalate/fluoride tube (gray tube)
6. Nonadditive "clot" tubes (red stoppered or gel tubes)

Evacuated Tube System Order of Draw

Purpose: Avoid possible test result error due to cross contamination from tube additives.

1. Blood culture tubes or bottles (for sterile procedures)
2. Tubes without additives (e.g., red stopper)
3. Tubes with additives:
   • Coagulation studies, citrate tube (e.g., light blue stopper)
   • Gel separator tube (red/gray or gold stopper)
   • Heparin (green stopper)
   • EDTA (lavendar stopper)
   • Other additives (gray stopper)

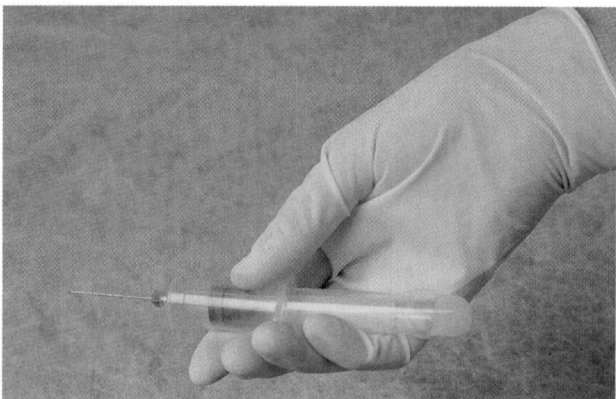

Figure 40-21   Proper hand position to hold an evacuated tube system.

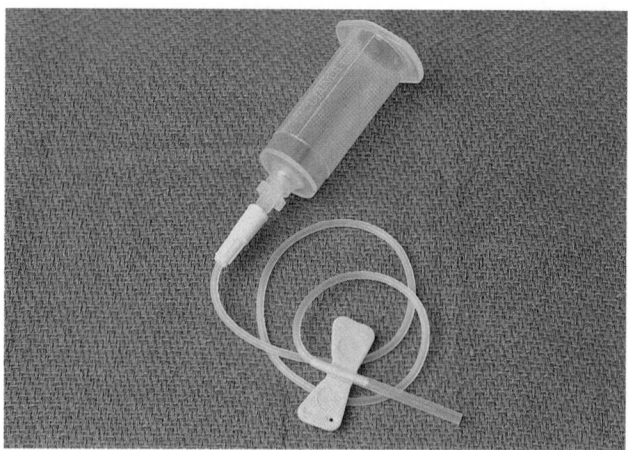

Figure 40-22   Butterfly needle assembly.

Butterfly Collection System

A system that combines benefits of the syringe system and the evacuated tube system is the butterfly collection system. The butterfly collection system has on one end a 21, 23, or 25 gauge needle with attached plastic wings. Six or twelve inches of tubing leads from the needle. On the other end of this tubing is a hub that can attach to a syringe. A needle covered by a rubber sleeve can also be attached to the tubing. The covered needle screws into an evacuated tube holder (Figure 40-22).

The butterfly system is used for small veins that are difficult to puncture with the evacuated tube system and standard evacuated tube system needle. The system also facilitates drawing from veins that have a tendency to collapse. The winged needle of the butterfly needle will slide into a small surface vein in the back of the hand, wrist, or foot. Instead of entering the vein at the usual 15 degree angle, the winged needle is inserted at approximately a 5 degree angle and then threaded into the vein. This procedure anchors the needle in the center of a small vein that is inaccessible by other methods. If the patient moves, the tubing gives flexibility so the needle will stay anchored and not pull out of the vein. The butterfly collection set works well on children that have small veins and the tendency to move while blood is being collected.

The system also gives the adaptability of initiating a draw with a syringe and then finishing it with the evacuated tube system. A syringe can be filled for procedures that require a syringe sample. It can then be removed, and the evacuated tube system can be attached for multiple tube collection. Although the butterfly collection system has many benefits, it is not used for all collections. It is much more expensive than the needle system. The additional expense is unnecessary for the majority of venipunctures.

Patient Reactions

Patients can have a variety of reactions to having their blood drawn. The medical assistant must anticipate these reactions and respond appropriately as quickly as possible. The most common patient reaction is pain. The patient will indicate that the venipuncture is painful. Slightly reposition the needle and then loosen the tourniquet. Loosening the tourniquet often helps because the tourniquet may be pinching the arm and causing discomfort rather than the needle. Avoid deep, probing venipunctures because they may go deeply into the arm and get too close to the nerves. If the pain persists, discontinue the venipuncture.

Other possible patient reactions and the medical assistant's appropriate responses are shown in Table 40-5.

The Unsuccessful Venipuncture

When a blood sample cannot be obtained, it may be necessary to change the position of the needle. Rotate the needle half a turn. The bevel of the needle may be against the wall of the vein. If the needle has not penetrated the vein far enough, advance it further into the vein. Advance it only slightly; a small change may mean the difference between a failed and a successful venipuncture. If the needle has penetrated too far into the vein, pull back a little. Always withdraw the needle slowly when the venipuncture has been unsuccessful. The blood often may start coming just as it seems the needle is ready to come out of the skin. The tube used may not have sufficient vacuum. Try another tube before withdrawing the needle. Methods of vein stimulation are shown in Table 40-6.

Probing the site is not recommended. Probing is painful to the patient and may cause a hematoma. Never attempt a venipuncture more than two times. If a blood

TABLE 40-5   PATIENT REACTIONS TO BLOOD DRAWS

Patient Reaction	Medical Assistant Response
1. Syncope (fainting)	Immediately remove the needle and stop the patient from falling. Lower the patient's head and arms. Wipe the patient's forehead and back of the neck with a cold compress if necessary. Pass an ammonia inhalant 4 to 5 inches away from the patient's nose (the patient will respond by coughing). If the patient still does not respond, notify a physician, move the patient to the floor, and place a pillow under the patient's legs.
2. Nausea	If a patient becomes nauseated, apply cold compresses to the patient's forehead. Give the patient an emesis basin, and have facial tissues ready if the nausea does not diminish. Deep slow breathing through the mouth may help.
3. Insulin shock/ hypoglycemia	The first signs of insulin shock are a cold sweat and pallor similar to the signs of syncope. The patient becomes weak and shaky, sudden mental confusion may follow, and it appears as though the patient's personality changes instantly. Call the physician if the patient loses consciousness.
4. Convulsions	The patient loses consciousness and exhibits violent or mild convulsive motions. Do not try to restrain the patient. Move objects or furniture out of the way to prevent the patient from striking objects and being hurt. Help the patient to the floor and into a reclining position. The patient usually recovers within a few minutes. Notify the physician about the patient's reaction. The physician will determine when to release the patient.
5. Cardiac arrest	The patient lapses into unconsciousness, has no pulse or respirations, the eyes are dilated, and there may be a blue or gray skin tone. Start cardiopulmonary resuscitation (CPR) immediately to avoid patient death. Only persons certified to do CPR can perform this procedure. Immediately notify the physician.

TABLE 40-6   METHODS OF VEIN STIMULATION

1. Position the patient's arm lower than the patient's heart.
2. Reapply the tourniquet.
3. Massage the arm from wrist to elbow.
4. Tap sharply at the venipuncture site with your fingers. This will cause the veins to dilate.
5. Use a blood pressure cuff in place of the tourniquet.
6. Warm the venipuncture site with a warming device or a warm washcloth (not hotter than 42°C).

diagnosis, the blood specimen may need to be redrawn to confirm the results. This is accomplished by either retesting the specimen or collecting another sample. This will either reconfirm that the correct patient was drawn and/or that the patient's test results changed significantly.

Factors Affecting Laboratory Values

There are numerous variables that can affect laboratory test results. The specimens are tested by analytical

sample cannot be obtained after two attempts, perform a microcollection (e.g., capillary puncture) if possible. Otherwise have another person attempt the draw. Notify the patient's physician if two medical assistants have been unsuccessful and a microcollection is not possible.

Criteria for Rejection of a Specimen

The primary goal of the medical assistant is to provide an acceptable specimen for laboratory testing as required by the physician. There are certain general criteria that must be met for a specimen to be acceptable. If the criteria are not met, the specimen is rejected and another venipuncture of the patient must be performed.

Table 40-7 lists quality assurance controls for specimen collection and processing. The list is not all inclusive. The type of specimen that is acceptable and the volume required are determined by the procedure ordered. The quality control checks done by the laboratory may indicate the results are valid. If the results do not agree with what the physician believes is the patient's

TABLE 40-7   QUALITY ASSURANCE FOR SPECIMEN COLLECTION AND PROCESSING

1. Each specimen must have its own label attached to the specimen's primary container.
2. Each specimen must have the test to be performed written on the label (CBC, Cholesterol, and so on).
3. Labels must have the patient's complete name and identification number.
4. Specimens in syringes with needles still attached are unacceptable.
5. All specimens must be in the appropriate anticoagulant.
6. Blood collection tubes with anticoagulant must be at least 75 percent full. All blood collection tubes for coagulation testing must be at least 90 percent full.
7. Uncoagulated blood specimens must be free of clots.
8. Certain tests require specimens to be free of hemolysis and lipemia, a milky appearance due to lipids.
9. The specimen may need to be recollected if the results do not agree with what the physician believes is the diagnosis of the patient.

instruments that give accurate and precise results. These results will accurately reflect what is wrong with the patient only if the specimen is collected correctly. A correctly collected specimen is the responsibility of the health care worker performing the collection procedure. Patient physiological factors may also contribute to inaccurate results. Other factors that can alter results are shown in Table 40-8.

Certain specimens must be chilled immediately after collection (Table 40-9). Place the blood tube into ice as it is withdrawn from the evacuated tube holder. Any delay in icing the specimen will alter test results. The longer the delay, the greater the change.

The medical assistant is not the only person who can affect test results. The patient can knowingly or unknow-

TABLE 40-9	EXAMPLES OF COMMON TESTS REQUIRING CHILLING OF THE SPECIMEN
Ammonia	
Catecholamines	
Gastrin	
Lactic acid	
Parathyroid hormone (PTH)	
pH/blood gas	

ingly alter the results by certain actions. An example of this occurs when a patient has had a cup of coffee but claims not to have had anything to eat or drink. The patient is often under the misconception that black coffee without sugar will not be a problem. Coffee and smoking affect the metabolism and can affect the test results.

CAPILLARY PUNCTURE

Venipuncture is the most frequently performed phlebotomy procedure, but it is not the procedure of choice in all circumstances. An alternative to venipuncture is capillary puncture, also known as dermal puncture or skin puncture.

Capillary puncture is the method of choice with two types of patients: when patient blood volume is a concern, such as with infants, and when vein access is difficult, such as with burned or scarred patients. Capillary puncture should not be used when a patient is edematous, dehydrated, or has poor peripheral circulation.

Composition of Capillary Blood

Blood obtained via capillary puncture is a mixture of blood from arterioles, venules, capillaries, and interstitial fluid. In most instances, a capillary puncture specimen most resembles arterial blood. Warming the site prior to puncture increases the blood flow as much as sevenfold. There may be significant differences between specimens obtained by capillary puncture and those collected by venipuncture. For example, the glucose level may be increased in capillary blood, while the potassium, calcium and total protein levels may be decreased. It is therefore important to always note on the specimen when capillary blood has been obtained.

Capillary Puncture Sites

The usual site for capillary puncture in adults and children is the fingertip (Figure 40-23). In adults, the ring finger is often selected because it usually is not callused. In infants, the lateral or medial plantar surface of the heel

TABLE 40-8	FACTORS AFFECTING LABORATORY RESULTS
Factor	**Effect**
Blood alcohol	When drawing a specimen for blood alcohol testing, a nonalcohol-based antiseptic should be used to clean the venipuncture site. The cleansing alcohol may falsely elevate the test result.
Diurnal rhythm	Some specimens must be drawn at timed intervals because of medication or diurnal (daily) rhythm. The exact time of collection must be noted on the specimen.
Exercise	Strenuous short-term exercise can make the heart work harder and increase the heart enzymes. Long-term exercise such as that performed by highly trained runners can cause erroneous results due to runner's anemia.
Fasting	Patient not in fasting state when fasting is required. Results of tests will not be accurate.
Hemolysis	Destruction of red blood cell membrane and release of intercellular contents into serum/plasma can be caused by: not allowing alcohol to air dry at venipuncture site, using a needle that is too small (less than 22 gauge), forcing the blood into a vacutainer tube from a syringe, or shaking the vacutainer tube instead of mixing by gentle inversion when mixing tubes with additives.
Heparin	Incorrect heparin used that interferes with tests being run on patient.
Stress	In children, violent crying before a specimen is collected can raise the WBC count.
Tourniquet on too long	Hemoconcentration, change in chemical concentration.
Volume	Not enough blood will cause a dilution factor, which can change the size of the cells and therefore produce a variation in test results.

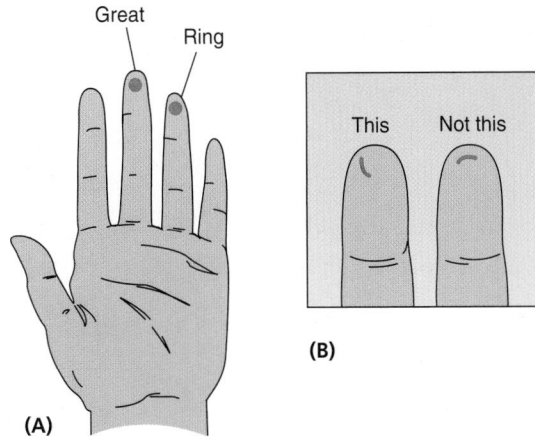

Figure 40-23 (A) Capillary blood collection sites. (B) Correct direction of capillary puncture.

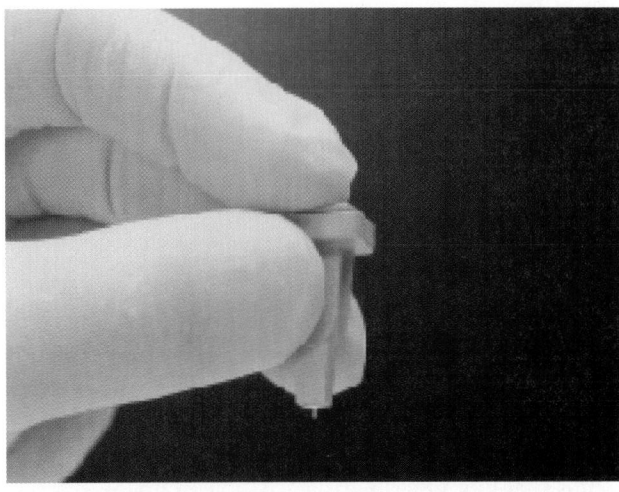

pad is usually used, and the procedure is often called a heelstick. The heelstick is most often performed when testing for Phenylketonuria (PKU), which is covered in detail in Chapter 44, Specialty Laboratory Tests.

Preparing the Capillary Puncture Site

The area selected for a capillary puncture must be carefully prepared. The puncture site will be warm if blood circulation is adequate. Coolness of the skin indicates decreased circulation. To increase circulation, the site may be gently massaged or a warm, moist towel or face cloth at a temperature not higher than 42°C may be used to cover the site for three to five minutes.

Alcohol-soaked gauze or cotton should be used to cleanse and disinfect the puncture site. The site should then be allowed to air dry. Residual alcohol at the puncture site results in hemolysis of the specimen, which may affect test results as well as cause a burning sensation to the patient. Betadine (povidone iodine) should not be used to clean the puncture site. Blood contaminated with iodine may falsely elevate certain blood chemistries.

Performing the Puncture

Gloves must be worn by the medical assistant when performing the puncture. The patient's hand and finger should be held so the puncture site is readily accessible. The puncture is made at the tip of the fleshy pad and slightly to the side (Figure 40-23). The skin near the chosen site should be pulled taut. If the tips of the fingers are heavily callused or thickened, a special lancet with a longer point may be used. The puncture should be performed in one quick steady motion. Capillary punctures are performed using semiautomated devices such as the disposable MICROTAINER® Brand Safety Flow Lancet®

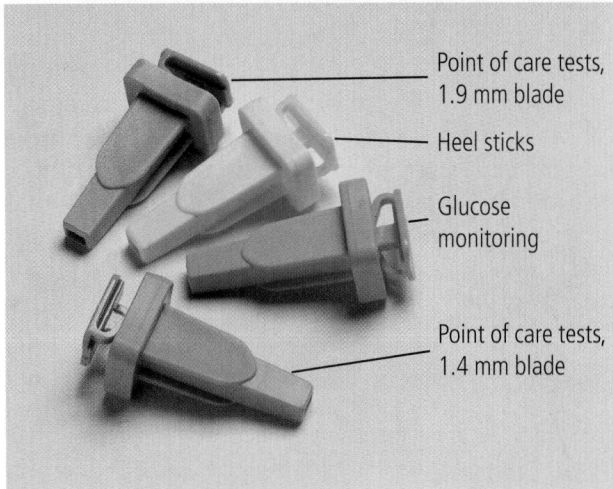

Figure 40-24 Microtainer® brand lancets are available in different types for various purposes. To use, hold lancet on skin and depress plunger with index finger to make puncture. Immediately release plunger while holding lancet on site. Discard lancet after use in biohazard container. (Courtesy of Becton-Dickinson Vacutainer Systems.)

(Figure 40-24). In the laboratory collection area, an acrylic safety shield can be placed between the patient and the medical assistant to protect the collector from blood splatters. Alternatively, safety glasses and a mask can be worn.

Collecting the Blood Sample

The first drop of blood is wiped away with dry, sterile gauze because it contains tissue fluid, which dilutes the blood drop and can also activate clotting. The second and following drops of blood are used for test samples. Depending on the tests to be performed, the blood may be collected in capillary tubes or other capillary collecting devices. Capillary tubes are glass or plastic tubes of small diameter.

It may be necessary to massage the finger to increase the blood flow. It is best to massage the whole hand, taking care not to apply direct pressure near the puncture site. Squeezing the fingertip should be avoided; this forces tissue fluid into the blood sample and dilutes it or may cause hemolysis. Do not use a scooping technique when collecting blood from the puncture site. Scooping can break the red blood cell membranes, leading to hemolysis. Allowing well-rounded drops of blood to form at the puncture site will aid in the collection process. If the flow of blood begins to slow, rewipe the puncture site with a sterile gauze pad (do not use alcohol). This will dislodge the platelet plug and cause the blood flow to increase.

The capillary tube should be held in an almost horizontal position, just tilted slightly downward. When the tip of the capillary tube is touched to the drop of blood, whether collecting directly from a patient's finger or from a collection tube, blood will enter the tube by capillary action because of the attraction between the liquid and the tube. Tubes should be filled two-thirds to three-quarters full (Figure 40-25). Usually, two to three tubes are filled from a capillary puncture. The capillary tubes are then sealed using either sealing clay or plastic caps (Figure 40-26). Manufacturer's instructions for the type of capillary tubes should be carefully followed.

Order of Draw

The order of draw for microcollection differs from that used in venipuncture. If multiple specimens are collected, EDTA specimens (lavendar caps) are collected first, then other additive specimens (green, gray caps) and lastly specimens that clot (red or gel caps).

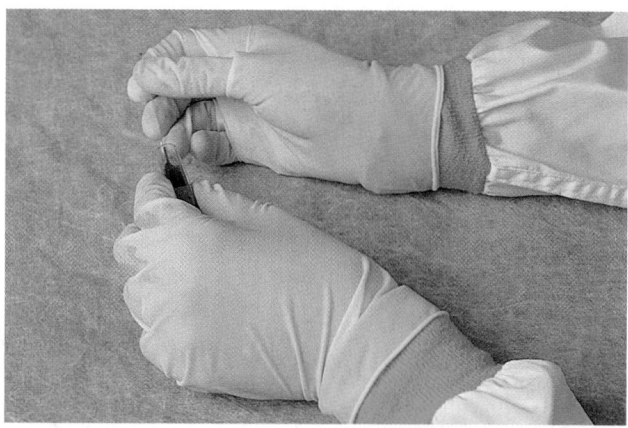

Figure 40-25   Filling a microhematocrit tube with blood by capillary action.

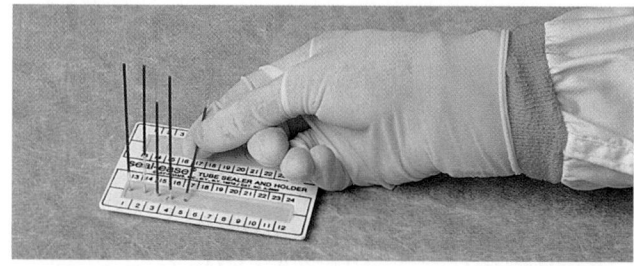

Figure 40-26   Sealing the microhematocrit tube with sealing clay.

In many ways the procedure for capillary puncture is similar to the other collection procedures discussed in this chapter, e.g., patient identification, safety precautions, specimen labeling. A detailed description of capillary puncture is found in Procedure 40-5.

Procedure 40-1   Finding a Vein in the Upper Arm

STANDARD PRECAUTIONS:

    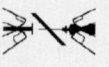

PURPOSE:
To obtain venous blood with limited discomfort to the patient.

EQUIPMENT/SUPPLIES:

Gloves	Gown or lab coat
Goggles and mask, if necessary	Tube holder
	Alcohol swab
Gauze	Tubes
Tourniquet	Bandage
Needle	Sharps container

PROCEDURE STEPS:

1. Identify the patient. Ask the patient's name and verify it with the computer label or identification number. If a fasting specimen is required, verify that the patient has not had anything to eat or drink.

2. Wash hands. Put on gloves, as well as safety glasses and mask if there is a potential for blood splatter.

(continues)

Procedure 40-1 (continued)

3. Apply tourniquet 3 to 4 inches above the venipuncture site. Apply tightly enough to stop blood flow but not so tight that blood flow in arteries is stopped. Refer to Figure 40-19.
4. Have the patient close the hand.
5. Place the patient's arm in a downward position.
6. Palpate the upper region of the arm, feeling for the median cubital, basilic, or cephalic vein with the tip of your index finger.
7. Feel for a soft bounce and a roundness to the vein. Follow the direction of the vein.
8. Feel the vein for its center and possibility of rolling.

9. After locating an acceptable vein, mentally map the location. Visualize the puncture site.
10. Clean the venipuncture site with a 70 percent isopropyl alcohol swab and complete the venous blood collection from the site.
11. If a vein cannot be found in the upper region of the arm, then the hand veins must be checked following the same procedure. The hand veins have a greater tendency to roll and venipuncture is more successful when a butterfly is used for hand vein collection.

Procedure 40-2 Venipuncture by Syringe Procedure

STANDARD PRECAUTIONS:

   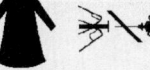 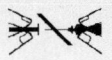

PURPOSE:
To obtain venous blood acceptable for laboratory testing as required by a physician.

SPECIMEN:
Venous blood collected to be aliquoted into evacuated tubes and/or special collection containers

EQUIPMENT/SUPPLIES:
Gloves	Tourniquet
Safety glasses and mask, if necessary	70% isopropyl alcohol swab
Syringe, varies in size	Gauze or cotton balls
Disposable needle for syringe, 21 or 22 gauge needle	Adhesive bandage or tape
	Sharps container
	Test tube rack
Evacuated tube(s) or special collection tube(s)	

PROCEDURE STEPS:
1. Position and identify the patient. Ask the patient's name and verify it with the computer label or identification number.
2. If a fasting specimen is required, verify that the patient has not had anything to eat or drink.
3. Wash hands.
4. Put on gloves, as well as goggles and mask if there is a potential for blood splatter.
5. Open the sterile needle and syringe packages, attaching the needle if necessary.
6. Prevent the plunger from sticking by pulling it halfway out and pushing it all the way in one time.
7. Select the proper tube(s) to transfer the blood to after collection.
8. Select a site and apply the tourniquet (Figure 40-27A).
9. Ask the patient to close the hand. The patient must not be allowed to pump the hand. Pumping of the hand will change the values of the laboratory tests being collected. Place the patient's arm in a downward position if possible.

(continues)

Procedure
40-2   *(continued)*

10. Select a vein, noting the location and direction of the vein. The median cubital vein is most commonly used.
11. Clean the venipuncture site with a 70 percent isopropyl alcohol swab in a circular motion from the center outward (Figure 40-27B).
12. Do not touch the venipuncture site.
13. Draw the patient's skin taut with your thumb. Place the thumb 1 to 2 inches below or above the puncture site (Figure 40-27C). This will anchor the vein.
14. With the bevel up, line up the needle with the vein and perform the venipuncture (Figure 40-27D).
15. Do not enter at the exact location at which the vein is felt. Enter the vein approximately ¼ inch below the vein location. The bevel of the needle must enter the skin at the point where the vein was palpated. Push the needle into the skin. A sensation of resistance will be followed by easy penetration as the vein is entered. This is known as feeling the "pop." Once this point is reached, stop and do not move.
16. Take the opposite hand and pull on the plunger of the syringe. Pull gently and only as fast as the syringe will fill with blood. Pulling too hard or fast will cause temporary collapse of the vein. If the vein does collapse, stop pulling on the plunger and let the vein refill with blood (Figure 40-27E).
17. Pull the plunger back until the desired amount of blood has been obtained.
18. Ask the patient to open the hand.
19. Release the tourniquet (Figure 40-27F).
20. Lightly place a sterile gauze square or cotton ball above the venipuncture site.
21. Remove the needle from the arm (Figure 40-27G).
22. Apply pressure to the site for 3 to 5 minutes. The patient may assist if able by elevating the arm above heart level (Figure 40-27H). The arm should be held in a raised, outstretched position. Do not allow the patient to bend the arm at the elbow. Bending the arm at the elbow to apply pressure may lead to a hematoma.
23. Aliquot blood into appropriate tube(s). Tubes should be held in a test tube rack. Puncture the stopper of the evacuated tube with the syringe needle and allow the blood to enter the tube until the flow stops. Mix if any anticoagulant is present.

(continues)

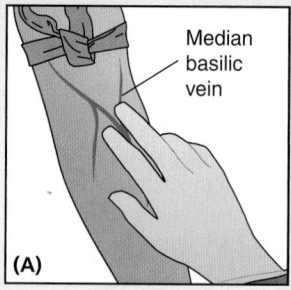
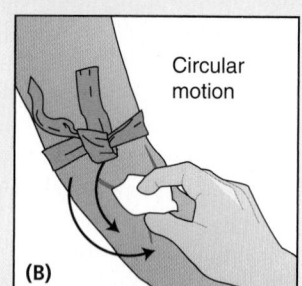
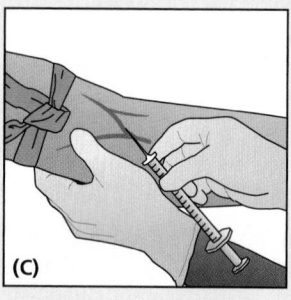
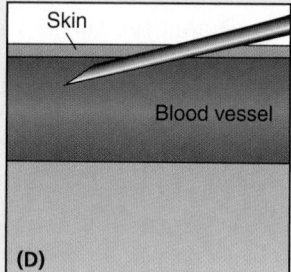
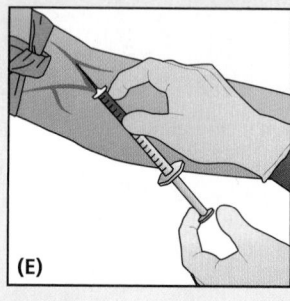
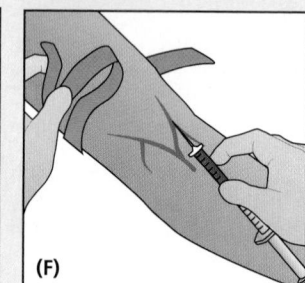
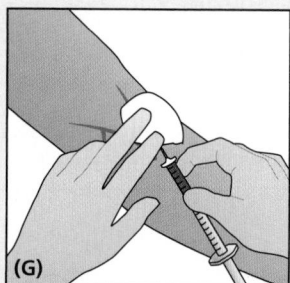
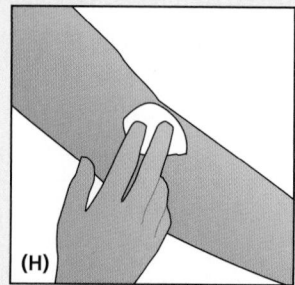

Figure 40-27   (A) Find vein and apply tourniquet.
(B) Apply alcohol and allow to air dry.
(C) Draw skin taut and insert needle.
(D) Needle entering the blood vessel.
(E) Withdraw blood slowly.
(F) Release tourniquet.
(G) Apply sterile pad before withdrawing needle.
(H) Have patient apply pressure to the site until clot forms.

Procedure

40-2 *(continued)*

24. Immediately discard the syringe and needle in the appropriate containers; e.g., needle to sharps container.
25. Discard the gauze and other waste in biohazard containers.
26. Label all tubes before leaving the examination room.
27. Apply an adhesive bandage (Figure 40-27I).
28. Remove and discard gloves and mask in a biohazard container.
29. Wash hands.
30. Thank the patient.
31. Document procedure.

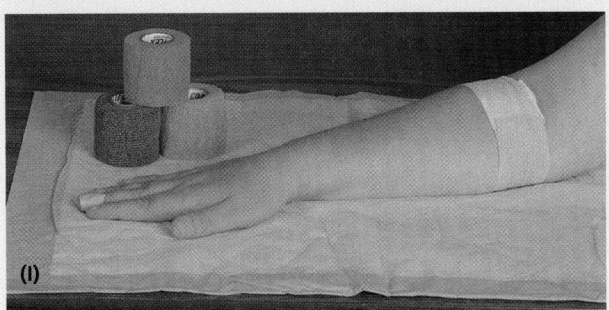

(I)

Figure 40-27 *(continued)* (I) Adhesive bandages for venipuncture are available in a variety of colors.

Procedure

40-3 **Venipuncture by Evacuated Tube System**

STANDARD PRECAUTIONS:

    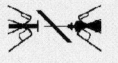

PURPOSE:
To obtain venous blood acceptable for laboratory testing as required by a physician.

SPECIMEN
Venous blood collected by evacuated tubes. Volume of blood dependent on size of tube and test requirements.

EQUIPMENT/SUPPLIES:

Gloves	Evacuated tube(s) or special collection tube(s)
Goggles and mask, if necessary	Tourniquet
Evacuated tube holder	70% isopropyl alcohol swab
Disposable needle for evacuated tube system, 20, 21, or 22 gauge needle	Gauze or cotton balls
	Adhesive bandage or tape
	Sharps container

PROCEDURE STEPS:
1. Position and identify the patient. Ask the patient's name and verify it with the computer label or identification number.
2. If a fasting specimen is required, verify that the patient has not had anything to eat or drink.
3. Wash hands.
4. Put on gloves, as well as goggles and mask if there is a potential for blood splatter.
5. Assemble equipment.
6. Break the needle seal. Thread the appropriate needle into the holder using the needle sheath as a wrench.
7. Before using, tap all tubes that contain additives to ensure that all the additive is dislodged from the stopper and wall of the tube.
8. Insert the tube into the holder until the needle slightly enters the stopper. Avoid pushing the needle beyond the recessed guideline, because a loss of vacuum may result. If the tube retracts slightly, leave it in the retracted position to avoid prematurely puncturing the rubber stopper.

(continues)

Procedure
40-3 *(continued)*

9. Apply the tourniquet.
10. Ask the patient to close the hand. The patient must not be allowed to pump the hand. Pumping of the hand will change the values of the laboratory tests being drawn. If possible, place the patient's arm in a downward position.
11. Select a vein, noting the location and direction of the vein.
12. Clean the venipuncture site with a 70 percent isopropyl alcohol swab.
13. Do not touch the venipuncture site.
14. Draw the patient's skin taut with your thumb. Place the thumb 1 to 2 inches below or above the puncture site (Figure 40-28). This will anchor the vein.
15. With the bevel up, line up the needle with the vein and puncture the vein. Remove your hand from drawing the skin taut. Grasp the flange of the evacuated tube holder and push the tube forward until the butt end of the needle punctures the stopper. Do not change hands while performing the venipuncture. The hand performing the venipuncture is the hand that holds the evacuated tube holder. The opposite hand manipulates the tubes.
16. Fill the tube until the vacuum is exhausted and blood flow into the tube ceases. This will assure the proper blood to anticoagulant ratio.
17. When the blood flow ceases, remove the tube from the holder. While securely grasping the evacuated tube holder with one hand, use the other hand to change the tubes. The rubber sleeve recovers the needle point, stopping the flow of blood until the next tube is inserted.
18. After drawing, immediately mix each tube that contains an additive. Gently inverting the tube 5 to 10 times provides adequate mixing without causing hemolysis.
19. Ask the patient to open the hand.
20. Release the tourniquet.
21. Lightly place a sterile gauze square or cotton ball above the venipuncture site.
22. Remove the needle from the arm. Be certain the last tube drawn has been removed from the holder before removing the needle. This prevents blood dripping from the tip of the needle.
23. Apply pressure to the site for 3 to 5 minutes. The patient may assist if able by elevating the arm above heart level to reduce blood flow. The arm should be held in a raised, outstretched position. Do not allow the patient to bend the arm at the elbow. Bending the arm at the elbow to apply pressure may lead to a hematoma.
24. Label all tubes at the patient's side before leaving the examination room.
25. Apply an adhesive bandage.
26. Remove and discard gloves and mask in a biohazard container.
27. Wash hands.
28. Thank the patient.
29. Document procedure.

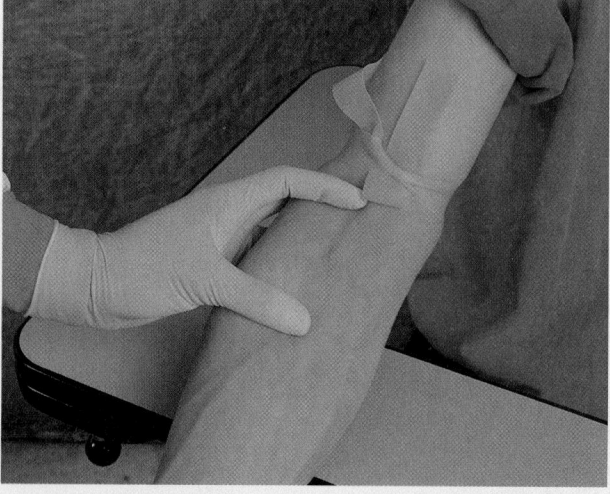

Figure 40-28   Pull the skin taut to prevent vein roll.

Procedure 40-4 Venipuncture by Butterfly Needle System

STANDARD PRECAUTIONS:

 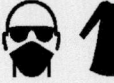 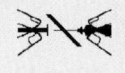

PURPOSE:
To obtain venous blood acceptable for laboratory testing as required by a physician.

SPECIMEN
Venous blood collected by butterfly needle system. Volume of blood dependent on size of tube and test requirements.

EQUIPMENT/SUPPLIES:

Gloves

Goggles and mask, if necessary

Evacuated tube holder

Butterfly needle system, 21, 23, or 25 gauge needle with or without luer adapter

Evacuated tube(s) or special collection tube(s)

Tourniquet

70% isopropyl alcohol swab

Gauze or cotton balls

Adhesive bandage or tape

Sharps container

PROCEDURE STEPS:

1. Position and identify the patient. Ask the patient's name and verify it with the computer label or identification number.
2. If a fasting specimen is required, verify that the patient has not had anything to eat or drink.
3. Wash hands.
4. Put on gloves, as well as safety glasses and mask if there is a potential for blood splatter.
5. Assemble equipment.
6. Open the package of butterfly needle system with evacuated tube luer adapter. The **luer** screws into the evacuated tube holder. The part inside the holder has a needle to puncture the tube top, the part outside the holder fits into a tubing port. Thread the luer needle into the holder.
7. Before using, tap all tubes that contain additives to ensure that all the additive is dislodged from the stopper and wall of the tube.
8. Insert the tube into the holder until the needle slightly enters the stopper. Avoid pushing the needle beyond the recessed guideline, because a loss of vacuum may result. If the tube retracts slightly, leave it in the retracted position.

9. Apply the tourniquet.
10. Ask the patient to close the hand. The patient must not be allowed to pump the hand. If possible, place the patient's arm in a downward position.
11. Select a vein, noting the location and direction of the vein.
12. Clean the venipuncture site with a 70 percent isopropyl alcohol swab.
13. Do not touch the venipuncture site.
14. Draw the patient's skin taut with your thumb and forefinger. Spread the thumb and forefinger 1 to 2 inches to each side of the puncture site.
15. Hold the wings of the butterfly with the bevel up. Line up the needle with the vein and perform the venipuncture. Remove your hand from drawing the skin taut. Grasp the flange of the evacuated tube holder and push the tube forward until the butt end of the needle punctures the stopper.
16. Fill the tube until the vacuum is exhausted and blood flow into the tube ceases. This will assure the proper blood to anticoagulant ratio. Due to air in the tubing, a loss of approximately 0.5 ml will result when collecting the initial evacuated tube.
17. When the blood flow ceases, remove the tube from the holder. While securely grasping the evacuated tube holder with one hand, use the other hand to change the tubes. The rubber sleeve recovers the point, stopping the flow of blood until the next tube of blood is inserted. Multiple draws require the same order of draw as an evacuated tube system draw.
18. After drawing, immediately mix each tube that contains an additive. Gently inverting the tube 5 to 10 times provides adequate mixing without causing **hemolysis**.
19. Ask the patient to open the hand.
20. Release the tourniquet.
21. Lightly place a sterile gauze square or cotton ball above the venipuncture site.
22. Remove the needle from the arm. Be certain the last tube drawn has been removed from the holder before removing the needle. This prevents blood dripping off the tip of the needle.
23. Apply pressure to the site for 3 to 5 minutes. The patient may assist if able by elevating the arm

(continues)

Procedure

40-4 *(continued)*

above heart level to reduce blood flow. The arm should be held in a raised, outstretched position. Do not allow the patient to bend the arm at the elbow. Bending the arm at the elbow to apply pressure may lead to a hematoma.

24. Label all tubes at the patient's side before leaving the examination room.
25. Apply an adhesive bandage.
26. Remove and discard gloves and mask in a biohazard container.
27. Wash hands.
28. Thank the patient.
29. Document procedure.

VARIATION TO THE PROCEDURE:

1. Draw with a butterfly system without a luer adapter.
2. Instead of threading the luer into the holder in step 6, attach a syringe.
3. Omit step 8.
4. In steps 15, 16, and 17, pull on the syringe instead of pushing the tube into the holder.
5. Aliquot blood into appropriate tubes as outlined in the syringe procedure.

Procedure

40-5 **Capillary Puncture by Fingerstick**

STANDARD PRECAUTIONS:

PURPOSE:

To obtain capillary blood acceptable for laboratory testing as required by a physician.

SPECIMEN:

Capillary blood collected by finger puncture. Volume of blood dependent on size of microcollection devices and test requirements.

EQUIPMENT/SUPPLIES:

Gloves
Goggles and mask, if necessary
70% isopropyl alcohol swab or pad
Microcollection tubes or capillary tubes
Lancet
Gauze
Adhesive bandage or tape
Sharps container

PROCEDURE STEPS:

1. Position and identify the patient. Ask the patient's name and verify it with the computer label or identification number.
2. If a fasting specimen is required, verify that the patient has not had anything to eat or drink.
3. Wash hands.
4. Put on gloves, as well as goggles and mask.
5. Assemble equipment.
6. Select puncture site on the palmar surface of the distal phalanx of the ring or middle finger. Do not use the side or tip of the finger. If necessary, warm site with a moist towel at a temperature not higher than 42°C for three to five minutes.
7. Clean the puncture site with a 70% isopropyl alcohol pad.
8. Allow the site to air dry.
9. Perform the puncture perpendicular to the fingerprint, holding the hand firmly to prevent sudden movement.
10. Using a clean gauze pad, wipe away the first drop

(continues)

Procedure

40-5 *(continued)*

of blood. Holding the finger in a downward position, apply gentle pressure to the finger. *Do not squeeze or milk the finger.*

11. Collect specimens using the proper order of draw.
12. Mix tubes with additives well.
13. Place a clean gauze pad on the puncture site and apply pressure until the bleeding stops.
14. Label all tubes at the patient's side before leaving the examination room.
15. Apply a bandage if necessary. Bandages are not

recommended for children under the age of two. Parents or guardian must be instructed to monitor the child carefully as the potential for ingestion of the bandage exists.

16. Remove and discard gloves and mask in a biohazard container.
17. Wash hands.
18. Thank the patient.
19. Document procedure.

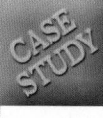

CASE STUDY 40-1

Inner City Health Care is short-staffed today and medical assistant Liz Corbin is feeling pressed for time. She has many tasks to complete, but first she must perform a venipuncture. She greets the patient, Wayne Elder, in a perfunctory manner, discouraging time-wasting conversation. Although Wayne appears apprehensive, he is not resistant, so Liz quickly assembles the necessary supplies, applies the tourniquet, and inserts the needle. While she is drawing his blood, Wayne faints.

CASE STUDY REVIEW

1. What should Liz do now?
2. What could Liz have done to prevent this situation from occurring?
3. In the future, what are some steps Liz can take to provide a positive experience for venipuncture patients?

SUMMARY

With a little practice, the medical assistant will become an expert at phlebotomy. The skills of phlebotomy cannot be learned primarily from a textbook; continuous practice will develop the skill to perfection. It may take months before the medical assistant feels comfortable and is able to obtain a sample without difficulty.

In all phlebotomy, safety is of the utmost consideration. Dispose of all sharps properly and separately from the noncontaminated trash. Proper handwashing between patients and wearing gloves, goggles, and masks with each phlebotomy will assure safety for both the patient and the medical assistant.

Proper specimen collection and handling of the specimen after collection by the medical assistant will assure that the patient obtains the most accurate result. The specimen must be treated in such a way that the integrity of the specimen is maintained. The quality of the sample must be the same when collected as when tested. Correct method of draw, order of draw, and the correct handling of the sample after collection will reduce the number of factors affecting the sample and give the most accurate result possible.

REVIEW QUESTIONS

Multiple Choice

1. Drawing blood with a 25 gauge needle increases the chance for:
   a. vein collapse
   b. hematomas
   c. hemoconcentration
   d. hemolysis

2. An anticoagulant is an additive placed in evacuated tubes in order to:
   a. dilute the blood prior to testing
   b. ensure the sterility of the tube
   c. make the blood clot faster
   d. prevent the blood from clotting

3. When collecting a blood sample with an evacuated tube system, the last tube drawn is withdrawn from the holder before removing the needle from the patient in order to:
   a. avoid hematoma at the venipuncture site
   b. avoid dripping blood out the end of the needle
   c. prevent clotting of the blood
   d. cause the blood to clot

4. Leaving the tourniquet on a patient's arm for an extended length of time before drawing blood may cause:
   a. hemoconcentration *stagnant blood.*
   b. specimen hemolysis
   c. stress
   d. bruising

5. The single most important way to prevent the spread of infection from patient to patient is:
   a. gowning and gloving
   b. handwashing
   c. always wearing masks
   d. avoid breathing on clients

6. Under standard precautions, all used needles are to be disposed of in the following manner:
   a. recapped
   b. discarded intact in a sharps container
   c. bent
   d. broken or cut off

7. When drawing multiple specimens in evacuated tubes, it is important to fill which of the following color-stoppered tubes first?
   a. light blue
   b. green
   c. lavender
   d. red

8. The anticoagulant of choice when drawing coagulation studies such as PT and APTT is:
   a. (red) no anticoagulant
   b. (light blue) sodium citrate
   c. (lavender) EDTA
   d. (green) heparin

9. When the medical assistant cannot perform a venipuncture successfully after two attempts, the medical assistant should:
   a. try at least two more times
   b. notify the physician
   c. ask another medical assistant to try
   d. request the test for the next day

10. If the blood is drawn too quickly from a small vein, the vein has a tendency to:
    a. collapse
    b. bruise
    c. disintegrate
    d. roll

Critical Thinking

1. A frightened patient begins crying when you enter the room to perform a venipuncture. How will you handle the situation? What is your responsibility to the patient? Why are your demeanor and appearance important in this type of situation?

2. Explain the difference between serum and plasma. Describe how serum and plasma samples are collected.

3. You are preparing to perform a venipuncture on a geriatric patient who has fragile veins. Which system will you use—a syringe and needle or an evacuated tube system? Why? How can vein collapse be avoided?

4. Discuss how clots are formed and what can be done to stop the clotting process.

5. You've calmed the crying patient and successfully drawn the patient's blood. What will you do next? Why is this step important? Describe the skills you have used.

6. The patient cries out in pain when you insert the needle into the vein. What will you do to make the patient more comfortable? If you decide to try another site, how will you locate it?

WEB ACTIVITIES

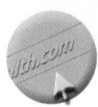

1. Visit the CDC and other government web sites for the most current information on Standard Precautions and proper protection during blood draws.

2. Search the keywords phlebotomy and puncture on the web. What organizations can you find that offer information for medical assistants?

REFERENCES/BIBLIOGRAPHY

Federal register, rules and regulations, 29 CFR part 1910.1030. (Vol. 56, 235). 1991, December 6.

Geller, S. J. (1992, March 3). *Effect of sample collection on laboratory test results.* ASCP Teleconference Series.

Hoeltke, L. B. (2000). *The complete textbook of phlebotomy* (2nd ed.). Albany, NY: Delmar.

National Committee for Clinical Laboratory Standards. (1991). *Protection of laboratory workers from infectious disease transmitted by blood, body fluids, and tissue* (2nd ed.). Approved Standard. NCCLS Document. M29-T2, Villanova, PA: National Committee for Clinical Laboratory Standards.

National Committee for Clinical Laboratory Standards. (1996). *Evacuated tubes and additives for blood specimen collection* (4th ed.). Approved Standard. NCCLS Document. H1-A4. Villanova, PA: Author.

National Committee for Clinical Laboratory Standards. (1998). *Collection, transport, and processing of blood specimen for coagulation testing and general performance of coagulation assays* (3rd ed.). Approved Guideline. NCCLS Document. H21-A3. Villanova, PA: Author.

National Committee for Clinical Laboratory Standards. (1998). *Procedures for the collection of diagnostic blood specimens by venipuncture* (4th ed.). Approved Standard. NCCLS document H3-A4. Villanova, PA: Author.

National Committee for Clinical Laboratory Standards. (1999). *Procedures and devices for the collection of diagnostic blood specimens by skin puncture* (4th ed.). Approved Guideline. NCCLS Document. H4-A4. Villanova, PA: Author.

Peek, G. J., Marsh, H., Keating, J., et al. (1990). The effects of swabbing the skin on apparent blood ethanol concentration. *Alcohol Alcoholism 25,* 639–640.

Tilton, R. C., Balows, A., Hohnadel, D. C., & Reiss, R. F. (1992). *Clinical laboratory medicine* (pp. 813–823). St. Louis: Mosby-Year Book.

Wedding, M. E., & Toenjes, S. A. (1992). *Medical laboratory procedures.* Philadelphia: F. A. Davis.

Chapter 41

HEMATOLOGY

KEY TERMS

Anisocytosis
Basophil
Centrifugal Hematology Analysis
Complete Blood Count (CBC)
Cyanmethemoglobin
Eosinophil
Erythrocyte
Erythrocyte Indices
Erythrocyte Sedimentation Rate
Erythropoietin
Hemacytometer (also spelled
    Hemocytometer)
Hematocrit
Hematology
Hematopoiesis
Hemoglobin
Hemoglobinopathy
Hypochromic
Impedance Principle
Leukocyte
Lymphocyte
Macrocytic
Microcytic
Monocyte
Neutrophil
Normochromic
Normocytic
Poikilocytosis
Polychromatic Stain
Thrombocyte

OUTLINE

OBJECTIVES

The student should strive to meet the following performance objectives and demonstrate an understanding of the facts and principles presented in this chapter through written and oral communication.

1. Define the key terms as presented in the glossary.

2. Describe the process of hematopoiesis.

3. Discuss how the clinical science of hematology and the CBC are used in the diagnosis and treatment of disease.

4. Compare the normal versus abnormal values of the CBC parameters.

5. Discuss how the hemoglobin and hematocrit are used to diagnose anemia.

6. Describe how the erythrocyte indices are used in the differential diagnosis of anemias.

7. Perform the calculations necessary to derive the erythrocyte indices MCV, MCH, and MCHC.

8. List the steps required to prepare and stain a differential white blood cell smear.

9. List the five types of normal white blood cells that can be seen on a stained blood smear and give the identifying characteristics of each.   (*continues*)

10. Describe the differences in the procedures for the Wintrobe and Westergren erythrocyte sedimentation rates.
11. Recognize the physiological reasons why the erythrocyte sedimentation rate varies with different states of health and disease.
12. List the two general types of automated hematology instruments used in the ambulatory care setting and describe their technology.
13. Perform the laboratory procedures included in this chapter in a manner acceptable for entry-level employment.

ROLE DELINEATION COMPONENTS

CLINICAL

Fundamental Principles

- Apply principles of aseptic technique and infection control
- Comply with quality assurance practices
- Screen and follow up patient test results

Diagnostic Orders

- Collect and process specimens
- Perform diagnostic tests

GENERAL (TRANSDISCIPLINARY)

Legal Concepts

- Document accurately
- Comply with established risk management and safety procedures

SCENARIO

The physicians in the office of Doctors Lewis & King MD often order hematological tests to assist them in diagnosing and treating patients. As she performs the tests in the physician's office laboratory, clinical medical assistant Audrey Jones uses her knowledge of hematology every day. Audrey is comfortable using an automated hematology analyzer or performing tests manually because she understands the purposes and procedures of the tests. She always follows all safety and quality control guidelines to protect herself and others and to ensure the accuracy of test results.

INTRODUCTION

Hematology is the study of the blood cells and coagulation in both normal and diseased states. The two main components of the blood are plasma (the liquid portion) and cells. Cells of the blood are also known as the formed elements of the blood. The study of hematology is usually limited to the cellular components of the blood and does not include the chemistry of the blood.

The cellular components of blood include **erythrocytes** (red blood cells), **leukocytes** (white blood cells), and **thrombocytes** (platelets). Blood has many different functions. These include the process of supplying nutrients and oxygen to all cells as well as the removal of the end products of metabolism. Blood is also involved in fighting infection as well as producing antibodies which are used in our immune systems for defense against foreign antigens.

Hematopoiesis is defined as the formation of blood cells (Figure 41-1). The process of hematopoiesis, as well as the blood-forming tissues of the body, is included in the study of hematology. In the embryo, hematopoiesis occurs in the yolk sac, liver, and spleen. After we are born, the primary site for the production of erythrocytes, granulocytes, and platelets is the bone marrow. Lymphocytes are also produced in the bone marrow, as well as in the lymph nodes. At birth, most of the bone marrow in the body is capable of producing blood cells. This process is confined to the bone marrow of the ribs, vertebrae, sternum, and iliac crest by the age of 20. Bone marrow that is producing cells is known as red marrow. As the area for hematopoiesis is reduced, the red bone marrow is replaced by yellow marrow, which is stored fat. When a physician collects a bone marrow sample in an adult, the site chosen for sampling is the sternum or the iliac crest.

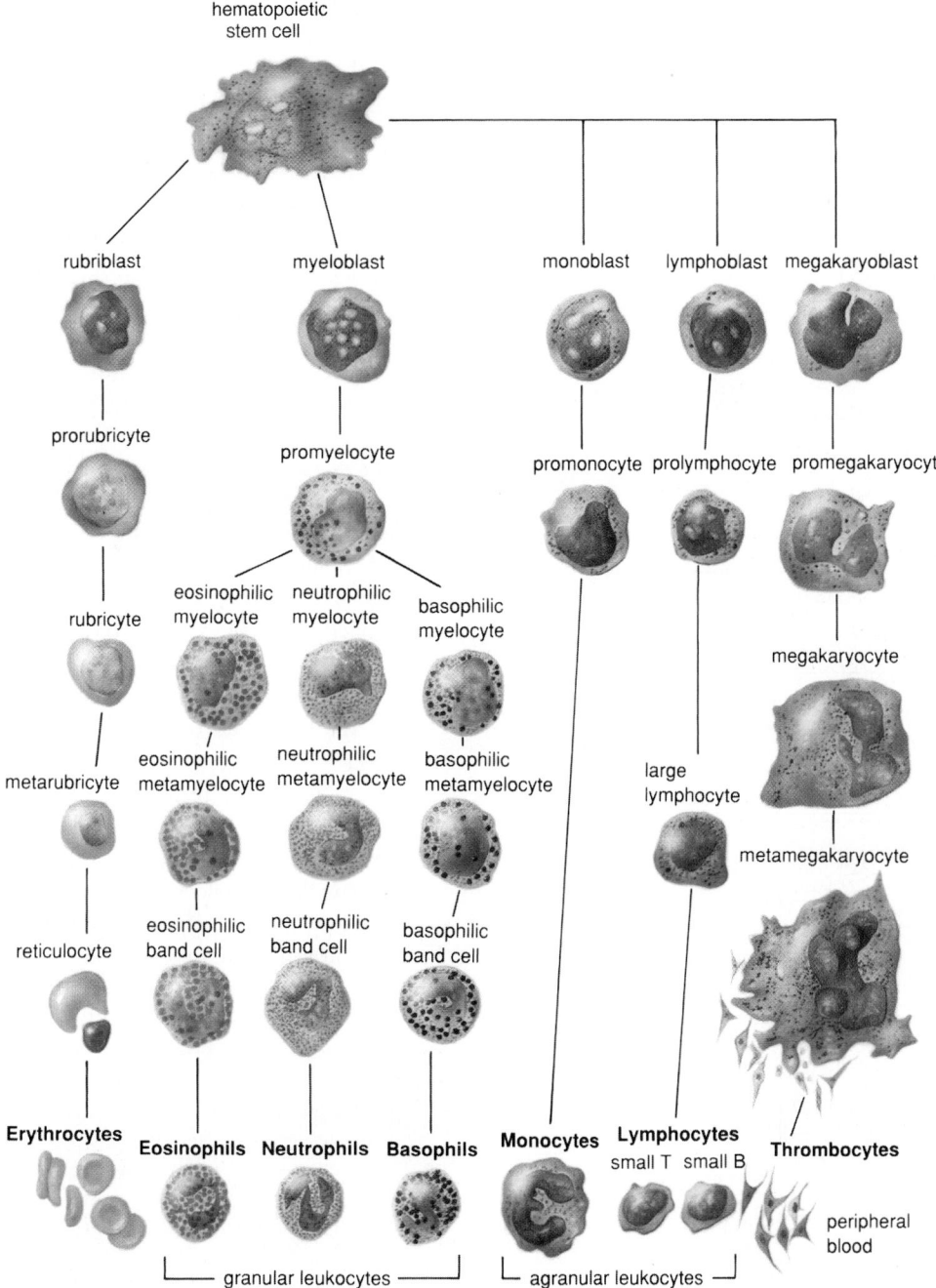

hematopoietic
stem cell

rubriblast

prorubricyte

rubricyte

metarubricyte

reticulocyte

Erythrocytes

myeloblast

promyelocyte

eosinophilic   neutrophilic
myelocyte   myelocyte
                                        basophilic
                                        myelocyte

eosinophilic   neutrophilic
metamyelocyte   metamyelocyte
                                        basophilic
                                        metamyelocyte

eosinophilic   neutrophilic
band cell   band cell
                                        basophilic
                                        band cell

Eosinophils   Neutrophils   Basophils

monoblast   lymphoblast   megakaryoblast

promonocyte   prolymphocyte   promegakaryocyte

megakaryocyte

large
lymphocyte

metamegakaryocyte

Monocytes   Lymphocytes
small T small B

Thrombocytes

peripheral
blood

└── granular leukocytes ──┘   └── agranular leukocytes ──┘

Figure 41-1   Hematopoiesis showing blood cells and platelet formation starting with hematopoietic stem cell.

HEMATOLOGICAL TESTS

Hematological tests are the second most common tests performed in the physician's office laboratory (POL). The most common test is the urinalysis. The cellular components of the blood may be affected by changes in either the blood-forming organs or in other tissues of the body. The study of these changes forms the basis of hematological tests performed in the POL.

Hematological tests performed in the clinical laboratory include:

- Hemoglobin
- Hematocrit
- White blood cell count (WBC)
- Red blood cell count (RBC)
- Platelet count
- Differential white blood cell count
- Erythrocyte sedimentation rate (ESR)
- Prothrombin time (PT)

The results of these hematological tests provide valuable information used by the physician in making a diagnosis, evaluating a patient's progress, and/or regulating further treatment.

The laboratory test ordered most frequently on blood in the ambulatory care setting is the complete blood count (CBC). The exact number of parameters included in the CBC will vary from laboratory to laboratory (Figure 41-2). The CBC generally includes:

- Hemoglobin determination
- Hematocrit determination
- White blood cell count (WBC)
- Red blood cell count (RBC)
- Differential white blood cell count

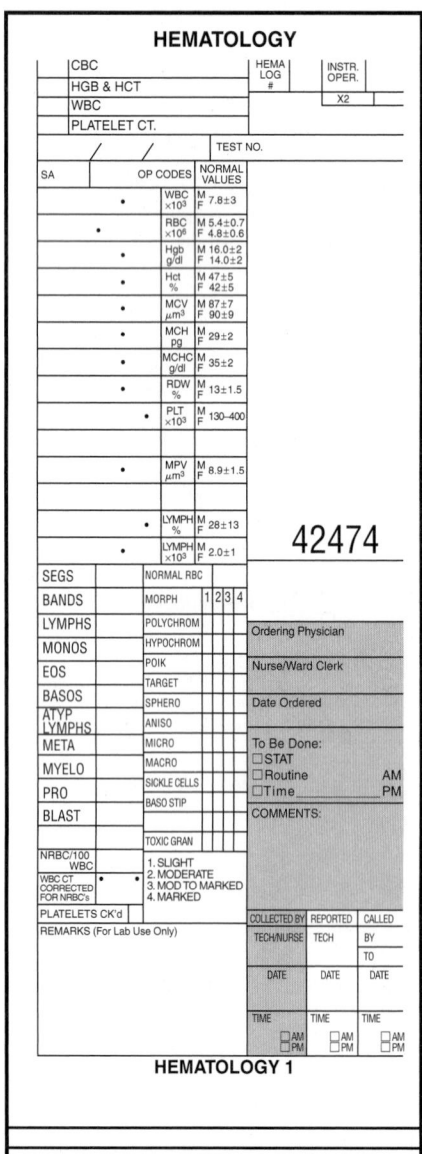

Figure 41-2 Hematology requisition form.

Erythrocyte indices are frequently included as a part of the complete blood count.

All of these tests can be performed by manual testing procedures or with an automated hematology analyzer. It is important to note that all automated hematology analyzers utilize a modification or adaptation of the manual methods. A complete understanding of each manual procedure will help you understand the automated methods.

Hemoglobin and Hematocrit Determinations

Hemoglobin and hematocrit tests are part of the complete blood count; however, they are frequently the only parameters of the CBC ordered by the physician. The abbreviations for hemoglobin and hematocrit are Hgb and Hct, respectively. Hemoglobin is the major component of the erythrocyte and serves as a transport vehicle for oxygen and carbon dioxide in the body. The hematocrit (packed red blood cell volume) is the ratio of the volume of packed red blood cells to that of the whole blood. Packed red blood cell volume is expressed as a percentage of the whole blood following centrifugation of the blood.

Hemoglobin is responsible for about 85 percent of the dry weight of the red blood cells. Hemoglobin is a conjugated protein composed of heme and globin. A single hemoglobin molecule consists of four globin chains with a heme group attached to each globin (Figure 41-3). The central ion of each heme group is an iron molecule.

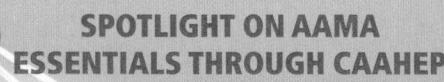

SPOTLIGHT ON AAMA ESSENTIALS THROUGH CAAHEP

- When required to perform hematology tests, the medical assistant should be knowledgeable in the skills necessary to perform the tests and sensitive to the patient's psychosocial needs and fears.

- By understanding methods used in hematology testing, the medical assistant will be better equipped to help the patient understand the procedures and to offer reassurance.

- It is important that the medical assistant remember to treat all patients with compassion and empathy when performing any type of hematology testing.

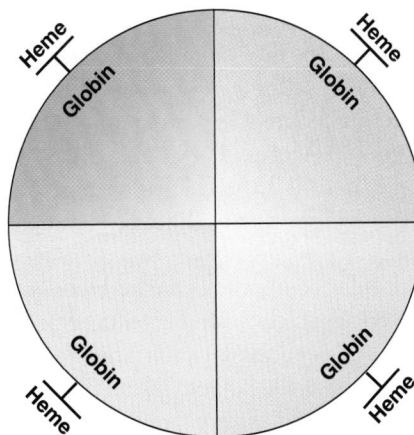

Figure 41-3 A normal hemoglobin molecule containing four globin chains with a heme group attached to each globin. One oxygen molecule can be transported by each heme group.

Synthesis of the heme portion of the hemoglobin molecule requires iron. The iron used in the synthesis of hemoglobin is normally absorbed in the duodenum of the small intestine following dietary intake. The daily iron requirement for an adult male is about 0.5 mg/day. A menstruating female requires about 2 mg/day.

As stated earlier, the major function of hemoglobin in the body is the transportation of oxygen to all the body cells. Hemoglobin carries 95 percent of all the oxygen to the cells and is responsible for transporting about 27 percent of the carbon dioxide produced by cellular metabolism back to the lungs where it is removed. The hemoglobin in the red blood cells also acts as a buffer system. This buffer system accounts for approximately 30 percent of the buffering capacity of whole blood.

The production of new red blood cells and consequently the formation of more hemoglobin is triggered by the hormone **erythropoietin**, which is produced in the kidney. This hematopoietic process is started when there is a decrease of available oxygen at the cellular level. Hgb A makes up the majority of normal hemoglobin found in the adult.

There are several forms of abnormal hemoglobin that are responsible for a group of diseases known as **hemoglobinopathies**. These abnormal forms of hemoglobin include hemoglobin S, hemoglobin C, and hemoglobin E. Hemoglobin S (Hgb S) is the most common abnormal form of hemoglobin observed in the laboratory. It is the form of hemoglobin that causes sickle cell anemia. When Hgb S molecules are subjected to certain conditions, they alter the physical structure of the red blood cells. The red blood cells assume a sickle shape, which makes it difficult, if not impossible, for the cell to pass through a capillary bed.

The most frequent hemoglobin disease seen in the ambulatory care setting is anemia, with iron deficiency anemia being the most common type. The laboratory findings of these individuals will be a normal or near normal hematocrit with a low hemoglobin value. The red blood cells of these individuals will be **hypochromic** because they lack hemoglobin. A decrease in available iron in the body is the most common cause of this type of anemia.

Hemoglobin values are determined by two methods: the specific gravity and **cyanmethemoglobin** methods. The specific gravity test is a procedure that utilizes different specific gravity solutions of copper sulfate. This is a screening technique used to determine the eligibility of blood donors; it is not an exact measurement method. The common way to measure hemoglobin levels in the ambulatory care setting is known as the cyanmethemoglobin method. This test is performed either by manual or automated methods. See Procedures 41-1 and 41-2.

The principle of the cyanmethemoglobin procedure is the same regardless of the method utilized. The red blood cells are lysed with a solution containing potassium ferricyanide and sodium cyanide which converts hemoglobin to cyanmethemoglobin. The cyanide solution is known as Drabkin's reagent and is sold under many brand names. Cyanmethemoglobin is a very stable compound, but it must be protected from light and excess heat. The pigmented solution of cyanmethemoglobin is read photometrically in a colorimeter or spectrophotometer at a wavelength of 540 nanometers (nm). The results are reported in grams per deciliter (g/dL). It is important to note that all forms of hemoglobin are converted to cyanmethemoglobin by this method except hemoglobin S.

CAUTION: The Drabkin's solution is poisonous. Precautions to observe when working with any reagents includes wearing gloves, working in a well-ventilated area, properly disposing of used reagents, wiping up all spills, and handwashing.

The normal reference values for hemoglobin vary according to both the age and sex of the individual (Table 41-1).

The hematocrit (packed red blood cell volume) is the ratio of the volume of packed red blood cells to that of the whole blood. Packed red blood cell volume is expressed as a percentage of the whole blood. This is achieved by centrifuging a prepared blood sample. It

TABLE 41-1	NORMAL HEMOGLOBIN VALUES OR REFERENCE RANGES BY AGE AND/OR SEX
Newborn	15–20 g/dL
Age three months	9–14 g/dL
Age ten months	12–14.5 g/dL
Adult female	12–16 g/dL
Adult male	13–18 g/dL

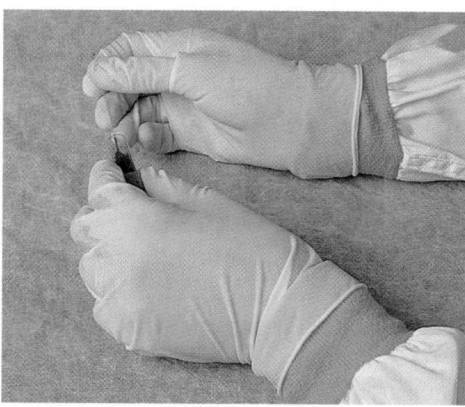

Figure 41-4 Filling a microhematocrit tube with blood by capillary action.

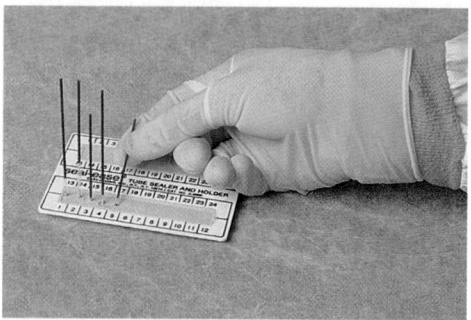

Figure 41-5 Sealing the microhematocrit tube with sealing clay.

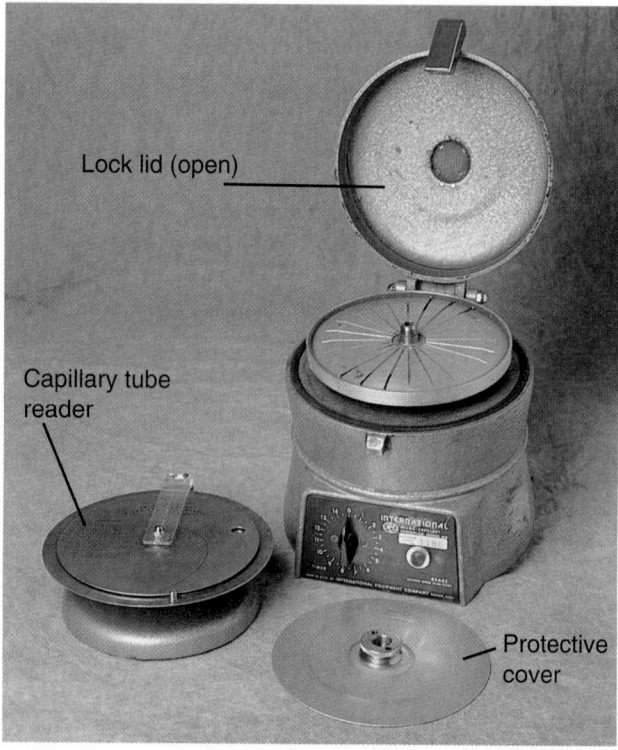

Figure 41-6 Microhematocrit centrifuge (right) with protective cover and lock lid (open) and a microhematocrit capillary tube reader (left).

can be performed using either a macrotechnique or a microtechnique. In the ambulatory care setting, the microtechnique is utilized. The test is called a microhematocrit (see Procedure 41-3) and requires only a couple drops of blood (Figures 41-4, 41-5, and 41-6). The macromethod is called the Wintrobe macrohematocrit. This method requires one milliliter (one cubic centimeter) of blood.

The cellular components of the blood sample separate into layers when they are centrifuged at high speeds (Figure 41-7). The cellular layers arrange themselves with the red blood cells at the bottom of the tube. White blood cells and platelets form a very thin layer called the buffy coat on top of the erythrocytes. The buffy coat has a whitish-tan appearance.

The white blood cell count of the sample can be estimated by measuring the buffy coat thickness. Each 0.1 mm of the buffy coat equals approximately 1,000 WBC/mm^3. Therefore, a buffy coat of 1 mm would equal a leukocyte count of approximately 10,000 WBCs/mm^3 and a 0.5 mm reading would equal 5,000 WBCs/mm^3. The cell counts may be reported in units of microliters (μL), which are equivalent to cubic millimeters.

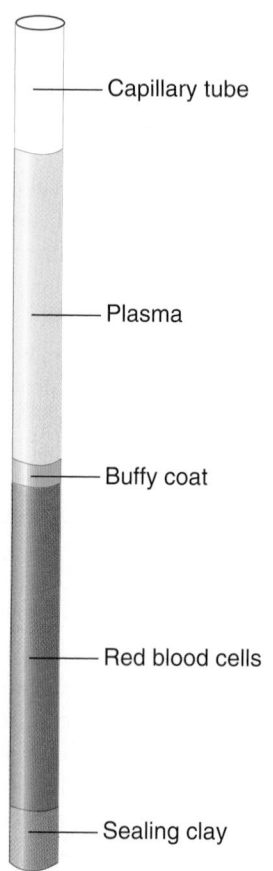

Figure 41-7 Diagram of packed cell column in the hematocrit showing separation of cellular components after centrifugation.

TABLE 41-2	NORMAL HEMATOCRIT VALUES OR REFERENCE RANGES BY AGE AND/OR SEX
Newborn	45–60%
One year old	27–44%
Adult female	36–46%
Adult male	40–55%

The normal values of hematocrit will vary according to the age and sex of the individual (Table 41-2).

Sources of error associated with the microhematocrit method include improper centrifugation, resulting in increased trapped plasma, and improper reading of the packed red cell volume, such as including the buffy coat layer.

CAUTION: The microhematocrit capillary tubes are made of thin glass and are easily broken. Care must be observed when handling these tubes. Gloves must be worn. Hold the tube horizontally with your finger held over the clean end of the three-quarters blood-filled capillary tube. Remove excess blood by wiping off the outside of the filled capillary tube. While holding your finger over the wiped-off collection end, carefully insert the clean end into the sealing clay. Do not exert excessive pressure. Do not contaminate the clay with blood. Self-sealing plastic microhematocrit capillary tubes are now available.

White and Red Blood Cell Counts

White blood cell counts and red blood cell counts can be performed using either a manual or automated method (see Procedures 41-4 and 41-5). All white blood cell counts and red blood cell counts performed in the POL utilize an automated method. It is important to note that all automated testing methods are based on a modification or adaptation of the manual methods. Performing the manual methods gives the student an opportunity to observe what occurs in the automated hematology instrument. The knowledge gained gives students a better understanding of what is really happening and they become better laboratory workers. In the past, blood-diluting pipettes were utilized when a white or red blood cell count was performed. These have been replaced by the Unopette® systems (Figure 41-8) when a manual blood cell count is performed in the medical laboratory.

Both the manual white blood cell count and the red blood cell count can be performed using a Unopette® system. Unopette® systems require that an exact amount of blood sample be diluted with a known volume of diluting solution. The diluted sample is mixed and transferred to a hemacytometer, where the cells are counted with the aid of a microscope. The normal reference values for leukocyte (WBC) counts and erythrocyte (RBC) counts vary according to both age and sex of the individual (Tables 41-3 and 41-4).

White Blood Cell Count Manual Dilution. When a manual white blood cell count is performed using a Unopette® kit, the diluting solution is an acetic acid solution. The solution will lyse the red blood cells and leave only the white blood cells and platelets (thrombocytes) intact.

The Unopette® method for performing a manual WBC count employs the same principle as the classical procedure that was utilized by the WBC diluting pipette method. The disposable blood-diluting Unopette® kit includes a prefilled reservoir of 0.475 mL, 3 percent acetic acid, a 25 μL capacity capillary pipette, and a pipette shield (Figure 41-8). This Unopette® unit gives a dilution of 1:20. Unopette® units are also available that will produce a 1:100 dilution. The diluted sample should stand for ten minutes to allow time for all of the red blood cells to be hemolyzed. The sample is stable for three hours after dilution if it is kept at room temperature.

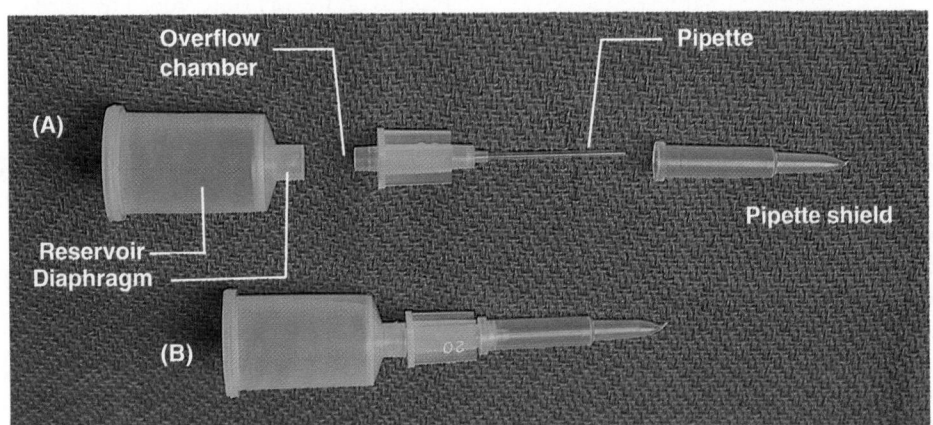

Figure 41-8 Parts of a disposable Unopette® blood-diluting unit: (A) Unassembled Unopette® unit. (B) Assembled unit.

Blood samples in either the white blood cell count or red blood cell count utilizing the Unopette® method may be collected directly from a capillary puncture. If a venipuncture sample is used, it should be collected in an EDTA (lavender) anticoagulant tube.

Red Blood Cell Count Manual Dilution. The manual red blood cell count is performed using the same procedure that was utilized with the white blood cell count. The method uses a pipette and a diluting solution. The diluting solution used with the RBC count is an isotonic salt solution also known as a Hayem and Gower, or Gower solution.

The Unopette® method for performing a manual RBC count employs the same principle as the classical procedure that was utilized by the RBC diluting pipette method. The disposable blood-diluting Unopette® unit includes a prefilled reservoir of 1.99 mL of diluent, a 10 μL pipette, and a pipette shield. The 10 μL pipette used with the 1.99 mL of diluent will give a dilution ratio of 1:200. It is best to perform the count immediately after the sample is diluted; however, the diluted specimen is stable for approximately six hours at room temperature.

CAUTION: The diluent used in the Unopette® RBC unit contains sodium azide which, if placed in an acid environment, can produce the extremely toxic compound hydrazoic acid. Care should be exercised when flooding or cleaning the hemacytometer and when discarding the diluent into the sink. Always dilute the solution with running water.

Both the WBC and the RBC manual counts are performed using a **hemacytometer** (Figure 41-9). The hemacytometer, also called a counting chamber, is a very precise piece of laboratory equipment which allows an exact volume of sample to be examined.

The hemacytometer utilizes a coverglass. Both the hemacytometer and coverglass must be completely clean, free of all dust, dirt, and grease. The process of filling the counting chamber is also known as flooding or charging.

Position the coverglass on the hemacytometer and be sure it covers both ruled areas on the counting cham-

When either a WBC or RBC count is performed using a hemacytometer, it is important that the sample be thoroughly mixed.

When a hemacytometer is filled with a Unopette®, the first two or three drops of diluted sample should be discarded before the counting chamber is flooded.

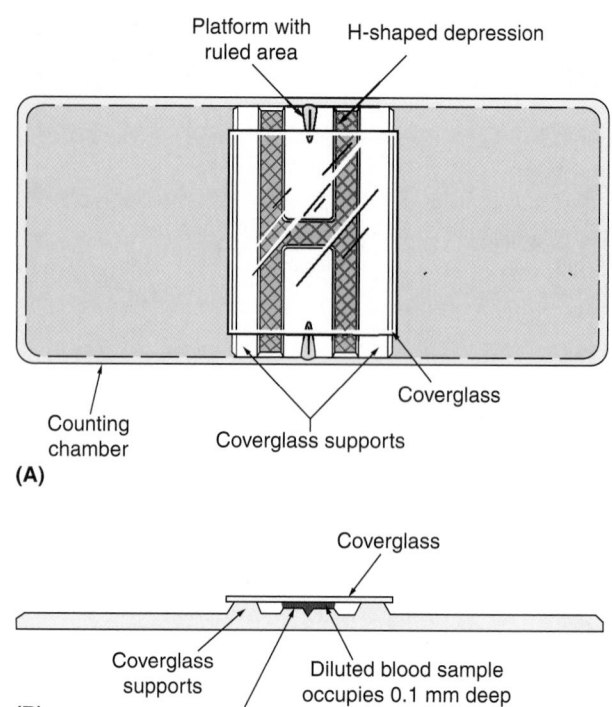

Figure 41-9 Hemacytometer: (A) Top view of hemacytometer with coverglass in place. (B) Side view with coverglass in place.

ber. Fill the chamber by letting the fluid from the Unopette® pipette flow evenly under the coverglass. The fluid should flow only on the platform of the hemacytometer. It *should not* flow into the H-shaped depressed areas (known as moats) that surround the platform. Most hemacytometers have a V-shaped trough to help in the flooding (charging) process. You will be able to see the fluid as it flows under the coverglass. If the hemacytometer is overflooded, it should be cleaned, dried, and the procedure should be repeated. After you have correctly flooded one side of the counting chamber, repeat the process on the opposite side. The filled counting chamber should stand for approximately two minutes to allow the cells to settle out of the fluid and stabilize before the count is performed (Figure 41-10).

Counting the WBC Sample Using Low-Power Magnification. The counting area on the hemacytometer when you are performing a WBC count is usually the four square millimeters indicated with the letter *W* (Figure 41-11). The count is performed using the low-power objective (10X). Remember that the total magnification observed when using the 10X objective is 100X. Magnification is the product of the power of both the objective and the eyepiece (ocular). The eyepiece on most microscopes is 10X; therefore, 10X × 10X = 100X.

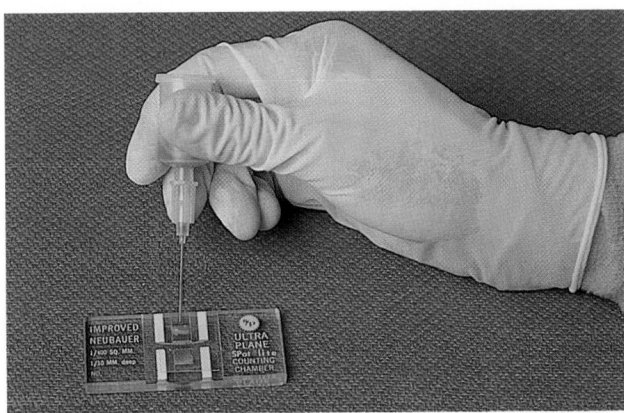

Figure 41-10 Filling the hemacytometer with a well-mixed diluted sample solution from a Unopette®.

Each of the four areas counted in the WBC area contains sixteen squares. The order followed to count the four areas is not really important; however, it is customary to start in the upper left-hand corner and move in a clockwise direction (Figure 41-12). All the cells in each of the four squares marked W are counted using the following rule: Cells that touch the lines on two sides of the area should be counted; cells that touch the other two sides should not be counted (Figure 41-13). This same rule applies when you are performing an RBC count. If the number of cells counted in each of the four groups of sixteen small squares varies by more than plus or minus ten, the count should be discarded. The counting chamber should be cleaned, dried, and filled with a fresh drop of well-mixed sample. Uneven distribution of cells on the counting chamber usually occurs because of a dirty hemacytometer and/or coverglass.

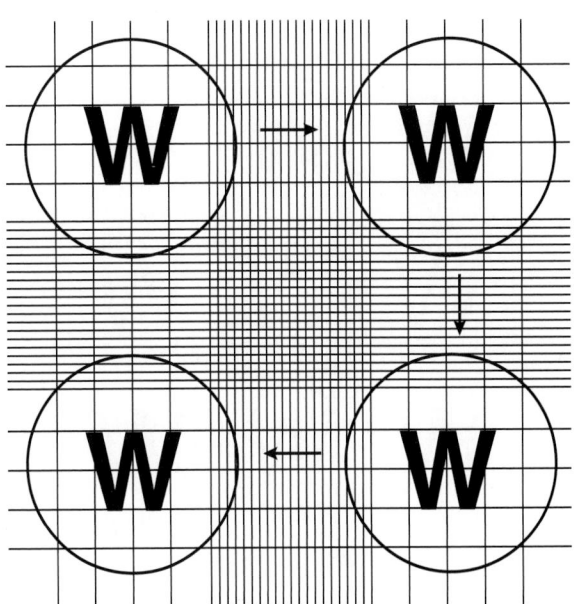

Figure 41-11 WBC counting areas marked with the letter *W*.

NOTE: If the white blood cell count is very low (below 3,000 cells/cu mm), it would be more accurate to count all nine square millimeters on each side of the counting chamber (Figure 41-14). The total would then be divided by nine instead of four. Using the larger area should increase the accuracy of the count.

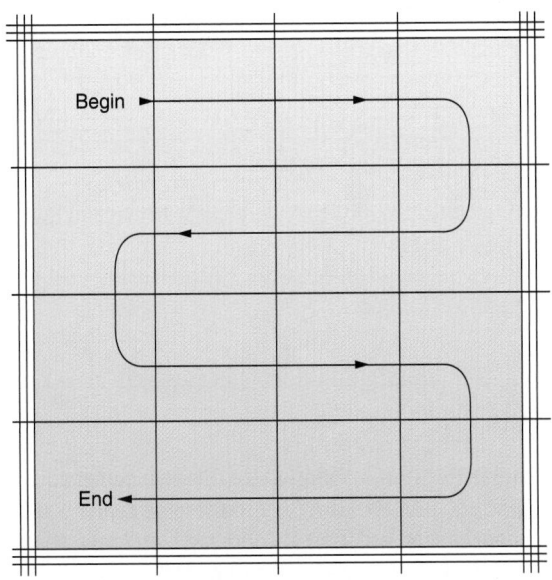

Figure 41-12 Counting pattern to follow when counting each of the one square millimeter areas of the hemacytometer.

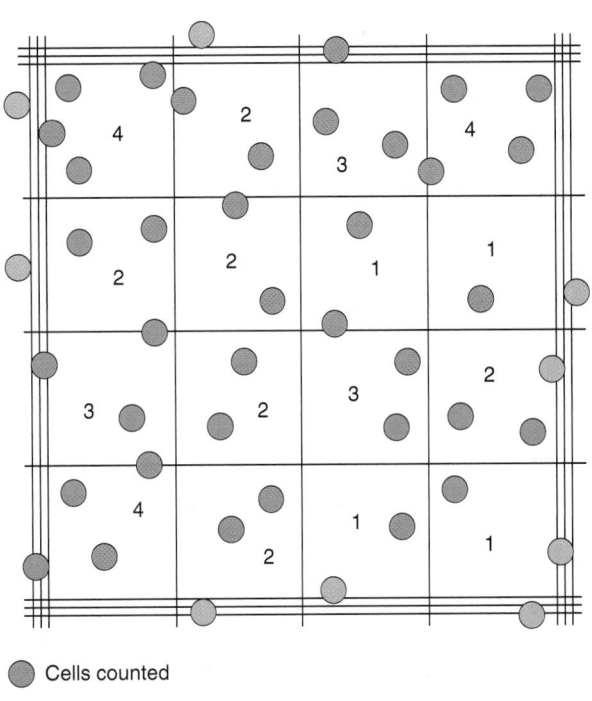

○ Cells counted

○ Cells not counted

Figure 41-13 Sample count in one square *W* area on one side of chamber. The purple cells and numbers shown denote the total number of cells counted in each square.

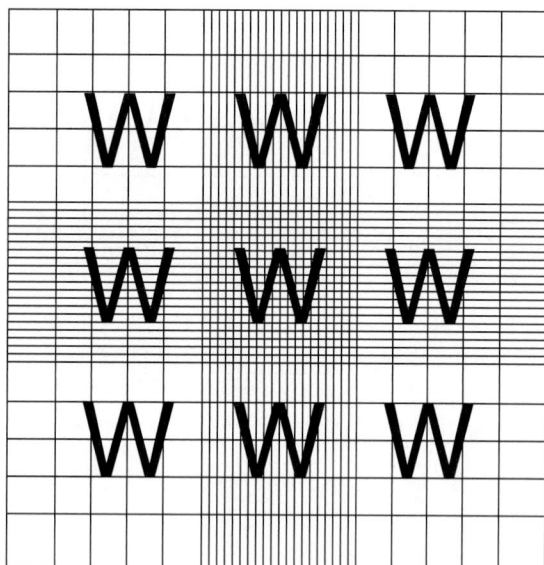

Figure 41-14 All nine large squares of the hemacytometer grid are used to count white blood cells when the count is low.

Calculating the White Blood Cell Count.

The total numbers of cells counted on both sides of the counting chamber are averaged. To calculate the number of white blood cells present in one cubic millimeter, the following formula is applied:

$$WBC/mm^3 = \frac{\text{average number cells counted} \times \text{depth factor} \times \text{dilution factor}}{\text{area counted (mm}^2)}$$

NOTE: The depth factor is always a value of 10 because the distance from the top of the platform of the hemacytometer to the bottom of the coverglass is 0.1 mm. To convert this value to 1 mm, it is multiplied by 10.

Counting the RBC Sample Using High-Power Magnification.

The area counted on the hemacytometer when performing a manual RBC count is usually one-fifth of a square millimeter. The procedure used to fill the hemacytometer for an RBC count is the same as that utilized in the WBC count. After the counting chamber is properly filled, it is allowed to settle for approximately two minutes. The RBC ruled area on the hemacytometer is first located using the low-power objective (10X). With the field in focus, change to the high-power objective (40X) and count the cells in the five RBC areas as indicated in Figure 41-15.

After counting the RBC area on one side of the counting chamber, repeat the procedure on the opposite side. The cells on the hemacytometer should be evenly distributed.

Example:

You perform a WBC count that has a dilution factor of 1:20 and you count the following number of cells. The cells are counted in the four *W* squares on the counting chamber.

1. Counting the cells:

	Side 1		Side 2
Square	Cells Counted	Square	Cells Counted
1	33	1	37
2	37	2	38
3	34	3	34
4	32	4	35
Total	136	Total	144

2. Calculating the average:
   a. 136 + 144 = 280
   b. 280 ÷ 2 = 140

3. Calculating the count:

$$WBC\ mm^3 = \frac{140 \times 10 \times 20}{4} = \frac{28,000}{4}$$
$$= WBC\ mm^3 = 7,000\ (or\ 7.0 \times 10^3)/mm^3$$

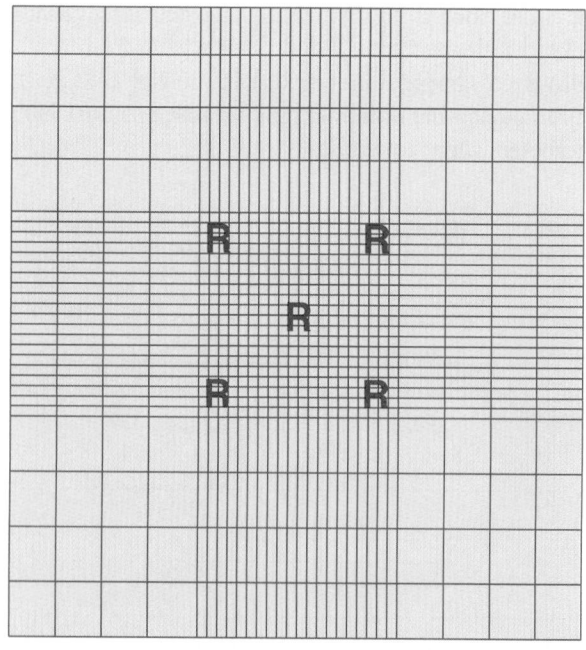

Figure 41-15 RBC counting area. The four corner squares and center square (labeled *R*) within the large center square on the hemacytometer are used to count red blood cells. These five areas equal one-fifth of a square millimeter.

TABLE 41-3 NORMAL LEUKOCYTE COUNTS

Leukocyte Count (Cells/mm³)

Age	Average	Reference Range
Newborn	18,000	9,000–30,000
One year	11,000	6,000–14,000
Six years	8,000	4,500–12,000
Adult	7,000	4,500–11,000

Example:

You perform an RBC count that has a dilution factor of 1:200 and you count the following number of cells. The cells are counted in the five *R* squares on the counting chamber.

1. Counting the cells:

Side 1		Side 2	
Square	Cells Counted	Square	Cells Counted
1	102	1	109
2	95	2	114
3	90	3	100
4	92	4	107
5	101	5	90
Total	480	Total	520

2. Compute the average:
   a. 480 + 520 = 1,000 cells
   b. 1,000 ÷ 2 = 500 average

3. Calculate the count:
   RBC mm³ = average number of cells × depth (mm) × dilution × area factor (mm)
   RBC mm³ = 500 × 10 (mm) × 200 × 5 (mm)²
   RBC mm³ = 500 × 10,000 (mm)³
   RBC mm³ = 5,000,000 or 5.0×10^6/mm³

The number of cells in each of the five small areas should not vary by more than twenty-five. If the variation is greater than twenty-five, it indicates an uneven distribution of cells. This count should be discarded, the counting chamber should be cleaned and dried, and the process repeated.

Calculating the Red Blood Cell Count. The total number of cells counted on both sides of the counting chamber are averaged. To calculate the number of red blood cells present in one cubic millimeter, the following formula is applied:

$$\text{RBC mm}^3 = \text{average number of cells} \times \text{depth}_{(mm)} \times \text{dilution} \times \text{area factor}_{(mm)}$$

The depth factor is always equal to 10 and the area factor in the RBC count is usually equal to 5. Remember that you usually count only one-fifth of a mm². To convert this to 1 mm², you must multiply by 5. The area factor in the formula can also be written as the denominator in the equation with a value of 0.20.

White Blood Cell Differential

The white blood cell (leukocyte) differential count is one of the most difficult tests to perform; it is also one of the most interesting. See Procedure 41-6. The reason it is so difficult is that there is no one way that a certain type of cell will always appear on a stained blood smear. The test is interesting because it provides the opportunity to visually examine all of the formed elements in the blood. It also enables the health care worker to see how the pathology of the patient is visible in the changes in the properties of

Some examples of blood cell changes associated with disease states are:

1. When a patient is experiencing an acute appendicitis, the white blood cell count will increase rapidly with a high percentage of neutrophils observed on the slide. There will also be an increase in the number of early or younger forms of these cells.
2. Patients who are suffering from a virus infection, especially adults, will frequently experience a reduction in white blood cells and the percentage of lymphocytes on the slide will increase. Patients with infectious mononucleosis will have increased numbers of lymphocytes, many of which will be atypical.
3. When patients have iron deficiency anemia, their differential slide will demonstrate red blood cells that show marked reduction in hemoglobin content. Their erythrocytes will appear hypochromic, lacking or low in color, because they lack the normal amount of hemoglobin in the red blood cell.

TABLE 41-4 NORMAL ERYTHROCYTE COUNTS

Age	Reference Range
Newborn	5.0 to 6.5×10^6/mm³
One year	4.0 to 5.0×10^6/mm³
Adult female	4.0 to 5.5×10^6/mm³
Adult male	4.5 to 6.0×10^6/mm³

the blood cells—both white cells and red cells—and how the types of cells will change with the pathology.

Making a Differential Blood Smear.

To perform a manual differential count, you must have a blood smear that has been stained. See Procedure 41-7. The most common way to make a differential blood smear is to use the two-slide or wedge method. The blood is spread out on the smear slide by using a second slide. This second slide is called the spreader slide.

The spreader slide should be held at a 30° to 35° angle. The greater the angle, the thicker the blood smear. If the angle is decreased during the end part of the spreading, the layer of cells on the smear slide will be very thin. A properly prepared blood smear has three distinct areas:

1. The heel of the smear, the area where the blood is too thick to examine properly
2. The feather edges of the slide where the smear is too thin and there are many holes or spaces between the cells
3. The body of the slide (between the thick area and the feather edge) where the cells are not overlaid and the smear does not have holes or large spaces between the cells

The smear slide should be allowed to air-dry and it should be stained as soon as it has dried. If the smear cannot be stained within a one-hour period after it is dried, it should be fixed to preserve the cells. Methyl alcohol is the fixative used to preserve blood smears.

Staining a Blood Smear.

Stains are applied to blood smears so that the formed elements may be more easily viewed and evaluated. A stained blood smear is evaluated in a procedure called the differential leukocyte count. This procedure is usually a part of the CBC (complete blood count). Stained smears may also be examined to detect and identify blood parasites such as those that cause malaria. A stained blood smear can provide important information regarding a patient's health. The evaluation of a blood smear often leads to the diagnosis or verification of disease.

Information gained during routine evaluation of blood smears may lead the physician to order special blood stains for further study. These special stains may be used to identify specific components of cells such as iron granules or nucleic acids. Bone marrow smears may be examined to evaluate blood cell production.

Types of Stains. The stains most commonly used to stain a blood smear for routine microscopic examination are called **polychromatic stains**. Polychromatic blood stains contain methylene blue, a blue stain, and eosin, a red-orange stain. Polychromatic stains are also known as Wright's or Giemsa's stains.

The staining method utilized to stain the blood smear may be the two-step method or the three-step method. In most ambulatory care settings, the three-step method (also called the quick stain method) is utilized because it is easier and faster, and does not require the rigid control of the two-step method.

Two-step Method. In the two-step method, the methylene blue, eosin, and fixative are combined into one solution, which is placed on the dried smear slide first. The slide is allowed to stain for one to three minutes and then a buffer is added to the stain. The two solutions are mixed and allowed to stand. The slide is then rinsed gently with distilled water and allowed to air-dry. The two-step method requires four to six minutes.

Three-Step, or Quick Stain, Method. The quick stain method requires less than one minute to complete. It is called the three-step method because the slide is dipped first in a fixative solution then into two separate staining solutions (Figure 41-16).

 CAUTION: The fixative solution contains methyl alcohol in concentration greater than 99 percent. This solution can be fatal or cause blindness if swallowed. The methylene blue and eosin staining solutions are aqueous (water) solutions.

The slide is dipped into each of the three solutions approximately five times, allowing one second for each dip. The excess solution is allowed to drain away and at the end of each process, the excess solution is removed by touching the end of the vertical slide onto a paper towel. The process is repeated for each of the solutions and then the slide is gently rinsed with water and allowed to air-dry before it is examined microscopically.

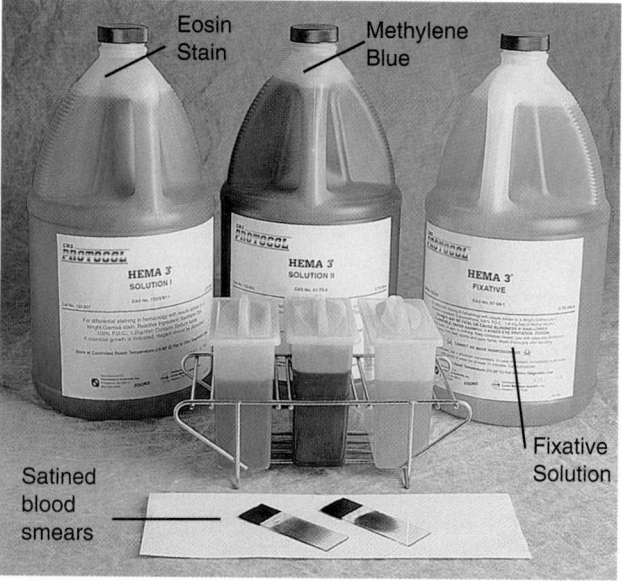

Figure 41-16 Hema-3 is a type of quick stain used in the ambulatory care setting.

Counting the Stained Differential Blood Smear. Cells are counted in the body area of the stained blood smear slides. The count usually consists of counting 100 white blood cells and determining the percentage of each of the five types. The characteristics of the white blood cells and the red blood cells are observed and noted. The relative number of platelets (thrombocytes) is noted on the lab report. When performing a differential leukocyte count, start in the thinnest area of the body portion of the slide and move in a serpentine pattern, making sure that cells are counted only once (Figure 41-17). The differential blood count is performed using the oil-immersion objective. Remember that this makes the total magnification 1,000X, because the oil-immersion objective is 100X and the eyepiece (ocular) is 10X.

The white blood cell features that must be studied to assist in the identification of the cell are: (1) the general size of the cell, (2) the nuclear characteristics, and (3) the cytoplasmic characteristics. The general size of the cell is determined by comparing it to the other types of cells on the slide as well as to the cells of the same type. Sometimes a single cell will be larger than the other cells of that type because it is younger. The characteristics of the nucleus that must be examined include shape, size, structure (such as dense or foamy), and color. The characteristics of the cytoplasm that must be examined and compared in the identification process include the amount, color, and types of inclusions.

It is very important that all of the preceding features of the cell be observed and studied during the identification and classification process. Probably the most common error made by beginners in white blood cell identification is that they let only one of these characteristics dominate their judgment when performing a differential count. The process of performing a correct differential leukocyte count requires a great deal of practice and study. It is imperative during the process to have access to a good blood cell atlas. *The Morphology of Human Blood Cells,* published by Abbott Laboratories, is an excellent reference.

Examination of a Blood Smear

The leukocytes on a stained blood smear can be divided into three groups: the myelocytic or granulocytic series (also called polymorphonuclear series), the lymphocytic, and the monocytic (Table 41-5; Figure 41-18). Mature cells in the granulocytic group have segmented nuclei and granules in the cytoplasm. The granulocytic group is further divided into three groups according to the types of granules in the cytoplasm. The three groups are the **neutrophil**, **eosinophil**, and **basophil**. The neutrophils are further indentified by the shape of the cell's nucleus. Mature cells have multiple nuclear lobes separated by a

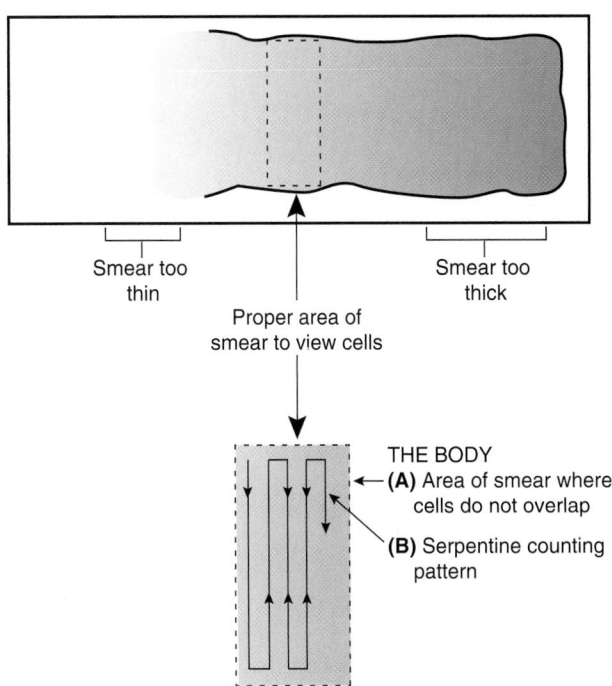

Figure 41-17 Proper area of slide to be viewed for differential count: (A) Close-up of proper body. (B) Counting pattern.

filament, hence the name segmented neutrophils (segs). Immature cells do not have distinct lobes, resulting in a nucleus that has a U shape. These cells are called band neutrophils (bands) (Figure 41-18 A and B). Eosinophils are easily recognized by the large red granules in the cell's cytoplasm (Figure 41-18E). Basophils are easily recognized by the large blue granules in the cell's cytoplasm (Figure 41-18F). The other two major divisions are the lymphocytic and monocytic divisions. Lymphocytes may be large or small in size. Table 41-6 and Figure 41-18 should be used in the process of identifying leukocytes on the stained blood smear.

After the leukocytes have been identified on the differential smear, the red blood cells and platelets (thrombocytes) are studied and evaluated. See Procedure 41-8. The average red blood cell is about 7.5 μm, which is slightly smaller than a small lymphocyte. Red blood cells that are about this size (7.5 μm) are called **normocytic**. Those

TABLE 41-5	LEUKOCYTE IDENTIFICATION GUIDE	
Divisions	**Cell Types**	**Polymorphonuclear Types**
I. Myelocytic, granulocytic, or polymorpho-nuclear	Neutrophil Eosinophil Basophil	Segmented cells Bands
II. Lymphocytic	Lymphocytes	
III. Monocytic	Monocytes	

TABLE 41-6	NORMAL VALUES FOR A DIFFERENTIAL LEUKOCYTE COUNT IN ADULTS

Neutrophil Bands: 3–5%
Neutrophil bands increase in appendicitis and many other diseases.

Neutrophil Segs: 54–62%
Segmented neutrophils increase in appendicitis and many other diseases. An elevation in neutrophils usually is indicative of an infectious disease.

Lymphocytes: 25–33%
Lymphocytes increase with infectious mononucleosis, lymphocytic leukemia, and many diseases of viral origin.

Monocytes: 3–7%
Monocytes increase in tuberculosis and monocytic leukemia.

Eosinophils: 1–3%
Eosinophils increase with allergic reactions, hay fever, and parasitic infections.

Basophils: 0–1%
Basophils increase in polycythemia vera, chicken pox, and ulcerative colitis.

that are larger are called **macrocytic** and those that are smaller are called **microcytic**. When the red blood cells on the differential slide show marked variation in size, this condition is called **anisocytosis**. The normal red blood cell has a round or slightly oval shape. If the shape of the red blood cells on the slide show marked variation, this is a condition known as **poikilocytosis**.

The red blood cell should contain hemoglobin that fills about one-half of the cell. The RBC is biconcave so most of the hemoglobin should be seen around the outer part of the cell. The central area of the RBC is pale. Red blood cells with the proper amount of hemoglobin are called **normochromic**. Those that do not have enough hemoglobin, that demonstrate too large of a pale central area, are called **hypochromic**.

The normal number of platelets observed on the differential smear averages about 10 per oil immersion field. The total platelet count can be estimated by counting the number of platelets in 10 fields and taking an average. The average number is then multiplied by 20,000. For example, if an average number of platelets is 15/oil immersion field, then the estimated total number of platelets is

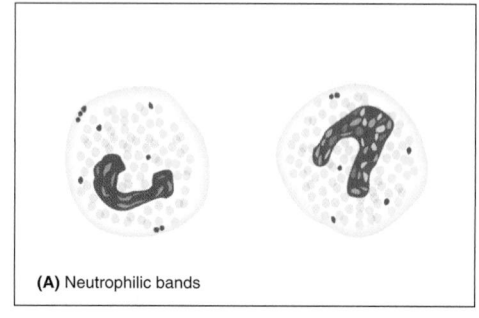

(A) Neutrophilic bands

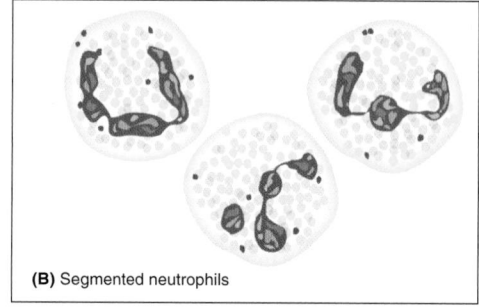

(B) Segmented neutrophils

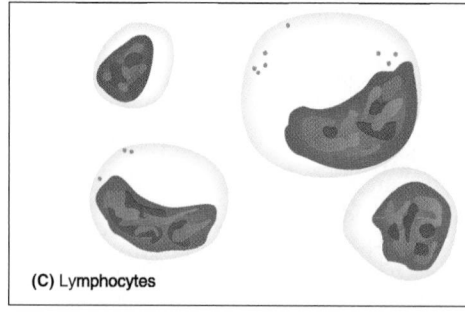

(C) Lymphocytes

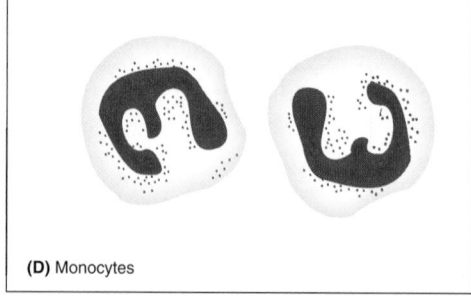

(D) Monocytes

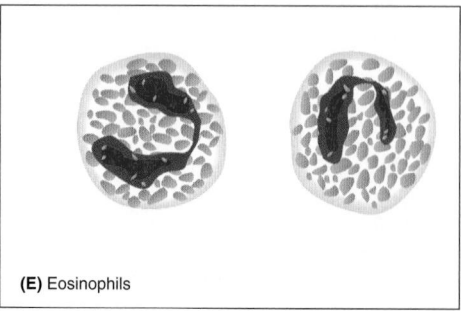

(E) Eosinophils

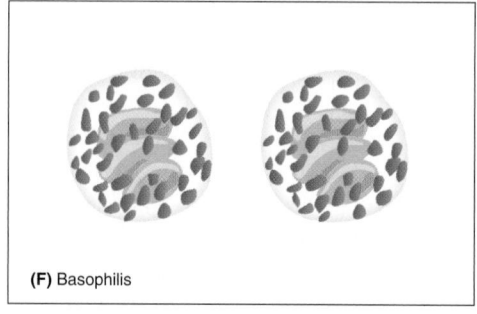

(F) Basophilis

Figure 41-18   Various divisions of leukocytes from a stained blood smear.

300,000/cm μL (15 × 20,000 = 300,000). The normal value for platelets (thrombocytes) is 140,000–400,000/cm μL. The differential count is performed automatically in most ambulatory care settings using an automated hematology instrument. This procedure is discussed later in this chapter.

Clinical Laboratory Improvement Amendment, 1988 (CLIA '88) Regulation Regarding White Blood Cell Differential Counts

- Laboratories that are certified for waiver-level testing only are not permitted to perform manual white blood cell differential counts.
- Laboratories with a moderate-complexity certification can perform a manual differential white blood cell count but may only identify and report normal cells.
- Laboratories certified to perform tests of high complexity can perform a manual differential white blood cell count and are permitted to identify and report both abnormal and normal cells.

See Chapter 38 for details on CLIA '88 regulations.

ERYTHROCYTE INDICES

The **erythrocyte indices** include the mean corpuscular (cell) volume (MCV), the mean corpuscular hemoglobin (MCH), and the mean corpuscular hemoglobin concentration (MCHC). These indices (plural for index) are calculations that provide information about the size of the red blood cells and the hemoglobin content. The blood parameters needed to calculate all three indices are the red blood cell count, the hematocrit, and the hemoglobin. The erythrocyte indices values are important in the diagnosis or classification and treatment of different types of anemia. Table 41-7 shows normal values for the erythrocyte indices.

Before the automated hematology instrument became commonly used in the ambulatory care setting, the

erythrocyte indices were not included as a part of the CBC because the red blood cell count was not an accurate measurement.

The following formulas are used to calculate the erythrocyte indices:

$$\text{Mean Corpuscular Volume (MCV)} = \frac{\text{Hematocrit}}{\text{RBC (in millions)}} \times 10$$

The result is reported in femtoliters (fL), a unit of volume 10^{-15} L, formerly reported in cubic microns (μm^3). This index gives the average volume of a red blood cell in the sample.

$$\text{Mean Corpuscular Hemoglobin (MCH)} = \frac{\text{Hemoglobin (in grams)}}{\text{RBC (in millions)}} \times 10$$

The result is expressed in picograms (pg), a micro microgram, or 1×10^{-12} g. This index estimates the weight of hemoglobin in a red blood cell of the sample.

$$\text{Mean Corpuscular Hemoglobin Concentration (MCHC)} = \frac{\text{Hemoglobin (in grams)}}{\text{Hematocrit}} \times 10$$

This result is expressed in grams/deciliter (g/dL). The MCHC is the average concentration of Hgb in a given volume of packed red blood cells (Hct).

Using Erythrocyte Indices to Diagnose

The MCH and MCV will be increased in megaloblastic anemias such as vitamin B_{12} and folate deficiency anemias. They will also be increased in acute blood loss anemia, chronic hemolytic anemias, aplastic anemias, hypothyroidism, and liver disease. The MCH and MCV will be decreased in hypochromic and microcytic anemias, including iron deficiency anemia, thalassemias, and occasionally in hyperthyroidism.

The MCHC will be increased in hereditary spherocytosis. It will be normal in macrocytosis. The MCHC will be decreased in iron deficiency anemia. The stained blood smear of a person with iron deficiency anemia will demonstrate red blood cells that are both hypochromic and microcytic.

ERYTHROCYTE SEDIMENTATION RATES (ESR)

The **erythrocyte sedimentation rate**, as the name implies, is a measurement of the rate at which the red blood cells in a well-mixed, anticoagulated blood sample will fall, or settle, toward the bottom when it is placed in a vertical tube. This test is commonly referred to in the

TABLE 41-7	NORMAL VALUES FOR THE ERYTHROCYTE INDICES
MCV	80–100 fL
MCH	27–33 pg
MCHC	32–36 g/dL

laboratory as a "sed rate." See Procedure 41-9. The ESR has been used for many years in the diagnosis and treatment of many disease states of the body. It is an inexpensive, accurate, and easy test to perform. Two factors that influence the sedimentation rate are the condition of the surface membrane of the red blood cell and changes in the level of fibrinogen in the plasma of the blood. During disease conditions in the body, the surface membrane of the red blood cell is altered, and this affects the rate at which the RBCs fall in the tube. Red blood cells will demonstrate this change even after the disease has subsided because RBCs have an average life of 120 days. For this reason, the ESR is a more accurate tool in diagnosing the onset of a disease than in checking the progress of treatment.

Fibrinogen is a plasma protein. The level, or concentration, of fibrinogen is altered during various disease states of the body.

Two ways to perform an ESR test are the Wintrobe method and the Westergren method. Both methods will provide the same information. Because of the simplicity in setting up the Westergren ESR, it has become the more widely used method in the ambulatory care setting.

Wintrobe Method

An EDTA venous blood sample is thoroughly mixed. With the use of a Pasteur pipette, the blood is transferred to a Wintrobe tube. The blood is added to the left zero mark at the top of the tube. It is important that no air bubbles are present in the blood column. The tube is placed exactly vertical in a rack and allowed to stand for exactly 60 minutes. The test is read by determining the number of millimeters (mm) the red cells have settled. The tube has a total capacity of 100 mm. The test is reported in mm/hr (Figure 41-19). Table 41-8 shows normal values for the Wintrobe method of ESR.

Westergren Method

The Westergren method differs from the Wintrobe method in that the blood sample is mixed with 3.8 percent sodium citrate solution before the tube is filled. The blood and sodium citrate are mixed and the tube is filled to the zero mark and placed exactly vertical in a rack. The tube is read after exactly 60 minutes, and the test is reported in mm/hr. Table 41-9 shows normal values for the Westergren method of ESR.

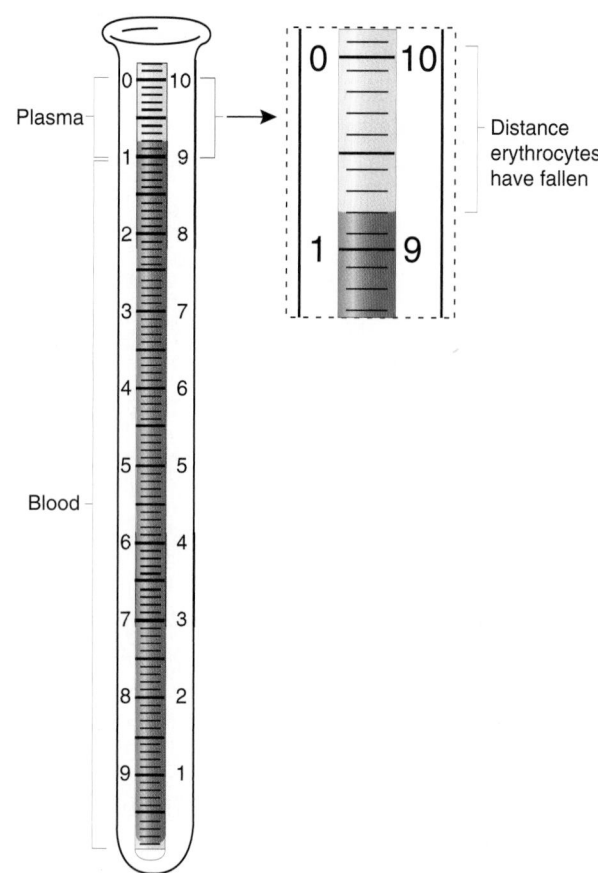

Figure 41-19   Wintrobe sedimentation tube showing settling of cells. The example shown illustrates a sedimentation of 8 mm.

The Polymedco company has produced a Sediplast® system to perform a Westergren ESR that is self-filling. It is a completely closed system that protects laboratory personnel from the risks associated with blood handling. The Sediplast® ESR System is shown in Figure 41-20.

The following guidelines should be followed when performing Wintrobe and Westergren ESR procedures to ensure accurate test results:

1. The tube must remain exactly vertical during the one-hour test time.
2. The test must be read at exactly 60 minutes (1 hour).
3. The counter on which the rack is placed must be free of vibrations.

TABLE 41-8	NORMAL VALUES FOR THE WINTROBE METHOD OF ESR	
Males	0–9 mm/hr.
Females	0–20 mm/hr.

TABLE 41-9	NORMAL VALUES FOR THE WESTERGREN METHOD OF ESR
Males (under 50)	0–15 mm/hr.
Males (over 50)	0–20 mm/hr.
Females (under 50)	0–20 mm/hr.
Females (over 50)	0–30 mm/hr.

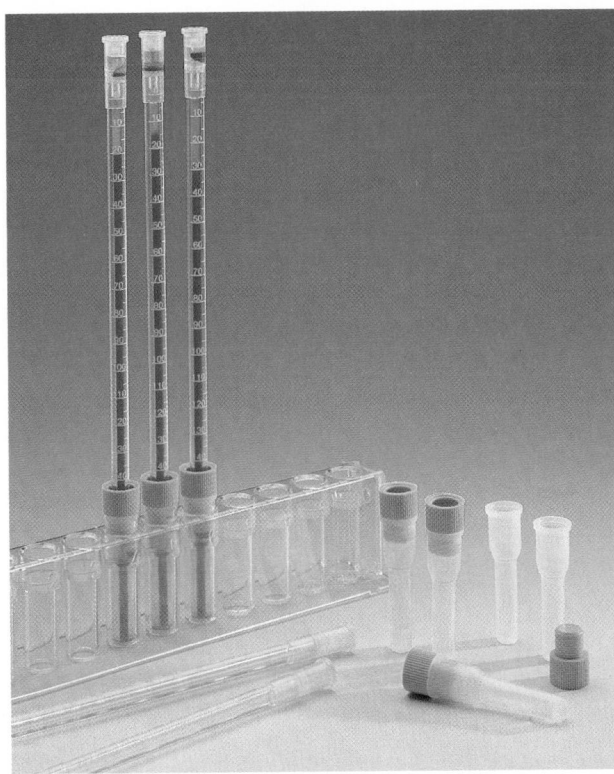

Figure 41-20 Sediplast® ESR System. The picture shows three filled tubes standing in the rack. Note the diluting vials with sodium citrate solution (right). (Courtesy of POLY-MEDCO Inc.)

4. The test should be set up within two hours after the blood is drawn.
5. The test should be conducted at room temperature.
6. The tube should not be placed in a draft, and it should not be exposed to direct sunlight.
7. The column of blood must be free of bubbles.

The erythrocytes in normal, nondiseased blood tend to remain suspended in the plasma. They do not aggregate (clump) together to form rouleaux. Rouleaux is a phenomenon where red blood cells form aggregates that look like rolls or stacks of coins (Figure 41-21).

This aggregate form causes the rate of sedimentation to increase. Red blood cells have membrane properties that tend to make them remain separated in the plasma. During certain diseased states, this repelling property is lost and the RBCs tend to aggregate.

Using the ESR to Diagnose

Erythrocyte sedimentation rates are increased in infections and inflammatory diseases, tissue destruction, and other conditions that lead to an increase in plasma fibrinogen. They are also increased with menstruation, pregnancy, malignant neoplasms, and multiple myeloma. With anemia, the ESR increases according to the severity of the condition.

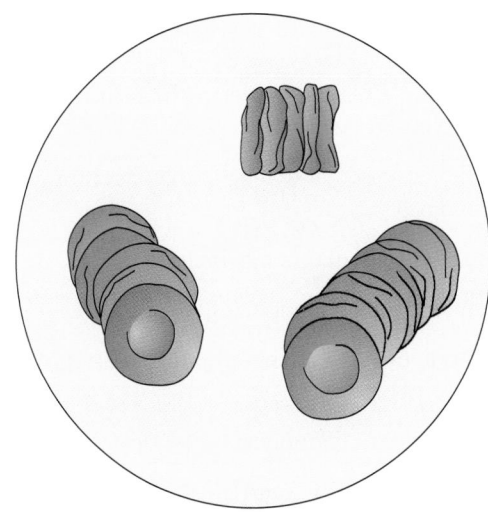

Figure 41-21 Erythrocytes forming rouleaux.

The ESR may be normal in osteoarthritis and in some cases of cirrhosis and malaria. The ESR values are decreased in polycythemia, spherocytosis, and sickle cell anemia.

AUTOMATED HEMATOLOGY INSTRUMENTATION AND QUALITY CONTROL

Most hematology tests performed in the ambulatory care setting today utilize some form of automated instrumentation. All procedures performed with automated instrumentation are modifications of manual methods. Automated hematology procedures have many advantages over the manual methods. They are faster, less expensive, simple to operate, and very accurate. The instruments can be calibrated and lend themselves to control testings. Most are equipped with printers that produce printed results. Many can store quality control results and print out quality control data summary sheets.

In addition to performing a wide variety of hematological tests, many automated hematology instruments also calculate part or all of the red blood cell indices and print the results. Some automated hematology instruments can be connected to other computers in the medical facility.

Semiautomated or completely automated hematology instruments can be purchased. The hematological parameters that are available on different automated office hematology instruments are:

- Red blood cell count
- White blood cell count
- Hemoglobin

- Hematocrit
- Platelet count
- Mean corpuscular volume (MCV)
- Mean corpuscular hemoglobin concentration (MCHC)
- Mean corpuscular hemoglobin (MCH)
- Percentage of granulocytes
- Granulocyte count (neutrophils, eosinophils, basophils)
- Percentage of lymphocytes/monocytes
- Nongranulocyte count (lymphocytes and monocytes)
- Mid-cell count (monocytes and band neutrophils)
- Percentage of mid-cells
- Lymphocyte count
- Percentage of lymphocytes
- Red blood cell distribution width (RDW)

The hematology instruments commonly utilized in the ambulatory care setting today employ two different principles of operation. One type takes the sample and makes appropriate dilutions before the sample is processed. The other type of instrument does not dilute the blood specimen but separates the sample into the different hematological values by centrifugation.

Hematology Instruments That Require Sample Dilutions

The type of technology utilized in the counting of particulate matter in the diluted sample is known as the **impedance principle** or resistance principle. A constant current is drawn across an electrolyte solution between two points. The blood sample is diluted with the same electrolyte solution. When the cells in the solution pass between these two points, they cause a change in the current flow at that point because they offer a resistance. The change in current flow produces an impulse which is counted as a cell. The various sizes of the cells can be interpreted by the instrument as different kinds of cells because they produce different amounts of resistance. Figure 41-22 shows an impedance hematology instrument that requires the operator to make manual dilutions. Fig-

ure 41-23 shows an impedance hematology instrument that is completely automatic. It pierces the rubber stopper of the blood sample, makes all of the necessary dilutions, reads the various parameters, and then self-cleans the instrument.

Hematology Instruments That Do Not Require Sample Dilutions

Centrifugal hematology analysis utilizes a nondiluted sample. Blood is drawn into a very precise capillary tube that has been treated on the inside with a special stain. This stain is picked up by the nuclei of the white blood cells. The tube is sealed and spun at very high speeds, causing the blood cells to separate into layers. These layers are read with the aid of a fluorescent microscope and a micrometer, which measures the thickness of the layer of each cell type.

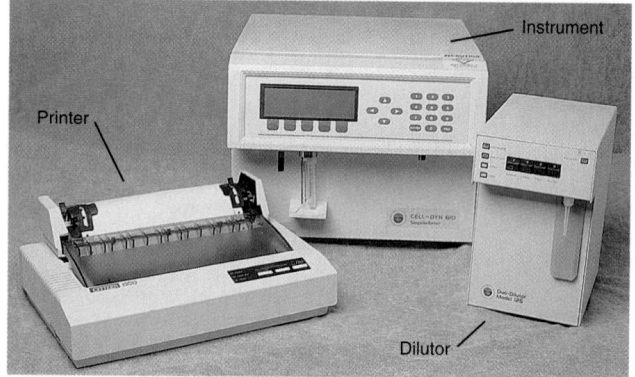

Figure 41-22 A semiautomated hematology instrument.

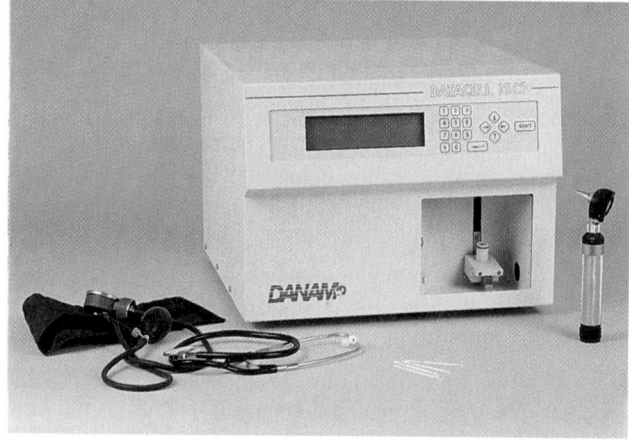

Figure 41-23 A completely automated hematology instrument.

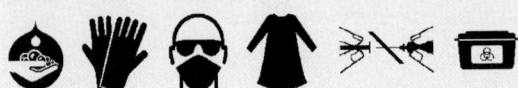

Hemoglobin Determination (Manual Method Using a Spectrophotometer)

STANDARD PRECAUTIONS:

PURPOSE:
Properly and safely perform a manual hemoglobin determination using a spectrophotometer to evaluate the oxygen-carrying capacity of the blood.

EQUIPMENT/SUPPLIES:
Gloves
Hand disinfectant
EDTA blood sample(s) or supplies for a capillary puncture
Spectrophotometer (540 nm wavelength)
Hemoglobin standard solution
Cuvettes
Laboratory stretch film
10% chlorine bleach solution
UNOHEME® hemoglobin system *or* supplies for manual hemoglobin:
  Graduated pipette, 5 mL, with pipetting aid
  Drabkin's reagent
  Test tubes, 5 mL capacity
  Micropipettor to deliver 20 µL volume and tips
  Biohazard container
NOTE: Consult operating manual for specific instructions for spectrophotometer.

PROCEDURE STEPS:
1. Wash hands and put on gloves.
2. Assemble equipment and materials.
3. Turn on spectrophotometer.
4. Set wavelength at 540 nm.
5. For UNOHEME® method proceed with 5a–g. For manual method go to step 6.
   a. Draw 20 µL of well-mixed EDTA anticoagulated blood into the UNOHEME® capillary pipette.
   b. Insert the capillary pipette into the UNOHEME® reservoir and draw the blood into the reagent. Rinse the capillary pipette several times taking care not to overflow pipette.
   c. Mix contents by swirling. Let sit five minutes.
   d. Transfer contents of reservoir to a cuvette.
   e. Place diluting fluid from an unused UNOHEME® reservoir into a cuvette labeled "blank."

f. Pipette 5 mL of a hemoglobin standard into cuvette labeled "Std."
   g. Proceed to step 7.
6. For manual method proceed with steps 6a–h.
   a. Label test tubes: blank, standard, and unknown (sample).
   b. Dispense 5.0 mL of Drabkin's reagent into blank and unknown tubes; dispense 5.0 mL of hemoglobin standard into standard tube.
   c. Mix blood sample for at least two minutes by hand or using mechanical mixer.
   d. Draw up 0.02 mL (20 µL) of blood with micropipette.
   e. Wipe excess blood from exterior of pipette with tissue.
   f. Dispense blood sample into the unknown (sample) tube.
   g. Mix contents of tube thoroughly and let stand for at least ten minutes (tubes can be mixed by inverting after placing laboratory stretch film over the top of the tube).
   h. Transfer contents of the tubes to cuvettes.
7. Place "blank" cuvette in the well of the spectrophotometer; set absorbance to zero following the manufacturer's instructions.
8. Place "standard" cuvette into the well of the spectrophotometer; read the absorbance and record the results.
9. Place "sample" cuvette (with UNOHEME® contents from step 5 or unknown from step 6) into the well of the spectrophotometer; read the absorbance and record the results.
10. Use the following formula to calculate hemoglobin concentration and record results:

$$\frac{A_{UNK}}{A_{STD}} \times Conc_{STD} = Conc_{UNK} \text{ (g/dL)}$$

11. Discard all specimens and contaminated materials into biohazard container.
12. Disinfect and clean equipment and return to proper storage.
13. Clean work area with surface disinfectant.
14. Remove and discard gloves into biohazard container and wash hands with hand disinfectant.
15. Document the results.

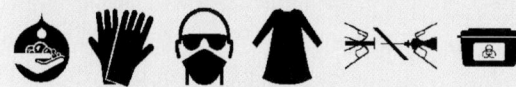

Hemoglobin Determination (Hemoglobin Analyzer)

41-2

STANDARD PRECAUTIONS:

PURPOSE:
Properly and safely perform an automated hemoglobin determination to evaluate the oxygen capacity of the blood.

EQUIPMENT/SUPPLIES:
Gloves
Hand disinfectant
10% chlorine bleach solution
Capillary puncture equipment or blood samples collected in EDTA
Hb-Direct™ System, HemoCue® System, or other hemoglobin analyzer with supplies appropriate for the analyzer
Biohazard container
Puncture-proof biohazard container for sharps
NOTE: Consult manufacturer's instructions for specific procedure.

PROCEDURE STEPS:
1. Wash hands and put on gloves.
2. Assemble equipment and materials for analyzer method.
3. Turn on instrument to warm up. Calibrate or standardize the instrument according to the manufacturer's directions.
4. Perform a capillary puncture (see Chapter 40) observing the Bloodborne Pathogen Standard. Wipe away the first drop of blood with a tissue or sterile cotton ball.
5. Collect blood from the puncture using a capillary or cuvette appropriate for the analyzer to be used. Avoid trapping air bubbles in the collection device.
6. Wipe excess blood from the outside of the collection device (if appropriate) being careful not to touch the open end of the device.
7. For the Hb-Direct™, complete steps 7a–d. For HemoCue®, go to step 8.
   a. Insert the filled capillary tube into a cyanmethemoglobin vial. Place cap tightly on vial

and invert gently five to ten times until capillary tube is empty of blood. (The light red reaction color is stable for five days at room temperature.)
   b. Let vial stand at room temperature for five minutes.
   c. Insert vial into the Hemoglobin Analyzer, using the following procedure (these steps should be followed closely to ensure that the capillary tube does not obstruct the analyzer light path):
      (1) Invert the vial slowly, then hold it horizontally for three seconds. As the vial is *slowly* returned to its upright position, the capillary tube should adhere to the upper side of the vial.
      (2) Position the vial so that the capillary tube is at the *back* of the vial.
      (3) Wipe fingerprints from the sides of the vial with a tissue.
      (4) Check that the reagent vial is tightly capped.
      (5) Insert the vial into the Hemoglobin Analyzer with the capillary tube positioned to the back of the vial.
      (6) Wait five seconds. Read the analyzer display. Check to ensure that the capillary tube has remained in the upper half of the vial.
   d. Read the hemoglobin concentration from the display and record. Proceed to step 9.
8. For HemoCue®:
   a. Insert the filled cuvette into the HemoCue® photometer within ten minutes of filling the cuvette.
   b. Read the hemoglobin value from the display and record.
9. Discard all contaminated materials into biohazard containers.
10. Return all equipment to proper storage.
11. Wipe counters with surface disinfectant.
12. Remove and discard gloves into biohazard container.
13. Wash hands with hand disinfectant.
14. Document the results.

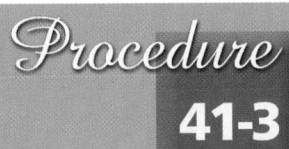

41-3 Microhematocrit

   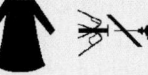

PURPOSE:
Properly and safely perform the microhematocrit procedure using a few microliters of blood in a capillary tube to separate the cellular elements of the blood from the plasma by centrifugation.

EQUIPMENT/SUPPLIES:
Gloves
Hand disinfectant
Capillary tubes, plain and with heparin
Acrylic safety shield
Precalibrated capillary tubes (optional)
Sealing clay or disposable plastic sealing caps (if not using self-sealing tubes)
Microhematocrit centrifuge and reader
Tube of anticoagulated venous blood (or commercially available simulated blood)
Paper towels or soft laboratory tissue
70% alcohol or alcohol swabs
Gauze or cotton balls, sterile
Blood lancets, sterile, disposable
Surface disinfectant or 10% chlorine bleach solution
Biohazard container
Puncture-proof biohazard container for sharps
NOTE: Consult the instruction manual for the centrifuge being used. Refer to the specific procedure being performed.

PROCEDURE STEPS:

1. Wash hands and put on gloves.
2. Assemble equipment and materials for capillary puncture and microhematocrit.

For direct specimen method, complete steps 3a–g. When utilizing a sample from a blood specimen tube, go to step 4.

3. Fill two capillary tubes from a capillary puncture.
   a. Perform a capillary puncture (see Chapter 40).
   b. Wipe away the first drop of blood.
   c. Touch one end of a heparinized capillary tube to the second drop of blood.
   d. Allow the tube to fill three-quarters full by capillary action. A slight downward angle of the

tube may be necessary (if using precalibrated tubes, fill to the line).
   e. Fill a second tube in the same manner.
   f. Wipe the outside of the filled capillary tube with soft tissue, if necessary, to remove excess blood.
   g. Seal the capillary tube by placing the clean end into the tray of sealing clay (the sealing clay will stay cleaner if the dry/clean end of the capillary tube is sealed). Proceed to step 5.
4. Fill two capillary tubes using a tube of EDTA anticoagulated blood (if not available, proceed to step 5):
   a. Mix the tube of blood thoroughly by gently rocking the tube from end to end a minimum of two minutes by mechanical mixer or fifty to sixty times by hand.
   b. Remove cap from the tube (with an acrylic safety shield placed between worker and tube).
   c. Tilt the tube so that blood is very near the top edge of the tube.
   d. Insert the tip of a plain capillary tube into the blood and fill three-quarters full by capillary action (if using precalibrated tubes, fill to the line). NOTE: Wipe the outside of the filled capillary tube with tissue, if necessary, to remove excess blood.
   e. Seal the tube by placing the clean end into the tray of sealing clay or by using a plastic sealing cap. If using self-sealing tubes, check to see that the plug expanded.
   f. Fill a second tube in the same manner.
5. Check to see if the interior sealing clay edge appears level in the tubes.
6. Place tubes into the microhematocrit centrifuge with *sealed* ends securely against the gasket (balance the centrifuge by placing the tubes opposite each other).
7. Fasten both lids securely.
8. Set the timer and adjust the speed if necessary.
9. Centrifuge for the prescribed time.
10. Allow the centrifuge to come to a complete stop and unlock the lid(s).
11. Determine the microhematocrit values using one of the following methods:
    a. A centrifuge that requires calibrated tubes and has a built-in scale:

(continues)

Procedure 41-3 *(continued)*

(1) Position the tubes as directed by the manufacturer's instructions.

(2) Read the microhematocrit value.

b. A centrifuge without a built-in reader:

(1) Carefully remove capillary tubes from centrifuge.

(2) Place tube on the microhematocrit reader provided.

(3) Follow instructions on the reader to obtain the microhematocrit value.

12. Average the values from the two tubes and record the microhematocrit.

13. Discard the capillary tubes and used lancets into a puncture-proof biohazard container for sharps.

14. Clean and return equipment to proper storage.

15. Clean the work area with surface disinfectant.

16. Remove and discard gloves into biohazard container and wash hands with hand disinfectant.

17. Wash hands with hand disinfectant.

18. Document the results.

Procedure 41-4 **White Blood Cell Count (Unopette® Method)**

STANDARD PRECAUTIONS:

   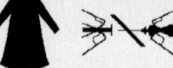

PURPOSE:

Properly and safely perform the white blood cell count using a self-contained system to determine the total number of white blood cells per cubic millimeter of blood.

EQUIPMENT/SUPPLIES:

Gloves
Surface disinfectant (10% chlorine bleach solution)
Tube of EDTA blood or supplies for a capillary puncture
Hand disinfectant
Unopette® WBC or WBC/Platelet system
Hemacytometer with coverglass
Hand tally counter
70% alcohol
Microscope
Lens paper
Acrylic safety shield or goggles and mask
Biohazard container
Biohazard container for sharps
NOTE: Following is a general procedure for the use of the Unopette® system. Consult the manufacturer's package insert for specific instructions.

PROCEDURE STEPS:

1. Assemble equipment and materials; obtain a Unopette® system for WBC or WBC/Platelet count.

2. Place a clean hemacytometer coverglass on a clean hemacytometer.

3. Pierce the diaphragm of the Unopette® reservoir with the pipette shield.

4. Set up acrylic safety shield or wear goggles and mask.

5. Wash hands and put on gloves.

6. Remove the shield from the pipette assembly. (Perform steps 7–14 with safety shield between you and the blood or blood solution.)

7. Fill the capillary pipette from a capillary puncture or from a tube of well-mixed EDTA blood.

8. Allow the blood to rise in the capillary until it automatically stops.

9. Wipe any excess blood from the outside of the pipette, being careful not to touch the tip with the tissue.

10. Squeeze the reservoir slightly, being careful not to expel any of the liquid.

11. Maintain pressure on the reservoir and insert the capillary pipette into the reservoir, seating the pipette firmly into the neck of the reservoir. Do not expel any of the liquid.

(continues)

Procedure
41-4 *(continued)*

12. Release the pressure on the reservoir, drawing the blood out of the capillary pipette and into the diluent.
13. Squeeze the reservoir gently three to four times to rinse the remaining blood from the capillary pipette. NOTE: Do not allow the blood-diluent mixture to flow out the top.
14. Swirl or turn the reservoir from side to side to gently mix the contents.
15. Let the reservoir sit for ten minutes (but no longer than an hour) to destroy the red blood cells.
16. Remove the pipette from the reservoir and insert it into the neck of the reservoir so that the pipette tip extends *upward* from the reservoir.
17. Thoroughly mix the contents of the reservoir. Invert the reservoir and gently squeeze to discard four or five drops onto paper towel or gauze.
18. Touch the tip of the pipette to the edge of the coverglass and counting chamber. Fill both chambers.
19. Place the filled hemacytometer into a Petri dish beside a damp cotton ball. Cover and let stand for ten minutes.
20. Carefully place the hemacytometer on the microscope stage and secure it.
21. Use the low-power (10X) objective to bring the ruled area into focus. Identify the nine white

blood cell squares.
22. Count the white blood cells lying within all nine squares, using the boundary rule.
23. Record the results.
24. Repeat the count, using the other side of the hemacytometer, and record the results.
25. Obtain the average count by adding the results from the two sides and dividing by two.
26. Calculate 10 percent of the average and add that to the average. Then multiply that total by 100 to get the number of white blood cells per cubic millimeter.
27. Place the hemacytometer and coverglass into the bleach solution for ten minutes, then rinse with water. Dry carefully with lens paper.
28. Discard any sharps into a puncture-proof biohazard container.
29. Return the tube of blood to the storage area or discard into biohazard waste. Discard the Unopette® assembly in the biohazard sharps container.
30. Return equipment to proper storage.
31. Clean the work area with surface disinfectant.
32. Remove and discard gloves into biohazard container.
33. Wash hands with hand disinfectant.

Procedure
41-5 Red Blood Cell Count (Unopette® Method)

STANDARD PRECAUTIONS:

    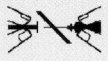

PURPOSE:
To count red blood cells.

EQUIPMENT/SUPPLIES:
Gloves
Hand disinfectant

Materials for capillary puncture, or blood sample, anticoagulated with EDTA
Hemacytometer with coverglass
Test tube rack or beaker to hold blood sample
Unopette® for RBC count (reservoir and pipette assembly)
Microscope
Lens paper
Alcohol (70% ethanol)

(continues)

Procedure

41-5 *(continued)*

Hand tally counter
Surface disinfectant or 10% chlorine bleach solution
Biohazard container
Biohazard container for sharps
Acrylic safety shield or goggles and mask
NOTE: Following is a general procedure for the use of the Unopette® system. Consult the package insert for specific instructions.

PROCEDURE STEPS:

1. Assemble equipment and materials. Set up acrylic safety shield or put on goggles and mask.
2. Place a clean hemacytometer coverglass over a clean hemacytometer.
3. Wash hands and put on gloves.
4. Puncture the diaphragm of the Unopette® reservoir. Hold the reservoir firmly on a flat surface with one hand and use the tip of the pipette shield to puncture the diaphragm. NOTE: The opening must be made large enough to easily accommodate the pipette.
5. Remove the shield from the pipette assembly.
6. Fill the capillary pipette from a capillary puncture or from a tube of well-mixed EDTA anticoagulated blood. The pipette will fill by capillary action and will stop filling automatically. NOTE: Keep pipette horizontal or at a slight (5°) upward angle to avoid overfilling.
7. Wipe excess blood from the outside of the capillary pipette with soft laboratory tissue. NOTE: Do not allow tissue to touch pipette tip.
8. Squeeze the reservoir slightly, being careful not to expel any of the liquid.
9. Maintain the pressure on the reservoir and insert the capillary pipette into the reservoir, seating the pipette firmly into the neck of the reservoir. Do not expel any of the liquid.
10. Release the pressure on the reservoir, drawing the blood out of the capillary pipette into the diluent.
11. Squeeze the reservoir gently three to four times to rinse the remaining blood from the capillary

pipette. NOTE: Do not allow the blood-diluent mixture to flow out the top.
12. Thoroughly mix the contents of the reservoir by gently swirling the reservoir and/or turning it side to side.
13. Withdraw the capillary pipette from the reservoir and insert it into the neck of the reservoir in reverse position (the pipette tip should now project upward from the reservoir).
14. Thoroughly mix the contents of the reservoir. Invert the reservoir and gently squeeze to discard four to five drops onto gauze or paper towel.
15. Fill both sides of the hemacytometer.
16. Carefully place the hemacytometer on the microscope stage and secure.
17. Use the low-power (10X) objective to bring the ruled area into focus.
18. Locate the large central square.
19. Carefully rotate the high-power (40X) objective into position and focus with the fine adjustment knob until lines are clear.
20. Adjust the light and/or condenser so that red blood cells are visible.
21. Count the cells in the four corner squares and one center square within the larger center square of the counting area, using the left-to-right, right-to-left counting pattern.
22. Record the results for each of the five squares (four corner and one center).
23. Repeat the count using the other side of the hemacytometer.
24. Use the worksheet to calculate the RBC count.
25. Record the result.
26. Disinfect the hemacytometer and coverglass.
27. Discard the specimen and disposable materials appropriately.
28. Return equipment to proper storage.
29. Clean work area with surface disinfectant.
30. Remove and discard gloves into biohazard container and wash hands with hand disinfectant.

Procedure 41-6

Preparation of a Differential Blood Smear Slide

STANDARD PRECAUTIONS:

   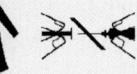

PURPOSE:
Properly and safely prepare an anticoagulated blood smear and a capillary blood smear by spreading blood on a microscopic slide, altering the form, structure, and distribution of cells (morphology) as little as possible, to microscopically view the cellular components.

EQUIPMENT/SUPPLIES:
Gloves
Hand disinfectant
Pencil
Microscope slides (1" × 3"), frosted end optional
95% ethyl alcohol
Laboratory tissue
Capillary tubes (plain and heparinized)
Slide drying rack
Hot water
Detergent
Distilled water
Methanol in covered staining (Coplin) jar
EDTA anticoagulated blood specimen (fresh)
Materials for capillary puncture
Surface disinfectant or 10% chlorine bleach solution
Biohazard container
Puncture-proof container for sharp objects

PROCEDURE STEPS:
1. Assemble equipment and materials.
2. Place a clean slide on a flat surface (be sure to touch only the edges of the slide with fingers). Write patient identification on the frosted area with a pencil.
3. Wash hands and put on gloves.
4. Obtain an EDTA anticoagulated blood sample (provided by the instructor).
5. Mix blood well and fill a plain capillary tube with blood.
6. Dispense a small drop of blood from the capillary tube onto the slide about one-half to three-fourths inch from the right end (if left-handed, reverse instructions) (Figure 41-24A).
7. Place the end of a clean, polished, unchipped spreader slide in front of the drop of blood at a

30°–35° angle. Spreader should be lightly balanced with fingertips (Figure 41-24B).
8. Pull the spreader slide back into the drop of blood by sliding gently along the slide until the blood spreads along three-fourths of the width of the spreader (Figure 41-24C).
9. Push the spreader slide forward with a quick steady motion (use other hand to keep slide from moving while spreader is pushed) (Figure 41-24D).
10. Examine the smear to see if it is satisfactory (Figure 41-24E).

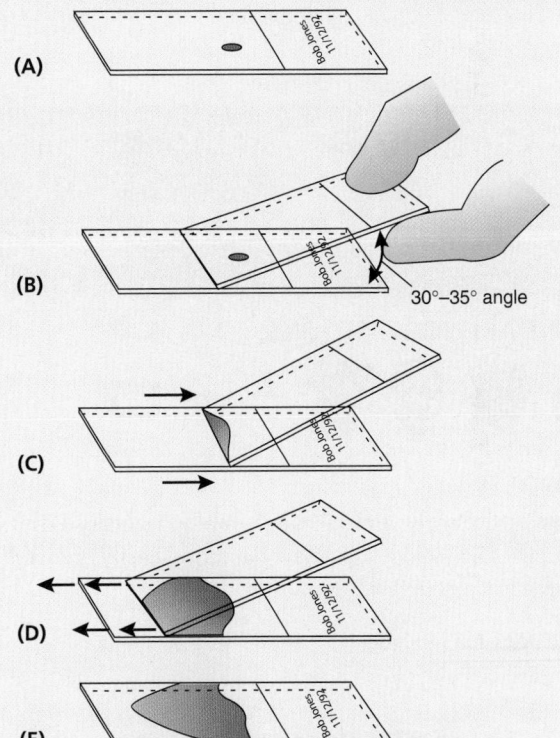

Figure 41-24 Making a blood smear for a differential white blood cell count using a spreader slide.
A. Position labeled end to right if you are right-handed, or to left if you are left-handed.
Place a small drop of blood on the slide.
B. Grasp the slide with your left hand to steady it.
C. Pull the spreader slide back into the drop of blood.
Let the blood spread along the back side of the spreader slide.
D. Quickly, without jerks, push the spreader slide to the left.
E. Allow the blood smear to air-dry before it is stained.

(continues)

Procedure
41-6 *(continued)*

11. Repeat the procedure until two satisfactory smears are obtained.
12. Allow the smear to air-dry quickly (stand slide on end in slide drying rack).
13. Place the dried smear in absolute methanol for thirty to sixty seconds to preserve the smear.
14. Remove the slide from methanol and allow to air-dry.
15. Store slide for staining.
16. Perform a capillary puncture, wipe away the first drop of blood, and fill one or two EDTA anticoagulated capillary tubes.

17. Prepare two blood smears from capillary blood, repeating steps 6–15.
18. Discard blood specimens appropriately or store for later use. Place contaminated materials into biohazard or sharps container.
19. Clean equipment and return to proper storage.
20. Clean work area with surface disinfectant.
21. Remove and discard gloves into biohazard container and wash hands with hand disinfectant.

Procedure
41-7   Staining a Differential Blood Smear Slide

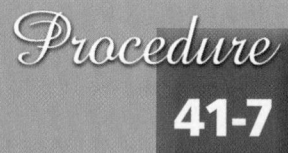

STANDARD PRECAUTIONS:

   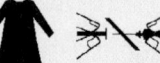

PURPOSE:
Properly and safely apply a stain to a blood smear so that the cells and structures may be more easily viewed through microscopic examination.

EQUIPMENT/SUPPLIES:
Gloves
Hand disinfectant
Blood smears, freshly prepared or preserved
Blood stain reagents:
  Wright's stain and buffer and/or
  commercial blood stain kit (quick stain)
Tube of EDTA anticoagulated blood (optional)
Staining rack
Immersion oil
Microscope
Lens paper
Forceps
Laboratory tissue
Lab apron or lab coat
Staining jars for quick stains

Surface disinfectant or 10% chlorine bleach solution
Biohazard container
Puncture-proof container for sharp objects
Slide storage box
NOTE: Stain characteristics may vary with stain lot. Follow the manufacturer's instructions for best results.

PROCEDURE STEPS:
1. Wash hands and put on gloves.
2. Assemble equipment and materials.
3. Prepare a blood smear (as in Procedure 41-6) or obtain a previously prepared, fixed smear.
4. Stain a blood smear by one of the following methods:
   a. Two-step method
      (1) Place the dried smear on the staining rack or on a flat surface, blood side up.
      (2) Flood the smear with Wright's stain but do not let stain overflow the sides of the slide.
      (3) Leave stain on slide one to three minutes (get exact time from instructor).
      (4) Add buffer, dropwise, to the stain until the buffer volume is about equal to the stain.

(continues)

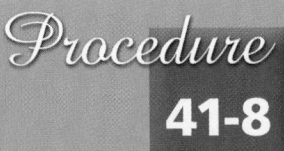

41-7 *(continued)*

   (5) Blow gently on the surface of the fluid to mix the solutions. A green metallic sheen should appear on the surface.

   (6) Allow buffer to remain on slide for two to four minutes (do not allow mixture to run off slide); get exact time from instructor.

   (7) Rinse thoroughly and continuously with a gentle stream of tap or distilled water.

   (8) Drain water from slide.

   (9) Wipe the *back* of the slide with a wet gauze to remove excess stain.

   (10) Stand smear on end to dry.

  b. Three-step method (quick stain)

   (1) Dip dry smear into solutions as directed by manufacturer's instructions (do not allow slide to dry between solutions).

   (2) Rinse slide (if instructed to do so).

   (3) Remove excess stain from the *back* of the slide with wet gauze.

   (4) Allow slide to air-dry by standing on end.

5. Place thoroughly dried slide on microscope stage, stain side up.

6. Focus with low-power (10X) objective.
7. Scan slide to find area where cells are barely touching each other (in feathered edge of smear).
8. Place a drop of immersion oil on the slide.
9. Rotate oil-immersion lens carefully into position.
10. Focus with fine adjustment knob only.
11. Observe erythrocytes; color should be pink-tan.
12. Observe leukocytes; nuclei should be purple; neutrophil granules should be pink-lavender.
13. Observe platelets; they should appear purple and granular.
14. Rotate the low-power (10X) objective into position.
15. Remove slide from microscope stage.
16. Clean oil objective thoroughly with lens paper.
17. Gently wipe oil from slide with soft tissue.
18. Clean equipment and return to proper storage.
19. Discard slides as instructed or store in slide box for use in Procedure 41-8.
20. Clean work area with surface disinfectant.
21. Remove and discard gloves into biohazard container and wash hands with hand disinfectant.

41-8   Differential Leukocyte Count

STANDARD PRECAUTIONS:

PURPOSE:
Properly and safely examine a stained blood smear to observe, identify, and record 100 leukocytes and "differentiate" the five types of leukocytes by size, nuclear characteristics, and cytoplasmic characteristics.

EQUIPMENT/SUPPLIES:
Gloves
Hand disinfectant

Stained normal blood smears
Microscope with oil-immersion objective
Immersion oil
Lens paper
Soft tissue or soft paper towels
Blood cell atlas; drawings or photographs and descriptions of stained blood cells
Tally counter or differential counter
Worksheet
Puncture-proof container for contaminated sharps
Surface disinfectant or 10% chlorine bleach solution

(continues)

Procedure

41-8   *(continued)*

PROCEDURE STEPS:

1. Wash hands and put on gloves.
2. Assemble equipment and materials.
3. Place stained smear on microscope stage and secure with clips.
4. Use the low-power (10X) objective to locate the feathered edge of the smear.
5. Bring the cells into focus using the 10X objective and coarse adjustment.
6. Scan the smear to find an area where the red blood cells are barely touching.
7. Place one drop of immersion oil on the smear.
8. Rotate the oil-immersion objective (97X or 100X) carefully into position.
9. Using the fine adjustment, focus until cells can be seen clearly.
10. Raise the condenser and open the diaphragm to allow maximum light into the objective.
11. Scan the slide to observe the leukocytes.
12. Study the smear; try to find and identify all five types of leukocytes.
13. Scan the smear to find platelets.
14. Scan the smear to observe red cells.
15. Repeat steps 3–14 until cells can readily be identified.
16. Repeat steps 1–10 using the same smear or a different one.
17. Count 100 consecutive leukocytes moving the slide or the movable stage so that consecutive microscopic fields are viewed; use the counting pattern illustrated in Figure 41-17.
18. Record on the worksheet how many of each type of leukocyte are seen.
19. Observe the red blood cells in at least ten fields. Note the hemoglobin content; record as normochromic or hypochromic. Look for any variation in shape.
20. Observe the red blood cell size. Record as normocytic, microcytic, or macrocytic. An approximation of the number of cells affected can be made by using a system of 1+ to 4+, or using small, medium, or large amount.
21. Observe platelets in at least ten fields:
    a. Note morphology.
    b. Estimate the number of platelets per oil immersion field: record as adequate, decreased, or increased, using the guide on the worksheet.
22. Rotate the low-power (10X) objective into place.
23. Remove the slide from the stage.
24. Using lens paper, clean the oil-immersion objective thoroughly.
25. Check the microscope stage and condenser for oil and clean with soft tissue if necessary.
26. Place the slide on its edge in a plastic slide box so oil can drain, or discard slide as instructed.
27. Clean remaining equipment and return it to proper storage.
28. Wipe work counter with surface disinfectant.
29. Remove and discard gloves into biohazard container and wash hands with hand disinfectant.

Procedure

41-9   **Erythrocyte Sedimentation Rate**

STANDARD PRECAUTIONS:

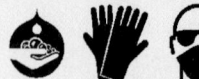 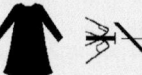 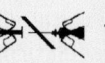

PURPOSE:
Properly and safely examine a blood sample by using either the Sediplast® (Westergren) or Wintrobe method to record the erythrocyte sedimentation rate.

(continues)

Procedure

41-9 *(continued)*

EQUIPMENT/SUPPLIES:
Gloves
Hand disinfectant
Sample of venous blood collected in EDTA
Sediplast® kit (or other ESR kit):
  sedivial and sedirack
  Sediplast® autozeroing pipette
  Pipette capable of delivering up to 1.0 mL
Wintrobe method:
  Wintrobe sedimentation tube (disposable or
    reusable)
  Wintrobe sedimentation rack
  Long-stem Pasteur-type pipette with rubber bulb
Timer
10% chlorine bleach solution
Biohazard disposal container
Acrylic safety shield or goggles and mask
Puncture-proof biohazard container for sharps
NOTE: Consult the manufacturer's package insert for
  specific instructions for the ESR kit being used.

PROCEDURE STEPS:
1. Wash hands and put on gloves.
2. Assemble equipment and materials.
3. Gently mix blood sample for two minutes.
4. Perform either method a (Sediplast® ESR) or
   method b (Wintrobe):
   a. Sediplast® ESR (modified Westergren)
      (1) Remove stopper on sedivial and fill to the
          indicated mark with 0.8 mL blood. Re-
          place stopper and invert vial several times
          to mix (or mix using pipette).
      (2) Place sedivial in Sediplast® rack on a level
          surface.
      (3) Gently insert the disposable Sediplast®
          pipette through the pierceable stopper
          with a twisting motion and push down
          until the pipette rests on the bottom of the
          vial. The pipette will autozero the blood
          and any excess will flow into the sealed
          reservoir compartment.
      (4) Set timer for one hour.
      (5) Return blood sample to proper storage. (If
          no laboratory work will be performed dur-

ing the incubation, remove gloves, discard
appropriately, and wash hands. Reglove
before handling test materials.)
      (6) Let the pipette stand undisturbed for
          exactly one hour and then read the results
          of the ESR: Use the scale on the tube to
          measure the distance from the top of the
          plasma to the top of the red blood cells.
      (7) Record the sedimentation rate:
          ESR (Mod. Westergren, 1 hr) = ___ mm
      (8) Dispose of tube and vial in appropriate
          biohazard container.
   b. Wintrobe method:
      (1) Place tube in Wintrobe sedimentation
          rack.
      (2) Check the leveling bubble to ensure that
          the Wintrobe rack is level.
      (3) Fill Wintrobe tube to the zero mark with
          well-mixed blood using the Pasteur pipette
          and being careful not to overfill.
          NOTE: Tube must be filled from the bottom
          to avoid getting air bubbles in the tube.
      (4) Set timer for one hour. Be certain the tube
          is vertical.
      (5) Return blood sample to proper storage. (If
          no other laboratory work is scheduled, re-
          move gloves, discard appropriately, and
          wash hands. Reglove before handling test
          materials.)
      (6) Measure the distance the erythrocytes
          have fallen (in mm): after exactly one
          hour, use the scale on the tube to measure
          the distance from the top of the plasma to
          the top of the red blood cells.
      (7) Record the sedimentation rate:
          ESR (Wintrobe, 1 hr) = ___ mm
      (8) Disinfect and clean equipment and return
          to storage.
      NOTE: If disposable equipment is used, dispose
      of in biohazard container.
5. Clean work area with surface disinfectant.
6. Remove gloves and discard into biohazard container.
7. Wash hands with hand disinfectant.

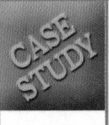

CASE STUDY 41-1

Today is busier than usual at Doctors Lewis & King. While she is performing an erythrocyte sedimentation rate for Jim Marshal, a patient in his late thirties, medical assistant Audrey Jones is called upon to help with another patient. She hurriedly places the sedimentation rack on top of an incubator in the sunlight by an open window and leaves to assist Dr. King.

CASE STUDY REVIEW

1. List two ways in which the test results may be affected.
2. What are the normal Westergren ESR values for males and females under 50 years of age?
3. What are the best conditions for an accurate test?

SUMMARY

Hematology tests are the second most frequently performed tests in the ambulatory care setting. Only the urinalysis is performed more frequently. Medical assistants must have a knowledge of hematology to accurately and efficiently perform the tests. The study of hematology includes hematopoiesis, which is the formation of the blood elements, as well as the hematological tests and their relationship to the pathology of the body.

This chapter has introduced the more common hematological tests that are performed in the ambulatory care setting, including all the parts of the complete blood count (CBC), the erythrocyte sedimentation rates methods, and the erythrocyte indices. All of these tests are utilized by the physician in the diagnosis and treatment of disease.

Most of the hematology procedures performed in today's ambulatory care setting utilize some type of automated instrumentation. Some automated hematology instruments require a diluted blood sample while others do not require a diluted sample. Both methods of automated instrumentation are discussed in the chapter.

CAUTION: Blood specimens used in the sampling of hematological procedures are biohazardous material. Be sure to follow Universal and Standard Precautions when you work with these specimens. Refer back to Chapter 22.

REVIEW QUESTIONS

Multiple Choice

1. Which of the following is *not* a cellular component of blood?
   a. erythrocytes
   b. leukocytes
   c. thrombocytes
   d. erythropoietin
2. The formation of blood is defined as:
   a. erythropoietin
   b. hematopoiesis
   c. mean corpuscular volume
   d. hemoglobinopathy
3. Sickle cell anemia, a hereditary disease, has which type of hemoglobin?
   a. hemoglobin S
   b. hemoglobin A
   c. hemoglobin E
   d. hemoglobin C

4. The volume of packed red cells compared to the total volume of the sample is calculated from which test?
   a. hematocrit
   b. hemoglobin
   c. MCH
   d. MCV
5. Manual blood cell counts are made using the:
   a. hemacytometer
   b. QBC
   c. nanometer
   d. spectrophotometer
6. The most common white cell type found in the granulocytic series is the:
   a. lymphocyte
   b. monocyte
   c. neutrophil
   d. basophil

7. The erythrocyte indices are used for the diagnosis, classification, and treatment of different:
   a. infections
   b. anemias
   c. inflammatory diseases
   d. neoplasms
8. Which hematological test result shows an increase with infections, inflammatory disease, pregnancy, and tissue destruction?
   a. hemoglobin
   b. MCV
   c. hematocrit
   d. ESR
9. The most frequent hemoglobin disease seen in the ambulatory care setting is:
   a. iron deficiency anemia
   b. sickle cell anemia
   c. leukemia
   d. anisocytosis

Critical Thinking

1. Describe three changes from normal, and their causes, that can be observed on a stained blood smear.
2. What hematological factors do the erythrocyte indices provide information about? List one example for each index in which a disease causes an elevation or decrease.

3. You are serving your externship in a local clinic. A physician has made a tentative diagnosis of appendicitis for a patient. In addition to the urinalysis, what single hematological test is most likely to confirm the diagnosis?
4. List the guidelines that must be followed in order to assure accurate sed rate results.
5. How is quality control maintained with automated hematology instruments? Refer to Chapter 38.

WEB ACTIVITIES

1. Visit the CDC's web site to review Standard Precautions required during blood collection.
2. Does the American Heart Association's web site offer parameters for different blood counts and hematology values? Are guidelines and tips on specimen collection outlined?

REFERENCES/BIBLIOGRAPHY

Henry, J. B. H. (Ed.). (1996). *Clinical diagnosis and management by laboratory methods* (19th ed.). Philadelphia: W. B. Saunders Company.

Palko, T., & Palko, H. (1996). *Laboratory procedures for the medical office*. Columbus, OH: Glencoe/McGraw-Hill.

Walters, N. J., Estridge, B. H., & Reynolds, A. P. (2000). *Basic medical laboratory techniques* (4th ed.). Albany, NY: Delmar.

Chapter 42

URINALYSIS

KEY TERMS

Acetest®
Acid/Base Balance
Amorphous
Bilirubin
Casts
Circadian Rhythm
Clinitest®
Creatinine
Critical Values
Crystals
Cultures
Glucose
Hematuria
Hyaline
Ictotest®
Ketoacidosis
Ketone
Leukocyte Esterase
Meniscus
Midstream Collection
pH
Quality Control
Reagents
Reagent Test Strip
Refractometer
Screening
Sediment
Specific Gravity
Supernatant
Tamm-Horsfall
Turbid
Urea
Urinalysis
Urinometer
Urobilinogen
Urochrome

OUTLINE

Urine Formation
   Filtration
   Reabsorption
   Secretion
Urine Composition
Safety
Quality Control
CLIA '88
Urine Containers

Urine Collection
   Urine Specimen Types
   Collection Methods
Examination of Urine
   Physical Examination of Urine
   Chemical Examination of Urine
   Microscopic Examination of Urine
     Sediment

OBJECTIVES

The student should strive to meet the following performance objectives and demonstrate an understanding of the facts and principles presented in this chapter through written and oral communication.

1. Define the key terms as presented in the glossary.
2. Explain the process of urine formation.
3. Discuss the importance of safety procedures and quality control when working with urine.
4. Describe the importance of proper collection and preservation of the random, midstream, clean-catch, and 24-hour urine specimens.
5. Identify the proper technique for examining the physical characteristics of a urine specimen.
6. Explain causes of abnormal physical characteristics of urine.
7. Describe methods for chemical examination of a urine specimen.
8. Explain the need to confirm abnormal results.
9. Describe the confirmatory tests for ketones, glucose, protein, and bilirubin.
10. Identify the proper method of preparing urine sediment for microscopic examination.
11. Identify normal and abnormal structures found during the microscopic examination of urine sediment.

CLINICAL

Fundamental Principles

- Apply principles of aseptic technique and infection control
- Comply with quality assurance practices
- Screen and follow up patient test results

Diagnostic Orders

- Collect and process specimens
- Perform diagnostic tests

GENERAL (TRANSDISCIPLINARY)

Legal Concepts

- Document accurately
- Comply with established risk management and safety procedures

Instruction

- Instruct individuals according to their needs

At Inner City Health Care, clinical medical assistant Wanda Slawson performs many urinalyses. Although urinalysis is a routine procedure, Wanda recognizes its importance as a diagnostic tool and she performs each test carefully to ensure accurate results. Wanda takes time to instruct patients in the proper collection procedures. She encourages patients to ask questions before collecting the urine sample and she provides written instructions for easy reference. When she performs the urinalysis, Wanda follows safety and quality control guidelines. By paying attention to the details of the procedure, Wanda does her best to ensure the quality of the urinalysis results.

INTRODUCTION

Examination of the urine (**urinalysis**) as a diagnostic tool for many diseases has been performed for centuries by medical practitioners. Urinalysis refers to the study of urine as an aid in patient diagnosis or to follow the course of disease. The urine examination is a routine part of most physical examinations.

The routine urinalysis is one of the most frequently performed procedures in the medical office laboratory. Many tests can be performed on one urine sample. This procedure is often ordered because urine is easily obtained, and much information about the body's metabolism may be gained from the results of this testing.

When physicians order a "routine urinalysis," they expect timely and accurate results. Results can indicate a systemic disease process and/or renal (kidney) or urinary tract disease.

Practice, experience, and attention to detail are the most important tools in achieving quality results. Following standard precautions when working with any body fluid is mandatory.

URINE FORMATION

Before discussing the analysis of urine, it is helpful to understand how urine is formed in the human body. The formation and excretion of urine is the principal way the body excretes water and gets rid of waste. These waste products, if not removed, rapidly can become toxic.

The kidney is a highly specialized organ that eliminates soluble (dissolved in water) waste products of metabolism. Urine is formed in the kidney and is excreted from the body by way of the urinary tract system (Figure 42-1). The kidney also regulates the fluid outside the cells of the body by eliminating certain fluids and returning other fluids, maintaining a careful balance (homeostasis). In this manner, the body is protected from dramatic changes in fluid volume, acidity and alkalinity (**acid/base balance**), composition, and pressure.

There are two kidneys, one on each side of the body. They are about 11 to 12 centimeters long and 5 to 6 centimeters wide. Kidneys are shaped like a lima bean with their concave border directed toward the midline of the body. The left kidney is slightly higher than the right.

Filtration

The kidney filters waste products, salts, and excess fluid from the blood. The filtering unit of the kidney is called the glomerulus. The part of the kidney that concentrates the filtered material is called the tubule. Together, the glomerulus and the tubule combine to form the nephron (Figure 42-2).

Most of the work of the kidney is done by the nephrons. There are approximately one million nephrons in each kidney. Each minute, more than 1,000 milliliters of blood flow through the kidney to be cleansed. In the glomerulus, certain substances are filtered out of the blood. The remaining filtrate then passes into the tubule where various changes occur. Substances filtered out from the body can include water, ammonia, electrolytes, **glu-**

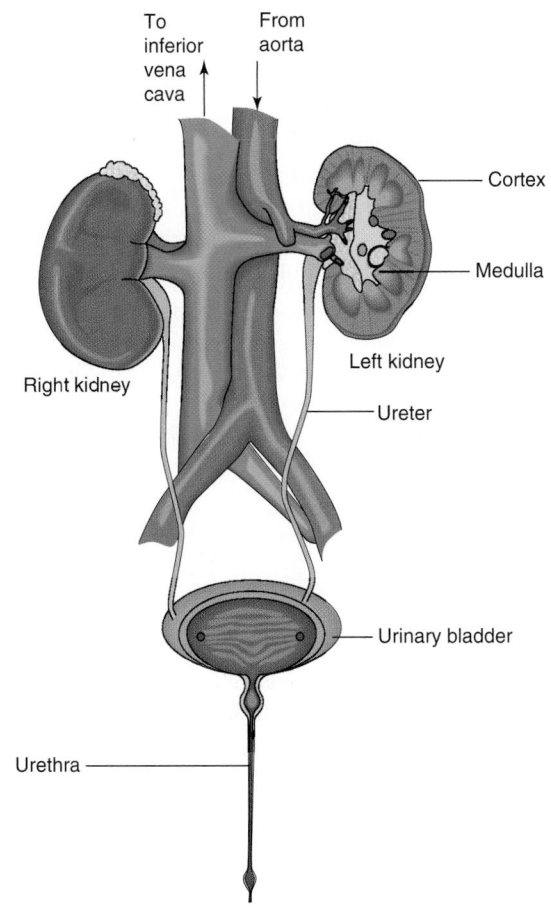

Figure 42-1 The urinary system.

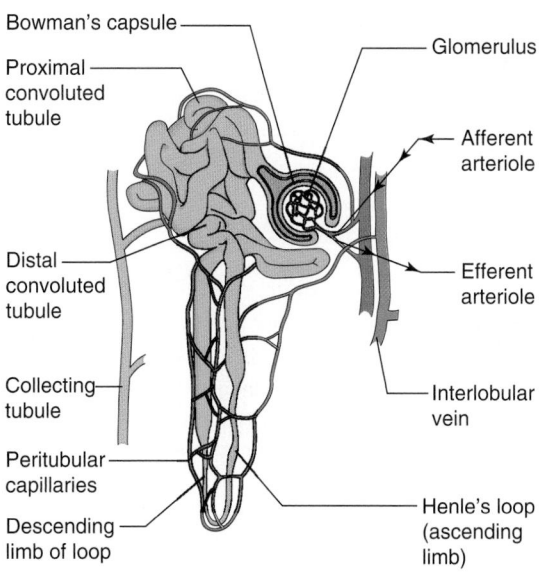

Figure 42-2 Parts of the nephron unit.

cose, amino acids, **creatinine**, and **urea**. These wastes leave the body in the eliminated urine.

For example, when diabetics have excess sugar in their blood, the body attempts to eliminate the excess glucose through the urine. Routine urinalysis testing will reveal the excess glucose, alerting the physician to the presence of too much glucose. Diabetes can be diagnosed in this manner, as well as determining that a diabetic is not taking enough insulin to control the glucose in the blood.

Reabsorption

While passing through the kidney, some substances may need to be reabsorbed by the blood. Approximately 180 liters of filtrate are produced daily by the body, but only 1 to 2 liters of urine are eliminated from the normally functioning human body. Therefore, much of the filtrate, including water, sodium, chloride, potassium, bicarbonate, glucose, calcium, and amino acids, is reabsorbed into the body.

Under normal conditions, blood cells and most proteins stay in the blood plasma because they are too large to pass through the walls of the capillaries of the glomerulus.

If blood cells and excess protein are found in the urine, the physician is alerted that the kidney is not filtering properly due to an irregular condition affecting the urinary tract.

As long as the concentration of glucose in the blood is below 180 mg/dL (milligrams per deciliter), the glucose will be completely reabsorbed. If the level increases above 180 mg/dL, the glucose is not reabsorbed. Substances such as glucose that are reabsorbed in relationship to their concentration in the blood are known as threshold substances. The needs of homeostasis call for sugar and protein to be almost completely reabsorbed, while other threshold substances such as creatinine, amino acids, potassium, sodium, and chloride are only partially reabsorbed.

Secretion

Near the end of the blood's journey through the kidney, specifically in the distal convoluted tubule, other substances that have not already been filtered are secreted into the urine. Such substances as hydrogen and ammonium ions may be secreted into the urine in exchange for sodium. Certain drugs in the blood at this point may also be secreted into the urine.

URINE COMPOSITION

After urine progresses through a healthy kidney, it is approximately 96 percent water and 4 percent dissolved substances, most of which come from either dietary intake or metabolic waste products. These substances are primarily urea, salt, sulfates, and phosphates. Abnormal constituents of urine include red and white blood cells, fat, glucose, casts, bile, acetone, and hemoglobin (Table 42-1).

TABLE 42-1	NORMAL AND ABNORMAL SUBSTANCES IN URINE
Normal	**Abnormal**
Urea	Bile
Uric acid	Blood
Creatinine	Fat
Sodium	Glucose
Potassium	Protein
Ammonium	White blood cells
Sulfate	Urobilinogen
Chloride	Microorganisms (bacteria and/or parasites)

Precautions To Use When Handling Urine Specimens

- Treat all specimens as if they were infectious, handling them with gloved hands.
- Avoid splashes or creation of aerosols when handling or disposing of urine specimens. Wearing face shields will prevent splashes from getting into the eyes, nose, or mouth.
- Process urine specimens as soon as possible.
- Store urine specimens appropriately in a designated refrigerator that contains no food or drink items.
- Dispose of urine appropriately, possibly in a special sink (run water to wash the specimen into the drain) or toilet.

When certain disease processes occur in the human body, the following changes in urine production and composition can occur:

- The amount of urine excreted can rise or fall
- Urine color can change
- Urine appearance can vary
- Urine odor can change
- Cells can be present in urine
- Chemical constituents in urine can change
- Urine concentration (specific gravity) may vary

SAFETY

Chapter 38 of this textbook covers the guidelines set up by government agencies to ensure the safety of everyone working in the health care field and for the protection of our environment. These guidelines are now referred to as standard precautions. Other terms used to describe care when handling infectious materials are transmission-based precautions and biohazard precautions.

QUALITY CONTROL

As in every area of the laboratory, every effort must be made by health care professionals to produce test results free from error. Much pressure is placed by regulatory agencies on facilities that perform laboratory tests such as urinalysis to maintain standards that will ensure reliable results. **Quality control** (QC) programs are an important part of urine testing to ensure accurate and reliable results for the patient. Quality control programs must be incorporated into every urine testing procedure. Because many of the tests are interpreted by visual examination, the quality control procedures are dependent on the expertise of the person performing the examination.

Testing protocols must be written out and available to personnel. Records of testing must be maintained. Equipment and instruments used for urine testing must be maintained and checked daily for proper calibration. If the instrument should require recalibration, the manufacturer's instructions are provided with the instrument.

Always be careful to perform the quality control procedures *exactly* as you perform the procedures on actual patient samples. Documentation of the performance of daily control testing must be kept for at least three years. With the advent of computer storage, the data can now be stored indefinitely. Commercially available urine control samples can be purchased from a number of manufacturers. Positive and negative controls should be run each day on all tests to be performed. Control results should be recorded on a daily log for easy access. The control samples should be stored as directed by the manufacturer.

CLIA '88

The regulations under the new Clinical Laboratory Improvement Amendments (CLIA) are discussed in Chapter 38. Several CLIA '88 regulations apply to the medical assistant performing urine testing. They include:

- Appropriate training in the methodology of the test being performed
- Understanding of urine-testing quality control procedures
- Proficiency in the use of instrumentation, being able to troubleshoot problems
- Knowledge of the stability and proper storage of **reagents** (substances involved in urine testing)
- Awareness of factors that influence test results
- Knowledge of how to verify test results

URINE CONTAINERS

The first step toward achieving proper results during laboratory testing is proper collection of the specimen to be tested. There are a variety of containers (Figure 42-3) used for urine collection, including nonsterile containers for random specimens (urinalysis), sterile containers for cultures (testing specimens for growth of bacteria), and 24-hour collection containers with added preservatives.

After specimen collection, the container must be labeled immediately with all the following information: patient's name, age, sex, identifying number, date, time of collection, and physician's name. These requirements may differ in various facilities. To prevent specimen mislabeling, the following procedures should always be followed. Specimen labeling should be done immediately following specimen collection. Never prelabel a specimen collection container. The only exception is when a patient is asked to collect a specimen on his or her own. Before the container is given to the patient, it should be labeled properly. If the patient cannot void, the container must be discarded immediately. This will prevent the container being used for some future patient collection. Always place the specimen label on the specimen collection container, never on the lid.

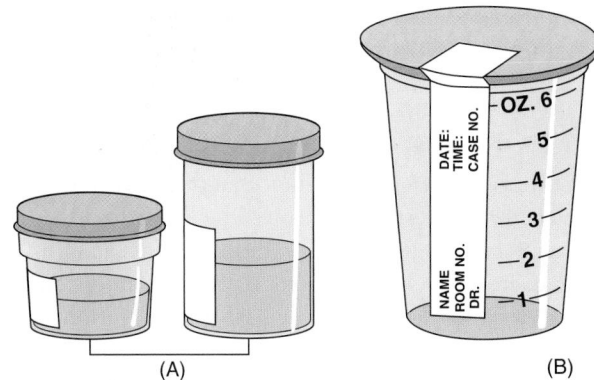

Figure 42-3 Urine collection containers: (A) Sterile. (B) Random.

Patients may have questions about how a specimen should be collected. The medical assistant must be able to give proper instructions using common terms that the patient will be able to understand. Most laboratories have containers made specifically for urine collection, but any container can be used for urinalysis testing as long as it is clean and dry. However, if the sample is to be cultured (tested for microorganisms), it must be collected in a sterile container. In some cases, catheterization, which is discussed later in this chapter, also is used.

URINE COLLECTION

Urine Specimen Types

Following are common types of urine specimens that might be ordered frequently by physicians.

Random (Spot) Specimen. Random (spot) urine samples are specimens that can be obtained at any time and are the most commonly collected specimens. Any random urine specimen can be used for routine urinalysis. However, a concentrated specimen is preferable to one that is dilute. The first morning void is typically the most concentrated specimen and is usually the specimen of choice for many urine tests.

Fasting/Timed Specimens. A fasting (going without food and drink) urine specimen is ordered less often than a random specimen. The physician may want to measure a urinary substance without interference from food intake. Some physicians may require an overnight fast. Others may ask the patient to have a meal and then urinate four hours later (that urine is not collected as the next voided specimen but is considered a *timed* specimen).

It is up to the medical assistant to give the patient proper instruction as to how to collect a fasting, or timed, specimen. Written directions given to the patient in addition to oral instructions are best. A regular urinalysis container can be used for a fasting specimen. It does not require a sterile container.

Twenty-Four-Hour Specimen. Urine varies in its concentration of certain substances at different times during any 24-hour period due to **circadian rhythm** and the intake of food and water. For instance, the amount of water excreted is highest from 10 A.M. to noon and 4 to 6 P.M. Chloride is in its highest concentration from noon to 2 P.M. Therefore, a 24-hour specimen is sometimes requested when quantitative tests (measuring the amount) for different substances are desired. The results of this type of collection then will be expressed in *units per 24 hours*. Some commonly tested substances include sodium, potassium, calcium, and creatinine.

The container used to collect this amount of urine should be of adequate size. Usually a one-gallon, dark-colored plastic bottle is used. For measuring some urine constituents, preservatives need to be added to the bottle before the collection begins. Without the preservative, these substances may break down and be impossible to quantify. Preservatives include thymol, toluene, and certain acids.

Urine collected over a 24-hour period of time is refrigerated between collections. After the collection is complete, it must be returned to the medical laboratory as soon as possible.

 Many 24-hour urine bottles contain preservatives. Some preservatives are strong acids or bases. As with all laboratory chemicals, the medical assistant and the patient should avoid contact between the preservative and the skin. Vapors must not be inhaled when adding the specimen to the container. In the patient's written instructions, there should be a warning about avoiding contact with preservatives.

Physicians sometimes choose to have a 2-hour or a 12-hour specimen instead of the usual 24-hour collection. All of the collection steps for a 24-hour specimen apply. Recording the time of day is very important (a 2-hour specimen is usually collected in the afternoon).

Collection Methods

In addition to ordering what type of urine specimen is desired (random, fasting, 24-hour), the physician might also order a certain type of collection method to collect the specific sample. These methods include random, clean-catch, midstream, and catheterization.

Random Collection. The patient simply urinates into a cup until the cup is fairly full. Patients often find collecting urine very awkward. In the process of collection, the specimen can become contaminated from such

---

Patient Teaching Tip

1. When giving a patient any type of instructions, make sure that the patient understands the importance of each step. Always provide written instructions as well. Emphasize that failing to follow the instructions will cause the results to be invalid, requiring another collection.
2. The patient begins a 24-hour collection by emptying the bladder and not keeping the specimen. The container is then labeled with the time of bladder emptying. Patients generally start the collection between 6 and 8 P.M., but any 24-hour period is acceptable.
3. Explain that each time the patient urinates within the 24-hour period, the urine is placed into the collection bottle.
4. Instruct the patient to refrigerate the bottle between urinations.
5. Explain to the patient that at the end of the 24-hour period, the patient should urinate and place the urine in the bottle. The exact time should be written on the label as the "ended" or "completed" time.
6. The most common errors in the 24-hour urine specimen collection are the inclusion of the first voided specimen and the discarding of one or more of the voided specimens during the 24-hour period. Be sure the patient understands these steps.

---

sources as epithelial cells (skin cells) around the genital area, bacterial contamination from the skin, excess mucus, or fecal contamination from the rectal area.

Clean-Catch Method. To avoid as much contamination as possible when collecting a specimen, physicians prefer that the patient cleanse the genital area before collection. The clean-catch order means that an antiseptic towelette is provided in addition to a urine container. Men cleanse the urethral opening with a single stroke of an antiseptic towelette. The stroke should be directed from the tip of the penis toward the ring of the glans. This should be repeated with another towelette.

Female patients should spread the outer vulval folds and cleanse the inner side of both folds with a single stroke from front to back. A second towelette is used to cleanse the urethral opening with a single front-to-back stroke. Female patients should also be instructed to notify the medical assistant if they are menstruating during the collection.

Midstream Collection. Sometimes a physician will order a midstream collection. After cleansing, the patient should begin to urinate into the toilet. The patient then stops the stream of urine and collects the next portion into a collection cup, voiding the final stream into the toilet. By this method, the initial urine stream will carry away any contamination left after cleansing. The midstream urine should be as free of contamination as possible.

Catheterized Collection. At times it is necessary to catheterize a patient. This procedure is performed by a physician or a health care worker specifically trained to do catheterizations.

A catheterization involves inserting a sterile tube directly into the bladder through the urethra. Samples obtained in this way are suitable for all urinalysis and microbiological procedures because they are not contaminated by the outside environment.

Due to the invasive action, this procedure can cause infection in the patient if not done correctly. Physicians order this method of collection only when other methods are contraindicated. A catheterization may be necessary when urine specimens collected by other methods continually test positive for bacteria.

EXAMINATION OF URINE

Urine should be examined in a fresh state, preferably while still warm if possible. However, urine usually cannot be tested immediately. If immediate testing is not possible, the urine should be refrigerated at about 4°C or stored on ice. The urinalysis should be performed as soon as possible, preferably within 2 hours. **Crystals** and **casts** begin to break down after 2 hours. Any time delay allows bacteria to multiply and can lead to inaccurate microbiology results.

The routine urinalysis procedure is composed of three parts:

- *Physical* examination of the urine
- *Chemical* examination of the urine
- *Microscopic* examination of urine sediment

 The medical assistant should remember to wash hands, put on gloves, and follow all of the safety guidelines when performing any of the following procedures. Some facilities require eye protection when pouring urine or any procedure where splashing urine into the eye could occur.

Physical Examination of Urine

When the medical assistant begins the process of performing a urinalysis, the first step is performing the physical examination. This examination consists of:

- Assessing the volume of the urine specimen, making sure that the specimen is sufficient for testing
- Observing and recording the color and transparency of the specimen
- Noting any unusual urine odor
- Measuring the specific gravity of the specimen

Specimen Volume. The first step in performing a urinalysis is to determine if the sample's volume is adequate for testing. Procedure 42-1 illustrates how initially to assess the volume of the urine specimen.

Urine Color. There is a wide range of color in normal urine, usually ranging from a pale yellow to a dark yellow or amber. The range of color usually is due to the concentration of the urine. A darker color generally indicates a more concentrated urine. The color (**urochrome**) comes from normal metabolic processes, the end products of which are deposited in the urine.

After assessing the adequacy of the urine volume, the medical assistant then observes and records the color of the urine, as in Procedure 42-2.

The diet and certain drugs can add substances to the urine that give it a specific color. The medical assistant should be familiar with some reasons for abnormally colored urine. For example, the most common cause of red urine is red blood cells, known as **hematuria**. Blood cells in urine may indicate bleeding in the urinary tract. The medication Pyridium is commonly used for bladder infections and gives urine a bright orange color. Table 42-2 lists several urine color variations and possible causes.

Urine Transparency. Urine transparency normally is not significant by itself. However, it may be helpful when included with the rest of the urinalysis information.

TABLE 42-2	URINE COLORS AND POSSIBLE CAUSES
Color	**Possible Cause**
Straw to yellow	Normal
Orange to amber	Concentrated urine
Colorless	Dilute urine
Deep yellow	Vitamin intake
Bright orange	Drugs, usually Pyridium
Orange-brown	Urobilin
Greenish-orange	Bilirubin
Smokey	Red blood cells
Wine red/reddish brown	Hemoglobin pigments
Green or blue	Methylene blue

Transparency of urine usually is recorded as clear, cloudy, hazy, or **turbid** (opaque), as in Procedure 42-3. These descriptive terms may vary in different facilities.

There are many causes of cloudy urine, most of which are considered normal. Cloudiness could be contributed to contamination from vaginal discharges, white blood cells, bacteria, or yeast. As urine cools, sometimes crystals form that also may give urine a cloudy appearance.

Urine Odor. With experience, the medical assistant will recognize certain odors in the urine that can indicate specific conditions. Odors, though not recorded on the final laboratory urinalysis report, should not be disregarded. For example, the urine of a diabetic who may have a condition known as **ketoacidosis** may have a sweet odor. Urine full of bacteria will have a foul odor that is easily recognized.

Urine Specific Gravity. **Specific gravity** is defined as the ratio of the weight of a given volume of a substance to the weight of the same volume of distilled water at the same temperature. Distilled water used as the reference point has been given the specific gravity value of 1.000. The specific gravity of urine indicates the concentrations of solids such as phosphates, chlorides, proteins, sugars, and urea that are dissolved in urine.

Variations in urine specific gravity can give the physician diagnostic information. In diabetes mellitus, glucose molecules will be very dense and give the urine a high specific gravity. The normal range of specific gravity for urine is from 1.003 to 1.035. Specific gravity is highest in the first morning samples because the urine is more concentrated.

Specific gravity is often tested by using either a urinometer or a refractometer. A **urinometer** is a calibrated, floating device. A **refractometer** measures the amount of light that is bent by particles suspended in a liquid. The two methods do not give exactly the same results but are close enough for most clinical applications. A specific gravity reading is also available in conjunction with chemical testing on some reagent strips.

Urinometer. A urinometer (Figures 42-4A and B) is made from a small glass tube weighted to float in a sample of urine (usually 15 mL). The glass tube has been calibrated, and the stem of the tube has been marked accordingly to read 1.000 at the bottom of the meniscus in distilled water at room temperature. The **meniscus** is the curvature that appears in a liquid's upper surface when the liquid is placed in a container. The medical assistant reads the specific gravity of the urine from the stem at the meniscus (Figure 42-4C). However, the temperature of the urine must be taken into account if it differs from 20

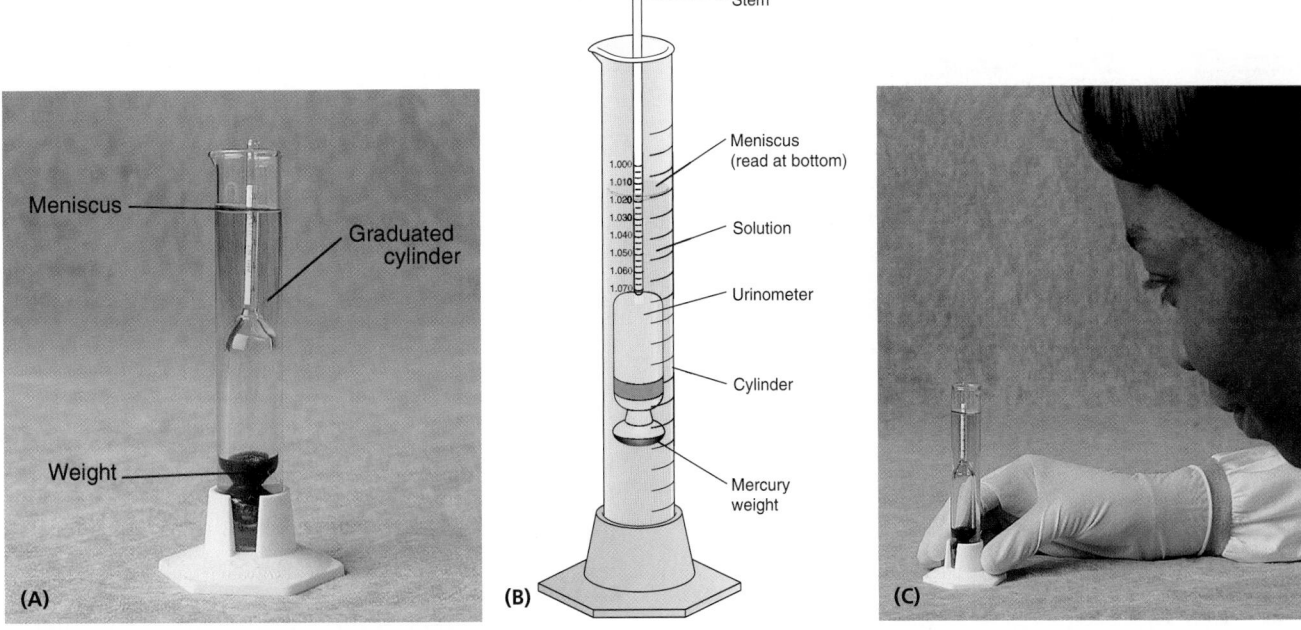

Figure 42-4 (A) Urinometer. (B) Urinometer parts. (C) The medical assistant reads the specific gravity of the urine from the urinometer stem at the meniscus.

degrees centigrade, which is normal room temperature. Add 0.001 to the reading for every 3 degrees above 20 degrees centigrade, and subtract 0.001 for every 3 degrees below 20 degrees centigrade. The buoyancy of a liquid changes with the temperature. The need for temperature correction can be avoided by allowing the sample of urine to come to room temperature.

Refractometer. The most common tool for determining the specific gravity of liquids is the refractometer (Figure 42-5). This instrument measures the refractive index of urine, which is the speed at which light travels through the air as compared to the speed at which it passes through urine. Light is slowed and therefore bent as it encounters particles—the more particles, the more bend. The bend can be used to determine the total number of particles and is not affected by the weight of the particles.

The refractometer reading is about 0.002 below that of the true specific gravity. This slight difference is more than made up for by the ease of using the instrument and the instrument's reliability. This instrument only needs a drop or two of urine, and the result does not have to be adjusted for temperature as long as the temperature is between 60° and 100°F. See Procedure 42-4.

Chemical Examination of Urine

After the physical testing of a urine specimen, the next step in urinalysis testing is chemical testing. This procedure once was complex, but today many manufacturers have made the task simple through a wide range of ready-

to-use reagents and the reagent test strip, or dipstick (Figure 42-6) as it is more commonly known.

A **reagent test strip**, or dipstick, is a narrow strip of plastic on which pads containing reagents for different reactions are attached. The pads have reagents to test for many metabolic processes, including kidney and liver functions, urinary tract infection, and pH balance. The reagent test strip is the primary tool used for chemical

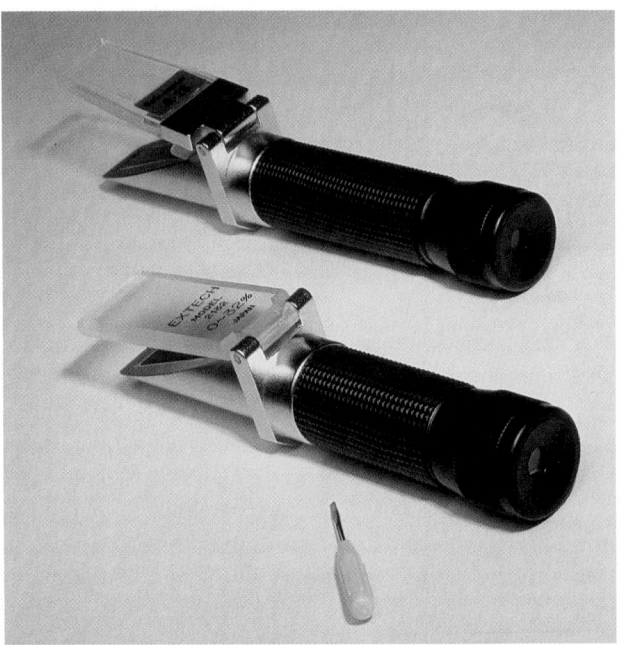

Figure 42-5 Refractometers.

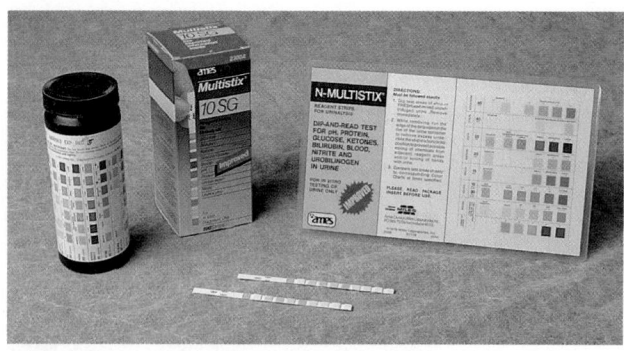

Figure 42-6 Multistix reagent strips with color-coded chart are used for chemical analysis of urine.

TABLE 42-3	CHEMICAL TESTING AVAILABLE ON URINE REAGENT TEST STRIPS
• Bilirubin	• Nitrites
• Blood	• pH
• Glucose	• Protein
• Ketones	• Specific gravity
• Leukocyte esterase	• Urobilinogen

examination of urine. Specific confirmatory tests or methods may be necessary based on the result of the reagent test strip. Table 42-3 lists some tests available on urine reagent strips.

Specific Reagent Test Strip Tests. *Bilirubin.* **Bilirubin** is a product of the breakdown of hemoglobin. Bilirubin in urine can indicate problems such as liver disease, hepatitis, and bile duct destruction. Bilirubin can break down in sunlight, so a urine sample should be protected from sunlight prior to testing for bilirubin.

Blood. Small amounts of blood (from blood cells or hemoglobin) can be detected by reagent strips. Urinary blood can indicate infection, urinary tract trauma, kidney bleeding, menses, and other conditions.

Glucose. A glucose test is added to a reagent strip to detect unsuspected diabetes or to check efficiency of insulin therapy in diabetics.

Ketones. **Ketone** bodies appear when excessive amounts of fatty acids are catabolized (broken down into simpler compounds) and when glucose availability is limited. Ketones occur during prolonged fasting.

Leukocyte. The **leukocyte esterase** test indicates white blood cells in the urinary tract, presumably attracted by invading bacteria.

Nitrites. The presence of urinary nitrites indicates the possibility of a urinary tract infection. Certain species of bacteria convert nitrates into nitrites, which are normally absent from urine.

pH. The **pH** test indicates the relative acidity or alkalinity of the urine. The urine has a pH range of 4.6 to 8.0, with a mean reading of 6.0. Starvation and ketosis increase urine acidity (pH reading goes below 7.0). Bacteria can make the pH alkaline (over 7.0), as can some drugs.

Protein. A small amount of protein is normal in the urine. Detectable amounts of protein in the urine indicate injury to the kidney, specifically to the glomerular membrane. Protein can increase during a high fever.

Specific gravity. Some reagent strips contain an indicator that turns various colors depending on the ion con-

centration of the urine. This test reads up to a 1.030 result.

Urobilinogen. **Urobilinogen** is a degradation product of bilirubin formed by intestinal bacteria. Increased levels of this substance suggest liver disease or bleeding disorders.

Reagent Test Strip Quality Control. Reagent test strips are easy to use, but the complexity of the chemical testing should not be overlooked. As with any chemical reaction, each test involves multiple steps that are sensitive to temperature, time, dilution, and other factors. Outdated strips or reagents should never be used. To get optimum results, a certain amount of care must be taken when handling and storing the reagent strips. They must not be exposed to moisture, volatile substances, direct sunlight, or excess heat. The strips should not be removed from their original container except at the time of use. Always follow the manufacturer's instructions for storage. Test results are represented by a color change. The test result is compared to a color chart on the label of the reagent test strip container. Employees performing this test should be tested for color blindness as many of the color changes are subtle.

Reagent test strips are ready to use directly from their container. Correct quality control procedures should be followed as required by CLIA '88 and the facility where the testing is performed. This usually includes using a quality control urine sample (with predetermined results). All that is needed for this testing are the strips, quality control specimen, and patient specimens. Procedure 42-5 explains how to perform a urinalysis chemical examination.

There are also automated urine analyzers (Figure 42-7A and B) capable of timing and reading the test strip. These instruments can be quite expensive and are not available in every laboratory. Today, automated urine analyzers are used more frequently as they are more accurate and cut down on human error.

When reporting results, it is important to use the proper units and terms as directed by your laboratory. An example of the sensitivity of the reagent strips is shown in Table 42-4 (there is variation in sensitivity among manufacturers).

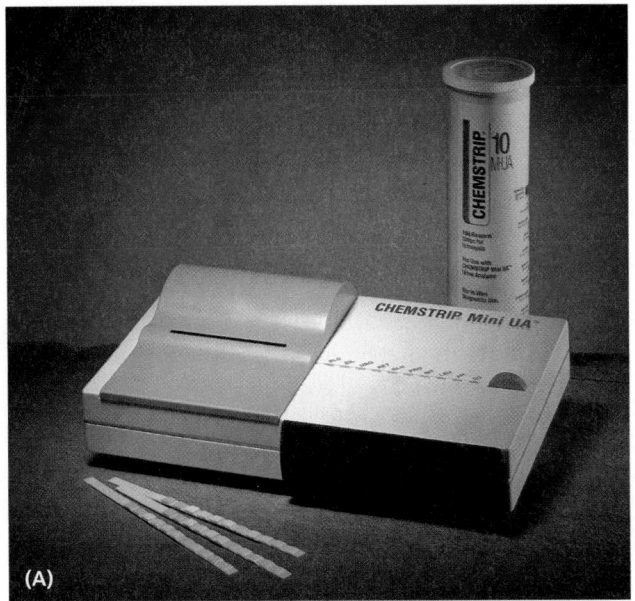

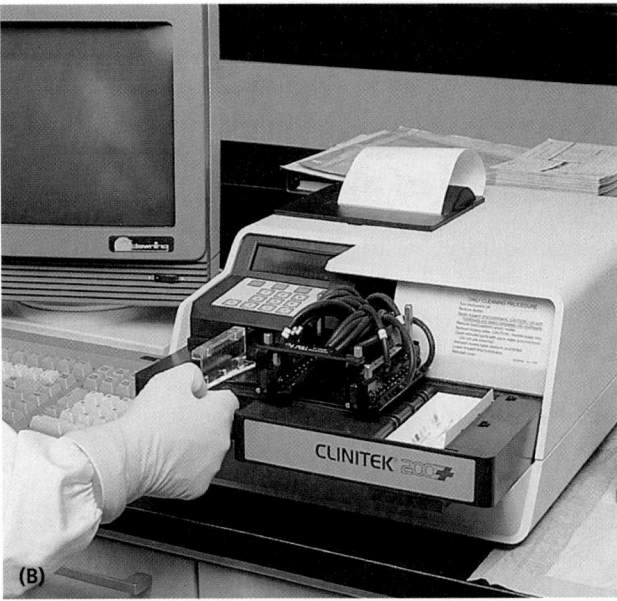

Figure 42-7   (A) The Chemstrip Mini UA Urine Analyzer is a semiautomated analyzer that provides accuracy and consistency of results when properly used. It is often used in laboratories where the volume of tests analyzed is less than forty strips per hour. (Courtesy of Boehringer Mannheim) (B) The Clinitek 200 semiautomated urine analyzer may be used in larger laboratories where there is a moderate to high volume of tests. Results are printed on a paper printout.

Confirmatory Testing. Since the reagent test strips are actually screening tests, some positive results must be confirmed with more sensitive and/or specific methods. The results of the dipstick test cannot be reported until positive results on the following tests are confirmed by the following methods. These tests include but are not limited to protein, ketones, bilirubin, and reducing sugars (to use when the glucose result is positive). Each laboratory will have a specific procedure for performing these confirmatory tests.

Protein. The most common confirmatory test for protein is the sulfosalicylic acid (SSA) test. It relies on

the precipitation of protein, causing turbidity (cloudiness) in the test tube when added to a sample of urine. Urine samples should be centrifuged and a clear supernatant used. The amount of precipitate found is roughly proportional to the protein concentration present. A negative test has no cloudiness; a trace amount is barely perceptible; a 1+ result is cloudy but not granular; a 2+ result is cloudy and granular; a 3+ result is heavy cloudiness with clumping; and a 4+ result is dense with large clumps. This is a qualitative method. A semiquantitative method is available by using a set of commercially available standards and comparing the turbidity of the patient sample to that of the standards.

Ketones. The Acetest® is a test for ketones that is available in tablet form. Ketones are produced during increased metabolism of fat. If ketones are present in urine, a drop of urine added to the tablet will produce a purple color (Figure 42-8).

TABLE 42-4	**REAGENT STRIP SENSITIVITY**	
Test	**Range**	**Normal Value**
pH	5–9	5–8
Protein	Negative to positive*	Negative
Glucose	Negative to >1,000 mg/dl	Negative
Ketone	Negative to >80 mg/dl	Negative
Bilirubin	Negative to large	Negative
Blood	Negative to large	Negative
Leukocyte Esterase	Negative to large	Negative
Nitrites	Negative to positive	Negative
Urobilinogen	0.2 to 8.0 mg/dl	2.0 mg/dl

*Note that positive results in a newborn for glucose, ketone, and protein are considered critical values and should be reported to the physician immediately.

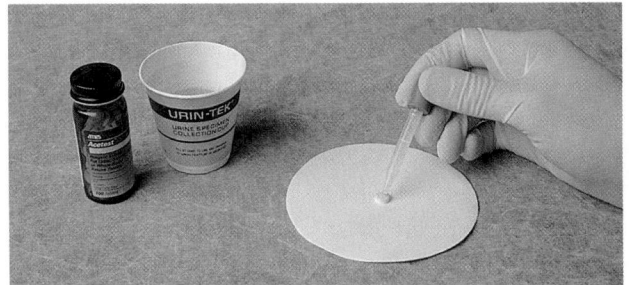

Figure 42-8   The Acetest® is a common test used to confirm the presence of ketones in urine.

Bilirubin. The **Ictotest**® is a specific test for bilirubin. It is approximately four times as sensitive as the reagent strip method. The test includes a tablet and an absorbent mat. If bilirubin is present, a purple color will develop when a urine drop is placed on the tablet.

Reducing sugars. The **Clinitest**® uses a prepared tablet and a color reaction comparison chart to help determine the quantity of sugar in the urine, as shown in Procedure 42-6. This test is used to detect reducing sugars (called reducing because these sugars give up electrons easily in chemical reactions) such as lactose and galactose, which are not detected by the glucose test on the reagent test strip. Screening for reducing substances is especially important in pediatric populations. The tablet used in the test contains copper sulfate, citric acid, sodium hydroxide, and sodium carbonate. The test is based on a copper reduction reaction known as the Benedict's test.

Microscopic Examination of Urine Sediment

In addition to the physical and chemical examination of urine, the medical assistant may also be required to perform a microscopic examination of a sample of urine after it has been centrifuged. The **sediment** (insoluble material) at the bottom of the centrifuge tube is used for the microscopic examination (see Chapter 39 for proper use of the microscope). The microscopic examination is helpful in determining kidney disease, disorders of the urinary tract, and systemic disease. It is particularly important that urine be freshly voided and examined as soon as possible to prevent deterioration of sediment components.

One of the most important items to have on hand when performing a microscopic urine examination is a urine color atlas. It takes years to be able to correctly identify abnormal components of urine. A color atlas should always be available to the medical assistant to help with identification.

Some laboratories make use of urine stains to add color to certain structures in the urine sediment. Sedistain® is an example of such a stain.

Sediment Components. Sediment is obtained by centrifugation of 10 to 15 mL of urine. The **supernatant** urine is carefully poured off, and the sediment in the tube is resuspended by shaking. A drop of sediment is then placed on a slide and examined microscopically.

When viewing a normal urine specimen, the medical assistant may see very little under the microscope. Squamous epithelial cells (Figure 42-9) may be seen, especially in women. These cells have no medical significance as they are skin cells continuously sloughed off into the urine.

They are generally reported as few, moderate, or many. If the physician sees many epithelial cells in the urine specimen, it is indicative that the specimen is contaminated.

Normal urine sediment can also contain a few red or white blood cells and a few bacteria resulting from external contamination. Clean-catch urine collecting techniques are designed to eliminate as much of this contamination as possible.

Abnormal Urine Sediment Cells and Microorganisms. The methods of reporting abnormal urine sediment may vary among health facilities. The medical assistant looks at the urine sediment microscopically to see if the specimen has one or more of the following components:

Red blood cells. Red blood cells appear as pale, light-refractive disks when seen under high power. Large amounts of red blood cells in urine (hematuria) indicate disease or trauma. These cells are counted in a microscopic field (high-power field or HPF) and reported as cells counted per HPF (e.g., 10/HPF).

White blood cells. A few white blood cells can appear in normal urine. More than a few white blood cells in urine often indicate a urinary tract infection. White blood cells are slightly larger than red blood cells, may appear granular, and have a visible nucleus (the red blood cell has no nucleus). Figure 42-10 shows both red and white blood cells in urine. White blood cells are reported in the same manner as red blood cells.

Renal epithelial cells. Renal epithelial cells (Figure 42-11) can indicate kidney disease if they are present in large numbers. They can be confused with both white blood cells and other epithelial cells. If these cells are suspected, they should be reviewed by a physician before reporting them. They are also reported in the same manner as white and red blood cells.

Bacteria. Bacteria can appear as tiny round or rod-shaped objects (Figure 42-12). Rod-shaped bacteria are generally easier to see as round bacteria may appear as **amorphous**, or shapeless, material. Bacteria can be reported as few, moderate, many, and loaded.

Yeast. Yeast cells (Figure 42-13) may be present in urine, possibly indicating a yeast infection in the urinary tract. Yeast cells are smaller than red blood cells but may appear similar to them. Yeasts are round and can be observed budding. To distinguish between yeast and red blood cells if there is a question, a drop of dilute acetic acid is added to the urine sediment. The red blood cells will lyse, but the yeast will not. The most common yeast found is *Candida albicans.* Yeasts are reported as the amount per high-power field.

Parasites. The most frequently seen parasite in urine is *Trichomonas vaginalis* (Figure 42-14). *Trichomonas*

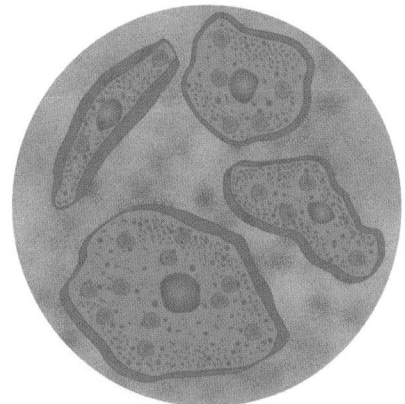

Figure 42-9   Squamous epithelial cells.

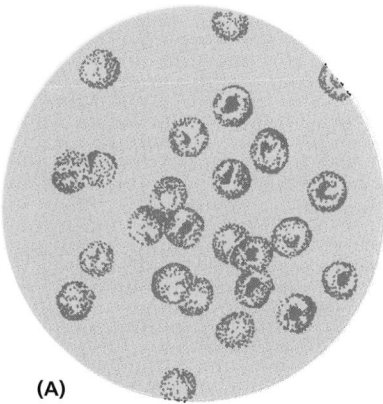

(A)   **(B)**

Figure 42-10   (A) White blood cells in urine. (B) Red blood cells in urine.

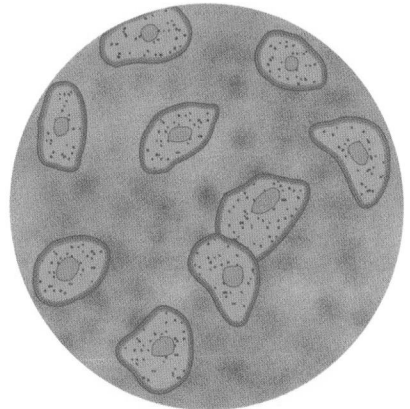

Figure 42-11   Renal epithelial cells.

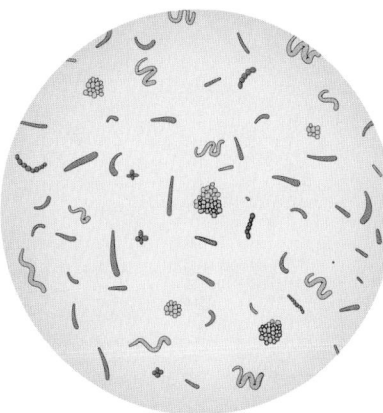

Figure 42-12   Bacteria in urine sediment.

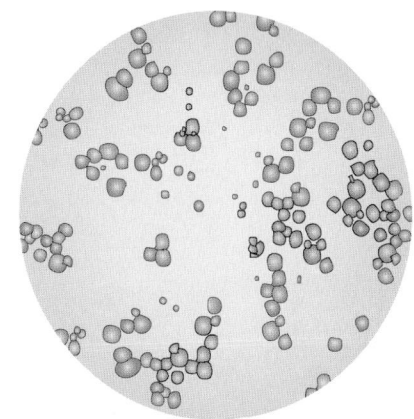

Figure 42-13   Yeast in urine sediment.

is a parasite that can infect the urinary tract. It is often recognized by the movement of its tail (flagella). Always check with a physician or someone more familiar with these organisms before reporting this organism.

Sperm. Sperm is reported only when seen in male urine unless specifically requested by a physician. Sperm have oval bodies with one long, thin flagella (Figure 42-15A).

Artifacts. Hair, fibers, baby powder, and oil are among the substances that may appear in urine sediment as a result of contamination during collection or later. If a structure cannot be identified using a good urine atlas, it probably is an artifact. A urine atlas will also show illustrations of artifacts. If in doubt, get an expert opinion (Figure 42-15B).

Crystals in Urinary Sediment. Crystals make up unorganized urine sediment. Since crystals are big, the tendency of the medical assistant is to pay attention to them. However, they are the most insignificant part of the urinary sediment; thus, they require little attention. These crystals include calcium phosphate, triple phosphate,

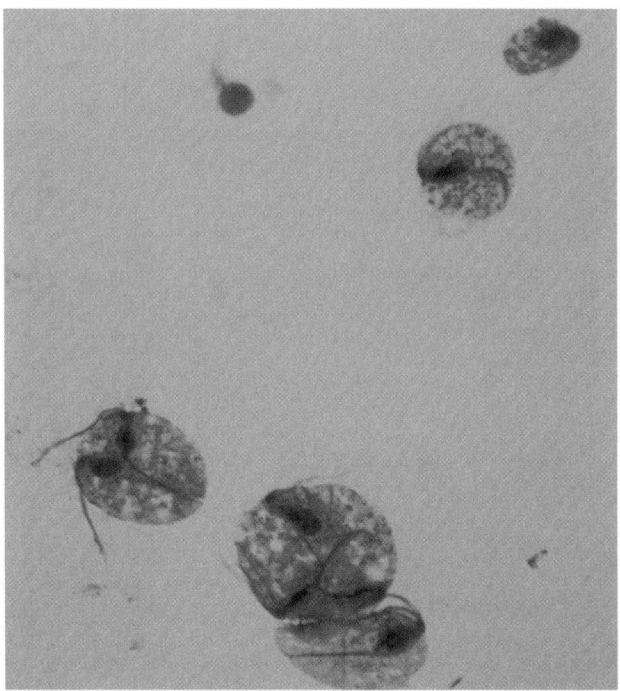

Figure 42-14   *Trichomonas* in stained urine sediment.

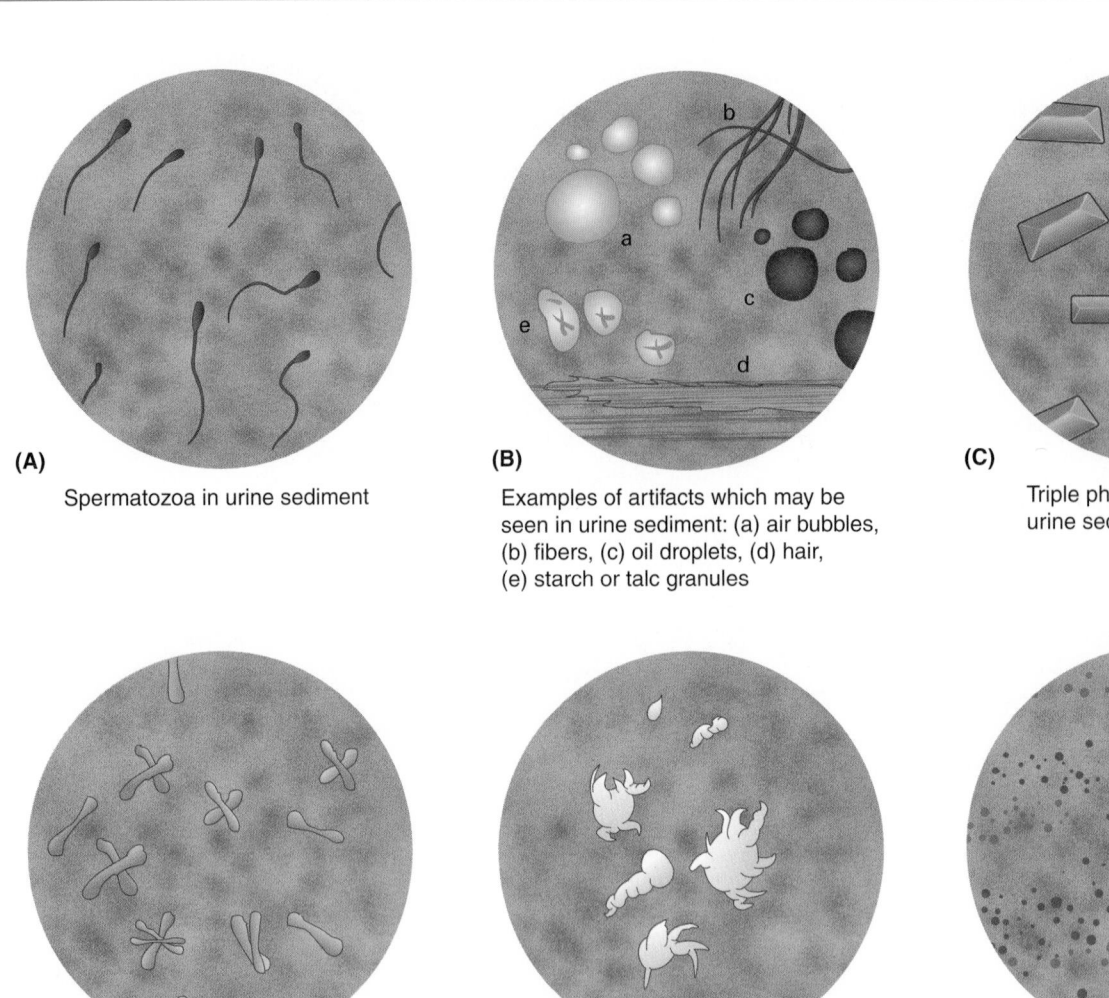

(A)   Spermatozoa in urine sediment

(B)   Examples of artifacts which may be seen in urine sediment: (a) air bubbles, (b) fibers, (c) oil droplets, (d) hair, (e) starch or talc granules

(C)   Triple phosphate crystals in urine sediment

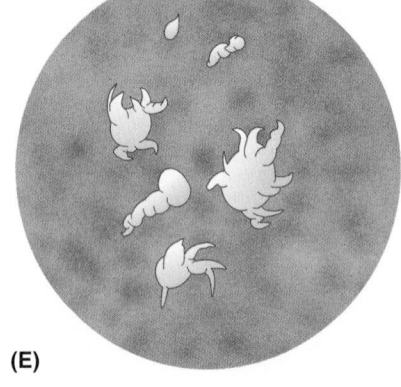

(D)   Calcium carbonate crystals in urine sediment

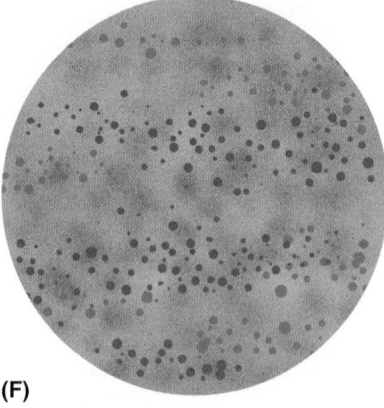

(E)   Ammonium biurate in urine sediment

(F)   Amorphous phosphates in urine sediment

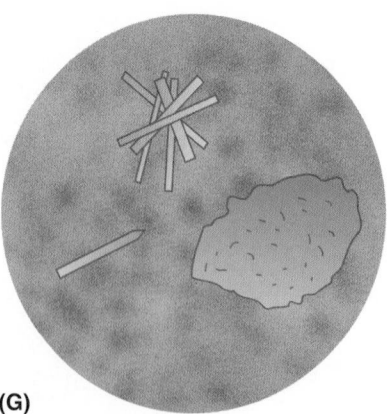

(G)   Calcium phosphate in urine sediment

Figure 42-15   Crystals and miscellaneous structures that can appear in urine.

calcium oxalate, amorphous phosphates and urates, and calcium carbonate. These crystals generally form as urine specimens stand, especially when refrigerated. Many laboratories do report these crystals. Refer to a urine color atlas to identify crystals. Figure 42-15 (C–G) illustrates several kinds of crystals that can be found in urine.

A few crystals in urine should be particularly noted if seen as they may indicate disease states. Uric acid, cystine, and sulfa drug crystals can indicate disease states. Refer to a urine atlas to observe the shape of these crystals.

Casts in Urinary Sediment. Casts are very important to see and identify in urine sediment. It takes a great deal of experience and expertise to recognize the many different kinds of casts that can be in sediment. When casts are suspected, the medical assistant should get an expert opinion before reporting their presence.

Casts are formed when protein accumulates and precipitates in the kidney tubules. The casts are then washed into the urine. Most casts are made from a particular type of protein called **Tamm-Horsfall** mucoprotein. Other proteins can also form casts. Serum proteins can form waxy casts. The presence of casts in the urine may indicate kidney disease.

Casts are cylindrical with rounded or flat ends. They are classified according to the substances observed inside them. Some casts may include debris as they are forming and may appear cellular or granular.

The most common cast seen in urine sediment is the **hyaline** cast. Rare hyaline casts can be seen in normal urine but increase with any kidney disease. They can also be seen as a result of fever, emotional stress, or strenuous exercise. Hyaline casts are nearly transparent and can be difficult to see under the microscope without some light adjustment.

Other types of casts include granular casts, containing remnants of disintegrated cells that appear as fine or coarse granules. Cellular casts may contain epithelial cells, red blood cells, or white blood cells. Figure 42-16 illustrates hyaline, granular, and cellular casts.

As mentioned before, identification of casts in urine takes an experienced eye. The medical assistant should always ask for assistance when identifying casts in urine sediment. See Procedures 42-7 and 42-8.

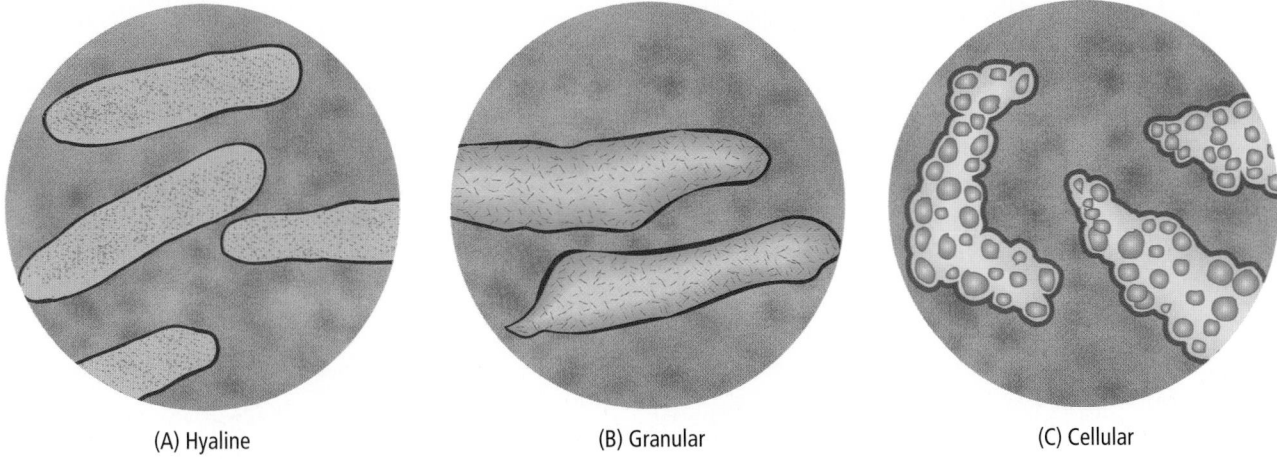

(A) Hyaline   (B) Granular   (C) Cellular

Figure 42-16 Casts in urine sediment.

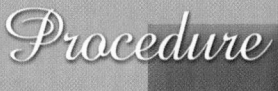

42-1   Assessing Urine Volume

STANDARD PRECAUTIONS:

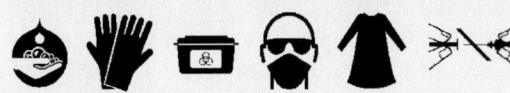

PURPOSE:
Determine and document the volume of a urine sample.

EQUIPMENT/SUPPLIES:

Gloves	Biohazard container
Graduated urine container	Antiseptic cleaner
Graduated cylinder	Laboratory report form

PROCEDURE STEPS:

1. Wash hands.
2. Put on gloves.
3. Assemble equipment and materials.
4. Follow all safety guidelines, being careful not to splash the urine sample. Wipe up all spills with antiseptic cleaner.
5. The sample must first be observed for proper labeling. Any unlabeled specimen is not tested. The medical assistant is required to determine whose urine is unlabeled. Then the patient is notified, and a new specimen is ordered. Guessing what urine belongs to which patient is not permissible.
6. After making sure that the urine container lid is tightly closed, mix the urine thoroughly.
7. If the container is not graduated, pour the urine into a suitable measuring device, such as a graduated cylinder.
8. The volume of the urine should be recorded in milliliters (mL); 10 to 12 mL is considered an adequate specimen. Some facilities do not require the recording of volume unless the quantity is insufficient.
9. In samples from 4 to 10 mL, the medical assistant should record the following comment on the results report: *"Interpret with caution. Quantity not sufficient for accurate quantitative analysis."* Some laboratories may not require this warning.
10. Samples of less than 4 mL (except for newborns) should be marked "QNS" (quantity not sufficient) and should not be tested. This policy also may differ from facility to facility.
11. After the volume is recorded on the laboratory report form, an aliquot (a smaller portion of the sample) may be used to continue the urinalysis. This aliquot should be placed in a standard urinalysis centrifuge tube.

42-2   Observing Urine Color

STANDARD PRECAUTIONS:

PURPOSE:
Observe and record the color of a urine specimen.

EQUIPMENT/SUPPLIES:

Gloves	Biohazard container
Urine specimen	Antiseptic cleaner
White card	Laboratory report form

PROCEDURE STEPS:

1. Wash hands.
2. Put on gloves.
3. Assemble equipment and materials.
4. Follow all safety guidelines, being careful not to splash the urine sample. Wipe up all spills with antiseptic cleaner.
5. Mix the urine specimen thoroughly.
6. Observe the color of the urine in a clear centrifuge tube. Use good light against a white background (a white card or sheet of paper will do).
7. Record the results on the laboratory report form.

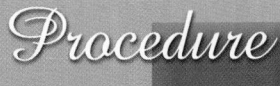

42-3   Observing Urine Clarity

STANDARD PRECAUTIONS:

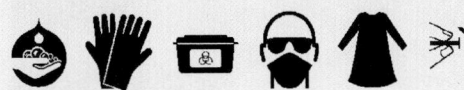

PURPOSE:
Observe and record the clarity of the urine specimen.

EQUIPMENT/SUPPLIES:

Gloves
Urine specimen in a
   centrifuge tube
White sheet of paper
   with print

Biohazard container
Antiseptic cleaner
Laboratory report form

PROCEDURE STEPS:
1. Wash hands.
2. Put on gloves.
3. Assemble equipment and materials.

4. Follow all safety guidelines, being careful not to splash the urine sample. Wipe up all spills with antiseptic cleaner.
5. Hold the centrifuge tube close to a printed sheet of white paper.
6. If you can clearly see the print on the paper, the specimen should be described as clear.
7. If the urine is slightly blurry, it might be described as hazy.
8. If the urine has cloudy material in it, describe it as cloudy.
9. If the urine is impossible to see through, it might be described as turbid.
10. Record the results on the laboratory report form.
11. Dispose of all biohazardous wastes in the biohazard container.

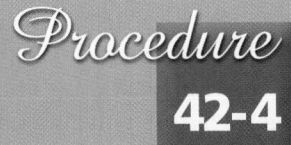

Using the Refractometer to Measure Specific Gravity

STANDARD PRECAUTIONS:

PURPOSE:
Measure and record the specific gravity of a urine specimen.

EQUIPMENT/SUPPLIES:

Refractometer
Urine sample
Gloves
Pipettes
Distilled water
5% saline solution

Lint-free tissues
Quality control
   urine sample
Biohazard container
Antiseptic cleaners
Laboratory report form

PROCEDURE STEPS:
1. Wash hands.
2. Put on gloves.
3. Assemble equipment and materials.
4. Follow all safety guidelines, being careful not to splash the urine sample. Wipe up all spills with antiseptic cleaner.
5. Quality control must be done on the refractometer before working with a urine specimen. This is done by checking the value of distilled water, which should read 1.000.
6. Clean the surface of the cover and the prism with a lint-free tissue moistened with distilled water. Wipe them dry.
7. Close the cover. Apply a drop of distilled water to the notched portion of the cover so that it flows over the prism (Figure 42-17).

(continues)

Procedure
42-4 **(continued)**

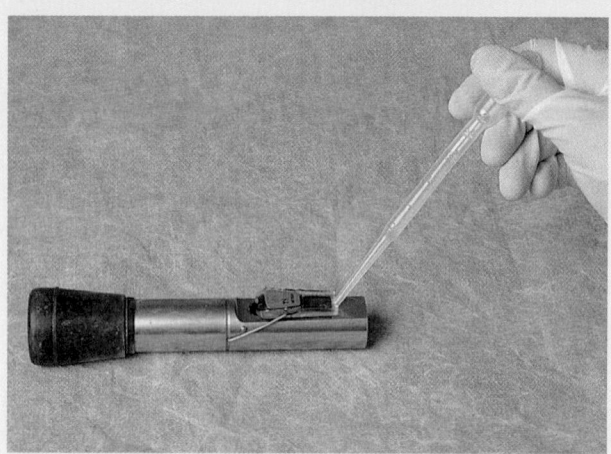

Figure 42-17 A pipette or dropper may be used to fill the refractometer with the urine sample.

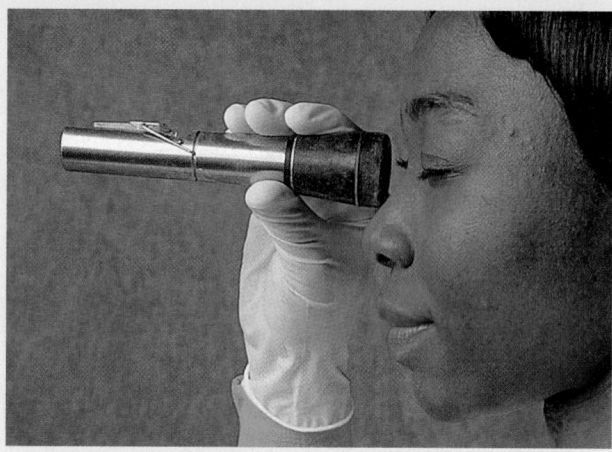

Figure 42-18 The medical assistant reads the refractometer to determine the specific gravity of the urine sample.

8. Tilt the instrument to allow light to enter. Read the specific gravity scale, which is the sharp dividing line between the dark and light areas (Figure 42-18). This reading should be at 1.000. If the reading is not 1.000, use a fresh sample of distilled water from another source.
9. Wipe the cover and prism between samples.
10. Next, test a sample of 5% saline solution, which should read 1.023 +/– 0.001. The instrument is now standardized. You are now ready to analyze quality control samples and patient samples. Use

the same method as in steps 1–9 and record your results on your quality control sheet.
11. Use the same procedure for each urine sample and record the result on the patient requisition.
12. Be sure to clean the area after finishing the procedure. Make sure any spills are cleaned with antiseptic solution. Make sure the refractometer is thoroughly cleaned with distilled water and a lint-free tissue. Dispose of all biohazardous waste in the biohazard container.

Procedure
42-5 **Performing a Urinalysis Chemical Examination**

STANDARD PRECAUTIONS:

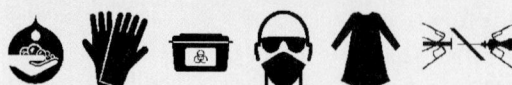

PURPOSE:
Detect any abnormal chemical constituents of a urine specimen.

EQUIPMENT/SUPPLIES:
Gloves
Dipsticks
Urine specimen
Biohazard container
Antiseptic cleaner
Laboratory report form

(continues)

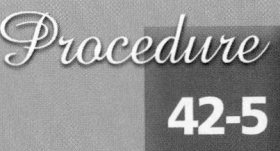

Procedure

42-5 (*continued*)

PROCEDURE STEPS:

1. Wash hands.
2. Put on gloves.
3. Assemble equipment and materials.
4. Follow all safety guidelines, being careful not to splash the urine sample. Wipe up all spills with antiseptic cleaner.
5. Mix the urine specimen thoroughly.
6. Remove a test strip from the container and replace the cap tightly (strips are adversely affected if the bottle is left open for long periods).
7. Immerse the strip completely in the uncentrifuged urine and remove it immediately (Figure 42-19A).
8. While removing the strip from the urine, run the edge of the strip against the rim of the container, tapping it lightly on the container to remove any excess urine (Figure 42-19B). RATIONALE: Excess urine can bridge the gap between reagent pads, causing inaccurate results.

9. Proper timing is essential for correct results. The proper time for each pad will be listed on the dipstick container.
10. Hold the dipstick close to the container, but do not touch it against the container. Compare the test areas to the proper area on the container and record the results (Figure 42-19C).
11. Record the results on the laboratory report form.
12. Discard the used reagent strips and other disposable items in the proper receptacles.

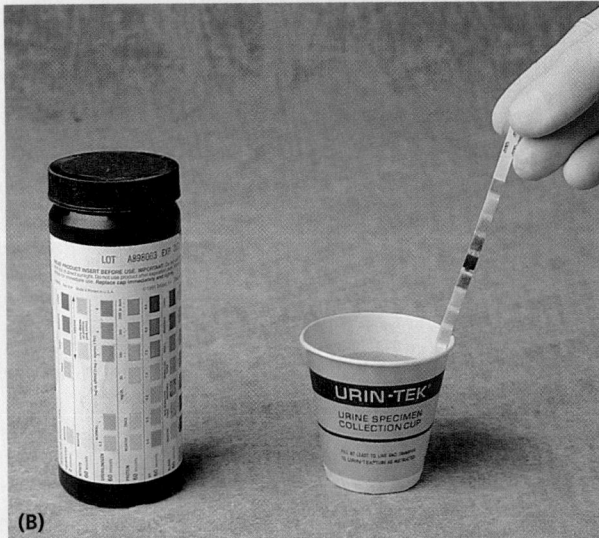

(B)

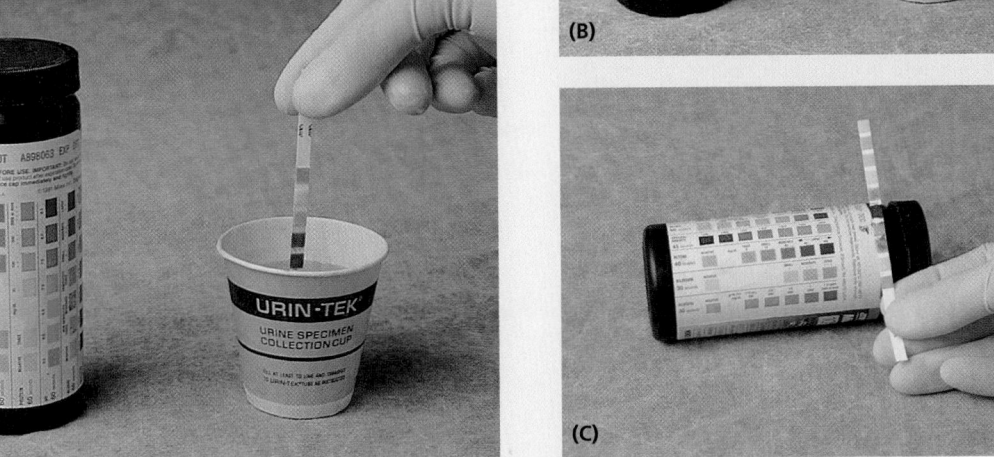

(A)

(C)

Figure 42-19 (A) Immerse the reagent strip in the urine sample. (B) After immersing the reagent strip, tap it lightly to remove excess urine. (C) Read the reagent strip by matching the color on the strip to a color on the container.

Procedure

42-6   Testing for Sugar in the Urine

STANDARD PRECAUTIONS:

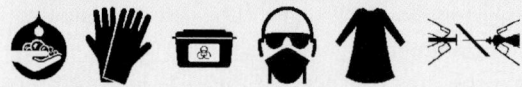

PURPOSE:

Perform a Clinitest on a urine specimen to detect reducing sugars.

EQUIPMENT/SUPPLIES:

Gloves	Disposable pipettes
Clinitest tablets	Biohazard container
Urine specimen	Antiseptic cleaner
Clean glass test tube	Laboratory report form
Distilled water	

PROCEDURE STEPS:

1. Wash hands.
2. Put on gloves.
3. Assemble equipment and materials.
4. Follow all safety guidelines, being careful not to splash the urine sample. Wipe up all spills with antiseptic cleaner.
5. Transfer 5 drops (0.3 mL) of urine into a clean glass test tube.
6. Add 10 drops (0.6 mL) of distilled water. Mix well, being careful not to splash the contents of the tube (Figure 42-20).
7. Drop one tablet into the tube. Watch the mixture while the complete boiling takes place.
   CAUTION: Do not touch the bottom of the tube. The bottom becomes very hot during the test reaction and can cause serious burns.
8. Do not shake the tube after adding the tablet until at least 15 seconds after the boiling stops.
9. At the end of the 15-second waiting period, gently shake the tube to mix. Do not touch the bottom of the tube as the heat of reaction is still present.
10. Compare the color of the liquid to the proper color chart. Ignore any color changes that occur after the waiting period.

11. There are two methods of reporting. One method is by percentage, and the other uses trace through 4+:
    ¼% or trace; ½% or 1+; ¾% or 2+; 1% or 3+; 2% or 4+
12. Urine containing more than 5% sugar will cause a rapid color change during the boiling. Observe closely during this time to detect a "pass-through" phenomenon in which the color changes from green to tan to orange to black or dark brown. If this happens, report as greater than 2% or 4+.
13. Record the results on the laboratory report form.
14. Dispose of all biohazardous waste in the biohazard container.
    NOTE: If a reducing sugar is present in the urine, the color changes from blue to green and then orange, depending on the amount of sugar present. This test is not specific for glucose, and many drugs may cause positive results. The Clinitest is not used for insulin monitoring.

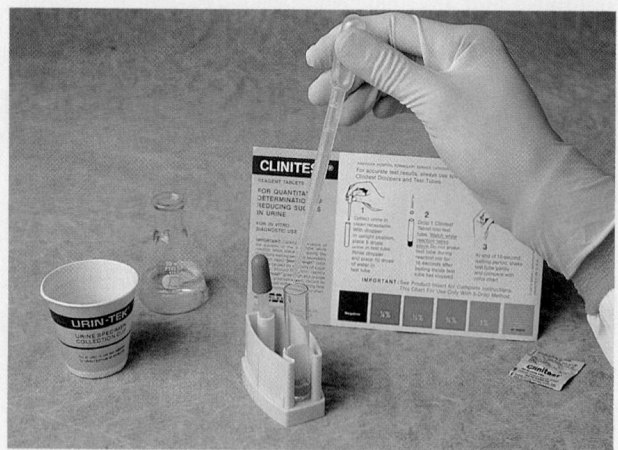

Figure 42-20   The Clinitest® confirmatory test.

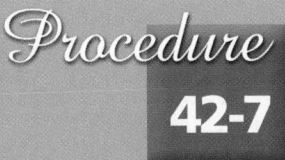

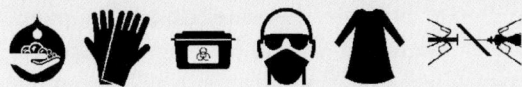

Microscopic Examination of Urine Sediment

STANDARD PRECAUTIONS:

PURPOSE:
Perform a microscopic examination of urine sediment.

EQUIPMENT/SUPPLIES:

Gloves	Centrifuge tube
Microscope	Urine sediment
Centrifuge	containing casts
Microscope slides	Urine atlas
Cover slips	Antiseptic cleaner
Disposable pipettes	Biohazard container

PROCEDURE STEPS:

1. Wash hands.
2. Put on gloves.
3. Assemble equipment and materials.
4. Follow all safety guidelines, being careful not to splash the urine sample. Wipe up all spills with antiseptic cleaner.
5. Obtain a urine specimen. The first morning specimen is preferred due to its concentration and pH, which tend to preserve the formed elements. The urine should be examined as soon as possible but may be refrigerated for a short time.
6. Mix the entire specimen well, then centrifuge a 10–15 mL aliquot (portion) at 1,500 revolutions per minute for 5 minutes.
7. After centrifugation, pour off the supernatant, leaving about 1 mL in the bottom of the centrifuge tube.
8. Tap or "flick" the bottom of the tube to resuspend the sediment in the remaining fluid.
9. Place a drop of the sediment on a microscope slide, carefully placing a coverglass over the drop of sediment.
10. Place the slide on the microscope stage and examine immediately. When examining urine sediment, it is important to keep the light subdued by lowering the condenser and to constantly vary the fine focus adjustment in order to view structures that are very faint. Again, proper light and focus adjustments take a great deal of practice.
11. Scan the sediment using a 100X (low power) magnification.
    NOTE: A 100X magnification is achieved by using the 10X objective lens, remembering that the ocular also is a 10X lens. 10X × 10X = 100X.
12. View 10 to 15 fields and around the edges of the drop for casts.
    NOTE: When using a cover slip, the casts can be forced to the edges.
13. Record the average number of each type of cast viewed per LPF (low-power field). It may be necessary to use the 40X objective (high power) to identify some of the casts. For example: If a type of cast is seen from two to four times in each field, report as 2–4 casts/LPF.
14. Scan the drop using a 400X (high power) magnification. Count and average the numbers of other formed elements in 10 to 15 fields.
15. Record the results on the laboratory report form.
16. Dispose of all biohazardous waste in the biohazard container. Be sure to clean off the microscopic lenses with lens paper. Wipe up all spills with antiseptic cleaner.

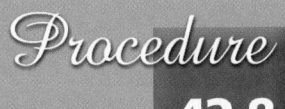

42-8 Performing a Urinalysis

STANDARD PRECAUTIONS:

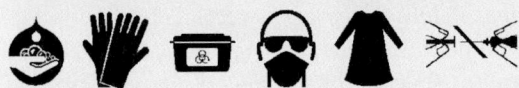

PURPOSE:
Perform a complete urinalysis, including the physical, chemical, and microscopic examination.

EQUIPMENT/SUPPLIES:

Gloves	Reagent strips (dipsticks)
Urine specimen	Control urine sample
Measuring cylinder	Urine atlas
Test tubes	Refractometer
Pipettes	(or urinometer)
Centrifuge tube	Distilled water
Centrifuge	Lint-free tissues
Microscope	Biohazard container
Microscope slides	Antiseptic cleaner
Coverglasses	Laboratory report form

PROCEDURE STEPS:
1. Wash hands.
2. Put on gloves.
3. Assemble equipment and materials.
4. Follow all safety guidelines, being careful not to splash the urine sample. Wipe up all spills with antiseptic cleaner.

PHYSICAL EXAMINATION:
5. Obtain a urine specimen. Measure the amount of the specimen in a measuring cylinder if there are no measurement markings on the specimen container. Make sure there is more than 12 mL of urine.
6. Mix gently and pour approximately 5 mL of urine into a test tube.
7. Observe and record the color of urine (straw, yellow, amber, red).
8. Observe and record the transparency of urine (clear, slightly cloudy, turbid).
9. Note unusual odors of the urine (not recorded).
10. Measure the specific gravity using either a refractometer or a urinometer.
    Refractometer: Place one drop distilled water on the glass plate and close. Look through the ocular and read the specific gravity from the scale. The reading should be 1.000. Then wipe the water

from the glass plate using lint-free tissues. Place one drop of urine on the plate, closing the plate. Look through the ocular, reading the specific gravity. Clean the glass plate with water and dry with a tissue. Record the results.
Urinometer: Pour 40 to 50 mL of distilled water into the glass cylinder (about three-fourths full). Insert the urinometer with a spinning motion. Read the specific gravity from the scale on the stem of the urinometer as it stops spinning. The reading should be 1.000. Rinse the equipment with distilled water. Repeat the procedure using a urine specimen. Clean the equipment carefully using detergent, rinsing thoroughly with distilled water, and drying carefully. Record the results.

CHEMICAL EXAMINATION:
1. Continue to wear gloves and use the same specimen as in the physical examination.
2. Test the urine control sample with a reagent strip. Dip the strip into the urine sample, moistening all pads.
3. Immediately remove the strip from the urine and tap it to remove excess urine.
4. Observe the reagent pads and compare colors to the color chart at appropriate intervals.
5. Record the results on a laboratory report form after properly disposing of the reagent strip.
6. If any tests are positive that need confirmation (protein, glucose, bilirubin, acetone), perform that test following the manufacturer's directions. Follow all safety precautions necessary.
7. Dispose of all biohazardous materials in a biohazard container.

MICROSCOPIC EXAMINATION:
1. Continue to wear gloves. Use the same urine sample. Follow all safety precautions necessary for this procedure.
2. Carefully pour 12 mL of specimen into a centrifuge tube. Centrifuge the specimen at 1,500 to 2,500 rpm for 5 minutes.
3. Carefully decant the supernatant and resuspend the sediment.
4. Pipette one drop resuspended urine sediment on a clean glass slide.

(continues)

Procedure
42-8 *(continued)*

5. Place a coverglass over the drop of urine.
6. Carefully place the slide under the microscope.
7. Under low power (10X), scan the slide with reduced light for casts. Refer to a urine atlas to refresh your memory about cast appearances.
8. Rotate to high power (40X and 45X objective).
9. Scan the slide and identify any blood cells, bacteria, yeast, parasites, and epithelial cells that may be seen.
10. Identify any crystals or amorphous deposits seen.

11. Record all the results on the laboratory report form.
12. Discard all biohazardous materials in the biohazard container.
13. Clean and return the equipment to proper storage, if necessary.
14. Clean the work area with disinfectant.
15. Discard gloves in the biohazard container.
16. Thoroughly wash hands with disinfectant soap.

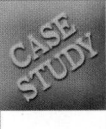

Annette Samuels came to Inner City Health Care today because she is experiencing frequent urination, itching, and burning when urinating. Dr. Rice ordered a urinalysis, which clinical medical assistant Wanda Slawson is performing. Wanda notes that the urine has a cloudy appearance and the dipstick tests positive for nitrites. Wanda confers with Dr. Rice, who instructs her to perform a microscopic examination of the specimen.

42-1

CASE STUDY REVIEW

1. Why does Dr. Rice want this specimen examined microscopically?
2. What should Wanda look for when she examines the specimen?
3. How should she report her findings?

SUMMARY

This chapter summarizes the basics of the urinalysis. Physicians order a variety of tests on urine to help them determine or rule out certain abnormalities in order to make a correct diagnosis and prescribe treatment.

Urine is formed as blood is filtered through the kidney. Substances such as by-products of metabolism, mineral excesses, cells, bacteria, parasites, crystals, and casts can be found in the urine during examination.

It is important for the medical assistant to:

- Understand the proper collection techniques for urine specimens. Medical assistants are often called upon to instruct patients in the proper collection procedures.

- Understand the safety guidelines involved with collecting and handling specimens, preservatives, and reagents. These guidelines must *always* be observed.
- Understand the importance of and the procedures for maintaining a consistent quality control program.
- Understand how to properly perform the urinalysis, following up with proper confirmatory tests when necessary.
- Understand and be constantly aware of factors that may interfere with the accuracy of a urinalysis.

REVIEW QUESTIONS

Multiple Choice

1. What safety guideline is important to follow during a routine urinalysis?
   a. use the same pipette for all patients' urine samples
   b. allow urine to sit at room temperature to ferment the urine properties
   c. once tested, urine can be disposed of by the janitorial service
   d. treat all specimens as if they were infectious
2. What are the three basic parts of a typical urine examination?
   a. volumetric, chemical, and macroscopic
   b. pathological, chemical, and confirmatory
   c. physical, chemical, and microscopic
   d. random, 24-hour, and catheterized
3. What is the specimen of choice for routine urinalysis?
   a. random
   b. clean-catch
   c. catheterized
   d. timed
4. A diabetic patient will normally have an excess of what substance in the urine?
   a. hemoglobin
   b. glucose
   c. insulin
   d. sodium
5. What is the most common way of doing a chemical analysis of urine in a physician's office?
   a. reagent strip test
   b. Clinitest®
   c. culture test
   d. Acetest®
6. Positive results for the following during chemical testing of newborn urine should be immediately reported to the physician:
   a. blood, pH, nitrates
   b. bilirubin, blood, leukocyte esterase
   c. pH, urobilinogen, specific gravity
   d. glucose, ketone, and protein
7. Confirmatory tests are done to:
   a. confirm negative results from initial testing
   b. confirm positive results from initial testing
   c. confirm urine volume
   d. confirm urine turbidity

8. What confirmatory urine test is done to test for evidence of incomplete fat metabolism?
   a. Clinitest®
   b. sulfosalicylic acid test
   c. Ictotest®
   d. Acetest®
9. Which substance or structure is automatically considered abnormal when found in urine?
   a. phosphates
   b. urea
   c. blood
   d. salt

Critical Thinking

1. What is the importance of proper urine collection?
2. How is a clean-catch urine sample collected?
3. What is a midstream urine specimen?
4. When is a urine preservative necessary?
5. Why is the first morning specimen preferred for routine urinalysis?
6. What would give a urine sample a cloudy appearance?
7. What is the normal specific gravity of urine?
8. If urine was kept at a temperature of 16° centigrade and specific gravity was performed, what adjustment, if any, would have to be made to the results?

WEB ACTIVITIES

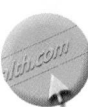

1. Search for CLIA information on the Internet. Are guidelines posted for specimen collection? When were these guidelines last updated?
2. Visit the CDC's web site and review the Standard Precautions that apply to urine collection and analysis.

REFERENCES/BIBLIOGRAPHY

Akron City Hospital Procedure Manual. (1996). Akron, OH: author.

Flynn, J., & Whitlock, S. (1997). *Delmar's clinical lab manual series: Urinalysis* (1st ed.). Albany, NY: Delmar.

Henry, J. B. (1996). *Clinical diagnosis and management by laboratory methods* (19th ed.). Philadelphia: W. B. Saunders.

Walters, N. J., Estridge, B. H., & Reynolds, A. P. (2000). *Basic medical laboratory techniques* (4th ed.). Albany, NY: Delmar.

BASIC MICROBIOLOGY

KEY TERMS

Aerobic
Aerosols
Anaerobic
Biochemical Tests
Broth Tubes
Check Cell Slides
Concentration Method
Counterstain
Culture
Decolorizer
Dermatophytes
DNA
Enterobacteriaceae
Expectorate
Fastidious Bacteria
Genus
Gram Stain
Holding Media
Immunosuppressed
Inoculate
Kirby Bauer
Lumbar Puncture
Microbiology
Mordant
Morphology
Mycobacteria
Mycology
Nematode
Normal Flora
Nosocomial
Ova
Parasitology
Pathogen

(continues)

OUTLINE

The Medical Assistant's Role in the Microbiology Laboratory
Microbiology
  Classification
  Nomenclature
  Cell Structure
Equipment
  Autoclave
  Microscope
  Safety Hood
  Incubator
  Anaerobic Equipment
  Inoculating Equipment
  Incinerator
  Media
  Refrigerator
Safety When Handling Microbiology Specimens
  Personal Protective Equipment
  Work Area
  Specimen Handling
  Disposal of Waste and Spills
Quality Control
Collection Procedures
  Specific Collection Requirements
Microscopic Examination of Bacteria
  Bacterial Shapes
  Dyes (Stains)

Simple Stain
Differential Stain
Acid-Fast Stain
Special Techniques
Potassium Hydroxide (KOH)
  Preparation
Culture Media
  Media Classification
Microbiology Culture
  Inoculating the Media
  Other Types of Streaking
  Primary Culture
  Subculture
Biochemical Tests
  Direct Tests
  Biochemical Tube Testing
Identification Systems
  Streptococcus Screening
    (Rapid Strep Testing)
  Packaged Systems
  Semiautomated and Automated
    Instruments
Sensitivity Testing
Parasitology
  Examination Methods
  Specimen Collection
  Common Parasites
Mycology

OBJECTIVES

The student should strive to meet the following performance objectives and demonstrate an understanding of the facts and principles presented in this chapter through written and oral communication.

1. Define the key terms as presented in the glossary.
2. Define microbiology, discussing classifications, and nomenclature relevant to the microbiology laboratory. *(continues)*

Petri Dish
Protozoa
Quality Control
Reagents
Sensitivity
Species
Stab Culture
Taxonomy
Tetrads
Virology
Wood's Lamp

OBJECTIVES (*continued*)

3. Describe bacterial cell structure.
4. List and describe the equipment used in the microbiology laboratory.
5. Explain how to safely handle microbiology specimens.
6. Describe the importance of and steps involved in quality control in the microbiology laboratory.
7. Explain the types of specimens collected for the microbiology laboratory and how they are collected.
8. List different types of stains used to microscopically observe microorganisms.
9. Perform a Gram stain.
10. List the different classifications of media used in the microbiology laboratory.
11. Describe how organisms are cultured onto various media.
12. Explain how biochemical testing is used to identify microorganisms.
13. Discuss identification systems used to identify bacteria.
14. Describe the significance of sensitivity testing.
15. List two parasites and two fungi that can be observed in the microbiology laboratory.

ROLE DELINEATION COMPONENTS

CLINICAL
Fundamental Principles
- Apply principles of aseptic technique and infection control
- Comply with quality assurance practices
- Screen and follow up patient test results

Diagnostic Orders
- Collect and process specimens
- Perform diagnostic tests

GENERAL (TRANSDISCIPLINARY)
Legal Concepts
- Document accurately
- Comply with established risk management and safety procedures

SCENARIO

To aid in diagnosing and treating patients, the physicians at Lewis and King MD order tests to identify disease-causing bacteria, fungi, viruses, and parasites. Some of these tests, such as the latex agglutination test for Group A Streptococcus, are performed in the office laboratory, while other tests are sent to a reference laboratory. Regardless of where the test will be performed, medical assistant Joe Guerrero follows all safety precautions when handling specimens. He checks the test manufacturer's or laboratory's procedures and carefully completes each step. By following all safety guidelines and test procedures, Joe ensures his and others' safety. He obtains a high-quality specimen for testing.

INTRODUCTION

The field of **microbiology** encompasses the study of all microorganisms, living structures that can be seen only with the powerful magnification of a microscope. The word *microbiology* comes from the Greek words *micro* (small) and *bios* (living). The field of microbiology includes the study of such organisms as bacteria, fungi, viruses, parasites, and algae (Table 43-1).

Many medical textbooks in microbiology include extensive study of all of the preceding organisms, including lesser known species in each category. It is the goal of this chapter to introduce the student to the field of microbiology with emphasis on bacteria, fungi, and parasites. Safety while working with microorganisms in the laboratory is emphasized. The relationship of bacteria to diseases also is explored.

TABLE 43-1   BIOLOGICAL SCIENCES

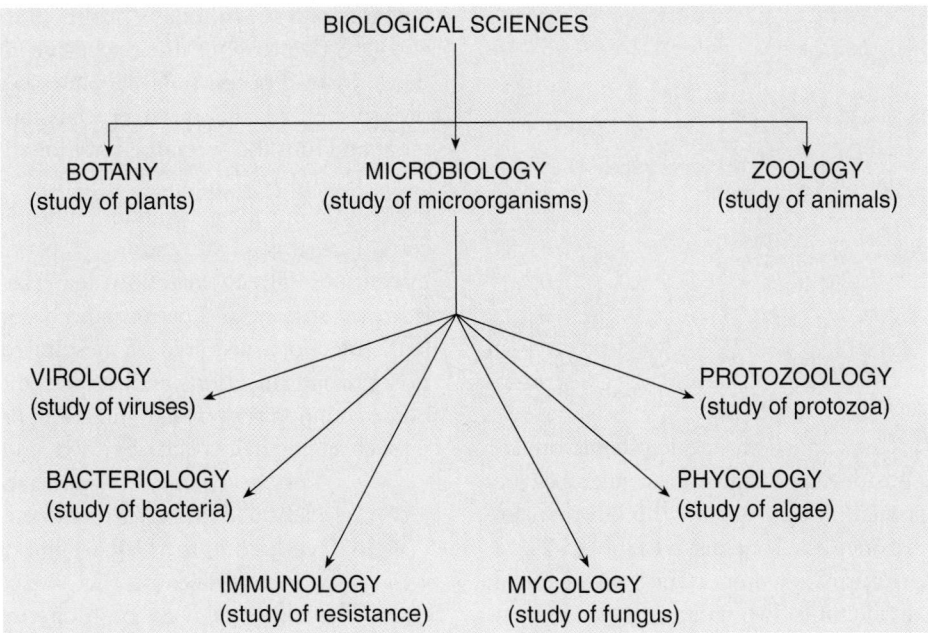

THE MEDICAL ASSISTANT'S ROLE IN THE MICROBIOLOGY LABORATORY

The role of the medical assistant in the microbiology laboratory may be to assist in isolating and identifying microorganisms that can cause harm and disease. A medical assistant might be asked to carefully smear a microscopic slide with body material that is suspected of being contaminated with bacteria. This slide is then stained in a special manner (described later in the chapter) and read under a microscope. The medical assistant may also place a sample of body secretions or excretions (urine, material from a sore throat, blood, sputum coughed up from the lungs, and so on) on special media to allow bacteria to grow. This is called a **culture**. The bacteria is usually allowed to grow at least twelve hours before the culture can be examined to identify the offending organism. In certain situations, a physician may request a **sensitivity** in addition to the culture. This is a test that will identify which antibiotic or antibiotics will effectively kill the microorganism identified as causing the infection.

In healthy individuals, several types of bacteria are found in various parts of the body. For instance, the throat has bacteria in it, called **normal flora**. These organisms are always present and help with the body's immune system. In disease, the causative microorganism is called a **pathogen** because it causes harm to the body.

The medical assistant's technique must be exact to avoid laboratory error. The medical assistant also must be assured the specimen for culture was taken with sterile supplies and brought to the laboratory in a reasonable amount of time. Delivery time of the specimen or culture may vary due to the type of specimen collected for culture. Some specimens may be refrigerated without harm. Some may be kept in **holding media**, media that will keep a specimen on a swab moist until it is cultured. These variations will be discussed later in specimen processing.

By doing the smear, culture, and identification through biochemical tests, the microbiologist can identify the organism and aid the physician in diagnosing and treating the patient. Most identification of organisms can be done successfully within 24 to 72 hours. Some organisms may take longer to grow. The acid-fast bacterium *Mycobacterium tuberculosis*, the causative organism of tuberculosis, may take longer; however, modern techniques are making it possible to identify this microorganism more rapidly.

MICROBIOLOGY

Classification

Taxonomy deals with the classification of living organisms. The scheme of naming organisms is based on similarities of structures. The current classification is based on a system devised by Carolus von Linne, a Swedish biologist. Although there are a number of classifications, there is no universal agreement on one particular system.

A common system divides living organisms into kingdoms. Prior to the discovery of the microscope in the sixteenth century, there were two known kingdoms,

TABLE 43-2   KINGDOM PROTISTA

I. Lower protists
   1. Prokaryotic—nuclear material not organized
     A. Bacteria
     B. Blue-green algae
II. Higher protists
   1. Eukaryotic—true nucleus
     A. Algae
     B. Slime molds
     C. Fungus
     D. Protozoa

animal and plant. A new kingdom of microscopic organisms, the *Protista*, was developed since most microbes are neither plant nor animal. The members of this kingdom are called *protists* and are one-celled organisms (Table 43-2).

The microorganisms of importance in medical microbiology are divided into two groups: the lower protists or *prokaryotes* (including blue-green algae and bacteria) and the higher protists or *eukaryotes* (including **protozoa**, algae, and fungi).

Nomenclature

The system used for naming bacteria is the binomial (two) nomenclature (system of names). Two Greek or Latin names are used, the first name being a **genus**, which is capitalized. The second name is the **species** name, which is not capitalized. These names may reflect a characteristic of a bacterium and/or names of places or persons associated with the discovery of the microorganism. For example, *Salmonella typhi* was discovered by an American microbiologist named Salmon. The bacterium causes typhoid fever.

Individuals who study bacteria are referred to as bacteriologists or microbiologists. These individuals have taken extensive courses in the field of microbiology. In most laboratories, clinical laboratory scientists or assistants help perform microbiology procedures. The job of these individuals is to quickly and efficiently identify the organism in a given culture that has been properly obtained and brought to the laboratory within a reasonable time frame.

Along with routine bacteriological cultures, many microbiology departments, especially in larger health care facilities, perform **parasitology** procedures for the identification of parasites; **virology** procedures for the identification of viruses; and **mycology** procedures for the identification of fungi. If an institution such as a clinic or physician's office laboratory is too small to properly identify many microorganisms, cultures often are sent to a ref-

erence laboratory. These laboratories are specialized laboratories set up with up-to-date equipment to handle large amounts of tests. In today's health care environment, it is cost-effective to centralize expensive and complex procedures. Instead of ten small laboratories each having their own specialized equipment, one laboratory buys the equipment and runs the specialized test for all ten laboratories.

The microbiology department works closely with the infection control department of a hospital to determine if certain organisms are causing infections throughout an institution. These infections can be acquired by an **immunosuppressed** patient and become a serious problem. Infections acquired in hospitals are referred to as **nosocomial** infections and should be closely monitored. Some common nosocomial infections are caused by bacteria such as Staphylococcus, Serratia, and monilia (a yeast).

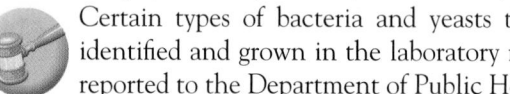 Certain types of bacteria and yeasts that are identified and grown in the laboratory must be reported to the Department of Public Health in your town or state because they are communicable diseases. These diseases vary from city to city and state to state. Some of the common bacteria that are reported are Salmonella, Shigella, and those organisms that cause sexually transmitted diseases (STDs), such as gonorrhea, syphilis, chlamydia, and herpes. The state and town you work in will have a list of reportable diseases that the clinic or physician's office laboratory will have posted.

Cell Structure

All living forms are alike in that their cells contain a nuclear material referred to as **DNA** (deoxyribonucleic acid, which carries special genetic information). The main structural difference of eukaryotes and prokaryotes is the arrangement of the nucleus. A eukaryote has a well-defined or true nucleus and is a higher form of microorganism. The prokaryote is a lower form of microorganism and has a simple nucleus that is not well-defined.

The bacterial cell, classified as a lower protist, is a single-celled organism with a cytoplasmic cell membrane, cell wall, and nucleus. The nucleus is not well-defined. The cell grows by taking in materials from the environment. After a certain amount of growth, the bacteria reproduce by division of the cell. Certain conditions are required for this reproduction to take place.

Figure 43-1 illustrates a basic bacterial cell. Not all bacteria possess flagella for motility, as some are not motile. Some bacteria can produce capsules around the outside of the cell, providing protection from antibiotic penetration and white blood cell attack. Some bacteria produce spores, an inactive state that can help bacteria resist chemicals, freezing, drying, radiation, and heating. Bacterial spores are so resistant they can live 150,000 years and can survive in dust.

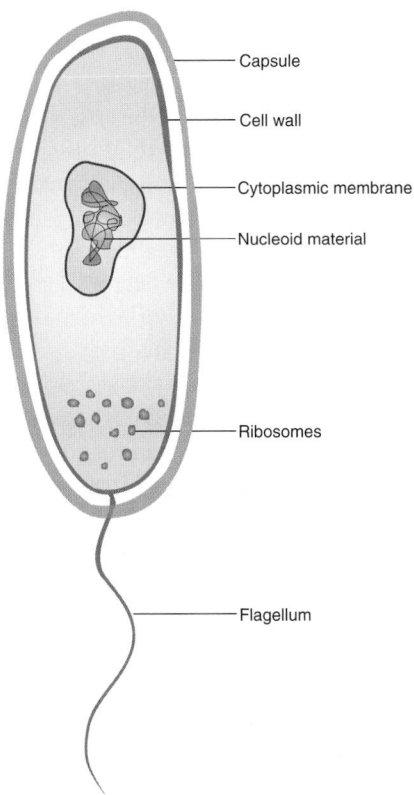

Figure 43-1 Basic bacterial cell.

EQUIPMENT

Basic equipment needed in a microbiology department of a clinic or a physician's office laboratory varies depending on the size of the facility. Most laboratories have some of the following equipment.

Autoclave

An autoclave (Figure 43-2) is used in the laboratory to sterilize equipment that may have been contaminated while processing specimens. It can be used to sterilize contaminated materials as well. The setting of 15 lb./sq. in. and a temperature of 121°C for 15 to 20 minutes is sufficient to kill infectious agents, spores, viruses, and contaminants. Small microbiology departments use a bench-top autoclave, and larger departments have a separate room with a large autoclave. Many laboratories no longer use autoclaves because of the use of presterilized and disposable equipment. Waste products are put into biohazardous bags and are disposed of by a service outside the health care facility.

Microscope

An important piece of equipment for the physician's office laboratory or clinic is the microscope. This instrument is used to view organisms that cannot be seen with

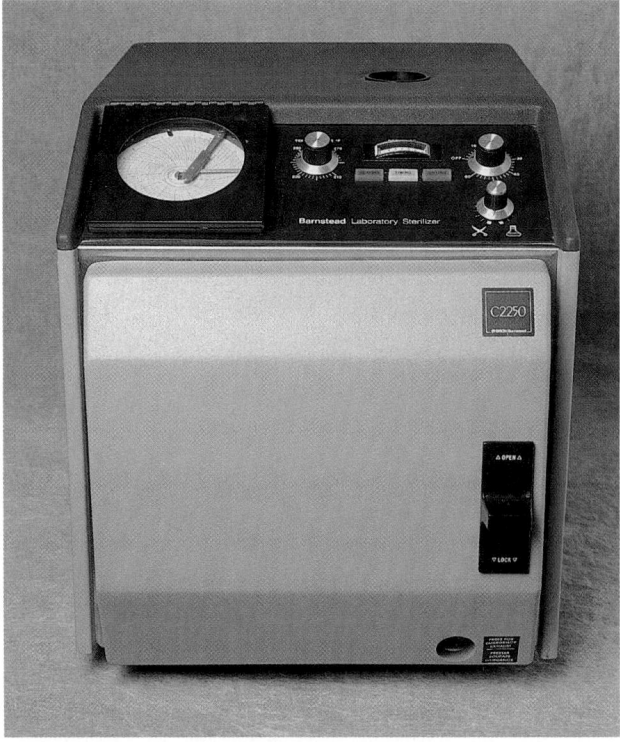

Figure 43-2 Small laboratory autoclave.

the naked eye on a prepared slide. Skill in using the microscope is necessary to gain information from studying the slide. The microscope is a delicate instrument and should be cared for properly as stated by the manufacturer. (Refer to Chapter 39, Introduction to the Medical Laboratory, for more information on the microscope.)

Safety Hood

Some laboratories, especially if they are culturing specimens with aerosols, will have a safety hood (Figure 43-3).

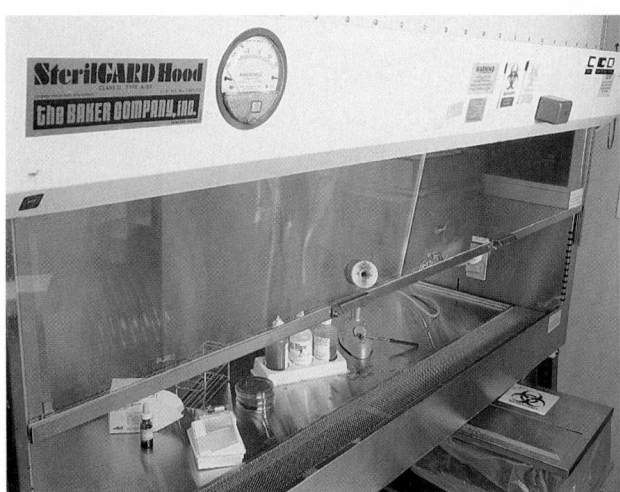

Figure 43-3 Laboratory safety hood.

Aerosols are airborne particles that can be released into the air when culturing. They are potentially dangerous if inhaled. By using the safety hood, the health care worker is separated from the specimen by a glass in front of the face, with fumes and aerosols suctioned into the hood. The use of a safety hood is mandatory when performing a culture on a specimen with a potential aerosol. Aerosols are particularly dangerous in fungus and mycobacterium cultures. It is a good idea to use the safety hood with foul-smelling specimens to minimize odors.

Incubator

The incubator is a cabinet that has a constant temperature of 35 to 37°C. Most organisms, whether **aerobic** (grow well in oxygen) or **anaerobic** (will not grow well or at all in oxygen), grow at these temperatures. Some bacteria, such as Yersina, grow at a lower temperature (26°C). A bacterium called Campylobacter requires a higher temperature (42°C). When working with these organisms, temperature requirements must be met for adequate growth.

Anaerobic Equipment

Certain types of cultures, such as deep wound cultures, could contain anaerobic pathogens. At the time of culturing, the medical assistant sets up some cultures in an oxygenated environment as well as an oxygen-reduced environment. Most laboratories post lists of cultures that need an anaerobic setup.

To grow anaerobic bacteria, the absence of oxygen is achieved by using something as simple as a candle jar (Figure 43-4) containing a lighted candle into which the inoc-

ulated petri dish is placed. When the cover is put on the jar the burning of the candle will use up the available oxygen and generate carbon dioxide. Organisms, such as *Neisseria gonorrhoeae*, which causes gonorrhea, need a high carbon dioxide atmosphere to survive. The use of a candle jar allows an easy collection and transport system that maximizes the recovery rate of certain microorganisms.

Another method of maintaining an anaerobic condition is a specialized jar called a gas pack jar (Figure 43-5). This jar contains a foil pack that, when activated, gives off carbon dioxide, decreasing the oxygen in the jar. Extensive culturing of anaerobes often is not performed by smaller laboratories. Anaerobic specimens are sent to reference laboratories better equipped to process them. Some small laboratories will perform a Gram stain on the suspected anaerobic cultures. The **Gram stain** is the most common stain used to observe the gross morphological features of bacteria and will be discussed later in this chapter.

Inoculating Equipment

An *inoculating loop* (Figure 43-6) is a piece of wire with a rounded end and a handle at the other end. The loop is used to **inoculate** organisms onto a culture medium in a plate or broth. If it is made of wire, the loop can be flamed to sterilize it before and after use. As an alternative, sterile plastic disposable loops can be used. These are one-time use and are disposed of in the biohazardous waste.

An *inoculating needle* (Figure 43-7) is similar to the loop but has a straight end. The needle is used when performing a **stab culture**. The needle is flamed, and the culture material is "stabbed" on the needle into medium in a tube. This technique is used for certain **biochemical tests** used for identification.

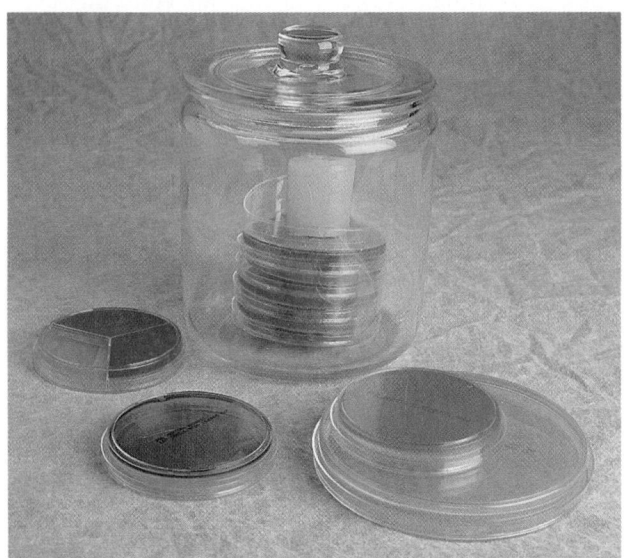

Figure 43-4   Candle jar with media for high CO_2 conditions.

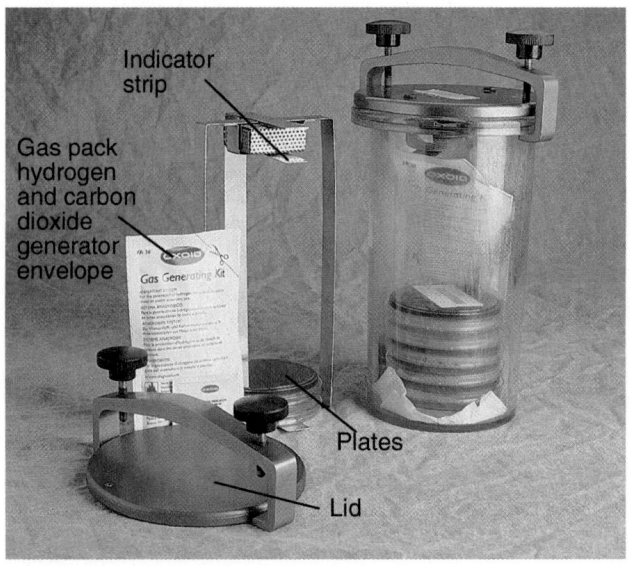

Figure 43-5   Gas pack anaerobic system.

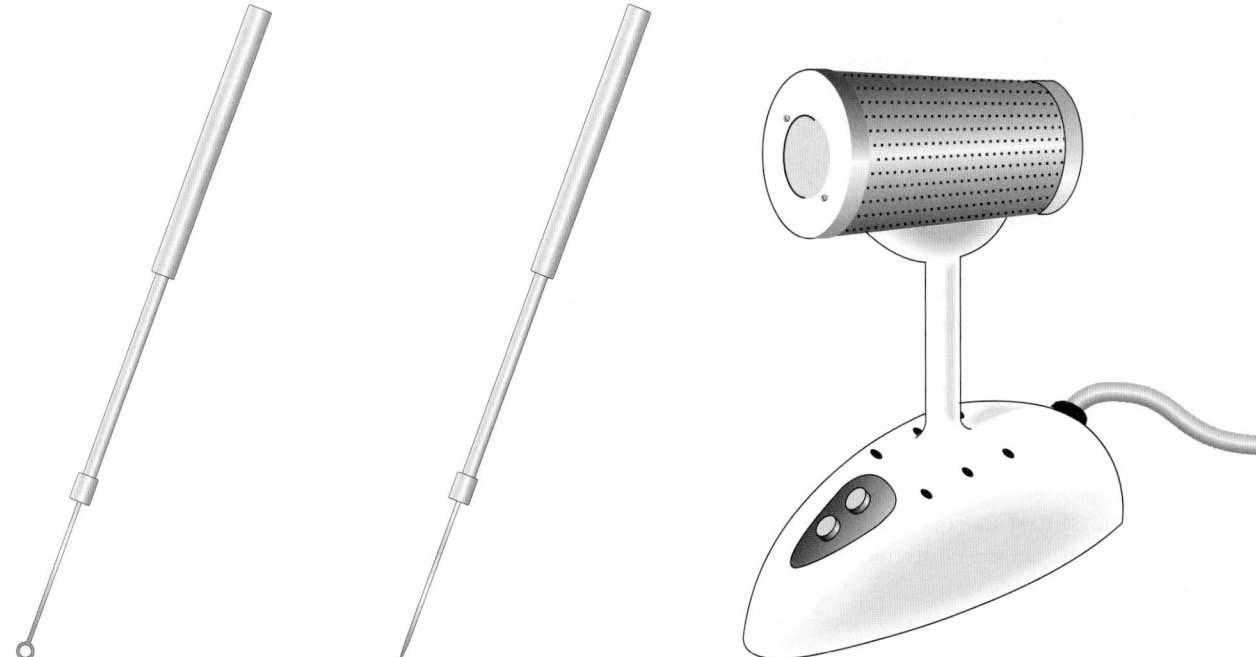

Figure 43-6 Inoculating loop. **Figure 43-7** Inoculating needle. **Figure 43-8** Electrical incinerator.

Incinerator

Incineration is the quickest method of sterilization. This can be accomplished by using an electrical incinerator (Figure 43-8) or a Bunsen burner (less popular today because of the open flame danger). When doing cultures, the inoculating needle or loop must be sterilized before and after it is used. This is done by placing the loop in the incinerator or passing through the flame of the Bunsen burner.

Media

Media in the microbiology laboratory refers to a host of substances used to foster the growth of bacteria. It is listed in this section of basic equipment (Figure 43-9), but will be explained in detail in the section about media.

Refrigerator

A refrigerator is needed to store certain materials, such as media and testing kits that need a temperature of 2 to 8°C. Food or drink should never be stored in the refrigerator with any specimens, kits, or media.

SAFETY WHEN HANDLING MICROBIOLOGY SPECIMENS

 Safety should be practiced in every area of the clinical laboratory at all times. Microbiology specimens can be dangerous because of potential pathogens. Following safety rules will reduce danger to all personnel concerned. Some important safety measures follow. A detailed discussion can be found in Chapters 22 and 38.

Personal Protective Equipment

Personal protective equipment should be worn at all times when processing microbiology specimens. It should be removed when leaving the work area. When processing microbiology specimens, the medical assistant wears a

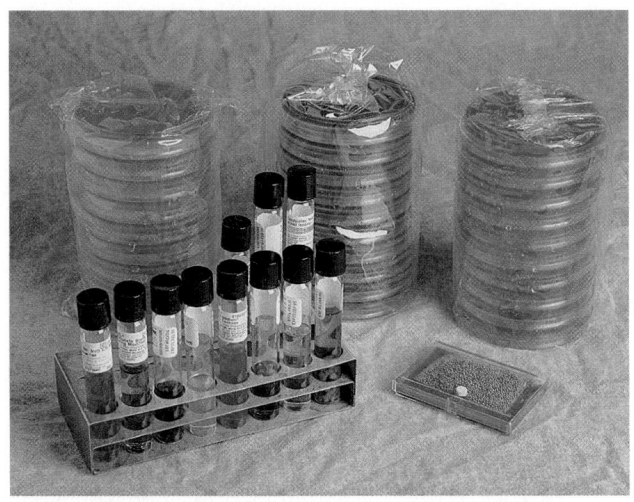

Figure 43-9 Various types of media tubes and plates.

buttoned laboratory coat or apron, safety goggles, and gloves. At times, personnel performing microbiology testing will work behind a shield or use a safety hood to avoid inhalation of aerosol pathogens and to avoid splashes and spatters of blood and/or body fluids.

There is never any eating, smoking, drinking, or putting objects into the mouth while working with microbiology specimens or in the laboratory area itself. Contact lenses should not be touched nor should makeup be applied. The practice of washing hands several times should be a habit. Washing hands after glove removal is important.

Work Area

The bench area where specimens are processed and set up should be cleaned with a strong germicide before and after daily use or immediately following a spill. Pathogens could be present where microbiology specimens are cultivated. This area should be dust-free and clean at all times.

Care should be taken not to have a cluttered work area. If using burners or incinerators, caution should be practiced to avoid body burns or fires.

Specimen Handling

Microbiology specimens will be brought to the physician's office laboratory or clinic to be processed, so the medical assistant should look for leaks and contamination on the outside of the transporting containers. It is a good practice always to wear gloves when receiving specimens. Most specimens will arrive in an "outside" plastic bag to avoid danger to laboratory personnel. When sending specimens to an outside laboratory to be cultured, it is important to use the appropriate container to avoid contamination of others. If there is a possibility of an aerosol specimen, the specimen must be cultured under a safety hood. All specimens should be handled as if they were contaminated. (Refer to Chapters 22 and 38 concerning standard precautions.)

Disposal of Waste and Spills

Most facilities will have a plan for disposal of dangerous biohazardous waste that should be strictly followed. Biohazardous waste generally is placed in red biohazard-marked bags (Figure 43-10). Most clinics or physician's office laboratories employ an outside agency to dispose of waste. It is extremely important that biohazardous waste is not placed with the regular waste and disposal guidelines are followed.

If a spill should occur, follow the agency's or employer's rules. Remember to disinfect with a 5 percent phenol or a 10 percent bleach solution.

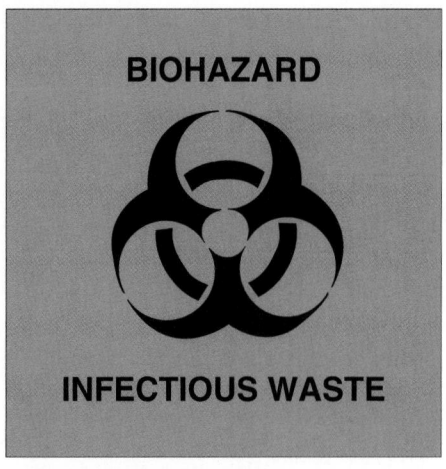

Figure 43-10 Biohazard symbol.

QUALITY CONTROL

Quality control is practiced in all areas of the clinical laboratory. The microbiology department has equipment, media, and reagents that need quality control checks periodically. Employees in the microbiology laboratory are also checked for accuracy by quality control programs. The following list details some measures that are a part of a quality control program in the microbiology laboratory:

- All equipment with temperature controls should be monitored daily.

- The microscopes should be cleaned and kept dust-free.

- All staining reagents should be checked with known **check cell slides**, which are preinoculated with known organisms, to determine the accuracy. This check is done when a new kit is received or a new batch of dyes are made.

- Testing for microorganism identification is often accomplished with the use of a special kit. When using kits for different tests, the positive and negative controls must be run at all times. Before use, the expiration date should be checked.

- Media of all types should not be used past the shelf life and should be stored at the proper temperatures and checked for growth with known organisms for quality control. All laboratories should have a specific list of bacteria to use on various media to test for growth.

- A procedure manual with all standard operating procedures written down should be updated periodically. All chemicals or reagents with material safety data sheets (MSDSs) should be available to reference when working with something with which one is not familiar.

Many microbiology laboratories subscribe to associations that periodically send unknown samples to be set up and identified. This is known as proficiency testing. The laboratory is then graded on its performance, to make sure technique is correct.

COLLECTION PROCEDURES

When a physician needs an identification of an organism that is causing infection, he or she orders a culture from that site. Before a culture is processed, it first should be checked to see if it was collected properly, delivered within a reasonable period of time, and collected in sufficient quantity. The results of the culture will depend on the quality of the original specimen. All specimens obtained for identification of infectious organisms must be taken from the site of the infection, not the surrounding area. Figure 43-11 lists methods of transmission for many common communicable diseases.

Once the specimen is collected correctly, it should be placed in the appropriate container and brought to the laboratory soon after collection. Many organisms, if not

Disease	How Agent Leaves the Bodies of the Sick	How Organisms May Be Transmitted	Method of Entry into the Body
Acquired immuno-deficiency syndrome (AIDS)	Blood, semen, or other body fluids, including breast milk	Inoculation by use of contaminated needles or by direct contact so that infected body fluids can enter the body	Transplacentally to embryo or fetus Nursing at breast
Cholera	Excreta from intestinal tract	As in typhoid fever	As in typhoid fever
Diphtheria	Sputum and discharges from nose and throat Skin lesions	Direct contact Droplet infection from patient coughing Hands of nurse Articles used by and about patient	Through mouth to throat or nose to throat
Gonococcal disease	Lesions Discharges from infected mucous membranes	Direct contact as in sexual intercourse Towels, bathtubs, toilets, etc. Hands of infected persons soiled with their own discharges Hands of attendant	Directly onto mucous membrane Through breaks in membrane
Hepatitis A, viral	Feces	As in typhoid fever	As in typhoid fever, rarely by blood transfusion
Hepatitis B, viral and delta hepatitis	Blood and serum-derived fluids, including semen and vaginal fluids	Contact with blood and body fluids	Transfusion Exposure to body fluids including during hetero- or homosexual intercourse
Hepatitis C	Blood	Transfusion Parenteral drug use Laboratory exposure to blood	Infected blood Contaminated needles

(continues)

Figure 43-11 Methods of transmission of some common communicable diseases. (From *Taber's Cyclopedic Medical Dictionary* [17th ed.], by C. L. Thomas [Ed.], 1993, Philadelphia: F. A. Davis Company. Reprinted with permission.)

Disease	How Agent Leaves the Bodies of the Sick	How Organisms May Be Transmitted	Method of Entry into the Body
		Health care workers exposed to blood, i.e., dentists and their assistants, and clinical and laboratory staff	
Hookworm	Feces	Direct contact with soil polluted with feces Eggs in feces hatch in sandy soil Feces may also contaminate food	Larvae enter through breaks in skin, especially skin of feet, and after devious passage through the body settle in the intestine
Influenza	As in pneumonia	As in pneumonia	As in pneumonia
Leprosy	Uncertain, may be from lesions Bacilli found in nodules that may break down, forming lesions	Uncertain, probably nasal discharges of untreated patients	Uncertain, probably via upper respiratory tract and broken skin
Measles (rubella)	As in streptococcal sore throat	As in streptococcal sore throat	As in streptococcal sore throat
Meningitis, meningococcal	Discharges from nose and throat	Direct contact Hands of nurse or attendant Articles used by and about patient Flies	Mouth and nose
Mumps	Discharges from infected glands and mouth	Direct contact with persons affected	Mouth and nose
Ophthalmia neonatorum (gonococcal infection of eyes of newborn)	Purulent discharges from the eye	Direct contact with infected areas as vagina or infected mother during birth Other infected babies Hands of doctor or nurse Linens	Directly on the conjunctiva
Pneumonia	Sputum and discharges from nose and throat	Direct contact Hands of caretaker Articles used by and about patient	Through mouth and nose to lungs
Poliomyelitis	Discharges from nose and throat, and via feces	Direct contact Hands of caretaker or attendant Rarely in milk	Through mouth and nose

(continues)

Figure 43-11   *(continued)*

Disease	How Agent Leaves the Bodies of the Sick	How Organisms May Be Transmitted	Method of Entry into the Body
Rubeola	Secretions from nose and throat	Droplet spread from nose or throat by direct contact with nasal or throat secretions Airborne spread is possible	Through mouth and nose
Streptococcal sore throat	Discharges from nose and throat Skin lesions	Direct contact Hands of caretaker Articles used by and about patient	Through mouth and nose
Syphilis	Infected tissues Lesions Blood Transfer through placenta to fetus	Direct contact Kissing or sexual intercourse Contaminated needles and syringes	Directly into blood and tissues through breaks in skin or membrane Contaminated needles and syringes
Tetanus	Excreta from infected herbivorous animals and man	Soil, especially that with manure or feces in it Dust, etc. Articles used about stables	Directly into bloodstream through wounds (organism is an anaerobe and prefers deep, incised wound)
Trachoma	Discharges from infected eyes	Direct contact Hands, towels, handkerchiefs	Directly on conjunctiva
Tuberculosis, bovine		Milk from infected cow	As in tuberculosis, human
Tuberculosis, human	Sputum Lesions Feces	Direct contact such as kissing Droplet infection from person coughing with mouth uncovered Sputum from mouth to fingers, thence to food and other things Soiled dressings	Through mouth to lungs and intestines From intestines via lymph channels to lymph vessels and to tissues
Typhoid fever	Feces and urine	Direct contact with food, water, articles, or insects contaminated with feces, or urine from patients	Through mouth via infected food or water and thence to intestinal tract
Whooping cough	Discharges from respiratory tract	Direct contact with person affected	Mouth and nose

Figure 43-11 (*continued*)

placed in a holding or transport medium to keep them viable (alive), will die if not kept moist. Transport media can have a moistening agent to keep the specimen from drying out. This media is then disposed of and not reused.

If a specimen comes into the laboratory in an improper container or has not been brought in within a reasonable period of time soon after collection, it should be rejected and another specimen obtained. The container in which the specimen has been placed should be sterile, and the right type should be used for a specific culture (Figure 43-12). Sterile containers are used for most collections, with the exception of stool collection containers, which do not have to be sterile. Culturette cultures are from swabs and should be kept moist. This system is a plastic tube that has a sterile swab used to collect the specimen and then placed back into the tube. Once in the tube, an ampule containing Stuart medium or another medium is squeezed, releasing the fluid to keep the swab moist.

The laboratory's success in isolating the causative pathogens depends on the following factors:

1. Proper collection from infection site
2. Collection of specimen during infection period
3. Sufficient amount of specimen
4. Appropriate specimen container
5. Appropriate transport medium
6. Specimen labeled properly
7. Specimen brought to the laboratory in a minimal amount of time

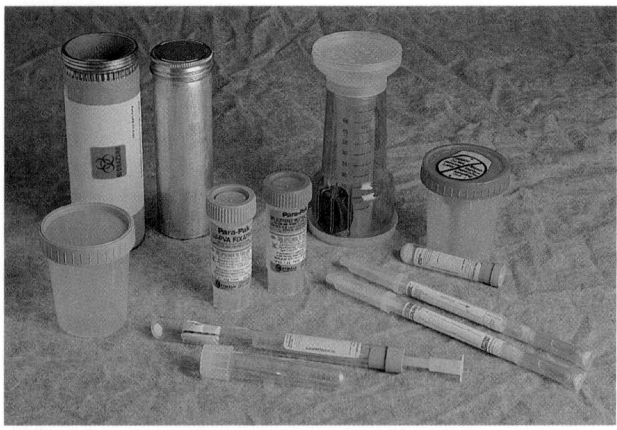

Figure 43-12 Various collection and transport containers for bacteriological specimens.

8. Specimen collected before the administration of antibiotics
9. Specimen inoculated onto proper media and placed in correct atmosphere to ensure growth

When collecting specimens, it is important that the medical assistant carefully follow procedures designated by the health care facility. Everyone handling specimens should wear gloves to protect themselves from leakage of the container and contamination with a pathogenic organism.

Specific Collection Requirements

Urine. Patients should be instructed to obtain a clean-catch urine in a sterile container. A clean-catch midstream specimen is obtained by first cleaning the genital area and then urinating midstream into a specimen container. Details of this procedure are found in Chapter 42. Patients should be given strict instructions so that a quality specimen for culturing can be obtained.

Sometimes a catheterization is done to collect the urine for culture. The urine must be collected into a sterile container if obtained by this method.

Throat. A specimen for throat culture is obtained by using a sterile tongue depressor to hold the patient's tongue down. With a sterile swab, have the patient say "ah." Gently swab the back portion of the throat and tonsils (if present). Avoid swabbing the sides of the mouth and tongue. Place the specimen swab in a sterile tube for delivery to the laboratory.

Taking a Throat Culture. Explain to the patient that a throat culture is necessary to identify certain organisms. Be sure to tell the patient that there might be some momentary discomfort in obtaining the specimen, and answer all questions about the process of obtaining the specimen. See Procedure 43-1.

SPOTLIGHT ON AAMA ESSENTIALS THROUGH CAAHEP

● A medical assistant taking a specimen or a secretion from a patient needs to be sensitive to the potential embarrassment the patient may experience from submitting to the collection process.

● By explaining the purpose and value of a specimen collection, the medical assistant can do much to allay the patient's fears.

● A calm and professional attitude displayed by a medical assistant while explaining the collection of such specimens as sputum and stool can often mean the difference between obtaining a useful specimen and a contaminated one.

The specimen is taken directly from the affected area with a sterile swab and distributed over the agar in a petri dish of clear plastic. Many physicians obtain, incubate, and read their own cultures for the patient's convenience and to maintain efficiency in the ambulatory care setting (Figures 43-13 and 43-14).

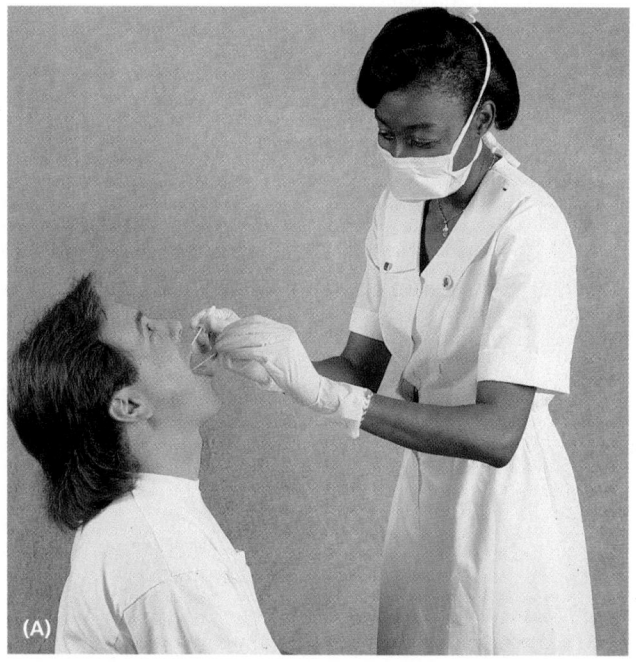
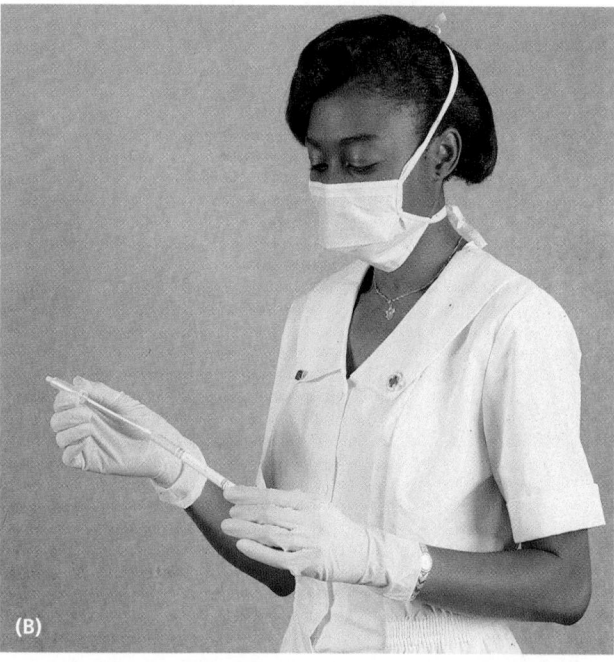

Figure 43-13 (A) The medical assistant obtains a throat culture using a commercially available sterile swab and culture tube with growth medium. Note the medical assistant wears gloves and mask. (B) After swabbing patient's throat for a culture, the medical assistant replaces swab into culture tube. A laboratory requisition form will be attached to the labeled tube and sent to the laboratory.

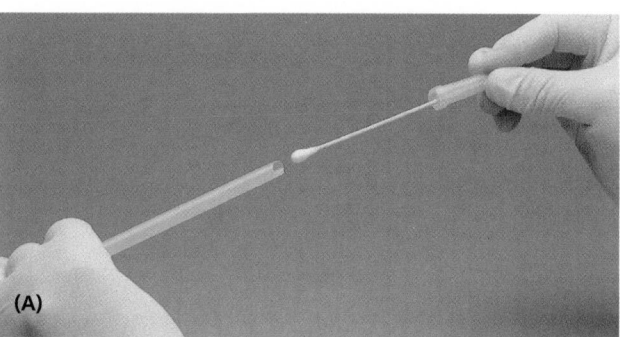
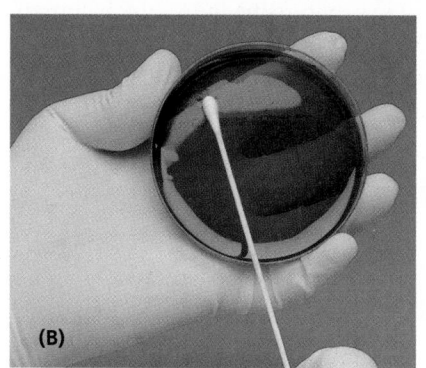
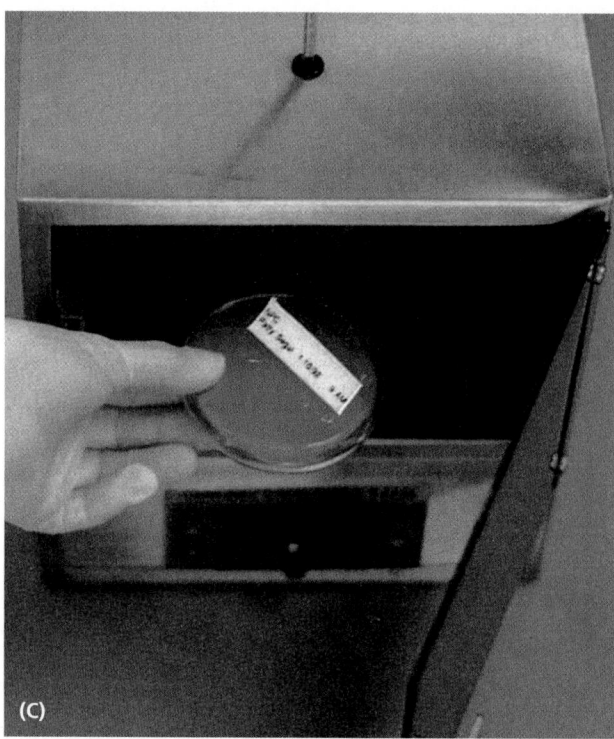

Figure 43-14 (A) The swab with specimen is put into transport container with culture media for laboratory analysis. (B) The medical assistant smears the culture plate with specimen from the swab; it is then streaked as shown in Procedure 43-6. (C) The culture plate is placed in an incubator with agar side up.

Patient Teaching Tip

As you obtain throat cultures from patients, you may want to give them some helpful advice concerning their condition. Generally when a person has a sore throat, it is associated with other respiratory symptoms as well. The following suggestions may provide some relief from discomfort and help them toward better health.

1. Advise patients to drink plenty of liquids (fruit juices) and to eat sensibly from the basic food groups.
2. Urge patients to get extra rest and dress comfortably (according to the weather/temperature outside).
3. Suggest use of gargles or throat lozenges (or both) to relieve painful sore throat.
4. Remind them to avoid tobacco/smoking.
5. Instruct them to cough/sneeze into tissue and discard into proper waste container wherever they are to prevent the spread of microorganisms.
6. Remind them not to eat or drink from another person's plate or glass and to use disposables at home when there is illness.

Nose. A nasal-pharyngeal swab may be requested with a throat culture. This is collected with a swab on a thin wire. A separate swab may be used for each nostril. The patient tilts back the head, and each swab is gently inserted into each of the nostrils. The swab is then placed into a sterile tube for transport to the laboratory.

Wound. When culturing a wound, a sterile needle might be used to aspirate pus-filled fluid from the wound, or a swab is used. It is important to get the swab deep into the wound without touching the surrounding skin. Specimens for wound cultures often are placed in anaerobic transport medium, especially if the wound is not superficial.

Sputum. To collect this specimen correctly, the patient should cough deeply and **expectorate** into the sterile container. The specimen should be a morning specimen and placed into a special container designed to protect all who handle the specimen from contamination. (Refer to Procedure 30-26.)

Stool. Stool specimens are brought to the laboratory for various tests. If the stool is to be examined for **ova** or parasites, the specimen should be as fresh as possible. Special containers often are used for ova and parasites.

For bacterial cultures of stool material (as well as for ova and parasites), several different specimens may be sent for testing at different times. The collection containers for stool cultures do not have to be sterile, but they must be clean and have a tight-fitting lid. Patients should be instructed to be careful not to contaminate the specimen with urine since urine may alter the results of the stool culture.

Cerebrospinal Fluid (CSF). The physician obtains cerebrospinal fluid by doing a **lumbar puncture.** (Refer to Procedure 30-32.) The fluid generally is dispersed in several departments of the clinical laboratory. Generally, the fluid goes first to the microbiology laboratory for a culture before it becomes contaminated by doing other tests. If a culture cannot be set up immediately, the tube should be placed in an incubator or left at room temperature. Refrigeration of spinal fluid can kill two common meningitis-causing bacteria, *Haemophilus influenzae* and *Neisseria meningitidis.*

Blood. Human blood is free from bacteria in a healthy human. If blood does become contaminated with bacteria, septicemia (septic blood infection) can result. Blood cultures are collected by the same means as regular blood collection, with special considerations to avoid any contamination of the blood. A variety of collection devices are available for collecting blood cultures, all requiring careful sterile techniques.

MICROSCOPIC EXAMINATION OF BACTERIA

There are usually two procedures involved in properly identifying bacteria: the microscopic examination and the culture. The microscopic examination involves viewing stained or unstained bacteria through the microscope. (See Procedure 43-2.)

Culturing is a means of isolating a disease-causing microorganism for identification. A specimen is obtained and placed in a culture medium, which contains nutrients comparable to human tissue to encourage growth of microorganisms. The medium is agar, a gelatinlike substance, mixed with nutrients.

Bacterial Shapes

Each genus of bacteria has a characteristic shape. A knowledge of the shapes of bacteria helps in identification (Figure 43-15). Bacteria have three basic shapes:

1. *Cocci.* Cocci are round in shape, occurring in clusters, pairs, singles, and **tetrads.** They are nonmotile microorganisms. (They do not move on their own accord.)

(A) Cocci (round)

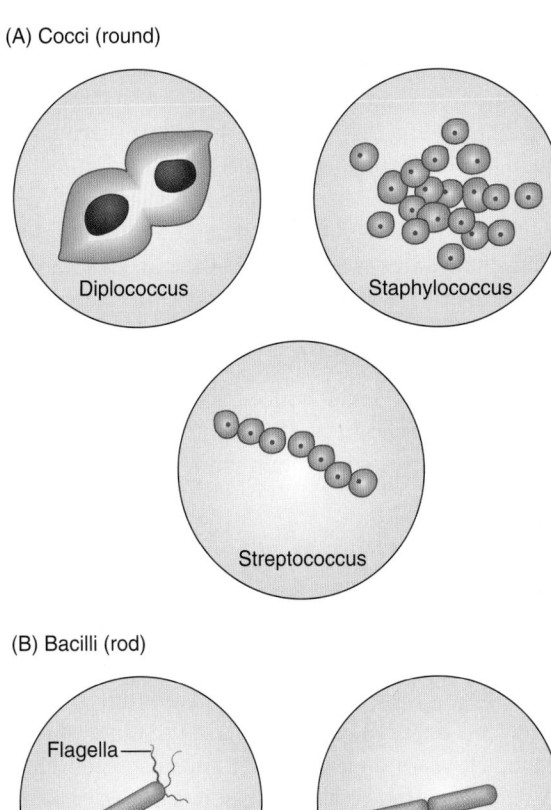

(B) Bacilli (rod)

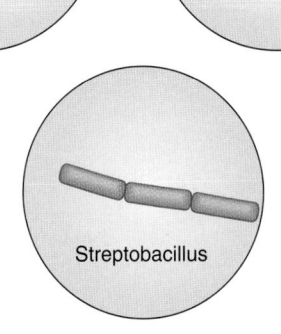

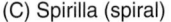

(C) Spirilla (spiral)

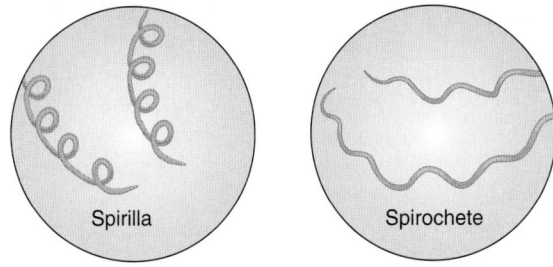

Figure 43-15 Three types of bacteria.

2. *Bacilli.* Bacilli are rod-shaped and can have rounded, straight, or pointed ends. Some bacilli have flagella that give bacteria motility (movement). Most bacteria are the shape of bacilli.
3. *Spirilla.* Spirilla are spiral-shaped bacteria that have one too many turns. Most spirilla are motile.

The microscopic examination produces information that is often needed to identify bacteria. However, biochemical reactions and the sensitivity pattern (how the organisms respond to antibiotics) are also needed to make the full identification.

Dyes (Stains)

The dyes used in microbiology are derived from coal tar. These dyes are acidic or basic and impart a color to the microorganism. Basic dyes carry a positive ion and stain structures that are acidic in nature. Methylene blue, a common stain, is a basic dye and binds to the DNA and RNA of the cell. An acid dye carries a negative ion and stains structures that are basic in nature such as cytoplasmic structures. An example of an acidic dye is safranin. Several different types of stains are used depending upon what test is ordered (Table 43-3).

Simple Stain

A simple stain uses a single stain on a fixed slide for a given period of time. A simple stain will show the arrangement and structure of the bacterial cell. It is fast, taking no more than three minutes to stain, but does not give much information.

Differential Stain

A differential stain is more complex than a simple stain. It is known as a differential stain because the stain result varies. A common differential stain is the Gram stain.

TABLE 43-3	STAINS AND THEIR USE
Stain	**Example**
Simple	Carbolfuchsin
	Gentian violet
	Methylene blue
	Safranin
Differential	Gram
	Acid-fast (Ziehl-Neelsen, Kinyoun)
Special	Capsule (Welch negative)
	Flagella (Leifson)
	Nuclei (Feulgen)
	Spore (Doerner)

The Gram stain uses a primary stain, a decolorizer, and a counterstain.

The Gram stain was developed in 1884 by Dr. Hans Christian Gram. More than 100 years later, this famous stain is still in use with little variation. This staining procedure differentiates bacteria by their Gram stain ability of being either negative or positive. A bacterium is Gram negative or positive by the nature of the cell wall and the ability of it either to retain or lose color through decolorization. This identification of Gram-positive or Gram-negative aids in identification of an organism. Gram-positive bacteria have a lower lipid (fat) content and are not decolorized as compared to Gram-negative bacteria, which have a higher lipid content and are readily decolorized.

The reagents used in the Gram stain are gentian or crystal violet, a purple stain that is the primary stain. Iodine, which acts as a mordant, holds the purple stain. Alcohol-acetone is the decolorizer that removes the purple color. Safranin is the red counterstain. When stained according to the manufacturer's directions, the Gram-positive bacteria stain purple, and the Gram-negative bacteria stain pink. Sometimes an organism will appear Gram-variable. This is found with Gram-positive organisms that have been exposed to acidic media, that are often old and lose their ability to retain the gentian violet, or the proper procedure has not been followed. See Procedure 43-3 and Figure 43-16.

The Gram stain is one of the most important procedures in the microbiology laboratory, giving valuable information by identifying Gram-positive bacteria such as *Staphylococcus* and *Streptococcus* or Gram-negative bacteria such as *E. coli* and Proteus.

The morphological arrangement, shape, and Gram-stain characteristic will begin to help identify the bacteria. Sometimes this is all the physician needs to know to start treatment for a pathogenic organism. For example, the bacteria causing gonorrhea (*Neisseria gonorrhoeae*) is a distinctive organism, having a characteristic diplococci shape that resembles a coffee or kidney bean. These organisms are found in and outside of white blood cells and can be identified by a Gram stain.

Acid-Fast Stain

Another differential stain, which is often referred to as a specific stain, is the acid-fast stain. This stain is either differential or specific in that it allows microscopic examination of acid-fast organisms, or mycobacteria. This group of organisms does not respond well to the Gram stain and is difficult to stain under ordinary circumstances due to a waxy capsule cell wall that resists staining. See Table 43-4 for examples of diseases caused by acid-fast organisms.

To stain these organisms, heat or a powerful dye is used in the procedure to stain the bacteria. The bacteria, once stained, resist decolorization with an acid alcohol,

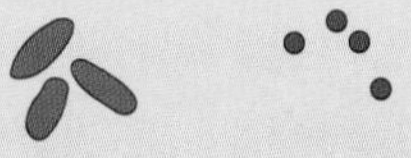

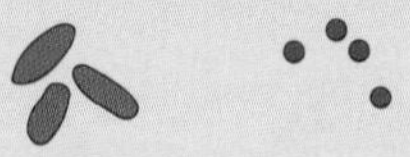

Step	Time	Procedure	Result
1	one minute	Primary stain: Apply crystal violet stain (purple) ↓ Rinse slide	All bacteria stain purple
2	one minute	Mordant: Apply Gram's iodine ↓ Rinse slide	All bacteria remain purple
3	three to five seconds	Decolorize: Apply alcohol ↓ Rinse slide	Purple stain is removed from Gram-negative cells
4	one minute	Counterstain: Apply safranin stain (red) ↓ Rinse slide	Gram-negative cells appear pink-red; Gram-positive cells appear purple

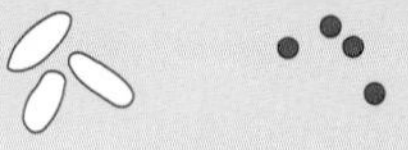

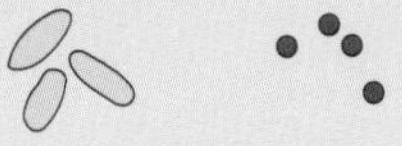

Figure 43-16   Steps in the Gram stain procedure.

TABLE 43-4	SOME ACID-FAST ORGANISMS	
Genus	**Species**	**Disease**
Mycobacterium	Tuberculosis	Tuberculosis (TB)
Mycobacterium	Leprae	Hansen's disease (leprosy)
Mycobacterium	Kansasii	Pulmonary disease
Mycobacterium	Avium-intracellulare complex	AIDS-related pulmonary disease

giving them the acid-fast name. The bacteria that causes tuberculosis is an acid-fast organism.

Two methods commonly used to stain acid-fast organisms are the Ziehl-Neelsen stain, shown in Procedure 43-4, which uses heat, and the Kinyoun stain, a cold method that does not include a heating process. Either of these stains is satisfactory.

Special Techniques

There are several special situations when more than the Gram stain or the shape and arrangement of an organism is needed to aid in the identification. Such situations would be the demonstration of the presence of flagella, spore, capsule, or nuclei of cells. The technique of these stains can be found in a detailed microbiology text.

There also are microscopic examinations of organisms in a living state, without staining. Characteristics that can be studied by this method include motility, shape, and arrangement of organisms. This technique requires the microorganisms to be in a liquid suspension.

For vaginal secretions, a swab of the vaginal discharge is placed in a sterile tube containing 1 mL of nor-mal saline and mixed. Then the suspension is viewed under a microscope. For stool or other bacterial specimens, a small amount of specimen is mixed with a drop of normal saline, then viewed under a microscope. These methods are known as the wet mount preparation and the hanging drop preparation. Refer to Procedure 43-5.

The wet mount preparation is a valuable diagnostic tool in determining the cause of vaginosis. Bacterial vaginosis is identified by the presence of "clue cells," epithelial cells covered by coccobacillary bacteria. Motile trichomonads are seen in case of *Trichomonas vaginalis*. The presence of pseudohyphae indicates a yeast infection. In many cases an accurate diagnosis can be made from the wet mount preparation, thus making more complex techniques unnecessary.

Potassium Hydroxide (KOH) Preparation

Another type of wet preparation is using 10 percent solution of potassium hydroxide in a wet preparation for the study of fungi and spores. The slide is prepared by using fragments of human hair, skin, or nails that could have fungus. These fragments are placed on a slide with a drop of 10 percent KOH and a coverslip on top. The KOH will clear debris. The slide should sit at room temperature for about one-half hour before examination for debris settlement.

The direct examination of specimens is best viewed with a phase or dark-field microscope rather than a bright-field microscope due to reduced illumination. If using a bright-field microscope, lower the condenser to reduce transmitted light. Proper disposal of these specimens is important as the organisms are alive and possibly pathogenic.

Table 43-5 is a listing of microscopic findings for several pathogens under direct microscopic examination.

TABLE 43-5	DIRECT MICROSCOPIC EXAMINATION OF CULTURE AND INFECTIOUS BACTERIA		
Specimen	**Procedure**	**Microscopic Findings**	
Cerebrospinal fluid	Gram stain	Haemophilus	Small Gram-negative pleomorphic bacteria
		Neisseria meningitides	Gram-negative diplococci
		Streptococcus pneumoniae	Gram-positive diplococci
	Gram stain Hanging drop	Listeriosis	Gram-positive nonsporing bacillus
Eye	Gram stain	Various Gram-positive and Gram-negative organisms	
Feces	Gram stain Direct mount Iodine	WBCs	Gram-positive bacteria Motility Ova and parasite *(continues)*

TABLE 43-5 *(continued)*

Specimen	Procedure	Microscopic Findings	
Genital	Gram stain	Neisseria gonorrhoeae	Gram-negative Intracellular diplococci
		Gordnerella vaginalis	Clue cells
		Chancroids	Small Gram-negative bacilli
	Darkfield Microscope	Syphilis	Coiled spirochetes
	Direct mount	Trichomonas	Darting Flagellates
	Direct 10% KOH	Yeast	Budding yeast forms
Skin	Direct 10% KOH	Fungus infection	Hyphae, mycellium, and spores
Sputum	Gram stain	Various Gram-negative and Gram-positive organisms	
	Acid-fast test	Acid-fast bacilli	
	Direct	Fungal infections	Hyphae, mycellium, and spores
Throat	Fluorescent Microscope	Strep infection	Fluorescent cocci in chains
Urine	Gram stain	Various bacterial organisms and yeast	
Wound	Gram stain	Gas gangrene	Gram-positive bacillus with spores
		Cellulitis	Various Gram-negative and Gram-positive organisms
	Direct mount	Fungal infections	Hyphae, mycellium, and spores

CULTURE MEDIA

After the proper collection of the specimen, the material collected must be inoculated on a proper culture medium. This is necessary for growth and eventual identification of an organism.

The results of culture, the growing of an organism on special media in the laboratory, are only as reliable as the method used in collecting the specimen. In addition, growth requirements of different organisms must be considered, such as moisture, temperature, oxygen, carbon dioxide, and essential nutrients. Organisms that are sensitive to drying must be put into transport medium immediately after collection to prevent loss of viability. Some bacteria require a specialized medium to grow and multiply. These are called **fastidious bacteria**. Aerobic bacteria grow only in the presence of oxygen. Anaerobic bacteria live and grow in the absence of oxygen. Examples of some common bacteria and their growth requirements are illustrated in Table 43-6.

When specimens are collected for the laboratory, the microorganism's growth requirements must be considered. No matter how good the specimen, if an anaerobic organism is kept in an aerobic atmosphere while being transported to the reference laboratory, it will probably not survive. Special anaerobic transport systems must be used.

Neisseria gonorrhoeae, the causative agent of the sexually transmitted disease (STD) gonorrhea, requires special media and an atmosphere of reduced oxygen and increased carbon dioxide. Therefore, the specimen must be collected from the patient and immediately placed on a special media in a reduced oxygen atmosphere.

Laboratory personnel who send bacterial specimens to a reference laboratory must be familiar with the trans-

TABLE 43-6   SOME COMMON BACTERIA AND THEIR GROWTH REQUIREMENTS

Organism	Disease	Medium	Oxygen Requirements
Streptococcus	Strep Throat	Blood agar	$\downarrow O_2, \uparrow CO_2$
Neisseria gonorrhoeae	Gonorrhea	Chocolate agar, modified Thayer-Martin (MTM)	$\downarrow O_2, \uparrow CO_2$
Staphylococcus	Infections, boils	Blood agar	O_2
Escherichia coli	Urinary tract infections	Blood agar, eosin methylene blue (EMB), MacConkey's	O_2

port media the reference laboratory provides. The reference laboratory should provide a procedure manual that explains how and when to use the various microbiology transport systems.

Media can be a solid, liquid, or semisolid substance that has the required nutrients to support the growth of bacteria. Such ingredients include vitamins, sugar, salt, minerals, and amino acids. Some media have the addition of special products like egg, potato, meat, milk, blood, and dyes.

The solid form of media is called agar. Agar has an appearance similar to gelatin. When heated, agar is a liquid; when cooled, it solidifies. Agar is poured into a **petri dish** (a plastic dish used to grow bacteria) so the bacteria can be studied for gross **morphology** (form and structure). Agar can also be placed in tubes.

Semi-solid media is made by adding less agar. Media in a liquid broth form is stored in tubes called **broth tubes** and allows for the observation of gas production, change in pH, and odor. Figure 43-7 shows many different types of media that can be used to identify bacteria. Media can be purchased already prepared, or it can be produced from ingredients in the laboratory. Charts listing the proper media to set up for specific types of cultures generally are prominently displayed in the set-up area of most microbiology laboratories.

Media Classification

There are several classifications of media, including:

- *Basic.* Basic media is used for general purposes and does not contain added nutrients. It will support the growth of many Gram-negative and Gram-positive organisms.

- *Differential.* Differential media contains substances that alter the appearance of some types of organisms and not other types. An eosin methylene blue (EMB) plate for lactose and nonlactose fermenters is an example of differential media. The lactose fermenter can use lactose and looks different on the agar.

- *Selective.* Selective media supports the growth of one type of organism, while inhibiting the growth of another. This is done by the addition of either a salt, dye, chemical, or antibiotic. A hektoen enteric (HE) plate for the growth of salmonella and shigella is a selective type of media.

- *Enriched.* This type of media contains substances that inhibit certain bacteria from growing. This media works well with cultures from sites that possess normal flora, like the throat. The normal flora is inhibited and pathogenic bacteria are encouraged to grow. Blood agar and chocolate agar are examples of enriched media.

All media that is used should first be checked with known organisms for quality control and for contaminants. The manufacturer will usually suggest a list of organisms for a quality control check. A check for contaminants involves a thorough visual check of the plate before using it. It is also important to store media according to the manufacturer's direction. *Never use outdated media.*

Table 43-7 lists common media by classification and use and Table 43-8 is a listing of media that might be selected for specific sources. All laboratories vary slightly in their recommendations of media to set up on specimens.

TABLE 43-7   COMMON MICROBIOLOGY MEDIA BY CLASSIFICATION AND USE

Type	Name	Use
Basic	Trypticase agar Trypticase broth	Supports the growth of most organisms
Differential	Blood agar MacConkey Eosin methylene blue (EMB)	Supports the growth of Streptococcus and Staphylococcus; demonstrates hemolysis Certain Gram-negative organisms Escherichia coli
Selective	Salmonella and Shigella (SS) Hektoen Phenylethyl alcohol Mannitol salt Selenite (GN) broth Thayer Martin Thioglycollate broth	Gram-negative Salmonella and Shigella Enteric organisms Inhibits Gram-negative growth Promotes growth of Staphylococcus Promotes growth of enteric organisms Promotes growth of Neisseria species Promotes growth of anaerobes
Enriched	Loefflers Chocolate Lowenstein Jensen	Promotes growth of Corynebacterium Promotes growth of Haemophilus species Promotes growth of mycobacteria

TABLE 43-8   COMMON SPECIMENS, SUSPECTED PATHOGENS, MEDIA RECOMMENDATIONS

Specimen Source	Potential Pathogens	Blood agar	Choc.	EMB	MacConkey	SSHE	Selenite	Thayer Martin	Thio.	CO_2
Eye/Ear	Neisseria gonorrhoeae Haemophilus species Staph. aureus Strep. pyogenes Pseudomonas aeruginosa Moraxella species	x	x	x	x			x	x	x
CSF	Neisseria meningitidis Strep. pneumoniae Haemophilus influenzae	x	x						x	x
Throat	Strep. pyogenes	x								x
Sputum	Strep. pneumoniae	x								
Urine	E. coli Klebsiella Proteus Pseudomonas aeruginosa Enterococcus	x		x	x					
Wounds	Staphylococcus Streptococcus Enterobactericae Anaerobic bacteria	x	x	x	x				x	x
Stool	Salmonella Shigella			x	x	x	x			
Stool	Pathogenic E. coli Yersinia species									
Vaginal	Neisseria gonorrhoeae	x	x					x		x

MICROBIOLOGY CULTURE

Inoculating the Media

After selecting the right medium for the culture and observing the specimen to make sure it is properly collected, the specimen is then inoculated onto the medium. If the specimen is on a swab, the swab is rolled directly onto the upper quadrant of the agar plate. If the specimen is a sputum or liquid, it is inoculated onto the plate with a loop.

The inoculum is spread back and forth in a sweeping motion with a flamed loop or needle. This is done to dilute the bacteria to obtain isolated colonies. The loop or needle should be cooled before streaking the bacteria. A hot loop will damage the agar, kill bacteria, and cause aerosols to form. To cool, touch it to the inside lid of the petri dish or stab into part of the media that is not inoculated. Never wave the loop or needle in the air to cool as this will contaminate it.

After the agar plate has been inoculated and properly labeled, it should be turned upside down and placed in the proper environment for growth. By turning the agar upside down, any condensation that forms from bacterial growth will be on the inside lid.

Liquid broths and agar slant tubes have screw caps. These caps must not be screwed on too tightly due to gas production by some organisms that can break the tube. See Procedures 43-6, 43-7, and 43-8.

Other Types of Streaking

Other types of streaking include the lawn streak. This streaking technique is used to place an organism over an entire area of an agar plate for sensitivity testing. The bacteria is spread over the entire plate using a swab (Figure 43-17), streaking over the entire area several times from different angles. After the streaking has been completed, disks saturated with different antibiotics are placed equidistant throughout the streaked area.

The colony count is a streaking technique much like the lawn technique. This technique is used to plate urine cultures. A special calibrated urine loop is used to make the first streak, followed by a second streak that goes across the entire length of the initial streak. Then another

Figure 43-17 Lawn or spread streak.

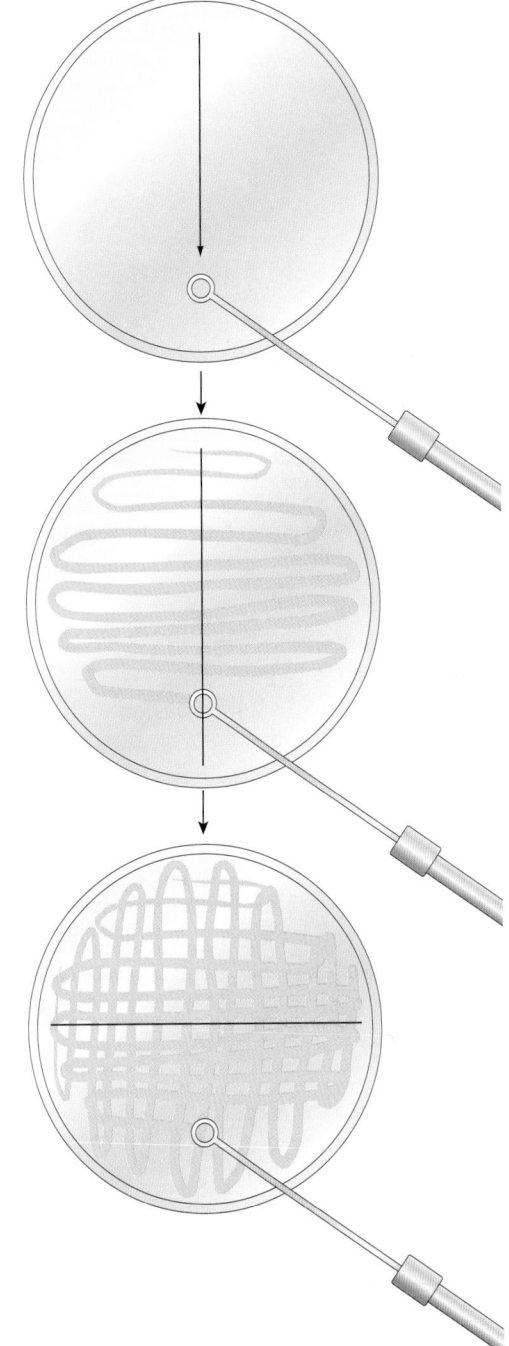

complete streaking is placed over the original streaks after rotating the plate (Figure 43-18). This method of using a calibrated loop to get a more accurate inoculation gives the physician an idea of how many colonies of bacteria are present.

Every laboratory will use slightly different ways of performing the basic streaks. The important factor is to use good aseptic techniques so there is no contamination from outside organisms, and all organisms that are streaked out are isolated enough to further test if necessary.

Primary Culture

After the media has been incubated for 24 to 48 hours, the initial or primary culture is read. The agar is observed for gross colony characteristics on the agar surface. In identifying the characteristics, the following aspects of the bacterial colonies are observed: size, shape, color, elevation, density, consistency, hemolytic versus nonhemolytic (if grown on blood agar), odor, and pigment production. Colonies that are hemolytic will utilize blood on a blood agar plate, while nonhemolytic colonies will not. By assessing the various characteristics, the microbiologist is able to make an initial identification of what bacteria are present. These characteristics are useful in the selection of various biochemical tests and differential media to make a final identification.

Specialized skill is required to examine an agar plate for colony characteristics. In many laboratories, these tasks are left to the microbiology professional staff. The medical assistant in these instances may be asked to set up and incubate the cultures, but not read the results.

The observation of the growing bacteria is made under a bright direct light by tilting the plate at various angles to see all characteristics. Often, a dissecting microscope or hand lens is used for better observation. On the

Figure 43-18 Colony count streak.

initial culture, the pathogens are mixed in with the normal flora in the first quadrant streaks, and it takes a trained eye to separate them.

Subculture

When working with bacterial cultures, there can be more than one pathogen growing in the culture. For instance, a wound culture may have both Gram-positive and

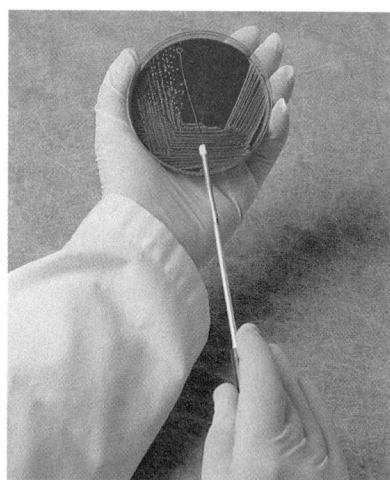

Figure 43-19 Suspicious pathogens are removed from one plate and streaked onto appropriate media to produce subcultures.

Gram-negative organisms growing. In order to identify each organism, these bacteria must be separated to other media. It is also necessary at times to separate the pathogenic bacteria from the normal flora, as in the throat and sputum cultures. Some initial cultures do achieve excellent isolation without having to subculture.

A pure culture is set up by using an inoculation loop or needle and picking the suspicious pathogen and streaking it onto the appropriate media for growth (Figure 43-19). This new plate will have only one type of organism present and from this plate biochemical tests can be set up. This step takes an additional 24 hours for the new subcultures to grow.

BIOCHEMICAL TESTS

In order to report to the physician exactly what organisms are causing patient infection, further testing may be necessary. Through the Gram stain, it is determined that the organism is either Gram-positive or Gram-negative. Initial growth on plates gives the microbiologist an impression of the colonies of the bacteria, and sometimes this is enough for identification if the bacteria has distinctive colonies. But most bacteria have similar characteristics on the initial plates. Further testing is needed to determine both the genus and species of the organisms. Table 43-9 illustrates a flowchart with biochemical testing as one of the final identification steps in this process.

Usually, laboratories will have a set procedure of tests to run when identifying certain genuses and species. Some organisms are much easier to identify than others. For example, the organism that causes strep throat will be obvious on blood agar. The *Beta Streptococcus, Group A* organism will use the red blood cells in the agar and produce a clear colony. Confirmation of this organism can be

TABLE 43-9   FLOWCHART OF SPECIMEN FOR IDENTIFICATION

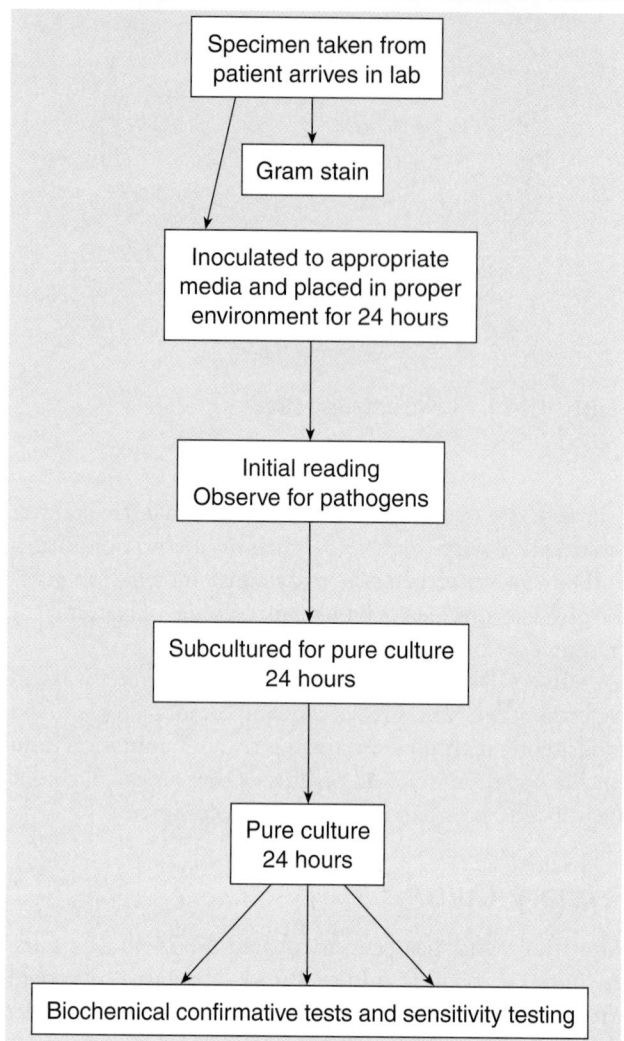

done rapidly with a specialized kit. Direct testing on isolated colonies has become very popular in today's health care environment due to the demand for immediate results.

Direct Tests

The following tests are done with immediate results. The directions included with the product by the manufacturer must be followed carefully.

- *Bile solubility. Streptococcus pneumoniae* is a Gram-positive coccus that can cause serious pneumonia. When a few drops of sodium desoxycholate are placed on these colonies, the colonies will lyse and disappear.

- *Catalase.* Colonies of Staphylococcus will foam (effervesce) when placed on a slide with a drop or two of hydrogen peroxide (catalase). This indicates hydrogen gas and is a positive test for staphylococcus species. Streptococcus organisms do not effervesce with catalase, although their colonies may look like Staphylococcus.

- *Coagulase*. Staphylococcus colonies that are coagulase-positive will clump when placed on a slide with rabbit plasma. Some Staphylococcus colonies are coagulase-negative. Different antibiotics may be used for coagulase-positive and coagulase-negative Staphylococci.

- *Indole*. Bacteria that possess the substance tryptophanase will react with Kovac's reagent to produce a red color (positive test). This test is also called the spot indole test.

- *Cytochrome Oxidase*. Certain bacteria will produce a blue-purple color when colonies are placed on a strip saturated with cytochrome oxidase.

- *Motility*. Some bacteria have motility and some do not. A direct microscopic examination can result in the observation of organized movement and the determination that the organism is motile.

These direct simple tests can be performed to make a final identification on some organisms or to give an indication as to what additional tests should be performed. Some highly sophisticated microbiology laboratories are now using high-tech systems that produce rapid identification results for many bacteria. (See Identification Systems section later in this chapter.) The identification techniques that follow will eventually be outdated with the increased demand for immediate results.

Biochemical Tube Testing

Identification of many bacteria can be facilitated by placing isolated colonies in a variety of tube media to determine how the bacteria will react. **Enterobacteriaceae**, a large group of Gram-negative bacteria, grow readily on many types of media. Many of these bacteria colonize the human intestinal tract and cause no problems. However, colonizing bacteria can cause problems if introduced into a susceptible site (the lung, spinal fluid, and so on) of a compromised host. Tube media often is used to help in the identification of Enterobacteriaceae, as well as other types of bacteria. Listed below are a few of the many tube media options available for bacterial identification. A larger, more complete list can be found in medical microbiology reference textbooks.

- *Triple Sugar Iron Agar (TSI); Kligler Iron Agar (KIA).* These complex carbohydrate media test the characteristic reactions of specific bacteria to various chemicals, especially the enterobacteriaceae. TSI contains lactose, glucose, sucrose, an iron salt, and indicators. KIA contains lactose, glucose, an iron salt, and indicators. The tubes are allowed to solidify on a slant. Several reactions can be observed in the bottom (butt) of the slant, as well as on the slant surface itself. The carbohydrate reaction in the butt and slant, the gas production of hydrogen and hydrogen sulfide, and pH change can be observed (Figure 43-20).

- *Citrate.* Only organisms that can utilize citrate as the sole source of carbon will react in this media.

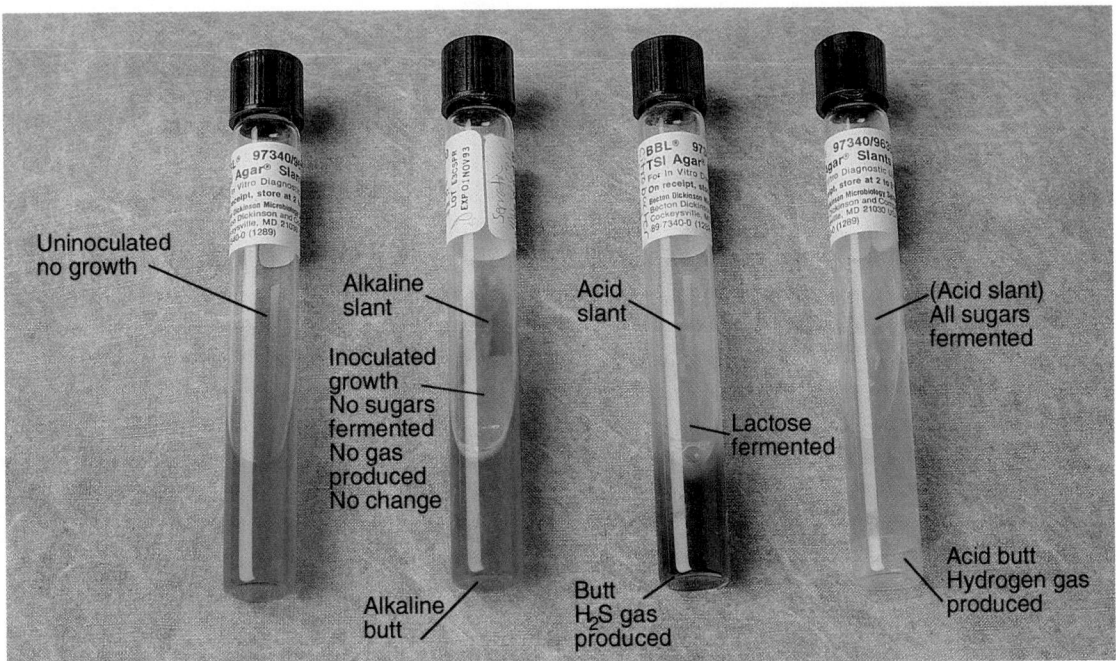

Figure 43-20 Triple sugar iron (TSI) agar.

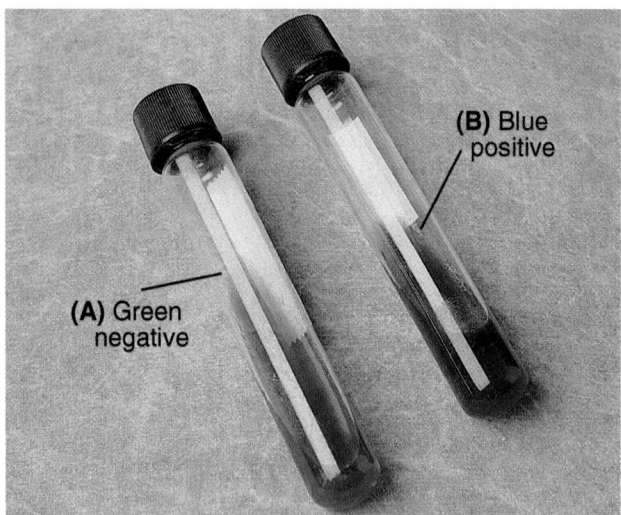

Figure 43-21   Citrate tubes: (A) E. coli. (B) Citrobacter Klebsiella.

TABLE 43-10	RECOMMENDED DIFFERENTIAL CHARACTERISTICS OF VARIOUS BACTERIA FOR IDENTIFICATION
Pathogen	**Biochemical Test**
Staphylococcus	Coagulase Mannitol Catalase
Streptococci	Catalase
Strep. pneumoniae	Bacitracin disk Bile esculin Quelling Bile solubility Camp test
Neisseria	Oxidase activity
Moraxella	CTA carbohydrate (maltose, sucrose, glucose, lactose)
Enterobacteriaceae	Lactose fermentation Oxidase activity H_2S production Decarboxylase activity Motility IMVIC reaction Urease
Nonfermentative Gram-negative bacilli	Oxidase activity Motility Indole Urease Growth on Mac Pigment production
Haemophilus	Enriched media with X and V factor Catalase Required CO_2 for growth Oxidase

The media is Simmons citrate agar with bromthymol blue as an indicator. The agar is made as a slant. When an organism has utilized citrate, the media turns from green to blue (Figure 43-21).

● *Urease Production.* Organisms that have the enzyme urease will break down the substance urea, producing ammonia and a pink-red color in the medium.

● *Bile Esculin.* This test is based on an organism's ability to break down the substance esculin in the presence of 1 percent to 4 percent bile. Some Streptococci organisms give a positive bile esculin reaction, seen as a blackened color on the media.

Table 43-10 is a listing of common pathogens and biochemical tests that might be used to help in their identification. Some tests are listed that are not explained in this text. Refer to a medical microbiology reference textbook for information on such tests.

IDENTIFICATION SYSTEMS

The age of high technology and computerized equipment has also made inroads into microbiology laboratories, clinics, and physician's office laboratories. Every day, traditional methods of identifying bacteria are being replaced by rapid identification tests, packaged systems (kits), and automated systems.

Rapid test systems give a quick identification, are economical, and allow physicians to start treatment sooner. A system is considered rapid if the physician can receive an answer while the patient is still in the physician's office.

Streptococcus Screening (Rapid Strep Testing)

There are a number of instant or rapid test kits on the market to identify Group A Streptococcus (also known as Beta Hemolytic Streptococcus Group A), the causative agent of a serious sore (strep) throat. It is very important to identify this Gram-positive Streptococcus as soon as possible because the bacteria can do serious damage (i.e., kidney and heart valve damage) if not treated with antibiotics immediately.

One test kit out today is based on the principle of enzyme immunoassay (EIA). This test is very sensitive and eliminates false positive tests. The directions should be strictly followed to produce an accurate test result. The results are based on color development of a spot on the test filter. Test results are available in minutes.

A latex agglutination test for Group A Streptococcus is based on an antigen and antibody agglutination. A throat swab is placed directly on the antibody coated slide, and the presence of a positive test is seen by the appearance of agglutination (clumping). Although these tests are quick and convenient, the following rules should be strictly followed:

1. Use the correct swab in taking the throat cultures. Some cottons and chemicals on the swab will interfere with test reagents.
2. Always run positive and negative control along with the actual test.
3. Read and understand directions before starting the test.
4. Never use outdated kits and materials.
5. Observe all safety guidelines.

If a patient has symptoms of an infected throat and the slide test is negative, the physician will also order a regular throat culture to make sure there is no infection present. Latex kits can give false readings, and it is best to follow up with the throat culture. Table 43-11 lists "Rapid Strep" kits approved for CLIA '88 waived testing.

Packaged Systems

Packaged systems are identification systems that have multiple tests within the container. These systems are used for identification of such microorganisms as anaerobic bacteria, enterobacteriaceae, and yeasts. These systems have replaced the many test tubes filled with various biochemicals.

Multitest media systems that will identify the Enterobacteriaceae bacteria include:

- *Enterotube®*. The Enterotube is a pencil-shaped chamber with eight compartments from which eleven reactions can be determined. To inoculate, unscrew each end of the tube. One end will have a wire needle for inoculation and the other end a small handle. To inoculate, touch the needle end to an isolated colony. With a slow rotary motion, pull the handle of the wire back through the chambers and out of the tube. Reinsert the wire into the first four compartments for anaerobic conditions. Also pull the plastic sleeve over these compartments. Incubate horizontally for 18 to 24 hours at 37°C. Add Kovac's reagent to the indole chamber of the tube and 10% ferric chloride to the phenylalanine chamber. This is best done with a hypodermic needle directly into the chamber. Read the reactions according to the manufacturer's directions, convert to a four-digit number, and compare the number to the organism in the code book (Figure 43-22).

- *API® System*. The API System consists of a plastic strip with twenty small cupules that are filled with a bacterial suspension for inoculation. The cupules contain dehydrated substrates for specific tests. There is an incubation tray to put the strip in with

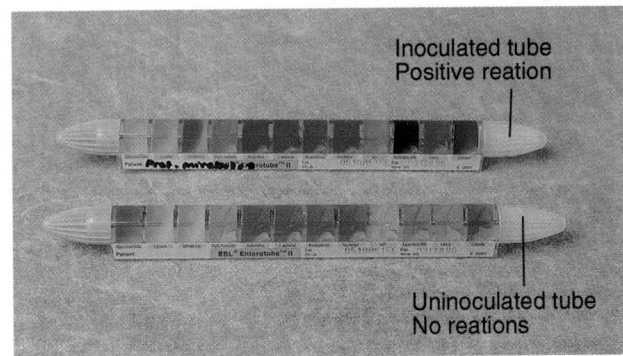

Figure 43-22   Enterotube.

TABLE 43-11	LIST OF WAIVED TESTS FOR *STREPTOCOCCUS, GROUP A (STREP A)*	
Manufacture	**Kit Name**	**Specimen**
Abbott	Signify Strep A Test	Direct from throat swab
Applied Biotech	SureStep Strep A	Direct from throat swab
Becton Dickinson	LINK 2 Strep A (II)	Direct from throat swab
Bianax	NOW Strep A Test	Direct from throat swab
BioStar Acceava	Strep A Test	Direct from throat swab
Genzyme	Contrast Strep A	Direct from throat swab
Jant Pharmacal	AccuStrip Strep A	Direct from throat swab
Mainline Technology	Mainline Confirms Strep A Dots Test	Direct from throat swab
Meridian Diagnostics	ImmunoCard STAT Strep A	Direct from throat swab
Quidel	QuickVue In-Line One-Step Strep A Test	Direct from throat swab
SmithKline	ICON Fx Strep A Test	Direct from throat swab
Wyntek Diagnostics	OSOM Strep A Test	Direct from throat swab

Reference: CLIA '88 Test Categorization List as of April 26, 1999. This list changes rapidly. For the most current listing, refer to the CDC website at www.cdc.gov.

a loose-fitting lid. Some cupules are overlaid with oil to reduce oxygen. The tray is incubated for 5 to 6 hours for the rapid test or 18 to 24 hours at 37°C. The tests are read visually as positive or negative and converted to a seven-digit number that corresponds to a bacterial organism in the code book. There are also API strips for the identification of yeasts, anaerobic organisms, and nonfermentative Gram-negative bacilli (Figure 43-23).

- *r/b System®*. This system consists of four constricted tubes called Beckford tubes. These four tubes contain eight types of biochemicals in media that will determine fourteen characteristic reactions. The medium above the constriction is a slant for aerobic reactions and the medium below the constriction is for anaerobic conditions. The tubes are inoculated with an inoculating needle for stabbing to the bottom and streaking to the top. They are incubated in an upright position at 37°C for 18 to 24 hours. The color changes in the tubes are compared to the color chart provided by the manufacturer.

There are several other packaged systems on the market. Selection of specific systems depends on the volume of work and cost for the particular size laboratory.

Semiautomated and Automated Instruments

The microbiology department of the clinical laboratory has been among the last departments to become automated. The nature of reading cultures has not lent itself well to automation until the past few years. Now systems such as ALADIN® and Vitek® are known as "walk-away" systems, where the microbiologist sets up the machine, and the work is done automatically. Semiautomated systems such as Biolog® and MicroScan® require more interaction between the microbiologist and the instrument. These automated and semiautomated systems are expensive and are used in high-volume laboratories.

SENSITIVITY TESTING

Antibiotic sensitivity testing often is ordered on the pathogenic organisms recovered from the culturing process. By setting up an antibiotic sensitivity test, the laboratory can identify which antibiotics destroy the pathogen, and the physician will be able to set up antibiotic treatment for the patient. Today's health care environment demands that this information be made available to the physician as soon as possible. Automated systems mentioned in the previous section are designed to produce this information as rapidly as possible.

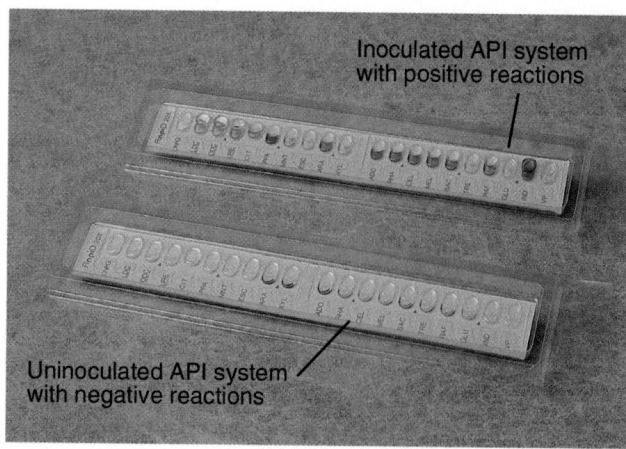

Figure 43-23   The API System identifies Gram-negative bacilli.

A traditional manual method of performing sensitivity testing is the **Kirby Bauer** method. It involves placing antibiotic disks on top of an inoculated plate. The plate is incubated for up to 24 hours. The pathogen will grow closely around a disk if the antibiotic is not destroying the organism. However, if an antibiotic will destroy the pathogen, there will be no growth at all around the disk. An obvious zone will be apparent.

To set up the Kirby Bauer test, a bacterial suspension of the isolated organism is compared to a barium sulfate standard to be sure that it is not too concentrated. A large Mueller Hinton plate is lawn streaked with a swab. The antibiotic disks are placed on the agar and gently pressed down for contact.

After 18 to 24 hours of incubation, the disk zones are measured with a metric ruler. Zones are measured for (R) resistant organisms (those the antibiotic cannot destroy), (I) intermediate (the organism is partially destroyed), and (S) sensitive (the organism is destroyed by the antibiotic).

The type of antibiotics used will vary depending on the organism that is grown. Zone sizes for R, S, and I will vary and the manufacturer's guidelines should be followed (Figure 43-24). As related to antimicrobial agents, bacteria are categorized as susceptible, moderately susceptible, or resistant to the antimicrobial agent. Definitions of these categories for various bacteria are published by the National Committee for Clinical Laboratory Standards. Refer to M2-A7, *Performance Standards for Antimicrobial Disc Susceptibility Tests*, 7th edition (2000); M7-A5, *Methods for Dilution Antimicrobial Susceptibility Tests for Bacteria That Grow Aerobically*, 5th edition (2000); M100-S10, Supplemental tables for M2-A7 and M7-A5; M11-A4, *Methods for Antimicrobial Susceptibility Tests for Anaerobic Bacteria*, 4th edition (1997).

There are several automated and semiautomated systems that utilize the antibiotic in several concentra-

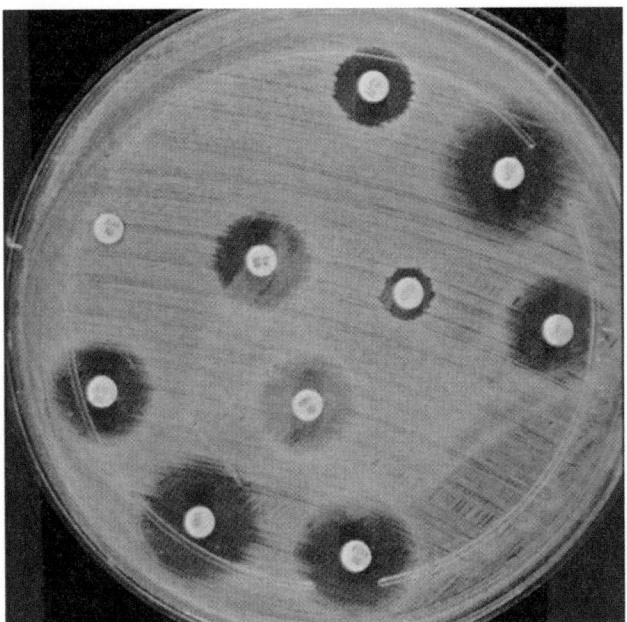

Figure 43-24 Zones of inhibition in an agar diffusion method of sensitivity testing.

tions against the isolated pathogen. The instrument prints out the most effective antibiotics. These systems are efficient and give results in a shorter period of time, but they are costly.

PARASITOLOGY

With the age of travel and more public awareness, we are beginning to see more parasitic infections. The field of parasitology is a vast one with many different types of parasites. They range from extremely small microscopic ones to those that are large and macroscopic in size. Parasites have varying life cycles. The degree of severity of illness depends on which parasite enters the human body and infects it. Parasites can be found in the blood, urine, or feces. The more common ones are found in the feces.

The study of parasitology in the clinic or physician's office laboratory is usually limited. Different geographical areas have different types of parasites that are seen. Resettled immigrant populations may be infected with a parasite previously unseen in a geographic area. World travelers can also bring back rare parasitic infections from their adventures.

Examination Methods

There are several methods used to examine parasites. They can be examined in permanent stained slides. (Refer to Procedures 43-2 and 43-3.) This type stains the parasite and provides a permanent record of the parasite seen. Another microscopic method is the direct wet mount.

(Refer to Procedure 43-5.) It is the examination of the feces in a suspension of saline or formalin applied in a thin layer on the slide.

The **concentration method**, either by flotation or sedimentation, is a procedure done to have a better view of the protozoa or ova in a specimen. In the sedimentation method, the parasites are found in the bottom layer of the test tube. In the flotation method, the parasites are found on the top layer. These procedures are not commonly performed in a physician's office laboratory. More detailed information can be found in a medical microbiology reference textbook.

One of the most common methods of fecal specimen examination for parasitic identification in a clinic or physician's office laboratory is the direct wet mount slide. The permanent stained slide and fecal concentration take more time and are done in the microbiology department of a hospital or reference laboratory.

Specimen Collection

Fecal specimens for identification of ova and parasites should be collected in wide-mouth containers with a tight lid to prevent leakage. The container should be put in a biohazard transport bag to avoid contamination and sent for examination immediately. The patient should be instructed not to contaminate the specimen with urine because it could interfere with testing. Special vials containing formalin are also available for ova and parasite testing that are preferred by some laboratories.

The laboratory procedure for collection and processing of the parasite specimen should be strictly followed to provide an accurate testing of the specimen. The collection time of the specimen should be followed as directed by the physician. Three specimens may be ordered over a specified period of time. Physician's offices will have specific instructions and containers with a preservative in them when an ova and parasite examination is requested.

When the specimen is sent for testing, it should be labeled correctly with the patient's name, date, and time of the specimen. It is important to know if the patient has been traveling, to what area of the world, and what is suspected by the physician to help aid in identification.

Before the microscopic examination is done, a description of the gross appearance of the stool should be recorded. The specimen should be checked for color, consistency, blood, and mucous. When working with the fecal specimens, all safety procedures should be followed and gloves should be worn at all times. The specimen should be disposed of by the procedures set forth by the clinic or physician's office laboratory using standard precautions and OSHA guidelines.

Common Parasites

Some of the more common parasites identified in the physician's office laboratory are *Enterobius vermicularis*, the causative organism of pinworm infection, and *Trichomonas vaginalis*, a parasite that infects the urogenital tracts of men and women.

Enterobius vermicularis. This **nematode** (round worm) is found worldwide, predominantly in children. The adult worm is shaped like a pin, wide at one end and pointed at the other end. The female worm is larger than the male. Infection with pinworm can cause severe itching, irritability, and insomnia, depending upon the severity of the infection. The adult female worm migrates to the anus at night, depositing ova (eggs) that cause itching during

hatching. At times, the adult worm can be found around the anus and on the stool. The adult worm measures approximately 7 to 12 mm long (Figure 43-25A). The egg is the infectious stage of the parasite (Figure 43-25B).

To diagnose the presence of the parasite, either the adult worm or ova has to be located in the specimen. A negative test should be confirmed by as many as six negative tests performed. The test is performed by taking a cellophane tape swab and placing the sticky side down to the skin around the anal area. The tape is placed on a slide and brought to the laboratory for examination (Figure 43-26).

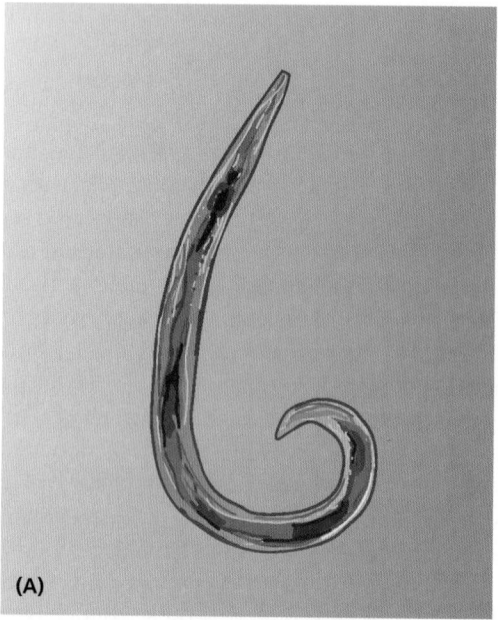

(A)

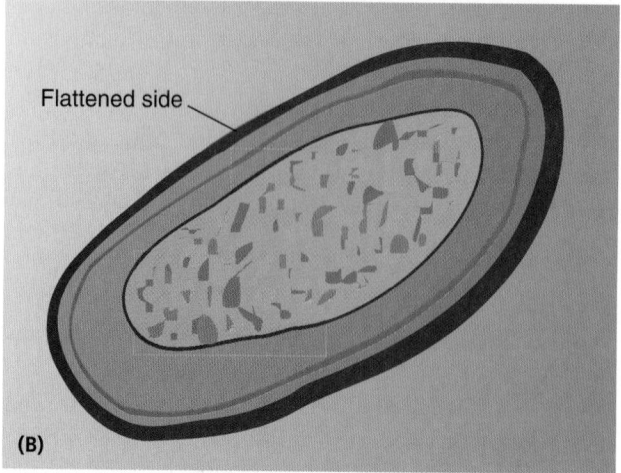

Flattened side

(B)

Figure 43-25 (A) Adult pinworm, *Enterobius vermicularis*. (B) *Enterobius vermicularis* egg (pinworm egg) at the infectious stage.

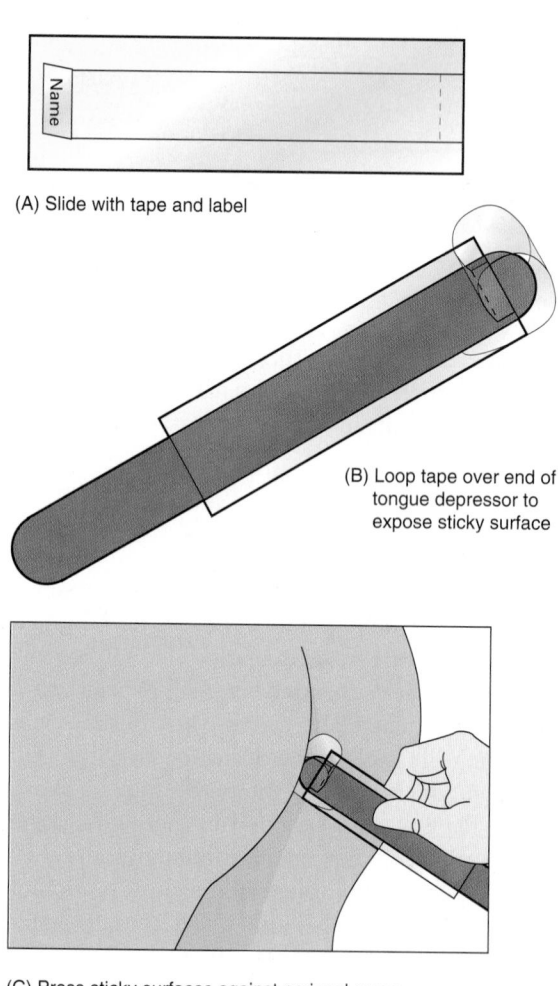

(A) Slide with tape and label

(B) Loop tape over end of tongue depressor to expose sticky surface

(C) Press sticky surfaces against perianal areas

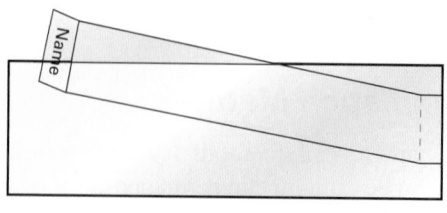

(D) Replace tape

Figure 43-26 Technique for preparing and using a cellophane tape swab.

Trichomonas vaginalis. This parasite is found in both men and women, but its presence is five times higher in women (men can harbor the organism for years without symptoms). The organism belongs to the flagellate (possesses flagella) class and is extremely motile. Infection with this flagellate causes a purulent yellowish-green discharge and dysuria. The organism is recovered from the discharge or urine and is transmitted sexually.

The trichomonad is recovered in a wet preparation slide of spun urine or vaginal secretion mixed with a drop of saline. (Refer to Procedure 43-5.) The specimen should not be contaminated with fecal material that could contain *Trichomonas hominis*, another flagellate. The prepared slide is examined under the low and high objectives of the microscope to observe the motility and morphology of the parasite (see Figure 42-14). There are also test kits and fluorescent stains used to diagnose this parasite.

MYCOLOGY

The field of mycology and the infections that cause fungi are extensive. Most identification and sensitivities testing for fungal organisms take place in larger laboratories and specific reference laboratories. Identification of two of the common fungal infections can be made quickly in the clinic or physician's office laboratory.

The genus Candida has several species that cause yeast infections in the body. Candida species are also pres-ent in the environment around us. They present a particular problem in the health care setting where they can cause serious nosocomial infections. Equipment can be easily contaminated with Candida organisms.

Yeast infections commonly are found on the moist areas of the body and in the subcutaneous tissue. An infection with yeast can range from mild to serious. *Candida albicans* is the causative agent of vaginal yeast infections. The specimen is examined microscopically for the characteristic budding yeast forms. (Refer to Procedure 43-5.) If the specimen is fluid and clear, it is placed on a slide with a drop of saline. If the specimen is thick, it should be mixed with 10 percent potassium hydroxide (one drop) on the slide to clear away debris. Once the specimen is prepared, it is microscopically examined.

Another group of significant fungi that sometimes can be generally identified are the **dermatophytes**. These fungi cause infections on the hair, skin, and nails. The microscopic structure of these fungi is very detailed. Some of the fungi that cause dermatophytic infections can be diagnosed using a **Wood's lamp**. This is a lamp with an ultraviolet light. Some dermatophytes will fluoresce (glow brightly) under this light.

Mycotic infections can also be identified through culture and kit identification systems. Fungi can produce heavy aerosols and should be processed and observed under the safety hood.

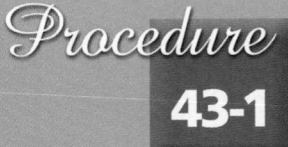

Procedure 43-1 Procedure for Obtaining a Throat Culture

STANDARD PRECAUTIONS:

PURPOSE:
To obtain secretions from the nasopharnyx and tonsillar area in order to incubate for means of identifying a pathogenic microorganism.

EQUIPMENT/SUPPLIES:
Tongue depressor
Culture tube with applicator stick or commercially prepared culture collection system
Label and requisition form
Gloves and mask

PROCEDURE STEPS:
1. Explain procedure to patient.
2. Have patient in sitting position. Adjust good light source.
3. Wash hands. Gather equipment.
4. Apply mask and gloves.
5. Remove sterile applicator from culture tube.
6. Ask patient to open mouth widely.
7. Depress tongue with tongue depressor.
8. Swab the back of throat and the tonsillar area.
   RATIONALE: Be certain to obtain a good sample of secretions or exudate from the very back of the throat paying special attention to red, raw, or with pustules.

(continues)

Procedure 43-1 *(continued)*

NOTE: On occasion separate cultures from each side of the throat may be taken per the physician's direction.

9. Remove applicator stick and place in culture tube(s).
10. Remove tongue blade and discard in biohazard waste container.
11. Push the applicator stick into the culture medium until the medium compartment is punctured and medium is released. RATIONALE: This keeps sample alive because medium contains nutrients similar to human tissue.
12. Ensure patient comfort.
13. Label culture tube(s) and send to outside laboratory or process the specimen according to agency policy.
14. Remove gloves and mask.
15. Wash hands.

Procedure 43-2   **Preparing a Bacteriological Smear**

STANDARD PRECAUTIONS:

PURPOSE:
Prepare a bacterial suspension for staining to examine bacteria microscopically.

EQUIPMENT/SUPPLIES:

Gloves	Loop or swab
Laboratory coat	Organism to be examined
Goggles (barrier shield or face shield can also be used)	Heat
	Stain rack
	Tray
Clean glass slide	Stains
Distilled water	

PROCEDURE STEPS:
1. Wash hands.
2. Put on personal protective equipment.
3. Assemble equipment and materials.
4. Apply a thin film of bacteria using a sterile or flamed loop or rolling a swab onto the surface of the slide, making a smear about the size of a nickel. If the bacteria is in a liquid suspension, apply directly to the slide; if not, add a drop of sterile water to the slide first.
5. Allow the bacteria to air-dry completely.
6. After the slide air dries, it is ready to be heat fixed. To heat fix the slide, pass it through the flame two or three times. This step is an important one. RATIONALE: If heat fixing is omitted, the bacteria will wash off in the staining process when water is applied. Avoid too much heat fixing because it can distort cells.
7. Allow the slide to cool before staining.

CAUTION: Use all safety precautions and make sure the suspension is air-dried before applying heat so that bacteria does not splatter.

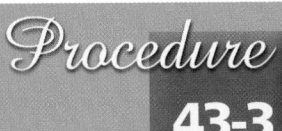

Procedure 43-3 Gram Stain

STANDARD PRECAUTIONS:

PURPOSE:
View organism microscopically to differentiate Gram-negative or Gram-positive bacteria through staining technique.

EQUIPMENT/SUPPLIES:

Gloves	Paper towels
Laboratory coat	Bibulous paper
Goggles (barrier shield or face shield can also be used)	Prepared bacteriological smear
	Heat
Distilled water in beaker or plastic squeeze bottle	Gram stain kit or individual Gram stain reagents
Loop or swab	Staining tray and rack

PROCEDURE STEPS:

1. Wash hands.
2. Put on personal protective equipment.
3. Assemble equipment and materials.
4. Flood the fixed smear with crystal violet for the manufacturer's recommended time period, usually one minute.
   NOTE: All bacteria cells will be purple.
5. Rinse the stain off the smear with a gentle stream of water from a beaker or plastic squeeze bottle.
6. Tilt the smear to remove excess water.
7. Flood the smear with Gram's iodine for the recommended time. RATIONALE: The iodine is a mordant that will hold the crystal violet to the Gram-positive bacteria.
   NOTE: All bacteria cells are still purple.
8. Rinse the smear as in steps 2 and 3.
9. Hold the smear by the short edge using forceps. Add the acetone-alcohol decolorizer by squeeze bottle or pasteur pipette until purple no longer runs off the slide.
   CAUTION: It is important to decolorize no longer than a few seconds to prevent over-decolorization.
   NOTE: Gram-positive bacteria remain purple; Gram-negative cells have no color.
10. Rinse the smear immediately to remove the decolorizer; tilt the slides to remove excess water.
11. Counterstain the smear by flooding the smear with safranin for the recommended time.
    NOTE: Gram-negative bacteria cells now have pink color.
12. Rinse the smear, tilt to remove excess water; wipe the back of the smear with paper towel to remove stain; stand smear on end or blot between sheets of bibulous paper to dry.

Procedure 43-4 Ziehl-Neelsen Stain

STANDARD PRECAUTIONS:

PURPOSE:
Identify acid-fast and non-acid-fast organisms.

EQUIPMENT/SUPPLIES:

Gloves	Loop or swab
Laboratory coat	Heat
Safety hood	Ziehl-Neelsen stain reagents (carbolfuchsin, acid alcohol and methylene blue or malachite green)
Barrier shield	
Face shield or goggles	
Glass slide	
Organism	
Distilled water	Staining rack and tray

(continues)

Procedure 43-4 *(continued)*

PROCEDURE STEPS:

1. Wash hands.
2. Put on personal protective equipment.
3. Assemble equipment and materials.
4. Place a prepared smear on a staining rack and apply heat, staining with carbolfuchsin. Apply heat under the smear until steaming. *Do not let the stain dry on the smear*; generously apply the carbolfuchsin.
5. Wash off the carbolfuchsin with *distilled* water. CAUTION: Do not flood with water when the smear is still very hot as it will crack.
6. Decolorize with acid alcohol about two minutes until no more stain is in the washing. All acid-fast organisms will retain the carbolfuchsin, which is red.
7. Wash off with distilled water.
8. Apply a counterstain of methylene blue or malachite green for 30 seconds. The counterstain will stain all the non-acid-fast material that did not retain the carbolfuchsin. These organisms will appear green or blue (Figure 43-27).
9. Wash off the smear with distilled water and air-dry completely. The smear can also be dried for several hours on a heat block.

CAUTION: All safety precautions for the microbiology laboratory should be followed. This smear should be prepared under a safety hood.

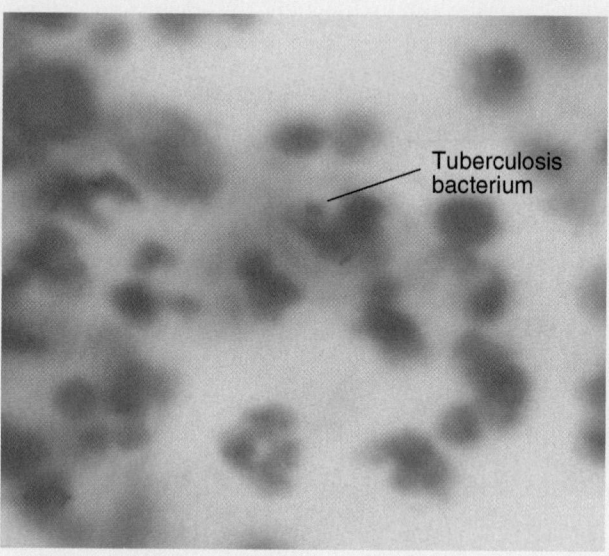

Tuberculosis bacterium

Figure 43-27   These non-acid-fast organisms have turned blue after the Ziehl-Neelsen stain.

Procedure 43-5 **Wet Mount and Hanging Drop Slide Preparations**

STANDARD PRECAUTIONS:

PURPOSE:
Prepare a slide for viewing live organisms for motility and identifying characteristics.

EQUIPMENT/SUPPLIES:

Gloves	Coverslips
Laboratory coat	Petroleum jelly
Clean glass slide	Dropper
Glass slide with concave well	Bacterial suspension

PROCEDURE STEPS:

1. Wash hands.
2. Put on personal protective equipment.
3. Assemble equipment and materials.

Wet Mount Preparation

4. Place a drop of the bacterial suspension on a clean glass slide (Figure 43-28A).
5. Place petroleum jelly around the edges of the coverslip (Figure 43-28B).

(continues)

Procedure

43-5 *(continued)*

6. Place a coverslip with the petroleum jelly on top of the bacterial suspension. RATIONALE: This cuts down on air currents and keeps the slide from drying out.
7. After the smear is prepared properly, it can be observed microscopically at any power (Figure 43-28C).

Hanging Drop Slide Preparation

8. The bacterial specimen is placed in the center of the coverslip with petroleum jelly around the edges of the coverslip (Figure 43-29A).

9. The slide is inverted and the concave well of the slide is placed over the coverslip (Figure 43-29B).
10. The slide is carefully turned right side up for examination (Figure 43-29C).

CAUTION: All laboratory safety precautions should be followed. Extreme caution should be followed. The organisms involved in this procedure are alive, not having been killed by heat fixation.

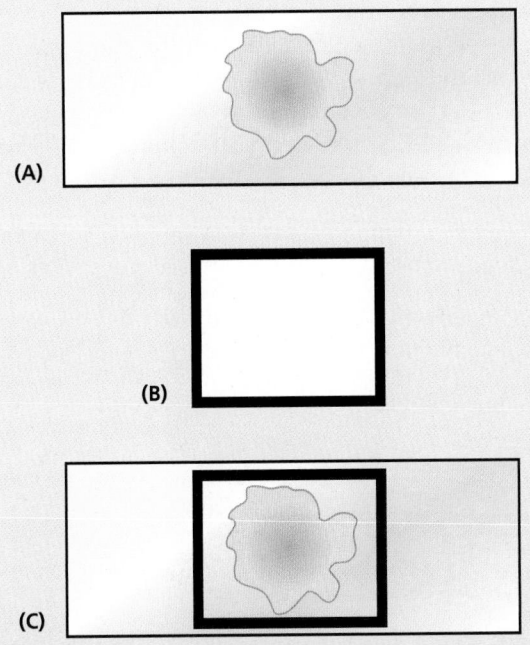

Figure 43-28 (A) Specimen placed on a glass slide. (B) Coverslip with petroleum jelly on edges. (C) Coverslip placed directly on top of slide with specimen.

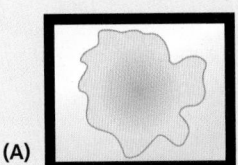

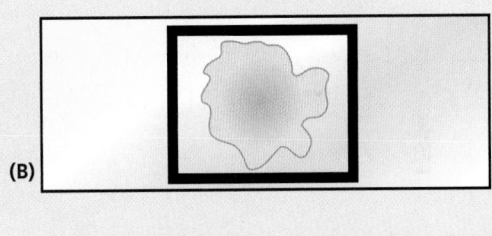

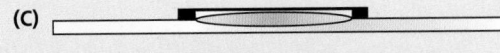

Figure 43-29 (A) Specimen placed on coverslip. (B) Slide placed over coverslip. (C) Slide turned right side up for examination.

Specimen Inoculation and Dilution Streaking

STANDARD PRECAUTIONS:

PURPOSE:
Inoculate solid media to study bacterial growth on agar.

EQUIPMENT/SUPPLIES:
Gloves
Laboratory coat
Plates
Barrier shield
Face shield or safety glasses
Heat
Blood agar
Inoculating loop
Bacterial specimen

PROCEDURE STEPS:
1. Wash hands.
2. Put on personal protective equipment.
3. Assemble equipment and materials.
4. Flame the loop (if a metal loop is used) and allow to cool. Apply the specimen to the plate with the sterile flamed loop or the specimen's swab. Once the specimen is applied, flame the loop again (Figure 43-30).
5. Use the loop to spread through the first streak and streak, turning the plate. Flame the loop.
6. Use the loop to spread through the second streak and streak, turning the plate.
7. Use the loop to spread through the third streak. Flame the loop.

CAUTION: All safety precautions for the microbiology laboratory should be followed. All cultures should be plated under a safety hood.

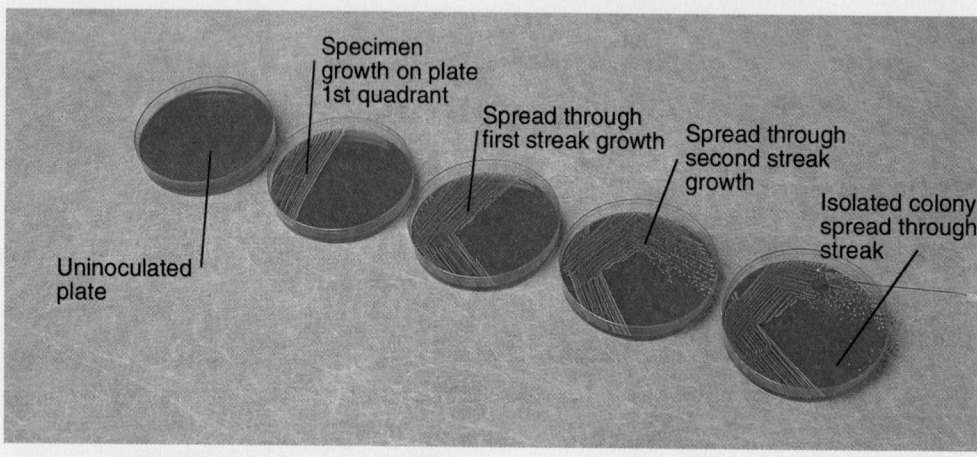

Figure 43-30   Stages of dilution streak.

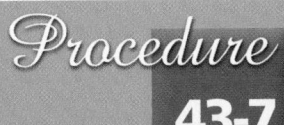

43-7 Broth Tube Inoculation

STANDARD PRECAUTIONS:

PURPOSE:
Inoculate liquid media to observe bacterial growth.

EQUIPMENT/SUPPLIES:

Gloves   Broth
Laboratory coat   Inoculating loop
Barrier shield   Liquid specimen
Face shield or goggles   Heat

PROCEDURE STEPS:

1. Wash hands.
2. Put on personal protective equipment.
3. Assemble equipment and materials.
4. Flame the loop. If disposable loop, do not flame!
5. Pick up the specimen carefully with the inoculating loop.
6. Slant the tube at a 30 to 40 degree angle and touch a loop to the inside of the tube just above the agar. When the tube is placed in an upright position, the inoculation will be submerged (Figure 43-31).
7. Then gently mix the tube. RATIONALE: To inoculate liquid media for bacterial growth.

CAUTION: All safety precautions for the microbiology laboratory should be followed. Certain cultures should be plated under a safety hood.

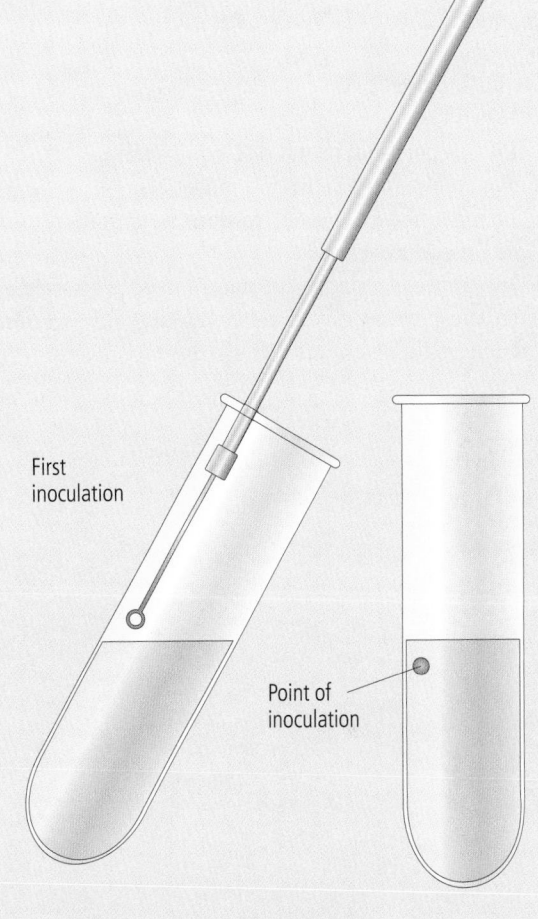

Figure 43-31   Broth tube inoculation.

43-8 Deep Inoculation/Slant

STANDARD PRECAUTIONS:

PURPOSE:
To study motility and biochemical reactions in slant media.

EQUIPMENT/SUPPLIES:
Gloves
Laboratory coat
Barrier shield
Face shield or goggles
Inoculating needle

(continues)

Procedure
43-8   *(continued)*

Deep agar or slant
Heat
Isolated bacteria

PROCEDURE STEPS:

1. Wash hands.
2. Put on personal protective equipment.
3. Assemble equipment and materials.
4. Using a needle, inoculate slant as in steps 4 and 5 of Procedure 43-7.
5. Inoculate the slant tube with a needle by stabbing to the bottom of the tube, making sure to flame the needle before and after this procedure.

6. For the slanted portion of the agar, use a needle to streak an "S" motion up the slant (Figure 43-32A).
7. The stab made deep in the agar can show whether or not the organism can move through the agar (motile) or just grow right around the stab (non-motile). The streak on the slant gives the bacteria a surface on which to grow. Some slants and deeps have biochemicals in them that change colors with different chemical reactions with the growing bacterial colonies (Figure 43-32B).

CAUTION: All safety precautions for the microbiology laboratory should be followed. Certain cultures should be plated under a safety hood.

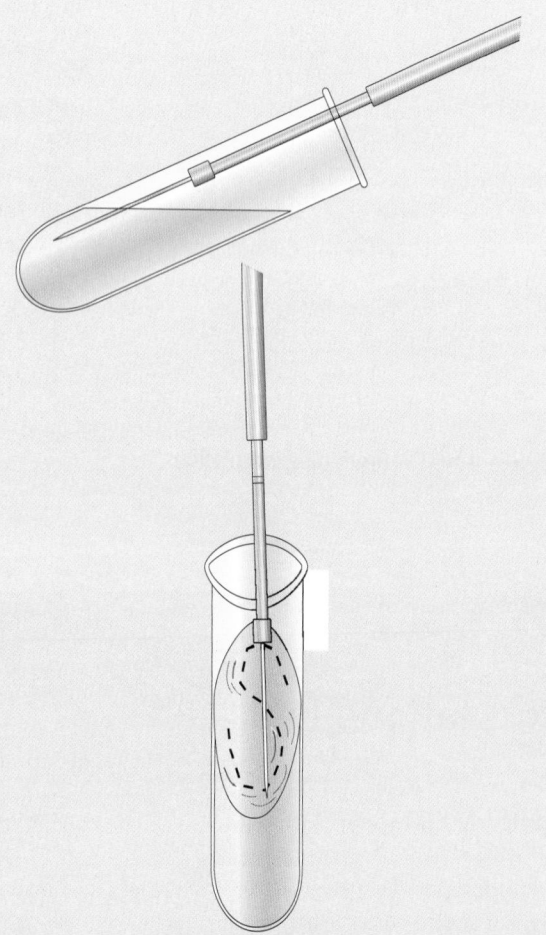

(A)

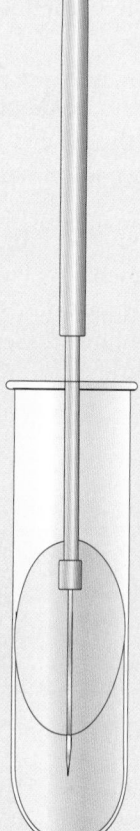

(B)

Figure 43-32 (A) Slant inoculation. (B) Deep inoculation.

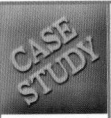

CASE STUDY 43-1

Mary O'Keefe has brought her three-year-old son Chris to the office of Doctors Lewis and King with a temperature of 102°F and an extremely sore and red throat. He is irritable and crying. After examining Chris, Dr. King orders a STAT latex agglutination test for Group A Streptococcus. Medical assistant Joe Guerrero has a difficult time acquiring the throat swab for the test due to Chris's condition. The test is run, and the results are negative.

CASE STUDY REVIEW

1. What are some reasons the test is negative?
2. What other procedure can be done to diagnose strep throat?
3. How would the test in question 2 be set up?

SUMMARY

The field of microbiology is vast. There are many microorganisms that are pathogenic and can cause serious infection in patients. The successful culturing and identification of such organisms is an important aspect of the successful treatment of patients. All specimens that are processed in the physician's office laboratory should be handled carefully, and all safety guidelines should be followed.

In order for the pathogen to be identified correctly, the utmost care must be taken in obtaining the culture. Sterile equipment must be used by the health care worker. When the culture is processed, the correct microscopic examination, media, incubation, and confirmatory tests must be used correctly to identify the pathogen.

Often a sensitivity test will be requested along with the culture. The information from this test will guide the physician in selecting the appropriate treatment for the patient.

Physicians' office laboratories vary in the type and number of cultures that are performed on the premises and those that are sent out to be performed in a reference laboratory. It is important to provide the best care for the patient by doing only those tests that a laboratory can reasonably handle given equipment and personnel limitations.

In addition to performing bacterial identification, some physician's office laboratories perform parasitology and mycology tests on a limited basis. When performing parasitology tests, it is important to obtain the proper specimen in the correct manner. When performing mycology tests, it is important to work under a safety hood to minimize the risk of exposure to spores from the fungal specimens.

Of utmost importance is the careful following of safety and quality control guidelines. These procedures help ensure patient and health care worker safety, as well as the integrity of test results.

REVIEW QUESTIONS

Multiple Choice

1. A structure that is *not* found on bacterial cells is the:
   a. nucleus
   b. ribosome
   c. spore
   d. cell wall
2. The proper sequence of staining in the Gram stain is:
   a. crystal violet, alcohol, Gram's iodine, safranin
   b. crystal violet, safranin, alcohol, Gram's iodine
   c. crystal violet, Gram's iodine, alcohol, safranin
   d. safranin, iodine, alcohol, Gram's iodine

3. An example of a nonselective media would be media that:
   a. contains a substance that alters the appearance of some organisms
   b. will support the growth of all organisms and does not alter their appearance
   c. supports the growth of one type of organism and inhibits the growth of other types of organisms
   d. identifies the biochemical activity of some organisms

4. When a CSF culture cannot be set up immediately, it should be placed in the incubator or remain at room temperature as opposed to being placed in the refrigerator because some organisms are affected by a low temperature. An example of this type of organism would be:
   a. *Beta streptococci*
   b. *Neisseria meningitidis*
   c. *Streptococcus pneumoniae*
   d. *Staphylococcus aureus*
5. The enterobacteriaceae are:
   a. Gram-positive organisms that include staphylococcus and streptococcus species
   b. fungal organisms that are easily identified in the laboratory
   c. Gram-negative organisms that commonly reside as normal flora in the intestinal tract but can cause infection
   d. common agents of sore throats
6. A culture from a knee wound on a young child showed a yellow creamy colony on blood agar. Given the following results, what is the most likely organism?
   Catalase—positive   Mannitol—positive
   Taxo A—negative   Coagulase—positive
   a. *Streptococcus pneumoniae*
   b. *Beta streptococcus*
   c. *Staphylococcus aureus*
   d. *Alpha streptococcus*
7. The best method of taking a specimen for the recovery of anaerobic organisms is to:
   a. swab deep and place into an anaerobic container
   b. aspirate purulent fluid and place into a test tube
   c. swab around the wound and place into an anaerobic container
   d. take as any other specimen for culture

Critical Thinking

1. Name two ways to identify whether an organism is motile.
2. If the iodine step was forgotten in a Gram stain, what color would the colonies appear?

3. Define an aerosol and explain how protection is provided when working with an aerosol.
4. What color is an acid-fast organism on a Ziehl-Neelsen stain?
5. Identify one potential pathogen and list the specimen source, media for culture, microscopic appearance, and the disease it causes.
6. A patient is given a requisition slip for a stool culture, ova and parasite examination. How would you instruct this patient to collect the specimen?
7. Explain why pinworm specimens are collected at a certain time of the day.

WEB ACTIVITIES

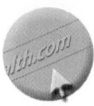

1. Visit the Centers for Disease Control and Prevention's website and other websites to review guidelines on Standard Precautions and use of personal protective equipment.

REFERENCES/BIBLIOGRAPHY

Barnett, M. (1992). *Microbiology laboratory exercises short version* (1st ed.). Dubuque, IA: Wm. C. Brown.

Baron, E. J., & Finegold, S. M. (1990). *Bailey and Scott's diagnostic microbiology* (8th ed.). St. Louis, MO: Mosby-Year Book Inc.

Garcia, L. S., & Bruckner, D. A. (1988). *Diagnostic medical parasitology* (1st ed.). New York: Elsevier.

Grover-Lakomia, L., & Fong, E. (1999). *Microbiology for health careers* (6th ed.). Albany, NY: Delmar.

Howard, B. J., Keiser, J. F., Smith, T. F., Weissfeld, A. S., & Tilton, R. C. (1994). *Clinical and pathogenic microbiology* (2nd ed.). St. Louis, MO: Mosby-Year Book Inc.

Koneman, E. W., Allen, S. D., Janda, W. M., Schreckenberger, P. C., & Winn, Jr., W. C. (1992). *Color atlas and textbook of diagnostic microbiology* (4th ed.). Philadelphia: J.B. Lippincott.

Morello, J. A., Mizer, H. E., & Wilson, M. E. (1991). *Laboratory manual and workbook in microbiology applications to patient care* (4th ed.). Dubuque, IA: Wm. C. Brown.

Walters, N. J., Estridge, B. H., & Reynolds, A. P. (2000). *Basic medical laboratory techniques* (4th ed.). Albany, NY: Delmar.

SPECIALTY LABORATORY TESTS

KEY TERMS

ABO Blood Group
Agglutination
Antibody
Antigen
Antiserum
Bilirubin
Blood Urea Nitrogen
Cholesterol
Choriocarcinoma
Cushing's Syndrome
Diabetes Mellitus
Ectopic Pregnancy
Enzyme Immunoassay
Epstein-Barr Virus (EBV)
Guthrie Screening Test
Hemolytic Anemia
Heterophile Antibodies
High-Density Lipoprotein (HDL)
Human Chorionic Gonadotropin
  (hCG)
Hydatidiform Mole
Hyperglycemia
Hypoglycemia
Infectious Mononucleosis
Insulin
Latex Beads
Low-Density Lipoprotein (LDL)
Mantoux Test
Phenylketonuria (PKU)
Purified Protein Derivative (PPD)
Rh Factor
Semen
Tine Test
Triglycerides
Tuberculosis
Wheal

OUTLINE

OBJECTIVES

*The student should strive to meet the following performance objectives and demonstrate an
understanding of the facts and principles presented in this chapter through written and oral
communication.*

1. Define the key terms as presented in the glossary.
2. List the three main precautions to be observed during all tests and
   the collection of samples included in this chapter.   (*continues*)

OBJECTIVES (*continued*)

3. Collect samples and perform and interpret all tests included in this chapter.
4. Discuss factors to be considered when evaluating test results.
5. Discuss transmission, incubation period, and symptoms of EBV infectious mononucleosis.
6. List the blood group antigens and antibodies found in each of the four ABO groups and the Rh factor.
7. Explain the cause of PKU and the symptoms caused by untreated PKU.
8. Indicate normal and elevated levels of phenylalanine and the dietary restrictions to be observed by PKU patients.
9. Discuss the cause of tuberculosis and some major characteristics of *Mycobacterium tuberculosis*.
10. Discuss the role of insulin in the regulation of blood glucose levels.
11. List and discuss differences between the normal values for fasting blood glucose, two-hour postprandial glucose, and the glucose tolerance test.
12. Explain the importance of cholesterol and triglyceride testing to identify patients at high risk for coronary heart disease.
13. Give the average values of cholesterol for adults, children, infants, and newborns.
14. Give the acceptable level of LDL in persons with or without coronary heart disease and discuss the role of HDL and LDL in coronary heart disease.
15. Give the normal values of urea nitrogen for adults, children, infants, and newborns and discuss the significance of elevated blood urea levels.

ROLE DELINEATION COMPONENTS

CLINICAL

Fundamental Principles

- Apply principles of aseptic technique and infection control
- Comply with quality assurance practices
- Screen and follow up patient test results

Diagnostic Orders

- Collect and process specimens
- Perform diagnostic tests

(*continues*)

SCENARIO

Audrey Jones, CMA, has worked at Doctors Lewis and King for over five years. In that time, Audrey has become proficient in obtaining specimens from patients for various laboratory tests. Audrey enjoys the work and finds it extremely challenging. She also realizes that communicating with patients to help them understand why their specimens are necessary for testing is just as important as being skillful in collecting and testing the specimens. Audrey has found that when she explains the reason the specimen is needed in terms patients can understand, they are often less fearful, which helps them relax. This can be especially helpful when collecting blood specimens.

INTRODUCTION

An increasing number of tests are performed in the ambulatory care setting, many of them by the medical assistant. In order to meet these new demands, the medical assistant must have a strong background in a variety of areas including medical terminology, laboratory safety procedures, and specimen collection. Because many procedures require collection of a blood specimen, the medical assistant must also be an excellent phlebotomist. Good record-keeping and communications skills round out the requirements. A quality control program is necessary to assure that the results are accurate and reliable. This will require a commitment on the part of the medical assistant to maintain the highest standards throughout the process.

A variety of specialty tests are covered in this chapter, including testing for pregnancy, infectious mononucleosis, blood types, semen analysis, phenylketonuria (PKU), tuberculosis, blood glucose, cholesterol, triglycerides, and blood urea nitrogen (BUN).

PREGNANCY TESTS

Pregnancy tests are used when pregnancy is suspected. Pregnancy tests may also be used to rule out pregnancy before prescribing birth control pills, X-ray studies, certain antibiotics or other drugs, and for females who are to undergo surgery.

Pregnancy testing is based on detection of human chorionic gonadotropin (hCG), a hormone secreted by the placenta that can be detected in the serum or urine of pregnant women as early as five days after conception. During pregnancy, hCG levels peak at about eight weeks, then drop to lower but detectable levels for the remainder of the pregnancy.

Commercial/Home Pregnancy Tests

A variety of accurate and easy-to-use commercial tests are available for use in the medical office. Manufacturers of pregnancy test kits have designed them to be sensitive, easy to perform and interpret, and to give rapid results. Pregnancy tests are one of the few tests available for purchase as an over-the-counter product. However, results of tests performed at home should be confirmed by a laboratory test using appropriate controls.

Testing Methods

Two testing methods using urine are discussed in this section: the slide test or agglutination inhibition test and the modified enzyme immunoassay (EIA). Diagnosis of pregnancy is made using these test results in conjunction with a physical examination including a pelvic exam by a physician. Serum pregnancy testing requires special equipment and is not usually performed in the medical office.

A positive reaction to any pregnancy test does not necessarily indicate a normal pregnancy. Detection of hCG can also indicate such abnormal conditions as an ectopic pregnancy, a developing hydatidiform mole of the uterus, choriocarcinoma, or cancer of the lung, stomach, pancreas, colon, or breast.

Quality Control. Kits must be stored and used at the temperature directed by the manufacturer. Most kits contain a built-in control; however, appropriate positive and negative urine controls must always be run with patient specimens. Kits and/or reagents must not be used after the expiration date. Manufacturer's instructions must be rigorously followed for the particular test used.

Slide Test or Agglutination Inhibition Test

The slide test is based on inhibition of agglutination (clumping) of hCG-coated latex beads. The hCG

Precautions for Pregnancy Testing

1. Use a clean container for collection of the urine specimen. Disposable containers are preferred. Detergent residue on nondisposable containers may interfere with test results.
2. The first-voided morning urine has the highest concentration of hCG and is the preferred specimen. If this is not available, a urine specimen with a specific gravity of at least 1.010 is acceptable.
3. If the specimen cannot be tested immediately, it may be stored at 4°C for up to twenty-four hours. Both urine and serum specimens may be used with some test kits; other kits use only one or the other.
4. Allow refrigerated urine specimens and test reagents to come to room temperature.
5. If using the slide test procedure:
   A. Avoid cross contamination with other urine specimens.
   B. Use a new stirrer for each test.

antiserum (antibody against hCG) is added to urine on a microscope slide. If hCG is present in the urine, an hCG/anti-hCG complex forms between the antiserum and the patient's hCG. Next, an antigen reagent containing latex beads coated with hCG is added to the mixture. If the hcG/anti-hCG complex formed, then there is no hCG antiserum available to react with the latex beads, and agglutination will *not* occur. Negative agglutination indicates positive pregnancy. Positive agglutination of the latex beads indicates negative pregnancy (Figure 44-1).

Enzyme Immunoassay (EIA) Test

The enzyme immunoassay (EIA) is a more complex procedure than precipitation or agglutination. The test can be designed in several different ways, but it always involves an antigen, an antibody specific for the antigen, and a second antibody conjugated to an enzyme. The test may be designed to detect a particular antibody in a patient's serum or to detect an antigen in a patient specimen.

Numerous tests are based on variations of the EIA. New technologies have been developed called membrane

EIAs. In these tests, most of the reagents are incorporated into an absorbent membrane, which is enclosed in plastic. When the sample (serum or urine) is added, it migrates through the membrane, reacting with the reagents and forming a color. Many of these tests are simple to set up and interpret even though the technology is complex. Examples of membrane EIAs include over-the-counter pregnancy test kits and tests for group A *Streptococcus*.

Enzyme immunoassays for hCG vary in design, but have some features in common. Most have the reagents incorporated into an absorbent membrane within a self-contained test unit, which may look like a plastic slide, a reagent strip, or a test cylinder. Tests may require the addition of the sample only or the addition of the sample and reagents to the test unit (Figure 44-2). Procedure 44-1 shows how to perform the enzyme immunoassay or agglutination inhibition test for pregnancy.

INFECTIOUS MONONUCLEOSIS

Infectious mononucleosis (IM) is a contagious disease that may have vague clinical symptoms and can mimic

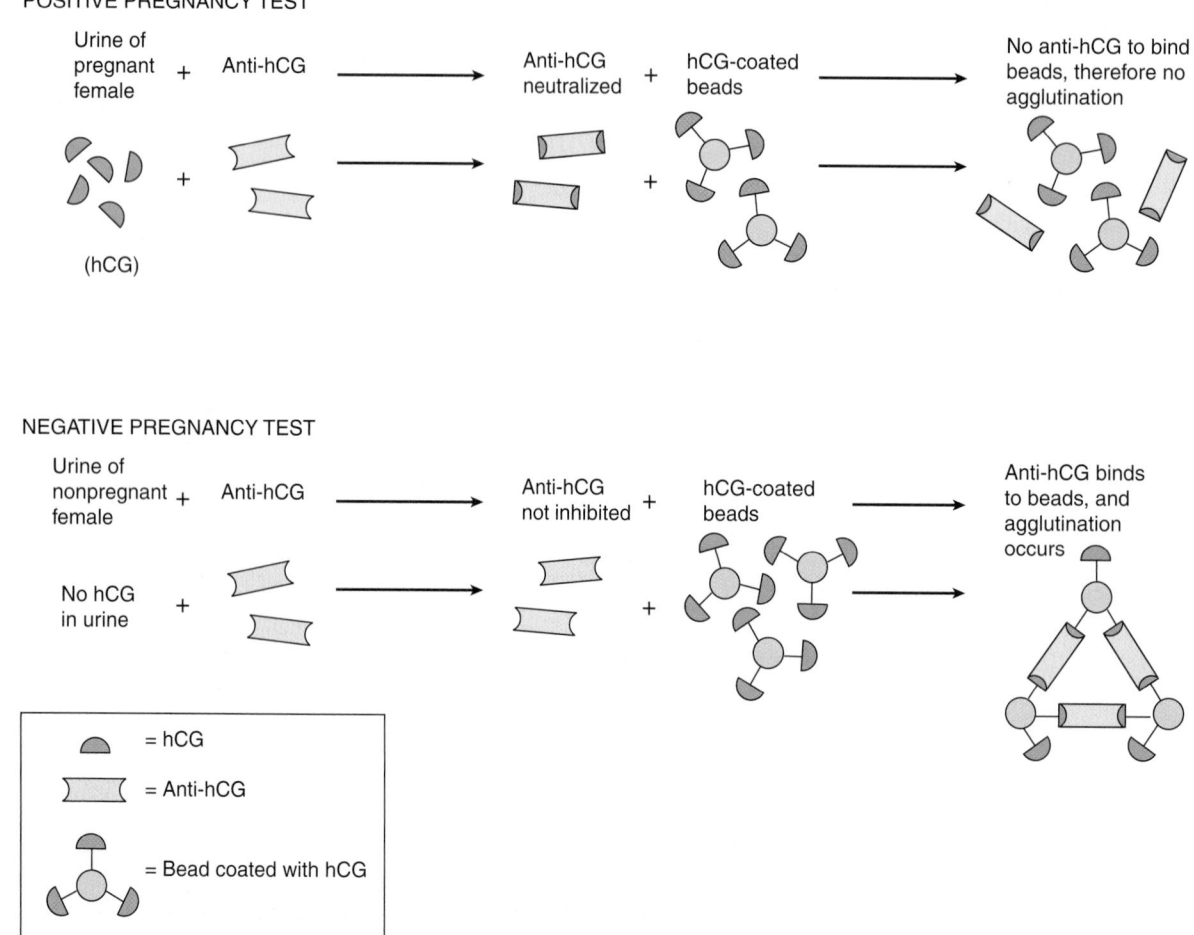

Figure 44-1   Principles of agglutination inhibition test for hCG.

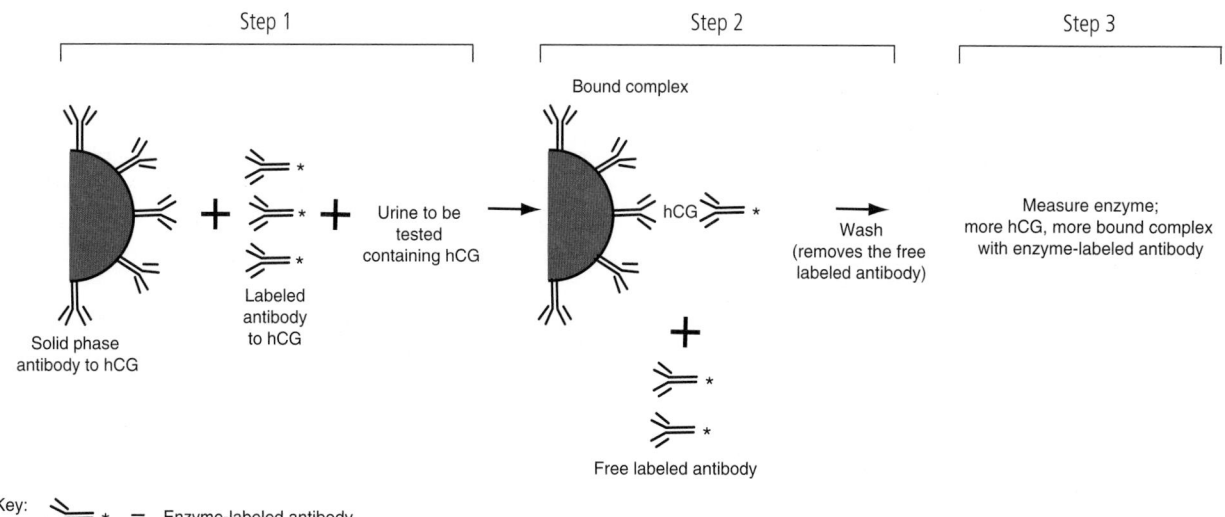

Step 1 Step 2 Step 3

Bound complex

Urine to be tested containing hCG

Solid phase antibody to hCG

Labeled antibody to hCG

hCG

Wash (removes the free labeled antibody)

Measure enzyme; more hCG, more bound complex with enzyme-labeled antibody

Free labeled antibody

Key: * = Enzyme-labeled antibody

Figure 44-2 EIA test for hCG.

other diseases. Serological tests are often the basis for an early diagnosis of the disease and may also be used to follow the course of the disease.

Infectious mononucleosis is commonly called "mono" or "kissing disease." The disease is a result of infection of the lymphocytes by the **Epstein-Barr virus (EBV)**. EBV is common in our population. By five years of age approximately 50 percent of the population are infected, increasing to 90 to 95 percent in adults. After the primary infection, the virus establishes a lifelong latency. The infectious virus may be isolated from saliva for several months, while antigens may be detected for life. In addition to causing infectious mononucleosis, EBV has been implicated in other diseases such as African Burkitt's lymphoma (a lymphoma of the lower jaw), nasopharyngeal carcinoma (NPC), and chronic fatigue syndrome.

Transmission of EBV

Transmission of EBV infectious mononucleosis is primarily by saliva which is why it is often referred to as "the kissing disease." EBV may also be spread by the sharing of drinking glasses and less often by blood transfusion. The disease is moderately contagious and is transmitted approximately 10 to 38 percent of the time in close social groups. In the home or in the hospital, careful handwashing will help prevent transmission of the virus.

Symptoms of Mononucleosis

Mononucleosis is seen most often in children and young adults. Incubation may vary from 4 to 50 days, however 7 to 14 days is the average. Infection in younger children is usually asymptomatic or manifests minor symptoms such as pharyngitis, otitis media, bronchitis, and other upper respiratory discomforts.

Classic symptoms usually occur when the primary infection is delayed until the second decade of life. It is the 15- to 25-year-old age group in which infectious mononucleosis is most often observed. Symptoms usually begin with a fever and swollen glands lasting for 3 to 5 days. Over the next 7 to 20 days the patient may develop a headache, malaise, chest pain, a cough, tonsillitis, a rash, soft, swollen lymph nodes, and a swollen spleen. Symptoms usually persist for 2 to 4 weeks and in more serious cases may last for more than a month.

Treatment of Mononucleosis

Because there are currently no effective drugs available for EBV infectious mononucleosis, treatment is primarily supportive. Although a vaccine is not yet available, some important work in that direction is ongoing.

Diagnosis of Infectious Mononucleosis

In order to properly diagnose IM, hematological and serological test results must be considered along with the clinical symptoms.

Hematological Test for Infectious Mononucleosis. The hematological test for IM includes a white blood cell count and evaluation of the patient's lymphocytes. In IM, a lymphocytosis, or increase in lymphocytes, usually occurs and large numbers of lymphocytes (greater than 20 percent) have an unusual or atypical appearance. Atypical lymphocytosis has a 95 percent specificity for patients with EBV mononucleosis, but is relatively insensitive for diagnosis. Because of this, serological testing is the method of choice for diagnosis of IM.

Serological Test for Infectious Mononucleosis. Persons with IM produce antibodies called heterophile antibodies by the sixth to tenth day of the illness. **Heterophile antibodies** are antibodies that react with similar antigens in more than one species. They are usually of the IgM class.

Detection of heterophile antibodies combined with the hematological and clinical findings provide the basis for the diagnosis of IM. The serological test is usually positive after the first week of illness. However, if test results are negative, the test should be repeated after a week if clinical symptoms are still present.

Slide Test for Infectious Mononucleosis

The most common serological test used for IM is a rapid slide test, which tests patients' serum for the presence of heterophile antibodies. The slide test gives quick, reliable results and is simple to perform. Tests are also available that detect antibodies to Epstein-Barr virus, the cause of IM.

Several commercial kits are available to test for IM. Most kits are based on agglutination principles and are adaptations of the Davidsohn differential test for heterophile antibodies, a cumbersome, time-consuming test. Colorimetric immunoassay kits for IM are also available from several manufacturers. Examples of IM kits include Color Slide® II Mononucleosis Test by Seradyn, BBL®

Monoslide™ Test by Becton Dickinson, Monospot® Slide Test by Meridian Diagnostics, and Monosticon Dri-Dot® by Organon Teknika Corporation.

Serological kits for infectious mononucleosis usually provide all the necessary reagents, materials, and controls. The laboratory must provide only the specimen to be tested, which is usually a small sample of the patient's plasma or serum, or a drop of capillary blood.

Performing the Slide Agglutination Test for IM. The principles for each manufacturer's test are the same; however, the instructions for the specific kit used should be strictly followed. The procedure for detecting the heterophile antibodies of IM described in this example is based on the Monospot® test by Meridian Diagnostics.

The test is performed using a glass slide that has two squares (I and II) etched on the slide. The reagent and patient sample are mixed thoroughly and a drop of indicator cells (horse erythrocytes) is added to a corner of each square using the capillary pipette provided in the kit (Figure 44-3).

The serum and reagent I are mixed using at least ten stirring motions with a clean wooden applicator stick. The indicator cells are then blended in so that the entire surface of the square is covered. The contents of square II are mixed in the same manner as square I (Figure 44-4).

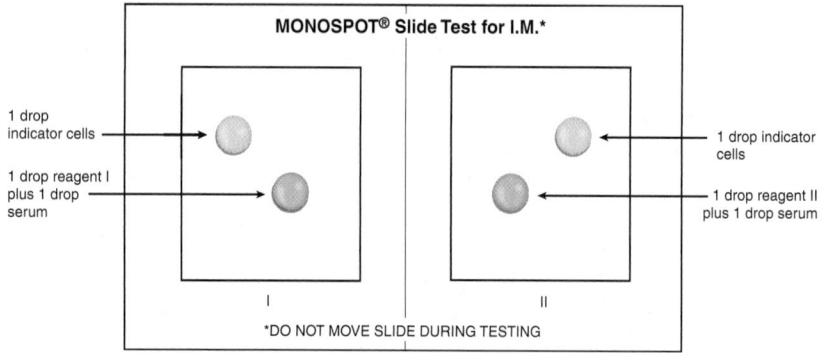

Figure 44-3   Monospot® slide with reagents added.

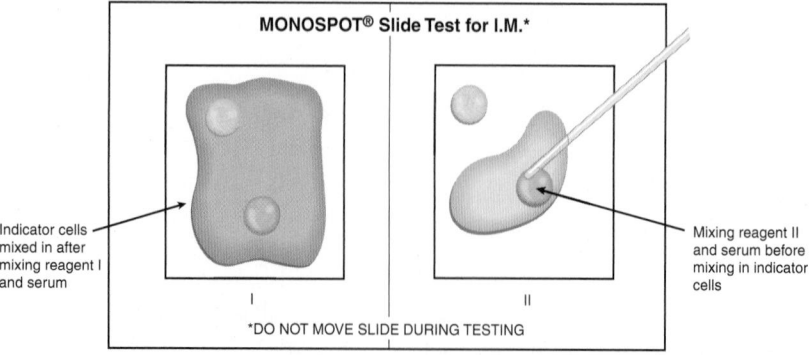

Figure 44-4   Mixing reagents on Monospot® slide using wooden applicator.

Do not use the contaminated applicator stick used to mix reagent I.

A timer is started as soon as mixing is completed and the slide is observed for one minute for agglutination of the horse cells. During this time, the slide should not be moved or picked up. At the end of one minute, the results are recorded and interpreted. Positive and negative serum controls provided with the kit should be tested in the same manner to ensure that all reagents are reacting properly.

Interpreting Results of Slide Test for IM. The presence or absence of heterophile antibodies of infectious mononucleosis will be indicated by the presence or absence of agglutination, as indicated in Table 44-1. See Procedure 44-2 for the steps involved in performing a slide test for infectious mononucleosis.

BLOOD TYPING: ABO BLOOD GROUPS AND RH FACTOR

Blood typing is based on the presence or absence of certain antigens on the surface of red blood cells (RBC). These antigens are carbohydrate molecules that react with antibodies specific to them to cause agglutination of the RBCs. Antibodies are protein molecules that are found in serum; they are also referred to as immunoglobulins (Ig). When RBC antigens and antibodies react, they cause the RBCs to agglutinate. This process is called hemagglutination. Hemagglutination reactions are used in the typing of blood. The two major categories of blood typing are for the **ABO blood group** and the **Rh factor**. Figure 44-5 illustrates how red blood cells are tested for blood type.

The ABO and Rh systems place certain restrictions on how blood may be transfused from one individual to another. Depending on their blood type, persons with a particular RBC antigen may have antibodies against the other type or types (Table 44-2). An incompatible blood transfusion results when the antigens of the donor RBCs react with the antibodies of the recipient RBCs. This is a potentially life-threatening situation, varying in severity from mild fever to anaphylaxis with severe intravascular hemolysis. Although ABO and Rh typing does not completely rule out the possibility of reaction, it greatly reduces the chances.

ABO Blood Typing

ABO blood typing is determined by the presence or absence of two major antigens, A and B. All people have one of the four blood group categories: A, B, AB, or O. People with group A RBCs have A antigens, group B RBCs have B antigens, group AB RBCs have antigens for

TABLE 44-1	INTERPRETATION OF MONOSPOT® TEST RESULTS
Positive Test	**Negative Test**
Agglutination pattern is stronger on the left side of the slide (square I) than on the right side of the slide (square II).	A. Agglutination pattern is stronger on the right side of the slide (square II) than on square I. *or* B. No agglutination appears in either square. *or* C. Agglutination is equal in both squares of the slide.

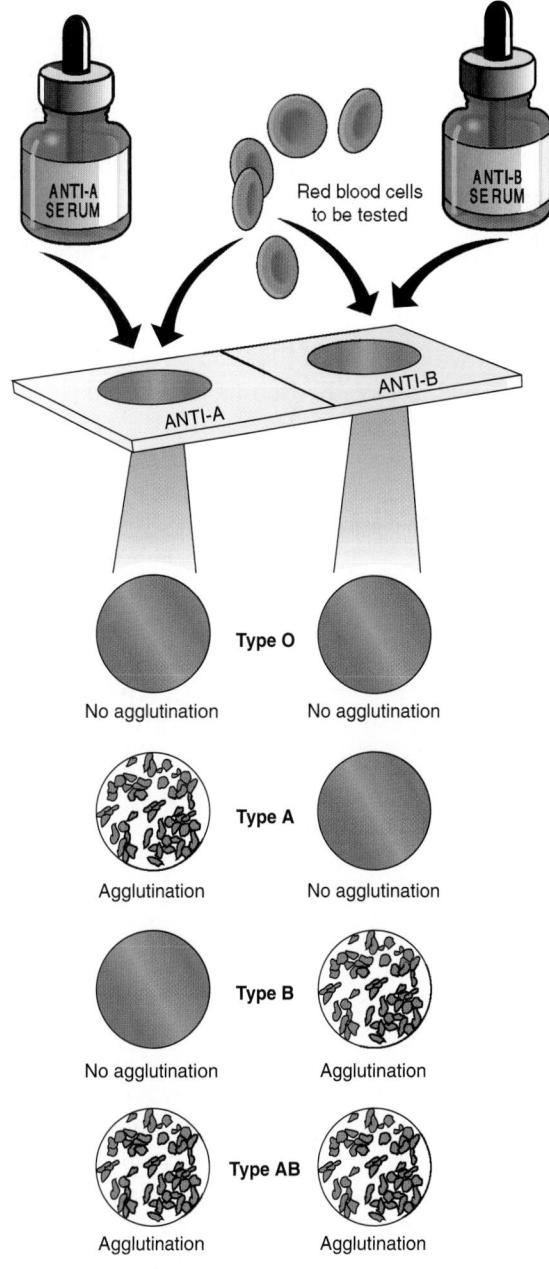

Figure 44-5 Blood typing ABO groups.

TABLE 44-2	ANTIGENS AND ANTIBODIES IN ABO AND RH BLOOD SYSTEMS	
Blood Group/Type	**Antigen on RBC**	**Serum Antibodies**
O (Universal donor)	None	Anti-A and Anti-B
A	A	Anti-B
B	B	Anti-A
AB	A and B	None
Rh+	D	No anti-D*
Rh–	D	No anti-D*

*There are no naturally occurring antibodies to the Rh system.

both A and B, and group O RBCs lack both A and B antigens. Naturally occurring antibodies to the other antigen types are found in the serum.

ABO type may be determined by the slide or tube method. The tube method is now most often used for blood typing.

Rh Blood Typing

Rh typing is routinely performed along with ABO typing. The Rh system is named for the rhesus monkey used in experiments that led to its discovery. The Rh factor is found on the surface of RBCs. People possessing the Rh factor are said to have Rh positive (Rh+) blood. Those without the Rh factor have Rh negative (Rh–) blood.

About 85 percent of North Americans are Rh positive, 15 percent Rh negative. Neither Rh negative nor Rh positive people have naturally occuring Rh antibodies in their blood. However, if an Rh negative individual receives a transfusion of Rh positive blood, he or she will develop antibodies to it. The antibodies take two weeks to develop. Generally, there is no problem with the first transfusion. However, if a second transfusion of Rh positive blood is given, the accumulated Rh antibodies will clump with the Rh antigen of the blood being received. Therefore, both blood type and Rh factor must be taken into account for safe and successful transfusions.

Blood typing is also performed on pregnant patients to determine the mother's blood type. In situations where the mother is Rh negative or type O, it is necessary to determine the father's blood type as well. If his blood is Rh positive or types A or B or AB, the mother's blood should be further tested for the presence of Rh antibodies. If the test is negative, then there is no risk to the fetus. A negative test should be repeated at weeks 30 and 36. If the test is positive, then the mother has been immunized by the Rh factor of the fetus and has produced antibodies referred to as anti-D (D is a major factor in the Rh group). A positive reaction also means that maternal hemolysis of fetal RBCs can occur. This condition is also called hemolytic disease of the newborn (HDN). The severity of

hemolytic anemia can be determined by evaluation of the quantity of bilirubin in the amniotic fluid. Fortunately, most cases of HDN can be prevented by administering RhoGAM to the Rh negative mother. RhoGAM is a concentrated solution of anti-D. When injected into the mother, RhoGAM will prevent her from producing the anti-D antibody. The injection must be administered within 72 hours after delivery of an Rh-positive baby or termination of pregnancy.

SEMEN ANALYSIS

With the progression of managed health care, more primary care physicians are performing semen analysis in their offices to determine sperm cell counts before referring patients to fertility specialists. Examination of semen is also performed as part of a complete fertility workup, to evaluate the effectiveness of a vasectomy, to determine paternity, and to substantiate rape cases.

When semen analysis is performed as part of a fertility workup, the procedure involves macroscopic and microscopic analysis of seminal fluid for determination of total sperm count, percent of motility, presence of agglutination, and percent of normally formed sperm cells (Table 44-3). All individuals will have variable sperm counts; therefore a single analysis is insufficient. To achieve a reasonable estimate of these factors, the seminal analysis should be repeated at least three times over a two-month

TABLE 44-3	REFERENCE VALUES FOR SEMEN ANALYSIS
Parameter	**Normal Range**
Appearance	White, viscid, opaque
Volume	1.5–5 mL
pH	7.12–8.00
Total count	50–200 million
% normal sperm	At least 80%
% motility	At least 60%

period. A complete analysis will also include an evaluation of the partner's cervical secretions and sperm survival. This involves determining the ability of sperm to penetrate the mucus and maintain motility.

Vasectomies are evaluated about six weeks after surgery. If sperm are seen at that time, then the effectiveness of the procedure is questionable and a follow-up analysis is required.

Semen Composition

Semen is a composite solution produced by the testes and the accessory male reproductive organs. It consists primarily of spermatozoa suspended in seminal plasma. Because there is considerable variation in composition between different portions of the fluid as ejaculated, it is important to collect the entire sample.

Altering Factors in Semen Analysis

Many factors can alter the results of semen analysis. Several drugs such as Cytoxan (cyclophosphamide) and nitrogen mustard lower sperm count. So may orchitis (inflammation of the testes), testicular atrophy, testicular failure, and obstruction of the vas deferens. Cigarette smoking is associated with a decrease in the volume of semen, while coffee drinking results in increased sperm density and an increase in the percentage of cells with abnormal morphology. Fever may temporarily suppress the count. Although research suggests that consumption of alcohol does not affect sperm function as measured by semen analysis, the patient is instructed to avoid alcohol for several days prior to testing as a precaution.

Although research suggests that fertility is most closely correlated with motility and morphology, men with very high (> 200 million/mL) or very low (≤ 20 million/mL) counts are likely to be infertile. Patients with aspermia (no sperm) or oligospermia (low sperm count, ≤ 20 million/mL) should be endocrinologically evaluated for pituitary, testicular, adrenal, or thyroid abnormalities.

Procedure 44-3 gives the steps for analyzing semen.

PHENYLKETONURIA (PKU) TEST

Phenylketonuria (PKU) is an inherited condition in which the amino acid phenylalanine is not metabolized, causing urine to have a mousy or musty odor. It is important that all newborns be tested for PKU because progressive mental retardation, tremors, and loss of muscle coordination can result if the condition is allowed to go untreated. Diagnosis must be made early so that a low-phenylalanine diet can begin immediately. Although the phenylalanine-restricted diet will prevent mental retardation, it will not cure the underlying condition. Routine screening of newborns for PKU is mandatory in most states and may be performed in the hospital or the medical office. The medical assistant's role is to properly explain the procedure to the infant's parents and collect the blood specimen for analysis.

Excess phenylalanine can be detected in blood or in urine. Normal levels of phenylalanine are less than 2 mg/deciliter (dL); more than 4 mg/dL is considered elevated. The **Guthrie screening test** is used to evaluate blood and is considered more accurate than urine tests. Phenylalanine can be detected in the blood of infants with PKU after three to four days on a breast milk or formula milk diet. Testing of breast-fed infants is delayed a few days due to the lack of phenylalanine in colostrum, the first breast milk. Colostrum is produced for the first two to three days after birth and is rich in antibodies, protein, and calories. True breast milk production begins after this time. Urine testing can detect PKU in infants who are at least 6 weeks of age and is usually done at the first checkup. A positive urine test is followed up with a blood test. Positive results from either blood or urine testing are confirmed by measuring serum phenylalanine and tyrosine levels. Infants with PKU have increasing phenylalanine levels (> 4 mg/dL) and decreasing tyrosine levels (< 0.6 mg/dL).

Patient Teaching Tip

The following instructions should be given to male patients when a semen sample is required for analysis:

1. Advise the patient to avoid consumption of alcohol for several days prior to the test. He should also avoid ejaculation for three days prior to collection of the semen sample.
2. Provide the patient with instructions and a container. The entire sample should be collected in a clean, dry, glass bottle that has been labeled, dated, and timed. The sample is collected by masturbation or interrupted coitus at home or may be collected at the medical office of the laboratory. Never collect the specimen into a condom.
3. Specimens for complete fertility analysis collected outside the laboratory must be brought to the laboratory within 30 minutes. Postvasectomy specimens should be brought to the laboratory within one hour of collection.
4. The sample must be transported to the laboratory at 37°C (98.6°F). Low temperature during transport will decrease the motility of sperm.

Patient Teaching Tip

Infants who test positive for PKU require a restricted-phenylalanine diet for normal development to occur. Instruct the mother to provide a low-phenylalanine diet. This will include a suitable milk substitute such as Lofenalac™, and later the addition of strained, low-protein foods. Blood and urine testing will continue to monitor the special diet.

Women of reproductive age who have PKU and want to have children must be instructed to begin a restricted-phenylalanine diet prior to conception to reduce the risk of damage to the fetus. Remaining on a general diet poses a high risk of producing a mentally retarded infant.

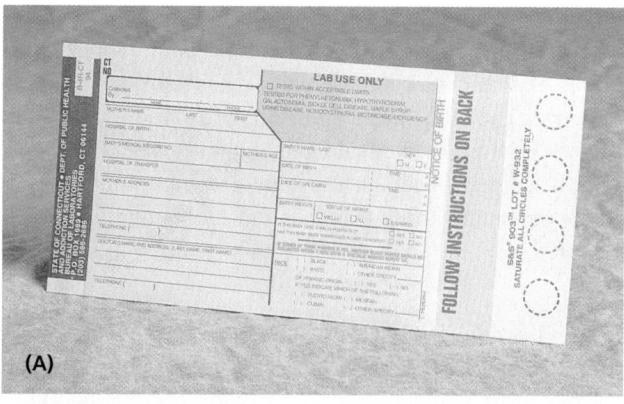

(A)

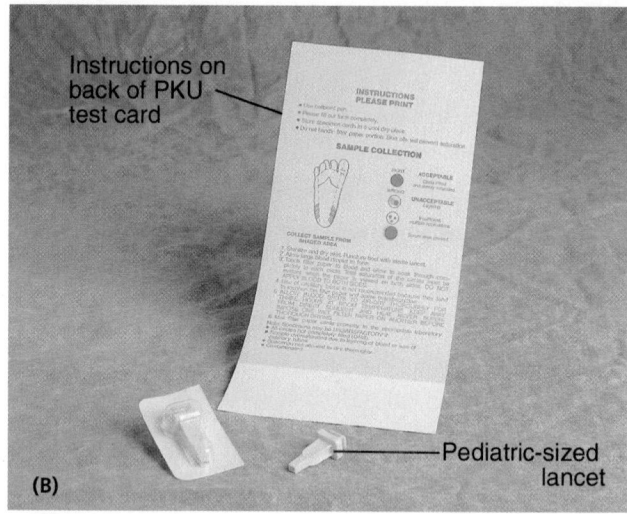

Instructions on back of PKU test card

Pediatric-sized lancet

(B)

Figure 44-6   (A) A filter paper test card is used to collect samples of infant's blood to screen for PKU. (B) Pediatric-sized lancets are available to limit the depth of the puncture when obtaining the blood sample from the infant. The back of the filter paper test card provides detailed instructions on performing the test and completing the card for testing.

Blood Testing for PKU

The Guthrie test was developed to screen for phenylalanine in the blood and is usually performed prior to the discharge of infants from the hospital. However, with managed care and the trend toward very short hospital stays for newborns, many pediatrician offices are now performing this test. Capillary blood is collected from a heel stick onto a "filter paper" test card and sent to the laboratory for testing. Patient, physician, and test information along with the blood samples are placed directly on the lab test card which is typically provided by most State Departments of Health (Figure 44-6). See Procedure 44-4, Obtaining Blood Sample for Phenylketonuria (PKU) test. Refer to Chapter 40 for proper capillary puncture technique.

Factors that May Influence the Guthrie Test

1. Feeding problems such as vomiting may result in a false negative reaction.
2. Failure to ingest sufficient phenylalanine—testing prior to three to four days of the beginning of a milk diet—will result in a false negative reaction.
3. Premature infants may give false positive test results due to a delay in the development of certain liver enzymes.
4. If either the mother (if breastfeeding) or the child is taking drugs such as salicylates, aspirin, or antibiotics, they may interfere with the test results.

Urine Testing for PKU

Urine testing can detect PKU in infants who are at least 6 weeks of age and is usually done at the first checkup and on infants who are on low-phenylalanine diets due to a previous positive test for PKU. Procedure 44-5 gives the steps to obtain a urine sample for the PKU test.

A positive urine test should be followed up with a blood test for PKU.

TUBERCULOSIS: *MYCOBACTERIUM* AND TB TESTING

Despite efforts to control its spread, **tuberculosis** infections are on the increase in the United States and around the world. Latent infection with tuberculosis is estimated in approximately 10 million United States residents and 2 billion persons worldwide. Because tuberculosis morbidity is on the rise, increasing 14 percent from 1985 to 1993 (*Nursing*, 1995) more patients are screened for the disease now than ever before. The Advisory Council for Elimination of Tuberculosis, an independent group of TB-control experts, recommends screening all patients who fall into high-risk groups. High-risk patients include those infected with the HIV virus, those who have had close contact with someone who has active TB, and those living or working in high-risk gathered settings (such as health care facilities, correctional facilities, and homeless shelters).

Cause of Tuberculosis

Infectious tuberculosis is caused by the small, rod-shaped bacterium, *Mycobacterium tuberculosis*. This aerobic bacterium is nonmotile and has a high content of lipid in its cell wall making it difficult to stain using basic aniline dyes. For this reason, the Ziehl-Nielson method was developed and is used as a tool for identification of mycobacteria. Mycobacteria will retain the red stain in the presence of acid alcohol and are therefore referred to as "acid-fast." Other bacterial species stain blue. Refer back to Chapter 43 for additional information on the Ziehl-Nielson stain.

Resistance in Mycobacteria

Mycobacteria exhibit an unusual degree of resistance on many fronts. They are able to tolerate drying and the effects of many disinfectants. Mycobacteria also show resistance to most antibiotics, making these infections very difficult to treat. To help overcome bacterial resistance to antimicrobial agents, patients take two or three drugs for a period of six to nine months. Mycobacteria are, however, susceptible to heat and are killed in milk by pasteurization (62°C for 30 minutes).

Transmission of Infectious Tuberculosis

Infectious tuberculosis is highly contagious. Seventy-five percent of new cases occur by inhalation of cough-produced airborne droplets from symptomatic or asymptomatic persons. Crowded conditions contribute to this transmission. Tuberculosis is often associated with poverty and is often seen in prisons and mental health hospitals. Occasionally, transmission through the skin or the GI tract may occur. A recent increase in tuberculosis is related to the rise in AIDS.

Diagnosis of Tuberculosis

One factor that complicates the diagnosis of tuberculosis is the fact that Mycobacteria are slow growers in the laboratory taking anywhere from 30 to 60 days. The average for *Mycobacterium tuberculosis* is 14 to 21 days with best growth in the laboratory on Lowenstein-Jensen agar. This means that isolation, identification, and diagnosis may take up to eight weeks. Recently, DNA probe technology for the identification of *Mycobacterium* species has been developed for the medical laboratory. The major advantage of these probes is rapid identification, within 1 to 2 hours.

Patients exhibiting a positive or questionable **purified protein derivative (PPD)** reaction should have a chest X ray to examine for tubercles, and a sputum sample should be stained to search for acid-fast rods. The presence of acid-fast rods in the sputum confirms active tuberculosis. Reasons for a positive reaction to PPD are varied. First and most obvious is that the patient has an active case of tuberculosis. Persons with an old, inactive case will also give a positive skin test as will persons who have been vaccinated with BCG. BCG (the bacille of Calmette and Guerin) is a vaccine made from live, avirulent M. *bovis*. The vaccine is used in Europe to help prevent childhood cases of tuberculosis. Persons who receive BCG will give a positive skin reaction for a minimum of four years, much longer in many cases.

Screening for Tuberculosis: Skin Testing

Screening for tuberculosis may be performed as part of a routine medical examination or as a prerequisite for school or employment. In states where medical assistants can legally perform injections, they may be responsible for administration and interpretation of the skin test. The most accurate method used is the **Mantoux test**. The **tine test**, which is a multiple-puncture test, may still be used in some areas but is no longer recommended by the American Academy of Pediatrics. Both the Mantoux and the tine methods use tuberculin, which is also referred to as PPD. PPD stands for purified protein derivative, and is a filtrate of tuberculin cultures that are used for skin testing. Persons who have been exposed to tuberculosis will develop a hypersensitive response to PPD resulting in the formation of an induration. An induration is a hard, red spot on the skin that is the result of sensitized lymphocytes migrating to the site of the injection. It is important to keep in mind that a positive skin test does not distinguish between active or inactive cases of tuberculosis. Again, a positive skin test will require further diagnostic testing including an X ray for lung lesions and an acid-fast stain of sputum to examine for the presence of *Mycobacterium tuberculosis*. Because of the severity of the reaction, do not administer the skin test to persons who have had a positive reaction in the past.

The Mantoux Test

In the Mantoux test, 0.1 mL of 5 TU (toxin unit) strength PPD is injected intradermally using a 1.0 mL tuberculin

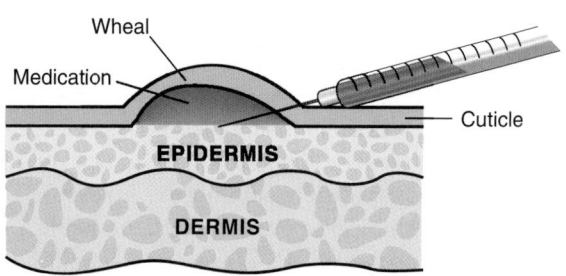

Figure 44-7 A raised wheal will form when the PPD is properly administered with an intradermal injection.

syringe. A short (⅜–½″), 26 or 27 gauge needle is used. Care must be taken to inject the PPD so that a **wheal** forms (Figure 44-7). If the injection is too deep, it will be impossible to read the wheal. If the injection is too shallow, the PPD may leak onto the skin. Either of these two errors would invalidate the test results. It is also very important to draw exactly 0.1 mL of the PPD as too much or too little would also lead to erroneous test results.

Choosing a Site to Administer the Mantoux Test.

To select a site for the Mantoux test, locate a site approximately 3 to 4 inches down from the bend of the arm on the anterior side. Avoid areas with excess hair, visible blood vessels, or scar tissue. The chosen site should be cleaned with alcohol and allowed to dry prior to administering the PPD.

SPOTLIGHT ON AAMA ESSENTIALS THROUGH CAAHEP

- When assisting pediatric patients, one way the medical assistant can gain the patient's trust and put him or her at ease is to make a game out of the procedure.

- Being aware of a patient's modesty and sensitivity while he or she is being examined will help to establish a positive rapport and help the patient to get through the examination in an expeditious manner.

- Often, taking a few moments to hold a patient's hand or talk to him or her before an examination will help to alleviate excessive fears and undue stress the patient may be experiencing.

BLOOD GLUCOSE

Glucose is the principal and almost exclusive carbohydrate found circulating in blood. It may also be detected in urine, cerebral spinal fluid, and semen. Glucose serves as an energy source for the body. Excess glucose is converted into glycogen for short-term storage in the liver and muscle cells, and as adipose tissue for long-term storage. Tests for blood glucose levels are commonly performed in the medical office. The results are used to screen for carbohydrate disorders such as **hypoglycemia** (low blood glucose level), **hyperglycemia** (high blood glucose level which occurs in **diabetes mellitus**), and liver dysfunction. A variety of testing methods have been developed to diagnose, evaluate, and monitor abnormalities in carbohydrate metabolism. They include the fasting blood sugar, the two-hour postprandial blood sugar, and the glucose tolerance test. All are briefly discussed here.

Blood glucose concentrations rise after a meal and are regulated by the action of several hormones including **insulin** and glucagon. Both insulin and glucagon are produced by the pancreas. Insulin is secreted by pancreatic cells in response to increased glucose levels and aids with the entry of glucose into cells for conversion into energy. Insulin is also required for proper storage of glucose (which is first converted into glycogen) in the liver and in muscle cells. Glucagon is secreted by the pancreas when blood sugar levels drop and triggers the breakdown of glycogen to help raise and regulate blood sugar levels.

Fasting Blood Glucose

Evaluation of fasting blood glucose levels is commonly used to screen for diabetes mellitus. Diabetes mellitus is a type of carbohydrate disorder characterized by insulin deficiency (or no insulin) and a state of hyperglycemia.

The normal fasting value of glucose ranges from 70–110 mg/100 mL (mg/dL). Refer to Table 44-4 for reference glucose values. 120 mg/dL of glucose is the dividing point between normal and hyperglycemic individuals.

Patient Teaching Tip

In preparation for the test, the patient should be instructed to fast for 12 hours (except for water). A fasting blood sample is usually collected in the morning to minimize inconvenience to the patient. Certain drugs such as oral contraceptives, salicylates, diuretics, and steroids may alter the results so the physician may restrict their use for two to three days prior to the test.

TABLE 44-4 REFERENCE VALUES FOR BLOOD GLUCOSE LEVELS

Test	Glucose Concentration (mg/dL)
Fasting	
Serum	70–110
Whole blood	60–100
2-hour postprandial	≤ 110
Glucose Tolerance (oral, serum)	
Fasting	70–110
1 hour	20–50 above fasting
2 hour	5–15 above fasting
3 hour	fasting level or below

Values vary slightly between laboratories depending on testing method used.

Generally, truly elevated glucose levels indicate diabetes mellitus. Other causes of hyperglycemia include **Cushing's syndrome** and acute stress response. Elevated blood glucose levels should be further evaluated using the glucose tolerance test.

Two-Hour Postprandial Blood Glucose

The two-hour postprandial (after eating) evaluation of blood glucose levels is used to screen for diabetes and to monitor insulin dosage. After fasting from midnight the night before, the patient eats a prescribed meal containing 100 grams of carbohydrate or consumes a 100-gram glucose test load solution such as Glucola®. Two hours later a blood specimen is collected and tested for glucose concentration. Glucose levels will return to or fall below the fasting level within two hours in nondiabetic individuals. Diabetic patients will have glucose levels of 140 mg/dL or higher. Elevated glucose levels should be further examined using the glucose tolerance test.

Glucose Tolerance Test

The glucose tolerance test provides more detailed information used to assess insulin response to glucose and to diagnose diabetes.

Patient Teaching Tip

The patient should be instructed to eat a high carbohydrate diet (300 g/day) for three days prior to the glucose tolerance test and to fast for 12 hours prior to collection of the blood specimen.

Fasting blood and urine specimens are drawn and evaluated for glucose level. If the results indicate hyperglycemia, the physician should be notified immediately. Hyperglycemia after fasting is abnormal and not an appropriate condition for further loading with additional glucose and may be dangerous to the patient. If glucose levels fall within the normal reference values, then the test may continue.

After providing the fasting urine and blood specimens, the patient consumes a glucose test solution containing 1.75 grams of glucose/kilogram of body weight, or the standard adult dose of 100 grams. Blood and urine specimens are typically collected at thirty minutes, one hour, two hours, three hours (and sometimes six hours) after ingestion of the glucose solution and are tested for glucose level. These measurements help determine the patient's ability to deal with increased glucose. During the test, the patient must not ingest anything except water. The patient must also abstain from smoking, as smoking acts as a stimulant and increases blood glucose levels.

During the second and third hours of the test, the patient may experience weakness, slight faintness, and perspire. These are all normal symptoms. If, however, the patient develops a headache, faints, or displays irrational speech or behavior, she may be experiencing hypoglycemic shock and the physician should be notified immediately.

The blood glucose level of nondiabetic patients usually peaks thirty to sixty minutes after consumption of the test load at 160–180 mg/dL and returns to the fasting level after two to three hours. Diabetic patients will still have elevated glucose levels at the end of the test.

Automated Methods of Glucose Analysis

Several types of glucose analyzers are available that are suitable for physician's office laboratories (POLs) or small clinical laboratories. Many of these operate on the principle of reflectance photometry and use adaptations of the enzymatic methods of glucose analysis. One example of an instrument suitable for small laboratories is the HemoCue® blood glucose analyzer.

Several small, inexpensive, handheld glucose meters are also made and are designed for home use by diabetics. Most of these are suitable for use in point-of-care (POC) testing or in physician's offices (Figure 44-8).

Glucose controls may be purchased from the instrument manufacturers to check instrument performance. It is always necessary to use test materials that are made for a particular instrument only with that instrument.

All of these analyzers are designed to be easy to use and to give rapid results. In general, better accuracy and precision (reproducibility) is obtained with the analyzers

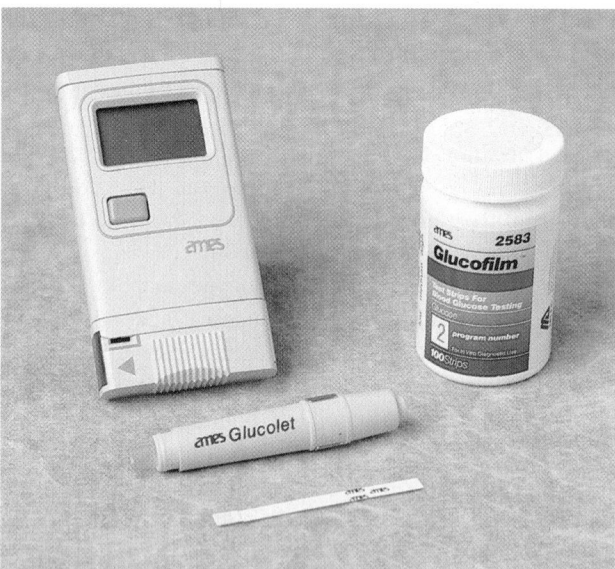

Figure 44-8   A variety of handheld glucose analyzers are now available for home and office use. These analyzers have become less expensive; however, the cost of the strips needed for the tests used can be expensive especially if used three times a day as recommended by most manufacturers. These analyzers do allow diabetics to safely test and track their blood glucose levels to help control diabetes.

designed for laboratory use than with the handheld photometers. With all instruments, it is necessary to use consistent proper specimen collection and testing technique to avoid variations in results.

Photometry Analyzers. The HemoCue® Blood-Glucose system is a compact glucose analyzer based on the principle of photometry. The system consists of a compact photometer and disposable microcuvettes. The self-filling microcuvette automatically draws up 5 µL of blood from a capillary puncture into its reaction chamber. The micro-

cuvette is then placed into the holder and pushed into the photometer. The glucose concentration in mg/dL is displayed within 45 to 240 seconds (Figure 44-9). This system is ideal for POLs and POC testing because of the stability of calibration and the minimum operator training required.

Reflectance Photometry Analyzers. Several glucose analyzers are available that are based on reflectance photometry. Blood from a fingerstick, serum, or plasma is applied to the reagent area of a test strip. The glucose in the sample reacts with the reagents in the pad(s) causing a color to form. The more glucose present in the sample, the darker or more intense the color. At the appropriate time, the strip is inserted into the test chamber and light is directed onto the test area. The amount of light reflected from the colored test area is measured by the photometer and converted to a digital readout showing the glucose concentration in mg/dL or mmol/L. Most instruments give results in one to three minutes. Instructions included with the test strips must be followed carefully for reliable test results. See Procedure 44-7, Measurement of Blood Glucose Using an Automated Analyzer.

Testing Profiles

Glucose testing may be part of a general profile chemistry test which can be useful in giving an overall view of an individual's state of health, especially when used in conjunction with other tests. Glucose testing may also be performed as part of a specific chemistry profile (renal profile) to determine the function of a particular biological system (Figure 44-10). The renal profile helps determine normal or abnormal function of the kidney. Another test in the renal profile of tests is the BUN, which is discussed later in this chapter.

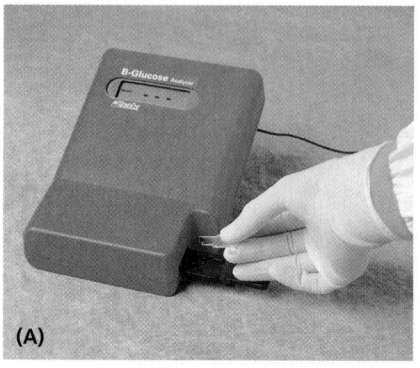
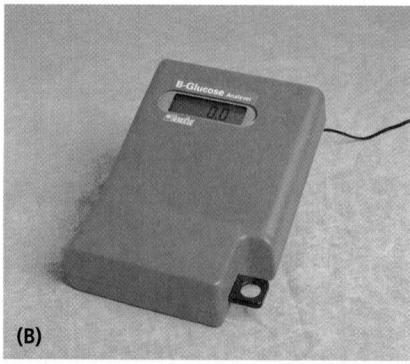
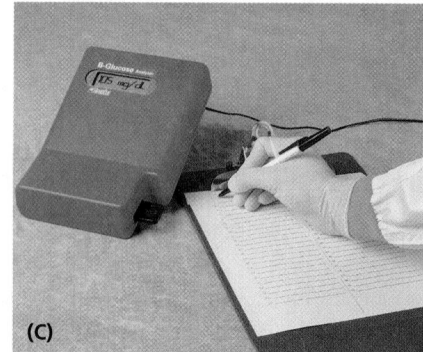

Figure 44-9   HemoCue® Blood-Glucose System: (A) A blood specimen is placed on the microcuvette, inserted into its holder, and pushed into the photometer. (B) Specimen is allowed to remain in analyzer until test is complete. (C) Glucose concentration is displayed in mg/dL after 45 to 240 seconds.

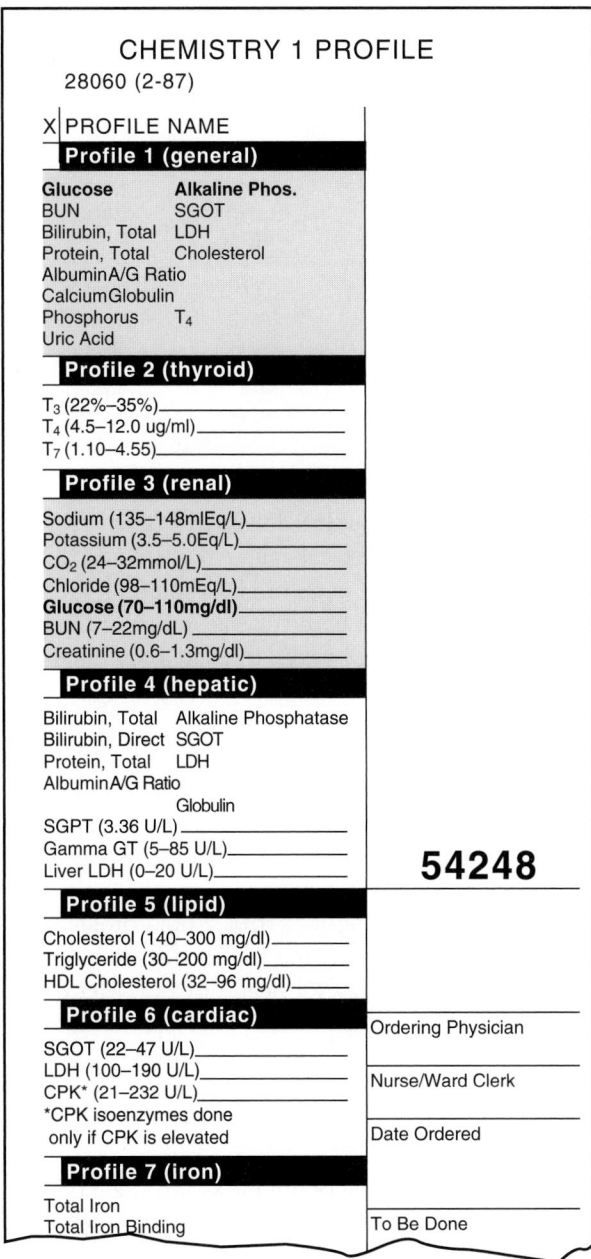

Figure 44-10 Example of a laboratory requisition form for chemistry profile tests. On this sample lab form, glucose testing is part of the general chemistry tests (Profile 1) and the renal tests (Profile 3).

Glycosylated Hemoglobin

Glycosylated hemoglobin (Hb A_1c) determination is a blood test that measures how well the glucose level has been controlled over the past four to six weeks versus the conventional blood test which shows only current day status. Physicians can use this test to determine if diabetics are consistently adhering to their diet and health guidelines or are adhering to their diet only for a day prior to their office visit.

Glycosylated hemoglobin is a stable molecule formed when sugar and hemoglobin bind together on the RBC. An elevated finding of glycosylated hemoglobin indicates poor glucose control in the assessment of glucose in the diabetic patient.

CHOLESTEROL

Cholesterol is a fatty compound that is essential for many vital life functions and is a normal constituent of blood. It is a steroid alcohol and a saturated fatty acid. Although it is required for life, cholesterol is not a necessary part of the diet. Sufficient quantities are manufactured by the body from carbohydrates and other fats. Because cholesterol has been linked to coronary artery disease, an increased interest in cholesterol levels and diet has developed. Typical cholesterol values for various age groups are shown in Table 44-5. To help reduce the risk of coronary artery disease, nutritionists and agencies such as the American Heart Association and the National Cholesterol Education Program advise that fats make up no more than 30 percent of the total intake of calories daily, and that the concentration of cholesterol in blood not exceed 200 mg/dL. Cholesterol of 240 mg/dL or above is considered to present a high risk of heart disease. Cholesterol levels between 200 and 239 mg/dL are considered borderline.

The Chemistry of Cholesterol

The cholesterol molecule consists of carbon, hydrogen, and oxygen. Most of the carbon atoms in the molecule are arranged into rings, rather than into long hydrocarbon chains as in most other lipids. A hydroxyl group (OH) attached to one of the carbon rings is what makes cholesterol an alcohol. Cholesterol is also a saturated, fatty acid. Saturated refers to the number of hydrogen atoms attached to the molecule. The more saturated the fat, the harder it is at room temperature. Fats of animal origin, for example, butter and animal fat, are saturated and are solid

TABLE 44-5	REFERENCE VALUES FOR TOTAL BLOOD CHOLESTEROL		
Age (years)	Range* mg/dL	Males mg/dL	Females mg/dL
0–19	120–230	—	—
20–29	120–240	235	220
30–39	140–270	265	240
40–49	150–310	280	265
50–59	160–330	300	320

*The upper limits of ranges are not necessarily the desired levels, but represent levels found in the U.S. population.

at room temperature. Monounsaturated and polyunsaturated fats are liquid at room temperature. Research into coronary artery disease has shown that saturated fats tend to raise levels of blood cholesterol. Monounsaturated fats (olive and peanut oils) do not change blood cholesterol levels and polyunsaturated fats (corn, safflower, sunflower, and many fish oils) tend to lower those levels.

Functions of Cholesterol

The human body is efficient at manufacturing cholesterol. Most cells are capable of doing so, especially the liver, the adrenal cortex, the testes, and the ovaries. All of the preceding cells, with the exception of the liver, use cholesterol to manufacture steroid hormones. Additionally, cholesterol is an important component of bile and cellular membranes. Although the body is very efficient at making cholesterol, it is not as easily degraded and may accumulate in the body and reach dangerous levels.

In addition to what the body produces, humans take in additional cholesterol through the ingestion of meat, eggs, and dairy products. The liver metabolizes cholesterol to its free form, which is then bound to lipoprotein and transported through the blood. Over time, excess cholesterol in the diet can result in a gradual increase of cholesterol concentration in the plasma. Increased concentrations of cholesterol in the plasma can rise to pathogenic levels. Some of the excess is stored in the liver while some is deposited on the walls of blood vessels (atherosclerosis) Atherosclerosis of the coronary arteries is the most common cause of acute myocardial infarction (heart attack).

Lipoproteins and Cholesterol Transport

Two kinds of lipoprotein are involved in the transport of cholesterol: **high-density lipoprotein (HDL)** and **low-density lipoprotein (LDL)**. Cholesterol bound to HDL is transported to the liver where it is excreted in the form of bile. HDL is sometimes referred to as good cholesterol. LDL cholesterol is deposited in the tissues as fat and inside the walls of blood vessels, and is referred to as bad cholesterol. High levels of LDL are associated with an increased risk of coronary artery disease. Persons with coronary artery disease should have levels of less than 160 mg/dL

Patient Teaching Tip

The patient is instructed to eat a low-fat diet for two weeks before the test, ending with a twelve- to fourteen-hour fast prior to collection of the blood sample.

TABLE 44-6   REFERENCE RANGES FOR HDL AND LDL CHOLESTEROL

| | HDL | | LDL |
Age (years)	Male Range mg/dL	Female Range mg/dL	Male and Female mg/dL
0–19	30–65	30–70	50–170
20–29	30–65	36–78	60–170
30–39	30–59	33–77	70–190
40–49	25–61	40–81	80–190
50–75	29–72	38–91	80–210

LDL while those without the disease should have levels of less than 180 mg/dL. Typical values for HDL and LDL are shown in Table 44-6. Levels of HDL and LDL are influenced by many factors, both genetic and environmental. It is possible to raise HDL levels through a combination of weight loss, a diet low in saturated fats, exercise, and cessation of smoking.

Blood cholesterol may be reported as total cholesterol or as total cholesterol and the HDL and LDL fractions. Cholesterol screening is used to help identify patients that are at a high risk for heart disease. See Procedure 44-8, Cholesterol Testing.

Cholesterol testing is part of a lipid profile which also evaluates lipoproteins and triglycerides to help identify patients at a high risk for heart disease. Refer back to Figure 44-10, which shows tests performed for lipid profiles on the lab form.

TRIGLYCERIDES

Triglycerides are a type of lipid found in the blood that serve as a source of energy. Fatty acids and glycerol from the diet are converted into triglycerides by the liver. When triglyceride levels in the blood are excessive, they are deposited in tissues as adipose tissue (Table 44-7). Triglycerides are transported within the bloodstream by low-density lipoproteins (LDL) and very low-density lipoproteins (VLDL).

Many factors influence serum triglyceride levels; several of these are listed in Table 44-8. Serum triglyceride

TABLE 44-7   REFERENCE VALUES FOR TRIGLYCERIDES

Age	Male	Female
Adults/Elderly	40–160 mg/dL	35–135 mg/dL
0–11 years	30–108 mg/dL	32–114 mg/dL
12–19 years	36–163 mg/dL	41–128 mg/dL

TABLE 44-8 FACTORS THAT INFLUENCE SERUM TRIGLYCERIDE LEVELS

Factors that Increase Concentration	Factors that Decrease Concentration
Pregnancy	Fasting
Estrogens, oral contraceptives	Ascorbic acid, clofibrate
Ingestion of fatty food	Uncontrolled diabetes mellitus
Ingestion of alcohol	Hyperthyroidism
Gout	Malnutrition

Patient Teaching Tip

Instruct the patient to remain on a stable diet for two weeks prior to collection of a blood specimen for triglyceride testing. The patient must also fast for the last 12 to 16 hours and avoid consumption of alcohol for 48 hours prior to the test.

concentration will rise moderately after ingesting a meal containing fat, peaking 4 to 5 hours later. Elevated concentrations of triglycerides are associated with an increased risk of coronary and vascular disease.

BLOOD UREA NITROGEN (BUN) TEST

The blood urea nitrogen (BUN) test measures the concentration of urea in blood. The amount of urea in blood reflects the metabolic function of the liver and the excretory function of the kidneys. Most renal diseases result in inadequate excretion of urea from the body; therefore, elevated concentrations of urea appear in the blood. BUN is one of several tests that are used to screen for renal disease and is especially useful for evaluating glomerular function.

Excess protein in the diet is not stored in the body but is metabolized (catalyzed) for energy production. Urea is the nitrogenous end-product of protein catabolism and is produced in the liver. It is deposited in the blood and carried to the kidneys for excretion. Surplus urea is measured as blood urea nitrogen, or BUN. Normal values of urea vary but in adults range between 8–25 mg/dL (see Table 44-9); concentrations above 100 mg/dL indicate serious impairment of renal function. Many factors other than renal disease may cause changes in urea concentration and should be considered in the process of diagnosis (Tables 44-10 and 44-11). Automated equipment is available to measure serum urea nitrogen.

TABLE 44-10 FACTORS THAT INFLUENCE SERUM UREA NITROGEN CONCENTRATION

Factors that Increase Urea	Factors that Decrease Urea
Kidney disease	Pregnancy
High-protein diet	Low-protein diet
Steroid use	Poor hepatic function
Urinary obstruction	Malnutrition
Dehydration	Overhydration
Gastrointestinal bleeding	
Enlarged prostate	
Diabetes	
Heart failure	
Shock	
High fever	
Infection	

TABLE 44-11 DRUGS THAT INFLUENCE SERUM UREA NITROGEN CONCENTRATION

Drugs that Increase Urea Concentration	Drugs that Decrease Urea Concentration
Tetracyclines	Streptomycin
Thiazide diuretics	Chloramphenicol
Allopurinol	
Aminoglycosides	
Cephalosporins	
Chloral hydrate	
Cisplatin	
Furosemide	
Guanethidine	
Indomethacin	
Nephrotoxic drugs: aspirin, methicillin, vancomycin, etc.	
Methotrexate	
Methyldopa	
Rifampin	
Spironolactone	

TABLE 44-9 UREA NITROGEN REFERENCE VALUES

	Concentration of Urea in mg/dL
Adults (slightly higher in elderly)	10–20
Infants and children	5–18
Newborns	3–12

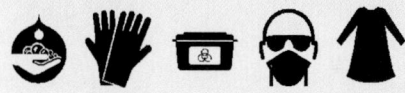

Procedure 44-1   Pregnancy Tests

STANDARD PRECAUTIONS:

PURPOSE:

To perform the enzyme immunoassay or agglutination inhibition test to detect hCG in urine to determine positive or negative pregnancy results.

EQUIPMENT/SUPPLIES:

Gloves
Hand disinfectant
Urine specimen
Stopwatch
Surface disinfectant (10% chlorine bleach solution)
Biohazard container
hCG negative urine control
hCG positive urine control
Pregnancy test kit for enzyme immunoassay (EIA) and/or the agglutination inhibition pregnancy test. Kits should include slide or test unit, dispensers, reagents, and so on.

PROCEDURE STEPS:

1. Wash hands and put on gloves.
2. Assemble all equipment and supplies.
3. Perform a modified enzyme immunoassay test for hCG following the manufacturer's instructions (if not available, skip to step 4).

   a. Obtain test kit materials, reagents, and urine specimen. Allow all materials to reach room temperature.
   b. Apply urine to the test unit using dispenser provided (Figure 44-11).
   c. Wait appropriate time interval (use stopwatch to time test).
   d. Apply first reagent/antibody to test unit using dispenser provided.
   e. Rinse unreacted reagent from unit after appropriate time.
   f. Apply color reagent/substrate to test unit.
   g. Observe color development after appropriate time interval.
   h. Stop reaction.
   i. Record results. Consult manufacturer's package insert to interpret test results (Figure 44-12).
   j. Repeat steps 3a–i using both positive and negative urine controls.
   k. Proceed to step 5.
4. Perform an agglutination inhibition test for hCG following the manufacturer's instructions.
   a. Obtain slide test kit, reagents, and urine specimen.
   b. Place one drop of antiserum in the center of the circled area of slide.

(continues)

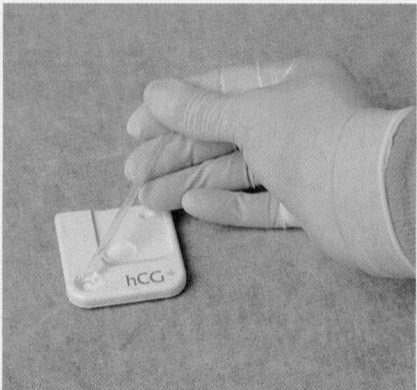

Figure 44-11   A drop of urine is placed in the urine test unit.

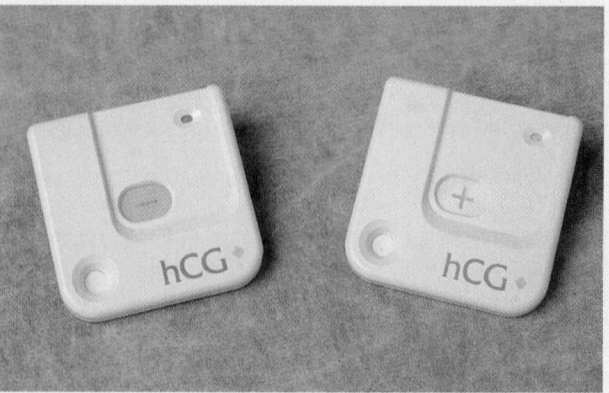

Figure 44-12   The package instructions will specify how the test is to be interpreted. The most common interpretation is with a negative sign (left) and positive sign (right).

Procedure
44-1 *(continued)*

c. Dispense one drop of urine beside the drop of antiserum.

d. Mix urine and antiserum with stirrer provided.

e. Rock the slide in a figure-eight motion for the appropriate time, usually one to two minutes (use stopwatch to measure time).

f. Apply one drop of well-mixed indicator particles to mixture on slide.

g. Mix indicator particles with antiserum-urine mixture and spread the mixture over the entire circled area of the slide using a stirrer.

h. Rock slide slowly in a figure-eight motion for the appropriate time, usually one to two minutes.

i. Observe slide for agglutination at the end of the time interval and record the results (no agglutination = positive; agglutination = negative). Refer to Figure 44-13.

j. Repeat steps 4a–i using positive and negative urine controls.

5. Disinfect reusable equipment by soaking in 10% chlorine bleach solution a minimum of ten minutes. Wash and rinse thoroughly.

6. Discard disposable supplies into biohazard container.

7. Dispose of specimen as instructed.

8. Clean work area with surface disinfectant.

9. Remove gloves and discard into biohazard container.

10. Wash hands with hand disinfectant.

11. Document procedure.

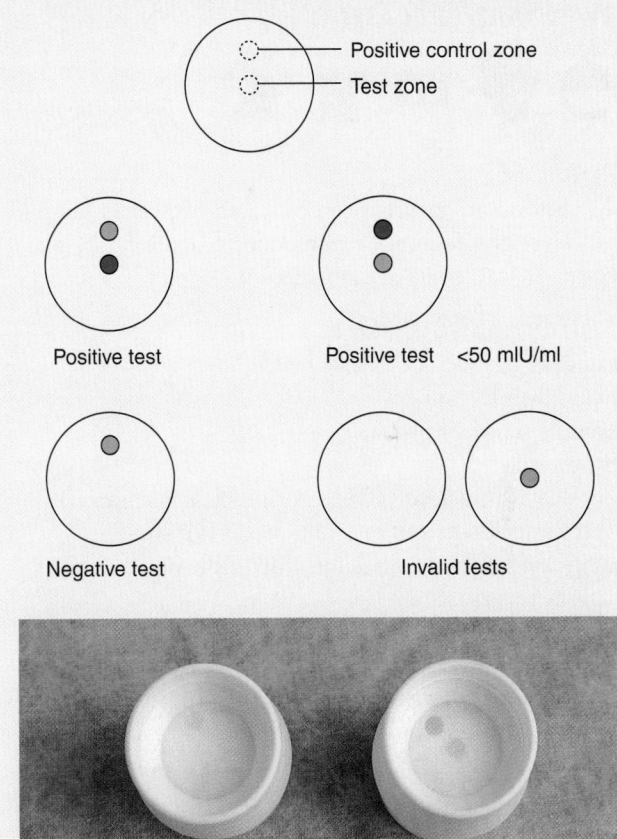

Figure 44-13 Illustration and photograph of positive and negative results with ICON II® hCG test.

Procedure 44-2   Slide Test for Infectious Mononucleosis

STANDARD PRECAUTIONS:

PURPOSE:

To perform an accurate test of serum or plasma sample to detect the presence or absence of heterophile antibodies of infectious mononucleosis.

EQUIPMENT/SUPPLIES:

Gloves
Hand disinfectant
Sample serum or plasma
Stopwatch
Surface disinfectant (10% chlorine bleach solution)
Test kit for infectious mononucleosis (kit should include instructions, slide, disposable pipettes, stirrers, reagents)
Biohazard container
NOTE: The procedure given is for Monospot® test by Meridian Diagnostics. Package insert should be consulted before the test is performed. If another kit is used, the specific manufacturer's instructions should be followed.

PROCEDURE STEPS:

1. Wash hands and put on gloves.
2. Assemble all equipment and supplies. Allow all materials to come to room temperature.
3. Place the Monospot® slide on a flat work surface.
4. Mix the reagent vials several times by inversion.
5. Fill the capillary pipette to the top mark:
   a. Place the rubber bulb on the end of the capillary pipette with the heavy black line.
   b. Insert the pipette into the vial of indicator cells.
   c. Allow the pipette to fill by capillary action to the top mark.
6. Place the index finger over the hole in the bulb and squeeze gently to dispense half the cells (10 µL) on a corner of square I of the slide (the level of the cells should now be at the lower mark on the pipette).

7. Deliver the remaining cells (10 µL) to a corner of square II.
8. Place one drop of thoroughly mixed reagent I in the center of square I.
9. Place one drop of thoroughly mixed reagent II in the center of square II.
10. Add one drop of serum to the center of each square using the disposable plastic pipette provided.
11. Use a clean applicator stick to mix reagent I with the serum using at least ten stirring motions and avoiding touching the indicator cells.
12. Blend in the indicator cells in square I with the applicator stick using no more than ten stirring motions and spread the mixture over the entire surface of the square.
13. Repeat steps 11 and 12 using reagent II in square II, using a clean applicator stick.
14. Start the stopwatch upon completion of the mixing of both squares.
15. Do not pick up or move the slide.
16. Observe for agglutination at the end of one minute (no longer) without moving the slide or picking it up.
17. Record the agglutination in each square and interpret the results. If the agglutination pattern is stronger in square I than in square II, the test is positive for the heterophile antibody of infectious mononucleosis. Any other combination of reactions is negative.
18. Record test results as positive or negative.
19. Repeat the test procedure (steps 3–18) using positive and negative control sera.
20. Discard contaminated materials into biohazard container.
21. Dispose of specimen appropriately and disinfect reusable materials by soaking in 10 percent chlorine bleach solution for at least ten minutes. Wash and rinse thoroughly.
22. Clean work area with surface disinfectant.
23. Remove gloves and discard into biohazard container.
24. Wash hands with hand disinfectant.
25. Document results.

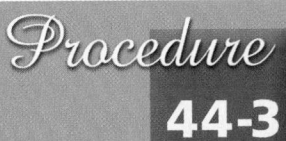 *Procedure*

44-3 **Analyzing Semen**

STANDARD PRECAUTIONS:

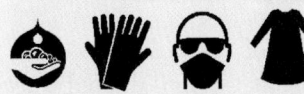

PURPOSE:
To analyze semen to determine total sperm count, percent of motility, and percent of normally formed sperm cells.

EQUIPMENT/SUPPLIES:
Gloves
10 mL graduated cylinder
pH test paper (approximate range: 6.1–10.0)
Automatic pipette
Hemacytometer
Diluting fluid
Sodium bicarbonate
Distilled water
Slides and coverslips
Petri dishes
Microscope
Coplin jar

PROCEDURE STEPS:
Macroscopic Examination

1. Wash hands and apply gloves.
2. Assemble all equipment and supplies.
3. Measure the specimen volume in a graduated cylinder.
4. Measure the pH using pH test paper.
5. Evaluate the viscosity:
   a. Upon collection, the gel-like specimen liquifies within 30 minutes and forms a translucent but viscous fluid. This is the result of the action of various enzymes contained in seminal fluid.
   b. As the specimen is poured into the cylinder, viscosity can be determined. A normal specimen will not appear watery or clumped and will pour in droplets. Some laboratories give a 0 to 4 rating to viscosity: 0 (watery) to 4 (clumped).
6. Remove gloves and wash hands.
7. Document results.

Microscopic Examination

1. Wash hands and apply gloves.
2. Assemble all equipment and supplies.
3. Mix semen specimen.
4. NOTE: Motility should be observed within 3 hours of collection.
   Place one drop of liquified specimen on a glass slide and cover with a coverslip. Examine for motility. Initially, 70–80% of the spermatozoa should be actively motile. Agglutination of sperm should be noted. Agglutination should be described by the orientation of the sperm sticking to each other: head to head, tail to tail, or other combinations.
5. Sperm count:
   a. Using automatic pipettes, make a 1:20 dilution of sample with sodium bicarbonate solution. Mix well.
   b. Fill both sides of the hemocytometer (also used for red and white cell counts) and allow the sperm to settle for 5–10 minutes.
   c. Count the sperm in 2 large WBC squares or 5 RBC squares. To calculate:
      If 5 RBC squares used:
      Count number of sperm × 1 million = sperm per milliliter
      If 2 WBC squares used:
      Count number of sperm × 100,000 = sperm per milliliter
6. Morphology: sperm are evaluated on the appearance of their tail and head in a stained preparation by a pathologist or trained technologist.
   a. Prepare two slides using the technique to make a blood smear. Do not allow the slides to air dry. Immediately immerse both slides into a coplin jar containing 95% alcohol.
   b. Deliver the slides to the pathologist to view for morphology.
7. Remove gloves and wash hands.
8. Document results.

Procedure 44-4   Obtaining Blood Specimen for Phenylketonuria (PKU) Test

STANDARD PRECAUTIONS:

PURPOSE:

To obtain a blood specimen using a PKU test card or "filter paper" to determine phenylalanine levels in newborns who are at least 3 to 4 days old.

EQUIPMENT/SUPPLIES:

Gloves
PKU filter paper test card and mailing envelope
Alcohol swabs
Cotton balls
Sterile pediatric-sized lancet
Biohazard waste container

PROCEDURE STEPS:

1. Wash hands and put on gloves.
2. Identify the infant. Explain the purpose of the test and the procedure to the parents. Discuss the feeding pattern of the infant prior to beginning the procedure. RATIONALE: Certain antibiotics, aspirin, or vomiting problems may cause false results.
3. Select and clean an appropriate puncture site (Figure 44-14).
4. Grasp the infant's foot taking care not to touch the cleansed area. Make a puncture approximately 2–3 mm deep in the infant's heel making sure the infant's lateral, or side, portion of the heel pad is used. A pediatric-sized lancet, which limits the depth of puncture, should be used (Figure 44-15). If possible, recent puncture sites should always be

avoided. Refer to Chapter 40, Phlebotomy: Venipuncture and Capillary Puncture.

5. Wipe away the first drop of blood with a cotton ball. RATIONALE: The first drop is diluted with alcohol and should not be collected for the test.
6. To collect blood for the test, press the back side of the filter paper test card against the infant's heel while exerting gentle pressure on the heel (Figure 44-16). The drop of blood should be large enough

(continues)

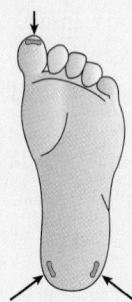

Figure 44-14   Capillary blood collection sites on an infant's foot. The most common site is the side of the infant's heel pad.

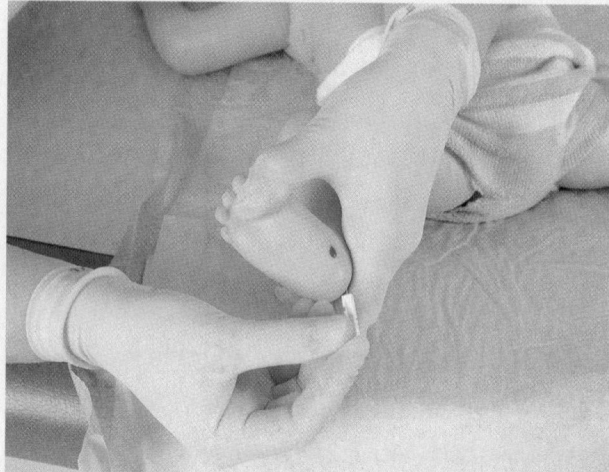

Figure 44-15   The infant's leg should be held securely with the nondominant hand and arm, while the dominant hand uses a pediatric lancet to perform a capillary heel stick.

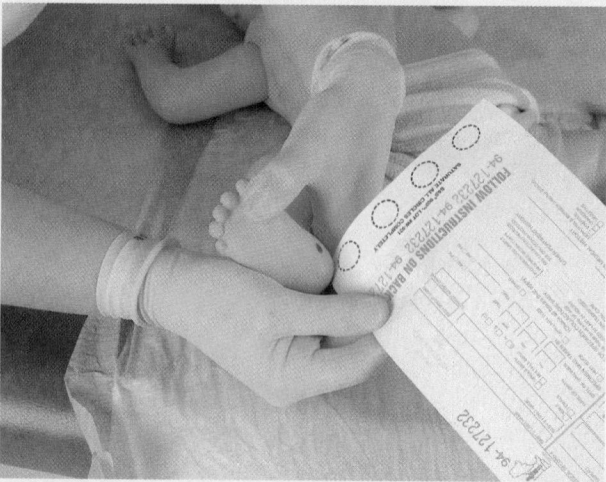

Figure 44-16   Drops of blood are transferred from the capillary puncture to all circles on the filter paper test card.

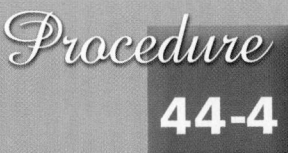

Procedure 44-4 *(continued)*

to completely fill and soak through the circle. *Do not* layer the multiple blood drops within a single circle. Completely fill all of the circles on the test card. RATIONALE: Failure to do so will require a retest.

7. Hold a cotton ball or gauze pad over the puncture and apply gentle pressure until the bleeding stops.

8. Properly dispose of all waste in biohazard container.

9. Remove the gloves and wash hands.

10. Allow the PKU test card to completely dry on a nonabsorbent surface at room temperature. This will take about two hours. If collecting more than one card, *do not* lay one card on another when drying. This could cause cross-contamination of blood between the cards.

11. After the test card is dry, put on gloves and complete the PKU test card with all patient and physician information.

12. Place the test card in the mailer envelope and send it to the laboratory within two days.

13. Remove gloves and wash hands.

14. Document the procedure in the patient's medical record. When test results are returned, these should also be placed in the patient's medical record.

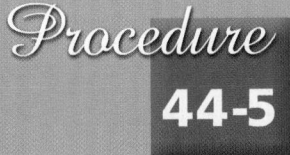

Procedure 44-5 Obtaining Urine Specimen for Phenylketonuria (PKU) Test

STANDARD PRECAUTIONS:

PURPOSE:
To obtain a urine specimen using the diaper test or the Phenistik test to determine phenylalanine levels in newborns who are at least 6 weeks old.

EQUIPMENT/SUPPLIES:
Gloves
10% ferric chloride for the diaper test
or
Phenistik for the Phenistik Method Test
Biohazard waste container

PROCEDURE STEPS:
1. Identify the infant. Verify that the infant is at least 6 weeks of age. Explain the purpose of the test and the procedure to the parents.

2. Wash hands and apply gloves.
3. Follow one of the two following procedures:
   Diaper Test:
   Apply several drops of 10% ferric chloride to a diaper that contains fresh urine. Development of a green color indicates a positive test.
   Phenistik Test:
   Dip the Phenistik test strip into fresh urine or press it against a diaper containing fresh urine. Development of a green color indicates a positive test.
4. A positive urine test should be followed up with a blood test.
5. Properly dispose of all waste in a biohazard waste container.
6. Remove gloves and wash hands.
7. Document the procedure and results in the patient's medical record.

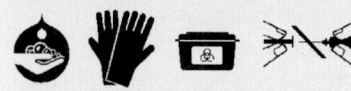

Procedure
44-6   Mantoux Test

STANDARD PRECAUTIONS:

PURPOSE:
To safely and accurately inject 0.1 mL of intermediate strength (5 TU) purified protein derivative (PPD) intradermally to present an indurated wheal to determine if an active or inactive tuberculous infection is present.

EQUIPMENT/SUPPLIES:
Gloves
Goggles
Tuberculin syringe
Short (⅜–½″) 26 or 27 gauge needle
PPD (5 TU strength)
Alcohol
Cotton balls or gauze
Sharps container
Biohazard waste container

PROCEDURE STEPS:
1. Wash hands and put on gloves and goggles.
2. Identify the patient and explain the procedure.
3. Select the site approximately 3 to 4 inches from the bend of arm on the anterior side.
4. Clean the site with alcohol and allow surface to dry. Do *not* touch the site after cleaning. If the site is touched, recleaning will be necessary.
5. Use a 1.0 mL tuberculin syringe fitted with a ⅜–½″, 26 or 27 gauge needle. Draw 0.1 mL of 5 TU strength PPD into the syringe.
   CAUTION: Be careful to draw the correct amount of PPD into the syringe.
   RATIONALE: Too much or too little PPD will cause erroneous results.
6. Hold the patient's forearm just under the chosen site to prevent movement during the injection (Figure 44-17A).
7. Slowly inject the PPD intradermally into the skin of the anterior portion of the arm to form a wheal approximately 6–10 mm (Figure 44-17B). A small amount of blood at the puncture site will not interfere with the test results. Do not rub the injection site.

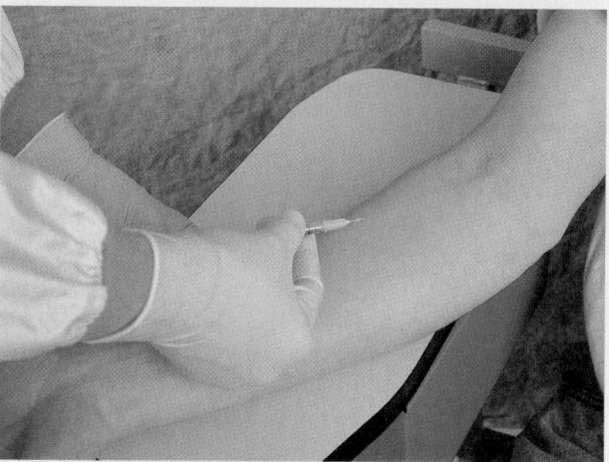

Figure 44-17A   The syringe should be at a 10 to 15 degree angle to allow the needle to penetrate the dermal layer of skin. If the injection is too deep, it will be impossible to read the wheal.

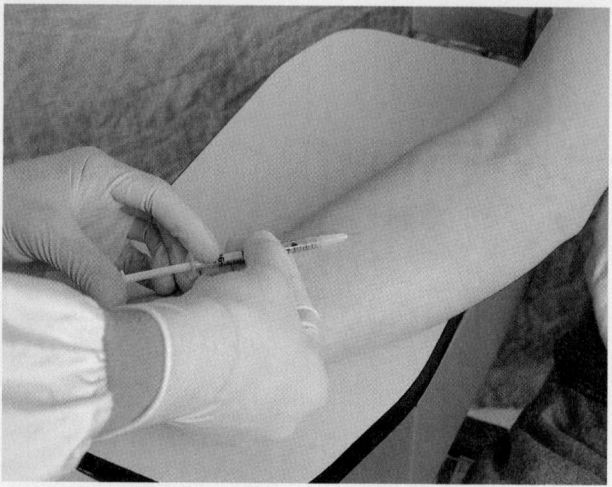

Figure 44-17B   It is important to inject the PPD slowly since absorption in this area is slow. If the medication is injected too fast, it may leak onto the skin and invalidate the test.

8. Dispose of the syringe and needle in a sharps container.
9. Watch the patient carefully and notify the physician immediately of any adverse reactions to the medication.

(continues)

Procedure

44-6 *(continued)*

10. Instruct the patient to return within 48–72 hours of the injection for test interpretation.
11. Remove gloves and wash hands.
12. Document procedure in the patient's medical record.

When patient returns for test interpretation:

13. Wash your hands and bend the patient's arm at the elbow. Inspect the injection site. Gently rub a finger across the induration to evaluate its size, then measure in millimeters (Figure 44-18).
14. Read the test according to Figure 44-19. Questionable results will require retesting. Document the test results in the patient's medical record.

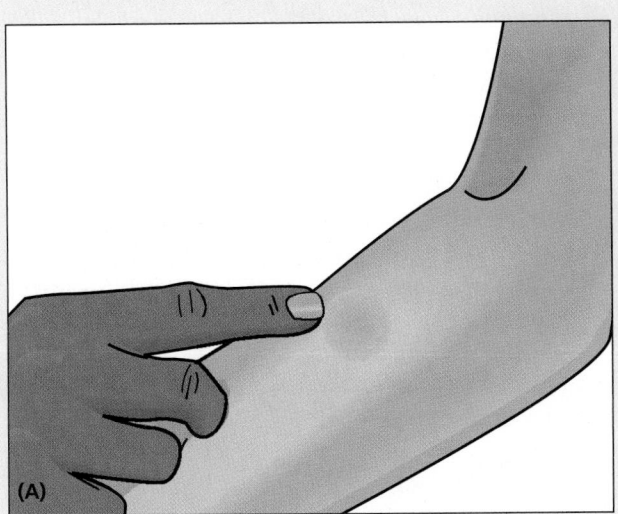
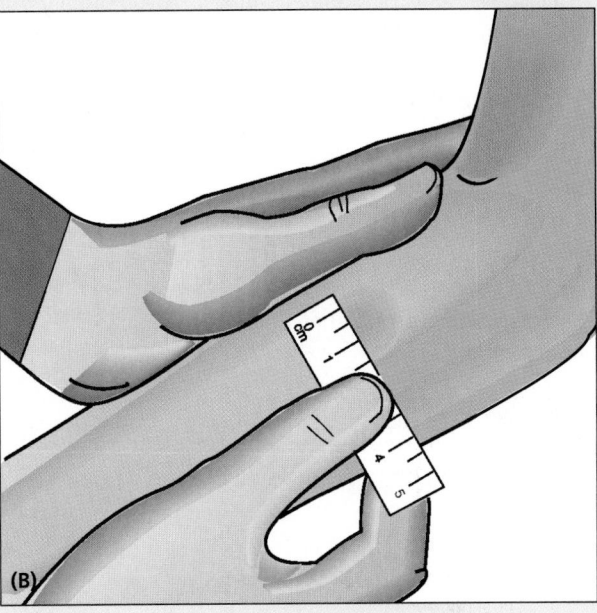

Figure 44-18 Gently inspect and measure the size of induration in response to tuberculin test 48 to 72 hours after administration.

Induration

(A) **Positive reaction** for past or present infection: 10 mm or more of induration

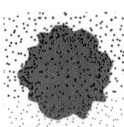

(B) **Doubtful reaction:** 5–9 mm
(In persons who are suspected to have been exposed to TB an induration of 5–9 mm is considered suspicious. Further diagnostic testing should follow.)

(C) **Negative reaction:** without induration or less than 5 mm.

Figure 44-19 The results of an induration are read as shown. A positive result should be communicated immediately to the physician.

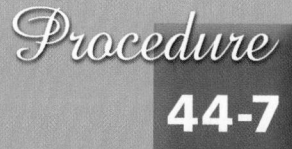

Measurement of Blood Glucose Using an Automated Analyzer

Procedure 44-7

STANDARD PRECAUTIONS:

PURPOSE:

To analyze blood glucose at timed intervals following the patient's ingestion of a standard glucose dose to aid in the diagnosis and management of diabetes or in the management of hypoglycemia.

EQUIPMENT/SUPPLIES:

Gloves
Goggles
Sterile lancet
Alcohol swabs or 70% alcohol and cotton balls
Glucose analyzer

Control solutions for glucose analyzer
Test strips for glucose analyzer
Laboratory tissue

PROCEDURE STEPS:

1. Review the manufacturer's manual for the specific glucose analyzer being used. Turn on the analyzer.
2. Clean the work area and assemble all materials and supplies.
3. Wash hands.
4. Put on gloves and goggles.
5. Record the control ranges, control lot number, and test strip lot number.
6. Perform the check test and the control test according to the manufacturer's instructions. If both tests are within range, proceed to the glucose test. Repeat both tests if either is out of acceptable range.

To perform the glucose test:

1. Remove a test strip from the bottle and replace the lid.
2. Perform a capillary puncture (refer to Chapter 40).
3. Apply a large drop of blood to the test strip.
4. Blot the test strip with tissue after the time interval recommended by the manufacturer.
5. Insert the test strip into the test chamber.
6. After the appropriate time interval has passed, read the glucose concentration.
7. Document the results.
8. Remove gloves and wash hands.
9. Properly dispose of all waste in a biohazard waste container.

Cholesterol Testing

Procedure 44-8

STANDARD PRECAUTIONS:

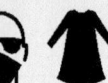

PURPOSE:

To determine the total cholesterol level to aid in diagnosis of coronary artery disease.

EQUIPMENT/SUPPLIES:

Gloves
Blood collecting equipment
Pipettes with disposable tips
Chlorine bleach
Commercial kit for manual determination of cholesterol
Controls and standards
Marking pen
Biohazard container

PROCEDURE STEPS:

1. Assemble all necessary equipment and materials.
2. Wash hands; apply gloves and goggles.
3. Obtain a blood sample from the patient, either by fingerstick or venipuncture, depending on the manufacturer's instructions (refer to Chapter 40).
4. Follow the manufacturer's instructions to perform the cholesterol test.
5. Properly dispose of all waste in biohazard container.
6. Document results.

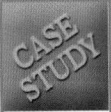

Anna Preciado, CMA, a clinical medical assistant at Doctors Lewis and King, has performed many venipunctures during her training at college, throughout her internship, and since her employment with Lewis and King. She has not, however, drawn a heelstick specimen from an infant since she was in college and even then she typically practiced on a doll. With more mothers and infants leaving the hospital so soon after the birth of the baby, she noticed that the practice is now scheduling infants for PKU tests. Anna is concerned and somewhat nervous about obtaining a PKU blood specimen from an infant.

CASE STUDY REVIEW

1. What course of action should Anna take to prepare herself for performing a procedure that she has not done in several years?
2. Should Anna simply tell the office manager or one of the physicians that she is not capable of obtaining the blood specimen?
3. Once Anna feels she is technically ready to perform the PKU blood test, what should she do to assure that the procedure goes well?

SUMMARY

A number of rapid test kits and automated methods are available for use in the ambulatory care setting by the medical assistant. For all of the tests discussed in this chapter, it is important for the medical assistant to have a basic understanding of the principles involved and the proper sampling procedures required. Safety procedures and standard precautions must be observed at all times and include the proper disposal of infectious materials and reagents. Gloves and goggles are always used when obtaining samples and while performing the actual test. Careful documentation by the medical assistant will help the physician in the diagnosis of the patient.

REVIEW QUESTIONS

Multiple Choice

1. The slide test for pregnancy and the detection of the hormone hCG is the same as the test method based on:
   a. agglutination inhibition test
   b. modified enzyme immunoassay
   c. antigen-antibody reaction
   d. color reaction
2. In addition to pregnancy, a positive hCG test can be found in the following pathological conditions *except*:
   a. ectopic pregnancy
   b. hydatidiform mole of the uterus
   c. pelvic inflammatory disease
   d. cancer of the lung
3. If a urine sample for a pregnancy test cannot be tested immediately, it may be stored in the following way for 24 hours:
   a. room temperature 25°C
   b. body temperature 37°C
   c. frozen
   d. refrigerated at 4°C
4. The kissing disease is synonymous with the disease:
   a. tuberculosis
   b. infectious mononucleosis
   c. hemolytic anemia
   d. hypoglycemia
5. Serum or blood would be the *specimen of choice* for all but the following test:
   a. ABO typing
   b. testing for the Epstein-Barr virus
   c. cholesterol
   d. hCG hormone
6. All but one of the following are correct statements about blood type:
   a. type A RBCs have A antigens on the cell
   b. type B RBCs have B antigens on the cell
   c. type O RBCs have A and B antigens on the cell
   d. type AB RBCs have both A and B antigens on the cell

7. Which of the following is a *true* statement about the Rh factor?
   a. Rh factor is a rare blood type
   b. Rh factor is present on all red blood cells
   c. Rh factor was discovered from rhesus monkeys
   d. People without the Rh factor on their RBCs have naturally occurring antibodies called anti-D in their plasma.

8. When instructing a patient in the correct collection of a specimen for semen analysis, all of the following should be considered *except*:
   a. avoid the consumption of alcohol several days before the test
   b. collection of semen into a condom is unacceptable
   c. specimen should be transported to the laboratory at 37°C within 30 minutes of collection
   d. avoid the consumption of fats several days before the test

9. Testing for phenylketonuria (PKU) is done on:
   a. newborns
   b. children 1 to 3 years of age
   c. teenagers
   d. adults over 40

10. The best site location for a tuberculin Mantoux test is:
    a. back of the hand
    b. forearm 3 to 4 inches from bend of arm
    c. ½″ above the back of the knee
    d. upper part of the arm in the deltoid muscle

11. A patient with hypoglycemia would have a blood glucose level of:
    a. 50–70 mg/dL
    b. 70–110 mg/dL
    c. 110–150 mg/dL
    d. 150–200 mg/dL

Critical Thinking

1. Why is the first-voided morning urine the preferred specimen for a pregnancy test?
2. In addition to causing infectious mononucleosis, in what other diseases has EBV been implicated?
3. Why is it necessary to repeat the seminal analysis three times over a two-month period?
4. List three reasons for a positive skin test for tuberculosis.
5. What factors may alter the results of a blood glucose measurement?

6. How can you distinguish between the diabetic and nondiabetic patient based on the results of the two-hour postprandial glucose evaluation?
7. Discuss the relationship between saturated fats and coronary artery disease.
8. What is the function of triglycerides in the body?
9. What instructions should the patient be given in preparation for a triglyceride evaluation?
10. What is the source of urea in the blood?

WEB ACTIVITIES

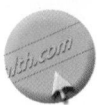

1. Search the CDC's and other government websites for information on infectious diseases such as mononucleosis.
2. Use search engines to research some of the conditions discussed in this chapter, such as phenylketonuria and tuberculosis.

REFERENCES/BIBLIOGRAPHY

Avey, A. M. (1993). TB skin testing: How to do it right. *American Journal of Nursing, 93,* 42–45.

Braun, M. M., Cote, T. R., et al. (1993). Trends in death with *tuberculosis* during the AIDS era. *Journal of the American Medical Association, 269,* 2865–2869.

Kaiser Permanente, Southern California Region. (1993). *Guide to laboratory services.* [Brochure].

Marshall, J. (1993). *Fundamental skills for the clinical laboratory professional.* Albany, NY: Delmar.

Meyers, R. (1989). *Immunology: A laboratory manual.* Dubuque, IA: Wm. C. Brown Publishers.

Pagana, K., & Pagana, T. (1992). *Mosby's diagnostic and laboratory test reference.* St. Louis: Mosby-Year Book, Inc.

Reese, R., & Betts, R. (Eds.). (1991). *A practical approach to infectious disease* (3rd ed.). Boston: Little, Brown and Co.

Reiss, B., & Evans, M. (1996). *Pharmacological aspects of nursing care* (5th ed.). Albany, NY: Delmar.

Sherris, J. C. (Ed.). (1990). *Medical microbiology: An introduction to infectious disease* (2nd ed.). New York: Elsevier Science Publishing Co.

Walters, N. J., Estridge, B. H., & Reynolds, A. P. (2000). *Basic medical laboratory techniques* (4th ed.). Albany, NY: Delmar.

Wedding, M. E., & Toenjes, S. A. (1992). *Medical laboratory procedures.* Philadelphia: F. A. Davis Company.

Wyngaarden, J. B., Smith Jr., L. H., & Bennett, J. C. (Eds.). (1992). *Cecil textbook of medicine* (19th ed.). 2 vols. Philadelphia: W. B. Saunders.

Section

IV

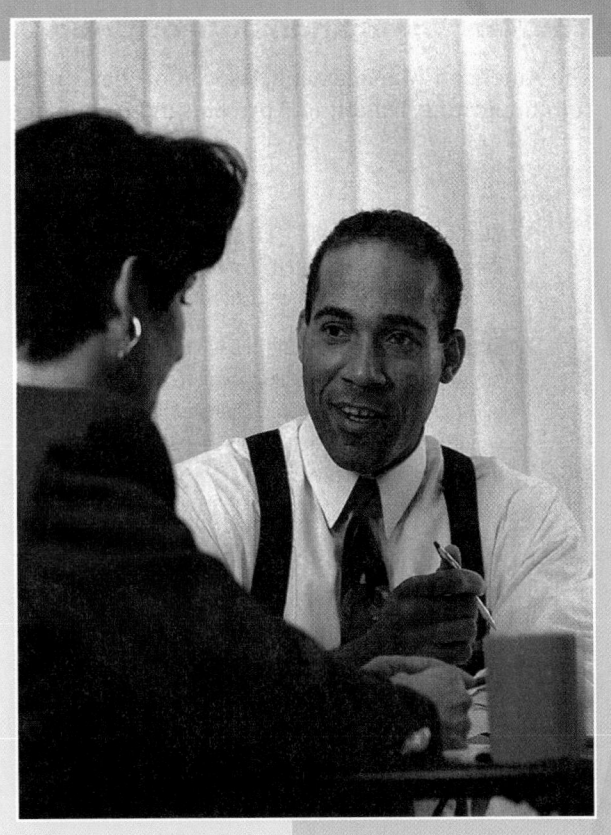

PROFESSIONAL PROCEDURES

OFFICE AND HUMAN RESOURCE MANAGEMENT

Chapter 45

THE MEDICAL ASSISTANT AS OFFICE MANAGER

KEY TERMS

Agenda
Ancillary Services
Benchmark
Benefit
Bond
Brainstorming
Charisma
Embezzle
Emulate
Externship
Fringe Benefit
"Going Bare"
Hierarchy
Internet
Itinerary
Liability
Malpractice
Marketing
Minutes
Negligence
Paradigm
Practicum
Procedures Manual
Professional Liability Insurance
Profit Sharing
Risk Management
Search Engine
Self-actualization
Shadow
Subordinate
Teamwork
Web Site
Work Statement

OUTLINE

The Medical Assistant as Manager
Qualities of a Manager
Management Styles
  People-oriented Personality
  Things-oriented Personality
  Idea-oriented Personality
  Other Management Styles
  Changing Styles for the Twenty-
    first Century
The Importance of Teamwork
  Getting the Team Started
  Using a Team to Solve a Problem
  Planning and Implementing a
    Solution
  Recognition
Supervising Personnel
  Staff Meetings
  Supporting Staff Members
Travel Arrangements
  Itinerary
Supervising Student Practicums
Time Management

Procedures Manual
  Organization of the Procedures
    Manual
  Updating and Reviewing the
    Procedures Manual
Marketing Functions
  Seminars
  Brochures
  Newsletters
  Press Releases
  Special Events
Record and Financial
  Management
  Payroll Processing
Facility and Equipment
  Management
  Inventories
  Equipment and Supplies
    Maintenance
Risk Management
Liability Coverage and Bonding

OBJECTIVES

The student should strive to meet the following performance objectives and demonstrate an understanding of the facts and principles presented in this chapter through written and oral communication.

1. Define the key terms as presented in the glossary.
2. Describe the qualities of a manager.
3. Identify three types of personalities and their management styles.
4. Differentiate between authoritarian and democratic management styles.
5. Discuss characteristics of managers and leaders.

(continues)

OBJECTIVES (continued)

6. Recall a minimum of four descriptions of managers/leaders for the new millennium.

7. List three benefits of a teamwork approach.

8. Discuss the importance of a meeting agenda.

9. List pieces of information that should be included in meeting minutes.

10. Identify the steps required to make travel arrangements.

11. Define the term itinerary and list important information the itinerary should contain.

12. List three methods of increasing productivity and efficient time management.

13. Describe the purpose of a procedures manual.

14. Describe the general concept of marketing and recall at least three marketing tools.

15. Describe the purpose and benefit of marketing.

16. Define records management, financial management, facility and equipment management, and risk management.

17. Describe the steps involved in payroll processing.

18. Describe liability coverage and what bonding means.

ROLE DELINEATION COMPONENTS

ADMINISTRATIVE

Practice Finances

- Process Payroll
- Manage renewals of business and professional insurance policies (adv)

GENERAL (TRANSDISCIPLINARY)

Professionalism

- Work as a team member
- Manage time effectively
- Prioritize and perform multiple tasks
- Facility planning (adv)
- Lead/motivate employees (adv)
- Plan and conduct staff meetings (adv)
- Train/orient employees (adv)

(continues)

SCENARIO

Marilyn Johnson has been employed by Doctors Lewis & King for the past eight years. Three years ago, she was promoted to the position of office manager when the facility added the second office for its associates in the next suburb. Marilyn has a baccalaureate degree in business administration. Her responsibilities at Doctors Lewis & King include various duties involving personnel, finances, and office efficiency.

INTRODUCTION

The skills and growing complexity of medical specialization have broadened the scope of employment options for the medical assistant. Many ambulatory health care facilities are turning to managed care as a means of ensuring consumer use of the appropriate level of care and to facilitate cost containment. This approach has created opportunity for medical assistants to advance to the office manager (OM) position based on individual facility needs.

In general, the office manager should have a minimum of an associate's degree. Large corporate settings may employ an OM and a human resource (HR) person with some crossover of responsibilities depending on the needs and organizational structure of the facility. Most HR positions require a minimum of a bachelor's degree with validation that the person has been accepted to an accredited master's program. The role of the medical assistant as a human resources manager is covered in Chapter 46.

Communication Skills
- Promote the practice through positive public relations
- Serve as liaison (adv)

Legal Concepts
- Comply with established risk management and safety procedures
- Follow employer's established policies dealing with the health care contract
- Follow federal, state, and local legal guidelines
- Maintain awareness of federal and state health care legislation and regulations
- Participate in the development and maintenance of personnel, policy, and procedure manuals
- Develop and maintain personnel, policy, and procedure manuals (adv)

Instruction
- Locate community resources and disseminate information
- Develop educational materials (adv)

Operational Functions
- Maintain supply inventory
- Evaluate and recommend equipment and supplies
- Supervise personnel (adv)
- Negotiate leases and prices for equipment and supply contracts (adv)
- Negotiate managed care contracts (adv)
- Create spreadsheets and input data (adv)
- Create databases and input data (adv)
- Perform computer searches (adv)
- Transmit and receive data and messages by Internet, e-mail, and web site (adv)

THE MEDICAL ASSISTANT AS MANAGER

The office manager of a medical office or ambulatory care facility is a role that can have vast and diverse responsibilities. In some offices, there may be one office manager and a separate human resources manager. In others, one person may be responsible for all duties that can fall under the role of office manager and human resources manager. This chapter covers the following office manager duties:

1. Create and update the office procedures manual
2. Supervise office personnel
3. Assist in improving work flow and office efficiencies (time management)
4. Prepare staff meeting agenda, conduct the meeting, and record minutes
5. Supervise the purchase, repair, and maintenance of office equipment
6. Supervise the purchase and storage of office supplies
7. Supervise the purchase and storage of controlled substances
8. Approve financial transactions and account disposition; generate financial reports as needed
9. Make travel arrangements and prepare an itinerary
10. Prepare patient education materials and arrange patient/community education workshops as needed
11. Arrange and maintain practice insurance and develop risk management strategies

QUALITIES OF A MANAGER

Qualifications of the manager will vary from office to office, however, some general requirements are common to any office setting. Attributes needed to perform as a high quality manager include but are not limited to the following:

- *People Skills.* The office manager must like people in general and enjoy working with them. Building confidence and self-esteem in others and being interested in promoting constructive relationships are essential qualities of the office manager. The ability to function as an effective team leader provides a role model for other staff members to emulate.

- *Truthfulness.* Lead by example! If an honest mistake is made, be the first to admit to the error and seek the best solution for preventing it from happening again. Respond honestly to requests. For example, two staff members ask for the same day off. The office manager will make the decision that only one member may have the day off and will review the policy manual to determine the appropriate criteria for designating who will have the request granted.

- *Fairmindedness.* It is important to always be fair with co-workers. Decisions that impact one fellow employee create a ripple effect. That is, you may have to make the same decision for another employee at another time. Decisions should be based, as much as possible, on the assumption that what is granted to one employee will be granted to others in similar situations. This approach will decrease the risk of being accused of playing favorites or being unfair.

- *Effective Communication Skills.* Communication skills include written and oral methods. The manager must communicate clearly, diplomatically, tactfully, and with respect for the feelings of others.

- *Organizational Skills.* Being organized includes being able to prioritize tasks, working efficiently and methodically. Know when and be willing to delegate tasks when others have the expertise and time to complete the task within the time lines.

- *Objectivity.* The manager must be able to view challenges without bias or prejudice. For example, when promotions are made, the office manager must be able to focus on the job description criteria and individual qualifications without introducing personal preference.

- *Problem-solving Skills.* The office manager must be a problem solver. This may include being creative and doing away with old **paradigms** and traditional approaches to solving a problem. When difficult issues arise, focus on the situation, issue, or behavior, not on the person. A discussion about solving the problem without laying blame is much more productive. Positive solutions may be more readily attained when discussing what was observed rather than what was told by someone else.

- *Technical Expertise.* The office manager should have a working knowledge of each procedure performed in the office, although it is not necessary to be the acknowledged technical expert. A good office manager is continually learning and encourages **subordinates** to seek opportunities to continue their education and advance their technical skills.

MANAGEMENT STYLES

There is a direct correlation between a person's personality and his or her management style. Three types of personalities and their management styles are discussed here (Institute for Management Excellence, 1998; Pyzdek, 1996).

People-oriented Personality

A team-oriented management style is most often used by people-oriented personalities. This personality is comfortable teaching, coaching, helping, communicating, advising, motivating, guiding, leading, and inspiring others. People-oriented managers tend to use the participatory management style by establishing and communicating the purpose and direction of the task and soliciting the participation of employees. These managers are leaders who use actions and words to show the way and inspire employees. They tend to coach by evaluating and advising, motivating and guiding.

SPOTLIGHT ON AAMA ESSENTIALS THROUGH CAAHEP

- Creating a positive office atmosphere helps to ease the patient's fears and feelings of helplessness.
- Training and supporting staff members in cultural diversity issues establishes a precedent for meeting the widely diverse needs of all patients.
- Being able to accept and offer criticism and to implement change are required attributes of a successful office manager.

Things-oriented Personality

Things-oriented personalities tend to have more process-oriented management styles. They are most comfortable with physical dexterity, building, constructing, modeling, remodeling, and working with tools or instruments. The autocratic management style is often used by this personality. Autocratic managers function on the premise that in most cases employees cannot make a contribution to their own work, and that even if they could, they wouldn't. Autocratic managers deal with this perception by using "carrots" and "sticks." The "carrot," in most cases, is a monetary incentive and the "stick" is docked pay for poor quality work.

Idea-oriented Personality

The innovation-oriented management style is most often employed by idea-oriented personalities. These managers are most comfortable working with ideas and information. Management by wandering around (MBWA) is often used by them to collect information that can then be used to generate new ideas and approaches to doing the job. MBWA users are observant and ask questions to get at the problem. Once the problem has been clearly identified they enjoy research, data collection, and then brainstorming sessions to arrive at solutions.

Other Management Styles

In some organizations the **hierarchy** is viewed as a "chain-of-command." The person in the topmost position on the organizational chart is the ultimate authority. This person may delegate authority to a subordinate who may, in turn, delegate authority to positions further down in the hierarchy. But these managers must possess complete knowledge of the work being done by their subordinates. This management style is often referred to as the authoritarian style. The manager holds all authority and responsibility and communicates from the top of the hierarchy down.

In the democratic management style, the person at the top of the organization holds final responsibility but also delegates authority to others by developing a shared vision of the goals and objectives of the organization. Communication is very active, flowing upward to higher authorities and downward to subordinates.

Changing Styles for the Twenty-first Century

Today, managers are often seen as administrators rather than leaders. An administrator is one who executes, directs, or manages affairs. A leader, on the other hand, is a person who shows the way or guides. As we move into the twenty-first century, office managers will be called upon to be leaders and possess leadership qualities.

A good leader is one who can inspire others by example. In the medical office setting, a leader has the ability to inspire employees in a direction that benefits the entire facility. A leader excels in achieving goals and therefore influences others to be goal setters and achievers as well. Managers become leaders by demonstrating on a daily basis that they believe in their vision for the organization. Leaders have **charisma**, that is, they motivate others and inspire allegiance and devotion. Table 45-1 contrasts some management and leadership characteristics. Table 45-2 contains suggested management techniques and a brief description of the managers and leaders of the new millennium. Notice the importance of leadership characteristics as opposed to management characteristics in these descriptions.

TABLE 45-1	MANAGEMENT AND LEADERSHIP CHARACTERISTICS
Management Characteristics	**Leadership Characteristics**
Punishment	Reward
Demands respect	Invites speaking out
Drill sergeant	Motivator
Limits and defines	Empowers
Imposes discipline	Values creativity
Bottom line	Vision
Control	Change
Hierarchy	Network
Rigid	Flexible
Automatic annual raises	Pay for performance
Dominates	Facilitates
Issues orders	Acts as role model
Demands unquestioning obedience	Coaches and mentors others
Knows all the answers	Asks the right questions
Not interested in new answers	Seeks to learn and draw out new ideas

Source: The Institute for Management Excellence. (1996, October). Managers vs. leaders. *Management vs. Leadership* [On-line]. Available: www.itstime.com/oct96b.htm.

THE IMPORTANCE OF TEAMWORK

The use of **teamwork** to improve the efficiency of the office may at first seem incongruent to your desire to improve office efficiency, since it seems that several people are now involved in solving a problem that you the manager should solve and explain. Teamwork builds morale and actually results in getting more accomplished with the resources you have because the team members

TABLE 45-2	DESCRIPTIONS OF MANAGERS AND LEADERS
Management by Coaching and Development (MBCD)	Managers see themselves primarily as employee trainers.
Management by Competitive Edge (MBCE)	Individuals and groups within the organization compete against one another to see who can achieve the best results.
Management by Decision Models (MBDM)	Decisions are based on projections generated by artificially constructed situations.
Management by Exception (MBE)	Managers delegate as much responsibility and activity as possible to those below them, stepping in only when absolutely necessary.
Management by Performance (MBP)	Managers seek quality levels of performance through motivation and employee relations.
Management by Styles (MBS)	Managers adjust their approaches to meet situational needs.
Management by Walking Around (MBWA)	Managers walk around the company, getting a "feel" for people and operations; stopping to talk and to listen.
Management by Work Simplification (MBWS)	Managers constantly seek ways to simplify processes and reduce expenses.

Source: The Institute for Management Excellence. (1996, October). Management styles. *Management vs. Leadership* [On-line]. Available: www.itstime.com/oct96.htm.

develop ownership of the solution to a problem and want to make it work. When it works, it flatters them and builds their esteem.

Efficiency of a team results from the collective working together to plan how to "work smarter" and how to dovetail tasks and support each other so that wasted effort is avoided. In order to achieve all of these things, a team must not only be given the responsibility and the authority to plan and execute their plan to solve a problem, but they must know your expectations for them. Sometimes this means that you, the office manager, must stick your neck out for them. They will reward you handsomely for doing so.

Getting the Team Started

A successful teamwork approach is not a mysterious event that just happens, it is the result of clear vision, specific goals, and a well-planned strategy on the part of the team leader. For teamwork to be successful, individual team members must understand and support the specifics of the problem they are being asked to solve. This is probably the most significant task of the team leader or the office manager. It is helpful in taking this important step to let the team develop its own work statement, for in this way they assume ownership of the goals and objectives you want them to achieve. The work statement frequently outlines specific tasks and their sequential order of accomplishment. Its purpose is to ensure that everyone is working toward the team goals and objectives.

A major pitfall at this stage may be diverse opinions which can lead to a work statement that does not meet the manager's goals and objectives for the team. It is your job as office manager to try to direct the team back to what you want them to work on without undermining their team spirit. Take care at this stage not to begin making assignments or to let team members start solving the problem until the work statement is complete. Under some circumstances it may be necessary for you, the office manager, to exercise your authority in defining the work statement, but be careful, as this approach could harm the team's collective spirit.

The next step in team development is to establish a timetable for achieving results and identifying the standards that must be maintained. Without a timetable a team feels no sense of urgency and tends to lose direction. You also have to paint a clear picture of the standards that must be maintained as you attempt to solve the problem. You should let the team develop both the standards as well as the timetable, but with your leadership and support.

Using a Team to Solve a Problem

Problem solution is the next step in team development. Some people call this stage brainstorming a solution.

Brainstorming is fun, but unless it is controlled by the leader, it will bog down into needless arguments and hurt feelings. In a successful brainstorming session everyone should feel free to contribute solutions to the problem without any consideration for practicality or flaws in the proposal. Only after everyone has had a chance to speak are the solutions looked at in terms of practicality and for technical correctness. At this point the team should not look at what is wrong with the solution, but what needs to be done to make it a workable solution.

Prioritization of the solutions comes next. In order to do this it is helpful to assign scores for impact on solving the problem and for changeability, or the difficulty in implementing a particular solution in your office environment. The result will be a list of solutions to the problem in descending order from the greatest impact on the problem with the least cost or difficulty in implementation. Do a needs assessment, remove oneself from the issue, and look at it from a different perspective. Benchmark (compare) your facility to other facilities and organizations to see how they accomplish tasks, compensate employees, and so on.

Planning and Implementing a Solution

The team should work out a detailed plan for implementation of the solution selected, including a schedule. Assignments should be made, resources of equipment and funds available to the team should be defined, and any remaining problems assigned to subteams that will function just as the primary team did in solving them. The team should continue to meet to discuss progress and to resolve additional problems that may occur.

Recognition

A successful team should not be disbanded until it is acknowledged for its efforts and physical recognition is given in the case of an important problem that was solved. In some cases, a dinner or luncheon is in order. This is the most important phase of team development, as it is responsible for developing a team spirit or sense of self-actualization within the organization. Once this spirit is implanted into an organization, it becomes infectious.

SUPERVISING PERSONNEL

Creating an atmosphere in which open and honest communication can take place is critical to supervising personnel. This type of communication may be encouraged through the establishment of regular staff meetings, with each staff member sharing ideas for improvement and areas of concern. Eliciting the help of others in problem-solving strategies will promote harmony (Figure 45-1).

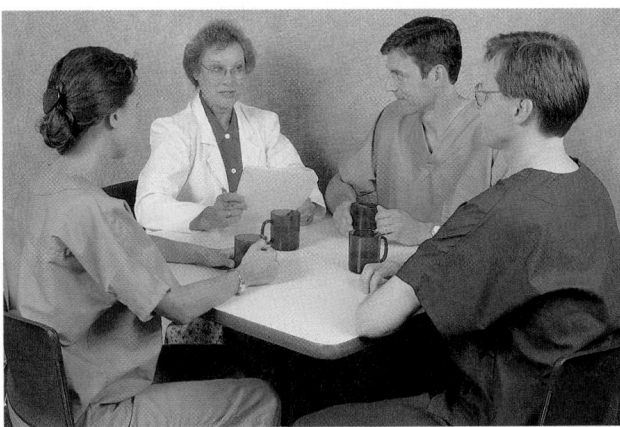

Figure 45-1 Consistently scheduled staff meetings can help office managers understand staff concerns as well as allow managers to communicate with the staff. This personal communication can help promote harmony among the health care team.

Staff Meetings

The office manager usually initiates the staff meeting idea and should officiate at such meetings. Failure of the office manager to be present may convey a message that the meeting is an event not worthy of attention. It is important that the office manager be familiar with basic parliamentary procedures. The purchase of books such as *Robert's Rules of Order* or *Parliamentary Procedure at a Glance* is an excellent investment.

Successful staff meetings are announced well in advance or on established time lines to enable the majority of the office personnel to attend. An **agenda** identifying the subjects to be covered during a given meeting should be issued prior to the meeting so that each attendee arrives prepared with input and/or questions relevant to the topics. Procedure 45-1 outlines the procedural steps for creating a meeting agenda. Figure 45-2 is a sample agenda. Each meeting should end with opportunity for nonagenda items to be discussed or suggested for inclusion in the next meeting. The meeting should have a fixed time to end.

A written record in the form of **minutes** should be maintained and sent to all team members regardless of whether they attended the meeting. This policy will keep all members informed about policy changes and decisions that impact the office operations. The minutes also trigger a reminder for any new procedures or revisions to be made in the procedures manual. See Chapter 15 for additional information related to agendas and minutes.

The first paragraph of the minutes should contain the following pieces of information:

- Kind of meeting (scheduled staff meeting, special meeting)

AGENDA

STAFF MEETING Wednesday, February 16, 2002
2:00 PM — Conference Room

1. Read and approve minutes of last meeting

2. Reports
   A. Satellite facility — Marilyn Johnson
   B. Patient flow — Joe Guerrero
   C.

3. Discussion of new telephone system

4. Unfinished Business
   A. Review new procedure manual pages
   B.

5. New Business
   A. Appoint committee for design of new marketing brochure
   B.

6. Open discussion and/or topics for next meeting's agenda

7. Set next meeting time

8. Adjourn

Figure 45-2 Sample meeting agenda.

- Name of the organization (Doctors Lewis & King)
- Date, time, and place of the meeting
- Names of those attending and who was the chair of the meeting
- Approval of previous minutes

The following paragraphs should address each of the agenda topics and include a brief summary of discussions, actions taken, name of person making any motions, the exact wording of the motion, and whether the motion was approved.

In addition to recording action plans under each agenda topic, it is desirable to summarize all action items agreed to in the meeting in one section of the minutes. This will facilitate easy access to information at a later date should it be required.

The last paragraph should include the date, time, and place of the next meeting and the hour of adjournment for this meeting. The person preparing the minutes should always sign them. A copy of the minutes should always be maintained in a book for easy reference.

Supporting Staff Members

The office manager may also be responsible for the following roles related to supporting staff employees. In large offices or clinics some of these responsibilities may be delegated to the human resources manager and are more fully covered in Chapter 46.

- Interview, hire, and terminate employees as delegated by the physician(s)/employer.

- Supervise or personally train employees. These responsibilities apply to new staff members as well as to updating current staff.

- Make weekly work schedules, vacation schedules, and determine how sick days will be covered effectively.

- Provide adequate staffing for employee absences.

- Establish probation periods within the legal boundaries of the employer and conduct performance evaluations as delegated by the physician(s)/employer.

- Establish increases and changes in the benefit package. These responsibilities should always be discussed with the physician(s)/employer first to be sure that the office manager is acting within the guidelines and scope of tasks delegated to that position.

TRAVEL ARRANGEMENTS

The office manager may be asked to make travel arrangements for physicians going on vacation or to conventions, symposiums, or out-of-town seminars and continuing medical education (CME) courses. If the physicians do a fair amount of travel or if they live in a metropolitan area, they may utilize the services of a travel agent. Attention to detail is extremely important in preventing travel disruptions.

Read carefully the instructions for completing registration forms, complete them, and mail them as quickly as possible to secure reservations to conventions, etc. Next make hotel and travel arrangements. General information regarding the physician's travel preferences should be maintained in a file folder and be referred to when making travel arrangements. Helpful information to maintain in this file includes:

- Name of travel agents used in the past (ranked by reputation and recommendation)

- Physician's or office credit card numbers

- Car rental preference
- Preferred airline, class of travel, seating choice
- Hotel/motel accommodations (bed size, suite, studio, connecting rooms, price range, amenities)
- Shuttle service

Next, contact the travel agent and identify the destination, date and time for departure and return, number traveling in party, and seating preference. A travel agent can also assist with rental car and hotel accommodations if needed. Take your time and pay attention to detail. When tickets are received, always check to see that all departure and arrival times match what is needed and that a confirmation number has been provided for car rentals and hotel arrangements. Procedure 45-2 outlines the procedural steps involved in making travel arrangements through a travel agent.

The Internet may be used to search for the lowest cost air, auto, and lodging reservations. The procedures do not require extensive knowledge of travel and airline reservation protocols. Searching for information on the **Internet** requires the use of a search engine if you do not already have a list of favorite travel **web sites**. A **search engine** is a special computer program available through your Internet service provider. With a search engine, you enter only the subject of your search and the engine will provide a list of web sites related to your subject. For example, if you are making travel arrangements you might access a search engine such as Lycos and key in the subject "air fares." The engine will return either a list of web sites or ask you to further refine your subject with suggestions such as cheap air fares, international travel, etc. Once you have refined your search, you may have choices such as Only-Travel. com, Expedia.com, or Priceline.com. Select the appropriate web site and follow its instructions.

Priceline.com and similar web sites are services that allow you to name the price you want to pay; Priceline finds a major airline willing to release seats on flights where they have unsold space. You need to have a reasonable idea of the price of the service you are trying to purchase; unreasonably low bids will just waste your time and effort. Procedure 45-3 outlines the steps for making travel arrangements via the Internet.

Itinerary

If you have utilized a travel agent in making the travel arrangements the agency will most likely provide several copies of the **itinerary**. An itinerary is a detailed plan for a proposed trip. The office should maintain one copy of the itinerary in case the physician must be reached for emergencies. The physician should have one copy to carry with him or her and a copy to leave with family members.

TRAVEL ITINERARY

James Whitney, MD
Inner City Health Care
400 Inner City Way
Seattle, WA 98400

Sept 15, 20--   INVOICE: 880133795

29 Sept 20-Friday
USAIR   6:30   Coach Class   Equip-Boeing 757 Jet
LV: Seattle   11:55P   Nonstop   Miles-2125   Confirmed
AR: Pittsburgh   7:23A   Elapsed time-4:28   Arrival Date-30Sept
                                             Seat-31C

30 Sept-Saturday
Alamo   1 Compact 2/4 DR   Drop-101CT   Confirmed
Pickup-Pittsburgh   Pittsburgh Airport   Chg-USD .00
Rate-   59.98   Baserate   Guaranteed   Extra Hr 10.00-UN
Phone-412-472-5060
                             Confirmation-1870649

01 Oct 20-Sunday
USAIR   1419 Coach Class   Equip-Boeing 737 Jet
LV: Pittsburgh   3:05P   Nonstop   Miles-2125   Confirmed
AR: Seattle   5:27P   Elapsed time-5:22
Lunch   Seat-20A

Ticket Number/s:
Whitney/James   35709334923   BA Card   461.00
      Air Transportation   416.36   Tax   44.64   TOTAL   461.00
                                              Sub Total   461.00
                                              Credit Card Payment   461.00-
                                              Amount Due   0.00

TICKET IS NON REFUNDABLE. TRIP INSURANCE IS AVAILABLE. RECONFIRM ALL FLTS 24 HRS PRIOR TO DEPARTURE

Figure 45-3 Sample travel itinerary.

You may need to develop the itinerary if you have made the travel arrangements via computer. Figure 45-3 shows a sample travel itinerary.

Important information to be included on any itinerary includes:

- Air travel: departure and arrival date and time, meals, airline name and telephone number, airport

- Car rental: name of provider, telephone number, confirmation number

- Hotel/motel: name, confirmation number, dates, telephone number

- Meeting location: name, address, room number, telephone number

SUPERVISING STUDENT PRACTICUMS

The student **practicum** is a transitional stage that provides opportunity for the student to apply theory learned in the classroom to a health care setting through practical, hands-on experience. Institutions accredited by the Committee on Accreditation of Allied Health Education Programs (CAAHEP) call this period **externship**. Some institutions may use the term *internship* and still others may operate through a co-operative education program. The number of hours for the practicum are predetermined along with criteria for site selection and tasks performed by the student.

The office manager should schedule an information interview with the extern student before the practicum begins. During this time a discussion of the expectations of the office manager and the extern may be established. A tour of the facility and introductions to key personnel aids the extern in feeling more comfortable the first day of "work."

Since the extern will be writing in medical records where correct spelling is mandatory or may be scheduling appointments and must write telephone numbers without transposition, some pretesting may be offered. By giving a spelling test of ten commonly used medical terms or verbally stating five telephone numbers for the extern to write down, an immediate evaluation is attained.

The office manager should directly supervise or identify someone else to supervise the extern. During the first few days of the practicum, the extern may simply **shadow** the supervisor, learning the routine, physician preference, and protocols for that particular office. As the extern begins to feel comfortable in the new environment, minimal tasks should be assigned. Based on the extern's ability to follow directions and perform tasks, increased skill-level tasks may be added.

The supervisor will supervise and evaluate the extern's progress; schedule activities that will provide experience in all aspects of medical assisting, including administrative, clinical, and laboratory procedures; maintain accurate records of attendance and hours "worked"; and communicate the extern's progress to the medical assisting supervisor from the educational institution. Procedure 45-4 provides steps for supervising a student practicum.

When working with externs, it is important to remember that they still have much to learn. When you take time to explain each step and to provide the rationale for each, students will learn more quickly. Demonstrating new and/or different techniques and approaches helps students by providing them with options that they may find more comfortable.

Remember that this type of learning is very stressful. The extern is not yet accustomed to communication with a "real" patient, let alone working with a physician. Your role as office manager is to reduce as much stress as possible for everyone concerned. Introduce the extern to the patient and ask the patient's permission to allow the student to perform a procedure. Many patients will be very tolerant when they realize the circumstances and will be quite cooperative.

TIME MANAGEMENT

Because medical office managers are responsible for numerous tasks and may experience many interruptions during the course of the day, it is important that they become disciplined and work well independently as well as with others. By focusing and pinpointing specific goals, which in turn may be translated into tasks to be completed during the workday, much can be accomplished.

Many office managers find it helpful to develop a "To Do" list on which tasks to be accomplished are listed. These tasks may be prioritized or simply listed as they come to mind or occur during the day. As each task is completed, it is crossed off. At the end of the day a sense of accomplishment is the reward for a clean list. Any tasks not yet completed may be prioritized and transferred to the next day's "To Do" list.

As much as possible, try to handle a paper only once. Read it, decide what action needs to be taken, and complete it. When responding to telephone calls, try also to bring closure to the call so that it is not necessary to make another call.

Do not procrastinate. Complete tasks as they arise whenever possible. Sometimes it takes longer to list a task on the "To Do" list and then have to rethink the solution than to just do it.

PROCEDURES MANUAL

The **procedures manual** provides detailed information relative to the performance of tasks within the facility in which one is employed. Each procedures manual should be designed for that specific office setting and should satisfy its requirements.

The procedures manual serves as a guide to the employee assigned a specific task and may also be useful in evaluating the employee's performance. If a temporary employee is assigned the task, the procedures manual will be invaluable in assuring that each procedure is completed as outlined.

The physician(s) and the office manager should have copies of the procedures manual and it should also be accessible to all employees. Copies of individual sections may be given to the employee responsible for the task; the employee should be instructed to follow these guidelines and told that they may be used as employee evaluation tools.

Organization of the Procedures Manual

It is best to use a loose-leaf binder with separator pages denoting each procedure. Many office managers find it helpful to divide the binder into administrative and clini-

Administrative Section	Clinical Section
Personnel Management	Physical Examinations
Communication	Infection Control
(oral and written)	Collecting Specimens
Patient Scheduling	Laboratory Procedures
Records Management	Surgical Asepsis
Financial Management	Emergencies
Facility and Equipment	
Management	

Figure 45-4 Many offices find that dividing the procedures manual into tabbed sections helps organize the material. A table of contents for the manual can also help locate information easily.

cal sections with subdivisions for each primary task performed (Figure 45-4).

To facilitate using the procedures manual, a consistent format should be developed and used throughout the manual. Each procedure should be a step-by-step outline or list of steps to be taken to complete a task as desired in that facility. Providing the rationale for a step, when appropriate, enhances the learning process, especially for new staff members. Procedure 45-5 provides steps for developing and maintaining a procedures manual.

Updating and Reviewing the Procedures Manual

When new procedures are added to the office routine, a new procedure page should be developed immediately. The new page is then useful as an educational tool or job aid while team members are learning new techniques.

An annual page-by-page review should be done to ascertain if each procedure is still being used and assure that each page is correct in each detail and satisfies all criteria established by the staff personnel. This contributes to an efficient office and gives all employees a sense of pride and satisfaction that they are performing within the scope of their training and to their greatest potential. The procedures manual should be reviewed by personnel performing the various tasks and their suggestions should be evaluated and incorporated into the revisions when appropriate. All new procedure pages and revisions should be dated (Rev. 02/15/02).

MARKETING FUNCTIONS

Effective communication skills are essential in the management of the ambulatory care setting. These skills are used by the office manager inside the ambulatory care setting to establish friendly, professional relationships with colleagues and patients. Communication is just as critical when relating to external audiences: other organizations, potential new patients, and community members. Developing relationships outside the office is often called marketing, a concept that office managers may utilize to enhance the image and visibility of an ambulatory care setting while also providing benefits to patients, potential patients, and the neighboring community.

In its broadest sense, **marketing** can be defined as the process by which the provider of services makes the consumer aware of the scope and quality of these services. While marketing is a tool traditionally used by for-profit organizations to promote and sell products and services, it has become increasingly acceptable among health care organizations, whether they are for- or not-for-profit.

Marketing functions and materials are diverse and can include seminars and workshops, patient education brochures, brochures that describe the ambulatory care setting and its scope of services, newsletters, press releases, and special events such as open houses or participation in community health care events. Depending on the size and resources of the medical office, the manager may choose to use all or some of these tools (Figure 45-5).

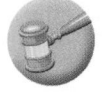 When producing written material and organizing events, it is essential that ethical guidelines be respected at all times. Marketing tools should be appropriate, in good taste, and designed to quietly enhance the reputation of the office. Cultural issues should always be considered. For example, patient education brochures for a practice with many Spanish-speaking patients should be produced in bilingual editions, with English on one side and Spanish on the other. Legal issues are important as well; when presenting material of a medical nature, it is extremely important that information be accurate and up-to-date.

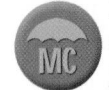 Effective marketing is a valuable tool for the office manager, especially as managed care calls on all health care professionals to become more competitive in order to survive. Marketing can increase visibility and credibility. The effective manager will enlist the talents and skills of the entire team in developing a marketing plan.

Seminars

As consumers become increasingly aware of lifestyle choices, they look to health care professionals for information and guidance. Seminars and workshops are useful vehicles for presenting health-related information; while expert advice can be given, there is also the opportunity for patients and health care professionals to interact.

Marketing Tool	Potential Uses and Value
Seminars	Can educate patients and provide good will in the community. All staff—administrative and clinical—can work as a team to organize, publicize, and deliver the seminars.
Brochures	Brochures are typically of two types: patient education brochures and brochures on office services. Can be simple 8 1/2" x 11" fact sheets, with text only, or more elaborate brochures folded to 4" x 9" that incorporate both text and graphics or photos. Both types of brochures are informative for patients and present a professional image of the ambulatory care setting.
Newsletters	Newsletters can be produced on a biannual or quarterly basis and can form the nucleus of a marketing program. Because they are versatile tools, they can include a wide range of information from health-related articles to staff introductions to insurance updates. They should be sent to individuals on the office's mailing list and be available in the reception area.
Press Releases	Periodic press releases on new equipment, new staff, and expanded or remodeled office space can be a vital link to the local community.
Special Events	Special events are an effective way to join with other community organizations to promote wellness. They can include participation in health fairs, cosponsorship of a charity event, or an open house on the premises to acquaint the community with new services or equipment.

Figure 45-5   Marketing tools and their use in a medical environment.

Seminars can be organized to meet patient and community needs. Some popular seminar topics include hypertension, diabetes, eating disorders, and exercise and weight management programs.

No matter what the topic area, the content should be oriented to the lay person's level of understanding, with a focused message and a delivery designed to maintain attention. Interactive seminars, which encourage audience participation, can be productive and enjoyable. Audiovisuals, such as projected slides, will provide visual reinforcement. Handouts, either from professional organizations or those produced by office staff, can elaborate on seminar content and help the participant review and remember what was said.

Brochures

Despite the promise of a paperless society, brochures continue to be valuable sources of information. In the health care setting, patients welcome a rack of brochures as a source of current, accurate background on medical issues. New patients also find that a brochure on office services will answer many questions about the practice, its philosophy, and its scope of services, and provide physician profiles.

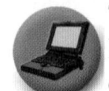Today, it is possible to produce a professional-looking brochure in the office using one of the computer programs that integrate text and graphics. If a brochure is produced in-house, it is important to consider writing, design, and production. Writing should be clear, to the point, and grammatically correct. Always proofread carefully before printing. Design should be kept simple; while computer programs offer sophisticated options, these are best left to experienced designers. Avoid the use of too many typefaces; choose a typeface and size for readability, and, if using artwork or photography, consider its reproduction qualities. Typically, brochures will be printed in one or two colors. Black or another dark ink is best for readability.

Often, a local printer will be able to advise the office manager on how to prepare a brochure or handout for printing. The simplest handouts can be quick-copied (a high-speed photocopy) on a white or lightly colored or textured stock. After printing, brochures should be made accessible to patients and other visitors in a rack or neatly arranged in piles (Figure 45-6). Occasionally, a brochure will be mailed; one that folds to 4" × 9" will fit into a standard #10 business envelope.

Patient Education Brochures. Like seminars, patient education brochures can address a variety of topics, including hypertension, diabetes, eating disorders, and exercise and weight management programs. When writing these brochures, always research material carefully, request permission for copyrighted materials, and present the information in a manner that is accessible to your patient population.

Office Brochures. A brochure on the practice can provide a wide range of information and will orient the new patient to the practice. One way to determine what information to include is to develop a list of frequently asked patient questions. Once this list is compiled, it can serve as the beginning of the brochure outline. Issues to consider might include:

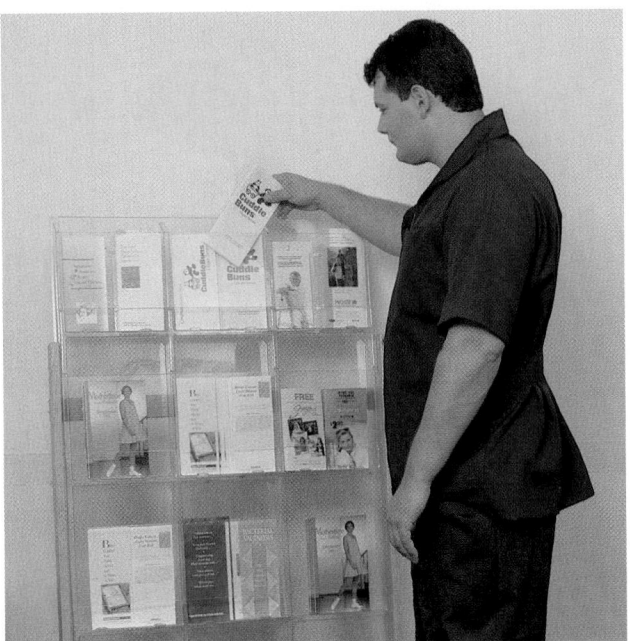

Figure 45-6   Brochures and handouts should be accessible and inviting to patients and office visitors.

- Brief history of the practice
- Brief resumes or credentials of physicians
- Philosophy of the practice
- Scope of services
- How to reach the practice in case of emergency
- Insurances accepted
- Rights of patients
- Policies regarding the release of information
- Scheduling information: How to schedule an appointment, cancellation policies
- Amenities on the premises such as parking, pharmacy, lab
- Location, map if necessary, and location of satellite offices

Newsletters

Newsletters are effective communication tools because they encourage regular contact with patients and other readers. Newsletters are a versatile medium, too; they can contain patient education articles, updates on staff changes, awards, information on insurance carriers, calendars of events, even recipes that are consistent with a healthful lifestyle.

Most newsletters can be written and produced in the office. Like brochures, they should be simple in design and format. An additional factor in newsletter production is mailing; an up-to-date database must be maintained, postal regulations must be followed, and the costs of mailing considered.

Press Releases

Press releases are simple, inexpensive marketing tools. Use them to announce new staff, promote a new service, or publicize a series of seminars. If a professional, courteous relationship is developed with the local press, most will be happy to receive and publish releases. When writing releases, always follow proper format, which includes a date of release, a contact person's name and telephone number, and a short headline. Releases are best kept to one double-spaced typed page. At the end of the release, type "30" or a number sign (#). Maintain an active list of local newspapers and editors' names so that you can mail or fax the release to the appropriate editor.

Special Events

While they can be time-consuming to organize and participate in, special events are rewarding, for they present an opportunity to interact with the community. They have high visibility, for often a group of community organizations will collaborate to cosponsor an event such as a walk-a-thon, blood pressure clinic, health fair for seniors, or wellness day for children and families. Sponsorship can be as simple as a donation to the cause; other times, staffing a booth or offering a service such as blood pressure checks is appropriate.

Like all marketing efforts, special events require organizational skills and teamwork, but they often result in heightened communication with the community and provide an educational service to patients and their families.

RECORD AND FINANCIAL MANAGEMENT

Physicians entrust a great deal of responsibility to their medical office managers. The daily payments received through the mail and office visits must be processed and prepared for banking. Office expenses must be processed and paid in a timely fashion to capitalize on any discounts available. Employee requirements and records such as Social Security records, Withholding Allowance Certificates (W-4 forms) (Figure 45-7) indicating the number of exemptions claimed, and Employment Eligibility Verification Forms (I-9) ensuring that all persons employed are either United States citizens, lawfully admitted aliens, or aliens authorized to work in the United States must be completed and filed with the appropriate federal agencies. Also, state and local tax records must be filed and maintained for each employee.

Form W-4 (2000)

Purpose. Complete Form W-4 so your employer can withhold the correct Federal income tax from your pay. Because your tax situation may change, you may want to refigure your withholding each year.

Exemption from withholding. If you are exempt, complete only lines 1, 2, 3, 4, and 7, and sign the form to validate it. Your exemption for 2000 expires February 16, 2001.

Note: *You cannot claim exemption from withholding if (1) your income exceeds $700 and includes more than $250 of unearned income (e.g., interest and dividends) and (2) another person can claim you as a dependent on their tax return.*

Basic instructions. If you are not exempt, complete the **Personal Allowances Worksheet** below. The worksheets on page 2 adjust your withholding allowances based on itemized deductions, adjustments to income, or two-earner/two-job situations. Complete all worksheets that apply. They will help you figure the number of withholding allowances you are entitled to claim. **However, you may claim fewer (or zero) allowances.**

Child tax and higher education credits. For details on adjusting withholding for these and other credits, see **Pub. 919,** How Do I Adjust My Tax Withholding?

Head of household. Generally, you may claim head of household filing status on your tax return only if you are unmarried and pay more than 50% of the costs of keeping up a home for yourself and your dependent(s) or other qualifying individuals. See line **E** below.

Nonwage income. If you have a large amount of nonwage income, such as interest or dividends, you should consider making estimated tax payments using **Form 1040-ES,** Estimated Tax for Individuals. Otherwise, you may owe additional tax.

Two earners/two jobs. If you have a working spouse or more than one job, figure the total number of allowances you are entitled to claim on all jobs using worksheets from only one Form W-4. Your withholding usually will be most accurate when all allowances are claimed on the Form W-4 prepared for the highest paying job and zero allowances are claimed for the others.

Check your withholding. After your Form W-4 takes effect, use Pub. 919 to see how the dollar amount you are having withheld compares to your projected total tax for 2000. Get Pub. 919 especially if you used the **Two-Earner/Two-Job Worksheet** on page 2 and your earnings exceed $150,000 (Single) or $200,000 (Married).

Recent name change? If your name on line 1 differs from that shown on your social security card, call 1-800-772-1213 for a new social security card.

Personal Allowances Worksheet (Keep for your records.)

A Enter "1" for **yourself** if no one else can claim you as a dependent . . . . A ____

B Enter "1" if:
- You are single and have only one job; or
- You are married, have only one job, and your spouse does not work; or
- Your wages from a second job or your spouse's wages (or the total of both) are $1,000 or less.

. . B ____

C Enter "1" for your **spouse.** But, you may choose to enter -0- if you are married and have either a working spouse or more than one job. (Entering -0- may help you avoid having too little tax withheld.) . . . . C ____

D Enter number of **dependents** (other than your spouse or yourself) you will claim on your tax return . . . . D ____

E Enter "1" if you will file as **head of household** on your tax return (see conditions under **Head of household** above) . E ____

F Enter "1" if you have at least $1,500 of **child or dependent care expenses** for which you plan to claim a credit . . F ____

G **Child Tax Credit:**
- If your total income will be between $18,000 and $50,000 ($23,000 and $63,000 if married), enter "1" for each eligible child.
- If your total income will be between $50,000 and $80,000 ($63,000 and $115,000 if married), enter "1" if you have two eligible children, enter "2" if you have three or four eligible children, or enter "3" if you have five or more eligible children G ____

H Add lines A through G and enter total here. **Note:** *This may be different from the number of exemptions you claim on your tax return.* ▶ H ____

For accuracy, complete all worksheets that apply.
- If you plan to **itemize or claim adjustments to income** and want to reduce your withholding, see the **Deductions and Adjustments Worksheet** on page 2.
- If you are **single,** have **more than one job** and your combined earnings from all jobs exceed $34,000, OR if you are **married** and have a **working spouse or more than one job** and the combined earnings from all jobs exceed $60,000, see the **Two-Earner/Two-Job Worksheet** on page 2 to avoid having too little tax withheld.
- If **neither** of the above situations applies, **stop here** and enter the number from line H on line 5 of Form W-4 below.

Cut here and give Form W-4 to your employer. Keep the top part for your records.

Form **W-4** Department of the Treasury Internal Revenue Service

Employee's Withholding Allowance Certificate

▶ For Privacy Act and Paperwork Reduction Act Notice, see page 2.

OMB No. 1545-0010 **2000**

1 Type or print your first name and middle initial — Last name	2 Your social security number
Home address (number and street or rural route)	3 ☐ Single ☐ Married ☐ Married, but withhold at higher Single rate. *Note: If married, but legally separated, or spouse is a nonresident alien, check the Single box.*
City or town, state, and ZIP code	4 If your last name differs from that on your social security card, check here. **You must call 1-800-772-1213 for a new card** . . . ▶ ☐

5 Total number of allowances you are claiming (from line H above **OR** from the applicable worksheet on page 2) 5

6 Additional amount, if any, you want withheld from each paycheck . . . . 6 $

7 I claim exemption from withholding for 2000, and I certify that I meet **BOTH** of the following conditions for exemption:
- Last year I had a right to a refund of **ALL** Federal income tax withheld because I had **NO** tax liability **AND**
- This year I expect a refund of **ALL** Federal income tax withheld because I expect to have **NO** tax liability.

If you meet both conditions, write "EXEMPT" here . . . . ▶ 7

Under penalties of perjury, I certify that I am entitled to the number of withholding allowances claimed on this certificate, or I am entitled to claim exempt status.

Employee's signature (Form is not valid unless you sign it) ▶ Date ▶

8 Employer's name and address (Employer: Complete lines 8 and 10 only if sending to the IRS.) 9 Office code (optional) 10 Employer identification number

Cat. No. 10220Q

Form W-4 (2000) Page 2

Deductions and Adjustments Worksheet

Note: *Use this worksheet only if you plan to itemize deductions or claim adjustments to income on your 2000 tax return.*

1 Enter an estimate of your 2000 itemized deductions. These include qualifying home mortgage interest, charitable contributions, state and local taxes, medical expenses in excess of 7.5% of your income, and miscellaneous deductions. (For 2000, you may have to reduce your itemized deductions if your income is over $128,950 ($64,475 if married filing separately). See **Worksheet 3** in Pub. 919 for details.) . . . 1 $

2 Enter:
- $7,350 if married filing jointly or qualifying widow(er)
- $6,450 if head of household
- $4,400 if single
- $3,675 if married filing separately

. . . . 2 $

3 **Subtract** line 2 from line 1. If line 2 is greater than line 1, enter -0- . . . . 3 $

4 Enter an estimate of your 2000 adjustments to income, including alimony, deductible IRA contributions, and student loan interest 4 $

5 **Add** lines 3 and 4 and enter the total (Include any amount for credits from **Worksheet 7** in Pub. 919.) . 5 $

6 Enter an estimate of your 2000 nonwage income (such as dividends or interest) . . . . 6 $

7 **Subtract** line 6 from line 5. Enter the result, but not less than -0- . . . . 7 $

8 **Divide** the amount on line 7 by $3,000 and enter the result here. Drop any fraction 8

9 Enter the number from the **Personal Allowances Worksheet,** line H, page 1 9

10 **Add** lines 8 and 9 and enter the total here. If you plan to use the **Two-Earner/Two-Job Worksheet,** also enter this total on line 1 below. Otherwise, **stop here** and enter this total on Form W-4, line 5, page 1 . 10

Two-Earner/Two-Job Worksheet

Note: *Use this worksheet only if the instructions under line H on page 1 direct you here.*

1 Enter the number from line H, page 1 (or from line 10 above if you used the **Deductions and Adjustments Worksheet**) 1

2 Find the number in **Table 1** below that applies to the **LOWEST** paying job and enter it here 2

3 If line 1 is **MORE THAN OR EQUAL TO** line 2, subtract line 2 from line 1. Enter the result here (if zero, enter -0-) and on Form W-4, line 5, page 1. **Do not** use the rest of this worksheet 3

Note: *If line 1 is* ***LESS THAN*** *line 2, enter -0- on Form W-4, line 5, page 1. Complete lines 4–9 below to calculate the additional withholding amount necessary to avoid a year end tax bill.*

4 Enter the number from line 2 of this worksheet 4

5 Enter the number from line 1 of this worksheet 5

6 **Subtract** line 5 from line 4 6

7 Find the amount in **Table 2** below that applies to the **HIGHEST** paying job and enter it here . . . . 7 $

8 **Multiply** line 7 by line 6 and enter the result here. This is the additional annual withholding needed . . 8 $

9 Divide line 8 by the number of pay periods remaining in 2000. For example, divide by 26 if you are paid every other week and you complete this form in December 1999. Enter the result here and on Form W-4, line 6, page 1. This is the additional amount to be withheld from each paycheck . . . . 9 $

Table 1: Two-Earner/Two-Job Worksheet

Married Filing Jointly				All Others			
If wages from LOWEST paying job are—	Enter on line 2 above	If wages from LOWEST paying job are—	Enter on line 2 above	If wages from LOWEST paying job are—	Enter on line 2 above	If wages from LOWEST paying job are—	Enter on line 2 above
$0 - $4,000	0	41,001 - 45,000	8	$0 - $5,000	0	65,001 - 80,000	8
4,001 - 7,000	1	45,001 - 55,000	9	5,001 - 11,000	1	80,001 - 100,000	9
7,001 - 13,000	2	55,001 - 63,000	10	11,001 - 17,000	2	100,001 and over	10
13,001 - 19,000	3	63,001 - 70,000	11	17,001 - 22,000	3		
19,001 - 25,000	4	70,001 - 85,000	12	22,001 - 27,000	4		
25,001 - 31,000	5	85,001 - 100,000	13	27,001 - 40,000	5		
31,001 - 37,000	6	100,001 - 110,000	14	40,001 - 50,000	6		
37,001 - 41,000	7	110,001 and over	15	50,001 - 65,000	7		

Table 2: Two-Earner/Two-Job Worksheet

Married Filing Jointly		All Others	
If wages from HIGHEST paying job are —	Enter on line 7 above	If wages from HIGHEST paying job are —	Enter on line 7 above
$0 - $50,000	$420	$0 - $30,000	$420
50,001 - 100,000	780	30,001 - 60,000	780
100,001 - 130,000	870	60,001 - 120,000	870
130,001 - 250,000	1,000	120,001 - 270,000	1,000
250,001 and over	1,100	270,001 and over	1,100

Privacy Act and Paperwork Reduction Act Notice. We ask for the information on this form to carry out the Internal Revenue laws of the United States. The Internal Revenue Code requires this information under sections 3402(f)(2)(A) and 6109 and their regulations. Failure to provide a **properly** completed form will result in your being treated as a single person who claims no withholding allowances; **providing fraudulent information may also subject you to penalties.** Routine uses of this information include giving it to the Department of Justice for civil and criminal litigation, to cities, states, and the District of Columbia for use in administering their tax laws, and for use in the National Directory of New Hires.

You are not required to provide the information requested on a form that is subject to the Paperwork Reduction Act unless the form displays a valid OMB control number. Books or records relating to a form or its instructions must be retained as long as their contents may become material in the administration of any Internal Revenue law. Generally, tax returns and return information are confidential, as required by Code section 6103.

The time needed to complete this form will vary depending on individual circumstances. The estimated average time is: **Recordkeeping** 46 min., **Learning about the law or the form** 13 min., **Preparing the form** 59 min. If you have comments concerning the accuracy of these time estimates or suggestions for making this form simpler, we would be happy to hear from you. You can write to the Tax Forms Committee, Western Area Distribution Center, Rancho Cordova, CA 95743-0001. **DO NOT** send the tax form to this address. Instead, give it to your employer.

Figure 45-7 The Form W-4 indicates the number of exemptions claimed by the employee for income tax purposes.

Payroll Processing

In some cases it is the office manager's responsibility to prepare payroll checks for each employee and record all deductions withheld. A W-2 form (Figure 45-8) summarizing all earnings and deductions for the year must be prepared for each employee by January 31 of each year. The Social Security Administration must receive a report of W-2 forms each year.

To comply with all governmental regulations, federal, state, and local, it is important that the office manager who processes payroll maintain complete, up-to-date records on every employee. This information should be gathered from new employees and updated every year and upon any change in employee status. Every employee file should contain social security number, number of exemptions claimed on the W-4 Form, the employee's gross salary, and all deductions withheld for all taxes including Social Security, federal, state, local, plus unemployment tax (where applicable), and disability insurance (where applicable).

In order to process payroll, the physician's office must have a federal tax reporting number, obtained from the Internal Revenue Service. In some states, a state employer number also is needed.

Preparing Payroll Checks. When preparing payroll checks, it is important to keep a record of all tax and insurance amounts deducted from an employee's earnings. Many ambulatory care settings that operate on a manual bookkeeping system find that the write-it-once system is the most efficient way to accurately maintain these records. Payroll records should include:

- Employee name, address, and telephone number
- Social security number
- Date of employment

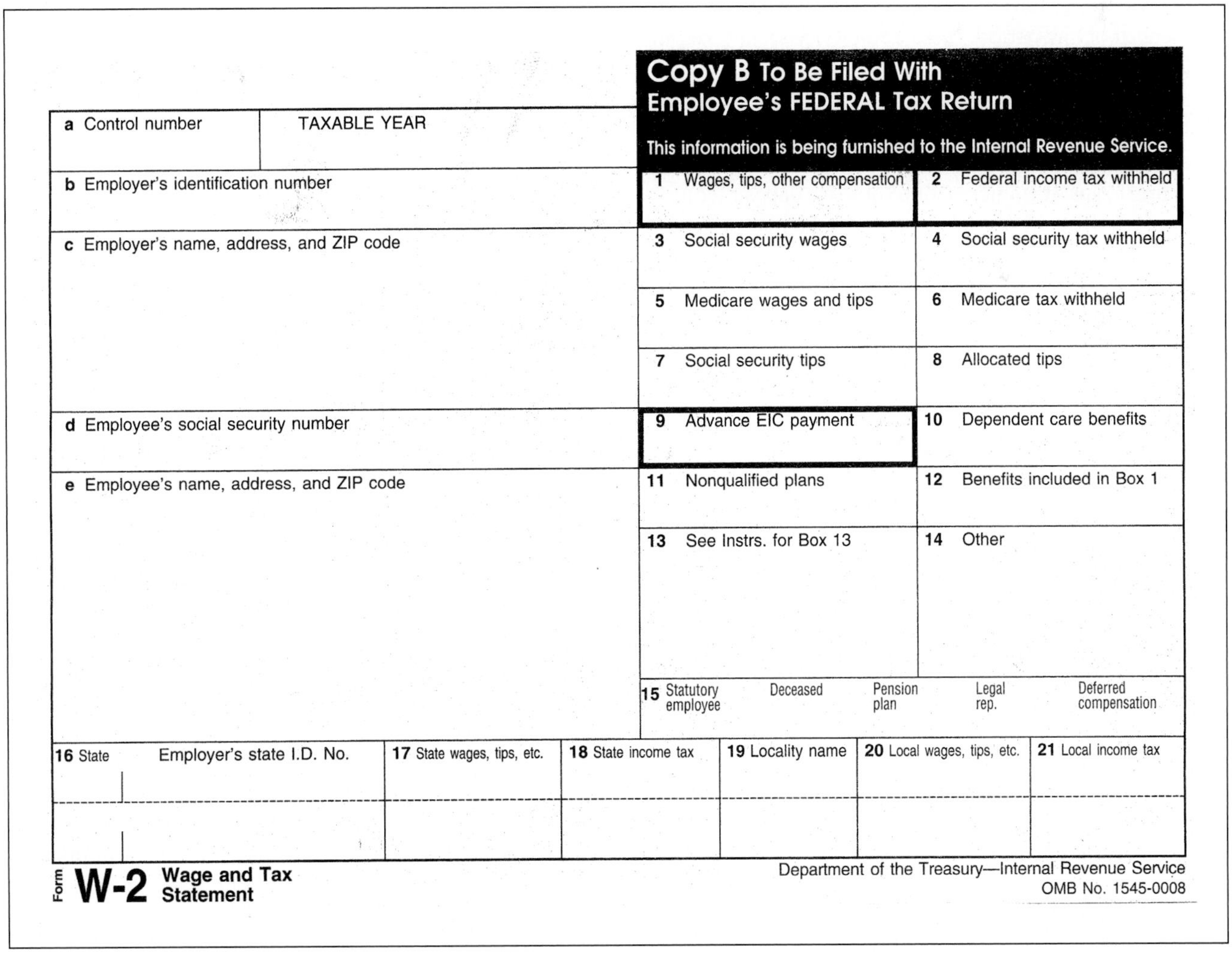

Copy B To Be Filed With Employee's FEDERAL Tax Return
This information is being furnished to the Internal Revenue Service.

a Control number | TAXABLE YEAR
b Employer's identification number
c Employer's name, address, and ZIP code
d Employee's social security number
e Employee's name, address, and ZIP code

1 Wages, tips, other compensation | 2 Federal income tax withheld
3 Social security wages | 4 Social security tax withheld
5 Medicare wages and tips | 6 Medicare tax withheld
7 Social security tips | 8 Allocated tips
9 Advance EIC payment | 10 Dependent care benefits
11 Nonqualified plans | 12 Benefits included in Box 1
13 See Instrs. for Box 13 | 14 Other
15 Statutory employee | Deceased | Pension plan | Legal rep. | Deferred compensation

16 State | Employer's state I.D. No. | 17 State wages, tips, etc. | 18 State income tax | 19 Locality name | 20 Local wages, tips, etc. | 21 Local income tax

Form W-2 Wage and Tax Statement
Department of the Treasury—Internal Revenue Service
OMB No. 1545-0008

Figure 45-8 The Form W-2 summarizes all earnings and deductions for the year and must be prepared for each employee by January 31.

Each paycheck stub should contain:

- Number of hours worked, including regular and overtime (if hourly)
- Date of pay periods
- Date of check
- Gross salary
- Itemized deductions for federal income tax, social security (FICA) tax, state taxes, city or local taxes
- Itemized deductions for health insurance, disability insurance
- Other deductions such as uniforms, loan payments, and so on
- Net salary (gross earnings minus taxes and deductions)

Figuring Taxes. When figuring federal income taxes and social security taxes, use the charts provided by the Internal Revenue Service. Federal tax is based on amount earned, marital status, number of exemptions claimed, and length of pay period. State and city or local taxes are typically a percentage of the gross earnings.

All federal and state taxes withheld must be paid on a quarterly basis to the appropriate government offices. These monies should be accompanied by the required reporting forms. It is important to observe deposit requirements for withheld income tax and social security and Medicare taxes. These requirements, which change frequently, are listed in the Federal Employer's Tax Guide, available from the U.S. Government Printing Office, Internal Revenue Service, or on-line at ftp://ftp.fedworld.gov/pub/irs-pdf/p15.pdf.

Managing Benefits and Other Responsibilities. Benefits, or additional remuneration to the salary earned by full-time employees, must also be managed and records maintained for each employee. Examples of benefits may include paid vacation, paid holidays, health/dental insurance, disability, profit-sharing options, and complimentary health care. Some ambulatory care settings may refer to all or some of these benefits as fringe benefits.

Other responsibilities of the office manager may include maintaining a personal file for each employee providing their history with the facility, application for their current position, evaluations, promotions, problems, awards, entitlements, legal forms required by state and federal agencies, and so on. All Occupational Safety and Health Administration (OSHA) data, hazard material training and documentation, cardiopulmonary resuscita-

tion (CPR) certifications, and continued education units (CEUs) must be recorded and maintained.

FACILITY AND EQUIPMENT MANAGEMENT

The physical plant or building must be observed and maintained with safety being a key ingredient. It should be the responsibility of each staff member to report to the office manager any facility repairs that require attention and suggest replacement or recommend new pieces of equipment as required by the practice to support the health care needs of its population.

The office manager is usually responsible for the maintenance of the office and may hire ancillary services to provide janitorial and laundry services, dispose of hazardous materials, and maintain aquariums or plants that may enhance the environment of the facility. The office manager must stress the importance of patient confidentiality at the close of each day. Ancillary services must not have access to confidential material.

Magazine subscriptions and health-related literature for the reception area are the responsibility of the office manager. Selections should be made carefully, keeping in mind the interests of the patients and their cultures. These materials should not be kept once they become dog-eared, torn, and outdated. The use of plastic protectors and appropriate storage shelving aid in keeping the area and materials tidy.

The office manager is also responsible for facility improvements including any necessary repairs, decorating and color scheme, and floor plan suggestions. The wise office manager does not make these decisions independently, but asks for suggestions from the physician(s) and staff members. Remember, the team-building approach adds a cohesive element to any office environment.

Inventories

All equipment in the facility must be inventoried and maintained. Documented files should be maintained for each piece of equipment. These files are maintained in a separate reference loose-leaf binder and may be divided into administrative and clinical categories. The binder may contain pocket pages in which copies of any warranties, service agreements/contracts, and instructions for use and maintenance may be placed. This binder should be accessible to anyone who may need to refer to its pages. It is also important that as new items or updated service agreements/contracts are purchased, the old ones are removed from the binder and replaced with the new items.

Equipment and Supplies Maintenance

The office storage areas should be well maintained, and each item should always be put back in its place with lids replaced properly to prevent any accidents. Medication storage requires special attention. Many medications must be stored at certain temperatures, kept dry, or stored in dark, airtight containers. Narcotics should always be stored in a locked cabinet. Require two individuals to sign off when narcotic supplies are used and maintain a daily inventory.

Laboratory equipment must be maintained and quality control measures utilized. Calibration checks are required for a number of pieces of equipment: sphygmomanometers and centrifuges to name two. Microscopes and various types of scopes used during physical examinations and specialty procedures contain light sources that must be checked before each use. A replacement supply of bulbs should be available. Refer to Safety and Regulatory Guidelines in the Medical Laboratory, Chapter 38, for more information on quality control and safety in the medical laboratory.

RISK MANAGEMENT

The office manager must practice **risk management**. The risk management process includes the identification, analysis, and treatment of risks within the medical office. The office manager should evaluate the practice to determine when potential risks are present and act to eliminate the risks or to prevent injuries from the risks.

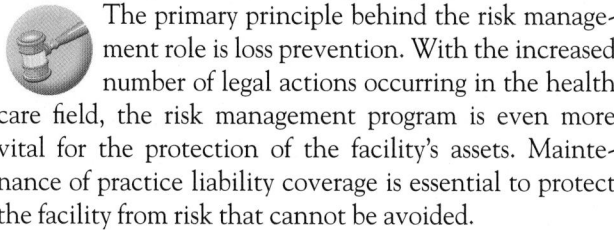

A comprehensive safety program is essential to risk management. This safety program is responsible for meeting the basic safety needs of patients, employees, and visitors. The manager will make sure that all safety guidelines and practices are followed throughout the office and that all staff members work within the scope of their training and qualifications.

The primary principle behind the risk management role is loss prevention. With the increased number of legal actions occurring in the health care field, the risk management program is even more vital for the protection of the facility's assets. Maintenance of practice liability coverage is essential to protect the facility from risk that cannot be avoided.

LIABILITY COVERAGE AND BONDING

Negligence is performing an act that a reasonable and prudent physician would not perform or failure to perform an act that a reasonable and prudent physician would perform. The common term used to describe professional **liability**, or legal responsibility, today is **malpractice**, a term that has negative connotations. It is much easier to prevent malpractice than to defend it in litigation so every effort should be taken to prevent negligence.

Insurance policies specifically designed to protect the physician's assets in the event a liability claim is filed and awarded in the patient's favor are available. Any physician not carrying such insurance is said to be **"going bare"** and would personally be responsible for any court costs, damages, and attorney fees if a malpractice suit were lost.

Practicing medical assistants should carry **professional liability insurance** for protection. Medical assistants who are members of the American Association of Medical Assistants (AAMA) have the option of purchasing personal and professional insurance through the organization at corporate rates.

Some physicians will carry the names of their employees on their policies. If this is the case, always ask to see the policy and verify that your name is printed on the policy—no name indicates no coverage. The manager may need to see that professional liability insurance has been purchased, all appropriate names are listed, and the premiums are paid in a timely fashion.

Professional liability insurance is important if the physician/employer is sued. In this event, the physician and the medical assistant could be named in the suit. If the case were lost, both the physician and the medical assistant could be liable.

Individuals who are responsible for handling financial records and money in the medical office may be bonded. A **bond** is purchased for a cash value in an employee's name which insures that the physician will recover the amount of loss in the event that an employee **embezzles** funds. It is the office manager or the human resources manager's responsibility to ask prospective employees if they are bondable. Individuals who are not bondable may not be the best candidates for the position.

Procedure 45-1 Preparing a Meeting Agenda

PURPOSE:
To prepare a meeting agenda, a list of specific items to be discussed and/or acted upon, in order to maintain the focus of the group and allow business to be transacted in a timely fashion.

EQUIPMENT/SUPPLIES:
List of participants
Order of business
Names of individuals giving reports
Names of any guest speakers
Computer and paper to print agendas

PROCEDURE STEPS:

1. Reserve proposed date, time, and place of meeting. RATIONALE: Ensure that the facilities are available for the meeting.

2. Collect information for meeting agenda by previewing the previous meeting's minutes for old business items, checking with others for report items, determining any new business items. RATIONALE: Ensure that all old and new business items have been identified.

3. Prepare a hard copy of the agenda and have it approved by chair of the meeting. RATIONALE: Confirmation by the chair of the agenda content ensures that agenda is correct and complete.

4. Send agenda to meeting participants two weeks in advance of the meeting. RATIONALE: Permits participants to prepare for the meeting by completing any tasks required and preparing any necessary documentation.

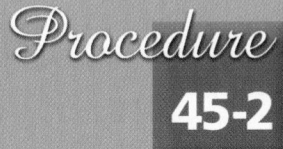

Procedure 45-2 Making Travel Arrangements

PURPOSE:
To make travel arrangements for the physician.

EQUIPMENT/SUPPLIES:
Travel plan
Telephone and telephone directory
Computer
Physician's or office credit card to pay for reservations

PROCEDURE STEPS:

1. Confirm the details of the planned trip: dates, time, and place for departure and arrival; preferred mode of transportation (plane, train, bus, car); number of travelers; preferred lodging type and price range; and whether travelers checks are required. RATIONALE: Confirming pertinent travel details ensure that correct arrangements will be made.

2. Make travel and lodging reservations by calling travel agent or using the computer for on-line ticket services. RATIONALE: Ensure that space for physician is reserved at desired times.

3. Pick up tickets or arrange for their delivery.

4. Check to see that ticket arrangements are accurate (dates, times, places).

5. Check to see that car rental and lodging accommodations are accurate and confirmed. RATIONALE: Avoid inaccuracies and confusion with schedule.

6. Make additional copies of the itinerary or create the itinerary if making arrangements via computer. The itinerary should list date and time of departures and arrivals, including flight numbers and seat assignments. Note mode of transportation to lodging (shuttle, bus, car, taxi). Include name, address, and telephone number of lodgings and meeting places.

7. Maintain one copy of the itinerary in the office file.

8. Give several copies of the itinerary to the physician. RATIONALE: Ensure that a copy is on file with the office and that there are sufficient copies for the traveler(s) and their families.

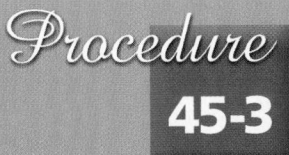

Making Travel Arrangements Via Internet

PURPOSE:
To make travel arrangements for the physician using the Internet.

EQUIPMENT/SUPPLIES:
Travel plan
Computer
Physician's or office credit card to pay for reservations.

PROCEDURE STEPS:
1. Confirm the details of the planned trip: dates, time, and place for departure and arrival; preferred mode of transportation (plane, train, bus, car); number of travelers; preferred lodging type and price range; and whether travelers checks are required. RATIONALE: Confirming pertinent travel details ensures that correct arrangements will be made.
2. Go to the computer and access the Internet.
3. Select a search engine to locate web pages under the subject "air fares." Web pages may provide links to air fares, auto reservations, and hotel/ motel reservations. Follow web page instructions for making arrangements. Review and copy confirmation of your transaction. RATIONALE: The Internet can be a time saver and cost-effective way of securing travel arrangements.
4. Pick up tickets or arrange for their delivery, if necessary. Tickets purchased on the Internet may be mailed or picked up at an airport, or they may be electronic tickets.
5. Make additional copies of the itinerary or create the itinerary. The itinerary should list date and time of departures and arrivals, including flight numbers and seat assignments. Note the mode of transportation to lodging (shuttle, bus, car, taxi). Include name, address, and telephone number of lodgings and meeting places.
6. Maintain one copy of the itinerary in the office file.
7. Give several copies of the itinerary to the physician. RATIONALE: Ensure that a copy is on file with the office and that there are sufficient copies for the traveler(s) and their families.

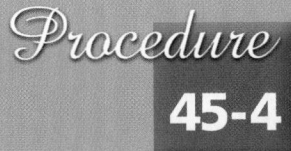

Supervising a Student Practicum

PURPOSE:
To prepare a training path for a student extern being assigned to the office. To make the involved office personnel aware of their responsibilities. To preplan which jobs the student extern performs and in what sequence they will be assigned. To make the externship successful by providing as much supervision and assistance as necessary.

EQUIPMENT/SUPPLIES:
None needed

PROCEDURE STEPS:
1. Review the clinical externship contract or agreement between your agency and the educational institution. RATIONALE: Guidelines and procedures are reviewed and refreshed in your mind.
2. Determine the amount of supervision the extern will require. RATIONALE: Prepares you to speak with the student and site supervisor regarding supervision.
3. Identify the supervisor who will be immediately responsible for the extern. RATIONALE: Establishes a person who knows he or she is to supervise the student and be responsible for the externship procedures.
4. Plan what tasks the extern will be allowed or encouraged to perform. RATIONALE: The office may or may not permit the student to perform

(continues)

Procedure 45-4 *(continued)*

invasive procedures. Determining tasks the student can and can not perform beforehand promotes a better relationship.

5. Create a schedule outlining the time the extern will be assigned to each unit. RATIONALE: Establishing a schedule keeps everyone appraised of what is happening and when.

6. Begin orientation for the extern as soon as he or she arrives at the office. Include a tour of the office and introduction to the staff. RATIONALE: Orients student and staff to each other and establishes guidelines for procedures.

7. Give the extern a copy of the Office Policy Manual and the work schedule for the entire externship. Answer any questions the extern might have. RATIONALE: Orients student and staff to each other and establishes guidelines for procedures.

8. Maintain an accurate record of the hours the extern works. Also log the date and reason for any missed days, late arrivals, or early dismissals. RATIONALE: Provides necessary documentation for the hours completed by the student.

9. Check with the extern frequently to be sure the extern is receiving meaningful training from the work experience. RATIONALE: Verifies that necessary training is being provided.

10. Consult physicians and staff members with whom the extern has worked for their opinion of the student's capabilities. Follow up on any problems that might be identified. RATIONALE: Verifies that necessary training is being provided.

11. Report the extern's progress to the medical assisting supervisor from the educational institution. This person usually visits once or twice each rotation. RATIONALE: Verifies that necessary training is being provided.

12. Prepare the student extern evaluation report from comments provided by the supervisor assigned and each employee who worked with the extern. RATIONALE: Provides necessary documentation for the externship experience.

Procedure 45-5 Developing and Maintaining a Procedures Manual

PURPOSE:
To develop and maintain a comprehensive, up-to-date procedures manual covering each medical, technical, and administrative procedure in the office, with step-by-step directions and rationale for performing each task.

EQUIPMENT/SUPPLIES:
Computer or electronic typewriter (electronic storage allows changes and revisions to be made easily)
Binder, such as a three-ring binder
Paper
Standard procedures manual format

PROCEDURE STEPS:
1. Write detailed, step-by-step procedures and rationales for each medical, technical, and administrative function. Each procedure is written by experienced employees close to the function and then reviewed by a supervisor and/or office manager. Rationales help employees understand *why* something is done. RATIONALE: Establishes consistent guidelines to be followed.

2. Collect the procedures into the Office Procedures Manual. RATIONALE: Provides a reference

(continues)

45-5 *(continued)*

guide with step-by-step instruction and examples where appropriate.

3. Store one complete manual in a common library area. Provide a completed copy to the physician/employer and the office manager. Distribute appropriate sections to the various departments. RATIONALE: Provides a reference guide with step-by-step instruction and examples where appropriate.

4. Review the procedures manual annually and add any new procedures, delete or modify as necessary, and indicate the revision date (Rev. 10/12/02). RATIONALE: Maintains current office protocols.

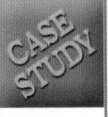

45-1

Dr. Lewis and Dr. King have requested sigmoidoscopy procedures to be scheduled for two different patients. The patients are scheduled. Both patients are put on a strict diet and pretest protocol for several days to prepare for the procedures. The day of the appointments, it is discovered that the two sigmoidoscopy procedures have been scheduled at the same time. The problem is that the office has only one sigmoidoscope available.

CASE STUDY REVIEW

1. Divide the class into two groups to discuss problem-solving solutions. Assume that rescheduling a patient is not an acceptable solution because of the patient's pretest protocol. The patients would be very upset if the procedure could not be performed due to a scheduling problem.

2. How could this problem have been avoided?

3. Both patients have been told about the scheduling problem and one is very upset and argumentative. What role should the office manager assume in this predicament?

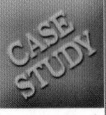

45-2

The office manager for Doctors Lewis and King has many leadership qualities and utilizes them effectively in her management style. She sets realistic goals and becomes a role model for subordinates to emulate. She empowers her subordinates and encourages creativity.

CASE STUDY REVIEW

1. Divide the class into small groups and ask them to brainstorm the pros and cons of this management style.

2. Discuss with your small group other management styles and your comfort level working under these management styles.

3. Within your group, develop a set of questions that might be asked at an interview to determine the management style of this manager prior to accepting employment.

SUMMARY

The office manager is the glue that holds the office together and keeps it running smoothly. When the manager sets a positive example for others, is considerate and aware of the diversity of others, a positive environment is created for teamwork. A teamwork approach enables the entire office to be more productive, provide the best health care, and foster an enjoyable work relationship.

The role of office manager varies greatly depending upon the size of the medical practice, the physician's trust in the manager's competency level, and the physician's comfort in delegating authority to others. An effective office manager is a tremendous asset to physicians. The personal and financial rewards are worthwhile to the medical assistant who desires a new dimension to explore and enjoys a challenge.

REVIEW QUESTIONS

Multiple Choice

1. The office manager should have a minimum of a (an):
   a. associate's degree
   b. bachelor's degree
   c. master's degree
   d. doctoral degree
2. When the office manager is too busy to perform a task, he or she should:
   a. refuse to do it
   b. delegate the task to someone who is knowledgeable
   c. put it off and do it when there is time later
   d. hope that no one will notice it did not get done
3. For teamwork to be successful, individual team members must:
   a. do as they are told by the office manager
   b. not ask why they are doing something a certain way
   c. understand and support the task
   d. think independently and solve the problem on their own
4. People-oriented personalities:
   a. are most comfortable with physical dexterity, building, construction, and working with tools or instruments
   b. are most comfortable working with ideas, information, and data
   c. are most comfortable teaching, coaching, helping, leading, and inspiring others
   d. use "carrots" and "sticks"
5. Meeting minutes:
   a. should address each agenda topic and include a brief summary of discussions, actions taken, name of each person making a motion, the exact wording of motions, and motion approval or defeat
   b. are a detailed plan for a proposed trip
   c. include information regarding mode of transportation and lodging reservations
   d. must follow parliamentary procedures

6. When working with externs, it is important to remember that:
   a. they should have expert knowledge about their field
   b. they do not need supervision when working with a patient
   c. they are very experienced with working on real patients
   d. they have much to learn
7. The procedures manual:
   a. is a detailed plan for a proposed trip
   b. provides detailed information regarding mode of transportation and lodging reservations
   c. provides detailed information relative to the performance of tasks within the health care facility
   d. summarizes action details of staff meetings
8. Which of the following statements is *not* correct regarding a student practicum?
   a. It is a transitional stage that provides opportunity for students to apply theory learned in the classroom to a health care setting through hands-on experience.
   b. It assumes that the student is an employee who does not need to be introduced to patients.
   c. It may require the student to shadow another medical assistant for a few days.
   d. It involves an evaluation of the student's progress.
9. Developing relationships outside the office is often called:
   a. marketing
   b. benchmarking
   c. advertising
   d. sales
10. Record and financial management involves all of the following *except*:
    a. payroll processing
    b. preparing payroll checks
    c. figuring taxes
    d. equipment and supplies maintenance

Critical Thinking

1. How would you, as the office manager, handle some-one who is spreading a harmful rumor about another employee in the office?

2. Discuss teamwork and the benefits of the teamwork approach.

3. How can the office manager promote open and hon-est communication?

4. This chapter identifies various management styles. Under which management style would you feel most comfortable working and why? Does this manage-ment style promote a teamwork atmosphere? Why or why not?

5. The student practicum can be a very stressful time for the extern. As an office manager, how can you help the extern feel more at ease the first day of "work"?

6. This chapter describes various tactics you can use to keep yourself organized, such as making a "To Do" list, handling a paper only once, and avoiding pro-crastination. Describe things that you do to keep yourself organized.

7. Describe how a procedures manual for a single-physician practice would differ from a procedures manual for a multi-physician practice.

8. Describe how a procedures manual could become outdated and need revision.

9. In what cases would a press release be used?

10. Explain why the primary principle behind the risk management role is loss prevention.

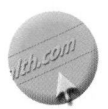

WEB ACTIVITIES

Use the web sites described in the text, or alter-native sites you know about, to plan a trip between two cities within the United States. Compare the fares for Sunday departure and Friday return dates with the fares for low volume days as obtained from the Priceline.com site. Also compare fares on flights purchased within one week of departure with fares on flights purchased a month prior to departure. Fol-low the instructor's instructions on completing and turn-ing in your results.

REFERENCES/BIBLIOGRAPHY

Colbert, B. J. (2000). *Workplace readiness for health occupations.* Albany, NY: Delmar.

Frew, M. A., Lane, K., & Frew, D. R. (1995). *Comprehensive medical assisting: Competencies for administrative and clinical practice* (3rd ed.). Philadelphia: F. A. Davis.

Institute for Management Excellence (June 1998). Linking personality with management style. [On-line]. Available: http://itstime.com/jun98.htm.

Lewis, M. A., & Tamparo, C. D. (1998). *Medical law, ethics, and bio-ethics for ambulatory care* (4th ed.). Philadelphia: F. A. Davis.

McConnell, C. R. (1998). *Case studies in health care supervision.* Gaithersburg, MD: Aspen Publishers.

Pyzdek, T. (1996). Management styles: Participatory manage-ment style. [On-line]. Available: http://www.qualityamerica.com/knowledgecente/articles/CQMStyle2.html.

THE MEDICAL ASSISTANT AS HUMAN RESOURCES MANAGER

KEY TERMS

Conflict Resolution
Educational History
Evaluation
Exit Interview
Involuntary Dismissal
Job Description
Letter of Reference
Letter of Resignation
Mentor
Networking
Overtime
Probation
Resumes
Salary Review
Work History

OUTLINE

OBJECTIVES

*The student should strive to meet the following performance objectives and demonstrate
an understanding of the facts and principles presented in this chapter through written and
oral communication.*

1. Define the key terms as presented in the glossary.
2. Describe the role of the human resources manager.
3. Explain the function of the office policy manual.
4. Identify methods of recruiting employees for a medical practice.
5. Discuss the interview process.
6. Describe appropriate evaluation tools for employees.
7. Recall procedures to follow when dismissing employees.
8. Identify items to keep in an employee's personnel record.
9. List and define a minimum of four laws related to personnel management.
10. Recall effective methods of resolving conflicts.

ADMINISTRATIVE

Practice Finances

- Manage personnel benefits and maintain records (adv)

GENERAL
(TRANSDISCIPLINARY)

Legal Concepts

- Follow federal, state and local legal guidelines

- Participate in the development and maintenance of personnel, policy and procedure manuals

- Develop and maintain personnel, policy and procedures manuals (adv)

Instruction

- Train and orient personnel (adv)

- Conduct continuing education activities (adv)

Operational Functions

- Supervise personnel (adv)

- Interview and recommend job applicants (adv)

Jane O'Hara, CMA, is the officer manager at Inner City Health Care. She also functions in the role of the human resources manager. Part of her responsibilities includes recruiting, hiring, training, and dismissing employees.

In one day Jane may meet with Dr. Rice to update the policy manual, place an advertisement in the local newspaper for a new medical assistant, welcome a new physician to the practice, being sure she completes all of the necessary forms, and meet with Karen Ritter to evaluate her salary.

INTRODUCTION

The medical assistant, while performing the tasks and assuming the responsibility of an office manager, also may function in the role of the human resources manager.

The title human resources manager is often reserved for an individual who manages a human resources department in a large, corporate setting. Many of the duties performed by this individual, however, may be performed in a sole proprietor's medical practice with only one or two employees.

TASKS PERFORMED BY THE HUMAN RESOURCES MANAGER

Tasks usually assigned to the human resources manager include determining job descriptions, hiring, training, and dismissing employees, and maintaining employee personnel records. But with today's quest for greater office efficiency and the tremendous increase in federal and state regulatory requirements, the skills required of a human resources manager have greatly broadened. Former responsibilities have been expanded to include writing the policy manual, planning employee evaluation, preventing and investigating discrimination

and harassment claims, and complying with regulatory agencies. The human resources manager also assists in providing training and educational opportunities for employees so they are up to date in all aspects of quality patient care.

Increasingly, human resource managers are expected to be able to support the organization's efforts that focus on productivity, service, and quality. In a climate in which there are too few persons for the positions to be filled, and the delivery methods for health care are changing almost daily, productivity, service, and quality are essential to a successful practice. It becomes the responsibility of the human resource manager to see that every employee's productivity level is high, that the service is A+, and that quality is at the highest level. Today's customers, the patients, will often choose their health care provider on the basis of service and quality.

The position of human resources manager now requires a higher level of education and experience to better grasp the legal and regulatory aspects of personnel management. The human resources manager also must have excellent people skills, a strong sense of fairness, and the ability to resolve conflicts. None of this is accomplished in a vacuum. It requires working in close cooperation with the office manager and the physician-employer(s).

This chapter discusses these responsibilities in groups of eight separate but overlapping functions:

1. Creating and updating the office policy manual
2. Recruiting and hiring office personnel
3. Orienting and training new personnel
4. Evaluating and planning salary review
5. Dismissing employees

6. Maintaining personnel records
7. Complying with all state and federal regulations regarding personnel
8. Planning/providing employee training and education

THE OFFICE POLICY MANUAL

The procedures manual described in Chapter 45 identifies specific methods of performing tasks. The policy manual provides more general guidelines for office practices.

Possible content of policy and procedure manual	
Policy Manual	**Procedure Manual**
General practices and policies of an office	Daily guide; step-by-step instructions for procedures

The policy manual will identify clear guidelines and directions required of all employees as well as define appropriate expectations and boundaries of the employment relationship. Having written policies means not having to determine a policy on a case-by-case basis. Policy manuals will vary by the size of the practice or problems to be addressed, but some topics include the mission statement of the practice, biographical data on each physician, employment policies, wage and salary policies, benefits to be awarded, and employee conduct expectations.

Establishing and stating the mission of the practice clearly identifies for employees the goals and objectives to be sought by each employee. Having biographical data of each physician helps employees to respond to queries from patients about a physician's training, education, and interests.

Employment policies might include statements on equal employment opportunity, job requirements for particular positions and to whom the person reports, recruitment and selection procedures, orientation of new employees, probation, and dismissal. Wage and salary policies should be in writing. How are employees classified, what are the working hours, how is overtime compensated, how are salary increases determined, what benefits (medical, retirement, vacation, holidays, sick leave) does the practice have? The answers to such questions are part of the policy manual. Employee conduct is another piece of the policy manual. Guidelines should be established about uniforms and appearance. Can an employee hold a second job outside the practice? Is smoking allowed? Are staff members responsible for housekeeping duties? A statement regarding the confidentiality of all information received in the practice is essential in this area of the policy manual.

Having a policy manual with clearly written directives helps employees understand the expectations and boundaries of the employment relationship. The policy manual should be reviewed with each new employee and updated on a regular basis. See Procedure 46-1 for details on developing and maintaining a policy manual.

RECRUITING AND HIRING OFFICE PERSONNEL

Before recruiting and hiring personnel to fill positions within the medical office, the human resources manager and physician-employer must know exactly what the role and responsibilities of the position are by having a job description for the position and follow a recruiting policy that is effective, fair, and observes all appropriate laws and regulations.

Job Descriptions

Before any position is filled, a **job description** must be in place. This is done cooperatively with the office manager and the physician-employer. Once the job qualifications are defined, the human resources manager can begin efforts to fill the position.

In daily operations most job descriptions are on file, but if the situation involves a new or greatly expanded office, a complete set of job descriptions is needed before recruiting can begin. Even when a written description is on file, it should be reviewed when a new employee is to be hired. The person who is leaving the position is often an excellent resource for the accuracy of the current job description and any changes that should be made.

The job description must include basic qualifications for the position and have enough information to provide both the supervisor and the employee with a clear outline of what the job entails (Figure 46-1). Necessary work experience, skills, education, and any special certification or licensure that is expected is to be identified in the job description. See Procedure 46-2 for details on preparing job descriptions.

Another important point with respect to the job description is that a review and update of the description should be done every year. Most jobs change constantly whether from a minor shifting of duties or the addition

JOB DESCRIPTION FORMAT

JOB TITLE:
Describes the job in one to three words; should be a title an employee can identify with and be proud of.
REPORTS TO:
Identifies position or person to whom the employee reports.
PURPOSE/OBJECTIVE:
A short statement outlining the purpose or mission of the job, explaining basically why this job exists; should make the person feel like an integral part of the whole organization.
RESPONSIBILITIES AND DUTIES:
Duties are statements that outline a particular function or task and identify what is being done; all statements are related to the work to be performed. Duties should identify the most predominant and significant tasks and convey a measure of frequency of occurrence. *Responsibilities* are simply names or titles for types of work areas. Duties are subsets of responsibilities.
WORK RELATIONSHIPS AND AUTHORITY BOUNDARIES:
When significant to the job, a statement describing the relationships and degree of interface of the job with internal and external groups.
POSITION REQUIREMENTS:
Education and experience that are required for the person to function in this capacity.

Figure 46-1   This sample format describes the main features of a job description with definitions for each feature. (From *Personnel Management Handbook*, 2nd ed., by Maryann Ricardo, The McGraw-Hill Companies, Inc. Copyright 1992. Reprinted with permission.)

of some new technical procedure or device. Without updating a job description, the wrong person may be recruited to fill a vacancy.

Recruiting

A major challenge facing the human resource manager today is recruitment. Medical assistants are listed in the top ten occupations with the fastest employment growth through 2006 according to the U.S. Department of Labor, Bureau of Labor Statistics. One reason for this demand is the aging of the U.S. population. It is estimated that over 80% of jobs are in the service industry, and all health care positions fit into that category. When physician-employers have been unsuccessful in recruiting qualified medical assistants, they have turned to contracting out some work, such as transcription and billing.

The human resources manager begins the recruitment process. Often a process called networking is a highly effective method of finding employees. **Networking** is a process in which people of similar interests exchange information in social, business, or professional relationships. For instance, the human resources manager may network with members of the American Association of Medical Assistants and express an interest in a new employee for a position that is open. Current employees are often an excellent resource because they may know of a qualified person who is looking for a position.

Checking with nearby universities, community, and technical colleges' medical assistant departments is another good resource. Employing a private or state placement agency is another possibility. While newspaper advertisements may generate many **resumes**, they are only marginally effective as a search tool. It is often far too time consuming to review the large volume of applications generated by this approach.

Preparing to Interview Applicants

Once several applicants have expressed interest in the position, preparation for the interview begins. The human resources manager should have a number of resumes to consider. Some may have already filled out a job application when they dropped off a resume. The resumes and applications can be reviewed together. Some important points to remember in reading resumes and applications follow.

Under **educational history**, look beyond the degree earned. Look for a good performance record at school and the kinds of supplemental education achieved. Does attendance at seminars and short-course training programs relate to your position needs? When reading a person's **work history**, make note of unexplained gaps in employment. You may want to ask specific questions in the interview. Has advancement been gained in each new position? Are the responsibilities and duties of the applicant's positions explained or will questions need to be asked of the prospective employee?

Look for information that indicates if this candidate really enjoys the kind of work setting you have. Is the applicant comfortable serving the infirm? Can you truly identify the level of skill from the descriptions or are the skills vague? The cover letter, if one is included, should address the specifics required of your position. Does the person display a negative or a positive attitude? Do not excuse any errors or unprofessional appearance in the job application or the resume. Each should be letter perfect. An individual who is careless in this respect is likely to be careless on the job.

Some applications will be set aside after using the preceding guidelines. With the remaining candidates, determine who is to be interviewed and make telephone calls to establish interviews. You may make note of the quality of speaking skills, especially if this person will be using the telephone on the job. Make an interview appointment date with only those who seem truly interested in the position during your telephone conversation.

The Interview

The interview is usually conducted by only one person if second interviews are anticipated. The physician-employer, office manager, or another employee may be present in either the first or the second interview, however. This is a decision made by the human resources manager and the physician-employer (Figure 46-2). The interviewer(s) will want to review the application and resume prior to the interview for particular points to ask the candidate. An interview worksheet is an excellent tool to use to make certain that you are fair and equitable with each candidate. The worksheet should provide enough room for notes taken during the interview.

Suggested items for the interview worksheet are:

- Applicant's name
- Telephone number
- Education and training

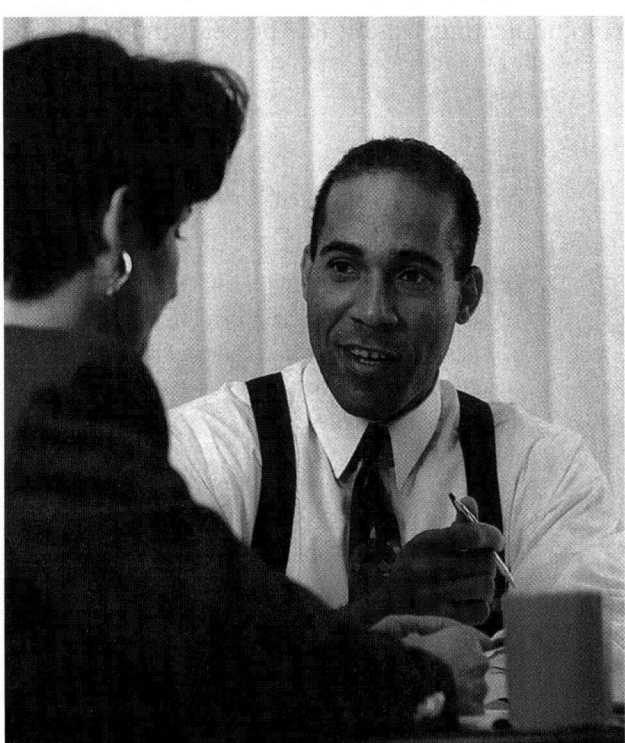

Figure 46-2 The interview can be conducted on a one-to-one basis with only the applicant and one staff member or with several staff members meeting with the applicant at once.

- Work experience
- Special skills
- Professional demeanor
- Voice and mannerisms specific to position
- Responses to questions
- Ability to problem solve when given a scenario
- Any health-related or work-related problems applicant discloses
- Interviewer's personal impressions and recommendations

Conduct interviews in a quiet and private setting. Do not schedule interviews back to back without time to collect your thoughts or to allow you to compare notes with others participating in the interview. Ask job-related questions such as Describe your last job. What did you like best about it? What did you like least? What is most important to you about a job? Describe your administrative and clinical skills. Figure 46-3 shows some sample questions. Let the applicant do the most of the talking.

Any questions related to age, sex, race, religion, or national origin are inappropriate. Inquiries about medical

General Questions
- What are your strengths and weaknesses?
- Why did you leave your last job?
- Identify what is most important to you in a job.

Questions Related to Work Relationships
- Describe an individual you have enjoyed working with.
- Explain how a conflict with a coworker was resolved.
- How would a coworker describe you?

Questions Related to Problem Solving
- Describe a work-related decision that made you very proud.
- Identify a task/procedure/assignment you could not do, and explain why.
- How do you approach a task when it seems mundane or boring?

Questions Related to Integrity
- If asked to do something illegal or unethical, what would you do?
- Tell us about a time when you broke a confidence.
- If you saw a coworker put a patient at risk, what would you do?

Figure 46-3 Common interview questions.

history, drug use, or arrest records may not be made. Keep your questions related to performance on the job. If you may want to bond this employee, you may ask candidates if they have been bonded before or are willing to be bonded. It may be best to leave salary discussions for a second interview, but it can also be helpful to determine if applicants' salary expectations are in line with what you can offer. A question such as What salary are you expecting? is appropriate. Do not make a job offer until all the candidates selected for interview have been interviewed, and do not prejudge someone on appearance or any other physical factor during or following the interview. Only the person's qualifications are to be considered.

At the close of the interview, let the applicant know when a decision will be made or whether a second interview will be conducted. A tour of the facility and introduction to key staff members may be offered, but are not necessary at the time of the first interview. Finally, thank the applicant for participating in the interview and being interested in the position.

Selecting the Finalists

Shortly after the final interview is complete, the human resources manager should compare notes with all the others involved in the interview to select the top candidates. This is done by comparing notes and impressions from the interviews and by taking into consideration the ability of a candidate to work with patients and colleagues having a variety of problems and cultural backgrounds. The next step is to check references of former employers, supervisors, coworkers, and teachers. A large corporate medical practice may even have a consent form each candidate is asked to sign that gives permission to check references and call former employers. You may need to recognize, however, that even with a release from a potential new hire, many organizations and businesses restrict the release of reference information to only name, dates of employment, and title of position served. Telephone checks for references are an excellent strategy since you receive an immediate response. If you stress confidentiality when you make the contact, it will be easier for the person to respond to your questions. Always check with more than one reference and former employer to get an accurate assessment of the candidate. A sample telephone reference check form is shown in Figure 46-4.

A checklist of questions to ask might include:

1. What were the dates of employment of (name of applicant) in your firm?
2. Describe the job performed.
3. Reason for leaving the job?
4. Strong points of the employee?
5. Limitations of the employee?

TELEPHONE REFERENCE CHECK FORM

Name of Applicant _____

Person Contacted _____

Position _____

Telephone Number _____

Relation to Applicant _____

1. I would like to verify some information given to us by (applicant's name) who is applying for a position with our organization. What are the dates of his employment with you?

   _____, 20___ to _____, 20___

2. What was the nature of his job?
3. What did you think of his work?
4. How did he get along with the other employees?
5. Did you see any difference in his job performance during the employment period?
6. What was his salary?
7. Why did he leave the job?
8. What are his strong points?
9. What are his limitations?
10. Please describe his attitude.
11. What degree of supervision did he need?
12. Could you comment on his attendance and dependability?
13. Were there any personal difficulties that you know of that may have interfered with his work?
14. Given the right opportunity, would you rehire him?
15. Is there anything else that we should know?

Reference call made by _____ Date _____

Figure 46-4 A telephone reference check form such as this one can help the interviewer ask consistent questions of several references. (From *Personnel Management Handbook,* 2nd ed., by Maryann Ricardo, The McGraw-Hill Companies, Inc. Copyright 1992. Reprinted with permission.)

6. Can you comment on attendance and dependability?
7. Any personal difficulties you were aware of that interfered with the work?
8. Would you rehire?
9. Anything else we should know about this candidate?

Offer the position when a first-choice candidate has been determined and indicate when a response is needed. Be prepared with a second-choice candidate should the preferred candidate respond negatively. At the time of the offer, the candidate should understand the salary offered, the starting date, the practice policies, and the benefits. When a candidate has accepted the position, a confirmation letter should be written that clearly spells out details discussed earlier. Give specific instructions on when and where the new employee should report the first day on the job. If practical, the employee should be given the policy and procedures manuals to read.

For the unsuccessful applicants, send a letter explaining that they are no longer being considered for the position and thank them for applying. Copies of these letters as well as the interview checklists should be kept for a minimum of six months should any questions arise regarding your choice of candidates. See Procedure 46-3 for details on interviewing.

ORIENTING AND TRAINING NEW PERSONNEL

Orienting and training new employees is the responsibility of both the human resources manager and the office manager who is most likely to work the closest with the new employee. It is common for a new employee to be placed on **probation** for sixty to ninety days during which time both the employee as well as supervisory personnel may determine if the environment and the position are satisfactory for the employee. Procedure 46-4 outlines how to orient and train personnel.

Important elements to orientation include the introduction of the new employee to other staff members, assigning a **mentor** who can respond to questions, and making the employee aware of the procedures to be performed in this new position. If the procedure's manual is detailed and accurate, this manual now becomes the daily "guide" for the new employee. Sometimes the individual leaving a position may still be present and is asked to assist in the orientation process. This is especially beneficial if there is a good working relationship between the employee who is leaving and the management of the practice. Depending upon the responsibilities of the new employee, a supervisor may be asked to monitor all procedures for a period of time for accuracy, safety, and patient protection. During the probation period, the employee should be officially evaluated by the human resources manager (see sample form in Figure 46-5). This **evaluation** becomes part of the employee's personnel record.

EVALUATING EMPLOYEES AND PLANNING SALARY REVIEW

It is very important that all employees know whether they are performing their job as expected and know how they can improve their performance if necessary.

PROBATIONARY EMPLOYEE EVALUATION FORM

Name_____

Hire Date _____

Job Title _____

Pay Rate_____ Supervisor _____

Do you recommend the employee continue in employment?
_____ Yes _____ No

Please state your reasons for whatever action you recommend. Use the guidelines below to make your decision.

1. Has the employee required more training than is normally needed for the job?
2. Has the employee grasped this job with very little training?
3. Is the employee performing at, above, or below (circle one) the standard for this job?
4. If below, when do you expect the employee to reach the standard?
5. Does the employee get along well with all staff members?
6. Has the employee maintained a good attendance record and a good work attitude?
7. Has the employee expressed any dissatisfactions?

_____ _____
Supervisor's Signature   Date

Figure 46-5 Sample probationary employee evaluation form. (From *Personnel Management Handbook*, 2nd ed., by Maryann Ricardo, The McGraw-Hill Companies, Inc. Copyright 1992. Reprinted with permission.)

Performance Evaluation

Not only is evaluation of employees necessary during the probation period, it is necessary for current employees as well. Evaluations should be performed no less than once a year on the anniversary of the hire date. Some human resources managers may wish to evaluate an employee more often, especially if a problem has surfaced in an evaluation.

The evaluation may take many forms; it can be formal or informal; it may involve more than one person. The results of the evaluation, however, must be a part of the employee's personnel record. For that reason, a formal evaluation is preferred. Many practices use a written evaluation that requires that the employee evaluate himself prior to meeting with the human resources manager (Figure 46-6). The human resources manager uses the same form for evaluation. During the meeting, notes are compared as the evaluation is conducted.

PERFORMANCE REVIEW FORM

_____   _____
Employee Name   Title

_____   _____
Supervisor   Department

TYPE OF REVIEW (Check One)

_____ Quarterly

_____ Annual

_____ Probation

_____ Other _____

Review Period Covered _____ to _____

PERFORMANCE DEFINITIONS

5 = Outstanding	Performance that is clearly superior, beyond the call of duty, or substantially above standard level. Seldom attained level of performance but achievable.
4 = Above Standard	Very commendable performance; exceeds the norm for the job.
3 = Standard	Competent and consistent performance; expected level of activity and performance for the job. Most often rating received.
2 = Below Standard	Performance needs improvement. This level of performance is unacceptable; needs improvement to meet the standards for the job. **Employee new to the job:** Performance might receive below standard rating due to lack of job knowledge and is expected to improve with experience. **Experienced Employee:** Performance is below acceptable level and requires direction and/or counsel.
1 = Unsatisfactory	Performance is unacceptable. Job activity is clearly and substantially lacking in quality, quantity, or timeliness. May also not be meeting cost or budget constraints. Needs much improvement to meet the standards for the job.

(office use only) EVALUATION SUMMARY Total I _____ + Total II _____	FINAL RATING: CHECK ONE (office use only) _____ Merit Increase Recommended _____ No Merit Increase—Satisfactory Performance/No Growth _____ No Merit Increase (Probationary/Special Evaluation) _____ No Merit Increase (Performance Probation) Re-evaluate in 90 Days for Unsatisfactory or in 180 Days for Needed Improvement

GENERAL PERFORMANCE RATING (PART I)

General Criteria	Rating	Comments Supporting Rating
1. **Patient Relations:** How well does the employee communicate a "we care" image to the patients, visitors, physicians, and fellow employees?		
2. **Work Responsibilities:** What is the quality of the employee's work relative to quality, quantity, and timeliness?		
3. **Teamwork:** Does the employee have a team spirit? Does the employee interact well with co-workers/supervisor/manager?		*(continues)*

Figure 46-6 Sample performance review form. *(Adapted from* Personnel Management Handbook, *2nd ed., by Maryann Ricardo, The McGraw-Hill Companies, Inc. Copyright 1992. Reprinted with permission.)*

General Criteria	Rating	Comments Supporting Rating
4. **Adaptability:** Is the employee open to change and new ideas? Does the employee remain flexible to changes in routine, workload, and assignments?		
5. **Personal Appearance:** How well does the employee maintain appropriate personal appearance, including proper attire, hygiene?		
6. **Communication:** Does the employee communicate well? Is information given and received clearly? Does he/she have good verbal and written skills?		
7. **Dependability:** Can the employee be relied upon for good attendance? Does the employee perform and follow through on work without supervisory intervention or assistance?		

Subtotal I _____ ÷ 7 General Criteria = _____

JOB-SPECIFIC CRITERIA RATING (PART II) (To be used with Job Description attached)

Responsibility and Standard	Rating	Comments Supporting Rating
Complete a section for each responsibility listed on the employee's job description.		

Subtotal II _____ ÷ _____ = _____
                                    # job duties

Contributions made since last review:

_____

_____

_____

Education or training received since last review:

_____

_____

_____

Action to be taken based on performance:

_____

_____

_____

Comments:

_____

_____

_____

_____	_____
Employee Signature	Date
_____	_____
Supervisor Signature	Date
_____	_____
Physician Signature	Date

Figure 46-6 *(continued)*

The climate of the performance evaluation should be comfortable and provide privacy (Figure 46-7). The meeting should be friendly, but the employee must sense the importance of the evaluation. Do not allow any disagreements to escalate into arguments during the evaluation. Without reading the employee's self-evaluation, ask the employee to tell about the self-assessment. Acknowledge the employee's point of view and identify when you agree or differ from the self-assessment. Be prepared to describe specific examples of positive performance and/or negative performance.

When negative performance is identified, ask the employee for possible solutions. Then a plan can be determined to alter the negative performance. In this way, a trusting atmosphere is established in that both of you are working together for a solution that will benefit the medical practice. Always look for and seek a win-win situation whenever possible. The action plan determined should then be evaluated at the next performance evaluation.

At the close of the evaluation, always express your confidence in the individual to make any changes necessary, offer assistance where needed, and thank the employee for participating. End any evaluation with a positive statement about some portion of the employee's performance.

There are occasions when reviews are performed more frequently than annually. A review would occur two to three months after a significant promotion to measure how things are progressing. Reviews occur more often when general performance falls well short of past efforts or a serious error in judgment has been made. This type of review may end with a reprimand, a warning to correct the problem by a given date, or possibly, immediate dismissal. Document any steps to be taken to correct a problem and any reason that is cause for dismissal.

Salary Reveiw

Although the practice is common in some areas, it may be better not to tie salary increases or bonuses with the annual performance evaluation. Conduct the **salary review** at the beginning of the new year separate from performance evaluations.

Salary review is important. Unfortunately, in smaller medical offices and ambulatory care settings, the review of salary may have to be raised by the employee. Physician-employers tend to forget that their employees have been with them for over a year without a raise or a discussion of financial reimbursement. If such is the case, it is perfectly acceptable for the employee to raise the issue on a yearly basis. However, the best approach is for the human resources manager to conduct salary reviews at the beginning or end of each calendar year.

Data should be collected prior to a salary review. The human resources manager should network with other

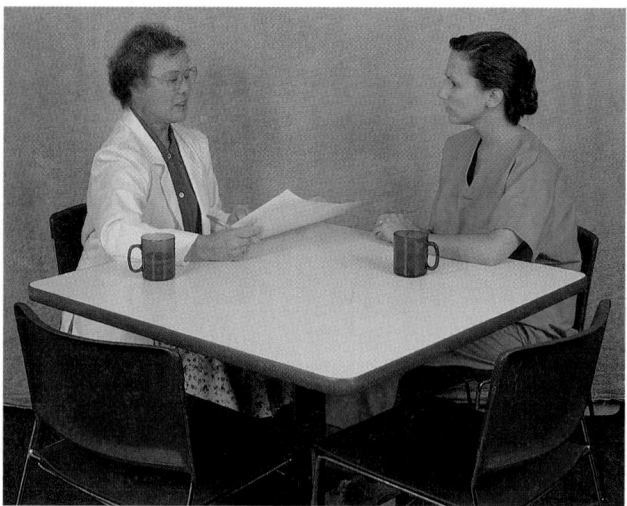

Figure 46-7 A comfortable, private setting encourages discussion during an employee evaluation.

human resources managers to determine wages and salaries for comparable individuals with comparable skills. Remember, also, that it is far more cost-effective to reward good employees with a salary increase than it is to train a new employee who commands a lesser salary than current employees. Reward employees well and provide benefits that encourage them to stay with the practice. Employees who stay with the practice for a long time not only fully understand how best to serve their physician-employers, they have established a relationship with patients that is very beneficial.

How much of a raise is to be awarded at the time of salary review is difficult to determine and will depend upon many factors which might include the profits of the year, the patient load, the workload, and the current cost of living.

The critical shortage of health care employees today is reflected in the shortage of medical assistants across the country. Newspapers advertising for individuals to work in the ambulatory care setting tell the story. A consideration worth mentioning is that often the salary does not match the education, experience, and special training required of someone working in the health care field. Educators often hear, "Why would I spend a year or more in education to be paid what I would make working in a fast food restaurant?" Because it is costly in time and resources to replace employees, it is best to invest that cost into a fair and just salary increase for valued employees.

DISMISSING EMPLOYEES

Most human resources managers do not enjoy rating the performance of other employees particularly when difficult topics are involved and it may be necessary to dismiss an employee. However, the written performance evaluation actually establishes the format for such a dismissal when necessary and is more likely to remove the emotion from the situation. **Involuntary dismissal** is still difficult when it is necessary.

Involuntary Dismissal

Involuntary dismissal results from two primary causes: poor performance or serious violation of office policies or job descriptions. When it becomes apparent to the human resources manager that the effectiveness of an employee is dropping well below expectations, it will be known in the review or a performance review may be called. The review allows the employee to be informed of the shortcomings, to explain any reasons for the present situation, and to determine a plan to alleviate the problem. If the problem is a serious one, probation is usually invoked and any lack of significant improvement in the time provided results in immediate dismissal.

When the problem is a violation of either office policy or procedures, both a verbal and a written warning are given to the employee. Involuntary dismissal follows if the situation persists. Dismissal may be immediate if the action is a serious violation of policy. Serious violations will depend upon the office practice, but some causes for immediate dismissal include theft, making fraudulent claims against insurance, placing the patient in jeopardy by not practicing safe techniques, and breach of patient confidentiality.

Some key points to keep in mind when dismissal is necessary are:

1. The dismissal should be made in privacy.
2. Take no longer than 10 minutes for the dismissal.
3. Be direct, firm, and to the point in identifying reasons.
4. Do not engage in an in-depth discussion of performance.
5. Explain terms of dismissal (keys, clearing out area, final paperwork).
6. Listen to employee's opinion and emotions; it is not necessary to agree.
7. Accompany the employee to their desk to pack their belongings.
8. Escort the employee out of the facility; do not allow to finish the work of the day.

Voluntary Dismissal

Other reasons for dismissal may be more pleasant. Changes in personnel occur for many good reasons and people voluntarily leave their jobs. They may relocate, seek advancement in another facility, or simply have personal reasons for leaving. These employees will give their manager proper notice and be able to turn their current projects and duties over to their replacements. They have time to say good-bye to their friends and leave with a good feeling about their employment.

Exit Interview

An **exit interview** is an excellent opportunity for the employee who voluntarily leaves a practice and the human resources manager to discuss the positive and negative aspects of the job and what changes might be made for a new person coming into the facility. A sample exit interview form is shown in Figure 46-8. It also allows the opportunity for the employee to ask for a **letter of reference** or to view the personnel file before leaving. In a voluntary dismissal, request a **letter of resignation** for the personnel file.

Any dismissal process, voluntary or involuntary, must include a statement in the personnel file. For involuntary dismissal, be certain that the reasons for the dismissal are well documented. Be honest, nonjudgmental, and do not allow emotions to escalate into hostility and anger. State only the facts in the personnel file; do not

---

EXIT INTERVIEW FORM

1. What did you like and dislike about the work you have been doing?
   (Including: support on the job; opportunity for personal growth; recognition and rewards)

2. What kind of people have you found the doctors, your immediate supervisor, and co-workers to be?
   (Including: attitude; fairness; scheduling and assignment of work; work expectations; technical competence; assistance and guidance available; team spirit)

3. What is your view of our management practices and policies?
   (Including: clarity and fairness of practice policies; communications; management and staff)

4. How have you felt about performance appraisals, your salary and benefits?
   (Including: adequacy of salary; regularity and fairness of appraisals)

5. What are your principal reasons for leaving the practice?
   (Including: primary dissatisfactions; job or personal changes)

6. In what areas do you feel we need to improve?

Interviewer signature: _____ Date _____

Employee signature: _____ Date _____

Figure 46-8 Sample exit interview form. (From *Personnel Management Handbook*, 2nd ed., by Maryann Ricardo, The McGraw-Hill Companies, Inc. Copyright 1992. Reprinted with permission.)

state opinion. Remember that employees have the right to view their personnel file at any time.

The physician-employer should always be informed of any dismissal as quickly as possible. Some will be involved in the actual dismissal process. A physician-employer is most likely going to be concerned about ongoing assistance in the practice and that a break not occur in quality care given to patients.

MAINTAINING PERSONNEL RECORDS

An important aspect of the responsibilities of the human resources manager is maintaining personnel records. All documentation and correspondence related to each employee from application to dismissal, from awards to reprimands including the formal reviews, must be kept in the confidential personnel file. Access to this file is limited to certain management personnel and the employee. Not all of these people are allowed to see the entire file. These files are usually kept for a period of three to five years.

This file also includes the kind of information normally maintained for payroll and business practices. That information includes name, address, and sex of employee. The position title, date of beginning employment, rate of pay (hourly or otherwise), total overtime pay, deductions or additions to wages, wages paid each pay period, and date of dismissal.

COMPLYING WITH PERSONNEL LAWS

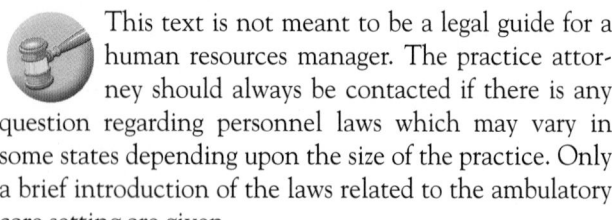

This text is not meant to be a legal guide for a human resources manager. The practice attorney should always be contacted if there is any question regarding personnel laws which may vary in some states depending upon the size of the practice. Only a brief introduction of the laws related to the ambulatory care setting are given.

Overtime must be addressed in each practice. Who is reimbursed for overtime and how is that reimbursement determined? Typically, medical receptionists and secretaries, insurance billers, medical transcriptionists, and medical assistants are likely to be paid overtime. Overtime pay at a rate of not less than one and one-half times the regular rate of pay after a forty-hour work week is standard. Each week stands alone and one week cannot compensate for another. If the practice does not want to be involved in overtime situations, require that any overtime be preauthorized in advance.

The Equal Pay Act of 1963 prevents wage discrimination for jobs that require equal skill, effort, and responsibility. The Civil Rights Act of 1964 prevents employers from discriminating against individuals on the basis of race, color, religion, sex, age, or national origin.

Sexual harassment violates Title VII of the Civil Rights Act. Steps must be taken to ensure that all employees are working in an atmosphere that is not hostile, where sexual gestures, the presence of pornographic or offensive materials, or obscene language are not allowed.

Employees have a right to expect safe working conditions. The Occupational Safety and Health Act (OSHA) was established to prevent injuries and illnesses resulting from unsafe or unhealthy working conditions. (Refer to Chapter 22 for detailed discussion of the standards and requirements, especially the section on blood-borne pathogens which went into effect in 1992.) Compliance with this law requires that each employee be aware of possible risks associated with chemical hazards and how to protect themselves. Since there are many of these hazards in a medical practice, compliance and protection for employees are extremely important, and training sessions should be held in this area.

The Immigration Reform Act requires employers to verify the right of employees to work in the United States. Documentation acceptable for verification is a Social Security card or birth certificate. The United States Department of Justice Immigration and Naturalization Service will provide instructions and a form for employees and employers to complete (Figure 46-9).

Employers cannot discriminate or condemn any full-time employee for jury duty. While the employer does not have to continue pay during jury duty, the employee cannot lose seniority, insurance, or other benefits. Many employers continue an employee's full pay during the time of service on a jury since the reimbursement for jury service is so small. This is a way to benefit your employees and encourage good citizenship.

This list is by no means comprehensive, but does include personnel regulations most likely to affect the medical practice. Any concerns should be directed to the practice's attorney.

SPECIAL POLICY CONSIDERATIONS

There are several other managerial issues that may arise in a medical office for which the office manager will have to plan. These can include policies for temporary employees, smoking, avoiding discrimination, and having a support system in place for employees who need physical or emotional help.

Temporary Employees

Temporary employees who may be employed for ninety days or less include students who are serving an internship

U.S. Department of Justice
Immigration and Naturalization Service

OMB No. 1115-0136
Employment Eligibility Verification

Please read instructions carefully before completing this form. The instructions must be available during completion of this form. **ANTI-DISCRIMINATION NOTICE.** It is illegal to discriminate against work eligible individuals. Employers **CANNOT** specify which document(s) they will accept from an employee. The refusal to hire an individual because of a future expiration date may also constitute illegal discrimination.

Section 1. Employee Information and Verification. To be completed and signed by employee at the time employment begins

Print Name: Last	First	Middle Initial	Maiden Name
Address *(Street Name and Number)*		Apt. #	Date of Birth *(month/day/year)*
City	State	Zip Code	Social Security #

I am aware that federal law provides for imprisonment and/or fines for false statements or use of false documents in connection with the completion of this form.	I attest, under penalty of perjury, that I am (check one of the following): ☐ A citizen or national of the United States ☐ A Lawful Permanent Resident (Alien # A_____) ☐ An alien authorized to work until ___/___/___ (Alien # or Admission # _____)

Employee's Signature	Date *(month/day/year)*

Preparer and/or Translator Certification. *(To be completed and signed if Section 1 is prepared by a person other than the employee.) I attest, under penalty of perjury, that I have assisted in the completion of this form and that to the best of my knowledge the information is true and correct.*

Preparer's/Translator's Signature	Print Name
Address *(Street Name and Number, City, State, Zip Code)*	Date *(month/day/year)*

Section 2. Employer Review and Verification. To be completed and signed by employer. Examine one document from List A OR examine one document from List B **and** one from List C as listed on the reverse of this form and record the title, number and expiration date, if any, of the document(s)

List A	OR	List B	AND	List C
Document title: _____		_____		_____
Issuing authority: _____		_____		_____
Document #: _____		_____		_____
Expiration Date *(if any)*: ___/___/___		___/___/___		___/___/___
Document #: _____				
Expiration Date *(if any)*: ___/___/___				

CERTIFICATION - I attest, under penalty of perjury, that I have examined the document(s) presented by the above-named employee, that the above-listed document(s) appear to be genuine and to relate to the employee named, that the employee began employment on *(month/day/year)* ___/___/___ and that to the best of my knowledge the employee is eligible to work in the United States. (State employment agencies may omit the date the employee began employment).

Signature of Employer or Authorized Representative	Print Name	Title
Business or Organization Name	Address *(Street Name and Number, City, State, Zip Code)*	Date *(month/day/year)*

Section 3. Updating and Reverification. To be completed and signed by employer

A. New Name *(if applicable)*	B. Date of rehire *(month/day/year) (if applicable)*

C. If employee's previous grant of work authorization has expired, provide the information below for the document that establishes current employment eligibility.

Document Title:_____ Document #:_____ Expiration Date (if any):___/___/___

I attest, under penalty of perjury, that to the best of my knowledge, this employee is eligible to work in the United States, and if the employee presented document(s), the document(s) I have examined appear to be genuine and to relate to the individual.

Signature of Employer or Authorized Representative	Date *(month/day/year)*

Form I-9 (Rev. 11-21-91) N

Figure 46-9 Employment Eligibility Verification, Form I-9.

from a local college practicing their skills for when they will be on the job. They should be reviewed every two to three weeks in cooperation with their college supervisor. Give them as much actual hands-on experience as possible; they are your future employees and the employees of your colleagues.

Smoking Policy

Smoking on the premises has become a greater concern in the past ten years. Many places of employment do not allow smoking at all. Some states and cities have laws that may govern this issue for you. When a policy is established, it should cover everyone—employers, employees, and patients. The objective is to have a policy that is workable and enforceable, promotes health, encourages employee morale and productivity, and sets examples for patients. A designated place for smoking may be necessary.

Discrimination

The Americans with Disabilities Act (ADA) establishes guidelines prohibiting discrimination against a "qualified individual with a disability" in regard to employment. Someone with a disability who satisfies the skills necessary for the job, has the experience, education, and any other job requirements, and who, with reasonable accommodation, can perform the job cannot be discriminated against. Employers often find that persons with disabilities are their finest employees. Of particular note for medical personnel is that persons with AIDS are included in the guidelines set forth by the ADA. Persons with AIDS cannot be discriminated against. It can be assumed that if you are providing a safe working environment and all employees follow the rules for standard precautions (see Chapter 22), that reasonable accommodation has been made for the person with AIDS.

Employees with Chemical Dependencies or Emotional Problems

Employees with chemical dependency or emotional problems are ill and are to be treated as such. The situation should be approached constructively rather than punitively. Make a commitment to the employee to assure that the employee is fit for and capable of quality patient care. The human resources manager and physician-employer must be able to recognize the problem when it exists and deal openly and honestly with the issue. If drug or alcohol treatment becomes necessary and an employee is temporarily suspended from employment, do not allow the

employee to return unless it is made certain the employee will not endanger herself or anyone else.

PROVIDING/PLANNING EMPLOYEE TRAINING AND EDUCATION

Health care changes daily; new procedures are established, a better technique is discovered for performing a particular task. Major changes regularly occur in medical insurance. Computer systems are updated or new software is added. A more sophisticated telephone system is installed to make certain patients are responded to promptly. New state or federal regulations demand additional training or compliance to safety regulations not previously necessary. New medications become available which physicians may prescribe and employees must understand. All this demands that employees receive a continuing and constant update in their area of employment.

Training and education may be done within the practice or outside the practice. When an employee is a member of a professional organization such as the American Association of Medical Assistants or the American Association of Medical Transcriptionists, many monthly meetings will include continuing education opportunities. Numerous seminars and conferences held throughout the country may be beneficial to employees. Local hospitals often have continuing education opportunities that might be beneficial. The human resources manager will keep abreast of these opportunities and encourage employees to attend. Any continuing education opportunity that may benefit the employee on the job and the medical practice itself should ideally be paid for by the physician-employer(s).

It is often best to provide training and education within the facility when the training necessary is very specific to the medical practice. For instance, training on new computer software is apt to be very specific to the particular setting. When sophisticated new equipment is purchased, companies often provide in-house training for the individuals who will be using the equipment. Take advantage of as many of those opportunities as are available and for as many of your employees as possible. When the training is quite expensive or time consuming, make certain one person receives the training. Then have that individual train others. Whenever possible, provide training outside of regular hours when patients are not being seen—before or after the office closes or during a lunch period. Always pay employees for any time served over their regular working hours.

Careful attention to continuing education and training for employees will pay for itself many times over

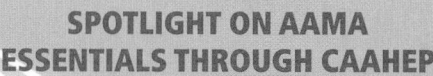

SPOTLIGHT ON AAMA ESSENTIALS THROUGH CAAHEP

● Conducting an exit interview with an employee who voluntarily leaves his or her position provides an atmosphere where the positive and the negative aspects of the position can be discussed. It can also identify what changes might be necessary when a new person fills the position.

● Part of being a good human resources manager is being able to solve conflicts between other employees, coworkers, supervisors, and physician-employers.

● Being able to acknowledge what stresses employees on the job will help to generate new ways or tasks to decrease or prevent stress.

again. The more confident and secure employees feel in the skills they are expected to perform, the more satisfied the practice's patients will be.

CONFLICT RESOLUTION

A good human resources manager will be a master at **conflict resolution**, solving problems between any two parties. The most difficult task is to prevent or solve conflicts that occur between employees or between employees and supervisors or physician-employers. Most conflict occurs because of poor communication or a misunderstanding, so effective communication is a goal for any manager.

Volumes of materials have been written about successful conflict management. One can probably never get enough material on the subject. Some guidelines that may be helpful in preventing and resolving conflicts follow:

● Listen to your employees. What do they say? What do they communicate nonverbally?

● Be prepared to temporarily assist an employee having a difficult time.

● Create a safe environment for an employee to admit a mistake.

● Manage by walking around and talking to your employees.

● Acknowledge the stressors of the job and compensate employees.

● Give ample verbal positive comments and pats on the back.

● Be honest with employees at all times.

● Provide office staff meetings in which employees can express their concerns.

● Treat employees fairly.

● Do not tolerate negative comments or actions among employees.

● Remember birthdays and special occasions with cards or small gifts.

● Provide small rewards when possible.

● Expect to work longer and harder than any employee.

● Have the physician-employer host a social lunch every 60 days.

● Keep employees informed of changes impacting them.

● Encourage an open door policy for concerns and complaints.

● Be a role model for all employees.

● Keep confidences.

● Encourage continuing education through workshops and seminars.

There is no end to such a list. A human resources manager who cares about each employee, who "carries water for the workers in the trenches," who administers fairly and honestly creates an environment where conflict will be at a minimum.

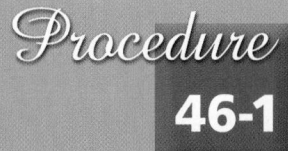

Procedure 46-1 Develop and Maintain a Policy Manual

PURPOSE:
To develop and maintain a comprehensive, up-to-date policy manual of all office policies relating to employee practices, benefits, office conduct, and so on.

EQUIPMENT/SUPPLIES:
Computer
Binder, such as a three-ring binder
Paper
Standard policy manual format

PROCEDURE STEPS:
1. Following office format, develop precise, written office policies detailing all necessary information pertaining to the staff and their positions. The information should include benefits, vacation, sick leave, hours, dress codes, evaluations, rules of conduct, and grounds for dismissal. RATIONALE: Well-defined policies clearly outlined for each employee are necessary for efficient and effective staff operations.
2. Identify procedures for reimbursing overtime, preventing discrimination and harassment, creating a safe working environment, and allowing for jury duty.
3. Include a policy statement related to smoking.
4. Identify steps to follow should an employee become disabled during employment.
5. Determine what employee opportunities for continuing education, if any, will be reimbursed; include requirements for recertification or licensure.
6. Provide a copy of the policy manual for each employee.
7. Review and update the policy manual regularly. Add or delete items as necessary, dating each revised page.

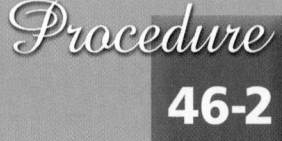

Procedure 46-2 Preparing a Job Description

PURPOSE:
To provide a precise definition of the tasks assigned to a job, to determine the expectations and level of competency required, and to specify the experience, training, and education needed to perform the job for purposes of recruiting and performance evaluation.

EQUIPMENT/SUPPLIES:
Computer
Paper
Standard job description format

PROCEDURE STEPS:
1. Detail each task that creates the job. RATIONALE: A detailed job description identifies clear expectations for each employee.
2. List special medical, technical, or clerical skills required.
3. Determine the level of education, training, and experience required for the position.
4. Determine where the job fits in the overall structure of the office.
5. Specify any unusual working conditions (hours, locations, and so on) that may apply.
6. Describe career path opportunities.

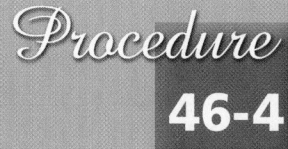

46-3 Interviewing

PURPOSE:
To screen applicants for training, experience, and characteristics to select the best candidate to fill the position vacancy.

PROCEDURE STEPS:

1. Review resumes and applications received.
2. Select candidates who most closely match the education and experience being sought.
3. Create an interview worksheet for each candidate listing points to cover.
4. Select an interview team; this team should always include the human resources or office manager and the immediate supervisor to whom the candidate will report.
5. Call personally to schedule interviews; this allows you to judge the applicant's telephone manners and voice.
6. Remind the interviewers of various legal restrictions concerning questions to be asked.
7. Conduct interviews in a private, quiet setting. RATIONALE: Careful interviewing of potential employees is an important step in hiring the best candidate for the position.
8. Put the applicant at ease by beginning with an overview about the practice and staff, briefly describing the job, and answering preliminary questions.
9. Ask questions about the applicant's work experience and educational background using the resume and interview worksheet as a guide.
10. Provide the most promising applicants additional information on benefits and a tour of the office if practical.
11. Applicant's general salary requirements may be discussed, but avoid discussion of a specific salary until a formal offer is tendered.
12. Inform the applicants when a decision will be made and thank each for participating in the interview.
13. Do not make a job offer until all the candidates have been interviewed.
14. Check references of all prospective employees.
15. Establish a second interview between the physician-employer(s) and the qualified candidate if necessary.
16. Confirm accepted job offers in writing, specifying details of the offer and acceptance.
17. Notify all unsuccessful applicants by letter when the position has been filled.

46-4 Orient and Train Personnel

PURPOSE:
To acquaint new employees with office policies, staff, what the job encompasses, procedures to be performed, and job performance expectations.

PROCEDURE STEPS:

1. Tour the facilities and introduce the office staff.
2. Complete employee-related documents and explain their purpose.
3. Explain the benefits programs.
4. Present the office policy manual and discuss its key elements.
5. Review federal and state regulatory precautions for medical facilities.
6. Review the job description.
7. Explain and demonstrate procedures to be performed and the use of procedure manuals supporting these procedures.
8. Demonstrate the use of any specialized equipment.
9. Assign a mentor from the staff to help with the orientation. RATIONALE: Without proper orientation and training, the best new employee can fail.

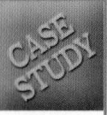

Bruce Goldman, CMA, has been with Inner City Health Care for one year. It is time for his first annual evaluation. The office manager, Jane O'Hara, gives Bruce a performance review form to complete before the formal evaluation. The following day, Bruce has an appointment to meet with Jane to discuss the evaluation. During the meeting, they discover they agree on most points.

46-1

CASE STUDY REVIEW

1. How should Jane handle discussing Bruce's frequent long lunches that extend beyond his scheduled lunch break time?

2. Would it be appropriate for Jane to ask a fellow CMA who works with Bruce to sit in to help her to evaluate him?

3. How should Jane end the formal evaluation?

SUMMARY

As you have seen from this discussion, human resources management is a challenge. It is, however, a rewarding one. While physician-employers are responsible for patients' physical care, the human resources manager is responsible for the employees in the organization. The human resources manager who is successful will manage these employees in a way that enables and encourages them to give the very best patient care possible. The medical assistant who has good communication skills and acquires additional training in human resources management will always have variety on the job and will have the satisfaction of watching a health care team run smoothly and efficiently.

REVIEW QUESTIONS

Multiple Choice

1. Human resources managers:
   a. need no special training for the job
   b. are responsible for hiring, training, and managing personnel
   c. usually work harder and longer hours than employees
   d. both b and c

2. The following questions may be asked in an interview:
   a. How old are you?
   b. Have you ever been arrested?
   c. Can you supply a birth certificate or a Social Security card?
   d. Do you plan to start a family soon?

3. Causes for immediate dismissal of an employee include:
   a. being late for work three times within a month
   b. theft, making fraudulent insurance claims
   c. placing a patient in jeopardy and breaching confidentiality
   d. both b and c

4. The most difficult tasks of the human resources manager may be:
   a. resolving conflicts between personnel and dismissing an employee
   b. evaluating employees and planning salary review
   c. planning for continuing education
   d. communicating with the physician-employer

5. The human resources manager will work closely with:
   a. the physician-employer
   b. the office manager
   c. all employees
   d. all the above

6. OSHA:
   a. requires employers to verify an employee's right to work in the United States
   b. protects employees who have disabilities from employment discrimination
   c. protects employees with chemical dependencies or emotional problems
   d. protects employees from unsafe or unhealthy working conditions

7. Conflict between employees:
   a. usually is the result of personality differences
   b. results when the manager is dictatorial
   c. usually is the result of poor communication or a misunderstanding
   d. is better ignored to allow employees to work it out
8. Employees receiving training or education necessary to the job:
   a. will seek that training after hours and not expect reimbursement
   b. will be continuous and constant in the health care field
   c. should always be paid for any time served over regular working hours
   d. both b and c
9. Personnel records:
   a. are usually kept for three to five years and may include payroll data
   b. are not available for everyone to view and must be kept confidential
   c. include all papers related to employment and personal data
   d. all the above
10. Dismissal:
    a. may be voluntary or involuntary
    b. should always be documented
    c. is a good time for an exit interview
    d. all the above

Critical Thinking

1. Discuss the importance of having employees participate in providing input to the job description.
2. How are references checked for prospective employees?
3. Discuss the advantages of having established policies and procedures for performance reviews.
4. How and when might physician-employers be directly involved in personnel matters?
5. You have an employee who gossips about other employees and is negative to everyone. She is otherwise an excellent employee. Plan a strategy to correct the situation.
6. You have just accepted a position to work in a larger more specialized clinic where you will be able to use skills you are not currently able to exercise. Identify two or three main points for a letter of resignation you will prepare.
7. An employee approaches you, the human resource manager, identifying that he/she has just become responsible for the care of an aging parent that may require occasional time away from work. You have no policy about how this absence should be treated. What kind of policy might be helpful? Where would you look for suggestions?
8. An exit interview form has been introduced in this chapter. Another simple form for an exit interview is to use the ABCs. A stands for "awesome." What do we do that is really good? B stands for "better." What could we do better in our organization? C stands for "change." What would you recommend we change? Discuss the merits of both forms for an exit interview.
9. Do a simple comparison of salaries in your community. Compare the hourly wages of a secretary, a medical assistant, a plumber, your automobile mechanic, and a person working in a fast-food restaurant. What conclusions can you make, if any?
10. What might physician-employers and human resource managers do to make certain they keep valued employees? Is salary really the most important issue?

WEB ACTIVITIES

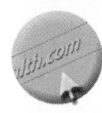

Research the World Wide Web for information about how to hire individuals. Consider http://www.ruf.rice.edu/~humres/Training/HowToHire as one resource for your search. Are there any differences in hiring for the medical profession as opposed to other types of businesses? What tips do you *not* find mentioned in the text?

REFERENCES/BIBLIOGRAPHY

Andress, A. A. (1996). *Manual of medical office management.* Philadelphia: W. B. Saunders Company.

Kinn, M. E., & Woods, M. A. (1999). *The medical assistant: Administrative and clinical* (8th ed.). Philadelphia: W. B. Saunders Co.

Mathis, R. L., & Jackson, J. H. (2000). *Human resource management* (9th ed.). Cincinnati, OH: South-Western College Publishing.

Ricardo, M. (1992). *Personnel management handbook* (2nd ed.). New York: McGraw-Hill, Inc.

Sullivan, D. (1992). *Effective management in nursing.* New York: Addison-Wesley.

ENTRY INTO THE PROFESSION

Chapter 47

PREPARING FOR MEDICAL ASSISTING CREDENTIALS

KEY TERMS

Accrediting Bureau of Health
  Education Schools (ABHES)
American Association of Medical
  Assistants (AAMA)
Certification Examination
Certified Medical Assistant (CMA)
Continuing Education Units (CEUs)
National Board of Medical Examiners
  (NBME)
Not current status
Recertification
Registered Medical Assistant (RMA)
Revalidation
Task Force for Test Construction

OUTLINE

OBJECTIVES

The student should strive to meet the following performance objectives and demonstrate an understanding of the facts and principles presented in this chapter through written and oral communication.

1. Define the key terms as presented in the glossary.
2. Differentiate between being certified and being registered.
3. Identify the benefits of certification and registration.
4. List the necessary qualifications to sit for the CMA certification examination.
5. List the necessary qualifications to sit for the RMA examination.
6. State when the CMA certification examination is offered and the registration deadlines.
7. State when the RMA examination is offered and the registration protocols.
8. Describe several methods for continuing education opportunities.
9. Explain when recertification/revalidation must take place.
10. Describe the procedure for recertification/revalidation.

**GENERAL
(TRANSDISCIPLINARY)**

Professionalism

- Enhance skills through
  continuing education

Legal Skills

- Recognize professional
  credentialing criteria

Dr. Ray Reynolds currently is the senior physician at Inner City Health
Care, a multi-physician urgent care center. When he began his practice
thirty-two years ago, however, he had a private practice and employed one
full-time and two part-time medical assistants. Dr. Reynolds felt the office
ran smoothly, except when an assistant had to be replaced. Retraining a new
person consumed a great deal of valuable time. Even if the new employee
came with experience from another medical office, the procedures still
required retraining.

Dr. Reynolds finds that when he needs to replace a medical assistant
now, he looks at the applicants' resumes and interviews only those
candidates who are certified medical assistants (CMAs) or registered medical
assistants (RMAs). The office is too busy to spend time training and
retraining new people.

INTRODUCTION

Thirty years ago medical assistants were trained on the job
by the practitioner for whom they were employed. Quality
control of training varied since there were no established
criteria for evaluating such training.

Hence, the certification examination was developed
by AAMA and the RMA examination was developed by

the AMT. Both examinations, along with methods of
continuing education and recertification, or revalidation,
establish criteria for evaluating training.

PURPOSE OF CERTIFICATION

Certification is intended to set a consistent minimum
standard for evaluating an individual's professional competence as a medical assistant. The **certification examination** is offered by the **American Association of
Medical Assistants (AAMA)**. Hiring physicians view
the credential as professional and an indication of entry-
level skills. Maintaining the credential demonstrates a
lifelong commitment to continuing education. The graduate medical assistant has a goal and challenge to which
to aspire, first by earning the credential, and second by
maintaining the credential through recertification.

Formal medical assistant education programs are
offered throughout the country in vocation-technical
high schools and colleges, proprietary schools, postsecondary vocational schools, community and junior colleges, and four-year colleges and universities. Medical
assistants may be trained on the job; however, physicians
recognize that their offices operate more efficiently with
professionally educated personnel.

PREPARING FOR THE
EXAMINATION

Preparation for the examination requires forethought,
scheduling, and discipline. It is important to plan well in
advance to ensure confidence and a positive test result,
earning your credential. If you are sitting for the examination immediately upon graduation, your preparation
time for the examination may only require two to three
months. If you have been out of school for some time or
your work experience has been very specialized, you may
need six to eight months to prepare for the examination.

During the forethought stage, determine the date
you want to sit for the examination. Check with the
appropriate Web site or make a telephone call to the
examination department to obtain the current application
form. The application form will contain information such
as dates, times, and locations of test sites, policies regarding
deadlines, incomplete applications, examination verification information, and information regarding study guides.

It is also important to consider looking for a study group or partner. The right study environment can be invaluable to your success for several reasons. First, it is important to select a study partner or group who shares your commitment to a successful outcome and who plans to sit for the examination near the same date you have selected. A study partner can also give you some accountability for keeping to the planned schedule.

Once it has been determined when and where you will sit for the examination and who your study partner, if any, will be, a meeting should be scheduled to discuss the review/study approach. It may be that your group will decide to review/study each subject provided in the Curriculum Content Outline accompanying the application. Other groups review/study only those areas in which they feel less confident. A plan that meets the needs of each group member and that all can agree to works best.

Meeting once or twice a week helps the group stay focused and on task. Independent study should be done throughout the week. During the independent study time, each group member may be asked to write 10 multiple choice questions relevant to the weeks' study topic. Answers to these questions should be on a separate page. Some find it helpful to also provide the rationale or textbook page number that supports their answer. When the group meets, a discussion of the study topic could take place and copies of the questions distributed for answering. The questions could then be corrected and discussion of any questionable or missed answers could take place.

Once a schedule has been established and agreed upon, discipline is required. It is critical that each group member spend time individually preparing for the next group meeting. Someone should be put in charge of each group meeting to keep the event from turning into a social time. To help with this, it is a good idea to set a specific time limit for the study/review session. If individuals want to visit after the session, they are free to do that without disrupting the purpose of the session. All members should be committed to being prepared and attending each scheduled review/study session.

REGISTERED MEDICAL ASSISTANT (RMA)

The American Medical Technologists (AMT), a national certifying body for health professionals, established the **Registered Medical Assistant (RMA)** credential in 1972. The RMA/AMT has its own bylaws, officers, local, state, and national organizations. Applicants for the RMA examination are graduates of schools accredited by the **Accrediting Bureau of Health Education Schools (ABHES)**, a regional accrediting commission, or other acceptable agency. Currently, there are over 52,000 RMAs certified by AMT. Registered medical assistants

SPOTLIGHT ON AAMA ESSENTIALS THROUGH CAAHEP

- Joining professional organizations, such as AAMA and AMT, and participating in the activities they afford, such as becoming certified or registered, helps a medical assistant to grow both personally and professionally.

- Obtaining certification or registration as a medical assistant requires a professional attitude, a high degree of understanding of medical assistant skills, and a positive approach to working with all types of patients and coworkers.

- A skilled and credentialed medical assistant should possess the ability to see beyond the complaining patient who may not be feeling well, and project a positive and professional caring attitude toward that patient.

and members of the AMT Registry are entitled to wear the RMA insignia.

AMT certification examinations are intended to evaluate the competence of entry-level practitioners. Content areas defined and validated by subject-matter experts, educators, and individuals working in their respective fields make up the test. Registration is granted in conjunction with other indicators of training and experience, since the tests provide only one source of information regarding examinee competence.

Examination Format and Content

The AMT registration examination consists of 200 to 210 multiple-choice questions. Examinees are required to select the single best answer; multiple answers for a single item are scored as incorrect. Test questions may require examinees to recall facts, interpret graphic illustrations, interpret information presented in case studies, analyze situations, or solve problems. The approximate percentages of questions in content areas are as follows:

1. General Medical Assisting Knowledge—42.5%
   - anatomy and physiology
   - medical terminology
   - medical law
   - medical ethics
   - human relations
   - patient education

2. Administrative Medical Assisting—22.5%
   - insurance
   - financial bookkeeping
   - medical secretarial-receptionist

3. Clinical Medical Assisting—35.0%
   - asepsis
   - sterilization
   - instruments
   - vital signs
   - physical examinations
   - clinical pharmacology
   - minor surgery
   - therapeutic modalities
   - laboratory procedures
   - electrocardiography
   - first aid

Application Process

The following criteria have been established for applicants sitting for the RMA Examination:

1. Applicant shall be of good moral character.
2. Applicant shall be a graduate of an accredited high school or acceptable equivalent.
3. Applicant must meet one of the following requirements:
   A. Applicant shall be a graduate of a
      - medical assistant program or institution accredited by an organization approved by the United States Department of Education
      - medical assistant program accredited by a Regional Accrediting Commission or by a national accrediting organization approved by the United States Department of Education
      - formal medical services training program of the United States Armed Forces
   B. Applicant shall have been employed in the profession of medical assisting for a minimum of five years, no more than two years of which may have been as an instructor in a postsecondary medical assistant program.
4. All applicants taking the AMT examination must pass to receive the Registered Medical Assistant (RMA) credential.

Application Completion and Test Administration Scheduling

The candidate should allow ample time for documentation to be completed before considering the scheduling of a test when submitting an application. It is the candidate's responsibility to keep abreast of the progress of the application and to aid in the timely response of references and employers. Tests may be scheduled *only* after applications are completed.

Examinations are administered throughout the year at testing center locations. Although most centers offer tests every week of the year, several locations administer tests only on specific days of the year. A complete and up-to-date list of sites will be forwarded when the candidate's application is approved. Most examinations may be scheduled within three days of application completion.

CERTIFIED MEDICAL ASSISTANT (CMA)

The American Association of Medical Assistants (AAMA) offers the certification examination. After successfully passing the certification examination, the **Certified Medical Assistant (CMA)** credential is awarded by the Certifying Board of the AAMA. The credential appears after your name and distinguishes you as a professional signifying achievement in a demanding career field.

CMAs are recognized by peers for their commitment to continued professional development. Survey results indicate that employers recognize the value of the credential by paying higher salaries and offering more benefits to CMAs. Broader career advancement opportunities and enhanced job security represent other benefits of certification. The CMA credential is a national credential and therefore is valid wherever the practitioner is employed within the United States.

Examination Format and Content

The CMA certification examination is a comprehensive test of the knowledge actually utilized in today's medical office. The content is drawn from an in-depth analysis of the numerous tasks medical assistants perform on a daily basis. The consultant for the examination is the **National Board of Medical Examiners (NBME)**, the same organization that develops licensure and specialty board examinations for physicians nationwide.

Examination questions are formulated by the Certifying Board's **Task Force for Test Construction**. This group is comprised of practicing medical assistants, physicians, and medical assisting educators from across the United States. Working with NBME, the Task Force updates the CMA examination annually to reflect changes in medical assistants' day-to-day responsibilities, as well as the latest developments in medical knowledge and technology.

The three major areas tested include:

1. *General medical knowledge:* terminology, anatomy, physiology, professionalism, communication, medicolegal guidelines/requirements
2. *Administrative knowledge:* typing and data entry, equipment, records management, screening and processing mail, scheduling and monitoring appointments, resource information/community services, managing physician's professional schedule and travel, managing the office, office policies and procedures, managing practice finances
3. *Clinical knowledge:* principles of infection control, treatment area, patient preparation and assisting the physician, patient history interview, collecting and processing specimens, preparing and administering medications, emergencies, first aid

Students must enroll as an AAMA member before their graduation date to be eligible for the reduced student rate. Once they are a student member they may stay at the student rate for one year after graduation if they don't choose to be an active or associate member and pay the higher dues amount. The additional year of membership at the reduced rate helps the recent graduate maintain membership while finding a job and getting established in a career.

Application Process

Candidates will want to read all instructions carefully before completing the application form. Incomplete or incorrect applications will not be processed and will be returned to the candidate. Postmark deadlines for applications, cancellations, and examination location changes are strictly enforced.

The examination is offered at over 250 test sites nationwide. A complete listing of the locations is included in the application. Applications are available from the AAMA Certification Department, 20 North Wacker Drive, Suite 1575, Chicago, IL 60606-2903 or telephone 312-424-3100 or e-Mail: certification@aama.ntl.org.

The appropriate application form must be completed and postmarked by October 1 for the January exam and by March 1 for the June exam.

The certification examination is scheduled from 9:00 AM to 1:00 PM the last Friday of January and the last Saturday in June.

It is recommended that the application be sent by certified mail, return receipt requested to verify delivery. The application must be typewritten or printed using black ink only. Be sure the application is signed and dated properly and the eligibility category section is completed appropriately.

Tear off the application page from the instruction pamphlet. Do not mail the instructions back with the application. Keep this information for future reference along with a copy of everything submitted, including a copy of your completed payment check or money order. If you are paying by VISA or MasterCard, provide the requested information at the top of the application.

A guide for the certification examination entitled *A Candidate's Guide to the AAMA Certification Examination* provides explanations of how to approach the types of questions used on the examination and tips on how to study for the content that will be tested. A sample 120-question examination is included.

Eligibility Categories and Requirements

You must fulfill one of the four eligibility categories to apply for the CMA examination. Figure 47-1 describes these requirements.

Grounds for Denial of Eligibillity

The following are grounds for denial of eligibility for the Certified Medical Assistant (CMA) credential, or for discipline of Certified Medical Assistants (CMAs):

- obtaining or attempting to obtain certification, or recertification of the CMA credential, by fraud or deception
- knowingly assisting another to obtain or attempt to obtain certification or recertification by fraud or deception
- misstatement of material fact or failure to make a statement of material fact in application for certification or recertification
- falsifying information required for admission to the CMA examination, inpersonating another examinee, or falsifying education or credentials
- copying answers, permitting another to copy answers, or providing or receiving unauthorized advice about examination content during the CMA examination
- unauthorized possession or distribution of examination materials, including copying and reproducing examination questions and problems.

Individuals who have been found guilty of a felon, or pleaded guilty to a felon, are not eligible to take the CMA Exam. However, the Certifying Board may grant a waiver based upon mitigating circumstances, which may include, but need not be limited to the following:

CATEGORY 1—CAAHEP GRADUATING STUDENT OR RECENT GRADUATE

Graduating students must have completed, by January 31 for the January test and by June 30 for the June test, formal training, including an externship, in a medical assisting program accredited by CAAHEP. If the student fails to complete the program by the required date, the exam will be considered invalid. Scores will not be released, and refunds will not be provided.

Requirement: Applications must be signed by the program director.

Recent graduates must take the exam within 12 months of graduation to qualify for the discounted fee.

Requirement: To verify completion, a photocopy of a diploma, certificate, associate degree, or official transcript must accompany the application, or the program director's signature must be obtained.

CATEGORY 2—CAAHEP GRADUATE

The candidate must be a graduate of a medical assisting program accredited by CAAHEP.

Requirement: To verify completion, a photocopy of a diploma, certificate, associate degree, or official transcript must accompany the application.

CATEGORY 3—ABHES GRADUATE WITH THE REQUIRED WORK EXPERIENCE

The candidate must have graduated from an ABHES accredited medical assisting program and have completed 12 months of full-time or 24 months of part-time health work experience under the supervision of a licensed health care provider, no later than the deadline date for the examination.

Requirements: (1) To verify graduation from an ABHES accredited medical assisting program, a photocopy of a diploma, certificate, associate degree, or official transcript must accompany the application. (2) To verify health care work experience, the candidate must submit documentation *on the employer's letterhead and signed by the employer* verifying 12 months of full-time or 24 months part-time health work experience under the supervision of a licensed health care provider. (School internship/externship or volunteer work experience does not meet the work experience requirement.) Such experience must be acquired *by the application deadline date.*

Full-time health work experience is defined as 30 or more hours per week. Part-time health work experience is defined as less than 30 hours per week.

CATEGORY 4—RECERTIFICANT

The candidate must be a Certified Medical Assistant applying for the CMA Examination to recertify his or her credential.

Requirement: A copy of the candidate's CMA certificate should accompany the application. (Contact the AAMA Certification Department if you are unable to locate your certificate. The month and year that you passed the CMA Examination will be required to research your records.)

Figure 47-1 CMA Eligibility Categories and Requirements through June 2001. (Source: *AAMA's CMA Examination.* AAMA Certification Department, Dept. 79-7999, Chicago, IL 60678-7999.)

- the age at which the crime was committed
- the circumstances surrounding the crime
- the nature of the crime committed
- the length of time since the conviction
- the individual's criminal history since the conviction
- the individual's current employment references
- the individual's character references
- other evidence demonstrating the ability of the individual to perform the professional responsibilities competently, and evidence that the individual does not pose a threat to the health or safety of patients

How to Recertify

Recertification of the CMA credential may be achieved by either reexamination or by the continuing education method. Recertification credits are evaluated on supportive documentation, and on their relevancy to medical assisting as defined by the AAMA Medical Assistant Role Delineation Study or the Content Outline for the Certification/Recertification Examination.

A total of 60 points is necessary to recertify the CMA credential. At least 20 points must be from AAMA continuing education units (CEUs). The remaining 40 points may be any formal credit (e.g., non-AAMA CEUs, contact hours, college credit) that has relevancy to medical assisting as defined by the AAMA Medical Assistant Role Delineation Study (shown in the appendices) or the Content Outline for the Certification/Recertification Examination. All 60 points may be from AAMA CEUs, but 20 *must be* from AAMA CEUs.

Continuing education courses are offered by local, state, and national AAMA groups. Guided study programs are also available through AAMA's "Quest for Excellence" program. *The Professional Medical Assistant,* the official bimonthly publication of AAMA, provides articles designated for continuing education units.

The CMA credentials must be recertified every five years. Certificates are current through December 31 of the fifth year following certification or recertification. For example, if you certified or recertified in 1996, your credential would hold current status through December 31, 2001. Failure to recertify will result in a **not current status.**

A CMA need not be a member of the AAMA, nor currently employed, in order to recertify. Figure 47-2 illustrates the Continuing Education Verification Form used to submit CEUs to AAMA for recertification. The entire recertification by continuing education instructions and application can be downloaded from AAMA's website (www.aama-ntl.org). Review of recertification applications can take up to 90 days. If all criteria are met, recertification is granted. The date that the application is postmarked to the AAMA Executive Office will be the date of recertification.

Upon meeting recertification requirements, the applicant receives a seal to affix to the original certificate. A Recertification Certificate is also available for purchase. AMT promotes continued education and **revalidation** of the RMA credential. Revalidation is processed through the American Medical Technologists Institute for Education (AMTIE) and is required on a five-year cycle. *Vital Signs,* a quarterly publication by AMT, is designed for registered medical assistants and students of ABHES schools.

The American Medical Technologists Institute for Education (AMTIE) offers STEP, a continuing education home-study program for healthcare practitioners. STEP is published in AMT's *Journal of Continuing Education Topics & Issues.* Health care practitioners may earn continuing education credit for reading articles, answering self-study questions, and returning answer sheets to the AMT office for scoring. AMT records credit earned and issues annual reports of STEP activities to program participants.

AAMA's CMA Recertification by Continuing Education
Continuing Education Verification Form

Name: Jane Doe   Social Security Number: 000-00-0000   Page Number: 1

Read the application instructions before completing this sheet. If additional space is needed, this form may be photocopied. You may use computer-formatted facsimiles of any part of this application. TYPE or neatly PRINT the information. On each page you use, enter your name, Social Security number, and the page number above. To convert credits to points, see How to Convert Credit to Recertification Points in the instructions. For information on how to determine the content category, refer to the section Content Areas Defined. Supportive documents must be attached to this form. Also attach a photocopy of your original certificate, if available. Do *not* send your original certificate.

1	2	3	4	5	6	7	8	9
Date of activity (m/d/y)	Sponsor (group or organization issuing the credit for the continuing education activity)	Program title	Amount and type of credit earned (eg, CEU, CME, contact hour or college credit)	Recertification points — AAMA CEUs	Other credit	Points per content area — Gen.	Adm.	Clin.
If using more than one page, copy the cumulative total for each column (5–9) from the previous page ☞								
7/3/98	AAMA	Adminis. the Medical Office	.4 CEU	4			4	
8/24/98	Trident Chapter	Medical Nutritional Needs	.6 CEU	6		6		
9/2/98	Eli Lily Co.	Aspects of Diabetes	.2 CEU		2			2
10/11/98	Tri-City Chapter	ICD-9-CM	.4 CEU	4			4	
11/17/98	AAMA	Quality Urinalysis Testing	.2 CEU	2				2
1/9/99	Administrative Seminars Inc.	Personnel Management	.8 CEU		8	8		
3/19/99	Riverside Hospital	Hepatitis In-service	1 Contact Hr.		1			1
4/24/99	South Carolina AAMA St. Soc.	Child Abuse	.4 CEU	4		2	1	1
6/21/99	U. of South Carolina	AIDS Awareness	2 Semester Hrs.		36	18		18
9/8/99	American Heart Association	CPR	4 Contact Hrs.		4	1		3
Total points in each column (5–9): (If using more than one page, copy the cumulative total for each column (5–9) to the top of the next page.)				20	51	27	17	27

Figure 47-2 Sample Continuing Education Verification Form for AAMA. (Source: *AAMA's CMA Examination.* AAMA Certification Department, Dept. 79-7999, Chicago, IL 60678-7999.)

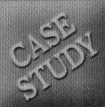

It is February, and Juan Estaban is beginning to research the procedures and requirements for taking the medical assisting certification examination. Juan is enrolled in a CAAHEP-accredited program.

47-1

CASE STUDY REVIEW

1. If Juan wants to take the examination in June, what is the procedure for applying?

2. Juan is setting up a study schedule. He plans to review course textbooks and tests, purchase a certification review study guide, and set up a study group. Set up a sample study schedule.

3. What criteria should Juan use when asking people to join his study group?

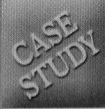

It is May, and Nancy McFarland, who graduated from an ABHES-accredited program four and a half years ago, is beginning to research the procedures and requirements for taking the medical assistant examination. Nancy completed her internship at Inner City Health Care and was hired to work there full-time (35 hours per week) when she graduated.

47-2

CASE STUDY REVIEW

1. If Nancy wants to take the exam in January, what is the procedure for applying?

2. Nancy is setting up a study schedule. She plans to review course textbooks and tests, purchase a study guide, and set up a study group. Develop a simple study schedule.

3. What criteria should Nancy use when asking people to join her study group?

SUMMARY

Many advantages for certification/recertification and registration have been discussed in this chapter. Although certification examinations are not legally required for practicing medical assistants, it is the goal of CAAHEP-accredited and ABHES-accredited institutions to encourage graduates to sit for and maintain their credentials.

Membership in the AAMA or in the AMT is also encouraged. In addition to the previously mentioned advantages of AAMA, other benefits such as receiving quarterly newsletters, *The Professional Medical Assistant* journal, credit card privileges, group insurance plans, legal advice, a loan program, and a discounted car rental program are available.

With nearly 400 local AAMA chapters and 51 affiliate state societies, there is the benefit of networking with others in the profession. As an information source for both professional and association issues, the executive staff at the AAMA's national headquarters is available to answer questions at a toll-free number (1-800-228-2262).

AMT currently has 37 chapters which meet regularly and allow networking with other Registered Medical Assistants plus other allied health professionals registered through the AMT, including phlebotomists, medical laboratory technicians, and dental assistants.

REVIEW QUESTIONS

Multiple Choice

1. The goal and challenge of each graduating medical assistant should be to:
   a. find employment
   b. have a good benefit package
   c. possess entry-level skills
   d. earn the CMA credential and maintain it

2. The certification examination is:
   a. a comprehensive test based on tasks medical assistants perform daily
   b. all true/false questions
   c. developed by the AMTIE
   d. developed by the NBME

3. Benefits from membership in a professional organization such as AAMA or AMT include all of the following *except*:
   a. discounted rates on legal representation
   b. legal advice
   c. nationwide networking opportunities
   d. professional journal publications
4. Recertification of the CMA credential options include:
   a. submit work experience
   b. reexamination or CEU method
   c. submit on-the-job training
   d. submit military training
5. Applications for the CMA exam must be postmarked by:
   a. October 1 for January exam and March 1 for June exam
   b. October 31 for January exam and March 31 for June exam
   c. September 30 for January exam and April 30 for June exam
   d. September 1 for January exam and April 1 for June exam
6. The RMA was established by the:
   a. ABHES
   b. CAAHEP
   c. AMT
   d. AAMA
7. Candidates who graduate from a medical assisting program that is not CAAHEP-accredited on the date of graduation, but is accredited by CAAHEP within 36 months of that date, are eligible to apply for the CMA exam under which category(ies)?
   a. Category 1
   b. Category 4
   c. Categories 3 or 4
   d. Categories 1 or 2
8. RMA examinations:
   a. are offered at Cogent testing center locations
   b. are offered twice a year
   c. are offered three times a year
   d. are offered six times a year

Critical Thinking

1. Describe the purpose and benefits of certification.
2. Identify the necessary qualifications for maintaining current CMA status
3. Identify the necessary qualifications for the certification examination as an RMA.

4. Differentiate between the methods of recertification for the CMA.
5. Identify several approaches to collecting CEUs.
6. List advantages of membership in a professional organization for medical assistants.

WEB ACTIVITIES

Using the World Wide Web, search your local and state AAMA or AMT web sites. Print and turn in to your instructor the location, meeting schedules, and any upcoming events planned for your state.

DOCUMENTATION

Upon successfully passing the Certification Examination and earning the CMA credential, one should begin to document all CEUs earned. Copies of the form illustrated in Figure 47-2 may be obtained from the AAMA for this purpose. It is important to have the following information for CEU documentation:

- complete date of the activity
- sponsor (group or organization issuing the credit for the CE activity)
- program title
- amount and type of credit earned (e.g., CEU, CME, contact hour or college credit)
- recertification points (AAMA CEUs or other credit)
- points per content area (general, administrative, clinical)

REFERENCES/BIBLIOGRAPHY

AAMA. (1997–1998). *AAMA certification/recertification examination for medical assistants*; January and June 2000 Application Instructions. Chicago: AAMA.

American Medical Technologists. [On-line]. Available: http://www.amt1.com.

Frew, M. A., Lane, K., & Frew, D. R. (1995). *Comprehensive medical assisting: Competencies for administrative and clinical practice*. Philadelphia: F. A. Davis Company.

Chapter
48

EMPLOYMENT STRATEGIES

KEY TERMS

Accomplishment Statements
Application/Cover Letter
Application Form
Bullet Point
Career Objective
Chronological Resume
Contact Tracker
Functional Resume
Interview
Power Verbs
References
Resume
Targeted Resume

OUTLINE

Developing a Strategy
  Self-Assessment
Job Analysis and Research
Budgetary Needs Analysis
Resume Preparation
  Resume Specifications
  Clear and Concise Resumes
  Accomplishments
  References
  Accuracy
  Resume Styles
  Vital Resume Information

Application/Cover Letters
Completing the Application Form
The Look of Success
  Personal and Professional Poise
The Interview Process
  Preparing for the Interview
  The Actual Interview
  Closing the Interview
Interview Follow-Up
  Follow-Up Letter
  Follow Up by Telephone

OBJECTIVES

The student should strive to meet the following performance objectives and demonstrate an understanding of the facts and principles presented in this chapter through written and oral communication.

1. Define the key terms as presented in the glossary.
2. List the steps involved in job analysis and research.
3. Describe a contact tracker and its usefulness.
4. Give three examples of accomplishment statements.
5. Differentiate chronological, functional, and targeted resumes.
6. Identify the purpose and content of a cover letter.
7. Demonstrate effective ways to anticipate and respond to an interviewer's questions.
8. Describe appropriate overall appearance and dress for an interview.
9. Identify the benefits of writing a follow-up letter.

**GENERAL
(TRANSDISCIPLINARY)**

Professionalism

- Project a professional manner and image
- Demonstrate initiative and responsibility
- Adhere to ethical principles

Communication Skills

- Use effective and correct verbal and written communications
- Recognize and respond to verbal and nonverbal communications

Eun Mee Soo is a graduate of a CAAHEP-accredited medical assisting program and recently passed the certification examination. She is now preparing her resume and beginning her job search. Eun Mee plans to move out of state (she always dreamed of moving north), so she will also be looking for a new apartment. All of these changes are a bit unsettling for Eun Mee. She is beginning to wonder if she should not relocate at this time but stay close to home until she feels more secure.

INTRODUCTION

So you are about to graduate from the medical assistant program! This time is often unsettling since many changes are occurring; the loss of security the classroom environment provided, loss of contact with fellow classmates, and loss of a structured schedule are just a few changes. Questions such as: Am I ready for my first job? How do I find a job? What do I say at the interview? begin to surface.

The focus on employment may represent apprehension and doubt or be sparked with anticipation and a sense of fulfillment. This chapter has been included to provide direction and to help answer some of the questions related to the job search.

DEVELOPING A STRATEGY

Positive thinking is one of the primary keys to success in planning your career and job search. Positive thinking leads to positive attitudes, positive feelings about yourself and others, and positive words and actions.

There is a job out there for you! Those individuals who are successful at finding that first job devote a minimum of forty hours per week at job strategy tactics. In other words, finding their first job is their first job. These individuals do not become discouraged by rejection, rather they learn from it and work harder for the next opportunity.

Self-Assessment

Perhaps the first place to begin the job campaign is with a self-assessment exercise. This exercise should stimulate your thought process related to the type of employment upon which you want to focus. Take a moment now to complete the exercise, Self-Evaluation Work Sheet (Figure 48-1).

JOB ANALYSIS AND RESEARCH

Begin to compile a list of potential employers in your immediate area or the geographical area in which you want to work. This may be accomplished by looking through the yellow pages of the telephone directory and/or the business listings. Select facilities that are within your geographic boundaries, provide the work setting and/or specialty you have selected, and appear to offer the basic guidelines you have established.

Now begin your research. Many offices have brochures available that describe their services, appointment scheduling, telephone policy, fees and insurance protocol, confidentiality issues, after-hours medical coverage, and mission statement or philosophy of practice criteria. Most of the larger medical centers offer community education series and prepare a calendar of events publication. Also found in these publications are articles on wellness issues, safety precautions, financial reports, and introductions of new procedures, equipment, and staff members. These documents are an excellent resource tool for learning more about a particular facility and should be studied carefully.

The computer can be of great value in your job search. There are multitudes of employment sites on the Internet and it is possible to search newspaper want ads for almost any large city you desire. The yellow pages are also on-line for most cities, permitting you to easily search for medical facilities that are in line with your goals and objectives.

It may also be helpful to develop your own list of "Hot Line" telephone numbers. Television and radio sta-

---

SELF-EVALUATION WORK SHEET

Respond to the following questions honestly and sincerely. They are meant to assist you in self-assessment.

1. List your three strongest attributes as related to people, data, or things.
   i.e.; Interpersonal skills related to people
   Accuracy related to data
   Mechanical ability related to things

   _____ related to _____
   _____ related to _____
   _____ related to _____

2. List your three weakest attributes as related to people, data, or things.
   _____ related to _____
   _____ related to _____
   _____ related to _____

3. How do you express yourself? excellent, good, fair, poor
   Orally _____ In writing _____

4. Do you work well as a leader of a group or team? Yes _____ No _____

5. Do you prefer to work alone and on your own? Yes _____ No _____

6. Can you work under stress/pressure? Yes _____ No _____

7. Do you enjoy new ideas and situations? Yes _____ No _____

8. Are you comfortable with routines/schedules? Yes _____ No _____

9. Which work setting do you prefer?
   Single-physician setting _____ Multiple-physician setting _____
   Small clinic setting _____ Large clinic setting _____
   Single specialty setting _____ Multi-specialty setting _____

10. Are you willing to relocate? _____ Willing to travel? _____

Figure 48-1   Self-evaluation work sheets can help determine a person's strengths, weaknesses, and preferences before the job search begins.

tions often share these numbers. By compiling these numbers into a list, you can efficiently make calls to determine if positions are open and the correct name and spelling of the person to whom the application should be addressed. A visit to your local employment agency may also provide additional resources. Remember to check for job openings on bulletin boards in laundromats, churches, health clubs, and any variety of locations. The Chamber of Commerce in your community may be another resource to consider. Journals and publications such as *The Professional Medical Assistant* (PMA) and your local AAMA chapter will be valuable resources to utilize. Network with professionals at every opportunity. Employers will often report employment opportunities to the Job Placement Center in the college campus or to your medical assistant instructors.

Competition in today's employment arena is very keen. Solicit all help possible as you search for that first job. Friends, relatives, and acquaintances provide the most successful leads to potential employment opportunities. Tell everyone you are looking for a job, the type of position, and the setting in which you would most like to work. Do not forget to tell your personal physician, ophthalmologist, and dentist about your employment goals. They have contact with other professionals who may need help and want to hire a medical assistant.

Direct contact with employers is the second most successful means of finding employment. It takes a lot of nerve and self-confidence to call on prospective employers unannounced or to pick up the telephone to call and ask if they are likely to be hiring medical assistants in the near future. This is an effective approach, however.

The third most effective way to gain employment is a combination of the methods previously discussed. For example, you are visiting the physician's office for an allergy injection. The medical assistant administering the injection asks how your classes are progressing and you share that you are about to graduate and are looking for an entry-level position. The medical assistant tells you that the office next door has a position open. After the injection, if you are dressed appropriately, you could stop in to inquire about the position and ask for an application form.

Don't overlook your externship facility if you participated in an externship program. Very frequently new MAs entering the job market are hired by the site where they did their externship. The site has had time to come to know them, their work ethic, and their knowledge. In addition the site has already invested time in some training so former externs are knowledgeable of the policies and procedures of the facility. Even if the site decides to advertise for the position and interview candidates, you will have an advantage over the other applicants provided your performance was good during your work there.

Review the reasons for employers not hiring shown in Figure 48-2. This figure lists the qualities employers want and do not want in an employee.

When you are serious about the job search and are giving forty hours per week to the process, you will contact numerous individuals. By devising some means of recording these contacts, their responses, and your action, you will not become confused or forget valuable information. A **contact tracker** such as the one suggested in Figure 48-3 may be helpful.

BUDGETARY NEEDS ANALYSIS

It is critical that you know just how much income is required to meet your living expenses. To accomplish this, begin to keep a diary of all purchases and payments. By reviewing your checkbook register you should be able to itemize basic expenditures; i.e., rent, utilities, payments (car, credit card), food, clothing, insurance, taxes, and so on. Once a monthly expenditure record is established, an estimate of the money required to live on may be calculated.

REASONS FOR EMPLOYERS NOT HIRING

Employers in business were asked to list reasons for not hiring a job seeker. Given in rank order (from most unwanted to least unwanted), the 15 biggest gripes are as follows:

1. Poor appearance (not dressed properly, poorly groomed).
2. Acting like a know-it-all.
3. Cannot express self clearly; poor voice, diction, grammar.
4. Lack of planning for work—no purpose or goals.
5. Lack of confidence or poise.
6. No interest in or enthusiasm for the job.
7. Not active in school extracurricular programs.
8. Interested only in the best dollar offer.
9. Poor school record (academic, attendance).
10. Unwilling to start at the bottom.
11. Making excuses, hedges on unfavorable record.
12. No tact.
13. Not mature.
14. No curiosity about the job.
15. Critical of past employers.

Figure 48-2   Reasons for employers not hiring. (Courtesy of Highline Community College, Counseling/Career Center, Des Moines, WA)

CONTACT TRACKER

	Company Name/Address	Telephone Number	Contact's Name	Resume Sent	Application/ Cover Letter	Application Form Sent	Follow-Up Phone	Follow-Up Letter	Result
1.									
2.									
3.									
4.									
5.									
6.									

Figure 48-3   A simple contact tracker such as this can help organize all communication you may have with potential employers.

RESUME PREPARATION

A **resume** is a summary data sheet or a brief account of your qualifications and progress in the career you have chosen. It is a useful tool for selling yourself and provides opportunity to describe your education, what you have done, and what you can do, and lists those who can vouch for your integrity and experience. A resume that is well thought out and written in such a way as to create interest in what you have to contribute to the employer may reward you with many interviews. During the interview your resume serves as a reference from which the interviewer may be prompted to ask questions.

Resume Specifications

The resume should be limited to one page in length. Keep a 1 to 1½ inch margin on all four sides of the page to create a picture-like frame. Capitalize major headings and single space between lines. Double space between sections. The use of **bullet point** lists instead of paragraphs aids the interviewer in gleaning key points quickly.

Select a high-quality bond stationery that is standard 8½ × 11 inches with a weight of between 16 and 25 pounds. This paper weight provides aesthetic benefit and will also accept the ink better resulting in a clean, sharp print resolution. Buff or ivory paper with matching envelope has the greatest eye appeal and distinguishes your resume from others.

Use a computer or word processor to produce your resume. It allows you the freedom to experiment with placement to create a picture-perfect resume or to individualize the resume for a particular position or facility.

Clear and Concise Resumes

Your resume must be short and easy to read and understand. Use statements that are positive and reflect confidence and portray you as a problem solver. Be sure that any information given within your resume or application form is not misleading or exaggerated. Leave out the word *I* when writing your resume. This is your personal resume and it is understood that you are referring to yourself.

Accomplishments

Use **accomplishment statements** if you have them from your externship or work experience. Accomplishment statements begin with **power verbs**, give a brief description of what you did, and the demonstrable results that were produced. Figure 48-4 provides a list of sample power verbs. Some accomplishment statement examples are: "Utilized computer skills to schedule and reschedule patient appointments" and "Demonstrated skills in setting up sterile trays and assisting with sterile procedures."

Accompanied	Billed	Computed	Demonstrated	Enumerated	Graded
Accumulated	Bought	Conducted	Deposited	Established	Graphed
Achieved	Budgeted	Conferred	Described	Estimated	Greeted
Acquired	Built	Constructed	Detailed	Evaluated	Headed
Administered	Calculated	Consulted	Determined	Examined	Hired
Admitted	Cashed	Contacted	Developed	Exchanged	Identified
Advised	Catalogued	Contracted	Devised	Exhibited	Implemented
Allowed	Changed	Contrasted	Diagnosed	Expanded	Improved
Analyzed	Charged	Contributed	Directed	Expedited	Improvised
Answered	Charted	Controlled	Discovered	Experienced	Increased
Applied	Classified	Converted	Dismantled	Fabricated	Indexed
Appointed	Cleaned	Convinced	Dispatched	Facilitated	Indicated
Appraised	Cleared	Coordinated	Distributed	Figured	Influenced
Arranged	Closed	Copied	Documented	Filled	Informed
Assembled	Coded	Corrected	Drew	Financed	Initiated
Assessed	Collated	Corresponded	Drove	Finished	Inspected
Assigned	Collected	Counseled	Earned	Fitted	Installed
Attached	Commanded	Created	Educated	Fixed	Instructed
Attained	Communicated	Debated	Employed	Formalized	Insured
Attended	Compiled	Decided	Encouraged	Formulated	Integrated
Authorized	Completed	Delegated	Engineered	Fulfilled	
Balanced	Composed	Delivered	Entertained	Generated	*(continues)*

Figure 48-4 These sample power verbs may help you define your previous job responsibilities.

Interpreted	Maintained	Overcame	Prompted	Related	Showed
Interviewed	Managed	Packaged	Proofread	Relayed	Sold
Introduced	Manufactured	Packed	Proposed	Renewed	Solicited
Inspected	Marked	Paid	Proved	Reorganized	Sorted
Inventoried	Marketed	Participated	Provided	Repaired	Stocked
Investigated	Measured	Patrolled	Published	Replaced	Stored
Invoiced	Met	Perfected	Purchased	Reported	Straightened
Issued	Modified	Piloted	Ran	Requested	Summarized
Judged	Monitored	Placed	Rated	Researched	Supervised
Justified	Motivated	Planned	Read	Responsible for	Supplied
Kept	Negotiated	Posted	Rearranged	Retrieved	Taught
Learned	Nominated	Prepared	Rebuilt	Revised	Telephoned
Lectured	Noted	Prescribed	Recalled	Routed	Tested
Led	Notified	Presented	Received	Scheduled	Trained
Licensed	Observed	Priced	Recommended	Secured	Transferred
Listed	Obtained	Printed	Reconciled	Selected	Transported
Listened	Opened	Processed	Recorded	Sent	Typed
Loaded	Operated	Procured	Reduced	Separated	Verified
Located	Ordered	Produced	Referred	Served as	
Logged	Organized	Programmed	Registered	Serviced	
Mailed	Outlined	Promoted	Regulated	Set up	

Figure 48-4   *(continued)*

References

Select a variety of **references** to be included on or with your resume. References may be listed on a separate sheet of paper that matches your resume. An individual who knows you or has worked with you long enough to make an honest assessment and recommendation regarding your background history is an excellent reference person. Use only nonrelated persons as references unless the work relationship has been formalized.

Choose references who are well-respected and are clear speakers and writers. No matter how much someone likes you and your work, it can hurt you if they cannot convey the information in a business-like manner. Professional references such as a former instructor, physician, externship supervisor, or fellow coworkers are excellent reference choices.

Always ask permission to use someone as a reference *before* the name is printed on the resume or reference list. You will want to verify the correct spelling of the reference's name, title, place of employment and position, and telephone number for prospective employers.

Help your references aid you in obtaining an interview and employment. A personal visit or telephone call to discuss your career objectives and how you plan to conduct your job search will be helpful. Ask for any suggestions they may have to offer. Provide them with a copy of your resume and cover letter. This helps them visualize the position for which you are applying and picture how you may benefit that employer.

Keep in touch with references. Check back to see who has called and how things went. Knowing what employers ask may produce some valuable pointers for your next letter, resume, or interview.

Finally, thank your references. They will appreciate knowing how you are doing and that you value their assistance.

Leave out "References Upon Request" if necessary to shorten your resume to save space. Employers know they can ask for references at a later date.

Accuracy

Proofread, proofread, and proofread your resume. Ask someone who is a good speller or your references to edit your resume. Then proofread it again yourself. Do not rely on your computer spell check; it does not differentiate between words such as to, too, two or here and hear. Eliminate repetition of information such as task descriptions. Summarize employment prior to ten years ago or leave it off if not relevant to the position you are seeking.

Resume Styles

Various resume styles have been developed, each having specific advantages and disadvantages. You will want to choose the style or combination of styles that best describes your strengths and ability to do the job. It may be to your advantage to check with the human resources department of the facility to which you are applying to see if there is a resume style preference.

Chronological Resume. The **chronological resume** is used by individuals who have job experience. The job history begins with the most recent experience first and concludes with the earliest experience at the bottom.

The chronological resume is advantageous when:

- The position is in a highly traditional field, such as teaching, law, or health care, where specific employers are of paramount interest

- You are staying in the same field as prior jobs

- Job history shows real growth and development

- Prior titles are impressive

The chronological resume is *not* advantageous when:

- Your work history is spotty

- You are changing career goals

- You have been in the same job for many years

- You are looking for your first job

Figure 48-5 is an illustration of a chronological resume.

Ashley Jackson
2031 Craig Street
Renton, Washington 98055
(206) 255-1365

WORK EXPERIENCE

September, 1996–Present   GROUP HEALTH COOPERATIVE
Direct support for a dermatology/surgery practice.
Patient preparation.
Medical and surgical asepsis.
Assist with sterile procedures.
Patient follow-up.

June, 1994–August, 1996   VALLEY INTERNAL MEDICINE
Clinical responsibilities.
Assisted with surgeries in ambulatory care setting.
Patient preparation.
Medical and surgical asepsis.
Assisted with sterile procedures.

March, 1994–June, 1994   VALLEY INTERNAL MEDICINE
Medical Assistant Externship
Administrative duties and clinical responsibilities utilizing all medical assisting skills, including patient induction, chief complaint, vital signs, patient preparation, EKGs, medical and surgical asepsis, and sterile procedures.

EDUCATION/CERTIFICATION

Associate in Applied Science degree, June, 1994, Highline Community College, Des Moines, Washington, 98198-9800.

Certified Medical Assistant, June, 1994.

Figure 48-5   Sample chronological resume.

Functional Resume. The **functional resume** highlights specialty areas of accomplishment and strengths. It allows you to organize these in an order that supports your work objective.

The functional resume is advantageous when:

- Your experience can be sorted into areas of function; i.e., administrative, clinical, supervisory
- You are changing careers
- You are reentering the job market after an absence
- Your career path or growth is not clear from a chronological listing
- You have had a variety of different, apparently unconnected work experiences

- Much of your work has been volunteer, freelance, or temporary
- You want to eliminate repetition of descriptions of job duties
- You have extensive specialized experience

The functional resume is *not* advantageous when:

- You want to emphasize a management growth pattern
- Your most recent employers have been highly prestigious and the specific employers are of paramount interest

A sample of a functional resume for a person reentering the job market is shown in Figure 48-6.

Joan Bishop
4320 Spraig Street
Renton, Washington 98055
(206) 255-2620

TEACHING:

Instructed community groups on issues related to child abuse.

Taught volunteers how to set up community program for victims of domestic violence.

Ran workshops for parents of abused children.

Instructed public school teachers on signs and symptoms of potential and actual child abuse.

COUNSELING:

Consulted with parents for probable child abuse and suggested courses of action.

Worked with social workers on individual cases, in both urban and suburban settings.

Counseled single parents on appropriate coping behaviors.

Handled pre-take interviewing of many individual abused children.

ORGANIZATION/COORDINATION:

Coordinated transition of children between original home and foster home.

Served as liaison between community health agencies and schools.

Wrote proposal to state for county funds to educate single parents and teachers.

WORK HISTORY:

1986–1990   Community Mental Health Center, Tacoma, Washington
            Volunteer Coordinator—Child Abuse Program
1990–1994   C.A.R.E.—Child-Abuse Rescue-Education, Trenton, New Jersey
            County Representative

EDUCATION:

1970   B.S. Sociology, Douglass College, New Brunswick, New Jersey

Figure 48-6   Sample functional resume; this style is useful for a person reentering the job market.

Targeted Resume. The targeted resume is best for focusing on a clear, specific job target. It should contain a career objective, and list your skills, capabilities, and any supporting accomplishments related to that objective. Graduating students will find this resume style enables them to list classes related to their career objective, grade point average, student awards, and achievements. This information adds substance to a resume when work experience is minimal and should be at the beginning of the resume since it is your most significant asset.

The targeted resume is advantageous when:

- You are very clear about your job target
- You have had a variety of experiences that appear unrelated to each other, but that include skills that you can use in a skills list related to your job target

- You can go in several directions and want a different resume for each
- You are just starting your career and have little experience, but know what you want and are clear about your capabilities
- You are able to keep your resume on a computer disk

The targeted resume is *not* advantageous when:

- You want to use one resume for several different applications
- You are not clear about your abilities and accomplishments

Figure 48-7 provides a sample of a targeted resume.

Ashley Jackson
2031 Craig Street
Renton, Washington 98055
(206) 255-1365

CAREER OBJECTIVE: To obtain a challenging position as a medical assistant in an ambulatory care/surgery facility.

ACHIEVEMENTS:
Certified Medical Assistant.
Graduate of an Accredited Medical Assistant Program.
Experienced in providing assistance with surgeries in an ambulatory care setting.
Excellent communication and interpersonal skills.

SKILLS AND CAPABILITIES:
Post-surgery patient follow-up.
Patient induction.
Vital signs.
Patient preparation.
EKGs.
Medical and surgical asepsis.
Sterile procedures.

WORK HISTORY:
September, 1996–Present	Group Health Cooperative, Seattle, WA, Surgical Medical Assistant.
June, 1994–August, 1996	Valley Internal Medicine, Renton, WA, Clinical Medical Assistant.
March, 1994–June, 1994	Valley Internal Medicine, Renton, WA, Externship Student/Trainee.

EDUCATION/CERTIFICATION:
Associate in Applied Science Degree, Highline Community College.
Certified Medical Assistant.

AFFILIATIONS:
American Association of Medical Assistants

Figure 48-7 Sample targeted resume; this style is useful when focusing on a specific job target.

Vital Resume Information

All resume styles must contain certain vital information about the job applicant. Essential information includes:

- Your full name, address including street number, city, state, and zip code.
- Your telephone number or a number where a message may be left. Always include the area code with the number.
- Your education. Begin with the most recent school attended and include the name, address, and graduation date with the diploma, certificate, or degree earned.
- Work experience. List company name and address. Do not underestimate the value of any job; relate transferable skills to your career objective.

APPLICATION/COVER LETTERS

The **application/cover letter** is a means of introducing yourself and submitting your resume to a potential employer with the goal of obtaining an interview. A well-written cover letter will highlight your qualifications and experience for employment and will enhance the information contained within your resume. The letter should follow a standard business style and should never be more than one page in length. It should be printed on the same paper as the resume.

Since this may be your first contact with a potential employer, the letter should sell you and describe your intentions regarding employment, display your personality, and create an interest in reading your enclosed resume.

Some guidelines to follow in writing the application/cover letter include:

1. Address your letter to a specific individual whenever possible. You may need to make a telephone call to obtain the name and correct spelling.
2. Keep the letter short, use correct grammar and spelling, and follow standard business letter format.
3. The first paragraph should state your reason for writing and focus the reader's attention.
4. The second paragraph should identify how your education, experience, and qualifications relate to the job and refer to the enclosed resume.
5. The last paragraph should close with a request for an interview.
6. Do not reproduce cover letters. An original letter should be sent to each individual.
7. The cover letter and resume should be mailed in a business size envelope that matches its contents or in an $8\frac{1}{2} \times 11$ manila envelope containing your return address.

A sample of an application/cover letter is shown in Figure 48-8A.

An alternate example of an application/cover letter using Information Mapping® to highlight and draw attention to specific information in your letter is shown in Figure 48-8B. This format is considered easier to read because the focus is on specific blocks of information. In addition, its uniqueness draws attention to your letter and resume and may result in your being selected when competition is keen.

COMPLETING THE APPLICATION FORM

Sooner or later during the job search you will be asked to complete an **application form**. How well you complete this task may be a key factor in obtaining an interview and/or that first job.

Reading through the application form questions, you may be tempted to write in "See resume" rather than repeat pertinent information already contained within your resume. Do not fall into this pitfall. Answer every item completely. Read all the directions carefully. Look for seemingly insignificant directions placed at the top or bottom of the page that state "Print Carefully," "Complete in Your Own Handwriting," or "Please Type." Employers may use this to assess your ability to read and follow directions.

If the application is to be handwritten, use black ink to complete the form. Black ink is considered legal and often is an indelible (permanent) ink and is more legible if the form must be duplicated. Concentrate when completing the form and be sure to print clearly and make no errors.

The current trend is toward on-line application forms. These forms are prepared by keying information into the appropriate spaces or blocks by using a computer. The completed forms may then be printed and mailed to the perspective employer or sent electronically. Sending electronically is increasingly the preferred method. All of the concerns relative to care in following instructions, providing complete and accurate information, and proofing the application for any errors before sending are applicable.

If you are asked to list experience but the application does not specify "paid experience," be sure to list any volunteer or externship experience that relates to the position you are seeking. Part-time employment can be important as an indicator of your willingness to work, your ability to serve the public, and your organizational skills.

You may be asked to complete the application form "on the spot." Plan ahead for this event and carry a completed copy of your resume, reference list, and

2031 Craig Street
Renton, Washington 98055
August 22, 20___

Sarah Molles, Manager
Seattle Group Health Cooperative
304 Fourth Avenue
Seattle, Washington 98124-1716

SUBJECT: SURGICAL MEDICAL ASSISTANT POSITION

Background I read your advertisement in the *Seattle Times* for a medical assistant to assist in a dermatology surgery practice. I meet the qualifications listed and would like to be considered for the position.

Qualifications I am a certified medical assistant graduated from a two-year accredited program. I have experience as a clinical assistant in an internal medicine clinic and have excellent communication and interpersonal skills.

Requested Action I would like to request an interview to discuss how I could be of value to your organization in the subject position.

Yours truly,

Ashley Jackson

Ashley Jackson

Enclosure, Resume

Figure 48-8(B)   Sample information mapped letter.

2031 Craig Street
Renton, Washington 98055
August 22, 20___

Sarah Molles, Manager
Seattle Group Health Cooperative
304 Fourth Avenue
Seattle, Washington 98124-1716

Dear Ms. Molles:

I read your advertisement in the *Seattle Times* for a medical assistant to assist in a dermatology surgery practice. I meet the qualifications listed and would like to be considered for the position.

I am currently a certified medical assistant graduated from a two-year accredited program. I have experience as a clinical assistant in an internal medicine clinic and have excellent communication and interpersonal skills.

I would like to request an interview to discuss how I could be of value to your organization in the subject position.

Yours truly,

Ashley Jackson

Ashley Jackson

Enclosure, Resume

Figure 48-8(A)   Sample application/cover letter.

application/cover letter with you. Information not included in your resume, such as which years you attended high school and your salary history, should also be carried with you. These documents should provide all the information needed to complete the application form and may be submitted with the application form. This demonstrates to the potential employer your seriousness and preparedness for finding a job.

THE LOOK OF SUCCESS

The look of success begins with the outward appearance. First impressions are lasting, so strive for a favorable, professional look from head to toe.

Hair should be clean, shiny, and healthy looking, and worn in an appropriate style for the ambulatory care setting. Long hair should be worn off the collar in perhaps a French braid or twist. Long hair that is worn on the shoulders or down the back has the potential for being caught in equipment. It also serves as a host for many airborne pathogens.

The skin should have a healthy glow. Consultation with a cosmetician may prove helpful in solving skin problems or provide opportunity for trying new products. A basic understanding of your personal skin type and selection of cosmetics that complement your skin tone aid in the presentation of a professional appearance. The natural look is most appropriate for the medical office.

Daily bathing, whether by soaking in a tub and using a loofah sponge or using a pulsating shower, cleanse and relax the body. If your skin tends to be dry, apply lotion or emollient cream to replace the natural oils depleted by the water. Many lotions, talcum powders, and deodorants are scented. Remember to use caution where perfumes and scents are concerned since many magnify when the body is under stress and the scent may be offensive or cause allergic reactions in others.

Bathe the feet, carefully washing between each toe, and take care to dry the feet completely. This aids in the prevention of fungal growth. To prevent ingrown toenails, trim the nails straight across rather than rounding the nails as you do the fingernails.

Fingernails should be manicured on a weekly basis. Nails should be short and oval shaped or have rounded corners. Cuticles should be softened by soaking the fingertips in warm water. Gently use an orange stick or a cotton-tipped swab and push the cuticle back. To prevent hangnails, apply cuticle oil as you gently push the cuticle back. Only clear nail polish should be worn in the ambulatory care setting. Nail polish that is chipped or cracked must be removed or replaced immediately as it creates crevices in which pathogens may hide, multiply, and be spread.

First impressions are lasting so make yours professional in all respects. Conservative business attire is appropriate. A tailored suit or a classic dress are effective in portraying a professional image. Pay attention to details such as your jewelry and shoe selection. Shoes should be polished and in good repair. They should fit properly and be comfortable and easy to walk in (Figure 48-9).

Personal and Professional Poise

When you feel well and know that you look good, you project a confident and professional appearance. In other words, you are professionally poised. Webster's dictionary defines poise as balance and stability; ease and dignity of manner. Personal poise combines all of the previously mentioned body appearances plus smoothness of movement and physical flexibility.

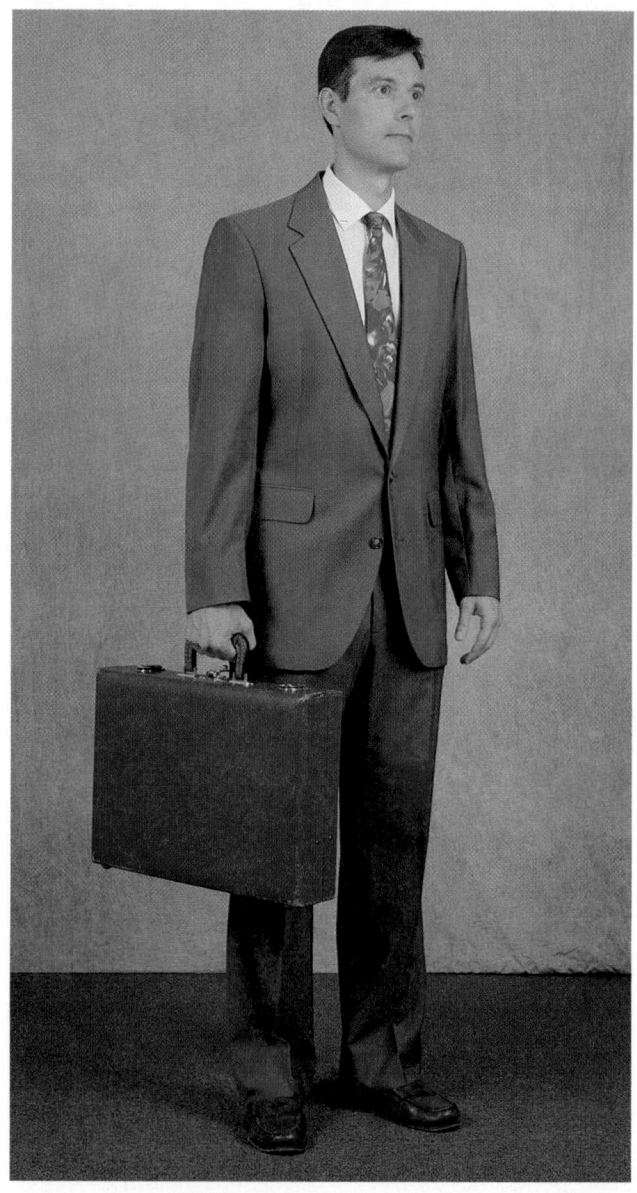

Figure 48-9   Medical assistant appropriately dressed and prepared for the interview.

THE INTERVIEW PROCESS

If your application/cover letter and resume have made a favorable impression with the organization, you may be invited for an interview. An interview is a meeting in which you and the interviewer discuss the employment opportunities within that particular organization. It will be the interviewer's responsibility to determine if you have the personality, education, and skills to perform the job. You, on the other hand, will be selling your qualifications and assessing if this is an organization in which you want to be employed.

Being well prepared for the interview will increase your self-confidence and ability to focus during the actual interview. Knowing that your application/cover letter, resume, and references all support your career goal and objectives allows you time to concentrate on interview preparation and presentation.

Preparing for the Interview

Before the interview takes place, you will want to study carefully the organization for which you are interviewing. Be prepared to relate your skills and interests to the needs of this organization. In other words, what can you contribute and why should they hire you? The interview is your opportunity to sell yourself and identify ways in which you can benefit the employer.

A copy of your resume and cover letter should be brought along to the interview just in case the interviewer can not locate the original or wants another copy. You should also have copies of letters of recommendation, a list of references, a copy of your transcript from the schools you attended, and copies of any certificates such as

AIDS training, First Aid, and CPR. These items should not be presented unless dictated by events that take place during the interview. You might also have with you the name of the interviewer and a copy of any questions you plan to ask the interviewer. A last minute review will refocus your thoughts before you go into the interview. You could also keep your list available for quick reference in the event that your mind goes blank when you are asked if you have questions.

In order to arrive five to ten minutes early, you may need to check a map for directions or make a trip the day before your interview. Try to travel about the same time as you would for the interview so you have an idea of the time it takes, traffic flow, construction areas encountered, and parking availability.

Introduce yourself confidently to the receptionist and identify by name the person you wish to see and the time of your appointment. Always arrive alone. The employer wants to see you and sense your self-reliance and responsibility. While you wait, try to relax and observe the office setting, other employees, what they are wearing, and their manner of conducting business. This may be helpful to you during the interview and in making a decision to work here.

The Actual Interview

When you enter an interviewer's office, think of yourself as a guest and take your cues from him or her. Most interviewers will introduce themselves and extend their hand. A firm handshake, responding by introducing yourself and smiling confidently convey a positive professional image. Remain standing until you are invited to be seated. Keep your personal items on your lap or place them on the floor near your chair. Do not invade the interviewer's territory by placing your things on the desk.

Sit erect in the chair with your feet flat on the floor or crossing only your ankles. Avoid nervous mannerisms while you speak and maintain good eye contact. Be natural and positive about the position, organization, and yourself. Present a professional image by using medical terminology when responding to questions or providing information. Observe the interviewer carefully for cues. Respond to questions completely, trying not to repeat yourself or give more information than was requested.

Be prepared for the kinds of questions that may be asked during the interview process. Ask yourself, "If I were the employer, what would I want to know about the applicant?" Figure 48-10 contains examples of standard questions asked by most employers. Consider how you would respond to each question.

Remember that the interviewer is asking questions to determine if you are qualified for the position and if you are the kind of person that will fit into the organization.

TYPICAL QUESTIONS ASKED DURING AN INTERVIEW

1. I see from your resume you graduated from _____ college. What did that college have to offer that others didn't?

2. What subjects did you enjoy the most and why?

3. What do you see yourself doing five years from now?

4. Tell me about yourself.

5. What do you consider to be your greatest strengths and weaknesses?

6. How do you think a friend or professor who knows you well would describe you?

7. What qualifications do you have that make you think you would be successful in this position?

8. In what ways do you think you can make a contribution to our organization?

9. What two or three accomplishments have given you the most satisfaction?

10. How well do you work under pressure?

11. Will you be able to work overtime occasionally?

12. Do you have any questions you would like to ask?

Figure 48-10   Knowing how you would answer some of these typical questions can prepare you for your interview.

Think before answering questions; try to provide the information requested in a positive and professional manner. *Listen* carefully so that you understand what information the question is requesting. *Ask* for clarification if you are uncertain. This demonstrates your ability to be open enough to ask questions when in doubt.

Closing the Interview

By observing the interviewer and listening carefully, you will be able to determine when the interviewer feels he or she has enough information about you to make a decision. Usually during the closing the interviewer will ask if you have any additional questions. This is your opportunity to collect information helpful in making a decision to accept or decline an offer. Your questions provide another opportunity to sell yourself, show that you have done your homework about the organization, and have listened carefully during the interview. Select three or four questions that will help you the most.

Questions about the organization are excellent choices. Examples might be:

- "What are the opportunities for advancement with this organization?"

- "I read that your organization has educational benefits. Could you explain briefly how that program works?"

- "You mentioned in-house training programs for employees. Could you give one or two examples?"

You may also have some questions about the job itself. Examples of these types of questions are:

- "Is this a newly created position? If so, what results are you hoping to see?"

- "Was the last person in this position promoted? What contributed to their advancement?"

- "What do you consider the most difficult task on this job?"

- "What are the lines of authority for this position?"

Do not use this question time to ask about salary, sick leave, vacations, or retirement benefits. At this point, your focus should be on the value and skills you can contribute to the organization. These questions may be asked during a second interview or when a position is offered.

Before you leave, thank the interviewer for taking time to discuss the position with you. If you definitely are interested in the position, ask to be considered as a candidate for the position. If follow-up procedures have not been explained, now is the time to ask when the final selection will be made and how you will be notified. A firm handshake as you leave, a pleasant smile, and confidence as you exit will leave a professional picture in the interviewer's mind.

INTERVIEW FOLLOW-UP

Following up after the interview is essential. This is the time to telephone your references to let them know the name of the organization and the person's name with whom you interviewed, something about the position, and your qualifications. Share any information that will help your references support you in obtaining the position.

Follow-Up Letter

Take time to write a follow-up letter to the interviewer a day or two after your interview. The letter should be written in standard business format and printed on the same paper as your application/cover letter and resume. Be sure that all spelling and grammar are correct.

The follow-up letter provides another opportunity to express your interest in the organization and the position. You can briefly emphasize the experience and skills you have to offer and again request being considered a candidate for the position.

Record the mailing date on your contact tracker and keep a copy of the letter in a file with other information about the organization. Figure 48-11 is a sample follow-up letter.

Follow Up by Telephone

Allow a few days for your follow-up letter to reach the interviewer. If you do not hear from the interviewer within a week or by the designated time established during the interview, you may telephone to ask if you are still being considered for the position or if a decision has been made.

Speak directly into the mouthpiece of the telephone using good diction and voice volume. Identify yourself and provide some information to aid the interviewer in recalling who you are. Perhaps mentioning the date you interviewed will suffice. Be polite and professional and remember to thank the individual for speaking with you. At the end of the conversation say good-bye and wait until they hang up before you break the connection. Log the telephone call and its response on your contact tracker for future reference.

2031 Craig Street
Renton, Washington 98055
August 28, 20--

Sarah Molles, Manager
Seattle Group Health Cooperative
304 Fourth Avenue
Seattle, Washington 98124-1716

Dear Ms. Molles,

Thank you for scheduling a personal interview with me last Wednesday, August 26, at 9:45 AM. I enjoyed discussing the medical assistant position open in one of your dermatology surgery practices. I would like to be considered for the position.

After talking with you, I feel my qualifications match closely with those you requested. My communication and interpersonal skills are excellent and a necessary ingredient for any medical assistant.

I look forward to hearing from you September 5 as you mentioned during the interview. If there are any questions I may answer, please telephone me.

Sincerely,

Ashley Jackson

Ashley Jackson
(206) 255-1365

Figure 48-11   Sample follow-up letter.

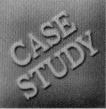

Eun Mee Soo is a recent graduate of an accredited medical assisting program and has no medical work experience except her externship at Inner City Health Care. Eun Mee has been employed part-time as a sales representative (clerk) in one of the city's prestigious clothing stores while she attended school.

48-1 CASE STUDY REVIEW

1. Which resume style would represent Eun Mee best and why?
2. What information should Eun Mee provide in the vital information section of the resume?
3. What is the purpose of an accomplishment statement? Provide an example of one that Eun Mee might use.

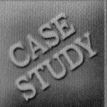

Doctors Lewis and King maintain a two-doctor family physicians' office. They are in need of a new medical assistant to take the place of one who will be leaving at the end of the month. They have established interviews with five applicants. Eun Mee Soo is the first candidate to be interviewed.

48-2 CASE STUDY REVIEW

1. Eun Mee enters the interview with some papers in her hand. What paperwork should she have brought with her?
2. Why should Eun Mee arrive five to ten minutes early for the interview?
3. How should Eun Mee enter the room?

SUMMARY

Finding your first job is your first job. How well you research, plan, prepare, and implement your tasks will make the difference between being hired or not being hired. Learn from each interview session. Listen to the questions that were asked and formulate answers that you feel would be appropriate for your next interview. Tell everyone you are looking for a job and solicit their help. Follow up on all leads and do not become discouraged.

Once you have been hired at that first job, continue your learning experience. Ask appropriate questions and try not to ask the same question a second or third time. Pay attention to details and learn individual preferences. Become a team player and look for ways you can help others. Carry your share of responsibility and do not be afraid to admit you are unfamiliar with certain aspects of the office. Employers need to know you can be trusted to work within the scope of your education and not beyond. Practice being an asset to your employer.

REVIEW QUESTIONS

Multiple Choice

1. The resume:
   a. is a summary data sheet or brief account of your qualifications and progress in your career
   b. is also known as a contact tracker
   c. always includes references
   d. is used to introduce yourself and identify qualifications

2. References:
   a. must always be listed on the resume
   b. should be a relative
   c. should be someone who likes you and your work but may not be a good communicator
   d. should be someone who knows you or has worked with you long enough to make an honest assessment of your capabilities and integrity

3. The targeted resume is advantageous:
   a. when prior titles are impressive
   b. when reentering the job market after an absence
   c. when you are just starting your career and have little experience
   d. when you have extensive specialized experience
4. The application/cover letter is:
   a. a detailed data sheet describing your vital information, education, and experience
   b. introduces you to a prospective employer and captures their interest in you as a candidate for the position
   c. lists individuals who can vouch for you
   d. should be lengthy and detailed
5. The interview:
   a. does not require much thought or preparation
   b. requires you to think before answering questions, listen carefully, and ask for clarification if uncertain of the question
   c. provides time to ask questions about salary, vacation, and benefits
   d. does not require any follow-up
6. Preparing for the interview:
   a. bathe yourself, groom your hair and fingernails, and wear clean and pressed conservative business attire
   b. allow adequate time to get to the interview
   c. prepare a packet to give the interviewer containing certificates, letters of recommendation, a list of references, and your list of questions
   d. a, b, and c
7. Job analysis should include:
   a. compiling a list of potential employers
   b. gathering information about employers in whom you have interest
   c. preparing a budgetary needs analysis
   d. all of the above
8. The best source for job search data is:
   a. the Internet
   b. friends and acquaintances
   c. the yellow pages and classified ads
   d. all the above
9. A frequently overlooked potential employer is:
   a. your personal health care provider
   b. your externship site
   c. the local hospital
   d. all of the above

10. You can impress the interviewer by:
    a. acting like you know it all
    b. having poise and good appearance
    c. showing flexibility by having no specific goals
    d. all of the above

Critical Thinking

1. Discuss the various resume styles and determine which style would be most suitable for you.
2. Discuss methods of researching a prospective employer.
3. Review Figure 48-2 and discuss the rationale behind each reason for employers not hiring.
4. Prepare a budget and discuss it with a classmate.
5. Collect and review numerous application forms.

WEB ACTIVITIES

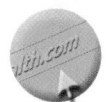

Select a location in the United States and use the Internet to research potential openings for medical assistants. Go to the Internet site Yahoo! [http://www.yahoo.com/] and research positions available at the location you have selected. Then research salaries for medical assistants in that area. If you have trouble working through the menu, select the site careers.yahoo.com and use the sections on job search and researching salaries to obtain the information. After you have completed these tasks, prepare an information packet on one of the facilities with a job opening for medical assistant. Include address, phone number, person to contact, and type of procedures performed at the location. You may need to do further Internet research to obtain some of this information. Follow the instructor's instructions on completing and turning in your results.

DOCUMENTATION

Copy or design your own contact tracker form and document all pertinent information regarding your job search contacts.

REFERENCES/BIBLIOGRAPHY

Yate, M. (1994). *Knock 'em dead the ultimate job seeker's handbook.* Holbrook, MA: Bob Adams, Inc.

Yate, M. (1993). *Resumes that knock 'em dead.* Holbrook, MA: Bob Adams, Inc.

GLOSSARY OF TERMS

abduction motion away from the midline of the body (Ch. 33).

ABO blood group genetically determined system of antigens found on the surface of erythrocytes. The population can be divided into four ABO blood groups: A, B, AB, and O (Ch. 44).

abortion expulsion of the products of conception before viability (Ch. 26).

abuse misuse; excessive or improper use, especially of narcotics or psychoactive drugs (Ch. 35).

accessibility making facilities or equipment available for use by any individual (Ch. 10).

accession record (numeric system) logbook used to assign numbers to correspondence or patients (Ch. 14).

accomplishment statements statements that begin with a power verb and give a brief description of what you did, and the demonstrable results that were produced (Ch. 48).

account aging process by which accounts are determined to be overdue (Ch. 20).

accounting system of monitoring the financial status of a facility and the financial results of its activities, providing information for decision making (Ch. 21).

accounts payable sum owed by a business for services or goods received (Ch. 17); also unwritten promise to pay a supplier for property or merchandise purchased on credit or for a service rendered (Ch. 21).

accounts receivable amount owed to a business for services or goods supplied (Ch. 17).

accounts receivable (A/R) ratio assets outstanding accounts receivable divided by the average monthly gross income for the past twelve months (Ch. 21).

accreditation process whereby recognition is granted to an educational program for maintaining standards that qualify its graduates for professional practice; to provide with credentials (Ch. 1).

accredited recognized as being outstanding (Ch. 4).

Accrediting Bureau of Health Education Schools (ABHES) entity accrediting institutions for the American Medical Technologists (Ch. 47).

Acetest® product used to test for the presence of abnormal amounts of acetone (ketones) in urine (Ch. 42).

acetone colorless, inflammable liquid. Found in the blood and urine of diabetics as a result of the breakdown of fatty acids (Ch. 38).

acid/base balance condition that occurs when the net rate at which the body produces acids or bases is equal to the net rate at which acids or bases are excreted (Ch. 42).

acquired immunodeficiency syndrome (AIDS) disorder of the immune system caused by a human immunodeficiency virus (HIV), a retrovirus that destroys the body's ability to fight infection. As the disease progresses, the individual becomes overcome by disorders, including cancers and opportunistic infections. There is no known cure for AIDS (Ch. 6, 22).

active listening received message is paraphrased back to the sender to verify the correct message was decoded (Ch. 4).

activities of daily living (ADL) activities usually performed during a typical day that involve caring for oneself, such as eating and brushing teeth (Ch. 33).

acupuncture treatment to relieve pain and disease by puncturing the skin with thin needles at specific points (Ch. 2, 3).

additive any material placed in a tube that maintains or facilitates the integrity and function of the specimen (Ch. 40).

adduction motion toward the midline of the body (Ch. 33).

adjustments increases or decreases to patient accounts not due to charges incurred or payments received (Ch. 17).

administer to give a medication (Ch. 35, 36).

aegis sponsorship or protection (Ch. 38).

aerobic organism that requires oxygen for growth (Ch. 43).

aerosols particles from potentially infectious materials that may be released in the air (Ch. 43).

afebrile without fever (Ch. 24).

agenda printed list of topics to be discussed during a meeting, sometimes giving time allocation (Ch. 15, 45).

agent person representing another (Ch. 7).

agglutination antigen-antibody reaction in which a solid antigen clumps with a solid antibody (Ch. 44).

airborne transmission spread of disease-causing microorganisms over long distances through the air (Ch. 22).

akinesia absence or loss of voluntary muscle movement (Ch. 30).

algorithm a special method for solving a specific kind of problem (Ch. 11).

alimentary canal digestive tract, made up of all the organs through which food passes throughout the body, from mouth to anus (Ch. 30).

aliquot part of the whole specimen that has been taken off for use or storage (Ch. 40).

allergy acquired hypersensitivity to a substance (allergen) that does not normally cause a reaction (Ch. 23, 31).

allied health professionals health care providers with a range of educational backgrounds and skills who support, complement, or assist physicians and who are a critical part of the health care team (Ch. 2).

allopathic method of treating disease with remedies that produce effects different from those caused by the disease itself. Most traditional physicians today are considered allopathic physicians (Ch. 3).

alveoli air sacs of the lungs that exchange carbon dioxide and oxygen (Ch. 30).

ambulation ability to walk (Ch. 33).

ambulatory care setting health care environment where services are provided on an outpatient basis. Ambulatory is from the Latin and means "capable of walking." Examples include the solo physician's office, the group practice, the urgent care center, and the health maintenance organization (Ch. 1, 2).

American Association for Medical Transcription (AAMT) nonprofit organization founded by medical transcriptionists to promote the profession (Ch. 16).

American Association of Medical Assistants (AAMA) premier organization dedicated to serving the interests of certified medical assistants (Ch. 47).

Americans with Disabilities Act (ADA) congressional act passed in 1990 to end discrimination against individuals with disabilities (Ch. 10).

amino acid basic structural unit of protein (Ch. 34).

amniocentesis surgical puncture of the amniotic sac to remove fluid for laboratory analysis (Ch. 22, 26).

amoebic dysentery infectious intestinal disease caused by amebas and characterized by inflammation of the mucous membrane of the colon (Ch. 22).

amorphous shapeless; possessing no definite form (Ch. 42).

amplified made larger or enlarged. The amplifier of the electrocardiograph enlarges the electrical impulse activity and the recording can be read more easily (Ch. 37).

amplitude amount, extent, size abundance, or fullness (Ch. 37).

anaerobic organism that needs little or no oxygen for growth (Ch. 43).

anaphylaxis hypersensitive state of the body to a foreign protein or drug (Ch. 35).

ancillary services professional occupational companies hired to complete a specific job (Ch. 45).

anesthesia loss of feeling or sensation; an anesthetic is any mechanism that causes anesthesia (Ch. 31).

angiogram series of X rays of a blood vessel(s) following injection of a radiopaque substance (Ch. 37).

anisocytosis marked variation in the size of cells (Ch. 41).

anomaly abnormality; marked deviation from normal (Ch. 26).

answering services services employed to answer the calls of an ambulatory care setting after hours; unlike an answering machine, a live operator answers the call and forwards it appropriately (Ch. 12).

antagonistic two entities that work against each other (Ch. 27).

antibacterial capable of destroying bacteria, often applied to a wound in the form of an ointment or cream (Ch. 31).

antibody specific chemical produced by B cells of the immune system in response to an antigen (Ch. 22, 44).

anticoagulant chemical in a blood tube that prevents the clotting of the blood by removing the calcium from the blood or by stopping the formation of thrombin (Ch. 40).

antigen substance such as bacteria or other agents that the body recognizes as foreign; the stimulus for antibody production (Ch. 22, 44).

antioxidant something that prevents oxidation (Ch. 34).

antiserum serum containing antibodies (Ch. 44).

antivirus program software program that identifies the signature of a computer virus and works to eliminate it from the computer system. Antivirus programs are useful only if updated by frequently downloading from the program supplier updates on new viruses. Antivirus programs are usually incapable of detecting a new type of virus (Ch. 11).

aphasia inability to communicate through speech or other methods. Often caused by brain dysfunction (Ch. 30).

apical pertaining to the apex of the heart. A site for measuring heart rate with a stethoscope (Ch. 24).

apnea cessation or absence of normal spontaneous breathing (Ch. 36).

appendicular skeleton skeleton that consists of the pectoral and pelvic girdles and the upper and lower extremities. The pelvic girdle attaches the upper extremities to the trunk (Ch. 30).

application/cover letter letter used to introduce yourself and your resume to a prospective employer with the goal of obtaining an interview (Ch. 48).

application form form devised by a prospective employer to collect information relative to qualifications, education, and experience in employment (Ch. 48).

applications software software that performs a specific data processing function (Ch. 11).

approximate to bring together the edges of a wound (Ch. 31).

arrhythmia deviation from the normal pattern or rhythm of the heartbeat (Ch. 24, 37).

arteriosclerosis hardening of the arteries caused by buildup of plaque, a deposit of fatty substances on the artery lining (Ch. 29).

articulating expressing oneself clearly and distinctly (Ch. 12).

artifact anything artificially produced (Ch. 37).

ascorbic acid   Vitamin C (Ch. 34).

asepsis   protecting against infection caused by pathogenic microorganisms (Ch. 3).

aseptic   freedom from any infectious material; absence of microorganisms (Ch. 30).

aspirate   to remove by suction (Ch. 22).

assay   analysis of a substance to determine constituents and relative proportion of each (Ch. 39).

assets   properties of value that are owned by a business entity (Ch. 21).

assignment of benefits   signing over of benefits by the beneficiary to another party (Ch. 18).

assistive device   any device used to help patients to walk (Ch. 33).

asymptomatic   without symptoms (Ch. 39).

ataxia   defective muscular coordination, primarily seen when attempting voluntary muscular movements (Ch. 25).

atrophy   decrease in size or ability of a part of the body due to disease, inactivity, or other condition (Ch. 33).

attribute   inherent characteristic (Ch. 1).

augment   to add or increase (Ch. 37).

auricle   The external ear, also called pinna (Ch. 30).

automated routing unit (ARU)   telephone system that answers a call and uses a recorded voice to identify departments or services (Ch. 12).

axial skeleton   consists of bones that lie around the center of the body (Ch. 30).

baccalaureate   degree of bachelor conferred by colleges and universities (Ch. 1).

balance   amount owed (N); to verify posting accuracy (V) (Ch. 17).

balance sheet   itemized statement of assets, liabilities, and equity; a statement of financial condition (Ch. 21).

bandage   nonsterile gauze or other material applied over a sterile dressing to protect and/or immobilize (Ch. 31).

bar code   black bars that are read by an optical scanner. The bar code option on the HCFA-1500 insurance claim form permits the physician name and address to be coded on the top right corner (Ch. 18).

barrier   obstacle that exists to protect an individual from contact with blood or other potentially infected materials. Called personal protective equipment (PPE), barriers include gloves, masks, face shields, laboratory coats, protective eyewear, and gowns (Ch. 22).

Bartholin gland   one of two small mucous glands located near the vaginal opening at base of labia majora (Ch. 26).

basal metabolic rate (BMR)   level of energy required when the body is at rest (Ch. 34).

baseline   known or initial measurement against which future measurements are compared (Ch. 24, 39); also, flat, horizontal line that separates the various waves of the ECG cycle (Ch. 37).

basic insurance   medical insurance that covers most physician fees, hospital expenses, and surgical fees according to the terms of the policy. The patient is usually responsible for a deductible (Ch. 18).

basophil   granulocytic white blood cell with dark purple cytoplasmic granules. It is the least common of the white blood cells (Ch. 41).

benchmark   making a comparison among different organizations relative to how they accomplish tasks, such as office computerization, organizing file systems, and employee remuneration (Ch. 11, 45).

beneficiary   person under a policy eligible to receive benefits (Ch. 18).

benefit   remuneration that is in addition to the salary (Ch. 45).

Betadine®   brand of povidone-iodine solution used as a skin antiseptic. Betadine is also available in a scrub (soap) solution (Ch. 31).

bias   slant toward a particular belief (Ch. 4).

bilirubin   orange-yellow pigment that forms from the breakdown of hemoglobin in broken down red blood cells. Bilirubin usually travels in the bloodstream to the liver, where it is converted to a water-soluble form and is excreted into the bile (Ch. 42, 44).

biochemical tests   tests that show biochemical properties and reactions of bacteria to achieve identification of microorganisms; often performed in solid and liquid media (Ch. 43).

bioethics   branch of medical ethics concerned with moral issues resulting from high technology and sophisticated medical research. Social issues such as genetic engineering, abortion, and fetal tissue research raise important bioethical questions (Ch. 8).

biohazard   material that has been in contact with body fluid and is capable of transmitting disease (Ch. 22).

biopsy   removal of a small piece of living tissue from an organ or other part of the body for microscopic examination to confirm or establish a diagnosis (Ch. 39).

bipolar   having two poles or processes (Ch. 37).

birthday rule   method to determine which of two or more policies covering a dependent child will be primary; that parent with the birthday falling first in the calendar year has the primary policy (Ch. 18).

bit   smallest unit of data a computer can process; eight bits make up a byte (Ch. 11).

blind copy   protects the privacy of e-mail. Other recipients cannot identify who else may have received the transmitted message (Ch. 15).

bloodborne   means of transmission of an infectious disease (such as HIV and HBV) via human blood (Ch. 22).

bloodborne pathogen   microorganism capable of causing disease found in blood or components of blood (Ch. 22).

blood urea nitrogen (BUN)   nitrogen in the blood in the form of urea. The level of nitrogen in the blood is an indicator of kidney function (Ch. 44).

body fluid   any secretion or excretion from the human body such as vaginal, cerebral-spinal, synovial, pleural, pericardial, peritoneal, amniotic, sputum, and saliva (Ch. 38).

body language   nonverbal communication that includes unconscious body movements, gestures, and facial expressions that accompany verbal messages (Ch. 4).

body mechanics practice of using certain key muscle groups together with correct body alignment to avoid injury when lifting or moving heavy or awkward objects (Ch. 33).

body substance isolation (BSI) type of precaution developed by a hospital that requires special handling of all bodily fluids (Ch. 22).

bond binding agreement with an employee ensuring recovery of financial loss should funds be stolen or embezzled (Ch. 45).

bond paper durable, strong paper usually used for correspondence (Ch. 15).

bradycardia (sinus) slow (below 60 beats per minute), but regular heartbeat (Ch. 24, 37).

bradypnea abnormally slowed respiratory rate (Ch. 24).

brainstorming process of developing ideas through a synergistic interaction among participants in an environment free of criticism (Ch. 45).

Braxton-Hicks irregular, intermittent, and painless uterine contractions; also known as false labor (Ch. 26).

breach of confidentiality unauthorized release of confidential information (Ch. 16, 19).

bronchi bifurcates from the trachea into each lung that terminate in the bronchial tubes (Ch. 30).

broth tubes tubes filled with a broth substance that will support the growth of certain microorganisms (Ch. 43).

bruits sound of venous or arterial origin heard on auscultation (Ch. 25).

BSA body surface area. A highly accurate method for calculating medication dosages for infants and children up to twelve years of age (Ch. 36).

bubonic plague infectious disease with a high fatality rate transmitted to humans from infected rats and ground squirrels by the bite of the rat flea (Ch. 3).

buccal relating to cheek or mouth (Ch. 35).

buffer words expendable words used while answering the telephone (Ch. 4, 12).

buffy coat layer of white blood cells and platelets that forms at the interface between the plasma and red blood cells in a tube of blood containing an anticoagulant (Ch. 40).

bullet points asterisk or dot followed by a descriptive phrase; helps the reader identify important points easily (Ch. 48).

burnout a state of fatigue or frustration brought about by a devotion to a cause, a way of life, or a relationship that failed to produce the expected reward (Ch. 5).

byte amount of memory needed to store one character (such as a letter or number). Computer memory and disk space are measured in kilobytes, megabytes, and gigabytes (Ch. 11).

calculi stones found in the urethra, bladder, ureters, or kidneys; an abnormality (Ch. 30).

calibration determination of the accuracy of an instrument by comparing the information provided with an accepted standard known to be accurate (Ch. 37, 38).

calorie unit of heat. The large Calorie (which is always capitalized) is used in discussion of human nutrition. The large Calorie is also expressed as the kilogram calorie (kcal), equal to 1,000 small calories (Ch. 34).

candida a species of yeast (Ch. 19).

cannula the blunting member in a Bio-Plexus Punctur-Guard® needle (Ch. 40).

capitation use of the number of members enrolled in a plan to determine salary of the physician; the physician is paid a fixed fee for each member no matter how many times that member is seen by the physician (Ch. 18, 19).

caption method of designation used on file guides (Ch. 14).

carbuncle necrotizing infection of skin and tissue composed of a cluster of boils (Ch. 30).

carcinoma in situ cancer that does not extend beyond the basement membrane (Ch. 26).

cardiac catheterization passage of a catheter into the heart through an arm or leg vein and blood vessels leading into the heart. The purpose is to obtain cardiac blood samples, detect abnormalities, and determine intracardiac pressure. Contrast medium can be injected and a coronary artery angiogram can be performed (Ch. 37).

cardiac cycle period from the beginning of one heartbeat to the beginning of the next succeeding beat, including systole and diastole. One complete heartbeat (Ch. 37).

cardiopulmonary resuscitation (CPR) combination of rescue breathing and chest compressions performed by a trained individual on a patient experiencing cardiac arrest (Ch. 9).

cardioversion conversion of a pathological cardiac rhythm (arrhythmia) such as ventricular fibrillation, to normal sinus rhythm (Ch. 37).

career objective expresses your career goal and the position for which you are applying (Ch. 48).

career orientation objective related to one's personal career goals or career growth (Ch. 40).

carotene Vitamin A (Ch. 34).

carrier person who harbors a pathogenic organism, and who is capable of transmitting the organism to others (Ch. 22).

cashier's check bank's own check drawn against the bank's account (Ch. 17).

casts tiny structures usually formed by deposits of protein or other substances on the walls of renal tubules; in urine, they can indicate kidney disease (Ch. 42).

catalyst substance that allows a chemical reaction to proceed at a much quicker rate and without as much energy input (Ch. 34).

catchment 40-mile radius of a military base where medical care is available to military dependents (Ch. 18).

catheterization insertion of a catheter tube into the body for evacuating fluids or injecting fluids into body cavities. In urinary catheterization, the tube is inserted through the urethra into the bladder for withdrawal of urine (Ch. 25).

cautery destruction of tissue by burning (Ch. 26, 31).

cell-mediated immunity the regulatory activities of T cells during the specific immune response (Ch. 22).

cellular telephones battery-operated portable telephones that are typically found in automobiles and other unfixed locations. One can receive and send messages from cellular phones (Ch. 12).

cellulose type of indigestible fiber made of carbohydrates found in plants (Ch. 34).

central processing unit (CPU) brain of the computer that performs instructions defined by software (Ch. 11).

centrifugal hematology analysis method of testing components of whole blood using centrifugation, fluorescent microscopy, and a micrometer (Ch. 41).

centrifuge device that spins tubes using centrifugal force to separate the fluid portion of blood from the formed elements (Ch. 40).

certification guarantees as being true or as represented by or as meeting a standard (Ch. 1, 47).

certification examination standardized means of evaluating medical assistant competency (Ch. 47).

certified check depositor's own check that the bank has indicated with a date and signature to be good for the amount written (Ch. 17).

certified medical assistant (CMA) a medical assistant who has successfully completed the AAMA's national certification examination and earned the status of being certified (Ch. 1, 47).

certified medical transcriptionist (CMT) recognized professional credential obtained through successful completion of both parts of the core certification examination administered by the MTCC at AAMT (Ch. 16).

cervical punch biopsy a biopsy of the uterine cervix using an instrument, the end of which is a punch (Ch. 26).

cesarean section delivery of fetus through surgical incision into the uterus (Ch. 26).

charge out-follow up system of processing requests for health information to ensure proper return of the information (Ch. 15).

charges fee for services rendered; increases balance due (Ch. 17).

charge slip form used to record services supplied and charges and payments for those services; functions as billing form for insurance reimbursement. Also known as an encounter form. See also **superbill** (Ch. 19).

charisma personality and appearance characteristics that influence people to support the person possessing it; magnetism (Ch. 45).

chart patient's file of medical history and treatment kept by the physician (Ch. 23).

chart notes (also called progress notes) physician's formal or informal notes about presenting problem, physical findings, and plan for treatment for a patient examined in the office, clinic, acute care center, or emergency department (Ch. 16).

check cell slides important part of quality control testing, where preinoculated slides with known organisms are used to test whether or not a stain procedure yields correct results (Ch. 43).

chemotherapeutic agents agents used in the treatment of diseases; the application of chemical reagents that are toxic to pathogenic microorganisms. Commonly used to describe agents (chemicals) used in the treatment of certain malignancies (Ch. 38).

Cheyne-Stokes regular pattern of irregular breathing rate often seen in children or may be seen in brain dysfunction (Ch. 24).

chief complaint (CC) specific symptom or problem for which the patient is seeing the physician today (Ch. 16).

chlamydia a bacteria that causes the most prevalent sexually transmitted disease (Ch. 26).

cholecalciferol Vitamin D (Ch. 34).

cholesterol sterol lipid that is widely distributed in animal tissues. Cholesterol is produced in the liver and is a component of bile (Ch. 44).

choriocarcinoma very rare malignant neoplasm, usually of the uterus or of an ectopic pregnancy. The exact cause is unknown (Ch. 44).

choroid layer highly vascular membrane covering the posterior of the eye between the sclera and retina (Ch. 30).

chronological resume resume format used when you have employment experience (Ch. 48).

circadian rhythm pattern based on a 24-hour cycle emphasizing the repetition of certain physiologic phenomena such as eating and sleeping (Ch. 42).

circumduction circular motion of a body part (Ch. 33).

civil law law related to actions between individuals (Ch. 7).

claim demand for payment; in this case it is a demand by the beneficiary to the insurance company for payment of medical expenses incurred during the effective dates of the medical policy (Ch. 18, 19).

claim register diary or register of claims submitted to each insurance carrier. When payment is received, the date and amount of payment is entered in the register (Ch. 19).

claustrophobia fear of being confined in any space (Ch. 32).

clinical chemistry analysis and study of blood, body fluids, excreta, and tissues in the diagnosis and treatment of disease (Ch. 39).

clinical diagnosis identification of a disease by history, lab studies, and symptoms (Ch. 23, 39).

clinical e-mail electronic messages sent to or by the physician's office regarding medical questions or advice (Ch. 15).

Clinitest® reagent tablet test that confirms the presence of reducing sugars in the urine (Ch. 42).

closed fracture uncomplicated fracture in which the bone does not break the skin (Ch. 30).

closed questions questions answered with a yes or no (Ch. 4).

clustering grouping together of nonverbal messages into statements or conclusions (Ch. 4); also, scheduling system where patients with similar complaints are seen for consecutive appointments, e.g., ear infections at 9:00, 9:30, and 10:00 A.M. with physical examinations at 1:00, 2:00, and 3:00 P.M. (Ch. 13).

cobalamin Vitamin B_{12} (Ch. 34).

coding process of marking data to indicate how information is to be filed (Ch. 14).

coenzyme substance that enhances a catalyst (Ch. 34).

cognition awareness with perception, reasoning, judgment, intuition, and memory (Ch. 29).

coinsurance that percentage paid by the company or that paid by the insured (Ch. 18).

collection agency outside establishment that collects outstanding debts (Ch. 20).

collection ratio gross income divided by the amount that could have been collected less disallowances (Ch. 21).

colonoscopy visual examination of the colon with a lighted scope (Ch. 30).

color coding method of filing utilizing colors to ensure quick filing and retrieval of records. Three common methods are Tab Alpha Code System, Alpha-Z System, and color-coded file folders (Ch. 14).

colposcopy visual examination of vaginal and cervical tissues using a colposcope following abnormal Pap smear. A magnifying lens and powerful lights are used (Ch. 26).

combination placement externship completed in more than one facility (Ch. 40).

comedone blackhead; usually the result of blocked sebaceous glands caused by acne (Ch. 30).

communicable contagious. Capable of being transmitted from one person to another either directly or indirectly (Ch. 22, 38).

communication cycle involves sending and receiving messages even when unconsciously aware of them (Ch. 4).

compensation overemphasizing of characteristics to make up for a real or imagined failure or handicap (Ch. 4).

competency legally qualified or adequate (Ch. 1).

complete blood count (CBC) battery of hematological tests consisting of hemoglobin, hematocrit, total white blood cell and red blood cell counts, differential white blood cell count, and the erythrocyte indices (Ch. 41).

compliance to act in accordance with conditions laid down (Ch. 1).

compounding combining two or more substances in definite proportions (Ch. 36).

concentration method method used in parasitology to identify parasites; consists of flotation and sedimentation methods (Ch. 43).

condenser directs the beam of light from the source to the specimen (Ch. 39).

conditions statements of the circumstances under which the objective will be achieved and with what supplies and equipment (Ch. 40).

condyloma a wart-like lesion of viral origin found on external genitalia or perianal region (Ch. 26).

confidentiality ethical and legal rules in regard to patient privacy (Ch. 12, 16).

confidentiality agreement when signed, the agreement signifies that the medical transcriptionist is committed to keep all patient information confidential (Ch. 16).

conflict resolution solving problems between coworkers or any two parties (Ch. 46).

congenital being born with; existing at time of birth (Ch. 26).

congruency the verbal message and the nonverbal message must agree (Ch. 4).

consecutive or serial filing numeric filing method where numbers are considered in ascending order using the entire set of figures (Ch. 14).

constrict to become smaller in diameter (Ch. 40).

consultation report document that reports the findings and/or advice of another physician requested to see a patient by the attending physician (Ch. 16).

contact tracker form used to keep track of employment contact information such as name of employer, name of contact person, address and telephone number, date of first contact, resume sent, interview date, follow-up information, and dates (Ch. 48).

contact transmission spread of disease-causing microorganisms by directly or indirectly touching the source of the infection or by touching an object or environmental surface (Ch. 22).

contaminate to make something unclean; often used to describe a sterile area being made "unsterile" or exposing a clean area to a pathogenic substance (Ch. 22, 31).

continuing education (CE) method of recertification of the certified medical transcriptionist credential (Ch. 16).

continuing education units (CEU) method for earning points toward recertification (Ch. 47).

continuous speech recognition (CSR) the process of direct conversion of spoken documentation into a written text, e.g., electronic version using a computer equipped with voice recognition software (Ch. 16).

contracting acquiring an infection from pathogens (Ch. 22).

contracture fibrosis of connective tissue in skin, fascia, muscle, or joint that prevents normal mobility of the related tissue or joint (Ch. 33).

contraindication any symptom or circumstance that indicates that the use of a particular drug is inappropriate when it would otherwise be advisable. For example, the use of alcoholic beverages is a contraindication when the drug Flagyl® is prescribed (Ch. 35).

control test test of a sample of known results to be used to compare with the results of a patient's sample (Ch. 39).

coordination of benefits (COB) the provision of an insurance contract that limits benefits to 100 percent of the cost (Ch. 18).

copayment payment required when seen by the physician (Ch. 18).

cost accounting determines what it costs for a practice to perform particular services (Ch. 21).

cost allocation process of taking costs from one area and allocating them to others (Ch. 20).

cost analysis procedure that determines the costs of each service (Ch. 21).

cost ratio formula that shows the cost of a procedure or service and helps determine the financial value of maintaining certain services (Ch. 21).

Council on Accreditation of Allied Health Education Programs (CAAHEP) national, voluntary, specialized, not-for-profit corporation (Ch. 40).

countershock application of an electric current to the heart directly or indirectly in order to alter a disturbance in cardiac rhythm (Ch. 37).

counterstain stain that is used in a staining process after the initial staining has been applied and rinsed off with a decolorizer (Ch. 43).

coupling agent an agent used when ultrasonography is used; enhances penetration of sound waves through tissue (Ch. 26).

crash tray or cart tray or portable cart that contains medications and supplies needed for emergency and first aid procedures (Ch. 9).

creatinine waste product formed in muscle that is excreted by the kidneys; elevated in blood and urine when kidney function is abnormal (Ch. 42).

credentialed testimonials showing that a person is entitled to credit or has a right to exercise official power (Ch. 1).

credit decreases balance due (Ch. 17).

credit bureau outside agency that provides information about a patient's credit history (Ch. 20).

crepitation grating sound heard on movement of ends of a broken bone (Ch. 9).

criminal law law related to wrongs committed against the welfare and safety of society as a whole (Ch. 7).

criterion level of acceptable performance (Ch. 40).

critical values test results that indicate a potentially life-threatening or greatly debilitating situation that must be reported to the physician immediately (Ch. 42).

cross-reference notation in a file to direct the reader to a specific record that may be filed under more than one name/subject, e.g., married name/maiden name or foreign names, where the surname is not easily recognizable (Ch. 14).

cryosurgery the destruction of tissue by application of extreme cold, silver nitrate, and carbon dioxide (Ch. 26).

cryotherapy use of cold to treat a physical condition (Ch. 33).

cryptorchidism undescended testicle (Ch. 28).

crystals found in normal urine sediment having no particular significance; a few should be noted as they may indicate disease states (Ch. 42).

culture social behavior patterns and beliefs (Ch. 6).

cultures microorganisms cultivated in a nutrient medium (Ch. 42, 43).

currency paper money (Ch. 17).

Current Procedural Terminology (CPT) standard codes for procedures and services. Used by most ambulatory care settings in encoding the claim form and recognized by most insurance carriers (Ch. 18, 19).

Cushing's syndrome hypersecretion of the adrenal cortex producing excessive glucocorticoids. The condition may be due to a tumor or hyperfunction of the anterior pituitary (Ch. 44).

cut placement of the tab on file folders (Ch. 14).

cyanmethemoglobin stable hemoglobin compound used to measure concentration of blood hemoglobin (Ch. 41).

cyanosis discoloration of the skin due to abnormal amounts of reduced hemoglobin in the blood caused by decreased oxygen and increased carbon dioxide in the blood (Ch. 25).

cycle billing method of spreading billing over the whole month instead of sending all bills at the end of the month (Ch. 20).

cystitis inflammation of the bladder (Ch. 29).

cytology science that deals with the formation, structure, and function of cells (Ch. 39).

cytoscopy visual examination of the urethra and bladder following insertion of a cytoscope, a lighted scope especially designed for the examination of these areas (Ch. 30).

database management software computer applications software designed for the manipulation of data within a database. This software allows for creation and editing capabilities, sorting capabilities, and comparing and summarizing activities (Ch. 11).

data input device any device capapble of converting hard copy, motion, temperature, position, or other analog signals into digital input for use by a computer (Ch. 11).

data output device device that converts digital data from a computer into hardcopy, motion, position, or other analog signals (Ch. 11).

data storage device device capable of permanently or temporarily storing digital data (Ch. 11).

data storage memory permanent memory not part of the motherboard. Utilizes any suitable data storage device. Can be read-only or read-write type of memory (Ch. 11).

day sheet form used with pegboard system to record daily patient transactions (Ch. 17).

debridement removal of dead or damaged tissue or foreign debris (Ch. 23).

declination form written formal refusal (Ch. 22).

decode to translate into language that is easily understood; to interpret (Ch. 4).

decolorizer substance used to remove the first stain applied in a differential staining process (Ch. 43).

deductible that amount of incurred medical expenses that must be met before the insurance policy will begin to pay (Ch. 18).

defendant person who defends action brought in litigation (Ch. 7).

defense mechanism behavior that protects the psyche from guilt, anxiety, or shame (Ch. 4).

defibrillation stopping fibrillation of the heart by use of drugs or by physical means (Ch. 37).

defibrillator a machine that delivers an electric current in order to alter a disturbance in cardiac rhythm (Ch. 37).

dementia impairment of intellectual function that is progressive and interferes with normal activities (Ch. 6, 29).

demyelination destruction of the nerve fibers; often a factor in multiple sclerosis (Ch. 30).

denial rejection of or refusal to acknowledge (Ch. 4).

deoxygenated blood that is high in carbon dioxide, low in oxygen, and pumped through the heart to the lungs where the carbon dioxide is exchanged for oxygen (Ch. 37).

depolarize process of reducing to a nonpolarized condition. Generation of an electrical current is enhanced. Electrical activity generated when the atria or ventricles contract (Ch. 37).

dermatitis inflammation of the skin characterized by redness, itching, and skin lesions (Ch. 22).

dermatophytes category of fungi causing infections of hair, skin, and nails (Ch. 43).

diabetes mellitus chronic disorder of carbohydrate metabolism characterized by hyperglycemia and resulting from inadequate production or utilization of insulin (Ch. 44).

diagnosis determination of disease or condition (Ch. 39).

diagnosis code numerical designation for a specific illness, injury, or disease; codes found in ICD-9-CM code book (Ch. 18, 19).

diagnosis-related groups (DRGs) classification of patients into categories based on primary diagnosis, procedure, and discharge status (Ch. 18).

diaphragm membrane separating the abdominal and thoracic cavities; functions in respiration (Ch. 12); also, a lens or other object that opens and closes to increase or decrease the amount of light on the object being illuminated (Ch. 39).

diastole one component of blood pressure measurement representing the lowest amount of pressure exerted during the cardiac cycle; the force exerted on the arterial walls during cardiac relaxation (Ch. 24, 37).

differential diagnosis diagnosis based on comparison of symptoms of similar diseases (Ch. 39).

digestion breaking down of food into smaller particles. It can be either physical or chemical (Ch. 34).

digital dictation dictation recorded directly into computers and managed by computers (Ch. 16).

dilate to enlarge in diameter (Ch. 40).

dilation expansion of an orifice or organ (Ch. 26).

direct payment payment made directly to the physician by the insurance company (Ch. 18).

disbursement to assign general ledger account information (account name or number) to a financial transaction (Ch. 17).

disinfection use of chemicals or boiling water to free an item from infectious materials but not their spores (Ch. 22).

dislocation displacement of a bone or joint from its normal position (Ch. 30).

dispense prepare and give out a medication to be taken at a later time (Ch. 35, 36).

displacement displacing negative feelings onto something or someone else with no significance to the situation (Ch. 4).

disposition temperament, character, personality (Ch. 1).

diuretic substance that causes less water to be reabsorbed by the kidney, and therefore causes water to be excreted from the body (Ch. 34).

DNA deoxyribonucleic acid; important nucleus material that carries genetic codes (Ch. 43).

doctrine principle of law established through past decisions (Ch. 7).

documentation providing factual support through written information (Ch. 22); also, written material that accompanies purchased software containing the information necessary for using the software appropriately; sometimes known as the manual (Ch. 11).

dorsiflexion moving the foot upward at the ankle joint (Ch. 33).

dosimeter a device for measuring X-ray output (Ch. 32).

double booking scheduling system where multiple patients are given an assigned appointment time, e.g., 9:30 A.M., to be seen by different office personnel at that time (Ch. 13).

dressing sterile gauze or other material applied directly to a wound to absorb secretions and to protect (Ch. 31).

droplet transmission method of spreading disease from respiratory secretions through the air. Spread is usually confined to within three feet of the infected patient (Ch. 22).

durable power of attorney for health care legal form that allows a designated person to act on another's behalf in regard to health care choices (Ch. 6, 7).

dysmenorrhea painful menses (Ch. 26).

dyspareunia painful intercourse (Ch. 26).

dysplasia abnormal development of tissue (Ch. 26).

dyspnea shortness of breath or labored/difficult breathing (Ch. 24).

dysuria painful or difficult urination (Ch. 30).

E codes ICD-9-CM codes for the external causes of injury, poisoning, or other adverse reactions that explain how the injury occurred (Ch. 19).

echocardiography noninvasive diagnostic method that uses ultrasound to visualize internal cardiac structure, including valves (Ch. 32).

eclampsia complication of pregnancy that includes general edema, hypertension, proteinuria, and convulsions (Ch. 26).

ectopic pregnancy pregnancy outside the uterus (Ch. 26, 44).

edematous abnormal accumulation of fluid in the tissues resulting in swelling (Ch. 40).

editing the process of manipulating text to avoid inaccuracies and inconsistencies within a document (Ch. 16).

educational history listing of places of learning and degrees or certificates earned (Ch. 46).

effacement thinning and shortening of the cervical canal during labor to permit passage of fetus (Ch. 26).

elective procedures those procedures not necessary for the health of the patient (Ch. 18).

electrocardiogram record of the electrical activity of the heart; showing P, QRS, and T waves (Ch. 37).

electrocardiograph instrument for recording the electrical activity of the heart (Ch. 37).

electrocardiography process of recording the electrical activity originating in the heart (Ch. 37).

electrode also known as a sensor. Used to conduct electricity from the body to the electrocardiograph (Ch. 37).

electrolyte conductor of electricity whose components are important in maintaining fluid and acid-base balance (Ch. 34, 37, 39).

electronic mail (e-mail) communications that are sent, received, stored, and forwarded on-line from computer to computer by means of a modem (Ch. 12, 15).

elimination removal of fecal waste from the body through the anus (Ch. 27).

emaciation state of being extremely lean (Ch. 30).

emancipated minor persons under age 18 who are financially responsible for themselves and free of parental care (Ch. 7).

embezzle to appropriate fraudulently to one's own use (Ch. 45).

Emergency Medical Services (EMS) Emergency Medical Services (EMS) system is a local network of police, fire, and medical personnel trained to respond to emergency situations. In many communities the system is activated by calling 911 (Ch. 9).

empathy ability to be objectively aware of and have insight into another's feelings, emotions, and behaviors, and to be aware of the significance and meaning of these to the other person (Ch. 1, 12, 29).

emphysema chronic pulmonary disease characterized by dilated and damaged alveoli (Ch. 24).

emulate imitate a characteristic of an individual in order to equal or surpass the original (Ch. 45).

encode (encoding) creating a message to be sent (Ch. 4).

endometriosis tissue that resembles the endometrium invades various locations in the pelvic cavity and elsewhere (Ch. 26).

endoscopy visual examination of body cavities with a lighted scope (Ch. 22, 30).

engineering controls physical or mechanical devices that isolate or remove health hazards from the workplace (Ch. 22).

enterobacteriaceae family of bacteria that contains genuses that are nonpathogenic and pathogenic to the intestinal and urinary tract (Ch. 43).

enunciation speaking clearly; articulating (Ch. 12).

envoy an electronic data exchange system that allows you to access patient eligibility information via modem (Ch. 18).

eosinophil granulocytic white blood cell with red eosin stained granules in the cytoplasm. It is elevated in cases of allergies (Ch. 41).

epidemiology field of science that studies the history, cause, and patterns of infectious diseases (Ch. 22).

epinephrine hormone also known as adrenaline. Epinephrine is manufactured as a chemical (pharmaceutical preparation) and is often mixed with local anesthetics for use as a vasoconstrictor in minor surgery (Ch. 31).

epistaxis nosebleed (Ch. 22).

Epstein-Barr virus (EBV) virus that is believed to be the cause of infectious mononucleosis and is implicated in such conditions as African Burkitt's lymphoma and nasopharyngeal carcinoma (Ch. 44).

equilibrium state of balance between opposing forces (Ch. 30).

ergonomics scientific study of work and space, including factors that influence worker productivity and that affect workers' health (Ch. 11).

erosion an eating away of tissue (Ch. 30).

erythema redness or inflammation of the skin or mucous membranes that is the result of dilatation and congestion of superficial capillaries (Ch. 30).

erythrocyte red blood cell, one of the formed elements of the blood (Ch. 40, 41).

erythrocyte indices three equations that provide information about the sizes and hemoglobin content of red blood cells. These include the MCV, MCH, and MCHC (Ch. 41).

erythrocyte sedimentation rate measurement of how far the red cells in a sample of blood fall in one hour (Ch. 41).

erythropoietin hormone that causes production of new red blood cells (Ch. 41).

esophageal varices tortuous dilation of the esophageal vein associated with any condition that causes obstruction of drainage from the esophageal veins into the portal vein of the liver. Seen in cirrhosis of the liver and alcoholism (Ch. 32).

established patient patient who has been seen previously in the office, with a pertinent history and medical information readily accessible in the chart (Ch. 13).

ethical conforming to accepted principles of right and wrong within a profession; see also ethics (Ch. 12).

ethics defined in terms of what is morally right and wrong; ethics will differ from person to person; often defined by a code or creed as in the Code of Ethics from the American Association of Medical Assistants (AAMA) (Ch. 8).

ethyl alcohol alcohol, used to make a solution (Ch. 38).

etiquette manners, politeness, proper behavior (Ch. 12).

eupnea normal breathing (Ch. 24).

evaluation assessment; significance or value of a situation (Ch. 40); also, assessment of an employee's job performance (Ch. 46).

eversion moving a body part outward (Ch. 33).

exclusive provider organization (EPO) a closed-panel PPO plan where enrollees receive no beneifts if they opt to receive care from a provider who is not in the EPO (Ch. 18).

excoriated abrasion of the epidermis by trauma, chemicals, burns, or other causes (Ch. 22).

excretion waste matter. The elimination of waste products from the body (Ch. 22, 38).

exit interview opportunity for departing employees to provide their positive and negative opinions of the position and facility (Ch. 46).

expectorate to bring up material from the lungs (Ch. 43).

expenses decreases in the owner's equity in a business caused by transactions involving asset outflows (Ch. 20).

expert witness individual with highly specialized knowledge and skills in a particular area who testifies to a standard of care (Ch. 7).

explanation of benefits (EOB) insurance report that is sent with claim payments explaining the reimbursement of the insurance carrier (Ch. 18, 19).

expressed contract written or verbal contract that specifically describes what each party in the contract will do (Ch. 7).

extension straightening of a body part (Ch. 33).

external respiration ventilation of the lungs when the exchange of oxygen and carbon dioxide takes place (Ch. 30).

externship transition stage between the classroom and actual employment; may also be referred to as internship or practicum (Ch. 1, 45).

extracellular pertaining to the environment outside of a body cell (Ch. 34).

exudate accumulated fluid in a cavity; an oozing of pus (Ch. 27, 31).

facial expressions various aspects of facial anatomy that send nonverbal messages (Ch. 4).

facilitate to make an action or process easier (Ch. 1).

Fair Debt Collection Practice Act 1977 federal law that outlines collection practices (Ch. 20).

fastidious bacteria bacteria that require a specialized medium to grow and multiply (Ch. 43).

fat-soluble   pertaining to substances that are hydrophobic and therefore dissolve better in fat (Ch. 34).

fax (facsimile)   machine that sends documents from one location to another by way of telephone lines (Ch. 12).

febrile   having a fever (Ch. 24).

Federal Register   federal government agency from which written CLIA '88 documents may be obtained (Ch. 38).

feedback   receiver's way of ensuring that the message that was understood is the same as the message that was sent (Ch. 4).

fenestrated drape   a type of drape with an opening, usually round, that can be placed with the opening over a particular body area; used in surgery and for proctological exams (Ch. 25).

field   basic data category within the database. Fields can be either numeric (numerals), alphanumeric (letters and numerals), logical, or memo (Ch. 11).

financial accounting   provides information for entities external to the practice; e.g., the federal government (Ch. 21).

firewall   software protection built into a computer system to prevent unauthorized access or hacking into a computer system and files (Ch. 11).

first aid   immediate (or first) care provided to persons who are suddenly ill or injured; first aid is typically followed by more comprehensive care and treatment (Ch. 9).

fiscal intermediary   local administrator for Medicare (Ch. 18).

fixed cost   cost that does not vary in total as the number of patients vary (Ch. 21).

flag   method of identifying a blank space or a question regarding dictator's meaning by attaching a note or marker to indicate the question (Ch. 16).

flexion   bending of a body part (Ch. 33).

floppy disk   portable read-write data storage device. It is storable and transferable between computers. Capacity is approximately 1.4 megabytes of data. Data is stored permanently until overwritten. Floppy drive unit is required to read-write data from disk (Ch. 11).

fluent   facility in the use of a language (Ch. 12).

fluoroscope   a device consisting of a screen; mounts separately or with an X-ray tube that shows the images of objects interposed between the table and the screen (Ch. 32).

folic acid   one of the B-complex vitamins (Ch. 34).

fomite   substance that absorbs and transmit infectious material, e.g., contaminated items such as equipment (Ch. 22).

footer   page formatting feature that allows for the bottom of all pages to be marked with keyed-in data. While the data is keyed in only once, it appears on every page in the document (Ch. 11).

forensic   pertaining to the law (Ch. 38).

form letter   letter containing the same content in the body but sent to different individuals (Ch. 15).

formaldehyde   colorless gas combined with methanol and used as a solution, such as a disinfectant, astringent, or a preservative for histologic specimen (Ch. 38).

fractures   break in a bone. There are several types of fractures, but all are classified as either open fractures or closed fractures (Ch. 9).

fraud   deliberate misrepresentation of facts (Ch. 19).

freelance MTs   self-employed medical transcriptionists (Ch. 16).

frenulum   of the tongue, a fold of mucus membrane located under the tongue attaching the tongue to the floor of the mouth (Ch. 24).

frequency   urinating frequently (Ch. 30).

friable   easily broken (Ch. 31).

fringe benefit   benefit above and beyond salary to which an employee may be entitled. Examples include health and life insurance, paid vacation, sick days, personal days, and tuition reimbursement for courses related to employment (Ch. 2, 45).

fulgaration   destruction by electric current (Ch. 26).

full block letter   major letter style in which all lines begin flush with the left margin. This style is suggested for offices desiring a contemporary-looking, efficient letter (Ch. 15).

fume hood   type of hood or barrier used in the laboratory to capture chemical vapors and fumes and move them away from health care workers and into a building's exhaust fan system (Ch. 38).

functional resume   resume format used to highlight specialty areas of accomplishment and strengths (Ch. 48).

furuncle   localized, suppurative staphylococcal skin infection originating in a gland or hair follicle (Ch. 30).

gait   manner or style of walking including rhythm and speed (Ch. 33).

gait belt   safety belt worn by the patient around the waist that provides a firm handhold for the caregiver when transferring the patient or when assisting in ambulation (Ch. 33).

galvonometer   mechanism in the electrocardiograph that changes the voltage into a mechanical motion for recording purposes (Ch. 37).

genetic engineering   alteration, manipulation, replacement, or repair of genetic material (Ch. 8).

genitalia   the reproductive organs, internal and external (Ch. 26).

genus   first Greek or Latin name given to a microorganism; always capitalized (Ch. 43).

geriatrics   the branch of medicine concerned with the problems of aging (Ch. 29).

gerontology   the scientific study of the problems associated with aging (Ch. 29).

gestation   period of development from fertilization to birth (Ch. 26).

gestures/mannerisms   movement of various body parts while communicating (Ch. 4).

gigabyte   1,000 megabytes of data (Ch. 11).

glucose   simple sugar that is a major source of energy in the human body; monitoring of blood glucose levels in urine and blood is a vital diagnostic test in diabetes and other disorders; also a test on a reagent strip (Ch. 39, 42).

glycogen   carbohydrate form used for storage of sugar in the body (Ch. 34).

goal   result or achievement toward which effort is directed (Ch. 5).

"going bare"   said of a physician who does not carry professional liability insurance (Ch. 45).

goniometer   instrument used to measure the angle of a joint's range of motion (Ch. 30, 33).

goniometry   measurement of joint motion (Ch. 33).

Good Samaritan laws   laws designed to protect individuals from legal action when rendering emergency medical aid, without compensation, within the areas of their training and expertise (Ch. 12).

Gram stain   most common stain used in microbiology to observe gross morphological features of bacteria; a differential stain, allowing differentiation between Gram-negative and Gram-positive organisms (Ch. 43).

graphics software   applications software used to create pictorial representations (Ch. 11).

gravidy   total number of pregnancies a woman has had regardless of duration, including a present one (Ch. 26).

guaiac   used to test for occult blood in feces (Ch. 30).

guide   device on file folders used to separate sections of file folders (Ch. 14).

Guthrie screening test   diagnostic test for the detection of phenylketonuria (PKU) (Ch. 44).

hacker   person who uses sophisticated software to gain unauthorized access to computer systems and files. Hacker gains access through use of a linked computer or a computer connected to the Internet (Ch. 11).

hard disk   read-write data storage device permanently attached to the computer cabinet containing the CPU. Data is stored permanently until overwritten. Capacity is approximately 20 gigabytes or more of data (Ch. 11).

hardware   physical equipment used by the computer system to process data (Ch. 11).

HCFA Common Procedure Coding System (HCPCS)   standardized coding system used to process Medicare claims (Ch. 19).

header   page formatting feature that allows the top of a page to be printed with identifying information. The data is only keyed in once, but appears on all pages in the document (Ch. 11).

Health Care Financing Administration (HCFA)   the national administrator of Medicare (Ch. 18).

health maintenance organization (HMO)   type of managed care operation that is typically set up as a for-profit corporation with salaried employees. HMOs "with walls" offer a range of medical services under one roof; HMOs "without walls" typically contract with physicians in the community to provide patient services for an agreed-upon fee (Ch. 2, 18).

Heimlich maneuver   abdominal thrusts designed to overcome breathing difficulties in patients who are choking (Ch. 9).

hemacytometer (also spelled hemocytometer)   precisely etched glass slide and coverslip used as a counting chamber for blood cells (Ch. 41).

hematemesis   vomiting blood (Ch. 30).

hematochezia   presence of bright red blood in feces (Ch. 30).

hematocrit   percentage of red blood cells within a specimen of anticoagulated whole blood (Ch. 41).

hematology   study of blood and the blood-forming tissues (Ch. 39, 41).

hematoma   accumulation of blood around the venipuncture site during or after venipuncture caused by the leakage of blood from where the needle punctured the vein (Ch. 30, 33, 40).

hematuria   abnormal presence of blood in urine, symptomatic of many disorders of the genitourinary system and renal diseases (Ch. 30, 42).

hemiplegia   paralysis of one side of the body (Ch. 33).

hemoconcentration   pooling of blood at the location of the venipuncture caused by leaving the tourniquet on the arm longer than one minute, resulting in inaccurate blood samples (Ch. 40).

hemoglobin   molecule with the red blood cell that transports oxygen (Ch. 41).

hemoglobinopathy   inherited disease resulting from the formation of an abnormal hemoglobin molecule (Ch. 41).

hemolysis   rupturing of the red blood cells during the process of blood collection. The serum or plasma becomes contaminated and has a reddish color (Ch. 40).

hemolytic anemia   anemia due to lysis of RBC (Ch. 44).

hemophilia   hereditary blood disease characterized by the blood's failure to clot, causing abnormal bleeding (Ch. 8).

hematopoiesis   formation of blood cells (Ch. 41).

heterophile antibody   antibody that reacts with other than the specific antigens as seen in infectious mononucleosis (Ch. 44).

Hibeclens®   brand of antiseptic soap solution (Ch. 31).

hierarchy   the order of significance or control; ranking of importance (Ch. 45).

hierarchy of needs   needs that are arranged in a specific order or rank; sequential arrangement. Associated with Abraham Maslow (Ch. 4).

high-density lipoprotein (HDL)   lipoprotein in the blood composed primarily of protein; removes cholesterol from peripheral tissues and transports them to the liver for excretion (Ch. 44).

histology   study of biopsied tissue samples for the determination of disease (Ch. 39).

history and physical examination report (H&P)   report of patient's history and physical examination to document reason for visit (Ch. 16).

history of present illness (HPI)   the chronological description of the development of the patient's illness (Ch. 16).

holding media   specific media used in the transport of microorganisms to support the life of the organisms until they can be put on nutrient medium in the laboratory (Ch. 43).

holistic   in medicine, used to identify a specific approach that treats the "whole" body, mind, and spirit (Ch. 2).

home-based MTs   medical transcriptionists employed by transcription services (Ch. 16).

homeostasis   state of equilibrium of internal environment (Ch. 34).

hospital-based laboratories   hospital-owned labs which perform most tests required by the hospital and local communities (Ch. 39).

human chorionic gonadotrophin (HCG)   hormone secreted by the trophoblast after fertilization of the ovum. It may be detected in the blood and urine of pregnant women (Ch. 26, 44).

human immunodeficiency virus (HIV)   AIDS virus; it is a retrovirus that ultimately destroys immune system cells (Ch. 6, 22).

human relations objectives   relate to improving communication and interpersonal skills (Ch. 40).

humoral immunity   immunity mediated by antibodies in body fluids such as plasma and lymph (Ch. 22).

hyaline   transparent, clear; hyaline casts are transparent and often hard to see in urine (Ch. 42).

hydatidiform mole   development of cysts and rapid growth of the uterus with bleeding (Ch. 44).

hydrogen peroxide   antibacterial solution that has a mechanical cleansing action (Ch. 31).

hydronephrosis   collection of urine in renal pelvis. This is caused by an obstruction and may result in a cyst. (Ch. 30).

hyperemesis gravidarum   severe nausea and vomiting during pregnancy with inability to eat; may lead to severe dehydration (Ch. 26).

hyperextension   position of maximum extension, or extending a body part beyond its normal limits (Ch. 33).

hyperglycemia   increased levels of blood glucose. Hyperglycemia does not necessarily mean that the patient is diabetic but may be an indication of prediabetes (Ch. 44).

hyperpnea   increased respiratory rate and depth as seen in exercise pain, fever, and hysteria (Ch. 24).

hypertension   blood pressure that is consistently above 140/90 (Ch. 24).

hyperthermia   body temperature above normal range; an unusually high fever (Ch. 29).

hyperventilation   ventilation rate that is greater than metabolically necessary, potentially leading to alkalosis (Ch. 24).

hypochromic   less color than normal (Ch. 41).

hypoglycemia   state of having a lower than normal blood glucose level (Ch. 40, 44).

hypotension   abnormally low blood pressure resulting in inadequate tissue profusion and oxygenation (Ch. 24).

hypothermia   extremely dangerous cold-related condition that can result in death if the individual does not receive care and if the progression of hypothermia is not reversed. Symptoms include shivering, cold skin, and confusion (Ch. 9, 29).

hypoventilation   decrease in respiration rate with shallow depth of respiration (Ch. 24).

hypoxemia   lack of oxygen in the blood (Ch. 36).

hysterosalpingogram   x-ray of uterus and fallopian tubes using a contrast medium (Ch. 26).

Ictotest®   confirmatory test for bilirubin (Ch. 42).

identification label   marking label placed on either the top or side edge of a file folder to indicate the proper designation for filing purposes (Ch. 14).

immune system   body's strong line of defense against invading microorganisms. The body recognizes foreign substances such as microorganisms and produces substances to fight them off. Antibodies, white blood cells, digestive enzymes, and resistance of the skin are some examples (Ch. 22).

immunity   ability of the body to resist specific pathogens and their toxins (Ch. 22).

immunoassay   measurement of reaction of antigen with specific antibody (Ch. 44).

immunoglobulins   family of proteins capable of acting as antibodies, thereby protecting individuals from pathogenic microorganisms; also, antibodies produced by the cells of the immune system (Ch. 22).

immunohematology   study of blood group antigens and antibodies; blood banking (Ch. 39).

immunology   the study of the components of the immune system and their function (Ch. 39).

immunosuppressed   referring to a patient whose immune system is unhealthy due to disease, medication, genetics, and so on; these patients can be particularly susceptible to attack by microorganisms (Ch. 22, 43).

impedance principle   method employed in hematology instrumentation that uses a diluted sample to measure resistance of an electrical current to formed elements in the blood (Ch. 41).

implied consent   consent assumed by the health care provider, typically in an emergency that threatens the patient's life. Implied consent also occurs in more subtle ways in the health care environment; e.g., when a patient willingly rolls up the sleeve to receive an injection (Ch. 7).

implied contract   contract indicated by actions rather than words (Ch. 7).

improvise   to make, invent, or arrange in an offhand manner (Ch. 1).

incinerate   to destroy by fire (Ch. 22).

income statement   financial statement showing net profit or loss (Ch. 21).

incompetence   legally, a person who is insane, inadequate, or not an adult (Ch. 7).

incontinence   uncontrollable loss of urine (Ch. 29).

independent physician association (IPA)   independent network of physicians in private practice who contract with the association to treat patients for an agreed-upon fee (Ch. 2).

index counter   measures the length of dictation on a cassette cartridge (Ch. 16).

indexing   selecting the name, subject, or number under which to file a record and determining the order in which the units should be considered (Ch. 14).

indirect statements   means of eliciting a response from a patient by turning a question into a statement of interest (Ch. 4).

infarction   area of tissue in an organ or part that becomes necrotic (dead) following cessation of blood supply (Ch. 37).

infection   invasion of pathogens into living tissue (Ch. 31).

infection control   methods to eliminate or reduce the transmission of infectious microorganisms (Ch. 22).

infectious agent   pathogen responsible for a specific infectious disease (Ch. 22).

infectious mononucleosis   acute infectious disease primarily affecting the lymphoid tissue caused by the Epstein-Barr virus (Ch. 44).

infectious waste   items that have come in contact with patient blood and/or body fluids. Contaminated items (Ch. 22).

inflammatory response body's defense against the threat of infection or trauma. Characterized by redness, pain, heat, and swelling (Ch. 22, 31).

information retrieval system system that allows electronic access to very large databases for the retrieval of information; e.g., Medlais and Medline (Ch. 11).

informed consent consent given by the patient who is made aware of any procedure to be performed, its risks, expected outcomes, and alternatives (Ch. 7, 31).

ingestion taking in of food, drugs, etc. into the body by mouth (Ch. 30).

inner-directed people people who decide for themselves what they want to do with their lives (Ch. 5).

inoculate to place colonies of microorganisms onto nutrient media (Ch. 43).

inspect to look carefully at the item to be filed to identify the key name, business, and subject the information relates to (Ch. 14).

insulin hormone secreted by beta cells of the islets of Langerhans of the pancreas essential for the proper metabolism of glucose (Ch. 44).

insurance abuse incidents or misrepresentations that are inconsistent with acceptable practice of medicine and lead to improper reimbursement, treatment that is not medically necessary for a disorder, or procedures that are harmful and/or of poor quality (Ch. 19).

integrate to incorporate into a larger unit; to form or blend into a whole (Ch. 1).

integrated delivery system a health care organization of affiliated provider sites combined under a single ownership that offers the full spectrum of managed health care (Ch. 18).

integrative medicine bringing together of two or more treatment modalities so they function as a harmonious whole; as seen in alternative forms of health care (Ch. 2).

integrity normal structure without damage (Ch. 40).

internal respiration passage of oxygen from the blood into the cells (Ch. 30).

International Classification of Diseases, 9th Revision, Clinical Modification (ICD-9-CM) standard diagnosis codes used to identify a patient's medical problem. Used by most ambulatory care settings in encoding the claim form and recognized by most insurance carriers (Ch. 18, 19).

Internet worldwide computer network available via modem that connects universities, government laboratories, companies, and individuals around the world (Ch. 11, 15, 45).

internship transition stage between classroom and employment (Ch. 1).

interview meeting in which you and the interviewer discuss employment opportunities and strengths you can contribute to the organization (Ch. 48).

interview techniques methods of encouraging the best communication between professionals and the patient (Ch. 4).

intravenous pyelogram X-ray studies of the kidneys, ureters, and bladder using a contrast medium (Ch. 28).

introjection identification with another person or with some object (Ch. 4).

invasive procedure surgical technique or procedure that penetrates healthy tissue. The potential for pathogenic microorganisms to enter the body exists (Ch. 22, 39).

inversion moving a body part inward (Ch. 33).

involuntary dismissal termination of employment based on poor job performance or violation of office policies (Ch. 46).

involution return of the uterus to normal size and shape after childbirth (Ch. 26).

ionizing radiation X-ray beams (Ch. 32).

ischemia local and temporary lack of blood to an organ or part due to obstruction of circulation (Ch. 37).

isoelectric having equal electrical potentials. It is represented on the ECG as the flat horizontal line, the baseline (Ch. 37).

isolation separating a patient with certain infections or communicable diseases from other individuals (Ch. 22).

isolation categories system of seven categories developed by the Centers for Disease Control (CDC) that isolates patients according to known infections. These categories have been condensed into three transmission-based precautions based on air, contact, and droplet routes of transmission (Ch. 22).

isopropyl alcohol 70 percent alcohol solution commonly used as a disinfectant (Ch. 31).

itinerary detailed written plan of a proposed trip (Ch. 45).

jargon words, phrases, or terminology specific to a profession (Ch. 12).

jaundice yellow discolorization of the skin and sclera caused by excess bilirubin in the blood (Ch. 22, 25).

Jaz® disk read-write data storage device. It is storable and transferable between computers. Capacity is approximately 1 to 2 gigabytes of data. Data is stored permanently until overwritten. Jaz drive unit is required to read-write data from the disk (Ch. 11).

job description outline of tasks, duties, and responsibilities for every position in the office (Ch. 46).

Joint Commission on Accreditation of Healthcare Organizations (JCAHO) commission established to improve the quality of care and services provided in organized health care setting through a voluntary accreditation process (Ch. 16).

ketoacidosis accumulation of ketones in the body, occurring primarily as a complication of diabetes mellitus; if left untreated, it could cause coma (Ch. 42).

ketone chemical compound produced during an increased metabolism of fat; also, test on a reagent strip (Ch. 42).

key (keyed) to input data by keystrokes on a computer, word processor, or typewriter (Ch. 15).

key unit first indexing unit of the filing segment (Ch. 14).

kinesics study of body language (Ch. 4).

Kirby Bauer manual sensitivity test involving streaking a plate of media with an isolated organism and applying antibiotic disks; the plate is later read to discern which antibiotics will destroy the organism (Ch. 43).

kit commercially packaged materials needed to perform laboratory tests (Ch. 38).

kwashiorkor   severe protein deficiency in infants and children (Ch. 34).

labyrinthitis   inflammation of inner ear or labyrinth (Ch. 9, 25).

lackluster   dull, lacking in sheen (Ch. 9).

Lamaze   technique consisting of breathing exercises to facilitate delivery (Ch. 26).

latex beads   tiny latex beads coated with antibodies or antigens that react with antigens or antibodies in the test sample in an agglutination reaction. The latex beads may be colored to make the reaction easier to visualize (Ch. 44).

lead   a conductor attached to an electrocardiograph. Consists of limb leads and chest leads (Ch. 37).

ledger   record of charges, payments, and adjustments for individual patient or family (Ch. 17).

lesion   injury or wound. A circumscribed area of tissue that has been altered pathologically (Ch. 22, 30).

letter of reference   letter usually written by an employee's past employer describing the employee's performance, attitude, or qualifications. This letter is presented to a potential employer when applying for a new job (Ch. 46).

letter of resignation   letter informing the current employer of the employee's decision to resign from a current position (Ch. 46).

leukocyte   white blood cell, one of the formed elements of blood (Ch. 40, 41).

leukocyte esterase   test on a reagent strip that indicates the presence of white blood cells in the urinary tract (Ch. 42).

leukorrhea   whitish or yellowish mucous discharged from the cervical canal or vagina. Usually normal unless there is an increase in amount or variation in color (Ch. 22).

liabilities   debts and financial obligations for which one is responsible (Ch. 21).

liability   legal responsibility (Ch. 45).

libel   false and malicious writing about another constituting a defamation of character (Ch. 7).

libido   sexual drive (Ch. 6).

license   permission by competent authority (the state) to engage in a profession; permission to act (Ch. 1).

licensure   granting of licenses to practice a profession (Ch. 1).

ligature   length of suture thread without a needle, used for tying off vessels during surgery (Ch. 31).

lipemia   excessive amount of fat (lipids) in the blood, resulting in a blood sample that has a milky appearance (Ch. 40).

liquid nitrogen   commonly and incorrectly referred to as dry ice, liquid nitrogen is a very volatile freezing agent used to destroy unwanted tissue such as warts (Ch. 31).

litigation   court action (Ch. 7).

litigious   prone to engage in lawsuits (Ch. 1).

living will   document allowing a person to make choices related to treatment in a life-threatening illness (Ch. 6).

lochia   discharge from the uterus of blood, mucus, and tissue during the period following childbirth (Ch. 22, 26).

long-range goals   achievements that may take three to five years to accomplish (Ch. 5).

low-density lipoprotein (LDL)   lipoprotein in the blood composed primarily of cholesterol. The cholesterol carried by LDL may be deposited in peripheral tissues and is associated with an increased risk of heart disease (Ch. 44).

luer   device that screws into an evacuated tube holder. The part inside the holder has a needle to puncture the tube top, the part outside the holder fits into a tubing port (Ch. 40).

lumbar puncture   surgical puncture of the lumbar area of the intervertebral spaces to aspirate cerebrospinal fluid for laboratory analysis (Ch. 22, 43).

lymphocyte   white blood cell with a dense non-segmented nucleus and lacking granules in the cytoplasm (Ch. 41).

macrocytic   term which describes a larger than normal cell (Ch. 41).

macro   a series of keystrokes that has been saved under a separate file name to be used and inserted repeatedly into a document or documents (Ch. 11).

macular degeneration   degeneration of the macula area of the retina caused by aging; a leading cause of visual impairment in people over 50, making it difficult to do fine work (Ch. 29).

mainframe computer   large computer system capable of processing massive volumes of data (Ch. 11).

major medical insurance   insurance that covers catastrophic expenses from illness or injury (Ch. 18).

major mineral   mineral that is required in large amounts by the body (Ch. 34).

malabsorption   inadequate absorption of nutrients from the intestinal tract (Ch. 30).

malaise   discomfort, uneasiness, or indisposition, often indicative of infection (Ch. 30).

malaria   acute infectious disease caused by the presence of protozoan parasites within the red blood cells; usually comes from the bite of a female mosquito (Ch. 22).

malpractice   professional negligence (Ch. 7, 45).

managed care   strategies designed to reduce the cost of health care by managing an insured's health care benefits (Ch. 2).

managed care operation   any health care setting or delivery system that is designed to reduce the cost of care while still providing access to care (Ch. 2).

managed care organization (MCO)   a health insurance organization that adheres to the principles of strong dependence on selective contracting with providers, the use of PCPs, prospective and retrospective utilization management, use of treatment guidelines for high cost chronic disorders, and an emphasis on preventive care, education, and patient compliance with treatment plans (Ch. 18).

managed competition   medical care in which physicians and hospitals compete for patients (Ch. 2).

managerial accounting   generates information to enable more efficient internal management (Ch. 21).

mandate   formal order to obey certain rules and regulations (Ch. 7, 38).

Mantoux test   test for tuberculosis involving the intracutaneous injection of PPD (Ch. 44).

marasmus   protein-calorie malnutrition seen in first year of life (Ch. 34).

marketing   process by which the provider of services makes the consumer aware of the scope and quality of those services. Marketing tools might include public relations, brochures, patient education seminars, and newsletters (Ch. 45).

masking   attempt to conceal or repress true feelings or the message (Ch. 4).

matrix   to establish an appointment matrix, a physician's unavailable time slots are marked with an X. Patients are not scheduled during those times (Ch. 13).

Mayo stand/instrument tray   portable metal tray table used for setting up small sterile fields for minor surgery and procedures (Ch. 31).

medical asepsis   clean and free from infection (Ch. 22, 38).

medical transcription   process that traditionally consisted of one person dictating and another writing the words in shorthand. Today, physicians typically dictate into a machine or recording device for transcription into a hard copy at a later time (Ch. 16).

medical transcriptionist certification commission (MTCC) credentialing program of the American Association for Medical Transcription (Ch. 16).

medical transcriptionist (MT)   one who transcribes dictation into written documents (Ch. 16).

Medicare allowable   the maximum amount Medicare will pay for each procedure or service performed (Ch. 18).

Medicare assignment   in exchange for accepting Medicare assignment, those physicians participating receive direct payment from Medicare and the physician agrees to write off any amount in excess of the Medicare Fee Schedule (Ch. 18).

Medicare Part A   benefits covering inpatient hospital and skilled nursing facilities, hospice care, and blood transfusion (Ch. 18).

Medicare Part B   benefits covering outpatient hospital and health care provider services (Ch. 18).

medigap policy   an individual plan covering the patient's Medicare deductible and copay obligations that fulfills the federal government standards for Medicare supplemental insurance (Ch. 18).

megabyte   one million bytes of data (Ch. 11).

melena   tarry stools due to blood in feces (Ch. 30).

memorandum   interoffice correspondence, usually referred to as a memo (Ch. 15).

meniscus   curvature appearing in a liquid's upper surface when a liquid is placed in a container (Ch. 36, 42).

menses   menstruation (Ch. 22).

mentor   person assigned or requested to assist in training, guiding, or coaching another (Ch. 46).

merge operation   word processing operation designed to produce form letters (Ch. 11).

message   content being communicated (Ch. 4).

metabolism   total of all changes, chemical and physical, that take place in the body (Ch. 34).

microbiology   branch of biology dealing with the study of microscopic forms of life (Ch. 39, 43).

microcomputer   personal or desktop computer. Also, a handheld or laptop model (Ch. 11).

microcyctic   term describing a smaller than normal cell (Ch. 41).

microorganism   microscopic living creature capable of transmission and reproduction in specific circumstances (Ch. 22).

microscopy   inspection with a microscope (Ch. 38).

midstream collection   urine sample collected in the middle of a flow of urine (Ch. 42).

minicomputer   one of the four categories of computers based on size: larger than a microcomputer and smaller than a mainframe (Ch. 11).

minor   person who has not reached the age of majority, usually 18 years (Ch. 7).

minutes   written record of topics discussed and actions taken during meeting sessions (Ch. 15, 45).

modalities   physical agents such as heat, cold, light, water, and electricity used to treat muscular or joint malfunction (Ch. 33).

modes of communication   speaking, listening, gestures, or body language, and writing. Also called channels of communication (Ch. 4).

modified block letter, indented   modified letter style with indented paragraphs. Paragraphs in this style of letter may be indented five spaces (Ch. 15).

modified block letter, standard   major letter style where all lines begin at the left margin with the exception of the date line, complimentary closure, and keyed signature. The exceptions usually begin at the center position or a few spaces to the right of center (Ch. 15).

modified wave   scheduling system where multiple patients are scheduled at the beginning of each hour, followed by single appointments every 10 to 20 minutes the rest of the hour (Ch. 13).

modulated   speech that varies in pitch and intensity (Ch. 12).

money market account   bank accounts that pay the highest interest rate (money-market rate) and permit writing a limited number of checks (Ch. 17).

monocyte   white blood cell without cytoplasmic granules that has a large convoluted non-segmented nucleus (Ch. 41).

monthly billing   method that sends all bills at the same time each month, usually on or around the 25th of the month (Ch. 20).

morbidity   number of cases of disease in a specific population (Ch. 22).

mordant   substance that causes dye to adhere to an object; iodine is a mordant in Gram stain (Ch. 43).

morphology   form and structure of an organism (Ch. 43).

mortality   the ratio of the number of deaths to a given population (Ch. 22).

motherboard   printed circuit board upon which the CPU, ROM, and RAM chips and other electronic circuit elements of a digital computer are frequently located (Ch. 11).

mounting   process of applying in sequence a portion of each of the twelve leads of the ECG recording onto a commercially prepared mounting form or plain sheet of paper as part of the patient's permanent record (Ch. 37).

moxibustion   ancient Chinese method of treatment that uses a powdered plant substance on the skin to raise a blister (Ch. 3).

multigravida   a woman who has been pregnant more than once (Ch. 26).

multiparous   pertaining to women who have had two or more pregnancies (Ch. 26).

muscle testing   method of testing the motion, strength, and task potential of a muscle or group of muscles, their tendons, and associated tissues (Ch. 33).

mycobacteria   special types of bacteria, also called acid-fast, that grow only on specialized media; tuberculosis is caused by a mycobacterium (Ch. 43).

mycology   study of fungi (Ch. 39, 43).

myringotomy   incision into the tympanic membrane; part of the treatment for otitis media (Ch. 27).

Nagele's rule   usual method for calculating expected date of birth (Ch. 26).

National Board of Medical Examiners (NBME)   consultants for the certification examination (Ch. 47).

nebulizer   instrument used to produce a fine spray of medication (Ch. 30).

negligence   failure to exercise a certain standard of care (Ch. 7, 45).

nematode   round worm (Ch. 43).

neonatal   pertaining to newborn (Ch. 26).

networking   process in which people of similar interests exchange information in social, business, or professional relationships (Ch. 46).

network interface   software, servers, and cable connections used to link computers (Ch. 11).

neutrophil   the most common type of granulocytic white blood cell (Ch. 41).

new patient   patient being seen for the first time in a medical office, on whom the office staff has not obtained a complete current medical history (Ch. 13).

niacin   one of the B-complex vitamins (Ch. 34).

nitrogenous   waste products in the blood indicating kidney disease (Ch. 30).

nocturia   increased voiding at night (Ch. 30).

nomogram   graph that shows the relationship among numerical values. Body surface area (BSA) of a patient can be estimated by its use (Ch. 36).

nonavailability statement   preauthorization for nonemergency civilian health care issued by the base commander when medical care required for a CHAMPUS eligible is not available at a government medical treatment facility within the patient's catchment area (Ch. 18).

noncompliant   failure to follow a required command or instruction (Ch. 7).

nonconsecutive filing   numeric filing method where numbers are considered in ascending order using subsets of figures within a number, e.g., in the number 574 19 2863: 2863 is unit 1, 19 is unit 2, 574 is unit 3 (Ch. 14).

noninvasive   procedures that do not require entering the body or puncturing the skin (Ch. 32, 37).

normal flora   microorganisms that are normally present in a specific site (Ch. 22, 43).

normal sinus rhythm   term used to describe the heart's rhythm when it is within the normal range (Ch. 37).

normocytic   term that describes a normal sized cell (Ch. 41).

no-show   patient who fails to keep an appointment without canceling the appointment with the office (Ch. 13).

nosocomial   hospital-acquired (Ch. 43).

not current status   effective January 2003, all CMAs employed or seeking employment must have current certified status to use the CMA credential (Ch. 47).

notary (notary public)   someone with the legal capacity to witness and certify documents; can take depositions (Ch. 17).

nullipara   a woman who has not carried a pregnancy to the stage of viability (Ch. 26).

nutrient   ingested substance that helps the body stay in its homeostatic state (Ch. 34).

nutrition   study of the bringing of nutrients into the body and how the body uses these nutrients (Ch. 34).

obfuscation   making things clouded or confused (Ch. 12).

objective   a patient sign that is visible, palpable, or measurable by an observer (Ch. 23); also, magnifying lens that is closest to the object being viewed with a microscope (Ch. 39).

obturator   tool that obstructs or closes a cavity or opening. The internal portion of an examination instrument that facilitates the entry of the instrument into the body; it is then withdrawn, permitting visualization of the internal area (Ch. 30).

occluder   instrument used to obstruct or close off an eye (Ch. 30).

occlusion   closure of a passage (Ch. 9).

oliguria   decrease in urine output (Ch. 30).

one-site placement   externship completed at only one facility (Ch. 40).

on-line   actively working on the Internet (Ch. 15).

open-ended questions   questions that encourage verbalization and response; questions that seek a response beyond a simple yes or no (Ch. 4).

open hours   scheduling system where patients are assigned a timeframe, e.g., 9:00 A.M. to 11:00 A.M., for arrival. They are then seen on a first-come, first-served basis within that time frame (Ch. 13).

ophthalmoscope   instrument for examination of the interior of the eye (Ch. 30).

optical character reader (OCR)   United States Postal Service's computerized scanner that reads addresses printed on letter mail. If the information is properly formatted, then the OCR will find a match in its address files and print a bar code on the lower right edge of the envelope (Ch. 15).

optical disk   portable and transferable read-write or read-only data storage device. Sometimes called a CD-ROM, CD-RW, or compact disk. Capacity is 1 to 8 gigabytes of data. Optical drive unit is required to read-write data from the disk (Ch. 11).

optic nerve   second cranial nerve that carries impulses for the sense of sight (Ch. 30).

orchiectomy   surgical excision of a testicle (Ch. 28).

orphan in typesetting, a term describing the situation in which a new paragraph begins on the last line of a printed page or column (Ch. 11).

orthopnea difficulty breathing in any position other than an upright position (Ch. 24).

oscilloscope an electronic device used for recording electrical activity of the heart, brain, and muscular tissues (Ch. 32, 37).

ossicle small bone; often refers to any of the three small bones of the ear (Ch. 30).

otoscope instrument used to examine the external ear canal and tympanic membrane (Ch. 30).

outer-directed people people who let events, other people, or environmental factors dictate their behavior (Ch. 5).

out guide or sheet card, folder, or slip of paper inserted temporarily in the files to replace a record that has been retrieved from the files (Ch. 14).

ova eggs of parasites (Ch. 43).

oval window opening in the middle ear. The base of the stapes, one of the ear ossicles, fits into this opening (Ch. 30).

overtime money paid at a rate of not less than one and one-half times the regular rate of pay after a forty-hour work week is completed (Ch. 46).

owner's equity amount by which business assets exceed business liabilities. Also called net worth, proprietorship, and capital (Ch. 21).

oxidation process of a substance combining with oxygen (Ch. 34).

oxygenated containing high levels of oxygen (Ch. 40).

oxytocin a pituitary hormone that stimulates the muscles of the uterus to contract, thus inducing labor (Ch. 26).

pagers also known as beepers. One-way paging systems often used inside hospitals and by physicians on call. Pagers only receive signals (Ch. 12).

palliative measures taken to relieve symptoms of disease (Ch. 22, 32).

pallor lack of color, paleness (Ch. 25).

palpate to search for a vein using the fingertips with a pressure and release touch (Ch. 40).

paradigm internalized example or pattern that may influence your perspective (Ch. 45).

parasitology study of organisms (parasites and/or their eggs) that live within or upon another organism and at the expense of that organism (Ch. 39, 43).

parasympathetic nervous system part of the autonomic nervous system that returns the body to its normal state after stress has subsided (Ch. 5).

parenteral injection of a liquid substance into the body via a route other than the alimentary canal (Ch. 22, 36).

parity carrying a pregnancy to the point of viability regardless of the outcome (Ch. 26).

partnership in this text, the collaboration of two or more physicians who share the costs and liabilities of a medical practice (Ch. 2).

parturition the process of giving birth (Ch. 26).

password a code word or number unique to a specific user. It is used to identify the user to authorize access to a database or specific computer system. The system administrator initially issues the password. Passwords must be changed frequently to prevent them from becoming known by unauthorized persons (Ch. 11).

patch modification to software to fix deficiencies in the software. Frequently downloaded from the software supplier's web site or from floppy disks provided by the supplier (Ch. 11).

patent open, not blocked (Ch. 26).

pathogen disease-producing microorganism (Ch. 22, 43).

patient service centers satellite lab facilities located in convenient areas for patients where specimens can be collected or dropped off (Ch. 39).

payee person named on check who is to receive the amount indicated (Ch. 17).

pegboard system most commonly used manual medical accounts receivable system (Ch. 17).

pelvic inflammatory disease infection of uterus, fallopian tubes, and adjacent pelvic structures; most common causes are gonorrhea and chlamydia; spread as sexually transmitted diseases (Ch. 26).

perception conscious awareness of one's own feelings and the feelings of others (Ch. 4).

perforation a hole caused by ulceration (Ch. 30).

performance objectives what is expected to be performed to demonstrate accomplishment (Ch. 40).

peripheral nerve nerves and ganglia away from the spinal cord (Ch. 30).

peritonitis inflammation of the peritoneum (Ch. 30).

pernicious anemia chronic anemia caused by lack of hydrochloric acid in the stomach; weakness, fatigue, tingling of extremities, and even heart failure can result; vitamin B_{12} injections are the treatment for this condition (Ch. 29).

personal computer also known as microcomputer (Ch. 11).

petri dish plastic dish into which agar is placed for the purpose of growing bacteria (Ch. 43).

petty cash small sum kept on hand for minor or unexpected expenses (Ch. 17).

petty cash voucher form used to record individual petty cash transactions (Ch. 17).

pH scale that indicates the relative alkalinity or acidity of a solution; measurement of hydrogen ion concentration (Ch. 42).

pharmacology study of drugs; the science concerned with the history, origin, sources, physical and chemical properties, and uses of drugs and their effects on living organisms (Ch. 35).

pharmacopeia book describing drugs and their preparation or a collection or stock of drugs (Ch. 3).

phenylketonuria (PKU) recessive, inherited disease in which the body is unable to oxidize phenylalanine to tyrosine (Ch. 44).

phlebotomy process of collecting blood (Ch. 22, 40).

physician-hospital organization (PHO) a business entity in which the hospital and selected physicians form a health care network for the purpose of contracting with managed care organizations (Ch. 18).

physician's directive another name for a living will (Ch. 6).

physicians' office laboratories (POL) laboratories within physicians' offices where common office lab tests are performed (Ch. 39).

placenta abruptio sudden and abrupt separation of the placenta from uterine wall (Ch. 26).

placenta previa placenta lies low in uterus and can partially or completely cover the cervical os (Ch. 26).

plaintiff person bringing charges in litigation (Ch. 7).

plantar flexion moving the foot downward at the ankle (Ch. 33).

plasma fluid portion of blood from a tube containing anticoagulant. This fluid contains fibrinogen (Ch. 40).

pluralistic (pluralism) society where there are several distinct ethnic, religious, or cultural groups that coexist with one another (Ch. 3).

poikilocytosis condition where red blood cells show marked variations in shape (Ch. 41).

point-of-service (POS) device device allowing direct communication between a medical office and the health care plan's computer (Ch. 19).

polychromatic stain stain containing both acid and basic dyes that is used to stain formed elements of the blood (Ch. 41).

polycystic situation of many (poly) or multiple cysts (Ch. 30).

polyp tumor with a stem found in nose, uterus, bladder, colon, or rectum (Ch. 30).

portfolio notebook or file containing examples of materials commonly used (Ch. 15).

position physical stance of two individuals while communicating (Ch. 4).

posting recording financial transactions into a bookkeeping or accounting system (Ch. 17).

posture relates to the position of the body or parts of the body; the pose taken while communicating (Ch. 4, 12).

potentiate to increase potency or action (Ch. 35).

power verbs action words used to describe your attributes and strengths (Ch. 48).

practice-based determined by the type of practice; a system of scheduling unique to the type of medical care provided (Ch. 13).

practicum transitional stage providing opportunity to apply theory learned in the classroom to a health care setting through practical, hands-on experience (Ch. 1, 45).

preauthorization obtaining an insurance carrier's consent to proceed with patient care and treatment. Unless authorization is obtained, insurance carriers may not pay benefits for specific problems (Ch. 18).

precipitate substance in the form of fine particles that separates from a solution if allowed to stand for a period of time (Ch. 36).

precordial pertaining to the area on the anterior surface of the body overlying the heart (Ch. 37).

pre-eclampsia a complication of pregnancy characterized by generalized edema, hypertension, and proteinuria (Ch. 26).

pre-existing condition illness, disease, or injury that occurred before the inception of the policy (Ch. 18).

preferred provider organization (PPO) organization of physicians who network together to offer discounts to purchasers of heath care insurance (Ch. 2, 18).

preferred provider physician who has signed a contract with a particular insurance carrier or HMO to provide care for a reduced rate in exchange for direct payment from the insurer (Ch. 18).

prejudice opinion or judgment that is formed before all the facts are known (Ch. 4).

prenatal time period between fertilization and birth (Ch. 26).

presbycusis progressive loss of hearing caused by the normal aging process (Ch. 29).

prescribe to order or recommend the use of a drug, diet, or other form of therapy (Ch. 35).

preservative chemical added to food to keep it fresh longer (Ch. 34).

primary care physician (PCP) primary care physician for a patient; all care is coordinated through the PCP (Ch. 18).

primary container container that directly contains the specimen (Ch. 40).

primigravida a woman pregnant for the first time (Ch. 26).

privileged confidential information that may only be communicated with the patient's permission or by court order (Ch. 16).

probate court court that administers estates and validates wills (Ch. 20).

probation period of time during which the employee and supervisory personnel may determine if both the environment and the position are satisfactory for the employee (Ch. 46).

problem-oriented medical record (POMR) a type of patient chart recordkeeping that uses a sheet at a prominent location in the chart to list vital identification data. Patient medical problems are identified by a number that corresponds to the charting; e.g., bronchitis is #1, a broken wrist is #2, and so forth (Ch. 4, 23).

procedure code numerical code signifying a specific medical procedure; codes found in CPT code book (Ch. 18, 19).

procedures manual manual providing detailed information relative to the performance of tasks within the job description (Ch. 45).

processed food food that is no longer in a whole, natural state; cooked or packaged with parts removed or ingredients added (Ch. 34).

professional liability insurance insurance policy designed to protect assets in the event a claim for damages resulting from negligence is filed and awarded (Ch. 45).

proficiency testing sample tests performed in a clinical laboratory to determine with what degree of accuracy tests are being performed. Testing samples are checked in the same manner as patient specimens (Ch. 38).

profile categories of groups of tests related by body system or body function (Ch. 39).

profit sharing sharing in the financial profits, gains, and benefits of an organization (Ch. 45).

progress notes (also called chart notes) physician's formal or informal notes about presenting problem, physical findings, and plan for treatment for a patient examined in the office, clinic, acute care center, or emergency department (Ch. 16).

projection act of placing one's own feelings upon another (Ch. 4).

pronation moving the arm so the palm is down (Ch. 33).

pronunciation saying words correctly (Ch. 12).

proofread to read a document to verify the accuracy of content and that correct grammar, spelling, punctuation, and capitalization were used (Ch. 15, 16).

proprietary privately owned and managed facility, a profit-making organization (Ch. 1).

prospective payment method of flat-fee pricing (Ch. 18).

prostaglandin modulator of biochemical activity in tissues (Ch. 26).

proteinuria protein in the urine (Ch. 30).

protozoa one-celled animals divided into four groups: amebae, flagellates, ciliates, and coccidia (Ch. 43).

pruritis itchiness (Ch. 35).

psychomotor retardation slowing of physical and mental responses; may be seen in depression (Ch. 6).

puerperium the period of time from the end of the third stage of labor until involution of uterus is complete, usually 3 to 6 weeks (Ch. 26).

pulmonary edema accumulation of serous fluid in the air vesicles and interstitial tissues of the lungs (Ch. 38).

purging method of maintaining order in the files by separating active from inactive and closed files (Ch. 14).

purified protein derivative (PPD) filtrate obtained from Mycobacterium cultures used for intradermal testing for tuberculosis (Ch. 44).

pyorrhea discharge of pus from the gums, around the teeth (Ch. 25).

pyrexia fever (Ch. 24).

pyridoxine Vitamin B_6 (Ch. 34).

pyuria pus in the urine (Ch. 30).

qualitative test analysis to identify quality or characteristics of components, such as size, shape, and maturity of cells (Ch. 39).

quality assurance (QA) process to provide accurate, complete, consistent healthcare documentation in a timely manner while making every reasonable effort to resolve inconsistencies, inaccuracies, risk management issues, and other problems (Ch. 16, 36).

quality control measures used to monitor the processing of laboratory specimens. Includes proper use, storage, handling, stability, expiration dates, and indications for measuring precision and accuracy of analytic processes (Ch. 38, 42, 43).

quantitative test analysis that can identify quantity or actual number counts such as counting the number of blood cells (Ch. 39).

radioactive emits rays or particles from nucleus (Ch. 32).

radiograph the film on which an image is produced through exposure to X-rays (Ch. 32).

radiolucent allowing X rays to pass through. A dark area appears on the radiograph (Ch. 32).

radionuclides atoms that disintegrate by emitting electromagnetic radiation (Ch. 32).

radiopaque impenetrable to X rays. A light area appears on the radiograph (Ch. 32).

radiopharmaceuticals radioactive chemicals used in testing the location, size, outline, or function of tissue, organs, vessels, or body fluids (Ch. 32).

rales abnormal bubbling or crackling sound heard by auscultation during the inspiratory phase of respiration (Ch. 24).

random access memory (RAM) a type of computer memory that can be written to and read from. The word *random* means that any one location can be read at any time. RAM commonly refers to the internal memory of a computer. RAM is usually a fast, temporary memory area where data and programs reside until saved or until the power is turned off (Ch. 11).

range of motion (ROM) amount of movement that is present in a joint (Ch. 33).

ratchets locking mechanisms on the handles of many surgical instruments (Ch. 31).

rationalization act of justification, usually illogically, that one uses to keep from facing the truth of the situation (Ch. 4).

read-only memory (ROM) permanently stored computer data that cannot be overwritten without special devices. Stores instructions required to start up the computer. Located on the motherboard (Ch. 11).

reagent chemical substance that detects or synthesizes other substances in a chemical reaction; used in laboratory analyses because it is known to react in a specific way (Ch. 39, 42, 43).

reagent test strip narrow strip of plastic on which pads containing reagents are attached; used in the urinalysis chemical examination to detect glucose, bilirubin, ketones, specific gravity, blood, pH, urobilinogen, nitrites, and leukocyte esterase (Ch. 42).

receiver recipient of the sender's message (Ch. 4).

recertification documentation admitted to support continued education for maintaining a professional credential (Ch. 16, 47).

record related fields, grouped together and organized in the same order (Ch. 11).

reference laboratories independent, regionally located labs used by hospitals for complex, expensive or specialized tests (Ch. 39).

references individuals who have known or worked with you long enough to make an honest assessment and recommendation regarding your background history (Ch. 48).

reference values also referred to as normal value, normal range, or reference range; range of values that includes 95 percent of test results for a normal healthy population (Ch. 39).

refractometer instrument that measures the refractive index of a substance or solution; used in the urinalysis physical examination to measure the urine specimen's specific gravity (Ch. 42).

registered medical assistant (RMA) credential awarded for successfully passing the AMT examination (Ch. 1, 47).

regression moving back to a former stage to escape conflict or fear (Ch. 6).

regulated waste any waste that contains infectious material that would pose a threat due to possible transmission of pathogenic microorganisms (Ch. 22).

rehabilitation medicine field of medical disciplines that seeks to restore an individual or body part to normal or near normal function following an illness or injury using physical and mechanical agents (Ch. 33).

reimbursement   payment (Ch. 38).

release mark   symbol, usually in the form of initials, a code, or a stamp, which indicates that material is ready to be filed (Ch. 14).

repolarization   re-establishment of a polarized state in a muscle following contraction (Ch. 37).

repression   coping with an overwhelming situation by temporarily forgetting it; temporary amnesia (Ch. 4).

requisition   request form sent with a specimen specifying tests to be performed on the specimen; most common tests are separated into logical categories with additional space for writing special requests (Ch. 38, 39).

rescue breathing   performed on individuals in respiratory arrest, rescue breathing is a mouth-to-mouth (using appropriate protective equipment) or mouth-to-nose procedure that provides oxygen to the patient until emergency personnel arrive (Ch. 9).

residual   amount of urine remaining in bladder immediately after voiding; seen with hyperplasia of prostate (Ch. 28).

resistance   ability of the immune system to resist or withstand an infectious disease (Ch. 22).

resource-based relative value scale (RBRVS)   basis for the Medicare fee schedule (Ch. 18).

resume   written summary data sheet or brief account of qualifications and progress in your chosen career (Ch. 46, 48).

retention   urine held in the bladder; inability to empty the bladder (Ch. 28).

retrolental fibroplasia   disease of blood vessels of retina in newborns (Ch. 36).

retrovirus   common name for some viruses that contain reverse transcriptase (Ch. 8).

revalidation   maintaining current RMA status (Ch. 47).

review of systems (ROS)   inquires about the system directly related to the problems identified in the history of the present illness (Ch. 16).

Rh factor   blood factor indicating the presence or absence of the Rh antigen on the surface of human erythrocytes (Ch. 44).

rhonchi   sounds during breathing similar to wheezes (Ch. 24).

rhythm strip   ECG recording of a single lead, usually lead II, that is used to determine the rhythm of the heart beat. An arrhythmia can more easily be seen in a rhythm strip because it is run longer per physician's request (Ch. 37).

riboflavin   Vitamin B$_2$ (Ch. 34).

ribonucleic acid (RNA)   nucleic acid in all living cells; sometimes takes the place of DNA in certain viruses (Ch. 8).

risk management   techniques adhered to in the ambulatory care setting that keep the practice, its environment, and its procedures as safe for the patient as possible. Proper risk management also reduces the possibility of negligence that leads to torts and malpractice suits (Ch. 7, 16, 45).

ROA   standard abbreviation meaning Received On Account (Ch. 17).

roadblocks (to communication)   verbal or nonverbal messages that block the communication cycle (Ch. 4).

rotation   turning a body part around its axis (Ch. 33); also, opportunity to spend two or three weeks in a variety of health care settings (Ch. 40).

salary review   informing the employee of their revised base pay rate (Ch. 46).

sanitization   cleaning or scrubbing contaminated instruments or fomites to remove tissue, debris, or other contaminants (Ch. 22).

saturated fat   fat that comes from an animal source and that contains more cholesterol than unsaturated fat, which comes from vegetable sources (Ch. 34).

scabies   infectious skin disease caused by the itch mite (Sarcoptes scabiei) which is transmitted by direct contact with infected persons (Ch. 22).

scleroderma   slowly progressing disease characterized by deposition of fibrous connective tissue in the skin and in internal organs (Ch. 25).

screen   in the medical office, determining who is calling and the reason for the call (Ch. 12).

screening   preliminary examination used to detect the most characteristic signs of a disorder that may entail further investigation (Ch. 42).

search engine   specialized computer program designed to find specific information on the Internet (Ch. 45).

secretion   substance produced by the cells of glandular organs from materials in the blood (Ch. 22, 38).

sediment   insoluble material that settles to the bottom of a liquid; material examined in the urinalysis microscopic examination (Ch. 42).

self-actualization   being all that you can be; developing your full potential and experiencing fulfillment (Ch. 5, 45).

semen   thick, viscid secretion discharged from the urethra of males at orgasm. It is a mixed product containing various fluids and spermatozoa (Ch. 44).

sender   the individual beginning the communication cycle (Ch. 4).

senile   mental and/or physical weakness sometimes associated with aging (Ch. 29).

sensitivity   test in which an organism is placed with antibiotics to determine which antibiotic will effectively kill the organism with the smallest dose (Ch. 43).

septicemia   invasion of pathogenic bacteria into the bloodstream (Ch. 3).

serum   liquid portion of blood obtained after blood has been allowed to clot (Ch. 9, 40).

server   computer with massive hard drive capacity that is used to link other computers together so that data can be shared by multiple users. A computer system in an ambulatory care facility are likely to be linked or networked with a central server (Ch. 11).

shadow   follow a supervisor or delegated subordinate in order to learn facility protocol (Ch. 45).

sharps   needles or scalpels or other sharp instruments that are capable of causing a penetrating or puncture wound of the skin (Ch. 22).

shingling   method of arranging charts in which sheets of paper are "shingled" up or across the page, with the most recent report placed on top of the previous one, giving access to the most current information first (Ch. 14).

shock   condition in which the circulatory system is not providing enough blood to all parts of the body, causing the body's organs to fail to function properly (Ch. 9).

short-range goals   long-range goals are dissected and reassembled into smaller, more manageable time segments (Ch. 5).

sickle cell anemia   an inherited disorder that may shorten life span (Ch. 26).

silver nitrate   caustic astringent antiseptic. As a weak liquid, it is applied to the eyes of newborns to prevent infections at birth. In the medical office, it is most often seen as a solid substance impregnated onto the end of a wooden applicator. Silver nitrate applicator sticks contain hydrochloric acid and other chemicals and are commonly used to cauterize small blood vessels in the nose or other mucous membranes (Ch. 31).

simplified letter   major letter style recommended by the Administrative Management Society that omits the salutation and complimentary closure. All lines are keyed flush with the left margin. In medical offices, this style is most often employed when sending a form letter (Ch. 15).

sitz bath   a bath to sit in (Ch. 31).

skills acquisition objective   concerned with the development of new on-the-job skills or learning new tasks or concepts (Ch. 40).

skills application/development objective   improvement and development of skills already learned (Ch. 40).

slack time   in the medical office, unscheduled time (Ch. 13).

slander   false and malicious words about another constituting a defamation of character (Ch. 7).

slang   nonstandard, often arbitrarily coined words used in casual speech (Ch. 12).

SOAP   acronym for patient progress notes based on subjective impressions (S), objective clinical evidence (O), assessment or diagnosis (A), and plans for further studies (P) (Ch. 14, 23).

sodium hydroxide   chemical used to chemically burn and destroy tissue; usually in a liquid state when used in minor surgery (Ch. 31).

sodium hypochlorite   household bleach (Ch. 22).

software   equivalent of a computer program or programs (Ch. 11).

sole proprietorship   medical practice that is owned by only one individual (Ch. 2).

sonographer   professionally trained individual capable of performing the ultrasound examination (Ch. 37).

sort   frequently used data processing operation that arranges data in a particular sequence or order (Ch. 11).

source-oriented medical record (SOMR)   a type of patient chart record keeping that includes separate sections for different sources of patient information, such as laboratory reports, pathology reports, and progress notes (Ch. 14, 23).

spamming   sending the same message to hundreds or thousands of e-mail addresses (Ch. 15).

species   second Greek or Latin name given to microorganisms; the species name is not capitalized (Ch. 43).

specific gravity   ratio of weight of a given volume of a substance to the weight of the same volume of distilled water at the same temperature; test often performed during the urinalysis physical examination (can also appear on the reagent strip) (Ch. 42).

spill kit   commercially packaged materials containing supplies and equipment needed to clean up a spill of a biohazardous substance (Ch. 22).

spirometry   test to measure the air capacity of the lungs (Ch. 30).

splint   any device used to immobilize a body part. Often used by EMS personnel (Ch. 9).

split keyboard   ergonomic keyboard; slanted to accommodate the natural position of the hands and support the wrists (Ch. 16).

sprain   injury to a joint, often an ankle, knee, or wrist, that involves a tearing of the ligaments. Most sprains are minor and heal quickly; others are more severe, include swelling, and may not heal properly if the patient continues to put stress on the sprained joint (Ch. 9).

spreadsheet software   computer applications packages that act as "number crunchers" because of their mathematical processing capabilities (Ch. 11).

sputum   substance from the respiratory tract expelled by coughing (Ch. 22).

stab culture   culture where the microorganism is stabbed into tubed solid media (Ch. 43).

standard   rules established to measure quality, weight, extent, or value (Ch. 22, 38).

standard precautions   precautions developed in 1996 by the Centers for Disease Control and Prevention (CDC) that augment universal precautions and body substance isolation practices. They provide a wider range of protection and are used any time there is contact with blood, moist body fluid (except perspiration), mucous membranes, or nonintact skin. They are designed to protect all health care providers, patients, and visitors (Ch. 9, 22).

STAT   abbreviation for the Latin *statim*, meaning immediate (Ch. 16).

status asthmaticus   severe episode of asthma that does not respond to ordinary treatment (Ch. 36).

statute   law enacted by a legislative body (Ch. 7).

statute of limitations   statute that defines the period of time in which legal action can take place (Ch. 20).

stertorous   snoring sound heard with labored breathing (Ch. 24).

stomatitis   inflammation of the mouth associated with radiation therapy. Can include swelling, redness, halitosis, ulcerations (Ch. 32).

strain   injury to the soft tissue between joints that involves the tearing of muscles or tendons. Strains often occur in the neck, back, or thigh muscles (Ch. 9).

stratum corneum   horny, outermost layer of the skin, epidermis, composed of dead cells converted to keratin that continually flakes away (Ch. 30).

stream   scheduling system where patients are seen on a continuous basis throughout the day, e.g., at 15-, 30-, or 60-minute intervals, each patient having a distinct appointment time (Ch. 13).

stress   body's response to change; can be manifested in a variety of ways, including changes in blood pressure, heart rate, and onset of headache (Ch. 5).

stressors   demands to change that cause stress (Ch. 5).

strictures   narrowing of a tube-like structure such as the esophagus or urethra (Ch. 31).

stridor   crowing sound heard on inspiration, the result of an upper airway obstruction (Ch. 24).

stylus   heated slender wire of the electrocardiograph that melts the wax off of the ECG paper during the recording (Ch. 37).

subjective   symptom that is felt by the patient but not observable by others (Ch. 23).

sublimation   redirecting a socially unacceptable impulse into one that is socially acceptable (Ch. 4).

subordinate   in an organization, a person under the direction of (reporting to) a person of greater authority (Ch. 45).

subpoena   written command designating a person to appear in court under penalty for failure to appear (Ch. 7).

subrogation   right of an insurer to collect monies it has paid out on behalf of its insured from another party (Ch. 18, 19).

superbill   billing the patient receives from the physician at the time of service delineating the visit, tests, diagnoses, charges, and when to return. See also **charge slip** (Ch. 17, 19).

supercomputer   fastest, largest, and most expensive of the four classes of computers currently being manufactured (Ch. 11).

supernatant   urine that appears above the sediment when centrifuged; poured off before sediment is examined in the urinalysis microscopic examination (Ch. 42).

supination   moving the arm so the palm is up (Ch. 33).

suppressed immune system   term used to describe an immune system unable to function normally due to the presence of a disease such as AIDS (Ch. 22, 38).

suppurative   producing or associated with the generation of pus (Ch. 27).

surgery cards   written reference for surgeries and procedures (Ch. 31).

surgical asepsis   procedures that render objects sterile; techniques to maintain sterile conditions during invasive procedures (Ch. 31).

surrogate   substitute; someone who substitutes for another (Ch. 8).

suture   surgical material or thread; may describe the act of sewing with the surgical thread and needle (Ch. 31).

swaged   a surgical needle attached to a length of suture material (Ch. 31).

symmetry   correspondence in shape, size, and position of body parts on opposites of the body (Ch. 25).

sympathetic nervous system   large part of the atuonomic nervous system that prepares the body for fight-or-flight (Ch. 5).

syncope   fainting (Ch. 9, 37).

systems software   software that provides instructions to the computer hardware; the operating system is the most common systems software (Ch. 11).

systole   one component of blood pressure measurement representing the highest amount of pressure exerted during the cardiac cycle; the force exerted on the arterial walls during cardiac contraction (Ch. 24, 37).

T cell   type of white blood cell that provides immunity (Ch. 22).

tachycardia   pulse rate greater than 100 beats per minute (Ch. 24).

tachycardia, sinus   abnormally rapid heartbeat greater than 100 beats/minute. A type of cardiac arrhythmia (Ch. 37).

tachypnea   abnormal increased rate of breathing (Ch. 24).

Tamm-Horsfall   mucoprotein secreted by the epithelial cells of the renal tubules (Ch. 42).

targeted resume   resume format utilized when focusing on a clear, specific job target (Ch. 48).

task force for test construction   committee of professionals whose responsibility is to update the CMA examination annually to reflect changes in medical assistants' responsibilities and to include new developments in medical knowledge and technology (Ch. 47).

taut   to pull or draw tight a surface, such as skin (Ch. 36).

taxonomy   classification of organisms into appropriate categories (Ch. 43).

Tay-Sachs   an inherited disease that is usually fatal (Ch. 26).

teamwork   persons synergistically working together (Ch. 45).

territoriality   represents the distance at which we feel comfortable while communicating with others (Ch. 4).

test cable   accessory device that attaches between the Holter monitor and the electrocardiograph to check for correct waveform and lack of artifact (Ch. 37).

tetrads   group of four similarly related entities (Ch. 43).

thalassemia   a hereditary anemia that may be fatal (Ch. 26).

therapeutic communication   use of specific and well-defined professional communication skills to create a feeling of comfort for patients even when difficult or unpleasant information must be exchanged (Ch. 4).

thermolabile   easily affected by heat (Ch. 22).

thermotherapy   use of heat to treat a physical condition (Ch. 33).

thiamin   vitamin B_1 (Ch. 34).

thixotropic separator gel   gel material capable of forming an interface between the cells and fluid portion of the blood as a result of centrifugation (Ch. 40).

thoracentesis   surgical puncture of the thoracic cavity to aspirate fluid (Ch. 22).

thrombocyte   (platelet) cellular fragment of megataryocyte; plays an important role in blood coagulation, hemostasis, and clot formation (Ch. 40, 41).

tickler file   system to remind of action to be taken on a certain date (Ch. 14).

tine test   skin test for tuberculosis (Ch. 44).

tinnitus   ringing or buzzing sound in the ear (Ch. 25).

titer   measurement of amount of antibody present against a particular antigen (Ch. 26).

tocopherol   vitamin E (Ch. 34).

tort   wrongful act that results in injury to one person by another (Ch. 7).

touch   physically making contact with others (Ch. 4).

tourniquet   device used to facilitate vein prominence (Ch. 40).

trace mineral   mineral required by the body in small amounts (Ch. 34).

tracing   graphic record usually of an event that changes with time as with the electrical activity of the heart (Ch. 37).

transcriber   device that makes it possible to transform voice recordings into a transcript or printed documents (Ch. 16).

transducer   device that converts one form of energy to another. During an ultrasound procedure, the transducer picks up echoes and converts them to electrical energy. The energy is transformed into a picture on a television monitor or printed on paper. Photographs of the image can be taken (Ch. 32, 37).

transient ischemic attack   temporary interference with blood flow to brain; may last only a few moments or several hours; neurological symptoms occur (Ch. 29).

transilluminator   instrument used to inspect a cavity or organ by passing a light through the walls (Ch. 28).

transmission   spread of infectious disease by direct contact, indirect contact, inhalation, ingestion, or bloodborne contact (Ch. 22).

transmission-based precautions   second tier of Centers for Disease Control and Prevention (CDC) guidelines that applies to specific categories of patients and that include air, contact, and droplet precautions. Transmission-based precautions are always used in addition to standard precautions (Ch. 22).

transurethral resection   removal of prostate tissue using a device inserted through the urethra (Ch. 28).

traveler's check   often used in place of cash when traveling; available in denominations of $10 to $100; requires a signature at place of purchase as well as signature at the time the check is used (Ch. 17).

triage   process to determine and prioritize patients' needs and the likely benefit from immediate medical attention. From the French *trier*, meaning "to sort" (Ch. 2, 9, 12, 13).

trichomoniasis   infestation with a Trichomonas parasite which may be transmitted through sexual intercourse (Ch. 22).

triglycerides   form of fat in the bloodstream that functions to store energy (Ch. 44).

trimester   three months; one-third of the gestational period of pregnancy (Ch. 26).

Truth-in-Lending Act   also known as the Consumer Credit Protection Act of 1968; an act requiring providers of installment credit to state the charges in writing and to express the interest as an annual rate (Ch. 20).

tuberculosis   infectious disease caused by the bacterium, *Mycobacterium tuberculosis* (Ch. 44).

turbid   opaque, lacking clarity (Ch. 42).

tympanostomy   placement of a tube through the tympanic membrane to allow ventilation of the middle ear; part of the treatment for otitis media (Ch. 27).

typhus (typhoid)   acute infectious disease that causes severe headache, rash, high fever, and progressive neurologic involvement. Prevalent where conditions are unsanitary and congested (Ch. 3).

ultrasonography   process of placing a handheld transducer against a body area to be tested. The transducer sends sound waves through the skin and the various internal organs. When echoes are formed and sent back the transducer converts them into electrical energy. This energy is transformed into a picture for a monitor, or printed on paper. Photographs of the images can be taken and become part of the patient's permanent record (Ch. 37).

ultrasound   use of high-frequency sound waves for therapeutic reasons to generate heat in deep tissue (Ch. 33).

Uniform Bill 92 (UB92)   unique billing form used extensively by acute care facilities for processing inpatient and outpatient claims (Ch. 19).

uniform resource locator (URL)   Web address that identifies and displays a particular Web page (Ch. 15).

unipolar   having or pertaining to one pole process (Ch. 37).

unit   each part of a name (business or person), words, or numbers that will be indexed and coded for filing (Ch. 14).

unit dose   premeasured amount of medication, individually packaged on a per-dose basis (Ch. 36).

universal emergency medical identification symbol   identification sometimes carried by individuals to identify health problems they may have (Ch. 9).

universal precautions   guidelines established by the Centers for Disease Control and Prevention (CDC) for the protection of health care workers from infectious diseases (Ch. 22).

urea   principal end product of protein metabolism (Ch. 42).

uremia   toxic condition of the blood caused by the kidneys' inability to filter waste products from the blood (Ch. 30).

urgency   the need to urinate immediately (Ch. 30).

urinalysis   examination of the physical, chemical, and microscopic properties of urine (Ch. 39, 42).

urinometer   device to measure specific gravity; consists of a float with a calibrated stem (Ch. 42).

urobilinogen   colorless compound produced in the intestine after the breakdown by bacteria of bilirubin (Ch. 42).

urochrome   yellow pigment that gives color to urine (Ch. 42).

urticaria   hives (Ch. 35).

usual, customary, and reasonable (UCR)   fee schedule often used by Medicare and some insurance carriers. *Usual* refers to the fee typically charged by a physician for certain procedures; *customary* is based on the average charge for a specific procedure by all physicians practicing the same specialty in a defined geographic region; and *reasonable* refers to the midrange of fees charged for this procedure (Ch. 17, 18).

utilization review organization   responsible for authorization of treatment, payment of claims, and performance of retrospective utilization review for an insurance plan (Ch. 18).

utilization review (UR)   review of medical services before they can be performed (Ch. 21).

V codes   ICD-9-CM codes representing either factors that influence a person's health status or legitimate reasons for contacting the health facility when the patient has no definitive diagnosis or active symptom of any disorder (Ch. 19).

vaccine pharmacologic agent capable of producing artificial active immunity (Ch. 22).

Vacutainer® brand of vacuum tube used in phlebotomy to obtain a venous blood sample for analysis (Ch. 22).

variable cost cost that varies in direct proportion to volume (Ch. 21).

vasoconstriction narrowing or constricting of blood vessels (Ch. 33).

vasodilation widening or dilating of blood vessels (Ch. 33).

vector a carrier of disease, usually an insect, that is the causative organism of disease from infected to noninfected individuals (Ch. 22).

venipuncture opening a vein to obtain a blood sample (Ch. 40).

vertigo the sensation of moving around in space; dizziness, light-headedness (Ch. 25).

vesicle blister or elevation on the skin (Ch. 30).

viable able to live, grow, and develop after birth; usually 24 weeks or greater than one pound (Ch. 26).

virology study of viruses (Ch. 43).

virulence an organism's relative power and degree of pathogenicity (Ch. 22).

viscosity degree of thickness of a liquid (Ch. 40).

vitiligo skin disorder characterized by smooth white spots on various areas of the body (Ch. 25).

volatile easily evaporated (Ch. 31).

voucher check check with detachable form used to detail reason check is drawn; commonly used in payroll checks (Ch. 17).

waiting period length of time defined in the insurance policy before the policy will begin to pay benefits for a pre-existing condition (Ch. 18).

waived (tests) used to describe a category of clinical laboratory tests that are simple, unvarying, and require a minimum of judgment and interpretation (Ch. 38).

watermark design incorporated in paper during the papermaking process that is visible when the paper is held up to the light (Ch. 15).

water-soluble pertaining to substances that are hydrophilic and therefore dissolve better in water (Ch. 34).

wave scheduling system where patients are scheduled for the first half hour of every hour and then seen throughout the hour (Ch. 13).

Web site a remote computer that stores World Wide Web documents consisting of Web pages (Ch. 45).

wheal slight elevation of skin that can be produced as a result of an intradermal injection (Ch. 36, 44).

wheezes high-pitched musical sound heard on expiration, often the result of an obstruction or narrowing of respiratory passages (Ch. 24).

widow in typesetting, a term describing the situation in which a line of text that is the end of a paragraph ends on a new page or column of printed text (Ch. 11).

Wood's lamp light source used to fluoresce certain fungal cultures; used to aid in the identification of dermatophytes (Ch. 43).

word processing software computer application that allows the user to format and edit documents before printing (Ch. 11).

work history outline of previous employment positions, employers, positions, duties, and responsibilities. Listed with the most recent position first (Ch. 46).

work practice controls measures used in the workplace that consist of physical equipment and mechanical devices to control employee exposure to bloodborne pathogens and other potentially infectious materials. Examples are sharps disposal containers, handwashing facilities, PPE, eyewash stations, and so on (Ch. 22).

work statement concise description of the work you plan to accomplish (Ch. 45).

World Wide Web (WWW) commonly known as the Web; composed of computers called servers that contain Web pages that may include text, pictures, sound, video, and links to other Web pages (Ch. 15).

wound a break in the continuity of soft parts of body structures caused by violence or trauma to tissues. In an open wound, skin is broken as in a laceration, abrasion, avulsion, or incision. In a closed wound, skin is not broken as in contusion, ecchymosis, or hematoma (Ch. 9).

wrist rest device used with flat keyboard to support the wrists (Ch. 16).

write-it-once system another name used to refer to the pegboard system (Ch. 17).

yellow fever acute infectious disease where a person develops jaundice, vomits, hemorrhages, and has a fever; caused mostly by mosquitoes (Ch. 3).

ZIP+4 standard Zip code including four additional digits that identify a postal delivery area. Mail will be processed more efficiently and effectively with the use of the ZIP+4 code in the address (Ch. 16).

Zip® disk portable read-write data storage device. It is storable and transferable between computers. Capacity is approximately 250 megabytes of data. Data is stored permanently until overwritten. Zip drive unit is required to read-write data from disk (Ch. 11).

COMMON MEDICAL ABBREVIATIONS AND SYMBOLS

a̅a̅	of each
AAMA	American Association of Medical Assistants
AAMT	American Association of Medical Transcription
ab	abortion
abd	abdomen
ABE	acute bacterial endocarditis
ABG	arterial blood gases
ABHS	Accrediting Bureau of Health Education Schools
ABO	blood groups
abs	absent
ac	before meals (ante cibum)
ac	acute
ACTH	adrenocorticotropic hormone
AD	right ear (auris dexter)
ADA	Americans with Disabilities Act
ADL	activities of daily living
ad lib	as desired
adm	admission
AFP	alpha fetal protein
AHD	arteriosclerotic heart disease
	atherosclerotic heart disease
AIDS	acquired immunodeficiency syndrome
AL	left ear (auris laevus)
alb	albumin
AM	before noon (ante meridiem)
AMA	against medical advice
	American Medical Association
AMI	acute myocardial infarction
amt	amount
ant	anterior
ante	before
A&P	anterior and posterior
	auscultation and palpation
	auscultation and percussion

aq	water
A/R	accounts receivable
ARU	automated routing unit
AS	left ear (auris sinistra)
ASA	acetylsalicylic acid
ASAP	as soon as possible
ASCAD	arteriosclerotic coronary artery disease
ASCVD	arteriosclerotic cardiovascular disease
	atherosclerotic cardiovascular disease
AU	each ear (aures unitas)
A&W	alive and well
Ba	barium
BaE	barium enema
BBB	bundle branch block
BC	birth control
BC/BS	Blue Cross/Blue Shield
BE	bacterial endocarditis
	barium enema
bid	twice a day
bil	bilateral
BM	basal metabolism
	bowel movement
BMR	basal metabolism rate
BP	blood pressure
BPH	benign prostatic hypertrophy
BS	blood sugar
	bowel sounds
	breath sounds
BSA	body surface area
BSI	body substance isolation
BSL	blood sugar level
BSN	bowel sounds normal
BSO	bilateral salpingo-oophorectomy
BSR	blood sedimentation rate
BUN	blood urea nitrogen

BW	below waist
	birth weight
	body weight
Bx	biopsy
C	Celsius
	centigrade
c̄	with
C1	first cervical vertebra
CA	cancer
	carcinoma
Ca	calcium
CAAHEP	Commission on Accreditation of Allied Health Education Programs
CAD	coronary artery disease
CAHD	coronary arteriosclerotic heart disease
caps	capsules
CAT	computerized axial tomography
CBC	complete blood count
CC	chief complaint
cc	cubic centimeter
CCU	coronary care unit
C&D	cystoscopy and dilation
CDC	U.S. Centers for Disease Control and Prevention
CE	continuing education
cerv	cervical
	cervix
CEU	continuing education unit
CHAMPUS	Civilian Health and Medical Program of the Uniformed Services
CHAMPVA	Civilian Health and Medical Program of the Veterans Administration
CHD	childhood disease
	congenital heart disease

CHD	congestive heart disease	DOB	date of birth	fl	fluid
	coronary heart disease	DOD	date of death	fl dr	fluid dram
CHF	congestive heart failure	DOE	dyspnea on exertion	fl oz	fluid ounce
CHO	carbohydrate	dos	dosage	FMP	first menstrual period
CIN	cervical intraepithelial	DPM	doctor of podiatric medicine	FP	family practice
	neoplasia	DPT	diphtheria, pertussis, and	freq	frequent
ck	check		tetanus	FSH	follicle-stimulating hormone
Cl	chlorine	DR	delivery room	ft	foot
cldy	cloudy	Dr	doctor	FTP	file transfer protocol
CLIA	Clinical Laboratory	dr	dram	fx	fracture
	Improvement	DRGs	diagnosis-related groups		
	Amendments	DSD	dry sterile dressing	G	gravida
cm	centimeter	dsg	dressing	g	gram
CMA	certified medical assistant	DT	delirium tremens	GB	gallbladder
CME	continuing medical education	DTR	deep tendon reflex	GC	gonococcus
CNS	central nervous system	D&V	diarrhea and vomiting		gonorrhea
C/O	complains of	DW	distilled water	GI	gastrointestinal
CO_2	carbon dioxide	D/W	dextrose in water	gm	gram
COB	coordination of benefits	dx	diagnosis	GP	general practice
COPD	chronic obstructive			gr	grain
	pulmonary disease	ea	each	grav	pregnancy
CPR	cardiopulmonary resuscitation	EBV	Epstein-Barr virus	GTH	gonadotropic hormone
CPT	Current Procedural Code	ECG	electrocardiogram	GTT	glucose tolerance test
CPU	central processing unit·	Echo	echocardiogram	gtt(s)	drop (drops)
crit	hematocrit		echoencephalogram	GU	genitourinary
CS	cerebrospinal	E. coli	*Escherichia coli*	GYN	gynecology
CS	cesarean section	ECT	electroconvulsive therapy		
C&S	culture and sensitivity	EDC	estimated date of confinement	h	hour
CSF	cerebrospinal fluid		or expected date of	HBP	high blood pressure
CSR	continuous speech		confinement	HCFA	U.S. Health Care Financing
	recognition	EDD	estimated date of delivery or		Administration
CT	computerized tomography		expected date of delivery	hCG	human chorionic
CVA	cerebrovascular accident	EEG	electroencephalogram		gonadotropin
CVP	central venous pressure	EENT	eyes, ears, nose, and throat	HCL	hydrochloric acid
CVS	chorionic villus sampling	eg	for example	HCPCS	HCFA Common Procedure
cx	cervix	EKG	electrocardiogram		Coding System
CXR	chest x-ray	elix	elixir	Hct	hematocrit
cysto	cystoscopic examination	EMG	electromyography	HCVD	hypertensive cardiovascular
	cystoscopy	EMS	emergency medical service		disease
		ENT	ear, nose, and throat	HEENT	head, eyes, ears, nose, and
DACUM	developing a curriculum	EOB	explanation of benefits		throat
DC	doctor of chiropracty	eos	eosinophil	Hgb	hemoglobin
D&C	dilation and curettage	EPO	exclusive provider	H&H	hemoglobin and hematocrit
DDS	doctor of dentistry		organization	HHS	U.S. Department of Health
DEA	U.S. Drug Enforcement	eq	equivalent		and Human Services
	Agency	ER	emergency room	HMO	health maintenance
dec	decrease	ERT	estrogen replacement therapy		organization
del	delivery	ESR	erythrocyte sedimentation rate	H/O	history of
diab	diabetic	EST	electroshock therapy	H_2O	water
diag	diagnosis	exam	examination	H&P	history and physical
diff	differential white blood cell	ext	extract	HPI	history of present illness
	count			HPV	human papilloma virus
dil	dilute	F	Fahrenheit	HR	human resource
disc	discontinue		female	hs	at bedtime
disp	dispense	fax	facsimile		hour of sleep
DM	diabetes mellitus	FBS	fasting blood sugar	ht	height
DNA	deoxyribonucleic acid	FDA	U.S. Food and Drug	hx	history
	does not apply		Administration	Hz	hertz
DNR	do not resuscitate	FH	family history		
DO	doctor of osteopathy	FHR	fetal heart rate	ICCU	intensive coronary care unit
DOA	dead on arrival	FHS	fetal heart sound	ICD	International Classification of
					Diseases, Adapted

ICD-9-CM	International Classification of Diseases, 9th revision, Clinical Modification
ICU	intensive care unit
ID	intradermal
I&D	incision and drainage
IM	internal medicine
	intramuscular
imp	impression
inf	infusion
inj	injection
I&O	intake and output
IPPB	intermittent positive pressure breathing
IUD	intrauterine device
IV	intravenous
IVP	intravenous pyelogram
JAAMT	*Journal of the American Association for Medical Transcription*
JAMA	*Journal of the American Medical Association*
JCAHO	Joint Commission on Accreditation of Healthcare Organizations
jt	joint
K	potassium
kg	kilogram
KOH	potassium hydroxide
KUB	kidney, ureter, and bladder
KV	kilovolt
L	liter
	left
l	length
LA	left atrium
	lactic acid
L&A	light and accommodation
lab	laboratory
lac	laceration
lap	laparotomy
lat	lateral
lb	pound
LBBB	left bundle branch block
LDL	low-density lipoprotein
LE	lupus erythematosus
liq	liquid
LLQ	lower left quadrant
LMP	last menstrual period
LP	lumbar puncture
LRQ	lower right quadrant
LUQ	left upper quadrant
L&W	living and well
lymphs	lymphocytes
M	male
m	meter
$\mathfrak{z}$	minim
MBCD	management by coaching and development

MBCE	management by competitive edge
MBDM	management by decision models
MBP	management by performance
MBS	management by styles
MBWA	management by wandering around
MBWS	management by work simplification
MCHC	mean corpuscular hemoglobin and red cell indices
MCO	managed care organization
MCV	mean corpuscular volume and red cell indices
MD	muscular dystrophy
	doctor of medicine
MDR	minimum daily requirement
med	medicine
mEq/L	milliequivalents per liter
mg	miligram
MH	marital history
	medical history
	menstrual history
MHx	medical history
MI	maturation index
	myocardial infarction
ml	milliliter
mm	millimeter
mm³	cubic millimeter
mmHg	millimeters of mercury
MMR	measles, mumps, and rubella
MOM	milk of magnesia
mono	mononucleosis
MP	menstrual period
MRI	magnetic resonance imaging
MS	mitral stenosis
	morphine sulfate
	multiple sclerosis
MT	medical technologist
	medical transcriptionist
MTCP	Medical Transcriptionist Certification Program
multip	multipara
MVP	mitral valve prolapse
NA	not applicable
NaCl	sodium chloride
narc	narcotic
NB	newborn
NBME	National Board of Medical Examiners
N/C	no complaints
ND	doctor of naturopathy
NEC	not elsewhere classified
neg	negative
NG	nasogastric
NGU	nongonococcal urethritis
NL	normal limits
NMP	normal menstrual period

noct	at night
non rep	do not repeat
NOS	not otherwise specified
NPO	nothing by mouth
NR	nonreactive
	no refill
	normal range
NS	nonspecific
	normal saline
	not significant
	not sufficient
N&T	nose and throat
N&V	nausea and vomiting
NVD	nausea, vomiting, and diarrhea
O	oral
	oxygen
	pint
O₂	oxygen
OB	obstetrics
OB-GYN	obstetrics-gynecology
OC	office call
	on call
	oral contraceptive
occ	occasionally
OD	drug overdose
	right eye (oculus dexter)
	doctor of optometry
OGTT	oral glucose tolerance test
OM	office manager
OOB	out of bed
OP	outpatient
O&P	ova and parasites
OPIM	other potentially infected material
OPV	oral poliovaccine
OR	operating room
ortho	orthopedics
OS	left eye (oculus sinister)
os	mouth
OSHA	U.S. Occupational Safety and Health Administration
OT	occupational therapist
	occupational therapy
OTC	over the counter
OU	both eyes (oculus unitas)
OURQ	outer upper right quadrant
OV	office visit
oz	ounce
P	phosphorus
	pulse
PA	posteroanterior
P&A	percussion and auscultation
PA	physician's assistant
PAC	phenacetin, aspirin, and codeine
	premature atrial contraction
Pap	Papanicolaou (smear, test)
para	number of pregnancies

para I	primipara	**pro-time**	prothrombin time	**sed rate**	sedimentation rate
PAT	paroxysmal atrial tachycardia	**PSA**	prostate-specific antigen	**segs**	segmented neutrophils
path	pathology	**PSRO**	Professional Standards Review Organization	**seq**	sequela
PBI	protein-bound iodine			**SF**	scarlet fever
pc	after meals	**PT**	physical therapy		spinal fluid
PCC	Poison Control Center		prothrombin time	**SG**	specific gravity
PCN	penicillin	**pt**	patient	**SH**	social history
PCP	primary care physician	**PTA**	prior to admission	**SIDS**	sudden infant death syndrome
PCV	packed cell volume	**pulv**	powder	**sig**	instructions, directions
PDR	*Physician's Desk Reference*	**PVC**	premature ventricular concentration	**sigmoid**	sigmoidoscopy
PE	physical examination			**SMA 12/60**	Sequential Multiple Analyzer (12-test serum profile)
peds	pediatrics	**px**	physical examination		
PEG	pneumoencephalography		prognosis		
PERRLA	pupils equal, round, regular, react to light, and accommodation	**q**	each; every	**SOAP**	subjective data, objective data, assessment, and plan
		q AM	every morning	**SOB**	shortness of breath
PET	positron emission transmission or tomography	**QA**	quality assurance	**sol**	solution
		qd	every day	**solv**	solvent
PH	past history	**qh**	every hour	**SOP**	standard operating procedure
	personal history	**q (2, 3, 4)h**	every 2, 3, or 4 hours	**SOS**	if necessary
	public health	**qid**	four times a day	**spec**	specimen
pH	hydrogen in concentration	**qn**	every night	**sp gr**	secific gravity
PHO	physician-hospital organization	**qns**	quantity not sufficient	**spont ab**	spontaneous abortion
		qod	every other day	**SR**	sedimentation rate
PI	present illness	**qs**	of sufficient quantity	**SS**	signs and symptoms
	pulmonary infarction	**qt**	quart	**s̄s̄**	one-half
PID	pelvic inflammatory disease	**R**	registration	**Staph**	Staphylococcus
PKU	phenylketonuria		right	**stat**	immediately
PM	after noon (post meridiem)	**RBC**	red blood cell	**STD**	sexually transmitted disease
	post mortem (after death)	**RBC/hpf**	red blood cells per high power field	**Strep**	Streptococcus
PMN	polymorphonuclear neutrophils			**subcut**	subcutaneous
		RBCM	red blood cell mass	**supp**	suppository
PMP	past menstrual period	**RBCV**	red blood cell volume	**surg**	surgery
PMS	premenstrual syndrome	**RBRVS**	Resource-Based Relation Value Scale	**sx**	signs
PNC	penicillin				symptoms
PO	postoperative	**REM**	rapid eye movement	**sym**	symptoms
po	by mouth	**resp**	respiration	**syr**	syrup
POB	place of birth	**Rh**	rhesus (factor)		
POMR	problem-oriented medical record	**Rh-**	rhesus negative	**T**	temperature
		Rh+	rhesus positive	**T₃**	tri-iodothyronine
POS	point-of-service plan	**RHD**	rheumatic heart disease	**T₄**	thyroxine
pos	positive	**RLQ**	right lower quadrant	**T&A**	tonsillectomy and adenoidectomy
poss	possible	**RMA**	registered medical assistant		
postop	postoperative	**RNA**	ribonucleic acid	**tab**	tablet
PP	postprandial	**R/O**	rule out	**TB**	tuberculin
PPB	positive pressure breathing	**ROA**	received on account	**tbs**	tablespoon
PPBS	postprandial blood sugar	**ROM**	range of motion		tuberculosis
PPD	purified protein derivative		read-only memory	**TC**	throat culture
PPO	preferred provider organization	**ROS**	review of systems		tissue culture
		RT	radiation therapy		total capacity
PPT	partial prothrombin time	**RUQ**	right upper quadrant		total cholesterol
preop	preoperative	**Rx**	prescription	**ther**	therapy
PRERLA	pupils round, equal, react to light and accommodation	**S**	subjective data (POMR)	**therap**	therapeutic
		s̄	without	**TIA**	transient ischemic attack
primip	woman bearing first child	**SA**	sinoatrial	**tid**	three times a day
prn	as the occasion arises, as necessary	**S&A**	sugar and acetone (urine)	**tinct**	tincture
		SBE	shortness of breath on exertion	**TLC**	tender loving care
procto	proctoscopy		subacute bacterial endocarditis	**TMJ**	temporomandibular joint
prog	prognosis	**SC**	subcutaneous	**top**	topically
PROM	premature rupture of membranes	**SE**	standard error	**TOPV**	trivalent oral poliovirus vaccine

TP	total protein	**URI**	upper respiratory infection	**WBC**	white blood cell
TPR	temperature, pulse, and respiration	**urol**	urology	**WC**	white cell
		URQ	upper right quadrant	**WDWN**	well developed, well nourished
tr	tincture	**URT**	upper respiratory tract		
trig	triglycerides	**URTI**	upper respiratory tract infection	**WHO**	World Health Organization
TSH	thyroid stimulating hormone			**WN**	well nourished
tsp	teaspoon	**USP**	United States Pharmacopoeia	**WNF**	well-nourished female
TUR	transurethral resection of the bladder	**UT**	urinary tract	**WNL**	within normal limits
		UTI	urinary tract infection	**WNM**	well-nourished male
tus	cough	**UV**	ultraviolet	**WO**	written order
T&X	type and crossmatch			**w/o**	without
		vac	vaccine	**wt**	weight
U	unit	**vag**	vagina		
UA	urinalysis		vaginal	**x**	multiply by
UB-92	Uniform Bill-92	**VD**	venereal disease	**XR**	x-ray
UCG	urinary chorionic gonadotropin	**VDRL**	Venereal Disease Research Library		
UCHD	usual childhood diseases			**YOB**	year of birth
ULQ	upper left quadrant	**vit**	vitamin	**yr**	year
ung	ointment	**vit cap**	vital capacity		
URC	usual, reasonable, customary	**vol**	volume		
urg	urgent	**VS**	vital signs		

Symbols

*	birth
†	death
♂	male
♀	female
+	positive
−	negative
±	positive or negative, indefinite
÷	divide by
=	equal to
>	greater than
<	less than
×	multiply by
#	number, pound
′	foot, minute
″	inch, second
℔	minum
ʒ	dram
℥	ounce
μ	micron
○	pint
@	at

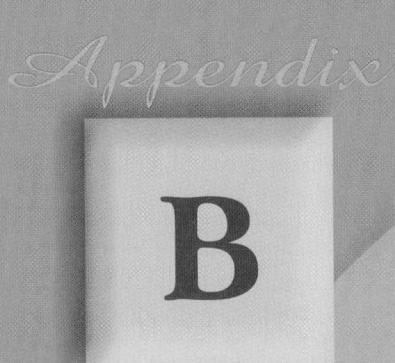

Top 200 Brand-Name Drugs by Retail Sales in 2000

Rank	Product	Total retail dollars (000)	Rank	Product	Total retail dollars (000)	Rank	Product	Total retail dollars (000)
1	Prilosec	$4,102,195	36	Synthroid	$649,256	71	Relafen	$351,595
2	Lipitor	3,692,657	37	Flovent	647,980	72	Serzone	349,127
3	Prevacid	2,832,602	38	Accutane	636,246	73	Cardura	344,406
4	Prozac	2,567,107	39	Flonase	618,714	74	Xalatan	340,492
5	Zocor	2,207,042	40	Avandia	617,629	75	Glucotrol XL	321,631
6	Celebrex	2,015,508	41	Ortho Tri-Cyclen	616,997	76	Detrol	319,193
7	Zoloft	1,890,416	42	Ultram	601,465	77	Seroquel	318,844
8	Paxil	1,807,955	43	Plavix	599,512	78	Humulin N	317,017
9	Claritin	1,667,347	44	Biaxin	588,366	79	Lotensin	316,922
10	Glucophage	1,629,157	45	Vasotec	584,418	80	Viracept	315,510
11	Norvasc	1,597,091	46	Pepcid	568,684	81	Avonex	313,114
12	Augmentin	1,584,397	47	Actos	550,674	82	Valtrex	311,102
13	Vioxx	1,517,993	48	Accupril	500,796	83	Allegra-D	310,369
14	Zyprexa	1,418,411	49	Enbrel	500,363	84	Adderall	307,423
15	Pravachol	1,203,474	50	Claritin D 24HR	493,420	85	Procrit	298,764
16	Premarin Tabs	1,146,808	51	Lamisil Oral	487,920	86	Claritin RediTabs	298,253
17	Neurontin	1,131,678	52	Ceftin	455,965	87	Cardizem CD	283,968
18	Oxycontin	1,052,771	53	Combivir	452,844	88	K-Dur 20	276,161
19	Cipro	1,023,657	54	Serevent	448,923	89	Diovan	270,144
20	Zithromax Z-Pak	961,579	55	BuSpar Dividose	434,023	90	Remeron	266,707
21	Risperdal	959,707	56	Prinivil	431,342	91	BuSpar	265,349
22	Wellbutrin SR	850,934	57	Coumadin Tabs	407,565	92	Zerit	264,738
23	Zestril	833,359	58	Claritin D 12HR	403,071	93	Hyzaar	264,128
24	Effexor XR	815,816	59	Evista	398,590	94	Ziac	258,299
25	Allegra	810,001	60	Cozaar	395,292	95	Zithromax Susp	252,501
26	Viagra	809,377	61	Nasonex	391,973	96	Miacalcin Nasal	245,241
27	Ambien	798,858	62	Diflucan	386,846	97	Sporanox	244,434
28	Depakote	758,329	63	Aricept	384,059	98	Lotrisone	243,440
29	Levaquin	753,711	64	Procardia XL	383,822	99	Lescol	238,343
30	Imitrex	747,631	65	Cefzil	382,250	100	Xenical	237,004
31	Zyrtec	739,543	66	Adalat CC	376,992	101	Betaseron	236,503
32	Celexa	737,487	67	Aciphex	372,138	102	Asacol	235,117
33	Prempro	711,798	68	Lotrel	353,784	103	Monopril	233,969
34	Fosamax	704,289	69	Toprol XL	353,725	104	Humulin 70/30	229,600
35	Singulair	676,515	70	Duragesic	352,934	105	Combivent	229,550

Rank	Product	Total retail dollars (000)	Rank	Product	Total retail dollars (000)	Rank	Product	Total retail dollars (000)
106	Flomax	$226,845	138	Plendil	$169,716	170	MS Contin	$125,606
107	Zofran	225,673	139	Proscar	166,868	171	Effexor	125,468
108	Axid	225,365	140	Levoxyl	164,919	172	Pulmicort Turbuhaler	122,785
109	Lamictal	221,847	141	Bactroban	163,939	173	Proventil HFA	121,417
110	Baycol	221,383	142	Daypro	163,783	174	Serostim	121,096
111	Topamax	219,865	143	Lanoxin	163,625	175	Clozaril	119,152
112	Mevacor	216,661	144	Alphagan	159,631	176	Gonal-F	119,096
113	Neoral	214,475	145	Diovan HCT	159,351	177	Arava	118,902
114	Neupogen	212,997	146	Amaryl	158,976	178	Lupron Depot	117,045
115	Famvir	205,223	147	Tricor	158,741	179	Vicoprofen Non-Inj	115,382
116	Epivir	205,172	148	Ortho-Cyclen	157,366	180	Covera-HS	115,239
117	Ortho-Novum 7/7/7	203,989	149	Humalog	157,153	181	Loestrin Fe 1/20	113,408
118	Azmacort	203,389	150	Arthrotec	152,530	182	Elocon	113,324
119	Luvox	199,293	151	Patanol	152,199	183	Skelaxin	113,307
120	Coreg	199,166	152	Vancenase AQ DS	150,883	184	Meridia	113,231
121	Zestoretic	198,956	153	Accolat	150,536	185	Nasacort AQ	112,518
122	Tiazac	198,727	154	Cellcept	150,193	186	Dovonex	110,975
123	Avapro	197,428	155	Copaxone	148,844	187	Catapres-TTS	109,703
124	Benzamycin	196,795	156	Zithromax	146,759	188	Zyrtec Syrup	109,389
125	Triphasil	196,589	157	Hytrin	145,267	189	Propulsid	107,279
126	Zomig	190,231	158	Casodex	143,906	190	Tequin	107,197
127	Rebetron 1200 Pen	189,843	159	Xanax	141,572	191	Rezulin	106,720
128	Imitrex Statdose	184,548	160	Tobradex	137,765	192	Rebetron 1000 Pen	106,624
129	Sustiva	183,008	161	Prograf	137,743	193	Stadol NS	105,637
130	Amoxil	176,847	162	Crixivan	137,645	194	Prevpac	105,011
131	Lovenox	175,402	163	Lo/Ovral 28	137,138	195	Loestrin Fe 1.5/30	103,323
132	Ditropan XL	174,058	164	Differin	136,023	196	Phenergan Supp	102,421
133	Atrovent Inh	174,018	165	DDAVP	133,016	197	Viramune	102,348
134	Zantac	172,662	166	Macrobid	131,419	198	Cosopt	102,212
135	Altace	172,308	167	Betapace	130,263	199	Estratest Tabs	101,697
136	Alesse-28	171,698	168	Ziagen	127,284	200	Prandin	100,310
137	Dilantin Kapseals	171,374	169	Zyban	126,122			

Top 200 Generic Drugs by Retail Sales in 2000

Rank	Product	Total retail dollars (000)	Rank	Product	Total retail dollars (000)	Rank	Product	Total retail dollars (000)
1	Hydrocodone/APAP	$935,093	16	Naproxen	$287,162	31	Methylphenidate	$172,863
2	Ranitidine HCl	690,854	17	Isosorbide Mononitrt	286,576	32	Amitriptyline	168,586
3	Atenolol	532,836	18	Carisoprodol	286,430	33	Trimethoprim/Sulfa	168,446
4	Lorazepam	530,084	19	Terazosin	286,378	34	Nifedipine ER	157,299
5	Albuterol Aerosol	501,115	20	Minocycline	278,055	35	Cimetidine	156,799
6	Alprazolam	489,753	21	Amoxicillin	252,789	36	Ipratropium Bromide	154,735
7	Propoxyphene-N/APAP	457,763	22	Ibuprofen	248,035	37	Hydrochlorothiazide	148,603
8	Cephalexin	399,055	23	Metoprolol Tartrate	230,657	38	Gemfibrozil	148,226
9	Tamoxifen	393,067	24	Furosemide Oral	227,718	39	Prednisone Oral	141,904
10	Clonazepam	351,304	25	Acetaminophen w/Cod	216,379	40	Methotrexate	132,550
11	Glyburide	333,348	26	Trimox	214,918	41	Captopril	129,457
12	Cartia XT	331,837	27	Acyclovir Systemic	209,307	42	Diclofenac Sodium	123,457
13	Albuterol Neb Soln	325,017	28	Cyclobenzaprine	192,847	43	Potassium Chloride	121,779
14	Verapamil SR	301,604	29	Warfarin	178,317	44	Clorazepate Dipot	117,470
15	Triamterene w/HCTZ	292,778	30	Trazodone HCl	173,623	45	Medrxyprgsterone Tab	113,414

Rank	Product	Total retail dollars (000)
46	Spironolactone	$113,240
47	Clindamycin Systemic	111,649
48	Doxycycline	110,567
49	Diltiazem CD	109,812
50	Estradiol Oral	109,688
51	Amiodarone	108,066
52	Enalapril	107,435
53	Hydroxychloroquine	105,895
54	Methylprednis Tabs	101,298
55	Diazepam	100,210
56	Cefaclor	99,915
57	Propranolol LA	98,875
58	Nitroglycerin	97,650
59	Clonidine	95,919
60	Pentoxifylline	95,402
61	Glipizide	93,619
62	Temazepam	93,513
63	Nortriptyline	91,972
64	Etodolac	90,898
65	Allopurinol	89,571
66	Diltiazem SR	89,489
67	Glyburide Micronized	79,195
68	Cefadroxil	76,442
69	Clobetasol	76,034
70	Morphine Sul Non Inj	74,084
71	Carbidopa/Levodopa	73,230
72	Orphenadrine Citrate	70,339
73	Naproxen Sodium	70,150
74	Nadolol	69,757
75	Oxycodone w/APAP	69,492
76	Benzonatate	68,749
77	Phentermine	68,626
78	Carbamazepine	67,842
79	Methylphenidate SR	67,025
80	Labetalol	66,498
81	Butalbital/APAP/Caf	65,896
82	Azathioprine	64,242
83	Prochlorperaz Mal	63,598
84	Propranolol HCl	62,698
85	Imipramine HCl	61,106
86	Methocarbamol	59,187
87	Metronidazole Tabs	58,338
88	Hyoscyamine	58,107
89	Neomycin/Polymx/HC	57,961
90	Metoclopramide	55,692
91	Doxepin	53,206
92	Cromolyn Sod Neb Sln	51,925
93	Tretinoin	51,616
94	Fluocinonide	51,573
95	Meclizine HCl	51,400
96	Piroxicam	51,077
97	Adipex-P	49,545

Rank	Product	Total retail dollars (000)
98	Dicyclomine HCl	$48,747
99	Indapamide	48,395
100	Prednisolone Oral	48,313
101	Octicair	47,988
102	Hydroxyzine	47,063
103	Bupropion	46,855
104	Nystatin Systemic	46,135
105	Triamcinln Acet Top	45,627
106	Baclofen	45,586
107	Ketoprofen	45,484
108	Sucralfate	45,451
109	Theophylline SR	44,118
110	Ticlopidine	43,870
111	Phenytoin Sodium Ext	43,299
112	Clozapine	43,091
113	Atenolol Chlorthal	43,068
114	Guaif/Phenylprop	43,027
115	Lithium Carbonate	42,933
116	Diphenoxylate w/Atro	42,844
117	Nitrofurantoin Mcroc	42,269
118	Penicillin VK	41,679
119	Oxybutynin Chloride	41,307
120	Butalbital Cmpd w/Cd	40,364
121	Hydrocortsn Valerate	39,458
122	Ery-Tab	39,313
123	Carbidopa/Levdpa ER	39,286
124	Diclofenac Potassium	38,006
125	Prednisolne Acet Oph	37,289
126	Promethazine/Codeine	37,253
127	Guanfacine HCl	36,569
128	Clomiphene Citrate	36,467
129	Timolol Maleate XE	36,124
130	Indomethacin	35,849
131	Timolol Maleate Oph	35,258
132	Sotalol	35,134
133	Desmopressin Acetate	34,621
134	Estropipate	34,373
135	Folic Acid	33,673
136	Sulindac	33,369
137	Bumetanide Non-Inj	33,250
138	Hydrocortison Top Rx	33,080
139	Polymyxin B/Trimeth	33,017
140	Albuterol Oral Liq	32,386
141	Oxazepam	32,333
142	Clindamycin Topical	31,721
143	Guaifenesin/Pseudoep	31,040
144	Phenazopyridine HCl	30,966
145	Ketoconazole Syst	30,812
146	Bisoprolol/HCTZ	29,235
147	Promethazine Tabs	29,058
148	Thioridazine HCl	28,833
149	Guaifenesin Rx	28,595

Rank	Product	Total retail dollars (000)
150	Doxazosin	$28,189
151	Diltia XT	27,569
152	Ketoconazole Topical	26,558
153	Levothyroxine	26,415
154	Dexamethasone Oral	26,304
155	Chlorhexidine Glucon	26,272
156	Desoximetasone	26,201
157	Bromocriptine	26,133
158	Enulose	26,002
159	Indomethacin SR	25,979
160	Haloperidol	25,865
161	Valproic Acid	25,856
162	Phenobarbital	25,548
163	Selegiline	25,384
164	Megestrol Tabs	24,555
165	Quinine Sulfate	24,441
166	Clotrimazole Top	24,320
167	Hydroxyurea	24,282
168	Naproxen EC	24,185
169	Lindane	24,164
170	Lonox	24,056
171	Nitroquick	24,030
172	Sulfasalazine	23,899
173	Cholestyramine	23,516
174	Digoxin	23,466
175	Triazolam	23,453
176	Acebutolol	23,093
177	Clomipramine HCl	22,853
178	Lactulose	22,593
179	Ibuprofen Liquid	21,880
180	Erythromycin Topical	21,769
181	Colchicine	21,372
182	Tobramycin Ophth	21,259
183	Hydroxyzine Pamoate	20,798
184	Ketorolac Oral	20,523
185	Isosorbide Dinitrate	20,205
186	Benztropine	20,203
187	Diclofenac Sodium SR	19,969
188	Diflorasone	19,534
189	Gentamicin Ophth	18,966
190	Diltiazem	18,792
191	Pentazocine/Naloxone	18,783
192	Naproxen Delayed Rel	18,730
193	Dipyridamole	18,696
194	Tetracycline	18,627
195	Probenecid	18,305
196	Methyldopa	18,283
197	Benzoyl Peroxd Acne	18,182
198	Nystatin/Triamcinoln	17,761
199	Erythromycin Ethylsc	17,383
200	Methadone HCl Non-In	17,188

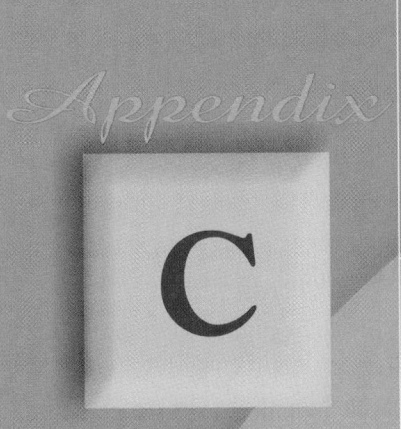

MEDICAL ASSISTANT ROLE DELINEATION CHART

Reprinted with permission of the American Association of Medical Assistants.

*Asterisk denotes advanced skill

ADMINISTRATIVE

Administrative Procedures

- Perform basic clerical functions
- Schedule, coordinate and monitor appointments
- Schedule inpatient/outpatient admissions and procedures
- Understand and apply third-party guidelines
- Obtain reimbursement through accurate claims submission
- Monitor third-party reimbursement
- Perform medical transcription
- Understand and adhere to managed care policies and procedures
- * *Negotiate managed care contracts (advanced)*

Practice Finances

- Perform procedural and diagnostic coding
- Apply bookeeping principles
- Document and maintain accounting and banking records
- Manage accounts receivable
- Manage accounts payable
- Process payroll
- * *Develop and maintain fee schedules (advanced)*
- * *Manage renewals of business and professional insurance policies (advanced)*
- * *Manage personnel benefits and maintain records (advanced)*

CLINICAL

Fundamental Principles

- Apply principles of aseptic technique and infection control
- Comply with quality assurance practices
- Screen and follow up patient test results

Diagnostic Orders

- Collect and process specimens
- Perform diagnostic tests

Patient Care

- Adhere to established triage procedures
- Obtain patient history and vital signs
- Prepare and maintain examination and treatment areas
- Prepare patient for examinations, procedures, and treatments
- Assist with examinations, procedures and treatments
- Prepare and administer medications and immunizations
- Maintain medication and immunization records
- Recognize and respond to emergencies
- Coordinate patient care information with other health care providers

GENERAL (TRANSDISCIPLINARY)

Professionalism

- Project a professional manner and image
- Adhere to ethical principles
- Demonstrate initiative and responsibility
- Work as a team member
- Manage time effectively
- Prioritize and perform multiple tasks
- Adapt to change
- Promote the CMA credential
- Enhance skills through continuing education

Communication Skills

- Treat all patients with compassion and empathy
- Recognize and respect cultural diversity
- Adapt communications to individual's ability to understand
- Use professional telephone technique
- Use effective and correct verbal and written communications
- Recognize and respond to verbal and nonverbal communications
- Use medical terminology appropriately
- Receive, organize, prioritize and transmit information
- Serve as liaison
- Promote the practice through positive public relations

Legal Concepts

- Maintain confidentiality
- Practice within the scope of education, training, and personal capabilities
- Prepare and maintain medical records
- Document accurately

- Use appropriate guidelines when releasing information
- Follow employer's established policies dealing with the health care contract
- Follow federal, state and local legal guidelines
- Maintain awareness of federal and state health care legislation and regulations
- Maintain and dispose of regulated substances in compliance with government guidelines
- Comply with established risk management and safety procedures
- Recognize professional credentialing criteria
- Participate in the development and maintenance of personnel, policy and procedure manuals
- * *Develop and maintain personnel, policy and procedure manuals (advanced)*

Instruction

- Instruct individuals according to their needs
- Explain office policies and procedures
- Teach methods of health promotion and disease prevention
- Locate community resouces and disseminate information
- * *Orient and train personnel (advanced)*
- * *Develop educational materials (advanced)*
- * *Conduct continuing education activities (advanced)*

Operational Functions

- Maintain supply inventory
- Evaluate and recommend equipment and supplies
- Apply computer techniques to support office operations
- * *Supervise personnel (advanced)*
- * *Interview and recommend job applicants (advanced)*
- * *Negotiate leases and prices for equipment and supply contracts (advanced)*

ANSWERS TO CASE STUDY REVIEWS

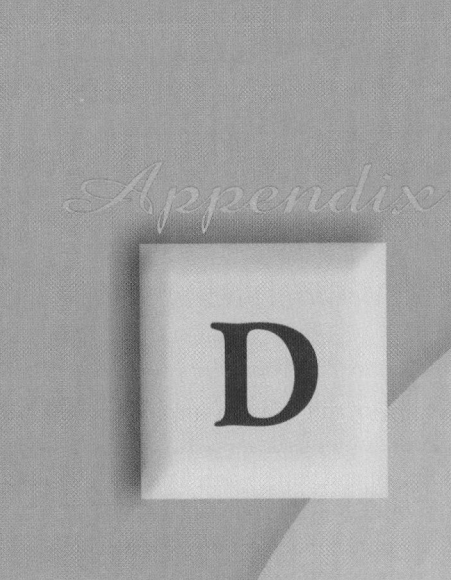

Chapter 5 Coping Skills for the Medical Assistant

Case Study 5-1

1. By being responsible, taking charge of the work environment, and being an inner-directed person, Ellen is more able to achieve her long-term goal of being an office manager. Certainly, she will learn by working closely with and observing Marilyn; there are also specific long-term, skill-building goals Ellen should set to give herself direction. If she gave herself three years to move into the office manager position, Ellen could set one long-term goal for each year. These might include (1) the first year, become proficient in all back-office clinical skills; (2) the second year, add front-office administrative tasks and skills; (3) the third year, begin to focus on office management.

2. Short-term goals break down long-term goals into smaller, more manageable time segments and will help Ellen more easily evaluate her progress. Short-term goals also provide a sense of periodic reward necessary to sustain motivation toward a long-range goal.

   Ellen should review her three long-term goals and determine what short-term goals they include. For example, the first year, Ellen wants to become proficient in all back-office clinical skills; short-term goals may include practicing accuracy when performing clinical duties and understanding which supplies are needed for which procedures. For her second-year goal of developing front-office administrative tasks and skills, Ellen may become proficient on the computer and learn the intricacies of scheduling patients. For the third-year goal that focuses on office management, Ellen can learn team-building skills and develop a procedures manual.

3. Ellen should take an active interest in her profession; she could attend seminars; speak with other medical assistants who are now office managers; read professional journals; and participate in professional organizations. This variety of exposure will enlarge Ellen's perspective and broaden her scope of information.

Case Study 5-2

1. Ellen is demonstrating the classic signs and symptoms of burnout, which include:
   a. she is a perfectionist
   b. she has a decreased sense of humor
   c. she displays frustration and irritability
   d. she is critical of herself and others
   e. she is physically and emotionally exhausted, yet continues to push herself
   f. her work has become a chore
   g. she feels like a failure if everything is not completed at the end of the day to her satisfaction

2. Ellen needs to take time for self-analysis by asking herself some hard questions. These questions must be answered truthfully and completely.

3. Ellen needs to institute some changes.
   a. List negative words or phrases often used, and then substitute neutral replacements.
   b. Create job diversity: Take a different route to work for a change; enter the office through a different door; change work routine where appropriate; investigate the possibility of a different work schedule.
   c. Become creative: Change work area décor by adding a new calendar; change family photo on desk, add a foliage or silk plant to the area.

d. Revisit short- and long-term goals, and make adjustments where necessary; be sure all goals are realistic and attainable.

e. Pay more attention to personal habits: Change eating habits; exercise more; get more rest and sleep; renew old friendships; go to lunch with coworkers.

f. Implement time management techniques.

g. Delegate responsibility to others who are capable.

Chapter 6 The Therapeutic Approach to the Patient with Life-Threatening Illness

Case Study 6-1

1. These questions are intended to help. In this culture, the family is deeply involved.

2. Having such a document would make it easier for everyone involved to know how much information should and can be shared with another.

3. Most all of this concern is related to the culture.

4. Have an honest discussion with everyone involved so it is clear to the staff how the patient would like to have information handled.

Case Study 6-2

1. Bruce should know that the human immunodeficiency virus (HIV) is transmitted between persons through sexual practices (sexual intimacy where body fluids might be exchanged); through direct blood-to-blood contact as in transfusions or needlestick injuries; and through intrauterine transmission. It is not transmitted through touching or other casual contact; AIDS is not an easily contracted disease.

2. AIDS patients and patients with the HIV virus often suffer extreme distress. Certainly, as a health care professional, Bruce needs to be sensitive to their needs and remember they may be both anxious and depressed. He should avoid being fearful and judgmental, but rather should be respectful toward patients with AIDS; while he should practice standard precautions, Bruce should also replace his fear with knowledge based on medical fact. He could be of assistance to HIV-infected or AIDS patients by referring them to support groups, social workers, legal advisors, and by helping the patient build coping skills.

3. Dealing with a large number of AIDS patients can be psychologically exhausting. While Bruce needs to combat his own prejudices, he also needs to be self-nurturing, not by withdrawing from AIDS patients but by giving himself a respite from time to time. If he routinely deals with AIDS patients, Bruce may benefit from a support group of his own that will help him build coping abilities.

Chapter 7 Legal Considerations

Case Study 7-1

1. It is critical that medical charts be kept current at all times. If the physician and medical assistant have maintained an accurate and up-to-date record of patient Boris Bolski's care, Joe can rely on the information in the chart to help him answer any questions. He should study the chart carefully.

Note: At all times, the patient's confidentiality must be respected. Typically, if the patient's attorney has issued the subpoena, the attorney will have the patient sign a release form. If the physician is subpoenaed by someone other than the patient's representative, the physician must be very careful about release of information and should proceed on a case-by-case basis. Certain records, because of their sensitive nature, may require a court order before being released.

2. Information in the chart should contain actual care rendered, dates that it was rendered, and charges made. Joe should note whether any comments were made on the chart that reflect patient input. Joe should also gather and review other material such as consent forms, insurance claim forms, and other documents related to patient care.

3. An expert witness is one who has the knowledge and experience to testify as to a reasonable and expected standard of care. Judges and jurors rely on the testimony of expert witnesses to understand the nature of medical information. Joe should answer questions in a factual way and in terms understood by the lay person.

Chapter 8 Ethical Considerations

Case Study 8-1

1. In most states, physicians and their employees are mandated to report all cases of suspected child abuse. Liz and Dr. Esposito must report the suspected abuse of Henry to the appropriate child protective agency.

2. and 3. Once the suspected abuse is reported, the responsible agency will respond to Henry's needs. However, in the meantime, Liz should take measures to protect and care for Henry, providing a safe environment if possible. While it may be difficult to do so, Liz should also view Juanita Hansen as a victim and seek treatment for her as well as for her son.

Chapter 9 Emergency Procedures and First Aid

Case Study 9-1

1. Wanda must first ascertain whether Annette is having trouble breathing. If she is, Wanda must direct her—and if necessary assist Annette—to receive immediate medical attention at the nearest hospital. If Annette says she is not having any breathing difficulty, Wanda should ask:

   - What are your symptoms?
   - Have you ever experienced an allergic reaction to an insect (specifically yellowjacket) sting before?
   - Do you have hives?
   - Are you experiencing any lightheadedness?
   - Do you have any itching either at the site of the sting or in other body locations?

   From these questions, Wanda needs to determine whether Annette is having a localized reaction, which can result in swelling, itching, and tenderness at the site of the sting, or a generalized reaction, which can be frightening for the patient and dangerous if it involves impairment of breathing functions.

2. If patients are allergic to an insect sting, it is possible that anaphylactic shock may ensue, which can lead to death. The patient must be directed to receive emergency care immediately, which will usually consist of the administration of epinephrine. If Annette must wait for EMS personnel, Wanda should stay with her over the telephone and calm her until EMS personnel arrive. For individuals who present at the ambulatory care setting with an apparent allergic reaction to a sting, the physician will prescribe epinephrine. Attempt to allay patient apprehension and monitor vital signs while waiting for EMS personnel to arrive.

3. Once Annette has received emergency treatment, Wanda can advise her to take certain precautions should she have another, and possibly more severe, reaction to an insect sting. For individuals with a known allergic reaction, the physician will prescribe epinephrine. These individuals should carry the epinephrine with them and self-inject, should they not be able to get immediate emergency care. The patient should then seek immediate emergency treatment. Advise all patients with known allergic reactions to be particularly careful when working or playing outdoors. Insects are not usually aggressive until their nests are approached; however, often these nests are not easy to detect and an individual may approach one without being aware of its presence. Patients with allergies to insects should always wear shoes out-of-doors, wear light-colored clothing, preferably with long sleeves and pant legs, look before taking a sip from a beverage when outdoors, and inspect lawn areas, shrubbery, and building walls periodically for evidence of nests of stinging insects.

Case Study 9-2

1. Because of the possibility that Mrs. Johnson is experiencing a myocardial infarction, Bruce should get a wheelchair and immediately take Mrs. Johnson into an examination room and notify Dr. Lewis. Bruce should help Mrs. Johnson onto the examination table, place her in semi-Fowler's position, loosen tight clothing, and take her blood pressure, pulse, and respirations. Bruce should activate EMS if Dr. Lewis directed him to. Because Mrs. Johnson is extremely anxious, Bruce must attend to her psychological needs.

2. The equipment, supplies, and medications that Dr. Lewis may want and need to be available for Mrs. Johnson are oxygen tank and mask, electrocardiograph, sphygmomanometer and stethoscope, and nitroglycerine, verapamil, and cardizem from the emergency cart.

3. Once the patient has been stabilized and Dr. Lewis has determined that Mrs. Johnson's symptoms are typical of angina pectoris, Bruce should continue to monitor Mrs. Johnson's vital signs and provide emotional support. He should notify the patient's family and remain with her until family members arrive to take Mrs. Johnson home.

4. Bruce can teach Mrs. Johnson and her family about the importance of using the prescribed form of nitroglycerin (sublingual tablets, transdermal patches) for angina attacks and the need to call Dr. Lewis if the nitroglycerin does not relieve symptoms. He can reinforce the need for regular exercise, a low-fat diet, stress reduction techniques, and no smoking.

Chapter 10 Creating the Facility Environment

Case Study 10-1

1. Audrey should greet the patient in a warm responsive manner and then assist Abigail Johnson to the extent she wants or needs assistance. In the examination room, privacy is especially important to patients. Space should be provided for patients to hang their clothes and undergarments. Mirrors are useful when

dressing. Rooms should be soundproof so that conversations are not overheard. Audrey can ask Ms. Johnson if she would like help disrobing. Staff should always knock before entering a room.

2. Environments that give patients as much control as possible are preferable. These empower patients and make them feel comfortable with the circumstances. Harmonious surroundings can be created with color, type of lighting, fresh, clean odors, and avoidance of unnecessary clutter and equipment.

3. Because Audrey is obviously sensitive to Ms. Johnson, this patient is likely to feel less nervous about her physical exam. Audrey's warm yet unobtrusive manner should put Ms. Johnson at ease and, in the end, create the circumstances in which patient and physician can honestly and openly communicate.

Chapter 11   Computers in the Ambulatory Care Setting

Case Study 11-1

1. To minimize injury from excessive computer use, computer equipment needs to be chosen, set up, and used properly. Walter should consider using alternative keyboards to reduce wrist strain, using screen glare protectors to deflect monitor glare, positioning monitors for individual comfort, and using chairs that offer lower back support.

   The student should sketch out a diagram indicating positioning of chair, monitor, and keyboard. Annotate the sketch to explain why elements are positioned a certain way. See Figure 11-8 for general guidelines.

2. Walter should give staff who use computers frequently a general set of guidelines to ensure quality work and worker safety. They should take frequent short breaks away from the computer screen; they should change their posture from time to time and develop a variety of comfortable postures; they should look away from the monitor when printing, etc.; they should pay attention to any pain and take corrective action at once. Table 11-1 provides more detail on ensuring staff safety.

3. The inexperienced medical assistant can more easily overcome computer timidity if encouraged to build skills gradually. Walter needs to seek a fine line between setting firm goals for staff computer literacy but not setting expectations too high too quickly. A series of training courses either on or off the job will help build familiarity both with the hardware and the

capabilities of the software. Staff should concentrate on learning one program at a time. Training after hours is preferable so center operations are not disrupted. When inexperienced users apply their skills in the workplace, they should have a "resource person" they can turn to as questions arise during computer use.

Case Study 11-2

1. Confidentiality is most likely to be jeopardized with the use of fax machines, computer-based medical records, electronic transfer of medical records, invasion by hackers, and inappropriate discussion of patient records.

2. *Fax machines*—Establish written protocols to ensure confidentiality is maintained. To do this, locate fax machines in restricted access areas under the supervision of someone with the authority to access sensitive data. Personnel should first sign a confidentiality statement and be trained in sending a fax correctly to ensure the proper recipient receives the fax. Protocols should also include guidelines on what to do if a fax is received by an unintended recipient.

   Computer-based medical records—The use of passwords is successful in controlling access to computer files and in providing an authentication mechanism. Development of a firewall to allow outside computers to access your computer while restricting access to your databases is essentially impossible. The office should not allow outside computers access to database computers and to communicate to an outside network or Internet while using a dedicated computer. Computer security protocols should be written, training should be provided to employees, and confidentiality statements should be signed by all personnel having exposure to computer-based medical records before access is granted.

   Electronic transfer of medical records—Follow the same procedures as computer-based medical records.

   Hackers—Medical records sent over the Internet to an external location can be intercepted by hackers and posted on the Web for all to read. Encryption programs may be employed when sensitive medical records must be transmitted via electronic means.

   Inappropriate discussion—All medical office employees should sign a confidentiality statement. During staff meetings, discuss the importance and ramifications of discussing confidential medical records via electronic methods.

3. Answers will vary.

Chapter 12 Telephone Techniques

Case Study 12-1

1. Triage is the act of evaluating the urgency of a medical situation. Because the young man is concerned about his mother's breathing, Audrey will automatically classify this call as a potential emergency. To gain additional information that will determine her actions, Audrey should ask the caller:

   - The patient's name and age
   - What happened to cause the situation
   - Briefly, the patient's medical background that may shed light on the current breathing problem
   - Whether the patient takes any regular medication
   - If there are any other symptoms

   Any breathing problems require emergency measures; after taking initial screening information, Audrey should inform Dr. Lewis, who will probably instruct Audrey to call 911 or the local emergency service to assist the patient as quickly as possible. Audrey will then follow up with the caller, and try to reassure him that help will be there as soon as possible. Once she has taken care of all urgent matters, Audrey should schedule a follow-up appointment for the patient with Dr. Lewis so he can ascertain the condition of the patient and determine the cause of the breathing difficulty.

2. Even though Audrey is not at the site, her Red Cross first aid and CPR training will give her the confidence to make difficult decisions under the pressure of time.

3. Audrey must be very careful not to give medical advice over the telephone, but only to triage the situation and help the caller assist the patient by making an appointment or by directing them to seek emergency assistance. In triaging, Audrey must always respect office procedures for handling emergency calls and act within the bounds of her training and expertise.

Case Study 12-2

1. Wanda will need to know the caller's name and telephone and ask if she can return a call once she has collected the requested information.

2. The purpose of the call-back verification procedure is to verify that the person requesting the medical information is, in fact, employed by Claussen-Mason Laboratories.

3. After the verification has been established and permission by Dr. King has been given, Wanda may release the required information and then document the call appropriately in the telephone log book.

Chapter 13 Patient Scheduling

Case Study 13-1

1. Any ambulatory care center must institute cancellation procedures in order to assure quality patient care; free up care time for other patients; and protect physicians from potential legal complications.

2. In order to treat a patient, the patient's cooperation is necessary. A regular pattern of cancellations or no-shows may indicate that the patient is not committed to assisting in treatment. Sometimes, a physician may decide to terminate treatment, in which case a letter terminating services and discontinuing care would be sent to the patient by certified mail. Because Rhoda Au is a long-term patient, the physician may try to speak to her personally to discover if there is a reason for the repeated cancellations.

3. Whether using a manual or computer method, a system must be developed so it is evident to staff making appointments that, due to cancellations, time is now available to schedule other appointments.

   In the manual system: Note changes on the appointment sheet of all appointments that were changed, canceled, or failed to show using the steps in Procedure 13-3.

   In the computer system: Software programs differ, but cancellations are typically performed by deleting the patient's name from the time slot; that time then reopens for other appointments.

   Whether using a computer or manual system, be certain to keep a record of all canceled appointments including patient name, date, and time. Also record canceled appointments on the patient chart.

Chapter 14 Medical Records Management

Case Study 14-1

1. Karen should first instruct Liz in the principles of the numeric filing system used by Inner City Health Care. In addition to instructing Liz in filing methodology, Karen also needs to impress upon her the

importance of maintaining up-to-date, easily accessible files. From a patient and physician point of view, good records enhance quality of care. Accurate files and documentation also are important should any litigation arise.

2. When filing any piece of documentation, Liz should follow these steps, which will enable her to efficiently process all written material.

- Inspect
- Index
- Code
- Sort
- File

3. If all active and inactive patient files are to be computerized, Karen and Liz will need to be familiar with computer use and then investigate medical software that meets the needs of Inner City Health Care. They should expect the transition to be a gradual one and should set a series of intermediate goals, such as: first, scan all inactive files for archival storage; second, scan or input active client files; third, develop a system for efficiently transferring chart data from manual notation to computer input; fourth, gradually computerize other records such as correspondence.

Chapter 15   Written Communications

Case Study 15-1

1. While style manuals vary in content, certain elements are critical. Also, Marilyn wants it to be as comprehensive as possible, so her outline of major headings might include:

- Introduction to the style manual
- The Lewis & King letter format
- A sample letter, noting standard elements that go into every letter
- Procedures for all outgoing correspondence
- Procedures for all incoming correspondence
- Commonly used medical terms
- Proofreading hints
- Writing tips
- Sample of form letters used by Lewis & King
- Summary of mail classes and services
- Summary of do's and don'ts in written communications

2. Marilyn can have medical assistants read a reference book on composition to educate them about usage and

style; she can encourage them to enroll in a business writing class; and she can help them build skills by giving manageable assignments that require an increasing level of ability.

3. After selecting the office letter style, Marilyn can identify standard components of any letter that leaves the offices of Lewis & King. These typically include:

- Date line
- Inside address of recipient
- Salutation
- Subject line
- Body of letter
- Complimentary closing
- Keyed signature and personal signature
- Reference initials, when applicable
- Enclosure notation, when applicable
- Carbon copy notation, when applicable
- Postscripts, when applicable
- Continuation page heading when the letter is more than one page

Chapter 16   Transcription

Case Study 16-1

Hospitals, multispecialty clinics, and solo physician practices offer competitive salaries and benefit packages. They may pay for professional memberships and registration fees for CE opportunities and an allowance for reference materials. The dictation from these settings encompasses a wide range of specialties, complexities, styles, and dialects. State-of-the-art equipment is often available so that new skills may be learned. There often are QA personnel to ask questions of and to obtain feedback on progress in document preparation.

Transcription services and home-based positions offer competitive pay rates and dictation from a wide range of specialties, complexities, styles, and dialects. There may be a more flexible work schedule available, with compensation based on production. There may or may not be QA personnel available.

Freelance MTs are in business for themselves. This environment offers the MT a sense of accomplishment and independence and the opportunity to work flexible hours. There may or may not be someone available to QA their work or answer questions when they get stuck. The freelance MT's earnings can be excellent if they are highly productive, transcribe accurately, and remain focused on building the business. At times there may be more work than can be readily handled and there may be slack peri-

ods with little to transcribe. Freelance MTs must maintain bookkeeping records and manage the business themselves or pay to have someone else handle the books.

Case Study 16-2

1. The physician dictated *upper lip* in the first sentence and *lower lip* in the last sentence. The MT does not know which is correct.

2. To verify which lip is correct, the MT will need to pull the patient's chart and read through the documentation or flag the document asking the physician to acknowledge which is correct. The physician would also have to check the chart, so it is probably best if the MT does this.

3. If the information can be verified before the document is printed, the correction can be made before printing the document. If the document has been flagged, the physician will verify the correct site. To make the correction, simply draw a single line through the error and write the correction above or below the error while preserving legibility of the error. The correction notation should also include the initials of the person entering the correction, the date, and reference to the lab report as a cross-reference.

Chapter 17   Daily Financial Practices

Case Study 17-1

1. Selecting an appropriate bookkeeping method, taking responsibility for banking, managing the purchase of supplies, and establishing a petty cash system are all topics that Joann should become familiar with. Marilyn will review with Joann all the daily financial practices as reviewed in this chapter, including:

• Discussion and determination of patient fees

• Credit arrangements

• Managing patient accounts using either a manual or computerized bookkeeping method

• Taking care of all banking procedures, including understanding different accounts, types of checks, making deposits, accepting checks for payment, writing checks, and reconciling a bank statement

• The activities involved in purchasing, including preparing the purchase order

• Establishing a petty cash fund

2. If Marilyn wants to institute computerized bookkeeping methods at Doctors Lewis & King, it may be helpful to have Joann begin the process of computerization while Marilyn continues to maintain accounts with the manual method. The computerization process is a gradual one and often the two systems must run side-by-side until the computer method is up and running and all personnel are familiar and comfortable with using the new system. As Joann is setting up the system, Marilyn can work side by side with her, teaching Joann about how accounts have been maintained manually; she will acquaint Joann both with the specifics of the office's daily financial practices and give her an understanding of the pegboard accounting method. At the same time, Marilyn will learn about the computer method by assisting Joann.

3. Part of daily financial practices includes accounts payable, or writing checks to pay bills, refund overpayments, and replenish petty cash. Joann must be careful about how she writes checks, making sure that they are legible, properly dated, include the name of the payee, the amount of payment in figures and words, and that the memo line is completed referencing the purpose of the check. The check stub must also be recorded to maintain an accurate record of payments made from the account. Before checks are sent, Joann should follow these rules:

• Check that numerical and written amounts agree.

• Check that everything is spelled correctly.

• Follow office procedure for having physicians or office manager approve and/or sign all checks.

• Determine that the check is made payable to correct payee, that the correct amount is paid, and that the current date is used.

Chapter 18   Medical Insurance

Case Study 18-1

	Total Charges	Allowed Charges
Office visit	$85.00	$80.00
Return visit	+65.00	+55.00
Total Charges	$150.00	$135.00
Less deductible	−100.00	−100.00
Subtotal	$50.00	$35.00
Apply 80% coinsurance	× 80%	× 80%
Insurance Payment	$40.00	$28.00
Patient Owes	$10.00	$7.00*

*(or $22.00 if physician does not accept assignment; $7.00 plus $15.00 disallowed by Medicare)

Chapter 19 Medical Insurance Coding

Case Study 19-1

Note: Students will need to look these codes up in ICD-9-CM and CPT code books. Answers here are based on 2000 code books.

1. The proper ICD-9-CM diagnosis codes for Mr. McKay are:

    787.0   nausea

    789.0   abdominal pain

2. The proper CPT procedure codes for Mr. McKay are:

    99204   new patient, extended office visit

    85031   CBC, complete

    82270   guaiac

    80061   lipid panel

    81000   urinalysis

3. When coding any claim form it is important that the medical assistant be as precise as possible, not guess, and not code what is not there. Coding must always correlate with the physician's notes in the chart; otherwise, fraud is committed and an ethical and legal principle violated.

Chapter 20 Billing and Collections

Case Study 20-1

1. Often, a quick telephone call may solve a collections problem, for the patient may have forgotten or misplaced the bill. No matter what the situation, a friendly tone is important. It is also critical to keep to the facts and remain tactful and pleasant. More is gained by remaining courteous than by assuming a threatening manner. In addition, legal rules and regulations apply to collection calls. A collection call should never be made in a way that is accusatory or that embarrasses the patient, for instance, by calling at the workplace.

2. If telephone collections are not effective, Ellen might send a series of letters once the account is 2 to 3 months past due. The first would ask the patient to pay the balance; the second, sent a month later, would again ask for immediate payment of the balance; the third would inform the client that the account is being assigned to a collection agency.

    The student should draft three letters and then compare them with the collections letters in Chapter 20.

3. If a patient has declared bankruptcy, Ellen may not send any statements nor make any attempt to collect delinquent accounts. In a bankruptcy, a physician's fee is likely to be one of the last to be paid because it is unsecured.

Chapter 21 Accounting Practices

Case Study 21-1

1. In reviewing fixed costs, the owners of Inner City Health Care would consider items that do not vary in total according to the number of patients. For example, these might include rent and/or mortgage, utilities, and the annual depreciation cost of equipment.

2. Variable costs will vary in direct proportion to patient volume. Variable costs will include items such as clinical supplies, laboratory fees, professional liability insurance, and the costs of billing and collections.

3. Utilization review, which is a review of service before it is performed, demands more accurate recordkeeping and documentation than ever before. Utilization review companies sell their services to employers and insurance carriers; these reviewers determine whether or not procedures or treatments are needed or will improve a patient's condition prior to the patient receiving medical services. If they decide a procedure or treatment is not needed, those services will not be covered by the insurance carrier. Thus, utilization review may affect the number of clinical procedures Inner City Health Care may perform and consequently its ultimate profitability. Also, if proper preauthorizations are not requested, Inner City may perform clinical procedures that the carrier may refuse to pay.

Chapter 22 Infection Control, Medical Asepsis, and Sterilization

Case Study 22-1

Include the following in an exposure control plan for blood and/or OPIM:

Exposure determination requires an employer to list all job classifications in which all employees in those jobs are exposed to blood and OPIM in the course of doing their job. Existing job descriptions can be used by the employer to identify the job categories that are at high risk for exposure to blood and/or OPIM. It is important that exposure determination be made without regard to the use of PPE.

The plan must consist of methods of compliance for prevention of exposure, hepatitis B vaccination, past exposure evaluation, communication of hazards to employees, documentation of the bloodborne standard, and a procedure for the determination of the events surrounding the exposure.

The written plan must be employee-accessible, updated at least annually, and modified when necessary and appropriate, especially to reflect a change in employee positions.

Case Study 22-2

By depriving pathogens of their growth requirements, they may be kept from causing an infection. This can be accomplished by providing good lighting since bacteria will die in direct light or sunlight; by providing or withholding oxygen according to the needs of the pathogen (aerobe or anaerobe); by lowering environmental temperature, pathogenic growth is reduced because they favor warm temperatures; and by keeping work surfaces dry, pathogenic growth can be inhibited because they need moisture to grow.

Chapter 23   Taking a Medical History, the Patient's Chart, and Methods of Documentation

Case Study 23-1

1. The medical assistant must be as thorough as possible while respecting the patient's privacy and help Adam understand that the medical history enables the physician to advise patients on how to prevent any future problems.

2. Joe should reassure Adam that patient information is confidential and that his mother has agreed to respect his privacy (since this is the case). Joe can also try to engage Adam in the medical history-taking by inviting Adam's perceptions, such as:

   • What do you expect from this exam?

   • What kind of treatment do you expect?

   Joe should also use his communication skills to get Adam to be responsive; if Joe can develop a relationship with Adam, Adam is more likely to be honest and Joe can be more effective in helping Adam analyze his social behaviors.

3. Joe should not be condemning or judgmental but should help Adam protect himself by following proper precautions. If Adam has come to respect and trust Joe, he is more likely to accept his opinion. Joe can give Adam some printed material to educate him about HIV infection; reading about the topic may encourage Adam to rethink some of his behaviors.

   Some techniques that Joe can use when dealing with sensitive topics include:

   • Asking these questions later in the interview;

   • Using direct eye contact;

   • Posing questions in a matter-of-fact tone;

• "Normalizing" the situation, e.g., saying, "Many students seem to do this. How does it affect you?"

Case Study 23-2

1. *personal data:* Harvey DiAntonio
   45 W. Smith Avenue
   Baltimore, MD 21208
   ph. 667-1870
   Insurance: BC/BS 211678756
   Major Medical—
   Diagnostic #4
   Referred by: Dr. Alan Byers
   DOB 07/08/1954

chief complaint: Severe "gripping" pain in the anterior mid-chest sometimes radiating to the abdomen, neck, and both arms.

present illness: Pain occurs with strenuous exercise, walking uphill, shaving, climbing stairs, after a heavy meal, during sexual intercourse. Pain lasts 20 minutes with each episode, does not stop when he ceases activity. Episode last week included dizziness, nausea, and fatigue. Episodes ongoing once or twice per month × 5 months.

past medical history: Essentially noncontributory. Has not had physical examination for eight years.

Surgeries: T & A, 1958
Appendectomy, 1964
Fractured rib L, 1984
Usual childhood diseases

Hospitalization:
Observation, 1962—Sinai Hospital
Dx bronchitis

family history: Both parents deceased, mother age 59—MI, father age 49 ? cause—brother living, hypertension—sister alive and well—two children alive and well (adolescents)

social history: Firefighter—pump operator—heavy exertion, smokes 1½–2 packs of cigarettes per day, overeats while on duty, hobbies—carpentry, music. Describes self as "fun-loving," "quick tempered," worries about finances. Eligible to retire, but prefers to remain working.

ROS: Well-nourished, well-developed male in no acute distress. Somewhat anxious. Wt. 198 pounds, BP 175/104—T. 98.6—P. 94 (reg.)

HEENT: normal
Neck   supple

Trachea	midline
Chest	normal in contour—calcium deposit L 6th rib noted on X ray, otherwise neg., probably due to old fracture.
Heart	presystolic gallop
Abdomen	negative
Extremities	negative
Genitalia	negative
Skin	negative
Neurological	negative
Laboratory	Hgb. 11.0 gm
EKG	presystolic atrial sounds, long P–R interval

Impression:

1. angina pectoris

2. anemia

3. hypertension

Plan: nitroglycerin tab sublingually as needed, watch quantity of food intake, low fat 1600 calories, 4 meals/day, avoid extreme cold, sleep 8 hours/night, avoid emotional upsets, no smoking, moderate alcohol intake.

Return in 2 weeks

Chapter 24 Vital Signs and Measurements

Case Study 24-1

1. A normal blood pressure reading for adults would have a systolic reading below 140 and a diastolic reading below 90. Herb's reading of 156/100 is considered hypertension, or a blood pressure that is above normal. Audrey should measure the patient's blood pressure again to confirm that a proper reading was taken. She should also confirm that the cuff size was correct, for a too small cuff can give an artificially high blood pressure reading.

2. Herb is obviously considering but having a difficult time implementing lifestyle changes. Audrey may find that educating Herb about diet and exercise may give him some information that will encourage him to make some changes in his lifestyle. While the high blood pressure may be due to a number of reasons, weight and smoking certainly can contribute to it. Audrey and Herb could pinpoint a long-term goal and then select a few manageable short-term goals to reduce Herb's weight, improve his circulation, and reduce his blood pressure.

3. In reviewing new resources, Audrey discovers that high blood pressure is now considered any reading over 140/90. Previously, she had learned that there were four categories of high blood pressure. In addition to learning new facts, Audrey also discovered the importance of periodically updating her base of information.

Chapter 25 The Physical Examination

Case Study 25-1

1. a. Observation or inspection
   b. Palpation
   c. Percussion
   d. Auscultation
   e. Mensuration
   f. Manipulation

2. Liz should know at least eight common positions that may be required of the patient during the physical examination.

   a. Supine or horizontal recumbent
   b. Dorsal recumbent
   c. Lithotomy
   d. Fowler's
   e. Knee-chest
   f. Prone
   g. Sims'
   h. Trendelenburg

3. Liz should know the basic components of an exam as observed by the physician and how each is an indicator of patient well-being.

   a. Patient appearance, including skin color, grooming, behavior. Patient appearance is also observed by the medical assistant during the patient history.
   b. Gait, including limp, dragging of one leg, balance, or a wide-based walk. Gait can indicate a problem with neurological functioning.
   c. Stature, including height and trunk and limb proportion.
   d. Posture; a person in pain may have postural abnormalities.
   e. Body movements, including both voluntary and involuntary movements.
   f. Speech, including loss of voice, difficulty speaking, using wrong speech patterns, and using words in the wrong order.
   g. Breath odors, which can indicate specific diseases such as diabetes or liver disease.
   h. Nutrition, to discover the cause of overweight or underweight conditions or edema.
   i. Skin and appendages, including abnormal skin color or skin conditions.

Case Study 25-2

1. Positioning and draping Mrs. Mason for a complete physical exam won't be different from any other patient who has a complete basic physical exam. Keep in mind Mrs. Mason's age and assist as necessary with positioning and draping. Protect her privacy while helping her to undress in preparation for the exam. Because Mrs. Mason has arthritis, she has limited mobility and needs assistance. Remain with her throughout and assist her onto the examination table and into the various positions for the exam.

    To position Mrs. Mason for the pelvic examination, she will not be able to assume lithotomy position due to her arthritic knees. The pelvic exam can be done with Mrs. Mason in either the dorsal recumbent or Sim's position.

    Be certain she is covered with a drape for warmth and privacy. A diamond shape placement of the drape for either dorsal recumbent or Sims' will facilitate viewing the pelvic area without undue patient exposure.

2. Because of Mrs. Mason's age and frail condition, special consideration should be given to her safety. Assist her on and off the table being certain at the conclusion of the exam that she remain seated on the edge of the exam table while you assess her readiness to get down from the table. Check blood pressure, pulse, and skin color before allowing her to step down. Help her to get dressed, remain with her throughout, and assist her into the physician's office and later out to the reception area to her waiting niece.

3. Since Mrs. Mason is experiencing vaginal spotting, Dr. King will perform a pelvic examination. Prepare the appropriate equipment and supplies necessary to do the pelvic exam.

Chapter 26   Obstetrics and Gynecology

Case Study 26-1

1. The initial prenatal visit is of utmost importance because it is a time for health promotion and patient education. A thorough history will be taken, and a physical exam will include abdominal, pelvic, vaginal, and breast examinations. Pelvic measurements are taken to be certain that Maria's pelvis size is sufficiently adequate to deliver her baby vaginally. Numerous laboratory tests are performed. Time will be spent promoting good health for mother-to-be and her fetus. Liz will stress the importance of healthy habits for Maria to practice. Such topics as proper nutrition, regular exercise, dental care, rest, and sleep will be addressed. Body changes and newborn and infant care

are discussed at this visit. The dangers of using alcohol, tobacco, and other drugs, either over-the-counter or prescription, are stressed.

2. Dr. King will watch for signs and symptoms of such diseases and conditions as the following:

Condition/Disease	Signs and Symptoms
Pre-eclampsia	Edema, hypertension, albuminuria, headache, vision changes, rapid weight gain
Hyperemesis gravidarum	Severe, unrelenting nausea and vomiting with possible dehydration
Vaginitis/STD	Vaginal discharge
Threatened abortion	Vaginal bleeding, abdominal pain, or cramping
Possible ectopic pregnancy	A one-sided pelvic or abdominal pain

There are other diseases and conditions pregnant women may experience as well as those listed. Dr. King will be on the alert for signs and symptoms of anything that seems to be out of the ordinary.

3. Some procedures and tests that may be done during the initial prenatal visit include:

   - Pelvimetry
   - Urinalysis
   - Complete blood count (CBC)
   - Rh factor
   - Blood type
   - Rubella titer
   - Hepatitis B and C
   - Venereal disease research laboratory (VDRL)
   - Pap smear
   - Gonorrhea and chlamydia cultures

4. Liz may include in her discussion with Maria the importance of good nutrition and what it entails, dental care, rest, relaxation, regular exercise, and sleep. She will caution Maria about drugs (alcohol, over-the-counter, prescription, tobacco, and street drugs) and their ability to cross over the placenta into the fetal circulation. Anticipated body changes, newborn and infant care, and breast-feeding are all part of patient education and health promotion that Maria will be taught.

Case Study 26-2

1. Rest for 24 hours after the procedure.

2. Do not lift heavy objects for approximately two weeks.

3. Leave vaginal pack in place for 24 hours or as directed by physician. Do not insert a tampon unless told to do so by physician.

4. Report any bleeding greater than an average menstrual period.

Case Study 26-3

1. An abdominal and pelvic examination will be done on Annette, therefore, a gynecological examination set-up will be necessary. There is a discharge, so a wet mount procedure will also be done.

2. Most likely the causative microorganism is trichomonas vaginalis. It is a parasite.

3. If the diagnosis is trichomonas, Dr. King is likely to prescribe medication by mouth (Flagyl) and treat both partners.

Chapter 27   Pediatrics

Case Study 27-1

1. Otitis media is an inflammation of the middle ear that frequently follows an upper respiratory tract infection in children. The eustachian tubes of a child are shaped differently than mature tubes. They are shorter and are more prone to having pathogens lodge and grow in the tubes. The infection can travel up the eustachian tube to the middle ear. Antibiotics are used to treat otitis media.

Case Study 27-2

1. When a child has an upper respiratory infection and is showing signs of possible otitis media, vaporizers and decongestants should be used to help prevent otitis media.

Chapter 28   Male Reproductive System

Case Study 28-1

1. First, a digital rectal examination will be done, then a prostate-specific antigen (PSA) blood test, a urinalysis, and a urine culture. Perhaps an intravenous pyelogram will be ordered also. The rectal examination allows Dr. Woo to palpate the prostate gland for enlargement. The PSA blood test measures the amount of a specific protein that is elevated in prostate cancer cases. If the PSA is within normal range, it can help rule out prostate cancer, although a

biopsy is necessary to confirm a diagnosis. A urinalysis and culture will show an infection that is not unusual with BPH. An intravenous pyelogram is helpful in determining kidney, ureter, and bladder damage from BPH.

2. The preliminary tests Dr. Woo might order are urinalysis, urine culture, and intravenous pyelogram.

Case Study 28-2

1. Dr. King's workup of Mr. Toomey will include an examination to determine if the testicle is painful, swollen, or inflamed. If there are none of these symptoms, Dr. King most likely will suggest Mr. Toomey have a biopsy of the mass in the right testicle. This will determine whether the lesion is benign or malignant.

Chapter 29   Gerontology

Case Study 29-1

1. Slower movements and decreased flexibility are due to changes in the muscles and joints. The muscles become weaker, and muscle fibers decrease in size and number. Loss of neurons that control muscle function results in slower movements. The wear and tear of everyday living causes worn out joints. Synovial fluid decreases leading to stiffness and immobility.

2. The activities of daily living (ADL) are affected by Mrs. Robinson's problems. It will be difficult or impossible to brush her teeth, comb her hair, use the toilet, feed herself, or bathe herself.

3. Dr. King might suggest some passive and active range of motion exercises to help increase her flexibility and decrease muscle stiffness. (See Chapter 33.)

Case Study 29-2

1. The number of taste buds decrease, and the sense of smell diminishes. Food tastes bland and unappetizing.

2. Dangers to watch for when taste and smell are no longer as acute are:

   • Accidentally eating spoiled food, which can cause food poisoning

   • Oversalting foods in an attempt to make it taste better

   • Weight loss and malnutrition may result

   • Gas leaks may go undetected causing loss of consciousness and death

   • The inability to hear a smoke alarm resulting in smoke inhalation, severe burns, or death from fire

Chapter 30 Examinations and Procedures of Body Systems

Case Study 30-1

1. The medical assistant's responsibilities include:
   a. Position the patient as requested by the physician.
   b. Clean and dry area to be casted. Note any bruises, swelling, or redness.
   c. Pad bony prominences.
   d. Provide correct width of stockinette for area.
   e. Provide correct width of webril.
   f. Place bandage in container of warm water for 5 seconds. Remove from water and gently squeeze out excess water.
   g. Assist physician with application of cast material.
   h. Comfort and reassure patient as needed.
   i. Give cast care instructions in writing.

2. a. Notify the physician if the following occur:
   - A bad odor coming from the cast
   - Numbness, tingling, severe pain, difficulty moving, severe swelling, cold fingers or toes
   - A burning sensation over a bony area
   - Bleeding or pink to red discoloration on the cast

   b. The following should be verbal and written instructions:
   - Allow casting material to dry by exposing it to air and keeping it uncovered, even at night. Applying pressure prior to drying can result in damage under the pressure area.
   - Elevate right arm to aid in reducing swelling and pain.
   - Observe fingers and toes for color and temperature changes, decreased sensation, and tingling. May indicate cast is too tight.
   - Do not place objects into cast to scratch irritated skin. A break in the skin will provide breeding ground for bacteria. Do not use cream or powder.
   - Do not get cast wet. This could cause malformation of the wrist and arm. Cover with waterproof covering when showering or bathing.
   - Clean cast with a damp cloth.
   - Use water-soluble marking pens if decorating the cast, allowing cast to breathe.
   - Do not cut or trim cast.

Case Study 30-2

1. Anita should be told the following:
   - Seal lips tightly around the mouthpiece.
   - Maintain good posture throughout the test.
   - Inhale deeply and quickly; exhale quickly and forcibly until no more air can be expelled.
   - Do no use bronchodilators for 24 hours before the test.
   - Maximum effort is required for accurate results.

Chapter 31 Assisting with Minor Surgery

Case Study 31-1

1. Wanda should try to gently educate the sisters about the cyst removal procedure in order to allay any apprehension. She will need to ask questions regarding Cele's general state of health and determine whether Cele has any known allergies. Wanda should note the date of Cele's last tetanus booster. Wanda will also need to explain the need for a signed consent form, which is standard protocol before any minor surgery. Costs are sometimes discussed but because the sisters are covered by Medicare and because Inner City accepts Medicare assignment, their only costs may be that of any prescription drugs.

2. The procedure should be fairly routine, especially because the cyst is not inflamed. However, the sisters still need to be instructed about what to expect during the procedure, approximately how long it will take, whether Cele needs to maintain a special diet before the procedure, and whether a special diet is needed after the procedure. If Dottie knows these specifics beforehand, she can shop and prepare for Cele's minor surgery, which will probably make her feel less nervous about being the caregiver.

3. Wanda should give Cele and Dottie specific wound care instructions. She should provide written as well as verbal instructions and tell the sisters to check regularly for symptoms of infection. Wanda should also provide a telephone number that Dottie can call both during and after hours. Wanda should call the sisters within the first postoperative day to check on Cele's condition. Wanda can also provide for a community agency, such as the Visiting Nurse Association, to check on the sisters and teach Dottie how to check for infection or help with any other problems that can arise.

Case Study 31-2

1. Patient preparation for excision of a nevus:
   a. Wash hands and greet patient.
   b. Offer restroom facilities.
   c. Escort to procedure area.

d. Check to see if patient followed preoperative instructions.

e. Review postoperative instructions.

f. Check for signed consent form.

g. Have patient remove clothing from waist up. Provide gown, drape, and pillow.

h. Position patient comfortably.

i. Prepare patient's skin for surgery.

2. Postoperative care for Letisha consists of:

a. Check vital signs.

b. Allow patient to rest if necessary. Remain with patient for her safety.

c. Assist patient off table and assist her to dress.

d. Review written instructions with Letisha and caregiver.

e. Schedule follow-up appointment.

f. Document postoperative instructions in patient's record.

3. The excised nevus will be carefully placed in a labeled biopsy container with a preservative (formalin). A laboratory requisition or request form will be attached to the specimen container. The specimen will be sent or taken to the laboratory, and documentation will be made in the patient's record.

Chapter 32 Diagnostic Imaging

Case Study 32-1

1. The purpose of the GI series is to study the esophagus, stomach, and small intestine for ulcers, tumors, hiatal hernia, and esophageal varices.

2. Preparation for GI series consists of:

The day prior to X ray: light evening meal, NPO after midnight.

The day of test: NPO postprocedure, increase fluid intake, take a laxative as prescribed.

Case Study 32-2

1. Mr. Brunnelle is told that the actual X rays belong to the hospital where they were taken and processed and although he has paid for them, they are not his. He can, however, have a copy of the radiologist's reports of the results of all of the X rays.

2. X rays are best left on-site so that they are accessible for future use to be compared with more recent films of the same body part. Also, this eliminates the possibility of their being lost if they were removed from the site at which they were taken.

Chapter 33 Rehabilitation and Therapeutic Modalities

Case Study 33-1

1. Before beginning any transfer, certain precautions must be observed:

- The equipment must be stable and firm. Lock the brakes of the wheelchair and be sure the examination table will not move during transfer.

- Check that there are no obstructions.

- Take small shuffling steps. Avoid crossing the feet.

- Adjust the transfer surface to about the same height as the wheelchair.

- Position the equipment on the patient's stronger side. Take advantage of the patient's assistance in lifting and moving.

- Always use a gait belt. Never lift the patient by the arms or under the armpits.

- Never have the patients put their arms around your neck.

- Both medical assistant and patient should wear nonslip footwear.

- Be sure the patient understands the process involved in the transfer.

- Practice good body mechanics.

2. For a one-person transfer, the medical assistant should follow the principles in (1) above and:

a. Place the wheelchair next to the examination table and lock the brakes.

b. Place the gait belt around the patient's waist.

c. Move the wheelchair footrests out of the way or remove if possible; have patient place feet on floor.

d. Position the stool in front of the examination table and as close to the wheelchair as possible.

e. Have patient move to edge of wheelchair; stand in front of patient with feet apart.

f. The medical assistant should bend at hips and knees, grasp the gait belt, and have patient place hand on armrests of wheelchair to push up. The patient can use his strong leg to push as well.

g. Have the patient step onto the stool with the foot closest to the table and pivot. His back is now to the examination table.

h. The patient should grasp the stool handle with one hand and place the other hand on the table.

i. Ease the patient onto the table and position as necessary.

j. Move the wheelchair and stool out of the way.

3. a. Position the wheelchair next to the examination table. Lock the brakes.

   b. Position the stool next to the wheelchair.

   c. Assist the patient to a sitting position. Place the gait belt snugly around patient's waist.

   d. Place your one arm under the patient's arm and around his shoulders, and the other arm under his knees. Pivot the patient so his legs are dangling over the side of the table.

   e. Move so you are directly in front of the patient.

   f. Grasp the patient by placing your hands under the gait belt. Plant your feet shoulder's width apart and bend your knees.

   g. Pull the patient slightly toward you so his feet come down onto the stool. Signal the patient to push off the table, grasping the stool handle for support.

   h. Have the patient step onto the floor with his strong leg and pivot so his back is to the chair.

   i. Have the patient grasp the armrests of the wheelchair.

   j. Lower the patient into the wheelchair and make him comfortable.

   k. Lower the footrests and place the patient's feet on them.

Case Study 33-2

Tell Mr. Schwarz to obtain a commercial ice pack or to use an ice bag for the ankle. A commercial pack is pliable and will conform to the shape of the ankle better than an ice bag. Cover the pack with a cloth before applying to the ankle. Leave in place about 30 minutes, and then remove and reapply for another 30 minutes. Report to the physician signs of redness or paleness of skin color, tingling, or increase in pain. Keep the leg elevated as much as possible, and continue ice pack application for about 24 hours.

Chapter 34   Nutrition in Health and Disease

Case Study 34-1

1. Wanda needs to gently educate Anita about the pregnant woman's need to increase various nutrients. Wanda could explain that during pregnancy the growth of the fetus, growth of the placenta, increase in adipose tissue, increased volume of blood, and growth of breast tissue all create the need for additional nutrients. Wanda should try to persuade Anita that pregnancy is an important time for both fetus and mother and that it is normal and healthy for the mother to gain weight.

2. The need during pregnancy is not just for extra calories but for specific nutrients, so Wanda should provide Anita with a range of foods that she can choose from, especially since Anita seems to be a picky eater. The foods should reflect the fact that protein requirements are nearly double during pregnancy; that vitamins are needed in higher quantities than usual; and that calcium, phosphorus, and iron are needed in such high quantities that a vitamin supplement is usually necessary.

3. Anita should be taught that her baby is more likely to be normal and healthy if she has good nutritional habits during her pregnancy. If the problem is one of not having access to healthy foods, the physician may prescribe a nutritional supplement in addition to the vitamin supplement Anita is probably taking. Wanda may want to gather some informational brochures that Anita can read and may even put her in touch with support groups that may encourage and support Anita in her pregnancy. Wanda could also review the list of important nutrients and their food sources and, together with Anita, compose a nutritious but easy-to-make menu.

Case Study 34-2

Mrs. Johnson's activity level, number of calories per day, and dosage of insulin would have to be considered. The diabetic diet consists of a specific number of grams of carbohydrates, protein, and fat. Various foods can be exchanged (derived from a food exchange list) to have a wide selection of foods that come from each of the basic five food groups.

The patient needs to know how to select the correct foods in the correct quantities, how to incorporate a daily exercise routine, and the importance of taking insulin at the appropriate time of the day. The overall goal is geared toward providing sufficient calories to maintain normal body weight, while providing adequate nutrition. Lifestyle is also taken into consideration as well as the patient's ability to comply with the prescribed diabetic diet. The prescribed amount of food should be eaten at prescribed times during the day. Meals should not be skipped.

Encourage the patient to learn more about diabetes by enrolling in a class about the disease at a local hospital.

Chapter 35   Basic Pharmacology

Case Study 35-1

1. Audrey should advise Maria to discard any medication—prescription or nonprescription—that is not used. Most medications lose their potency after a period of time and others become toxic. Maria should discard the leftover suppositories and buy a new supply.

2. Sometimes, an infection or other condition will clear up before a patient finishes all medication and the patient discontinues use. Audrey should tell Maria that in this and other cases, medication should be taken exactly as directed for the prescribed number of days, etc.

3. To discover whether another form of medication might be available for Maria's yeast infection, Audrey consults the PDR. She finds that medications are available that can be taken by mouth, intravenously, or applied topically but that the suppository is the most effective form. The student should consult the PDR to discover what Audrey learned during her research.

Case Study 35-2

Since Dr. King keeps controlled substances on the premises, Joe Guerrero, the certified medical assistant, has the legal responsibility to do the following:

1. Monitor the physician's DEA registration renewal date.

2. Maintain legally designated records.

3. Provide security for all drugs, in particular, controlled substances.

4. Provide security for prescription pads.

5. Destroy expired drugs and document properly.

6. Know and understand federal and state laws that regulate drugs including controlled substances.

Chapter 36   Calculation of Medication Dosage and Medication Administration

Case Study 36-1

1. The size syringe used would be a U-100 insulin syringe.

2. The medication label would indicate 100 units per milliliter. If you use the correct syringe, a U-100 syringe, and draw up 10 units of insulin, the correct dose will be accurately measured.

3. Route of administration for insulin is 90 degree angle with a SC needle. Specifics for insulin administration require that you (a) rotate your site for each injection, (b) give subcutaneously at 90 degree angle, (c) do not massage the injection site following administration, and (d) be certain that insulins are compatible before mixing together in the same syringe.

4. (a) Encourage her to attend diabetes education classes at local hospital or clinic. (b) Stress the importance of monitoring blood and urine for glucose levels. (c) Stress importance of adhering to the diet as prescribed by the physician. (d) Engage in regular exercise.

Case Study 36-2

1. BSA of child = 0.74

$$\frac{0.74(m^2)}{1.7(m^2)} \times \text{adult dose} = \text{child's dose}$$

$$\frac{0.74}{1.7} \times \frac{400}{1} = \text{child's dose}$$

$$\frac{0.74}{1.7} \times \frac{400}{1} = \frac{400 \times 0.74}{1.7} =$$

$$\frac{296}{1.7} = 173.55 \text{ or } 174 \text{ mg}$$

2. $\dfrac{\text{Desired}}{\text{On Hand}} \times \text{quantity} = \text{dose}$

$$\frac{174 \text{ mg}}{400 \text{ mg}} \times 1 \text{ ml} = \text{dose}$$

0.44 ml to be administered

3. Give 0.44 ml of erythromycin 400 mg/ml subcutaneously into the vastus lateralis muscle at a 45° angle using a 23–25 gauge ⅝ inch needle.

Chapter 37   *Electrocardiography*

Case Study 37-1

1. Call emergency medical services—911—for transport to the hospital emergency room. Under Dr. Rice's direction, Wanda would prepare to administer oxygen and other medications as directed, frequently check blood pressure and pulse, place patient in Semi-Fowlers position, assist Dr. Rice as needed, comfort and reassure the patient, and perform CPR if necessary.

2. Wanda can explain (using either hand-drawn pictures or an anatomical model of the heart) the location of the coronary arteries on the myocardium of the heart and their significance as the major supplier of oxygenated blood to the heart itself. She could explain that the lining of the arteries build up with fatty deposits that harden over time and begin to block the flow of blood to the heart. Blood flow to the heart muscle is diminished (especially during periods of increased activity) and the heart's muscle tissue responds by symptoms of pain or pressure beneath the sternum into the neck, jaw, shoulder and/or throat. Rest usually relieves the pain of angina. Pain that does not subside may indicate a complete obstruction of the coronary arteries. No blood flow to nourish the heart muscle results in a heart attack, a much more serious situation that requires immediate medical attention.

   Some strategies and healthy habits about which Wanda can remind Mrs. Johnson are (a) avoid tobacco, (b) take medications as prescribed, (c) report unusual symptoms or problems to Dr. Rice, (d) eat a low-fat, low-cholesterol, low-sodium diet, (e) exercise regularly with Dr. Rice's permission, (f) get adequate rest, (g) keep weight under control and at an acceptable level, (h) encourage family members to take a CPR course, and (i) practice stress reduction behaviors.

3. Some resources that can benefit Mrs. Johnson are:

   • American Heart Association. Educational materials to learn about arteriosclerotic heart disease, and ways to prevent and manage it.

   • American Diabetes Association. Educational materials and classes held in local clinics and hospitals regarding the relationship between diabetes and heart disease. Balance among exercise, diet, and insulin is stressed.

   • American Dietetic Association. Educational materials on proper diet for diabetic control and prevention of further fatty deposits on artery linings of the heart.

   • American Red Cross. Classes available to learn CPR. Patient and family members benefit from learning CPR in the event a patient suffers a myocardial infarction and goes into cardiac arrest.

   • Weight control centers such as Weight Watchers® to learn healthy eating and exercise behaviors for weight reduction and control. Portion control, low-fat, low-sodium food choices are stressed.

   • YWCA. Under Dr. Rice's direction, Mrs. Johnson could enroll in a regularly scheduled exercise class to strengthen her heart, lower blood cholesterol levels, and help reduce emotional stress. Yoga and/or meditation classes are also available for stress reduction.

Case Study 37-2

1. The symptoms that Mr. Matthews has been experiencing—palpitations, fast and slow heartbeats, and dizziness—are symptoms of cardiac arrhythmia. Since Mr. Matthews' resting ECG showed no evidence of arrhythmia, Dr. Abbott ordered a Holter monitor in order to record Mr. Matthews' cardiac activity for a 24-hour period. By going about his normal activities while wearing the monitor, should Mr. Matthews again experience similar symptoms, the monitor will pick up the abnormality.

2. Instructions to Mr. Matthews include:
   a. Keep a daily diary of all activities, symptoms, and emotions and note the time they occur.
   b. Do not shower or swim. The recording could be interrupted and the monitor damaged.
   c. Do not handle the electrodes. It could cause artifacts to occur.
   d. Do not remove recorder from its case.
   e. Do not use an electric blanket. It can cause interference, another artifact.
   f. Depress the event marker only briefly and when experiencing a significant symptom. Overuse of the marker can mask the ECG tracing.

3. Activities that should be recorded in the patient's diary include:
   a. Eating meals
   b. Sexual activity
   c. Medications taken
   d. Times of sleep
   e. Smoking
   f. Bowel movements
   g. Physical exercise

Chapter 39   Introduction to the Medical Laboratory

Case Study 39-1

1. No, because the accuracy of the test can be compromised by the patient not fasting.

2. Explain the purpose of the test and the importance of fasting to obtain accurate results. Give the patient written information about the diet. Have the patient repeat the instructions.

3. Perhaps enlist the help of a family member or friend.

Chapter 40   Phlebotomy: Venipuncture and Capillary Puncture

Case Study 40-1

1. Immediately remove the needle and stop the patient from falling. Lower the patient's head and arms. Wipe the patient's forehead and back of the neck with a cold compress if necessary. Pass an ammonia inhalant 4 to 5 inches away from the patient's nose. If the patient still does not respond, notify a physician, move the patient to the floor, and place a pillow under his legs.

2. Liz could have had Wayne lie down and used a pillow to help support his arm to keep it straight for easier venous access.

3. Take the time to ask patient about previous venipuncture experiences, put patient at ease, allay patient's fears, and persuade patient to allow blood to be drawn. Have patient assume the reclining position, which is best for apprehensive patients and patients who may faint.

Chapter 41   Hematology

Case Study 41-1

1. The test results may be affected in the following ways:
   - Falsely increased because of heat from incubator
   - Falsely increased because of vibrations from opening and closing the incubator door
   - Falsely increased due to heat from the sunlight
   - Falsely decreased due to low temperatures by the window during cool periods

2. Normal Westergren ESR values:
   - Males: 0–15 mm/hr.
   - Females: 0–20 mm/hr.

3. Test conditions should be controlled to avoid excessive heat or cold, drafts, and vibrations.

Chapter 42   Urinalysis

Case Study 42-1

1. To aid in the diagnosis of a urinary tract disorder. The presence of abnormal urine sediment cells and microorganisms can be determined when the specimen is examined microscopically.

2. Wanda should look for the presence of white blood cells, bacteria, yeast cells, or parasites.

3. WBC—report as cells per high-power field; e.g., 10/HPF; bacteria—report as few, moderate, many, loaded; yeast cells—report as amount per HPF; parasites—check with physician or someone else more familiar with these organisms before reporting.

Chapter 43   Basic Microbiology

Case Study 43-1

1. Possible reasons for a negative test: a good swab was not obtained, the sides of the mouth and tongue were swabbed by mistake; incorrect swab was used, could be cotton or contain a chemical that would interfere with the test; the test and materials were outdated; directions for the test were not followed; the child does not have strep throat.

2. A throat culture can be set up.

3. A proper throat culture is obtained by swabbing the back of the throat in the red area while trying to avoid the sides of the mouth and tongue. Set up a swab on a blood agar plate in CO_2 atmosphere.

Chapter 44   Specialty Laboratory Tests

Case Study 44-1

1. Anna should review the specific procedure in the office procedures manual to be sure she knows all aspects of the procedure. Anna should also let the office manager or one of the physicians know that she feels uncomfortable performing this procedure. They may be able to (1) review the procedure with Anna to give guidance and answer any specific questions; (2) they may actually accompany Anna while she does the procedure; or (3) they may perform the procedure with Anna attending. It is important to let your supervisor know of any concerns about performing clinical procedures. Inadequate or inaccurate performance can cause risks to patients and to the practice.

2. If the practice is relying on Anna to perform all clinical duties, Anna may not be as valuable to the practice if she is unwilling to perform procedures expected of her, within the scope of her training. Rather than telling her supervisor that she is not capable or willing to do the procedure, however, Anna should let them know she does not feel confident she knows the procedure well enough to do it correctly and she should let her supervisor know that she is *willing* to try with help.

3. Anna could help make the procedure an effective one by:
   a. making sure all necessary equipment and supplies are on hand and within easy access;
   b. making sure she knows *why* the test is necessary so that she can accurately explain the procedure to the parents, especially if they have questions. If Anna knows answers to their questions she will feel more confident;
   c. requesting the parents' assistance to hold and reassure the baby as much as possible;
   d. using a steady, quick, and accurate motion when actually performing the heelstick; a slow stick of the lancet will cause more distress to the infant and will not produce a better sample;
   e. realize and expect that the infant will cry when the heelstick is performed. Anna should not be upset by this and she should also let the parents know this will happen so they are not upset.

Chapter 45   The Medical Assistant as Office Manager

Case Study 45-1

1. Answers will vary, but the groups should discuss and incorporate the teamwork approach to plan and implement a solution.

2. The team previously should have identified the resources available and met to brainstorm possible problems that could occur and what their solutions might be.

3. The office manager should remain calm and try to keep the argument from escalating. Other patients may be present as well; they should not be disturbed. One of the duties of the office manager is to supervise personnel, so she would want to be supportive of the staff while being understanding of the patients' feelings.

Case Study 45-2

1. Answers will vary, but pros may include that this management style communicates purpose and direction of

tasks, solicits participation of others, inspires subordinates, encourages open communication, empowers others, serves as a role model, and is a continuous learner. Cons may include that she may be thought of as one who tattles to higher authorities.

2. Answers will vary.

3. Answers will vary.

Chapter 46   The Medical Assistant as Human Resources Manager

Case Study 46-1

1. Jane should be up-front with Bruce and state that it has been noticed that he frequently takes longer lunches than he is allotted. The two should work on an action plan to correct this situation, and a re-evaluation should be scheduled.

2. Although evaluations may involve more than the office manager or human resource manager and the employee, it probably would not be appropriate to involve the employee's peer or fellow worker. It may affect work relationships and cause hard feelings.

3. Jane should end the formal evaluation on a positive note by stating her confidence in the individual to make any changes necessary, offering assistance where needed, and thanking the employee for participating. End with a positive statement about some portion of the employee's performance.

Chapter 47   Preparing for Medical Assisting Credentials

Case Study 47-1

1. Juan must request the application from the AAMA Certification Department or the Program Coordinator and be sure to complete the correct application. Juan should read all the instructions carefully before completing the application form. The application must be free from errors and each item must be completed in full. The application must be postmarked by March 1 for him to be allowed to take the June examination.

2. Answers will vary, but here is one sample schedule:

   March—Form study group. Contact people to see if they are interested. Set up a regular meeting time at least one time per week. Purchase study guides.

   April—Increase study group meetings to two times per week. Begin to review course textbooks and tests.

May—Increase study group meetings to three times per week. Study independently two or three times per week also.

3. Juan should be careful to approach people he knows will take the examination seriously. He does not necessarily have to ask only those who are his friends.

Case Study 47-2

1. Nancy must be of good moral character and have graduated from an accredited high school or acceptable equivalent. Nancy must determine the appropriate requirement she satisfies and have been employed in the profession of medical assisting for a minimum of five years, no more than two years of which may have been as an instructor in a postsecondary medical assistant program.

2. Since most examinations may be scheduled within three days of application completion, Nancy should begin her study schedule several months prior to January to allow plenty of time to study each of the categories covered on the test.

3. Nancy should begin early to find a study partner(s). The study partner(s) should take the examination seriously and have a similar date in mind for sitting for the exam. The partner(s) should also agree to and be committed to the study schedule. Meeting once or twice a week helps keep the group focused. Independent study should be done throughout the week. During the independent study time, each group member could write 25 questions relevant to the weeks' study topic. When the group meets, a discussion of the study topic could take place and then copies of the questions distributed for answering. The questions could be corrected and discussion of any questionable or missed answers could take place.

Chapter 48   Employment Strategies

Case Study 48-1

1. The functional resume is probably the best resume style for Eun Mee to follow. The advantages of the functional style are that it allows areas of experience to be sorted into areas of function. This is useful when reentering the job market after an absence, when you have a variety of different, apparently unconnected work experiences, and when you have volunteer work experience.

2. Vital information should include full name, address including street number, city, state, and zip code, and telephone number including area code.

3. Accomplishment statements simply state your accomplishments and what you have done in previous employment settings. They are a way of tooting your own horn to help prospective employers realize your capabilities. Accomplishment statements should begin with power verbs and give a brief description of what you did and the demonstrable results that were produced. An example would be "During my experience as a sales representative, I serviced numerous customers who, as a result of my responsiveness to their needs, asked for me personally when they returned to the store for purchases."

Case Study 48-2

1. The candidate should bring an extra application, cover letter, resume, and reference sheet.

2. Arriving early will give Eun Mee time to collect her thoughts and become composed. It will also demonstrate good work habits to the employer: punctuality.

3. The candidate should wait patiently until the employer calls her in and wait for the employer's cues. The candidate should return a firm handshake and wait to be offered a seat.

INDEX

Delmar's Medical Assisting Administrative Skills CD-ROM
and
Delmar's Medical Assisting Clinical Skills CD-ROM

Set-Up Instructions

1. Insert disk into CD-ROM player.
2. From the Start Menu, choose *RUN*.
3. In the *Open* text box, enter **d:setup.exe** then click the *OK* button. (Substitute the letter of your CD-ROM drive for **d:**)
4. Follow the installation prompts from there.

System Requirements
Administrative Skills CD-ROM

166 MHz Intel Pentium processor or greater

Microsoft® Windows® 95, 98, NT4, 2000

32 MB of installed RAM

100 MB of available disk space

256-color monitor capable of 800 × 600 resolution

CD-ROM drive

Microsoft® Windows® compatible sound card

System Requirements
Clinical Skills CD-ROM

100 Mhz Intel Pentium

Microsoft® Windows® 95 or later

32 MB or more of RAM

Approx. 8 MB free disk space

SVGA monitor with 24-bit (16 million colors) display

4x or faster CD-ROM drive

Sound card and speakers

License Agreement for Delmar Thomson Learning Educational Software/Data

You, the customer, and Delmar Thomson Learning incur certain benefits, rights, and obligations to each other when you open this package and use the software/data it contains. BE SURE YOU READ THE LICENSE AGREEMENT CAREFULLY, SINCE BY USING THE SOFTWARE/DATA YOU INDICATE YOU HAVE READ, UNDERSTOOD, AND ACCEPTED THE TERMS OF THIS AGREEMENT.

Your rights:

1. You enjoy a non-exclusive license to use the software/data on a single microcomputer in consideration for payment of the required license fee (which may be included in the purchase price of an accompanying print component), or receipt of this software/data, and your acceptance of the terms and conditions of this agreement.

2. You acknowledge that you do not own the aforesaid software/data. You also acknowledge that the software/data is furnished "as is" and contains copyrighted and/or proprietary and confidential information of Delmar Thomson Learning or its licensors.

There are limitations on your rights:

1. You may not copy or print the software/data for any reason whatsoever, except to install it on a hard drive on a single microcomputer and to make one archival copy, unless copying or printing is expressly permitted in writing or statements recorded on the disk(s).

2. You may not revise, translate, convert, disassemble or otherwise reverse engineer the software/data except that you may add to or rearrange any data recorded on the media as part of the normal use of the software/data.

3. You may not sell, license, lease, rent, loan, or otherwise distribute or network the software/data except that you may give the software/data to a student or and instructor for use at school or temporarily at home.

Should you fail to abide by the Copyright Law of the United States as it applies to this software/data, your license to use it will become invalid. You agree to erase or otherwise destroy the software/data immediately after receiving note of Delmar Thomson Learning termination of this agreement for violation of its provisions.

Delmar Thomson Learning gives you a LIMITED WARRANTY covering the enclosed software/data. The LIMITED WARRANTY follows this License.

This license is the entire agreement between you and Delmar Thomson Learning interpreted and enforced under New York law.

This warranty does not extend to the software or information recorded on the media. The software and information are provided "AS IS."

Any statements made about the utility of the software or information are not to be considered as express or implied warranties. Delmar Thomson Learning will not be liable for incidental or consequential damages of any kind incurred by you, the consumer, or any other user.

Some states do not allow the exclusion or limitation of incidental or consequential damages, or limitations on the duration of implied warranties, so the above limitation or exclusion may not apply to you. This warranty gives you specific legal rights, and you may also have other rights which vary from state to state. Address all correspondence to Delmar Thomson Learning, Box 15015, Albany, NY 12212 Attention: Technology Department.

LIMITED WARRANTY

Delmar Thomson Learning warrants to the original licensee/purchaser of this copy of microcomputer software/data and the media on which it is recorded that the media will be free from defects in material and workmanship for ninety (90) days from the date of original purchase. All implied warranties are limited in duration to this ninety (90) day period. THEREAFTER, ANY IMPLIED WARRANTIES, INCLUDING IMPLIED WARRANTIES OF MERCHANTABILITY AND FITNESS FOR A PARTICULAR PURPOSE, ARE EXCLUDED. THIS WARRANTY IS IN LIEU OF ALL OTHER WARRANTIES, WHETHER ORAL OR WRITTEN, EXPRESS OR IMPLIED.

If you believe the media is defective, please return it during the ninety-day period to the address shown below. Defective media will be replaced without charge provided that it has not been subjected to misuse or damage.

This warranty does not extend to the software or information recorded on the media. The software and information are provided "AS IS." Any statements made about the utility of the software or information are not to be considered as express or implied warranties.

Limitation of liability: Our liability to you for any losses shall be limited to direct damages and shall not exceed the amount you paid for the software. In no event will we be liable to you for any indirect, special, incidental, or consequential damages (including loss of profits) even if we have been advised of the possibility of such damages.

Some states do not allow the exclusion or limitation of incidental or consequential damages, or limitations on the duration of implied warranties, so the above limitation or exclusion may not apply to you. This warranty gives you specific legal rights, and you may also have other rights which vary from state to state. Address all correspondence to Delmar Thomson Learning, Box 15015, Albany, NY 12212 Attention: Technology Department.